Native American Medicinal Plants

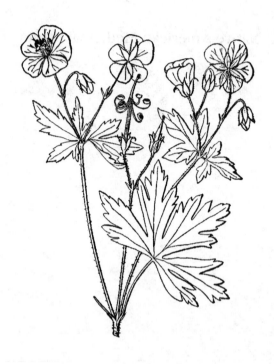

Native American Medicinal Plants

An Ethnobotanical Dictionary

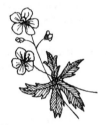

Daniel E. Moerman

Timber Press
Portland • London

This abridged work is based on the author's Native American Ethnobotany published by Timber Press Inc. in 1998.

Facts stated in this book are to the best of the author's knowledge true; however, the author and publisher can take no responsibility for any illness or damage that might result from use of the materials described herein.

Cover photograph courtesy of the Library of Congress.

The botanical drawings in this volume were obtained from the U.S. Department of Agriculture Natural Resources Conservation Service's PLANTS Database (http://plants.usda.gov, Baton Rouge, La.: National Plant Data Center). These drawings were originally published in *An Illustrated Flora of the Northern United States, Canada and the British Possessions* by N. L. Britton and A. Brown (3 vols., 1913. New York: Scribner's Sons) or in *Wetland Flora: Field Office Illustrated Guide to Plant Species* (Washington, D.C.: U.S. Department of Agriculture Natural Resources Conservation Service). The geranium drop capitals and other elements throughout were drawn by Jennifer Sontchi.

Published in 2009 by Timber Press, Inc.

The Haseltine Building	2 The Quadrant
133 S.W. Second Avenue, Suite 450	135 Salusbury Road
Portland, Oregon 97204-3527	London NW6 6RJ
www.timberpress.com	www.timberpress.co.uk

Printed in China

Library of Congress Cataloging-in-Publication Data

Moerman, Daniel E.
    Native American medicinal plants : an ethnobotanical dictionary / Daniel E. Moerman.
        p. ; cm.
    Abridged version of: Native american ethnobotany / Daniel E. Moerman. c1998.
    Includes bibliographical references and indexes.
    ISBN 978-1-60469-035-4 (hardback) — ISBN 978-0-88192-987-4 (pbk.) 1. Medicinal plants—North America—Dictionaries. 2. Materia medica, Vegetable—North America—Dictionaries. 3. Indians of North America—Medicine—Dictionaries. 4. Indians of North America—Ethnobotany—Dictionaries. 5. Ethnobotany—North America—Dictionaries. I. Moerman, Daniel E. Native American Ethnobotany. II. Title.
    [DNLM: 1. Indians, North American—North America—Dictionary—English. 2. Plants, Medicinal—North America—Dictionary—English. 3. Ethnobotany—North America—Dictionary—English. QV 13 M694na 2009]
    RS171.M64 2009
    615'.32103—dc22

                                                                                            2008050291

A catalog record for this book is also available from the British Library.

For Claudine, with love.

Contents

Preface

I am delighted to introduce an abridged edition of *Native American Ethnobotany* in a new format and with a new title: *Native American Medicinal Plants*. This volume contains the approximately 25,000 medicinal uses of some 2700 plant species from the original volume with the relevant references.

This is the most comprehensive and authoritative listing of Native North American plant use for medicines available anywhere. The medicines are used for everything from sore eyes to rheumatism, from kidney illnesses to love medicines, from panaceas to tonics. They represent uses from native peoples living all over North America, from the Arctic Eskimo to the Florida Seminoles, from the Canadian Algonquin to the southwestern Navaho and Hopi.

The original encyclopedia, *Native American Ethnobotany,* had a long history. In 1970, I was in the Sea Islands of South Carolina doing anthropological fieldwork for my Ph.D. dissertation in a rural black community. I was surprised to learn that sometimes when people were ill, they gathered various wild plants as medicines. Although I had not intended to do so, I began to inquire into the matter. In time, I had identified about 35 species of plants, from *Allium* to *Zanthoxylum*, which were so used. I then asked what seemed at the time to be a few simple questions: How had these people learned of these plants? Did it do any good to take them? Had anyone else ever used them, and if so, for what?

In asking these questions I found I was in the company of some of the great American students of ethnobotany of the past—Huron H. Smith, Francis Densmore, Melvin Randolf Gilmore, Matilda Coxe Stevenson, Gladys Tantaquidgeon, and many others. Their fascinating works, too often overlooked, were found with the help of reference librarians in the recesses of one library or another across the continent. Most of the works have long been out of print or were published in specialist journals and were very hard to find.

Once found, many of the works were difficult to use. Most were not indexed, or at least not very well indexed. To answer a seemingly simple question such as, Who used *Allium* and for what?, took hours of digging. I decided to try to coordinate the information. I bought a few hundred index cards, the kind with sorting holes around the edges, and started filling them in. Soon I had more cards than would fit on the sorting pin. I had to start new boxes of subcategories to store the cards. Once I dropped a stack of cards on the floor. It was very discouraging. Eventually I transferred the information to cards that could be fed into the hopper at the computing center at the University of Michigan–Dearborn. The material was then read into a database using the TAXIR (Taxonomic Information Retrieval) system available on the university computer.

In 1975, with a summer stipend from the National Endowment for the Humanities, I filled out thousands of code sheets with material from the works by Smith, Tantaquidgeon, and others. With funds provided by the university, I hired keypunch operators to produce the thousands of cards needed for computing. The first version of the database was published in 1977 as *American Medical Ethnobotany: A Reference Dictionary* (New York: Garland Publishing). That book included 1288 plant species from 531 genera from 118 families used in 4869 different ways in 48 different societies. There was no index, but each of the 4869 items appeared in the book four times—one list organized by genus, one by family, one by use, and one by tribe.

Even though that book had more than 500 pages, it was far from a comprehensive list of Native American medicinal plant use. I had not had time nor resources to code several other available sources (for example, Francis Elmore on the Navaho, Erna Gunther on the Northwest Coast peoples). And at the time there were no sources available on two major groups, the Cherokee and Iroquois. With the help of several reference librarians, I continued to add to my collection of ethnobotanical works, published and unpublished. Paul Hamel and Mary Chiltoskey's *Cherokee Plants and Their Uses* and James Herrick's monumental *Iroquois Medical Botany* appeared later in the 1970s (those two sources alone had more items in them, 4875, than all the rest of my original database).

Improvements in database technology and important grants from the National Endowment for the Humanities and the National Science Foundation helped further my work over the decades. *Medicinal Plants of Native America* was published in 1986 by the University of Michigan Museum of Anthropology and *Native American Ethnobotany* in 1998 by Timber Press. The latter includes plants used for other purposes, such as food and building, and it dwarfs the present volume in size.

This book incorporates all the parts of *Native American Ethnobotany* dealing specifically with medicinal uses, and is an effort to provide an affordable alternative for those especially interested in the uses of plants as medicine. Thus, the present volume brings my work on Native American plants full circle. I hope you will use it in good health.

Acknowledgments

So many people and organizations have contributed materially and otherwise to this project that it is not feasible to list them all. Foundations, universities, libraries and librarians, colleagues, students, friends, and family have all been indispensible to a project that took approximately 25 years to complete. Here I thank them all without naming any, for to name one would require me to name them all, and I would surely miss someone. Thank you all.

The current abridged edition was made possible by Neal Maillet of Timber Press, who conceived the project, and Lisa DiDonato Brousseau, who did most of the work. I deeply appreciate their confidence in this project.

Anthropologists are often and rightly criticized for taking from the lives of other people and not giving very much back. In a small effort to address that criticism, I decided some time ago to find funds sufficient to purchase a copy of the original book to give to each of the 1100 or so registered American Indian tribes and Canadian First Nations. With the help of many individuals and companies, we originally managed to give books to about half of the tribes. Then, Mike Balick of the New York Botanical Garden interested the Force for Good Foundation in the project. The foundation is funded by the Nu Skin Company of Provo, Utah, a cosmetics company with a rich corporate conscience. Their support allowed us to complete the project, sending copies of the book to all 1100 groups.

On a more personal level, my wife, Claudine Farrand, is a true partner. She provided context for this work by making life fun. My daughter, Jennifer Sontchi, did the lettered geranium illustrations seen throughout the book, and I thank her for them.

But our deepest debt is to those predecessors of ours on the North American continent who, through glacial cold in a world populated by mammoths and saber-toothed tigers, seriously, deliberately, and thoughtfully studied the flora of a new world, learned its secrets, and encouraged the next generations to study more closely and to learn more. Their diligence and energy, their insight and creativity, are the marks of true scientists, dedicated to gaining meaningful and useful knowledge from a complex and confusing world. That I cannot list them individually by name in no way diminishes my sense of obligation to them.

Plant Use by Native Americans

Native American peoples had a remarkable amount of knowledge of the world in which they lived. In particular, they knew a great deal about plants. There are in North America 31,566 kinds (species, subspecies, varieties, and so on) of vascular plants: seed plants, including the flowering plants (angiosperms) and conifers (gymnosperms), and spore-bearing plants, including the ferns, club mosses, spike mosses, and horsetails (pteridophytes). North America is defined here as North America north of Mexico as well as Hawaii and Greenland. American Indians used thousands of species of vascular plants as medicines. *Native American Medicinal Plants* also contains information on nonvascular plants (algae, fungi, lichens, liverworts, and mosses). The data for nonvascular plants are much less complete than those for vascular plants, however.

Native American Medicinal Plants includes information on medicinal plant use by Native American people. Most of the plants used are native to North America, but some are not. Some are plants that were introduced into North America—some perhaps in pre-Columbian times and others certainly thereafter—and became naturalized, growing spontaneously. Other plants are introductions that were kept in cultivation. The information in *Native American Medicinal Plants* documents plant usage no doubt dating back to very early times and passed down through generations as traditional knowledge, as well as innovations in response to much more recent plant introductions.

Plants Used as Drugs

There are more than 2500 species included in *Native American Medicinal Plants* that were used medicinally by Native Americans. The listing of Drug Usage Categories toward the end of this chapter defines the many sorts of medicinal use that appear in the Catalog of Plants. The ten plants with the greatest number of drug uses by Native Americans are: *Achillea millefolium*, common yarrow (359), *Acorus calamus*, calamus (221), *Artemisia tridentata*, big sagebrush (166), *Lomatium dissectum*, fernleaf biscuitroot (142), *Prunus virginiana*, common chokecherry (132), *Artemisia ludoviciana*, Louisiana sagewort (128), *Oplopanax horridus*, devil's club (128), *Juniperus communis*, common juniper (119), *Mentha canadensis*, Canadian mint (116), and *Urtica dioica*, stinging nettle (114).

The first thing people usually ask about American Indian medicinal plants is, Do they work? This, it turns out, is tricky question. The short answer is, Yes. The longer answer is more interesting. What does it mean to say that a medicine "works"? Essentially it means that the medicine has the effect that we want it to have, that it meets our expectations. This means that a drug that meets one person's expectations may not meet another's, and people may therefore disagree over whether the drug works. Such disagreements usually hinge on different conceptions of health or healing. This is to say that definitions of health and well-being are often cultural matters; they are rarely simple matters of fact.

Consider a case not from American Indian medicine but from the history of European medicine. In the European tradition as recently as the early twentieth century (and very often in many other medical traditions as well) people understood that illness was in part the result of certain kinds of imbalance in the body's humors. Certain humors (such as blood, bile, or phlegm) accumulated at the expense of others, and the healer's goal was to reestablish the proper balance. One common way to achieve this was to purge the sick individual, to cause him to vomit.

Consider also these similar cases. The Iroquois used *Lobelia inflata* to induce vomiting; they soaked the whole plant in cold water, which they drank. *Lobelia* has several English common names, among them emetic herb, vomit wort, and pukeweed. It contains a series of alkaloids, but the one probably responsible for its major actions on the human body is lobeline. Besides causing emesis, some species of Lobelia have been used as an expectorant in cough syrups. So, does it work? Well, a physician in the European tradition and an Iroquois healer could probably agree that *Lobelia* is an effective emetic—the drug works. But why do the Iroquois want to induce vomiting? They use this emetic to cure a sufferer of "tobacco or whiskey addiction." It is at this point that the Euro-American and the Iroquois may find themselves at odds, the latter saying it does work, the former saying it does not work. Euro-American medical theory does not, to my knowledge, contain any theory allowing that vomiting will cure people of addiction to cigarettes or whiskey. Similarly, the Cherokee, are reported to use *L. inflata* as an emetic (now we have triple agreement) to cure asthma (and now a triple disagreement). Whereas the Euro-American, the Iroquois, and the Cherokee are likely to agree on one dimension of these treatments (emesis), they may disagree about others. Asking about the effectiveness of a drug, then, is not a simple biological or medical issue but a complex problem of culture and meaning.

Issues of culture and meaning come in many different forms. For example, in all the thousands of listings in this book one will find only 55 items categorized as Cancer Treatment in the Catalog of Plants. Cancer is evidently a much more important disease in modern America than it was in native America. Why? The primary reason seems to be that Native American peoples did not suffer from cancer nearly as often as do modern Americans. Cancer is a relatively recent disease that is to some degree dependent on carcinogens, substances that "cause" or accelerate cancer. Most carcinogens are industrially manufactured artifacts like food colors, radioactive materials, and x-rays. An interesting exception is tobacco. Native Americans regularly used tobacco as a ceremonial smoke. A dozen or so people would occasionally share a bowl of tobacco in a pattern very different from the addicted smoking of Europeans and Euro-Americans (modern cigarettes are, of course, industrially manufactured products). The other significant carcinogen that is not an industrial product is sunlight. The differences in susceptibility to cancer caused by tobacco and sunlight in Native America and among modern Americans are matters of culture, and they seem to me to account for the general lack of cancer among Native American people, at least in the past, and therefore, the rarity of cancer treatments documented here.

In contrast to cancer treatments, one will find 523 treatments classified as Eye Medicine in the Catalog of Plants. The explanation for this is probably to be found in a similar cultural comparison: American Indians often lived in smoky houses. As the conditions that required treatment varied, so did the treatments available.

This cultural analysis does not mean that American Indian medicines are not valuable for modern conditions. Indians used *Podophyllum peltatum* (mayapple) for a broad range of things: as a cathartic, an insecticide, for rheumatism, and so on. Although it has been so reported, it seems very unlikely that they used mayapple as a cancer remedy. In Western medicine, a resin from the roots known as podophyllin is a common and moderately effective treatment for condylomata acuminata or venereal warts. Because some forms of venereal warts (caused by a virus) can be a precursor to cancer, this botanical remedy can be said to be a cancer cure. *Podophyllum peltatum* is also the basis for the production of etoposide, a semisynthetic derivative of podophyllotoxin, a chemical found in mayapple. Etoposide is widely used in the treatment of several forms of cancer.

Another interesting example of cross-cultural drugs is taxol, which is found in the leaves and bark of several species of yew of the genus *Taxus*. Native Americans used three species of Taxus for a broad range of things: antirheumatic, cold remedy, lung medicine, and so on. The Tsimshian Indians of British Columbia have been reported to use the plant "for internal ailments and cancer." *Taxus* has not traditionally been an important Western medicine but, as a result of screening of plant material at the National Cancer Institute in Washington, D.C., researchers investigated taxol as a possible cancer drug. Taxol, or paclitaxel, extracted from the bark of *Taxus brevifolia* is today used for treating cases of advanced breast or ovarian cancer.

Of course, just because taxol "works" for ovarian cancer does not mean it "works" for treating rheumatism, colds, or lungs, at least not in any very absolute sense. We must always consider the expectations and wishes of the people taking medicines. Usually, we take medicines when we "do not feel well." The goal is to "feel better." For example, say I am tired, sore, have a low fever, a sore throat, and a runny nose. Occasionally, a chill runs down my spine. I have not slept well for two days. My wife goes into the kitchen and makes a big pot of fresh chicken soup. It is rich and flavorful; the whole house smells warm and sweet. I eat a small bowl of the soup and along with it I eat a crusty piece of bread. I feel much better. An hour later I go to sleep and get some real rest. Are we to class chicken soup as an effective drug? Perhaps, but clearly this is different from, say, the matter of taxol and ovarian cancer. In the matter of chicken soup, much of the "effectiveness" of the treatment probably comes from the context within which the "cure" takes place. But the soup is an important part of that context and probably essential to it.

An interesting question is *why* plants have medicinal value. Plants produce a broad range of chemicals that serve a variety of purposes for the plants, some of which can be used by people to serve their own often different purposes. Phytochemists have classified plant chemicals as either primary or secondary: primary chemicals are those involved in the basic biochemistry of plant life, particularly photosynthesis; secondary chemicals are all the rest. Drugs generally belong to the class of secondary chemicals. Typically, in the past these secondary chemicals were thought not to be essential; they were considered to be the byproducts of primary processes or to be just random. More recently, as scientists have taken a more ecological approach to plant chemistry, the view of the function of secondary chemicals has changed. Plants seem to produce many chemicals that are biologically active, in other organisms as well as in themselves, to enhance their own survival. They may produce herbicides to inhibit the growth of competing plants. For example, salicylic acid (a naturally occurring chemical from which aspirin is made) is a water-soluble phytotoxin (plant poison) that washes off the leaves of willows (*Salix*) and other plants to the ground below, inhibiting the growth of competing plants. Juglone, produced by black walnut trees (*Juglans nigra*), does the same thing.

Plants also produce toxic or repellent chemicals that deter browsing by insects and other herbivores. Some familiar botanical insecticides are nicotine from tobacco (*Nicotiana*) and the pyrethrin found in chrysanthemums (such as *Dendranthema* and *Leucanthemum*). Pyrethrin is the active ingredient in common commercial insecticides. In certain cases, herbivores have adapted to these defenses. A well-known case is that of the monarch butterfly (*Danaus plex-*

ippus). The monarch larvae feed on milkweeds (*Asclepias*), which are very toxic to other animals and insects. The larvae ingest and sequester various cardiac glycosides throughout their bodies, thereby deterring birds from feeding on them. Humans, too, can use the cardiac glycosides of milkweed when they want to cause vomiting for whatever reason (recall the discussion above about pukeweed).

Similarly, pines (*Pinus*) are generally protected against a variety of insects and fungi by the pitch they exude from bark and leaves. Protection against insects is both physical (the sticky pitch drowns them) and chemical (the monoterpenes in pitch are toxic to many insects). Several kinds of bark beetles (such as *Dendroctonus* species), however, can detoxify these substances and even use them as pheromones that serve to attract a sufficiently large number of beetles to overcome the physical resistance of the tree—the tree's chemical defense is turned against itself. Similarly, people have used pine pitch as a disinfectant and for a broad range of other purposes as well. Both people and other creatures can occasionally find their own uses for the secondary chemicals that plants produce.

Some cases of animal use of plant secondary chemicals are straightforward. For example, it is reasonable enough to use pyrethrin to kill insects; that is probably what the chrysanthemums make them for in the first place. Similarly, it seems reasonable to expect that substances produced by plants to protect themselves against worms that eat their roots might turn out to be useful for treating intestinal parasites. Other cases are less obvious. Several different plants— birches (*Betula*), willows (*Salix*), wintergreen (*Gaultheria*), *Spiraea*—produce various salicylates, among them salicin and methyl salicylate, which are precursors for aspirin. Aspirin, or acetylsalicylic acid, is a semisynthetic drug, a modification of the natural precursors. The natural products do more or less what aspirin does, but aspirin is much less toxic than salicin. The natural salicylates have the advantage of being readily absorbed through the skin, and for that reason they are often used as the active ingredients in sports creams for stopping muscle pain. The chemical processes of the salicylates and guts are true for insects, too, which have similar chemicals to protect their guts from being digested. It is plausible to argue that the salicylates are also toxic to insects. Thus, the natural salicylates are probably herbicides that serve to reduce competition for growing space for the plants that produce them. But why should an herbicide stop headaches? This is a question without an obvious answer. In part, it is because no one is quite sure how aspirin or the other salicylates work in the first place. They apparently inhibit the production of prostaglandins. Prostaglandins are important chemicals involved in the processes of temperature regulation, inflammation, and pain; they also help maintain the mucous layer in the gut, preventing the stomach from digesting itself. This is apparently why aspirin can upset the stomach. But it is not at all clear why an herbicide should be an effective inhibitor of prostaglandin production. There are many other similar cases, all of which indicate how much we have yet to learn about human and plant physiology.

Problems and Paradoxes

It is usually not too difficult to make sense of American Indian medicinal plant use with analyses such as those described above. Often the drugs involve a secondary chemical that performs understandable functions for the plant. There are, however, limits to such rational interpretations. It is easy to find cases in which different peoples—sometimes even the same peoples— are reported to use the same plant, often prepared in the same or very similar ways, for quite opposite purposes. Consider these paradoxical cases:

The Woodlands Cree are reported to mix the fruit of *Arctostaphylos uva-ursi* (kinnikin-nick) with grease and give it to children as a treatment for diarrhea, whereas the Upper Tanana are said to eat raw kinnikinnick berries as a laxative.

The Hualapai are said to use a decoction of the leaves of *Eriodictyon angustifolium* (yerba santa) as a laxative, whereas the Paiute are reported to use the same formulation as a treatment for diarrhea.

The Iroquois reportedly use a decoction of the roots of *Silphium perfoliatum* (cup plant) as an emetic, whereas the Meskwaki use the root of the same plant to alleviate the vomiting and nausea that often accompany pregnancy.

The Cherokee are said to use an infusion of the bark of *Hydrangea arborescens* (wild hydrangea) as an antiemetic for children but are also said to also use the same thing to induce vomiting to "throw off disordered bile."

Similar cases can be found in which the same plant is used as both a stimulant and a sedative. There are even a few cases in which a plant is considered poisonous by one group, whereas another uses it as an antidote for poisoning.

How are we to account for such apparent contradictions? I believe there is much in medicine—any form of medicine—that resists logic, rationality, and explanation. For example, modern Western biomedicine has a long history of treatments once deemed essential that are now considered nonsense. Historians seem generally to agree, for example, that George Washington was bled to death by his physicians. It is likely that some of the treatments we use today will be ridiculed in a decade (as will some of their replacements in another decade). In addition, some physicians are better than others. The most highly trained physicians can make mistakes, as seen in many malpractice suits in our courts. There is no reason to believe that Native American physicians had a monopoly on accuracy. They doubtless made mistakes, too, and some of these mistakes are probably reported in the material in this book.

Some treatments that seem paradoxical may be homeopathic in some sense. The bulk of Western medicine is allopathic. In allopathy, disease is fought by using its opposite, or something that acts against the disease, such as an antibiotic. Homeopathy treats disease by prescribing drugs, usually in very small doses, that produce symptoms resembling the disease being treated. The logic of homeopathy underlies the practice of vaccination for smallpox or measles in which a controlled and attenuated case of an illness is induced to develop an immunity to a real infection. Thus, what one group recognized as a poison, another group may have recognized as a homeopathic treatment for poisoning.

Some of the seemingly paradoxical cases may be the result of confusion on the part of the Native Americans consulted, errors in understanding by the investigator, or both. Some errors in understanding may be due to mistranslation. It is unlikely that such errors are restricted to paradoxical cases—the potential of such errors in any case urges us to be careful with *all* the information gathered here.

These reservations do not undercut the real value of the information gathered in *Native American Medicinal Plants*. There is no doubt that Native Americans had a huge reservoir of real knowledge about the medicinal values of plants. But they were human beings who also made mistakes, who sometimes understood things wrongly or differently. That there may be some errors in the information gathered here does not make everything wrong. However, just because something has been reported does not make it true.

Appreciating the Common Knowledge of Our Past

There is an enormous amount of real human knowledge contained in *Native American Medicinal Plants*. The earliest evidence we have of human beings using plants for medicine comes from the Middle Paleolithic site of Shanidar in northern Iraq, dated about 60,000 years ago. People have been experimenting with nature since then (and perhaps before). People first came to the Americas about 15,000 years ago and have been studying the plants of the two continents ever since. Given that the floras of North America and China are remarkably alike, it is possible that the earliest Asian immigrants to North America saw recognizable plants when they got here. It is also possible that they brought useful plants with them either deliberately or accidently as weed seeds in their clothing.

Much of this accumulated knowledge of useful plants, slowly wrung from nature over millennia, has in a few centuries been lost, at least lost as a part of normal human life. There are specialists—anthropologists, ethnobotanists, phytochemists, pharmacognosists—who are aware of some portions of what this book contains. But in past times this was to a large degree the knowledge of ordinary people. Surely there were specialists, people who were more interested than others in these matters, and they may even have developed esoteric knowledge that they kept to themselves for personal profit. But generally this was normal human knowledge, part and parcel of everyday life. People walked in the world and saw plants they knew to be useful for treating various ailments. Their children learned of these matters as naturally as our children learn the names of baseball teams or athletic shoes or rock bands. In a world where one may buy a bottle of aspirin tablets at a grocery store for little more than the price of the bottle, there is not much need for people to be able to recognize willow, black birch, spiraea, or wintergreen as naturally occurring painkillers.

And I do not believe there is a need for anyone to give up on aspirin tablets and rely on willow twigs. One need not eat medicinal plants in order to appreciate them, any more than a birdwatcher needs to eat a curlew to enjoy it. But when one knows something of the medicinal uses people have made of thousands of the wild plants around us, the plants take on a new meaning, a new value greater than their beauty, their cooling shade, or their pleasant scent.

Sources of Information on Plant Usages

Native American Medicinal Plants is based on the research of hundreds of scholars. I accumulated the material over a period of more than 25 years. In that period, any time I saw an item containing useful information, I made a note of it. In addition, in 1993 I did an intensive search of the literature using traditional techniques such as reading bibliographies and using computerized search techniques.

The criteria for selecting a source to be included were fairly simple. First, the material had to be primary, that is, based on original work with Native Americans who used the plants. I excluded all secondary material based on prior published work. If I found an interesting secondary source, I examined its bibliography to identify original sources that had yet to be consulted. In a few cases the primary source was not written by the individual who actually did the fieldwork. For example, source 49 by Catherine Fowler is based on primary research done many years earlier by Willard Z. Park with the Northern Paiute, work that was not published at the time. As a second criterion, the source had to have reasonably clear scientific plant names, the plant identifications preferably having been made by professional botanists. Third, at least some of the information had to come from Native Americans living north of the Rio Grande. Fourth, information was coded only once even if it was published several times. In such cases I tried to use the earliest publication, but sometimes I used a later one if it had better plant identifications. The oldest source was published in 1840, the most recent in 1993.

Although I used sources in which care had been taken in plant identification, no doubt some plants were misidentified and thus misnamed. In some cases, what may have been recognized as one species at the time the plant was originally identified may now be recognized as two similar species. In addition, there is further work to do on the plants themselves. Apart from the matter of the accuracy of identification, the precision of identification in *Native American Medicinal Plants* depends on that in the original sources. For example, in some species different subspecies or varieties may be recognized. If one source reported a plant named only to the level of species and another source reported a plant to the level of subspecies or variety (or used a name that can be attributed to a particular subspecies or variety), then the usages will be listed in the Catalog of Plants under the species or under the subspecies or variety, respectively. Thus, the usages of *Quercus rubra* by the Cherokee were reported in two sources, and because the sources used plant names that can be determined to different levels of precision, some uses are reported under the entry for *Quercus rubra* and others under that for *Quercus rubra* var. *rubra*.

Drug Usage Categories

Some care needs to be exercised in the interpretation of certain drug usage categories. For example, there are a number of uses described for particular diseases, such as Cancer Treatment and Tuberculosis Remedy. Most of these disease categories have a minimum of 50 to 60 items (information about plants used in those ways) listed under them, and some are very large with hundreds or more. Some treatments for specific diseases without a category of their own are classified under Miscellaneous Disease Remedy. A few examples of such are treatments for diabetes, flu, and measles. But listed under one of the other major usage categories, Other, are usages not for a particular disease (such as flu) but for plants said to be used for treatments such as antibiotics, or for sunstroke, or for "strengthening veins."

Another subcategory is Unspecified. For example, a source may state that a plant is used as a medicine but reports nothing about the particular use. "The plant is used medicinally" would be a typical report classified under Unspecified. Unspecified is a large category, including 567 reports.

The following is a list of the drug usage categories listed in the Catalog of Plants:

Abortifacient. Designed to eliminate a pregnancy, induce an abortion, or "bring on a delayed period" (an emmenagogue); see also Contraceptive

Adjuvant. An item that is a subordinate element in medicines that helps them work or taste better

Alterative. Something that changes the character of one's system; this category is used only if the term *alterative* actually appears in the source

Analgesic. Relieves pain

Anesthetic. Reduces the sense of touch or pain

Anthelmintic. Used for the treatment of intestinal parasites

Anticonvulsive. Stops or prevents convulsions or fits

Antidiarrheal. Used to stop diarrhea

Antidote. Negates the effects of a poison; see also Poison

Antiemetic. Inhibits vomiting

Antihemorrhagic. Stops hemorrhage, especially internal bleeding; see also Hemostat

Antirheumatic (External). Used for rheumatism or arthritis and that is applied externally, for example, a liniment

Antirheumatic (Internal). Used for rheumatism or arthritis and that is taken internally, for example, aspirin

Basket Medicine. Makes people buy baskets; if a prospective buyer picks up a basket, he will not be able to let go and will pay the price asked

Blood Medicine. Designed to purify or influence the blood

Breast Treatment. Used to treat breasts

Burn Dressing. All types of dressings applied externally to burns

Cancer Treatment. Used to treat cancer or tumors; this category is used only if the word *cancer* explicitly appears in the source

Carminative. Relieves flatulence or "gas"

Cathartic. Causes evacuation of the bowels, a strong laxative; physic and purgative are synonyms of cathartic; see also Laxative

Ceremonial Medicine. Used as a part of ceremonies

Cold Remedy. Used for the relief or cure of colds

Contraceptive. Used to prevent pregnancy; see also Abortifacient

Cough Medicine. Used for the relief or cure of coughs

Dermatological Aid. Used to treat any conditions of the skin or hair: acne, dandruff, itching, etc.

Diaphoretic. Causes sweating

Dietary Aid. Affects the diet or hunger in a situation involving illness, usually used to increase the appetite of a sick person with no appetite or to decrease it

Disinfectant. Used to eliminate "infection," literal or otherwise

Diuretic. Causes urination; see also Urinary Aid

Ear Medicine. Used for earaches, deafness, or any other afflictions of the ear

Emetic. Causes vomiting

Expectorant. Promotes the ejection of mucus from the lungs, usually by spitting; see also Pulmonary Aid, Respiratory Aid

Eye Medicine. Used for any afflictions of the eye

Febrifuge. Used to reduce fevers

Gastrointestinal Aid. Used to treat distress of the digestive tract

Gland Medicine. Used for the treatment of irregular glands: swollen, suppurating, etc.

Gynecological Aid. Used to treat problems surrounding pregnancy and childbirth and other problems specific to women

Hallucinogen. Substance that induces hallucinations

Heart Medicine. Used for the treatment of heart problems

Hemorrhoid Remedy. Used for hemorrhoids or "piles"

Hemostat. Used to stop external bleeding; this category is also used for topical treatments for nosebleed; see also Antihemorrhagic

Herbal Steam. Used medicinally in a steam bath for various ailments

Hunting Medicine. Used to help a hunter find or capture prey

Hypotensive. Used to reduce blood pressure

Internal Medicine. Used for various internal ailments; these are frequently very vaguely described, for example, "decoction of flowers taken for internal disorders"

Kidney Aid. Used for kidney troubles and the treatment of "dropsy," an anachronistic term for edema that appears often in older ethnobotanical literature

Laxative. A mild treatment for constipation; see also Cathartic

Liver Aid. Used for the treatment of various liver disorders

Love Medicine. Used to procure love from another

Miscellaneous Disease Remedy. Used for a particular disease, one not categorized elsewhere, such as ague, grippe, or rabies

Narcotic. Produces sleep or stupor, a strong sedative; see also Sedative

Nose Medicine. Used for the treatment of various nose ailments; see also Hemostat

Oral Aid. Used for the treatment of various mouth disorders

Orthopedic Aid. Used for afflictions of the muscles or bones

Other. Used for various conditions and ailments that are not diseases and not categorized elsewhere, such as heat prostration, meanness, and sunstroke

Panacea. Used as a cure-all, a drug that will help any condition

Pediatric Aid. Drug specifically mentioned as a treatment for children

Poison. Substance that usually kills, injures, or impairs an organism; see also Antidote

Poultice. Held against the skin

Preventive Medicine. Prevents various ailments

Psychological Aid. Directed toward the mind and specifically toward issues of will or desire

Pulmonary Aid. Used for lung conditions; see also Expectorant, Respiratory Aid, Tuberculosis Remedy

Reproductive Aid. Used by males or females to facilitate successful reproduction

Respiratory Aid. Used to help breathing; see also Expectorant, Pulmonary Aid

Sedative. Reduces excitement or upset; see also Narcotic

Snakebite Remedy. Used for the treatment of snakebites

Sports Medicine. Used by athletes for various complaints or to enhance performance

Stimulant. Stimulates or wakes a person up

Strengthener. Used to increase strength

Throat Aid. Used for afflictions of the throat

Tonic. Used as a tonic for various ailments; only used when the term *tonic* is specifically mentioned in the source

Toothache Remedy. Used for toothaches as well as any other dental medicines

Tuberculosis Remedy. Used for the treatment of tuberculosis; this category is used only when the source specifically mentions *consumption, scrofula,* or *tuberculosis* (scrofula is a form of tuberculosis that affects the lymph nodes, especially of the neck); see also Pulmonary Aid

Unspecified. Used as an unspecified medicine or to treat unspecified illnesses; this category is used if the source states something such as "plant used as a medicine" but with no more specific information

Urinary Aid. Used for problems of the urinary tract and by men for sexual organ problems; see also Diuretic

Venereal Aid. Used for any venereal disease: gonorrhea, syphilis, etc.

Vertigo Medicine. Used for treating dizziness

Veterinary Aid. Used to treat diseases and injuries of animals

Witchcraft Medicine. Used for sorcery or magic

Native Americans

The names of Native American or American Indian groups is a complicated matter. Even the phrase *American Indian* is problematic, for it reflects the fact that Christopher Columbus and his followers were naive about the location of "India." Many people now seem to prefer the term *Native American*. But it is also the case that indigenous peoples were here long before the continents of the New World were named after the Italian navigator Amerigo Vespucci. In Canada, the generic term usually used is *First Nations*. Yet, the fact remains that many people have been quite happy with the term *Indian*. Consider, for example, the American Indian Movement of the 1960s. Because these names often have political significance, it is for all practical purposes impossible to refer generically to the indigenous population of the Americas without offending someone, but such is not the intention here.

There are similar problems with tribal names. A classic case is the name Eskimo. The word is, apparently, an English mispronunciation of a French mispronunciation of a Montagnais or Micmac word *ayashkimew*, which seems to have meant something like "eaters of raw meat," intended as a nasty insult. The Eskimo people generally call themselves Inuit or Innuit, meaning "people." (I am unaware of the Inuit name for the Micmac, but my guess is that it was equally insulting.) Such derived names are not always insults, however. The name Navaho or Navajo is a Spanish variation on a Tewa word meaning "large arroyo with cultivated fields," a place name. The Navajo name for themselves is Dene, meaning "people," but many Navajo also call themselves Navajo. Again, the names used to refer to particular Native American tribes can occasion political debate. Referring to one group by a term that means "people" implicitly asserts that other groups are something other than people, for example. Names used in *Native American Medicinal Plants* are not intended in any way to offend anyone. I have elected to use the names for peoples reported in the original sources. This means that material for "the same people" is sometimes listed under different designations, but rarely is it for the same people at the same time. There are 217 groups mentioned in *Native American Medicinal Plants*, as listed below. The reference numbers below correspond to the sources enumerated in the Bibliography, from which information on each of the peoples was obtained:

Abnaki. Saint François du Lac, about 100 miles (160 km) northwest of Montréal, Quebec (121)
Alabama. Located on a state reservation on the Trinity River in Polk County, Texas (148, 152)
Alaska Native. Alaska (71)
Aleut. On 17 Aleutian Islands that lie between the Alaska Peninsula and Attu, Alaska (6, 126, 163)
Algonquin. New England (18)
Algonquin, Quebec. Western Quebec (14)
Algonquin, Tête-de-Boule. Manouan, about 260 miles (420 km) north of Montréal, Quebec (110)
Anticosti. On the Ile d'Anticosti in the Saint Lawrence River, north of the Gaspé Peninsula, Quebec (120)
Apache. Various Apache groups live in Arizona and New Mexico (13, 27, 38, 100, 115)
Apache, Chiricahua & Mescalero. Chiricahua Apache ranged through western New Mexico, southeastern Arizona, and southward into Mexico; their eastern boundary began at the Rio Grande. The Mescalero Apache were principally located in New Mexico; the Rio Grande was their western boundary (28)

Apache, Mescalero. Southern New Mexico, western Texas, and northern Chihuahua, Mexico (10, 13)

Apache, Western. Fort Apache Reservation, Arizona (21)

Apache, White Mountain. White Mountain, Arizona (113)

Apalachee. In the sixteenth and seventeenth centuries, the Apalachee lived in Spanish Florida, what is now northern Florida and southern Georgia (67)

Arapaho. Between the Platte and Arkansas Rivers in eastern Colorado and southeastern Wyoming (15, 98, 100)

Atsugewi. North of the Sierra Nevada and south of the Pit River in northeastern California (50)

Bannock. Idaho (98)

Bella Coola. Near the mouth of the Bella Coola River, about 250 miles (400 km) north-northwest of Vancouver, British Columbia (62, 127, 158)

Blackfoot. Over the region of Montana, Alberta, and Saskatchewan. Blackfoot is a common spelling in Canada, whereas Blackfeet is more common in the United States (68, 72, 82, 95, 98, 100)

Cahuilla. Southern California (11)

California Indian. California (15, 98)

Carrier. Near Fort St. James and Anahim Lake in central and northern British Columbia (26, 75, 158)

Carrier, Northern. Near Hagwelget in northwestern British Columbia (127)

Carrier, Southern. Near Ulkatcho in northwestern British Columbia (35, 127)

Catawba. Along the Catawba River in the Carolinas (134, 152)

Chehalis. Central coast of Washington (65)

Cherokee. Throughout much of western North Carolina (particularly in Graham and Cherokee Counties) and in northwestern Georgia. There are also many Cherokees in Oklahoma (66, 105, 145, 152, 177, 178)

Cheyenne. Montana and Oklahoma (15, 63, 64, 68, 69, 82)

Cheyenne, Northern. Montana (68)

Chickasaw. Information in source 23 was collected by Gideon Lincecum between 1800 and 1835 in Mississippi. Most Chickasaws are now in Oklahoma (23, 152)

Chippewa. Also known as the Ojibwa, Chippewas are located in the upper Midwest and southern Ontario. Source 41 describes the Ojibwa of northern Minnesota, primarily the Leech Lake, Red Lake, and White Earth reservations but also including a consultant from the Bois Fort reservation. Source 43 describes the Ojibwa of northern central Minnesota and the Manitou Rapids Reserve in Ontario. Source 59 describes people from Pinconning and Lapeer, Michigan, and Sarnia, Ontario. Currently, many of these people refer to themselves as Anishininaabe, which means something like First People or Original People. See also Ojibwa

Choctaw. Saint Tammany Parish, Louisiana, on the northern shore of Lake Pontchartrain, is a center of the Choctaw region. Information in source 23 was collected by Gideon Lincecum between 1800 and 1835 in Mississippi (20, 23, 135, 152)

Chumash. Southern California (11)

Clallam. Olympic Peninsula, Washington (47)

Coahuilla. Southern California coast (9)

Cocopa. Southwestern Arizona and Baja California and Sonora, Mexico, generally along the lower Colorado River (52)

Comanche. The Comanche Indian Reservation is near Indiahoma, Comanche County, Oklahoma (24, 27, 84)

Concow. The Round Valley Indian Reservation is in Mendocino County, California, and stretches as a band about 60 miles (100 km) broad for 84 miles (135 km) along the coast, about midway between San Francisco and the Oregon border to the north (33)

Costanoan. In the Coast Ranges of central California, from San Francisco south to Big Sur and from the Pacific coast inland to the Diablo Range foothills (17)

Costanoan (Olhonean). Central California (97)

Cowichan. Southeastern coast of Vancouver Island, British Columbia (156, 160)

Cowlitz. South-central Washington (65)

Cree. From the Northwest Territories (12) through central Alberta and southwestern Saskatchewan (82) to Montana (68)

Cree, Alberta. Northern Alberta (126)

Cree, Hudson Bay. Hudson Bay region, Canada (78)

Cree, Woodlands. Saskatchewan (91)

Creek. Information from source 23 was collected by Gideon Lincecum between 1800 and 1835 in the original Creek homeland in Georgia. Most Creeks are today in Oklahoma (23, 145, 148, 152, 177)

Crow. A Siouan tribe living in southwestern Montana and northern Wyoming (15, 68)

Dakota. The Dakota, also known as the Lakota or Sioux, live on a number of reservations in Montana, the Dakotas, Nebraska, and Minnesota (57, 58, 82, 100). See also Lakota and Sioux

Delaware. Originally on the East Coast. Today, some live in Ontario but most are in Oklahoma (151)

Delaware, Oklahoma. Oklahoma (150)

Delaware, Ontario. Ontario (150)

Diegueño. Throughout southernmost California, notably on the Santa Ysabel Indian Reservation in San Diego County (11, 70, 74)

Eskimo. Across the Arctic regions of Alaska, Canada, and Greenland; also known as Inuit (126)

Eskimo, Alaska. Nelson Island, on the Bering Sea coast of the Yukon-Kuskokwim Delta, western Alaska (1), villages along the northern Bering Sea and Arctic Alaska (3), western and southwestern Alaska (106), and Kodiak, Alaska (126)

Eskimo, Arctic. Central Canadian Arctic and sub-Arctic (106)

Eskimo, Chugach. Southern Alaska, east of the Kenai Peninsula along the coast to Controller Bay, Alaska (126)

Eskimo, Inuktitut. Alaska, Canada, and Greenland (176)

Eskimo, Inupiat. Kotzebue in northwestern Alaska (83)

Eskimo, Kuskokwagmiut. Napaskiak, western Alaska (101)

Eskimo, Nunivak. Nunivak Island, Alaska (126)

Eskimo, Western. Lower Kuskokwim, Nunivak, and Nelson Islands on the western coast of Alaska (90)

Flathead. An Interior Salish tribe located in western Montana and Idaho, north of the Gallatin River, between the Rocky Mountains in the west and the Little Belt Range in the east (15, 68, 75, 82)

Gabrielino. Southern California (11)

Gitksan. Along the northern coast of British Columbia and along the Skeena River (35, 61, 62, 127)

Gosiute. In desert territory bordering the Great Salt Lake in Utah on the south and extending westward into eastern Nevada (31)

Great Basin Indian. Uintah-Ouray Reservation, Fort Duchesne, Utah (100)

Green River Group. South of Seattle, Washington (65)

Gros Ventre. An Algonquian tribe living in the Milk River area of northern Montana (15, 68, 98)

Haihais. Central coast of British Columbia (35)

Haisla. Central coast of British Columbia (35, 61, 62)

Haisla & Hanaksiala. Central coast of British Columbia (35)

Hanaksiala. Central coast of British Columbia (35)

Havasupai. Cataract Canyon, a side branch of the Grand Canyon in northwestern Arizona (13, 139, 171, 174)

Hawaiian. Hawaii (2, 94)

Heiltzuk. Central coast of British Columbia (35)

Hesquiat. Coast of British Columbia and Hesquiat Harbor, Vancouver Island, British Columbia (35, 159, 160)

Hoh. Near the mouth of the Hoh River on the western side of the Olympic Peninsula, Washington (114)

Hopi. Several villages on the Hopi Reservation in northeastern Arizona, which is surrounded by the Navajo Reservation (13, 27, 29, 34, 46, 115, 164, 174, 179)

Houma. Louisiana (135)

Hualapai. Northwestern Arizona (169)

Iroquois. Throughout upstate New York and in southern Quebec (73, 103, 118, 119, 170)

Isleta. The Isleta pueblo is located on the western bank of the Rio Grande, 12 miles (19 km) south of Albuquerque, New Mexico (27, 85)

Jemez. The Jemez pueblo is located on the Jemez River about 45 miles (72 km) northwest of Albuquerque, New Mexico (13, 27, 36, 85, 174)

Karok. Along the Klamath River in an area paralleling the California coast from above Bluff Creek in Humboldt County to Happy Camp in Siskiyou County (5, 97, 125)

Kawaiisu. East of Bakersfield in southeastern California (180)

Keresan. There are seven pueblos near Albuquerque, New Mexico, where the languages are classified as Keresan. The Eastern Keresan pueblos are Cochiti, San Felipe, Santa Ana, Santo Domingo, and Sia. The Western Keresan pueblos are Acoma and Laguna. All of these but Santa Ana and Santo Domingo are treated separately in this book (172). See also Keres, Western; Sia

Keres, Western. The Acoma and Laguna pueblos (147). See also Keresan

Kiowa. Southern plains near the Arkansas and Red Rivers (15, 166)

Kitasoo. Central coast of British Columbia (35)

Klallam. Southern shore of Vancouver Island, British Columbia, and the northern central Olympic Peninsula, Washington (65)

Klamath. Southern central Oregon (37, 97, 98, 140)

Koasati. Southeastern United States (152)

Koyukon. Huslia and Hughes, Alaska (99)

Kuper Island Indian. Kuper Island, southwest of Nanaimo, Vancouver Island, British Columbia (156)

Kutenai. Montana (68)

Kwakiutl. Northern Vancouver Island and north of Vancouver Island on the mainland coast of British Columbia (16, 156, 157)

Kwakiutl, Southern. Central coast of British Columbia and northeastern coast of Vancouver Island, British Columbia (157, 158)

Kwakwaka'wakw. Central coast of British Columbia (35)

Lakota. Also known as Dakota and Sioux. Standing Rock Reservation is located on the central border of North Dakota and South Dakota (88); Rosebud Reservation is in Todd County, South Dakota (88, 116). See also Dakota and Sioux

Luiseño. Southern California near San Juan Capistrano (11, 132)

Lummi. Northwestern border of Washington, near British Columbia (65)

Mahuna. Southwestern California (117)

Makah. Northwestern tip of the Olympic Peninsula, Washington (35, 55, 65, 160)

Malecite. New Brunswick, Canada (96, 137)

Mandan. North Dakota along the Missouri River near the mouth of the Heart River (15, 58)

Maricopa. South-central Arizona (27, 38, 81)

Mendocino Indian. Mendocino County, California, halfway between San Francisco and the Oregon border (33)

Menominee. Wisconsin (44, 128)

Meskwaki. Tama, Iowa (129)

Mewuk. Central California (97)

Micmac. Nova Scotia, Prince Edward Island, New Brunswick east of the St. John River, and part of the Gaspé Peninsula, Quebec (32, 96, 122, 133, 136, 168)

Midoo. Central California (97)

Miwok. The Sierra Nevada together with the western foothills and a relatively small portion of the adjacent Sacramento–San Joaquin Valley, California (8)

Modesse. Northern California (97)

Mohegan. Connecticut (25, 149, 151)

Montagnais. Throughout eastern Quebec, Lac-St.-Jean (19), the northern coast of the Gulf of St. Lawrence and the lower St. Lawrence River (133), and Labrador (149)

Montana Indian. Montana (15, 68)

Montauk. Eastern end of Long Island, New York (25)

Nanticoke. Delaware (149, 150)

Narraganset. Rhode Island (25)

Natchez. Lower Mississippi River (148, 152)

Navajo. Northern Arizona, northwestern New Mexico, and southeastern Utah (13, 27, 38, 45, 46, 76, 82, 85, 92, 113, 115, 142, 174)

Navajo, Kayenta. Northeastern Arizona, near Monument Valley (179)

Navajo, Ramah. Western New Mexico (165)

Neeshenam. Bear River, Placer County, California (107)

Nevada Indian. Nevada (98, 100)

Nez Perce. Along the lower Snake River and its tributaries in western Idaho, northeastern Oregon, and southwestern Washington (15, 68, 82)

Nitinaht. Southwestern coast of Vancouver Island, British Columbia, from near Jordan River to Pachena Point, extending inland along Nitinat Lake (55, 159, 160)

Nootka. Southwestern coast of Vancouver Island, British Columbia (146, 159, 160)

Nootka, Manhousat. Vancouver Island, British Columbia (160)

Nuxalkmc. Valley of the Bella Coola River, South Bentinck Arm, Tallio Inlet, and Kimsquit in western central British Columbia (35)

Oglala. South Dakota (58)

Ojibwa. Also known as the Chippewa, Ojibwas are located in the upper Midwest and southern Ontario. Source 4 describes the Ojibwa north of lakes Superior and Huron in Ontario. The Fort Bois Ojibwa described in source 112 live on a reservation 140 miles (225 km) northwest of Duluth, Minnesota. People described in source 130 live in northern Wisconsin. See also Chippewa

Ojibwa, South. Red Lake and Leech Lake, Minnesota (77)

Okanagan-Colville. The Okanagan occupied the Okanagan and Similkameen River valleys and the shores of Lake Okanagan on both sides of the U.S.-Canadian (British Columbia) border. The Colville are located on the Colville Reservation in northeastern Washington (62, 162). Okanagan is the Canadian spelling. See also Okanagon

Okanagon. The Okanagon are found on the Colville Reservation in Washington and on various reserves in British Columbia (104, 141, 153). Okanagon is the American spelling. See also Okanagan-Colville

Omaha. Nebraska (48, 56, 58)

Oregon Indian. Oregon (98)

Oregon Indian, Warm Springs. Warm Springs, north-central Oregon (87, 98)

Oto. Eastern Nebraska along the Platte River (58)

Oweekeno. Central coast of British Columbia (35)

Paiute. Generally in the Great Basin region, although some live in California and Oregon. People described in sources 15 and 104 are from Surprise Valley, California. Source 93 describes the Warm Springs Reservation, Oregon. The remaining sources (27, 98, 100, 144, 155) generally describe people living in Nevada.

Paiute, Northern. Western Nevada (49)

Papago. In desert regions south of the Gila River of Arizona and extending into Sonora, Mexico (13, 27, 29, 38, 81, 98, 123)

Pawnee. Missouri River region (58)

Penobscot. Northern New England and the maritime provinces of Canada. There is a Penobscot Reservation in Maine (133, 149)

Pima. Gila and Salt River valleys of southern Arizona (13, 27, 38, 81, 123)

Plains Indian. Montana (68, 82)

Poliklah. Northern California (97)

Pomo. Sonoma, Mendocino, and Lake Counties, California (7, 33, 54, 97, 98)

Pomo, Calpella. Northern California (33)

Pomo, Kashaya. Coast of Sonoma County, California (60)

Pomo, Little Lakes. Northern California (33)

Pomo, Potter Valley. Northern California (33)

Ponca. The Northern Ponca are located in Nebraska and South Dakota, whereas the Southern band is located in Oklahoma (58, 80)

Potawatomi. Wisconsin (131)

Puyallup. Southeastern side of Puget Sound, Washington (65)

Quileute. Western coast of the Olympic Peninsula, Washington (55, 65, 114)

Quinault. Southwestern coast of the Olympic Peninsula, Washington (65, 175)

Rappahannock. Virginia (25, 138)

Ree. Montana (15)

Round Valley Indian. Round Valley, 200 miles (320 km) north of San Francisco in northern California (33)

Saanich. Southeastern side of Vancouver Island, British Columbia (156)

Salish. North of Vancouver Island on the mainland coast of British Columbia (153, 156, 157, 159)

Salish, Coast. Northern central side of Vancouver Island and north of Vancouver Island on the mainland of British Columbia (156, 157)

Salish, Cowichan. Southeastern side of Vancouver Island, British Columbia (156, 160)

Samish. Northern coast of Washington, near the British Columbia border (65)

Sanpoil. South of the Columbia River in northeastern Washington (75, 109, 162)

Sanpoil & Nespelem. South of the Columbia River in northeastern Washington (109, 162)

Seminole. Southern Florida (145)

Seri. Isla Tiburon in the Gulf of California, Mexico (40)

Shasta. Along the Klamath River in northern California near the Oregon border (79, 97)

Shinnecock. Long Island, New York (25)

Shoshoni. Mostly in Nevada, but extending into Montana and central California (68, 82, 97, 98, 100, 155)

Shuswap. Southern interior plateau of British Columbia (75, 102, 153)

Sia. Sia (sometimes Zia) is a Keresan pueblo near Albuquerque, New Mexico (173). See also Keresan

Sikani. Headwaters of Peace River in British Columbia (127)

Sioux. Also known as the Dakota or Lakota; across the Great Plains from Minnesota to Wyoming and Montana (15, 68, 98, 130). See also Dakota and Lakota

Sioux, Fort Peck. The Fort Peck Reservation is in northern Montana (15)

Sioux, Teton. Wyoming and Montana (42)

Skagit. Northwestern Washington (65)

Skagit, Upper. Northern Cascade Range, Washington (154)

Skokomish. West-central side of Puget Sound, Washington (65)

Snake. Montana (15)

Snohomish. Northeastern side of Puget Sound, Washington (65)

Songish. Southeastern side of Vancouver Island, British Columbia (156)

Squaxin. South of Puget Sound, Washington (65)

Stony Indian. Montana (68)

Swinomish. Northern coast of Washington (65)

Tanaina. Near Anchorage, Alaska (126)

Tanana, Upper. Alaska between Anchorage and Fairbanks (86)

Tarahumara. Southern Arizona and northern Mexico (13)

Tewa. Near Santa Fe, New Mexico (13, 27, 34, 115)

Thompson. Southwestern British Columbia (75, 104, 141, 153, 161)

Tlingit. Southeastern coastline of the Alaska panhandle from Yakutat Bay to Cape Fox (65, 89, 126)

Tolowa. Northwestern California (5)

Tsimshian. Northern coast of British Columbia into the southeastern portion of the Alaska panhandle (35, 61, 62, 65)

Tsimshian, Coast. Central coast of British Columbia (35)

Tubatulabal. California (167)

Umatilla. Along the Umatilla and Columbia Rivers in Oregon (37, 75)

Ute. Western Colorado and eastern Utah (27, 29, 30, 37, 98)

Wailaki. Round Valley Reservation in Mendocino County, northern California (33, 98)

Walapai. Cataract Canyon, a side branch of the Grand Canyon in northwestern Arizona (13, 139, 171)

Washo. Near Lake Tahoe on the California-Nevada border (98, 100, 155)

West Coast Indian. West Coast of the United States (111)

Wet'suwet'en. East of the central coast of British Columbia (61)

Winnebago. Originally living near Green Bay, Wisconsin, they now occupy reservations in Wisconsin and Nebraska (58, 108)

Yana. Northern California (124)

Yavapai. Western Arizona (13, 51, 53)

Yokia. Ukiah, Mendocino County, northern California (33)

Yokut. Central California (97)

Yuki. Round Valley, Mendocino County, northern California (33, 39, 98)

Yuma. Lower Colorado River valley in Arizona (27, 29)

Yurok. Northwestern California (5)

Yurok, South Coast (Nererner). Northwestern California (97)

Zuni. The Zuni pueblo is about 40 miles (64 km) southwest of Gallup, New Mexico (13, 22, 27, 29, 113, 143)

Organization of Information

Scientific Plant Names

The information in *Native American Medicinal Plants* is organized in the Catalog of Plants alphabetically by the scientific names of the plants. Scientific plant names have a very particular form, for example, *Abies balsamea* for balsam fir. *Abies* is the genus and *balsamea* the species name, in combination called a binomial.

Some plant names are more complex. In some species, botanists recognize subspecies or naturally occurring varieties. Usually the rank of subspecies *or* variety is recognized in a particular species, but sometimes both ranks are used and then a subspecies may comprise more than one variety. For the purpose of completeness the subspecies (abbreviated here as ssp.) and variety (var.) names are both given in this book, for example, the full name of Pacific red elder, a plant used in a dozen or so ways by West Coast tribes, is *Sambucus racemosa* ssp. *pubens* var. *arborescens*.

When reference is made to an unknown species of a particular genus, the abbreviation "sp.," for species, is used. A source may have referred to one unknown species of a genus or more than one unknown species; "sp." is used here for both kinds of references.

Species that are known to result from hybridization have a multiplication sign added to their names, for example, *Apocynum ×floribundum*, formed by the hybridization *Apocynum androsaemifolium × A. cannabinum*.

Common Plant Names

Although a correctly identified plant can be assigned one, unique scientific name, a plant may have many common names. Unlike scientific names, there are no rules of nomenclature governing common names. Different people in the same place or people in different places have bestowed their own names on plants. Some plants do not have truly commonly used names at all. The common name included in the Catalog of Plants is not necessarily the one used by ethnobotanists reporting on usage. And because various ethnobotanists may have used different common names for the various usages of the plant, usually more than one common name appears in the original sources. When one is available, what has generally been chosen is a relatively standard common name established by the U.S. Department of Agriculture Natural Resources Conservation Service. The common names used by the various ethnobotanists are cross-referenced in the Index of Common Names, however, so that information on Native American plant use may be found even if one does not know the scientific name of the plant.

Unfortunately, with few exceptions the names applied to plants by Native Americans, their common names for the plants, have not been recorded in the sources and are not indexed. With so many Native American languages, it would require a separate, large book to treat the American Indian names of plants as comprehensively as their uses are cataloged here.

Ethnobotanical Information

Under each plant name, drug usages are divided alphabetically by tribe, all the names of which are listed in the previous chapter under Native Americans. Following the tribe name are all the medicinal uses of the plant, listed alphabetically according to the categories defined in the previous chapter under Drug Usage Categories.

The statements on usage are followed by an abbreviated reference, for example, (161: 140). The reference applies to all preceding statements, even if the reference is separated from the particular statement, for example, by the italicized name of a different usage category or the boldfaced name of a different tribe. The number preceding the colon refers to the source from which the information came, and sources are enumerated in the Bibliography. The number following the colon is the page number in that original source. When the original source used a plant name that differs from that adopted in the Catalog of Plants, the name used in the source is also given within the parentheses, for example, within the entry for *Brickellia eupatorioides* var. *eupatorioides*, (as *Kuhnia rosmarinifolia* 165:52). When differences are minor, however, such as insignificant differences in author citation, these other names are not given.

Two comprehensive Plant Usage Indexes are provided so that the information collected in the Catalog of Plants can be found in ways other than by plant name. In the Index of Tribes, the information is first arranged alphabetically by names of Native American groups, as listed in the previous chapter under Native Americans, and then alphabetically by drug usage. Plants are identified to the level of species in the Index of Tribes. If subspecies or varieties appear in the Catalog of Plants, check under those names, too, for all usages indexed. For example, one may look up Comanche and under Cold Remedy see that *Rhus trilobata* was used. The specific ethnobotanical information and the source from which the information was obtained may be found by turning to *Rhus trilobata* and *R. trilobata* var. *pilosissima* in the Catalog of Plants.

In the Index of Usages, plant genera are arranged alphabetically under the particular usage, as defined in the previous chapter under Drug Usage Categories. For example, one may look up Cold Remedy and see that *Rhus* was used by the Cahuilla, Cheyenne, Chippewa, Comanche, and Iroquois. The specific ethnobotanical information and the sources from which the information was obtained may be found by turning to *Rhus* in the Catalog of Plants and examining the Cold Remedy entries listed for all *Rhus* species.

Catalog of Plants

Abies amabilis, Pacific Silver Fir
Bella Coola *Eye Medicine* Liquid pitch mixed with mountain goat tallow and used for infected eyes. *Gastrointestinal Aid* Infusion of bark taken for stomach ailments. *Throat Aid* Liquid pitch mixed with mountain goat tallow and taken for sore throat. *Tuberculosis Remedy* Infusion of bark taken for tuberculosis. (158:197) **Haisla** *Tonic* Bark and other plants used as a tonic. *Unspecified* Bark and other plants used for "sickness." (61:152) **Hanaksiala** *Gastrointestinal Aid* Infusion of bark taken for stomach ulcers. *Hemorrhoid Remedy* Infusion of bark taken for hemorrhoids. (35:173) **Kitasoo** *Unspecified* Decoction of bark used medicinally. (35:316) **Nitinaht** *Internal Medicine* Infusion of crushed bark, red alder and hemlock barks taken for internal injuries. *Preventive Medicine* Boughs placed in fire and smoke inhaled to prevent sickness. (160:71) **Oweekeno** *Cold Remedy* Pitch boiled with grease or pitch and sugar and taken for colds. (35:68) **Thompson** *Cold Remedy* Pitch taken for colds. *Panacea* Pitch taken for any type of bad disease. *Tuberculosis Remedy* Poultice of pitch and buttercup roots used for tuberculosis. Pitch taken for tuberculosis. Decoction of boughs and/or bark taken for tuberculosis. *Unspecified* Decoction of branches taken as medicine. (161:97)

Abies balsamea, Balsam Fir
Abnaki *Dermatological Aid* Gum used to make various ointments. Gum used for "slight" itches. (121:164) *Disinfectant* Used as an antiseptic. *Panacea* Leaves made into pillows and used as a panacea. (121:155) *Unspecified* Needles and wood stuffed into pillows and used for good health. (121:163) Needles stuffed into pillows and used for good health. (121:164) **Algonquin, Quebec** *Dermatological Aid* Poultice of gum applied to open sores, insect bites, boils, and infections.

Gynecological Aid Needles used in a sudatory for women after childbirth and for other purposes. *Heart Medicine* Roots used for heart disease. *Laxative* Needles used to make a laxative tea. *Poultice* Needles used for making poultices. *Unspecified* Needles used in a sudatory for women after childbirth and for other purposes. (14:124) **Algonquin, Tête-de-Boule** *Cold Remedy* Sap chewed for colds. (110:118) **Anticosti** *Kidney Aid* Decoction of bark and bark from another plant taken for kidney troubles. Gum eaten for kidney pains. *Throat Aid* Infusion of sap used for sore throats. (120:64) **Chippewa** *Analgesic* Gum melted on warm stone and fumes inhaled for headache. (43:338) *Antirheumatic (External)* Decoction of root used as herbal steam for rheumatic joints. (43:362) *Dermatological Aid* Gum of plant with bear grease used as an ointment for the hair. (43:350) *Herbal Steam* Gum of plant melted on warm stone as herbal steam for headache. (43:338) Decoction of root sprinkled on hot stones and used as herbal steam for rheumatism. (43:362) **Cree, Woodlands** *Abortifacient* Pitch used for menstrual irregularity. *Cold Remedy* Infusion of bark and

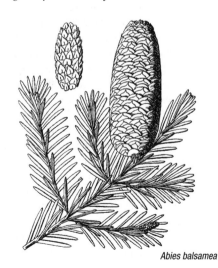

Abies balsamea

sometimes wood taken for colds. *Cough Medicine* Infusion of bark and sometimes wood taken for coughs. *Dermatological Aid* Pitch and grease used as an ointment for scabies and boils. Poultice of pitch applied to cuts. *Tuberculosis Remedy* Infusion of bark taken for tuberculosis. Decoction of pitch and sturgeon oil used for tuberculosis. (91:21) **Iroquois** *Antirheumatic (External)* Steam from decoction of branches used as a bath for rheumatism. *Antirheumatic (Internal)* Compound decoction taken for rheumatism. (73:269) *Cancer Treatment* Poultice of gum and dried beaver kidneys applied for cancer. (118:37) *Cold Remedy* Compound decoction taken for colds. (73:269) Infusion of gum and hot milk taken as an antiseptic for colds. (118:37) *Cough Medicine* Decoction taken straight or diluted with alcohol for coughs. *Dermatological Aid* Compound decoction applied to cuts, bruises, sprains, or sores. *Gynecological Aid* Steam from decoction of branches used as a bath for parturition. *Orthopedic Aid* Decoction used as wash and poultice applied to cuts, bruises, sprains, and sores. (73:269) *Tuberculosis Remedy* Compound decoction taken during early stages of consumption. *Urinary Aid* Used for bed-wetting. *Venereal Aid* Used for gonorrhea. (73:270) **Malecite** *Laxative* Juice used as a laxative. (96:244) *Unspecified* Pitch used in medicines. (137:6) *Venereal Aid* Infusion of bark used for gonorrhea. Infusion of bark, spruce bark, and tamarack bark used for gonorrhea. (96:257) **Menominee** *Adjuvant* Inner bark used as a seasoner for medicines. *Analgesic* Infusion of inner bark taken for chest pain. *Cold Remedy* Liquid balsam pressed from trunk used for colds. (128:45) *Dermatological Aid* Gum from plant blisters applied to sores. (44:132) *Pulmonary Aid* Liquid balsam pressed from trunk used for pulmonary troubles. *Unspecified* Poultice of fresh inner bark used for unspecified illnesses. (128:45) **Micmac** *Antidiarrheal* Buds, cones, and inner bark used for diarrhea. *Burn Dressing* Gum used for burns. *Cold Remedy* Gum used for colds. *Dermatological Aid* Gum used for bruises, sores, and wounds. *Gastrointestinal Aid* Cones used for colic. *Laxative* Buds used as a laxative. *Orthopedic Aid* Gum used for fractures. *Venereal Aid* Bark used for gonorrhea and buds used as a laxative. (32:53) **Montagnais** *Dietary Aid* Inner bark grated and eaten

to benefit the diet. (133:313) **Ojibwa** *Ceremonial Medicine* Needle-like leaves used as part of the ceremony involving the sweat bath. *Cold Remedy* Balsam gum used for colds and leaf smoke inhaled for colds. (130:378) *Cough Medicine* Plant used as a cough medicine. (112:244) *Dermatological Aid* Balsam gum used for sores and compound containing leaves used as a wash. *Diaphoretic* Needle-like leaves used as part of the medicine for the sweat bath. *Eye Medicine* Liquid balsam from bark blister used for sore eyes. *Stimulant* Leaves used as a reviver and used in compound as a wash. (130:378) **Ojibwa, South** *Cold Remedy* Bark gum taken for chest soreness from colds. *Dermatological Aid* Bark gum applied to cuts and sores. *Diaphoretic* Decoction of bark used to induce sweating. *Venereal Aid* Bark gum taken for gonorrhea. (77:198) **Penobscot** *Burn Dressing* Sap smeared over burns, sores, and cuts. *Dermatological Aid* Sap used as a salve for burns, sores, and cuts. (133:309) **Potawatomi** *Cold Remedy* Needles used to make pillows, believing that the aroma kept one from having a cold. (131:121) Fresh balsam gum swallowed for colds. *Dermatological Aid* Balsam gum used as a salve for sores. *Tuberculosis Remedy* Infusion of bark taken for "consumption and other internal affections." (131:68, 69)

Abies concolor, White Fir

Keres, Western *Antirheumatic (External)* Infusion of foliage used as a bath for rheumatism. *Antirheumatic (Internal)* Infusion of foliage taken for rheumatism. (147:24) **Paiute** *Dermatological Aid* Poultice of fresh pitch applied to cuts. *Pulmonary Aid* Decoction of needles and bark resin taken for pulmonary troubles. *Tuberculosis Remedy* Soft bark resin eaten or infusion of bark taken for tuberculosis. *Venereal Aid* Compound decoction of resin taken for venereal disease. **Shoshoni** *Dermatological Aid* Simple or compound poultice of warm pitch applied to sores or boils. *Pulmonary Aid* Decoction of needles and bark resin taken for pulmonary troubles. (155:30) **Tewa** *Dermatological Aid* Resinous sap from main stem and larger branches used for cuts. (115:38) **Washo** *Tuberculosis Remedy* Soft bark resin eaten or infusion of bark taken for tuberculosis. (155:30)

Abies fraseri, Fraser's Fir
Cherokee *Dermatological Aid* Used for wounds and ulcers. *Gastrointestinal Aid* Taken "to loosen bowels and cleanse and heal internal ulcers." *Gynecological Aid* Used for "falling of the womb," the "whites," and weak backs in females. *Kidney Aid* Burst blister, take ooze alone or with turpentine for "kidney trouble." *Laxative* Taken "to loosen bowels and cleanse and heal internal ulcers." *Pulmonary Aid* "Balsam for breast and lung complaints with pain, soreness or cough." *Urinary Aid* Used for urinary diseases. *Venereal Aid* Used for venereal diseases. (66:34)

Abies grandis, Grand Fir
Bella Coola *Eye Medicine* Compound of gum drawn on a hair across sore eyes. (127:50) Liquid pitch mixed with mountain goat tallow and used for infected eyes. (158:197) *Gastrointestinal Aid* Decoction of root bark or stem taken every day for stomach trouble. (127:50) Infusion of bark taken for stomach ailments. (158:197) *Throat Aid* Compound of gum from bark blisters warmed and taken for sore throat. (127:50) Liquid pitch mixed with mountain goat tallow and taken for sore throat. (158:197) *Tuberculosis Remedy* Decoction of root bark or stem taken every day for tuberculosis. (127:50) Infusion of bark taken for tuberculosis. (158:197) **Carrier, Southern** *Unspecified* Tree used as medicine. (127:50) **Chehalis** *Cold Remedy* Decoction of needles taken for colds. (65:19) **Gitksan** *Antirheumatic* (*External*) Poultice of compound containing bark applied for rheumatism. *Dermatological Aid* Poultice of compound containing bark applied to boils or ulcers. *Pulmonary Aid* Poultice of compound containing bark used as a chest plaster for lung hemorrhage. (127:50) **Green River Group** *Cold Remedy* Decoction of needles taken for colds. (65:19) **Hesquiat** *Dermatological Aid* Blister pitch mixed with oil rubbed on the hair and scalp because it smelled nice. Blister pitch mixed with oil rubbed on the scalp to prevent the hair from falling out. (159:41) **Karok** *Tonic* Infusion of needles taken as a tonic. (125:379) **Kwakiutl** *Ceremonial Medicine* Branches and pollen used in purification rites and ceremonies. *Cough Medicine* Decoction of pitch taken for coughs and tuberculosis. *Dermatological Aid* Pitch and grease eaten or rubbed

on sores and boils. *Laxative* Decoction of pitch taken as a tonic and laxative. Pitch and catfish oil taken for constipation. *Oral Aid* Root held in the mouth for gum boils and canker sores. *Tonic* Infusion of bark taken as a tonic to stay young and strong. *Tuberculosis Remedy* Decoction of pitch taken or pitch rubbed on chest and back for tuberculosis. (157:268) **Nitinaht** *Internal Medicine* Infusion of crushed bark, red alder and hemlock barks taken for internal injuries. *Unspecified* Boughs placed in fire and smoke inhaled to prevent sickness. (160:71) **Okanagan-Colville** *Cough Medicine* Decoction of bark taken for bad coughs. *Dermatological Aid* Needles dried, powdered, mixed with marrow, and used to scent the hair and keep from going bald. Bark dried, powdered, and rubbed on the neck and under the arms as a deodorant. *Dietary Aid* Pitch taken for a loss of appetite. *Gastrointestinal Aid* Pitch taken for ulcers. Decoction of bark taken for "bad stomachs" with loss of appetite and loss of weight. *Gland Medicine* Pitch mixed with deer marrow and applied externally each evening for goiter. *Other* Branch tips chewed for allergies caused by water hemlock. *Strengthener* Pitch taken for a general feeling of weakness. *Tuberculosis Remedy* Pitch taken for consumption. (162:23) **Okanagon** *Cathartic* Decoction of bark and gum taken as a physic. *Eye Medicine* Gum used for sore eyes. (104:41) **Saanich** *Dermatological Aid* Pitch mixed with venison suet and used for psoriasis and other skin diseases. Pitch made into a salve and used for cuts and bruises. (156:69) **Salish, Coast** *Dermatological Aid* Infusion of pounded root bark used for falling hair and dandruff. (156:69) **Shuswap** *Dermatological Aid* Poultice of soft pitch applied to sores. *Panacea* Decoction of bark taken for tuberculosis and other sickness. *Toothache Remedy* Hard pitch chewed to clean the teeth. *Tuberculosis Remedy* Decoction of bark taken for tuberculosis. (102:50) **Thompson** *Cathartic* Decoction of bark and gum taken as a physic. (141:462) *Cold Remedy* Pitch taken for colds. (161:97) *Eye Medicine* Gum used for sore eyes. (104:41) Decoction of bark used as a wash for sore eyes and gum used in corners of eyes. (141:462) *Panacea* Infusion of boughs taken for any illness. Pitch taken for any type of bad disease. (161:97) *Pediatric Aid* Branches thought to be of help to young girl under "magical spell." (141: 509) *Tuberculosis Remedy* Poultice of pitch and buttercup roots used for tuberculosis. Pitch taken for tuberculosis. *Unspecified* Decoction of branches taken as medicine. (161:97) *Venereal Aid* Very strong decoction of various plant parts taken for gonorrhea. (141:462) *Witchcraft Medicine* Branches thought to be of help to young girl under "magical spell." (141:509)

Abies lasiocarpa, Subalpine Fir

Blackfoot *Analgesic* Needle smudge smoke inhaled for headaches. (72:79) *Ceremonial Medicine* Plant burned as ceremonial incense. (95: 273) *Cold Remedy* Poultice of leaves applied for chest colds. (82:17) Poultice of plant applied for chest colds. (95:273) *Dermatological Aid* Needles used as a deodorant. (72:107) Infusion of needles mixed with grease and applied as a hair tonic. Needles packed into moccasins as a foot deodorant. (72:123) Leaves mixed with grease and used as hairdressing. Gummy secretions used on wounds as an antiseptic. (82:17) *Emetic* Infusion of resin taken as an emetic to clean the insides. (72:65) *Febrifuge* Poultice of leaves applied for fevers. (82:17) Poultice of plant applied for fevers. (95:273) *Oral Aid* Resin chewed for bad breath and pleasure. (72:123) *Pulmonary Aid* Gummy secretions taken for lung troubles. (82:17) *Stimulant* Needle smudge smoke inhaled for fainting. (72:79) *Tuberculosis Remedy* Infusion of needles taken for coughing up blood, a sign of tuberculosis. Needle smudge used to fumigate the patient with tuberculosis. (72:70) *Venereal Aid* Needle smudge used to fumigate those faces that were swollen from a form of venereal disease. (72:69) *Veterinary Aid* Needle smudge used to fumigate sick horses. Little bags of needles tied on a belt and hung around the horse's neck as a perfume. Infusion of bark given to horses for diarrhea. (72:87) Ground needles used in horse medicine bundles. (82:17) **Cheyenne** *Ceremonial Medicine* Needles burned as incense in ceremonies by persons afraid of thunder. *Stimulant* Plant used to revive a dying person's spirit. *Witchcraft Medicine* Burning needle smoke and aroma used to chase away bad influences (illness). (69:5) **Crow** *Ceremonial Medicine* Young twigs and leaves burned as incense in certain ceremonies. (15:5) *Cold*

Remedy Infusion of crushed needles taken for colds. *Cough Medicine* Infusion of crushed needles taken for coughs. *Laxative* Infusion of crushed needles used for constipation. **Flathead** *Dermatological Aid* Needles dried, pounded, mixed with deer grease, and used as a hair tonic. Needles, lovage roots, buckbrush leaves, and pinedrops boiled and used to make hair grow longer. Needles pounded and used alone or mixed with grease or marrow for skin diseases. Needles pulverized into baby powder and used for rashes from excessive urination. *Oral Aid* Needles pounded, mixed with lard, and used for bleeding gums. *Pediatric Aid* Needles pulverized into baby powder and used for rashes from excessive urination. (68:2) **Gitksan** *Cold Remedy* Decoction of bark or inner bark used for colds. *Cough Medicine* Decoction of bark or inner bark used for coughs. *Misc. Disease Remedy* Decoction of bark or inner bark used for flu. *Tonic* Decoction of bark or inner bark used as a tonic. (61:152) **Kutenai** *Dermatological Aid* Gummy bark secretions used for cuts and bruises. **Montana Indian** *Cold Remedy* Poultice of needles used for colds. Infusion of needles and resinous blisters used for colds. (68:2) *Dermatological Aid* Gummy secretion from the bark used as an antiseptic for wounds and ulcers. Plant applied to corns for easy removal. (15:5) Gummy bark secretions used as an antiseptic for wounds. *Febrifuge* Poultice of needles used for chest fevers. (68:2) *Pulmonary Aid* Gummy secretion from the bark taken for lung troubles. (15:5) **Okanagan-Colville** *Cough Medicine* Decoction of bark taken for bad coughs. *Dermatological Aid* Bark dried, powdered, and rubbed on the neck and under the arms as a deodorant. Needles dried, powdered, mixed with marrow, and used to scent the hair and keep from going bald. *Dietary Aid* Pitch taken for a loss of appetite. *Gastrointestinal Aid* Pitch taken for ulcers. Decoction of bark taken for "bad stomachs" with loss of appetite and loss of weight. *Gland Medicine* Pitch mixed with deer marrow and applied externally each evening for goiter. *Other* Branch tips chewed for allergies caused by water hemlock. *Strengthener* Pitch taken for a general feeling of weakness. *Tuberculosis Remedy* Pitch taken for consumption. (162:23) **Shoshoni** *Cold Remedy* Infusion of needles taken for colds. Infusion of resinous blisters taken for colds.

(98:37) **Thompson** *Cold Remedy* Pitch taken for colds. *Cough Medicine* Decoction of bark taken over a period of time for bad coughs. *Dermatological Aid* Poultice of pitch used alone for cuts or with Vaseline for sores. The pitch was smeared over injuries and covered with a bandage. In earlier times, animal fat was probably used in place of Vaseline Decoction of bark taken over a period of time for bruises. *Orthopedic Aid* Decoction of bark taken over a period of time for sprains. *Panacea* Pitch taken for any type of bad disease. *Tuberculosis Remedy* Inner bark eaten as a medicine for "shadow on the chest," the beginning of tuberculosis. It made the informant very sick with aching, flu-like symptoms, but after that, she did not develop tuberculosis. Poultice of pitch and buttercup roots used for tuberculosis. Pitch taken for tuberculosis. Decoction of boughs and/or bark taken for tuberculosis. *Unspecified* Decoction of branches taken as medicine. (161:97) **Wet'su-wet'en** *Cold Remedy* Decoction of bark or inner bark used for colds. *Cough Medicine* Decoction of bark or inner bark used for coughs. *Misc. Disease Remedy* Decoction of bark or inner bark used for flu. *Tonic* Decoction of bark or inner bark used as a tonic. (61:152)

Abies procera, Noble Fir
Paiute *Cold Remedy* Dried branches stored for use as a cold remedy. Crumbled leaves smoked for colds. Mashed leaves sewn into a sack placed around the child's neck "for colds." *Cough Medicine* Decoction of leaves taken as cough medicine. *Dermatological Aid* Dried branches stored for use as a deodorant. (as *A. nobilis* 93:45)

Abronia elliptica, Fragrant White Sand Verbena
Hopi *Pediatric Aid* Plant placed on child's head to induce sleep. (174:75) *Sedative* Plant placed on child's head to induce sleep. (174:36, 75)

Abronia fragrans, Snowball Sand Verbena
Keres, Western *Dietary Aid* Roots ground, mixed with corn flour and eaten to give one a good appetite and to make one fat. *Psychological Aid* Roots ground, mixed with corn flour, and eaten to keep one from becoming greedy. (147:24) **Navajo** *Dermatological Aid* Plant used for boils. (76:158)

Gastrointestinal Aid Plant taken to "remove the effects of swallowing a spider." (45:46) **Navajo, Kayenta** *Cathartic* Plant used as a cathartic. *Dermatological Aid* Plant used for insect bites. *Diaphoretic* Plant used as a sudorific. *Emetic* Plant used as an emetic. *Gastrointestinal Aid* Plant used for stomach cramps. *Panacea* Plant used as a life medicine. (179:21) **Navajo, Ramah** *Dermatological Aid* Cold infusion used as lotion for sores or sore mouth and to bathe perspiring feet. *Oral Aid* Cold infusion used as lotion for sores or sore mouth. (165:26) **Ute** *Gastrointestinal Aid* Roots and flowers used for stomach and bowel troubles. (30:32) **Zuni** *Gastrointestinal Aid* Fresh flowers eaten for stomachaches. (22:377)

Abronia turbinata, Transmontane Sand Verbena
Shoshoni *Dermatological Aid* Poultice of mashed leaves applied to swellings. (155:30)

Abronia villosa, Desert Sand Verbena
Paiute *Diuretic* Used as an urinary inducer. (98:41) **Shoshoni** *Burn Dressing* Poultice of mashed roots applied to burns. (155:30)

Abutilon incanum, Pelotazo
Hawaiian *Gastrointestinal Aid* Dried flowers eaten for gripping stomachaches. Flowers, root bark, and other plants pounded, resulting liquid heated and taken for stomachaches. (2:69)

Acacia koa, Koa
Hawaiian *Diaphoretic* Leaves spread out on the bed to cause the patient lying on them to sweat. *Pediatric Aid* Ashes of this and other plants applied to the mouth interior of infants for physical weakness. *Strengthener* Ashes of this and other plants applied to the mouth interior of infants for physical weakness. (2:46)

Acalypha virginica, Virginia Threeseed Mercury
Cherokee *Kidney Aid* Root used for "dropsy." *Misc. Disease Remedy* Root used for pox. *Urinary Aid* Root used for "gravel." (66:61)

Acamptopappus sphaerocephalus var.
hirtellus, Rayless Goldenhead
Kawaiisu *Analgesic* Mashed plant used as a salve for pain. (180:9)

Acer alba, White Maple
Micmac *Cough Medicine* Bark used as a cough remedy. (32:53)

Acer circinatum, Vine Maple
Karok *Love Medicine* Branches used by women as a love medicine. (125:385) **Thompson** *Antidiarrheal* Wood burned to charcoal, mixed with water and brown sugar, and taken for dysentery. *Misc. Disease Remedy* Wood burned to charcoal, mixed with water and brown sugar, and taken for polio. (161:145)

Acer glabrum, Rocky Mountain Maple
Blackfoot *Cathartic* Infusion of bark taken in the morning as a cathartic. (72:65) **Navajo, Ramah** *Panacea* Infusion of branches used for swellings, a "life medicine." (165:36) **Okanagan-Colville** *Hunting Medicine* Branch tied in a knot and placed over the bear's tracks while hunting to stop the wounded bear. (162:59) **Thompson** *Antiemetic* Decoction of wood and bark taken for nausea caused by smelling a corpse. (141:475) *Gynecological Aid* Decoction of sticks and saskatoon sticks taken to heal women's insides and stimulate lactation. The decoction was made either with two sticks each of saskatoon and rocky mountain ma-

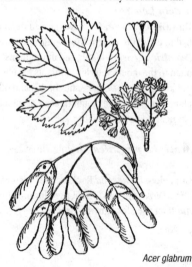

Acer glabrum

ple, or, for a stronger medicine, four sticks each and used after childbirth to heal women's insides and to stimulate the flow of milk for nursing. *Snakebite Remedy* Decoction of four straight, young sticks used as a wash or taken for snakebites. The informant could not recall whether the decoction was taken internally or used as a wash. (161:146)

Acer macrophyllum, Bigleaf Maple
Klallam *Tuberculosis Remedy* Infusion of bark taken for tuberculosis. (65:39) **Kwakiutl** *Dermatological Aid* Sticky gum from the spring buds mixed with oil and used as a hair tonic. (157:275) **Thompson** *Tonic* Raw sap used as a tonic in the olden days. (161:147)

Acer negundo, Box Elder
Cheyenne *Ceremonial Medicine* Wood burned as incense for making spiritual medicines. (68:4) **Meskwaki** *Emetic* Decoction of inner bark taken as an emetic. (129:200) **Ojibwa** *Emetic* Infusion of inner bark taken as an emetic. (130:353)

Acer nigrum, Black Maple
Ojibwa, South *Antidiarrheal* Decoction of inner bark used for diarrhea. "Arbor liquore abundans, ex quo liquor tanquam urina vehementer projicitur [A tree full of sap, which shoots out forcefully, just like urine]." (77:199)

Acer pensylvanicum, Striped Maple
Abnaki *Respiratory Aid* Used for bronchial troubles. (121:154) **Algonquin, Quebec** *Unspecified* Infusion of plant used as a medicinal tea. *Veterinary Aid* Plant eaten by a moose with a broken bone to aid its healing. (14:196) **Iroquois** *Emetic* Decoction of bark taken as an emetic. *Laxative* Compound decoction of bark taken as a laxative. *Orthopedic Aid* Decoction of bark applied as poultice for paralysis. (73:378) **Micmac** *Antihemorrhagic* Wood used for spitting blood. *Cold Remedy* Bark used for colds. *Cough Medicine* Bark used for coughs. *Kidney Aid* Wood used for kidney trouble. *Misc. Disease Remedy* Bark used for "grippe." *Orthopedic Aid* Unspecified plant parts used for "trouble with the limbs." *Venereal Aid* Wood used for gonorrhea. (32:53) **Ojibwa, South** *Emetic* Decoction of inner bark taken as an emetic.

(77:200) **Penobscot** *Antihemorrhagic* Compound infusion of plant taken for "spitting up blood." (133:311) *Dermatological Aid* Poultice of steeped bark applied to swollen limbs. (133:310) *Kidney Aid* Compound infusion of plant taken for kidney trouble. *Tonic* Compound infusion of plant taken as a tonic. *Venereal Aid* Compound infusion of plant taken for gonorrhea. (133:311)

Acer rubrum, Red Maple
Cherokee *Analgesic* Infusion of bark taken for cramps. *Antidiarrheal* Infusion taken for dysentery. *Dermatological Aid* Infusion taken for hives. *Eye Medicine* Inner bark boiled and used with water as wash for sore eyes. (66:44) Decoction of inner bark boiled to a syrup and used as a wash for sore eyes. (177:73) *Gynecological Aid* Compound infusion of bark taken for "female trouble" and cramps. *Misc. Disease Remedy* Hot infusion of bark given for measles. (66:44) **Iroquois** *Blood Medicine* Complex compound taken as a blood purifier. *Eye Medicine* Infusion of bark used as drops for sore eyes and cataracts. *Hunting Medicine* Decoction of plants used as a wash for traps, a "trapping medicine." (73:378) **Ojibwa** *Eye Medicine* Decoction of bark used as a wash for sore eyes. (130:353) **Potawatomi** *Eye Medicine* Decoction of inner bark used as an eyewash. (131:37) **Seminole** *Dermatological Aid*, *Hemorrhoid Remedy*, and *Orthopedic Aid* Decoction of bark used for ballgame sickness: sores, back or limb pains, and hemorrhoids. (145:269)

Acer rubrum var. *drummondii*, Drummond's Maple
Koasati *Dermatological Aid* Infusion of bark taken and used as a wash for gun wounds. (152:39)

Acer saccharinum, Silver Maple
Cherokee *Analgesic* Infusion of bark taken for cramps. *Antidiarrheal* Infusion taken for dysentery. *Dermatological Aid* Infusion taken for hives. *Eye Medicine* Inner bark boiled and used with water as wash for sore eyes. *Gynecological Aid* Compound infusion of bark taken for "female trouble" and cramps. *Misc. Disease Remedy* Hot infusion of bark given for measles. (66:44) **Chippewa** *Dermatological Aid* Bark boiled and used as a wash for old, stubborn, running sores. (59:136) **Iro-**

quois *Unspecified* Sap, thimbleberries, and water used to make a medicine. (170:142) **Mohegan** *Cough Medicine* Infusion of bark, removed from south side of tree, taken for cough. (149:269) **Ojibwa** *Venereal Aid* Infusion of root bark taken for gonorrhea. (112:232) **Ojibwa, South** *Antidiarrheal* Decoction of inner bark used for diarrhea. (77:198) *Diuretic* Compound decoction of inner bark taken as a diuretic. (77:199)

Acer saccharum, Sugar Maple
Iroquois *Blood Medicine* Complex compound used as a blood purifier. *Dermatological Aid* Compound decoction of leaves used as a wash on parts affected by "Italian itch." *Eye Medicine* Compound infusion of bark used as drops for blindness. (73:378) Sap used for sore eyes. (170:142) *Pulmonary Aid* Infusion of bark with another whole plant taken by forest runners for shortness of breath. (as *A. saccharophorum* 118:52) *Unspecified* Sap, thimbleberries, and water used to make a medicine. (170:142) **Mohegan** *Cough Medicine* Inner bark used as a cough remedy. (151:69, 128) **Potawatomi** *Expectorant* Inner bark used as an expectorant. (131:37)

Acer spicatum, Mountain Maple
Algonquin, Tête-de-Boule *Dermatological Aid* Poultice of boiled root chips applied to wounds and abscesses. (110:118) **Iroquois** *Antihemorrhagic* Compound decoction of roots and bark taken for internal hemorrhage. (73:377) *Gastrointestinal Aid* Plant used for intestinal diseases. (119:94) **Malecite** *Eye Medicine* Infusion of outside bark used for sore eyes. Poultice of outside bark used for sore eyes. (96:248) **Micmac** *Eye Medicine* Bark used for sore eyes. (32:53) **Ojibwa** *Eye Medicine* Infusion of pith used as a wash for sore eyes and pith used to remove foreign matter. (130:353) **Potawatomi** *Cough Medicine* Compound containing inner bark used as cough syrup. (131:37)

Achillea millefolium, Common Yarrow
Abnaki *Cold Remedy* Infusion of whole plant given to children for colds. (121:174) *Febrifuge* Used for fevers. *Misc. Disease Remedy* Used for grippe. (121:154) *Pediatric Aid* Infusion of whole plant given to children for colds. (121:174) **Algonquin,**

Quebec *Analgesic* Crushed leaves used as a snuff for headaches. *Cold Remedy* Used for colds. *Poultice* Leaves used for poultices. *Respiratory Aid* Used for respiratory disorders. (14:240) **Algonquin, Tête-de-Boule** *Analgesic* Decoction of leaves and flowers used for headaches. (110:118) **Bella Coola** *Breast Treatment* Leaves pounded, heated, and used for breast abscesses. (158:201) *Burn Dressing* Poultice of chewed leaves applied to burns. (127:65) Leaves pounded, heated, and used for burns. *Dermatological Aid* Leaves pounded, heated, and used for boils. *Pediatric Aid* and *Respiratory Aid* Poultice of leaves and eulachon (candlefish) grease applied to the chest and back of children for bronchitis. (158:201) **Blackfoot** *Analgesic* Infusion of plant taken or rubbed on the body to soothe the pain of gastroenteritis. (72:65) *Antirheumatic* (*External*) Poultice of chewed flowers applied to swollen parts. Infusion of plant applied to swellings. *Dermatological Aid* Infusion of plant applied to sores. (72:74) *Diuretic* Infusion of plant taken as a diuretic to pass the sickness with the urine. (72:69) *Gynecological Aid* Infusion of leaves taken when labor pains started and to ease the delivery. Infusion of leaves taken to expel the afterbirth. (72:60) *Liver Aid* Infusion of plant taken or rubbed on the body for liver troubles. (72:65) *Panacea* Infusion of plant rubbed on the body part affected by sickness. (72:69) *Throat Aid* Infusion of plant taken for sore throats. (72:70) *Veterinary Aid* Infusion of plant used as an eyewash for horses. (72:87) **Carrier, Southern** *Cold Remedy* Decoction of entire plant, except roots, taken for colds. *Dermatological Aid* Poultice of chewed leaves applied to swellings. *Orthopedic Aid* Poultice of chewed leaves applied to sprains. (127:65) **Chehalis** *Antidiarrheal* Decoction of leaves taken for the passage of blood with diarrhea. (65:49) **Cherokee** *Antihemorrhagic* Used for hemorrhages and spitting blood. *Dermatological Aid* Astringent leaves used for hemorrhages and bowel complaints. *Febrifuge* Infusion taken for fever. *Gastrointestinal Aid* Used for bowel complaints. *Gynecological Aid* Used for flooding. *Hemorrhoid Remedy* Used for bloody piles. *Respiratory Aid* Dried leaves smoked for catarrh. *Sedative* Infusion taken for restful sleep. *Urinary Aid* Used for bloody urine. (66:62) **Cheyenne** *Analgesic* Infusion of leaves and flowers taken for chest

pains. *Antiemetic* Infusion of fresh or dried plant taken for nausea. (69:17) *Cold Remedy* Infusion of leaves used for colds. (68:6) Infusion of fresh or dried plant taken for colds. *Cough Medicine* Infusion of fresh or dried plant taken for coughs. *Diaphoretic* Infusion of fresh or dried plant taken to cause perspiring. (69:17) *Febrifuge* Infusion of leaves used for fevers. (68:6) *Heart Medicine* Infusion of leaves and flowers taken for heart troubles and chest pains. *Hemostat* Crushed leaves placed in the nose for nosebleeds. *Respiratory Aid* Infusion of plant taken or leaves rubbed on body for respiratory diseases. *Throat Aid* Infusion of fresh or dried plant taken for tickling of the throat. *Tuberculosis Remedy* Infusion of plant taken or leaves rubbed on body for tuberculosis. (69:17) **Chippewa** *Analgesic* Decoction of leaves steamed and inhaled for headache. (43:336) *Dermatological Aid* Decoction of root applied to skin "eruptions." (43:350) *Herbal Steam* Decoction of leaves sprinkled on hot stones as herbal steam for headache. (43:336) *Stimulant* Dried chewed root spit onto limbs as a stimulant. (43:364) *Veterinary Aid* Decoction of leaves and stalk applied to horses as a stimulant. (43:366) **Clallam** *Cold Remedy* Infusion of leaves used for colds. *Gynecological Aid* Infusion of leaves used during childbirth. (47:199) **Cowlitz** *Dermatological Aid* Infusion of leaves used as a hair wash. *Gastrointestinal Aid* Decoction of roots taken for stomach troubles. (65:49) **Cree, Woodlands** *Analgesic* Infusion

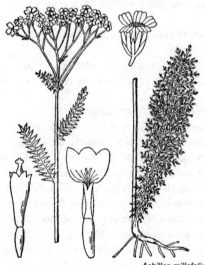

Achillea millefolium

of plant heads used to make a compress for head-aches. *Antihemorrhagic* Leaves chewed for bleed-ing. *Febrifuge* Infusion of plant heads used to make a compress for fevers. Decoction of roots taken for fevers. *Toothache Remedy* Decoction of roots taken or roots chewed for toothaches. (91: 23) **Creek** *Toothache Remedy* Plant used as tooth-ache medicine. (148:663) **Crow** *Burn Dressing* Poultice of plant used for burns. *Dermatological Aid* Poultice of plant used for boils and open sores. (68:6) **Delaware** *Kidney Aid* Infusion of plant used for kidney disorders. *Liver Aid* Infusion of plant used for liver disorders. (151:35) **Delaware, Oklahoma** *Kidney Aid* Infusion of whole plant taken for kidney disorders. *Liver Aid* Infusion of whole plant taken for liver disorders. (150:29, 74) **Flathead** *Antirheumatic (External)* Leaves boiled and used for aching backs and legs. *Cold Remedy* Infusion of leaves used for colds. *Dermatological Aid* Leaves crushed and used for wounds. *Disinfectant* Herb used as a disinfectant. *Febrifuge* Infusion of leaves used for fevers. (68:6) **Gitksan** *Throat Aid* Decoction of young plant or root gargled for sore throat. (127:65) **Gosiute** *Analgesic* Infusion of plant used for headaches. (31:360) *Antirheumatic (External)* Poultice of plant applied to joints affected by rheumatism. (31:350) Poultice of plant applied for rheumatism. *Dermatological Aid* Poultice of plant applied to bruises. *Gastrointestinal Aid* Infusion of plant used for biliousness. (31:360) **Haisla & Hanak-siala** *Unspecified* Plants placed on heated rocks and rising vapors used for unspecified illness. (35:220) **Hesquiat** *Analgesic* Leaves chewed and the juice swallowed for any kind of internal pain. *Cough Medicine* Leaves chewed and the juice swallowed for prolonged cough. *Gastrointestinal Aid* Leaves chewed and the juice swallowed for the stomach. *Internal Medicine* Leaves chewed and the juice swallowed for internal organs. (159:61) **Iroquois** *Analgesic* Infusion of roots or leaves used internally or externally for headaches. (73: 469) Plant chewed and poultice of leaves applied for neuralgia. *Anthelmintic* Infusion of leaves given to children with worms. *Anticonvulsive* Decoction of plants given and used as wash for babies with convulsions. *Antidiarrheal* Compound decoction of plants, bark, and roots taken for diarrhea. (73:470) Infusion of smashed plants taken for di-

arrhea. (73:471) Infusion of plant and seeds from another plant used for diarrhea. (118:64) *Anti-emetic* Decoction or infusion of plants, bark, and roots taken for vomiting. (73:470) Decoction of leaves, branches, and another plant taken for vom-iting and nausea. (118:64) *Antirheumatic (Internal)* Infusion of plants taken when "sore through the joints." *Blood Medicine* Compound decoction of plants, roots, and bark taken as a blood puri-fier. (73:470) *Emetic* Infusion of smashed plants taken as an emetic for sunstroke. (73:471) *Febrifuge* Infusion of leaves given to babies with any kind of fever. (73:469) Infusion of smashed plants taken for fever caused by sunstroke. (73:471) Poultice of plant applied and infusion of plant used for fevers. (119:103) *Gastrointestinal Aid* Plant used for "summer complaint" and decoction of plants taken for cramps. (73:470) Decoction of plant fragments taken for digestive cramps. (118: 64) *Misc. Disease Remedy* Plant used as a miscel-laneous disease remedy. (73:470) *Panacea* Infu-sion of leaves given to babies with any kind of sick-ness. *Pediatric Aid* Infusion of leaves given to babies with any kind of sickness or fever. (73:469) Compound decoction of stems given to children with diarrhea. Decoction of plants given and used as wash for babies with convulsions. *Stimulant* Cold infusion given and used as wash on uncon-scious person who had fallen. *Venereal Aid* Com-pound decoction of plants, roots, and bark taken for venereal disease. (73:470) Decoction of plant tops used as a wash on parts affected by gonor-rhea. (73:471) **Karok** *Dermatological Aid* Poul-tice of soaked stalks and leaves applied to wounds. (125:390) **Klallam** *Cold Remedy* Decoction of leaves taken for colds. *Dermatological Aid* Poul-tice of chewed leaves applied to sores. *Gynecolog-ical Aid* Decoction of leaves taken during child-birth. (65:49) **Kutenai** *Dermatological Aid* Leaves crushed and used for wounds. Decoction used for washing sores and other skin problems. *Disinfectant* Herb used as a disinfectant. (68:6) **Kwakiutl** *Antirheumatic (External)* Leaves used in a steam bath for rheumatism. *Cold Remedy* Poultice of leaves applied to the chest for colds. (157:278) *Dermatological Aid* Poultice of chewed leaves applied or compound rubbed on sores and swellings. (157:266) *Gynecological Aid* Poultice of leaves applied to chest for hardened breasts after childbirth. *Herbal Steam* Leaves used in a steam bath for rheumatism or general sickness. *Panacea* Leaves used in a steam bath for general sickness. (157:278) **Lakota** *Dermatological Aid* Poultice of dried and chewed plants applied to wounds and sores. (88:46) **Lummi** *Analgesic* Decoction of flowers taken for body aches. *Diaphoretic* Decoction of flowers taken to produce sweating. *Misc. Disease Remedy* Decoction of flowers taken to prevent mumps. (65:49) **Mahuna** *Toothache Remedy* Rolled leaves inserted into cavity of painful tooth. (117:24) **Makah** *Blood Medicine* Leaves chewed as a blood purifier. (55:322) Decoction of leaves taken to purify the blood. (65:49) *Cathartic* Leaves chewed "to clean one out." (55:322) *Diaphoretic* Raw leaves chewed by women to produce sweating at childbirth. (65:49) *Gynecological Aid* Plant taken by an expectant mother close to the time of birth for an easy delivery. Plant taken at the start of labor "to hurry the baby." (55:322) Decoction of leaves taken to heal the uterus after birth. Raw leaves chewed by women to produce sweating at childbirth. (65:49) *Other* Plant used like an antibiotic. *Throat Aid* Leaves chewed and the juice swallowed for sore throats. (55:322) **Malecite** *Dermatological Aid* Used as a liniment for bruises. *Orthopedic Aid* Used as a liniment for sprains. (96:244) **Mendocino Indian** *Analgesic* Infusion of leaves and flowers taken for headaches. *Dermatological Aid* Infusion of leaves and flowers used as a wash for bruises. *Eye Medicine* Infusion of leaves and flowers used as a wash for sore eyes. *Gastrointestinal Aid* Infusion of leaves and flowers taken for stomachaches. *Orthopedic Aid* Infusion of leaves and flowers used as a wash for sprains. *Tuberculosis Remedy* Infusion of leaves and flowers taken for consumption. (33:391) **Menominee** *Dermatological Aid* Poultice of dried, powdered leaves applied to swellings and sores. (44:132) Poultice of leaves used on children's rash and fresh tops used to rub on eczema. *Febrifuge* Infusion of leaves used for fevers. *Pediatric Aid* Poultice of leaves used for "the rash of children." (128:28, 29) **Micmac** *Antirheumatic (External)* Dried, powdered bark or green leaves rubbed over swellings. (168:25) *Cold Remedy* Herb used for colds. (32:53) *Dermatological Aid* Dried, powdered bark or green leaves rubbed over bruises. *Diaphoretic* Decoction of plant taken with milk to cause a

sweat for colds. (168:25) *Orthopedic Aid* Herb used for swelling, bruises, and sprains. (32:53) Dried, powdered bark or green leaves rubbed over sprains. (168:25) **Miwok** *Analgesic* Dried or green mashed leaves used for pain and used during influenza epidemic. Dried or green mashed leaves used for pain. *Cold Remedy* Infusion of leaves and flowers taken for bad colds. *Misc. Disease Remedy* Infusion of leaves and flowers used externally for influenza. (8:166) **Mohegan** *Dietary Aid* Cold, compound infusion taken as an appetizer. *Gastrointestinal Aid* Cold, compound infusion taken for the stomach. (149:266) Compound infusion of leaves taken as a stomach aid and to improve the appetite. (151:75, 128) *Kidney Aid* Infusion of plant taken for the kidneys. (149:269) Simple or compound infusion of leaves taken for kidney disorders. (151:69, 128) *Liver Aid* Infusion of plant taken for the liver. (149:269) Simple or compound infusion of leaves taken for liver disorders. (151:69, 128) **Montagnais** *Febrifuge* Infusion of plant used for fever. (133:315) **Nitinaht** *Cold Remedy* Decoction of plants taken for colds. *Panacea* Plants chewed and swallowed as "medicine for everything." (160:96) *Throat Aid* Leaves chewed and the juice swallowed for sore throats. (55:322) **Ojibwa** *Ceremonial Medicine* Florets smoked for ceremonial purposes. *Febrifuge* Florets placed on coals and smoke inhaled to break a fever. (130:362) **Okanagan-Colville** *Analgesic* Infusion of roots taken for headaches. *Antidiarrheal* Infusion of roots taken for diarrhea. *Antirheumatic (External)* Decoction of whole plant used as a bath for arthritic or rheumatic pains. *Cathartic* Decoction or roots and scarlet gilia leaves taken as a physic. *Cold Remedy* Infusion of roots taken for colds. *Dermatological Aid* Leaves and stems mixed with white clematis and witches'-broom branches to make a shampoo. *Gastrointestinal Aid* Infusion of roots taken for stomachaches. *Laxative* Decoction or roots and scarlet gilia leaves taken as a laxative. *Toothache Remedy* Roots mashed and applied to the tooth for toothaches. (162:74) **Okanagon** *Dermatological Aid* Decoction used as wash for chapped hands, pimples, rashes, and insect bites. *Eye Medicine* Decoction of whole plant used as a wash for sore eyes. *Snakebite Remedy* Decoction of plant used as a wash for insect or snake bites. *Tonic* Decoction of whole plant taken as a tonic. (as *Achilles mille-folium* 104:40) **Paiute** *Analgesic* Green plants smelled by old men for headaches. *Cold Remedy* Infusion of plant taken or green plants smelled for colds. (144:317) *Dermatological Aid* Poultice of crushed leaves applied to swellings. (87:196) Decoction of leaves and stems used as a liniment for skin sores. (144:317) *Eye Medicine* Cold infusion of leaves used as a wash for sore eyes. (87:197) *Orthopedic Aid* Poultice of crushed leaves applied to sprains. (87:196) *Toothache Remedy* Leaves chewed for toothache. (87:197) **Paiute, Northern** *Cold Remedy* Decoction of roots taken for chest cold. Roots dried and chewed raw for colds. *Cough Medicine* Leaves soaked and used for coughs. *Dermatological Aid* Poultice of pulverized roots applied to cuts and sores. *Diaphoretic* Leaves soaked and sprinkled on the hot rocks in the sweat bath. *Kidney Aid* Decoction of roots taken for kidney troubles. *Misc. Disease Remedy* Decoction of roots taken for flu. *Throat Aid* Root chewed and the saliva allowed to flow down the throat for sore throats. (49:128) **Potawatomi** *Stimulant* Flowers smudged on live coals to revive comatose patient. *Witchcraft Medicine* Flowers smudged on live coals to repel evil spirits. (131:47, 48) **Quileute** *Antirheumatic* (*External*) Poultice of boiled leaves applied to rheumatic limbs. *Febrifuge* Poultice of boiled leaves applied to rheumatic limbs for the fever. *Panacea* Decoction of leaves used as an aromatic bath for sick infants. *Pediatric Aid* Decoction of leaves used as an aromatic bath for sick infants. **Quinault** *Eye Medicine* Decoction of roots used as an eyewash. *Tonic* Decoction of roots taken as a general tonic. *Tuberculosis Remedy* Decoction of roots taken for tuberculosis. (65:49) **Saanich** *Cold Remedy* Young leaves chewed and juice swallowed for colds. *Throat Aid* Young leaves chewed and juice swallowed for sore throats. *Toothache Remedy* Poultice of leaves held in the mouth for toothaches. (156:80) **Salish** *Eye Medicine* Decoction of plants used for sore eyes. (153:293) **Shuswap** *Blood Medicine* Decoction of flowers and roots taken as a blood purifier. (102: 58) *Dermatological Aid* Infusion of leaves taken for poison ivy. (102:56) **Skagit** *Antidiarrheal* Decoction of leaves taken for diarrhea. **Snohomish** *Antidiarrheal* Decoction of leaves taken for diarrhea. **Squaxin** *Dermatological Aid* Poultice of

chewed leaves applied to sores. *Gastrointestinal Aid* Decoction of roots taken for stomach troubles. **Swinomish** *Other* Plant used as a bath for invalids. (65:49) **Thompson** *Antidiarrheal* Infusion of leaves given to children for diarrhea. Leaves chewed or infusion of leaves taken for dysentery. Infusion of roots or whole plant taken for diarrhea. *Antirheumatic* (*External*) Decoction of leaves and roots used for bathing arthritic limbs. Poultice of pounded roots used on the skin for sciatica. *Cold Remedy* Infusion of flowers taken in small quantities for colds. Infusion of roots or whole plant taken for colds. Leaves chewed or decoction of leaves taken for colds. Roots chewed or decoction of roots taken for colds. (161:166) *Dermatological Aid* Decoction of plant used as a wash for chapped hands, pimples, rashes, and insect bites. (as *Achilles millefolium* 104:40) Infusion of plant used as wash or powdered stem and leaf applied for skin problems. (141:460) Leaves and roots rubbed on sores. Poultice of mashed basal leaves used for cuts. (161:166) *Eye Medicine* Decoction of whole plant used as a wash for sore eyes. (141:460) *Gastrointestinal Aid* Infusion of roots or whole plant taken for bad stomach cramps. *Misc. Disease Remedy* Infusion of flowers taken in small quantities for influenza. *Orthopedic Aid* Leaves and roots rubbed on broken bones. *Panacea* Decoction of whole plant taken for any sickness. Decoction of plant used as a wash for any kind of sickness. *Pediatric Aid* Infusion of leaves given to children for diarrhea. (161:166) *Snakebite Remedy* Decoction of plant used as a wash for insect or snake bites. (as *Achilles millefolium* 104:40) Decoction of whole plant used as a wash for snakebites. (141:460) *Tonic* Decoction of whole plant taken as a tonic. (as *Achilles mille-folium* 104:40) Decoction of whole plant taken as a tonic "for slight indisposition." (141:460) *Toothache Remedy* Mashed root placed over a tooth for toothache. *Unspecified* Roots and stems considered "a good medicine." *Urinary Aid* Infusion of flowers taken in small quantities for bladder trouble. *Venereal Aid* Root used for venereal disease. (161:166) **Ute** *Dermatological Aid* Poultice of plant applied externally to bruises. *Panacea* Infusion of plant taken for cases of sickness. (30:32) **Winnebago** *Dermatological Aid* Infusion of herb used as a wash for swellings. *Ear Medicine* Wad of leaves or infusion put into ear for earache. (58:134) **Yuki** *Cold Remedy* Infusion of leaves and flowers taken for cold in the chest. *Respiratory Aid* Infusion of leaves and flowers taken for cold in the chest. (39:47)

Achillea millefolium var. *arenicola*, Common Yarrow

Pomo, Kashaya *Dermatological Aid* Mashed leaf juice used as a salve on sores. (as *A. borealis* ssp. *arenicola* 60:120)

Achillea millefolium var. *borealis*, Boreal Yarrow

Aleut *Analgesic* Infusion of leaves taken for pains in stomach, throat, chest, and muscles. *Cold Remedy* Infusion of leaves taken for colds, stomach pains, and throat pains. *Gastrointestinal Aid* Infusion of leaves taken for stomach pains and throat pains. *Hemostat* Leaves used as a coagulant for cuts and stuffed into nostrils for nosebleeds. *Throat Aid* Infusion of leaves taken for stomach pains, throat pains, and colds. *Tuberculosis Remedy* Infusion of leaves taken for consumption in post-Russian era. (as *A. borealis* 6:426) **Costanoan** *Dermatological Aid* Decoction of plant used as a wash for sores. Poultice of heated leaves applied to wounds to prevent swelling. *Gastrointestinal Aid* Decoction of plant taken for stomachaches. *Toothache Remedy* Heated leaves held in the mouth for toothaches. (as *A. borealis* 17:25) **Eskimo, Alaska** *Unspecified* Infusion of dried plants used for medicinal purposes. (as *A. borealis* 3:716) **Eskimo, Nunivak** *Unspecified* Infusion of dried plants used for its medicinal qualities. (as *A. borealis* 126:325) **Kwakiutl** *Dermatological Aid* Poultice of chewed or soaked and heated plant applied to swellings and sores. (as *A. borealis* 16:381)

Achillea millefolium var. *californica*, California Yarrow

Yurok *Eye Medicine* Used to wash or steam aching, sore eyes. (5:15)

Achillea millefolium var. *occidentalis*, Western Yarrow

Carrier *Antirheumatic* (*External*) Decoction of leaves and stems used as a bath for rheumatism. *Toothache Remedy* Crushed roots placed in the tooth for toothaches. (as *A. lanulosa* 26:85) **Cheyenne** *Antiemetic* Infusion of leaves taken for nausea. (as *A. lanulosa* 63:189) Infusion of green or dried leaves taken for slight nausea. (as *A. lanulosa* 64:189) *Cold Remedy* Infusion of leaves taken for colds. (as *A. lanulosa* 63:189) Infusion of green or dried leaves taken for colds. (as *A. lanulosa* 64:189) *Cough Medicine* Infusion of plants taken for coughs. (as *A. lanulosa* 63:189) Infusion of dried, pounded plant taken for coughs. (as *A. lanulosa* 64:189) *Throat Aid* Infusion of plants taken for tickling in the throat. (as *A. lanulosa* 63:189) Infusion of dried, pounded plant taken for tickling in the throat. (as *A. lanulosa* 64:189) **Cree, Woodlands** *Pediatric Aid* Flowers and wild mint flowers wrapped in a cloth, dipped in water, and used to remove teething gum pus. *Toothache Remedy* Decoction of roots and other herbs taken for teething-related sickness. Flowers and wild mint flowers wrapped in a cloth, dipped in water, and used to remove teething gum pus. (as *A. lanulosa* 91:22) **Great Basin Indian** *Dermatological Aid* Poultice of crushed, fresh plant applied to sores. *Laxative* Infusion of plant taken as a mild laxative. (as *A. lanulosa* 100:50) **Kawaiisu** *Snakebite Remedy* Dried, crushed, and powdered leaves applied to snakebite wounds. (as *A. lanulosa* 180:9) **Meskwaki** *Dermatological Aid* Decoction of stem and leaves used as a wash for "place on the body that is ailing." *Febrifuge* Infusion of leaves and blossoms taken for fever. *Misc. Disease Remedy* Infusion of leaves and blossoms taken for ague. (as *A. lanulosa* 42:210) **Montana Indian** *Cathartic* Infusion of herb used as a cathartic. (as *A. lanulosa* 15:5) **Navajo** *Dermatological Aid* Infusion of plant used as a wash for cuts and saddle sores. *Stimulant* Plant used in a "life medicine for impaired vitality." *Tonic* Plant used in a tonic. (45:79) **Navajo, Kayenta** *Analgesic* Plant used for headaches caused by weak or sore eyes. *Eye Medicine* Plant used in lotion for sore eyes caused from wearing ceremonial masks. *Febrifuge* Plant used as a fever medicine. (as *A. lanulosa* 179:44) **Navajo, Ramah** *Ceremonial Medicine* Plant used as a ceremonial emetic. *Emetic* Plant used as a ceremonial emetic. (as *A. lanulosa* 165:47) **Ojibwa** *Ceremonial Medicine* Compound containing flowering heads smoked for ceremonial purposes. *Dermatological Aid* Poultice of leaves ap-

Achillea sibirica •

plied to spider bite. (as *A. lanulosa* 130:362) **Paiute** *Analgesic* Poultice of fresh, mashed and boiled leaves applied to sprained ankle pains. Poultice of fresh, mashed leaves dampened with water applied with a cloth to tired, aching feet. (as *A. lanulosa* 93:118) Crushed green plant smelled for headaches. Decoction of leaves taken for headaches. Decoction of root taken for gas pains. Poultice of boiled, whole plant applied to pains or sores. Poultice of mashed leaves applied as a compress for headaches. *Antirheumatic (External)* Decoction of plant used as a liniment or wash for sores or rashes. *Blood Medicine* Decoction of plant taken as a blood tonic after childbirth. *Cold Remedy* Root chewed for colds. (as *A. lanulosa* 155:31–33) *Cough Medicine* Infusion of leaves taken as a cough medicine. (as *A. lanulosa* 93:118) *Dermatological Aid* Decoction of plant used as a liniment or wash for sores or rashes. Poultice of boiled, whole plant applied to sores. Poultice of mashed, green plant applied to swellings. Poultice of mashed leaves applied to swellings or sores. (as *A. lanulosa* 155:31–33) *Emetic* Infusion of yarrow taken as an emetic for tuberculosis and other respiratory diseases. (as *A. lanulosa* 93:118) *Eye Medicine* Strained decoction of leaves used as drops for sore eyes. *Febrifuge* Decoction of leaves used as a wash for fevers. *Gastrointestinal Aid* Decoction of root taken for gas pains. *Gynecological Aid* Decoction of plant taken as a blood tonic after childbirth. *Kidney Aid* Decoction of root believed to be good for the kidneys. (as *A. lanulosa* 155: 31–33) *Respiratory Aid* Infusion of yarrow taken as an emetic for respiratory diseases. *Toothache Remedy* Poultice of fresh, mashed roots packed around an infected tooth for the pain. (as *A. lanulosa* 93:118) Green leaves or roots used in various ways for toothaches. (as *A. lanulosa* 155:31–33) *Tuberculosis Remedy* Infusion of yarrow taken as an emetic for tuberculosis. (as *A. lanulosa* 93: 118) *Urinary Aid* Decoction of plant taken for bladder ailments. *Venereal Aid* Compound decoction of plant taken for gonorrhea. *Veterinary Aid* Decoction of plant used to disinfect cuts and saddle sores on horses. Poultice of boiled leaves applied to collar sores on horses. (as *A. lanulosa* 155:31–33) **Sanpoil** *Abortifacient* Decoction of stems and leaves used to cause abortion. *Cold Remedy* Decoction of root boiled until dark in color and taken while warm for colds. (109:218) **Shoshoni** *Analgesic* Crushed green plant smelled for headaches. Decoction of flower taken for stomachaches and used as a liniment for muscular pains. Decoction of leaves taken for headaches. Poultice of boiled, whole plant applied to pains or sores. *Anesthetic* Poultice of fresh roots applied to deaden pain so wound could be opened. Poultice of mashed, fresh roots applied as an anesthetic to painful wounds. *Antidiarrheal* Decoction of plant taken for diarrhea. *Antiemetic* Decoction of plant taken for upset stomach. *Antirheumatic (External)* Decoction of plant used as a liniment or wash for sores or rashes. (as *A. lanulosa* 155:31–33) *Carminative* Infusion of roots taken for gas pains. (as *A. lanulosa* 98:45) *Cold Remedy* Decoction of plant taken for colds. (as *A. lanulosa* 155:31–33) *Dermatological Aid* Poultice of whole plant applied for felon. (as *A. lanulosa* 98:43) Decoction of flower used as a wash for itching. Decoction of plant used as a liniment or wash for sores or rashes. Decoction of root used as a preliminary soak to help extract splinters. Poultice of boiled, whole plant applied to sores. Poultice of fresh roots applied to deaden pain so wound could be opened. Poultice of mashed leaves applied to swellings or sores. *Gastrointestinal Aid* Decoction of flowers taken for stomachaches or indigestion. Decoction of leaves taken for colic or dyspepsia. *Orthopedic Aid* Decoction of flowers used as a liniment for muscular pains. *Toothache Remedy* Green leaves or roots used in various ways for toothaches. **Washo** *Dermatological Aid* Poultice of mashed leaves applied to swellings or sores. (as *A. lanulosa* 155:31–33) **Zuni** *Burn Dressing* Blossoms and root chewed and juice applied before fire-eating or -walking. Poultice of pulverized plant mixed with water applied to burns. (as *A. lanulosa* 143:42)

Achillea sibirica, Siberian Yarrow
Cree, Woodlands *Oral Aid* Poultice of chewed roots applied to gum sores. *Pediatric Aid* Decoction of roots and other herbs taken for teething-related sickness. *Toothache Remedy* Decoction of roots and other herbs taken for teething-related sickness. (91:23)

Achlys triphylla, Sweet After Death
Cowlitz *Tuberculosis Remedy* Infusion of leaves taken for tuberculosis. **Lummi** *Dermatological Aid* Decoction of leaves used as a hair wash. *Emetic* Infusion of smashed plants taken as an emetic. (65:31) **Paiute** *Eye Medicine* Strained infusion of dried, shredded roots used as a wash for cataracts. (93:73) **Skagit** *Dermatological Aid* Decoction of leaves used as a hair wash. *Tuberculosis Remedy* Infusion of leaves taken for tuberculosis. (65:31) **Thompson** *Veterinary Aid* Decoction of roots used as a delousing wash for sheep. (161:186)

Aconitum columbianum, Columbian Monkshood
Okanagan-Colville *Poison* Plant considered highly poisonous. *Witchcraft Medicine* Used for witchcraft. (162:117)

Aconitum delphiniifolium, Larkspurleaf Monkshood
Eskimo, Inupiat *Poison* Roots considered poisonous. (83:140) **Salish** *Unspecified* Plant used as a medicine. (153:294)

Aconitum fischeri, Fischer Monkshood
Gosiute *Poison* Plant considered poisonous. (31:360)

Aconitum heterophyllum
Cree, Hudson Bay *Poison* Plant considered poisonous. (78:303)

Aconitum maximum, Kamchatka Aconite
Aleut *Poison* Plant possibly used at one time as a poison. (6:428)

Acorus calamus, Calamus
Abnaki *Carminative* Used for stomach gases. (121:154) Decoction of roots taken for stomach gas. (121:175) **Algonquin, Quebec** *Cold Remedy* Infusion of ground roots taken for colds. *Cough Medicine* Infusion of ground roots and chokecherry taken for coughs. *Gynecological Aid* Infusion of ground roots taken after childbirth and for symptoms of menopause. *Heart Medicine* Infusion of ground roots and pepperroot taken for heart disease. *Preventive Medicine* Carried on the person in order to avoid contracting a disease. (14:

135) **Blackfoot** *Analgesic* Rootstock ground, mixed with tobacco, and smoked inhaled for headaches. *Gastrointestinal Aid* Poultice of crushed rootstocks and hot water applied for cramps. *Pulmonary Aid* Poultice of crushed rootstocks and hot water applied to sore chests. *Throat Aid* Poultice of crushed rootstocks and hot water applied to sore throats. *Toothache Remedy* Poultice of crushed rootstocks and hot water applied to toothaches. (82:23) **Cherokee** *Analgesic* Root chewed for headache. *Anthelmintic* Used for worms. *Anticonvulsive* Infusion given to "prevent recurrent spasms." *Antidiarrheal* Root chewed and juice swallowed for diarrhea. *Carminative* Used for flatulent colic. *Cold Remedy* Root variously chewed or used in infusion for colds. *Dermatological Aid* Used for "white swelling." *Diaphoretic* Used as a diaphoretic. *Diuretic* Used as a diuretic. *Gastrointestinal Aid* "Possesses stimulant and stomachic virtues" and used for "gravel." *Kidney Aid* Used for yellowish urine and "dropsy." *Stimulant* "Possesses stimulant and stomachic virtues" and used for "gravel." *Throat Aid* Root chewed for sore throat. *Urinary Aid* Used for flatulent colic, "white swelling," worms, yellowish urine, and "gravel." (66:28) **Cheyenne** *Analgesic* Decoction of root taken for bowel pain. (63:42) Infusion of roots taken for bowel pain. (63:171) Infusion of root taken for bowel pain. (64:171) Plant smoked for headaches. *Ceremonial Medicine* Plant used in a sweat lodge ceremony. *Cold Remedy* Plant smoked or in-

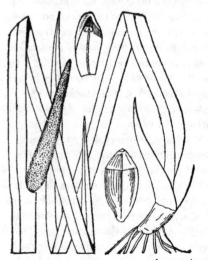

Acorus calamus

fusion of roots taken for colds. *Diuretic* Infusion of roots taken as a diuretic. (69:7) *Gastrointestinal Aid* Decoction of root taken for bowel pain. (63:42) Infusion of roots taken for bowel pain. (63:171) *Laxative* Infusion of roots taken as a laxative. (69:7) *Panacea* Chewed root rubbed on skin for any illness. (63:42) Root chewed and rubbed on the skin for any illness. (63:171) *Pediatric Aid* Bit of root tied to child's clothing to keep the night spirits away. (63:42) Root tied to child's dress or blanket to keep away the night spirits. (63:171) *Witchcraft Medicine* Bit of root tied to clothes to keep night spirits away from children. (63:42) Root tied to child's dress or blanket to keep away the night spirits. (63:171) Plant used to ward off ghosts. (69:7) **Chippewa** *Cathartic* Warm infusion of root taken as a physic by children and adults. (43:344) *Cold Remedy* Decoction of root taken or snuff of pulverized root used for colds. (43:340) Infusion of plants taken for colds. *Cough Medicine* Infusion of plants taken for coughs. (59:124) *Hunting Medicine* Decoction of roots used on fish nets as a charm. (43:376) *Pediatric Aid* Decoction of root taken and dried root chewed by children for toothache. Decoction of root used by children as a gargle for sore throat. (43:342) Infusion of root taken by children and adults as a physic. (43:344) *Respiratory Aid* Infusion of plants taken for bronchial troubles. (59:124) *Throat Aid* Decoction of root gargled by children and root chewed by adults for sore throat. *Toothache Remedy* Decoction of root taken or root chewed, especially by children, for toothache. (43:342) **Cree** *Gastrointestinal Aid* Rootstock ground, mixed with water, and taken for an upset stomach. *Throat Aid* Rootstock peeled, chewed, and liquid swallowed for sore throats. (82:23) **Cree, Alberta** *Hallucinogen* Root chewed for the hallucinogenic effects. *Stimulant* Root chewed for the stimulant effects. *Unspecified* Root chewed for the medicinal effects. (126:331) **Cree, Woodlands** *Adjuvant* Roots added to any decoction to improve medicinal action. *Analgesic* Poultice of powdered roots and yellow pond lily roots or cow parsnip roots applied for headaches. *Antihemorrhagic* Decoction of rootstocks used for coughing up blood. *Antirheumatic* (*External*) Poultice of powdered roots and yellow pond lily roots or cow parsnip roots applied to painful joints, applied for

muscle pain, and applied for rheumatism. Rootstocks used for sore muscles and rheumatic pains. *Cold Remedy* Rootstock chewed to prevent getting a cold after sweating during the winter. Roots smoked in a pipe for colds. Dried rootstock chewed for colds. *Cough Medicine* Rootstock chewed for coughs from colds. Dried rootstock chewed for coughs. *Dermatological Aid* Decoction of rootstocks used for rash from touching nettles or other irritating plants. Poultice of powdered roots and yellow pond lily roots or cow parsnip roots applied to flesh worms. Poultice of chewed rootstock applied to cuts. *Ear Medicine* Poultice of water softened rootstock applied to the ear for earaches. *Febrifuge* Rootstocks used for severe chill. *Gastrointestinal Aid* Grated rootstocks in water taken for stomachaches. Rootstocks used for upset stomachs. *Hemostat* Poultice of chewed rootstock applied as a styptic. *Orthopedic Aid* Decoction of rootstocks used for lower back pains. Poultice of powdered roots and yellow pond lily roots or cow parsnip roots applied to limb swellings. Rootstock used for facial paralysis. *Panacea* Grated rootstocks used as an ingredient in a many herb remedy for various ailments. *Pediatric Aid* Decoction of rootstocks used for sickness related to teething. *Pulmonary Aid* Decoction of rootstocks used for whooping cough. Decoction of rootstocks used for stabbing pains in the chest. *Throat Aid* Decoction of rootstocks used for sore throats. Dried rootstock chewed for sore throats. *Toothache Remedy* Decoction of rootstocks used for sickness related to teething. Poultice of chewed rootstock applied to aching teeth. *Venereal Aid* Decoction of rootstocks used for venereal disease. (91:24) **Dakota** *Carminative* Dried roots taken as a carminative. (57:359) Plant used as a carminative and decoction taken for fever. *Ceremonial Medicine* Blades of grass used as garlands in mystery ceremonies. *Cold Remedy* Rootstock chewed, decoction taken, or smoke treatment used for colds. *Cough Medicine* Rootstock chewed as a cough remedy. *Febrifuge* Decoction of plant taken for fever. *Gastrointestinal Aid* Infusion of pounded rootstock taken for colic. *Panacea* Rootstock regarded as a panacea. *Psychological Aid* Paste of rootstock rubbed on warrior's face to prevent excitement and fear. *Toothache Remedy* Rootstock chewed for toothache. (58:69, 70) **Delaware**

Abortifacient Infusion of roots used for suppressed menses. *Cold Remedy* Infusion of roots used for colds. *Cough Medicine* Infusion of roots used for coughs. *Gastrointestinal Aid* Roots used with sassafras roots for intestinal pains. (151:37) **Delaware, Oklahoma** *Abortifacient* Compound containing root taken for suppressed menses. *Analgesic* Compound containing root used for stomachache and intestinal pains. *Cold Remedy* Compound containing root taken for colds. (150:31, 74) *Cough Medicine* Infusion of root taken for coughs, colds, and suppressed menses. (150:31) **Delaware, Ontario** *Cold Remedy* Infusion of scraped root taken for colds. (150:31) **Iroquois** *Anthelmintic* Compound infusion of roots taken for tapeworms. *Blood Medicine* Compound infusion of roots taken as a blood remedy. (73:279) Infusion of plant and another plant given to children with poor blood circulation. (118:70) *Cold Remedy* Used for colds and sore throats from colds or singing. (73:279) *Dermatological Aid* Compound decoction taken for "boils around the abdomen of children." (73:278) *Ear Medicine* Decoction of roots used as drops in ear for earache. (73:279) *Emetic* Compound decoction of plant taken by women as an emetic for epilepsy. (73: 278) *Gastrointestinal Aid* Powdered roots and cold water taken when feeling bad after eating meals. *Misc. Disease Remedy* Infusion of powdered roots taken for grippe with chills. (118:70) *Pediatric Aid* Compound decoction taken for "boils around the abdomen of children." (73:278) Infusion of plant and another plant given to children with poor blood circulation. Infusion of roots and another plant given to children who scream during the night. *Respiratory Aid* Infusion of roots and roots from another plant used for hard respiration from lower chest pains. (118:70) *Throat Aid* Decoction of roots used as gargle for sore throat. (73:279) *Toothache Remedy* Root packed into hole of aching tooth to break up the tooth. Roots smoked and the smoke sucked into hollow tooth for toothache. *Witchcraft Medicine* Used for the detection of bewitchment. (73:278) **Lakota** *Cough Medicine* Roots chewed for coughs. *Hypotensive* Infusion of roots taken for high blood pressure. *Misc. Disease Remedy* Infusion of roots taken for diabetes. (88:48) *Orthopedic Aid* Infusion of pulverized roots and gun powder taken for arm and

leg cramps. (116:26) *Throat Aid* Roots chewed for sore throat. *Toothache Remedy* Roots chewed for toothache. (88:48) **Malecite** *Cold Remedy* Infusion of one root used for colds. *Preventive Medicine* Roots chewed to prevent disease. (96:249) *Unspecified* Used for medicines. (137:6) **Menominee** *Abortifacient* Compound decoction of root used for irregular periods. (44:133) *Analgesic* Root, a very powerful remedy, used for stomach cramps. *Cathartic* Root used as a "good physic for the whole system, clearing the bile and all." (128: 22, 23) *Cold Remedy* Root chewed or decoction of root used as cold remedy. (44:130) *Gastrointestinal Aid* Root used for stomach cramps. (128:22, 23) **Meskwaki** *Analgesic* Decoction of root taken for "a cramp expected in the stomach." (129:202) *Burn Dressing* Compound used for burns. *Cathartic* Plant used as a physic. (129:201, 202) *Cough Medicine* Decoction of root taken for cough. *Gastrointestinal Aid* Decoction of root taken for "a cramp expected in the stomach." *Tuberculosis Remedy* Decoction of root taken for tuberculosis. (129:202) **Micmac** *Cold Remedy* Root used for colds. *Cough Medicine* Root used for coughs. *Misc. Disease Remedy* Root used for cholera, smallpox, and other epidemics. *Panacea* Root and herb used for the prevention of disease in general and root used for disease in general. (32:53, 54) Plant used as a panacea. (133:316) *Pulmonary Aid* Root used for lung ailments, pneumonia, and pleurisy. (32:53, 54) *Unspecified* Roots chewed for medicinal use. (136:258) **Mohegan** *Abortifacient* Infusion of root taken for suppressed menses. *Analgesic* Infusion of root taken for stomach pains. (151:69, 128) *Antirheumatic (Internal)* Small pieces of root used for rheumatism. (151: 128) *Cold Remedy* Infusion of root taken for colds. *Panacea* Root chewed to insure good health and root carried to "ward off sickness." (151:69, 128) *Tonic* Complex compound infusion including sweetflag root taken as spring tonic. (149:266) **Nanticoke** *Cold Remedy* Infusion of root given to infants for colds. (150:55) *Gastrointestinal Aid* Root used as colic medicine. (150:55, 84) *Pediatric Aid* Infusion of root given to infants for colds. (150:55) **Ojibwa** *Analgesic* Root used for stomach cramps. *Cathartic* Root used as a quick acting physic. *Cold Remedy* Root used for cold in the throat. *Gastrointestinal Aid* Root used for stomach cramps. (130:355) *Heart Medicine* Used as a heart stimulant. (4:2247) *Hunting Medicine* Root and sarsaparilla root made into tea and used on gill nets to bring a fine catch of whitefish. (130:428) *Throat Aid* Root chewed for sore throat. Used to make a throat tonic for singers. (4:2247) Roots chewed for sore throat. (4:2309) Root used for "a cold in the throat." (130:355) **Omaha** *Carminative* Plant used as a carminative. (56:334) Plant used as a carminative and decoction taken for fever. *Ceremonial Medicine* Blades of grass used as garlands in mystery ceremonies. *Cold Remedy* Rootstock chewed, decoction taken, or smoke treatment used for colds. *Cough Medicine* Rootstock chewed as a cough remedy. *Febrifuge* Decoction of plant taken for fever. (58:69, 70) *Gastrointestinal Aid* Root chewed for stomach disorders. (48:584) Infusion of pounded rootstock taken for colic. *Panacea* Rootstock regarded as a panacea. (58:69, 70) *Tonic* Rootstock chewed as a tonic. (56:334) *Toothache Remedy* Rootstock chewed for toothache. (58:69, 70) *Veterinary Aid* Plant put into the feed of ailing horses. (48:584) **Pawnee** *Carminative* Plant used as a carminative and decoction taken for fever. *Ceremonial Medicine* Blades of grass used as garlands in mystery ceremonies. *Cold Remedy* Rootstock chewed, decoction taken, or smoke treatment used for colds. *Cough Medicine* Rootstock chewed as a cough remedy. *Febrifuge* Decoction of plant taken for fever. *Gastrointestinal Aid* Infusion of pounded rootstock taken for colic. *Panacea* Rootstock regarded as a panacea. *Toothache Remedy* Rootstock chewed for toothache. **Ponca** *Carminative* Plant used as a carminative. *Ceremonial Medicine* Blades of grass used as garlands in mystery ceremonies. *Cold Remedy* Rootstock chewed, decoction taken, or smoke treatment used for colds. *Cough Medicine* Rootstock chewed as a cough remedy. *Febrifuge* Decoction taken for fever. *Gastrointestinal Aid* Infusion of pounded rootstock taken for colic. *Panacea* Rootstock regarded as a panacea. *Toothache Remedy* Rootstock chewed for toothache. (58:69, 70) **Potawatomi** *Antihemorrhagic* Compound decoction of small amount of root taken for hemorrhage. *Respiratory Aid* Powdered root snuffed up nose for catarrh. (131:39, 40) **Rappahannock** *Gastrointestinal Aid* Chewed plant juice taken by older people for the stomach.

(138:29) Infusion given to children and babies for pains and stomach cramps. *Pediatric Aid* Infusion given to children and babies for fretfulness, pains, and stomach cramps. *Sedative* Infusion given to children and babies for fretfulness. (138:30) *Tonic* Chewed plant juice taken by older people as a tonic. (138:29) **Shinnecock** *Blood Medicine* Root nibbled "to dry your blood." *Oral Aid* Root dried, cooked in sugar, and eaten for the breath. (25:118) **Sioux, Fort Peck** *Abortifacient* Used to cause abortion. *Panacea* Root chewed and swallowed as a "cure-all." (15:5) **Winnebago** *Carminative* Plant used as a carminative and decoction taken for fever. *Ceremonial Medicine* Blades of grass used as garlands in mystery ceremonies. *Cold Remedy* Rootstock chewed, decoction taken, or smoke treatment used for colds. *Cough Medicine* Rootstock chewed as a cough remedy. *Febrifuge* Decoction of plant taken for fever. *Gastrointestinal Aid* Infusion of pounded rootstock taken for colic. *Panacea* Rootstock regarded as a panacea. (58:69, 70) *Tonic* Complex compound injected via bird wing bone for general health. (108:265) *Toothache Remedy* Rootstock chewed for toothache. (58:69, 70)

Acourtia microcephala, Sacapellote
Coahuilla *Cathartic* Decoction of plant taken to produce "a very quick passage of the bowels." (as *Perezia microcephala* 9:78)

Acourtia wrightii, Brownfoot
Hualapai *Dermatological Aid* Poultice of woolly "cotton" applied to open, bleeding wounds. (as *Perezia wrightii* 169:49) **Navajo, Kayenta** *Gynecological Aid* Plant used for difficult labor, a postpartum medicine. (as *Perezia wrightii* 179:49) **Pima** *Hemostat* Plant used as a styptic. (as *Perezia wrightii* 123:80)

Acrostichum danaeifolium, Inland Leatherfern
Seminole *Febrifuge* Infusion of plant taken and rubbed on the body for high fevers. (145:202)

Actaea pachypoda, White Baneberry
Blackfoot *Cold Remedy* Decoction of root used for colds and coughs. *Cough Medicine* Decoction of root used for coughs and colds. (as *A. eburnea*

95:275) **Cherokee** *Dermatological Aid* Infusion of root used for itch. *Stimulant* Infusion given "to relieve and rally a patient at point of death." *Throat Aid* Infusion of root used as a gargle. *Toothache Remedy* "Will kill teeth of young people if not careful with it." (66:55) **Chippewa** *Anticonvulsive* and *Pediatric Aid* Decoction of roots taken by children and adults for convulsions. (as *A. alba* 59:130) **Iroquois** *Urinary Aid* Decoction of roots taken when "a man urinates blood." (as *A. alba* 73:321) **Meskwaki** *Analgesic* Decoction of root taken for childbirth pain. *Gynecological Aid* Decoction of root taken for childbirth pain. *Stimulant* Root used to revive and rally a patient at the point of death. *Urinary Aid* Used as a genitourinary remedy for men and women. (as *A. alba* 129: 237, 238)

Actaea rubra, Red Baneberry
Alaska Native *Poison* Berries considered poisonous. (71:149) **Algonquin** *Analgesic* Used for stomach pains, in some seasons for males, other seasons for females. (18:142) **Blackfoot** *Cold Remedy* Decoction of roots taken for colds. *Cough Medicine* Decoction of roots taken for coughs. *Veterinary Aid* Decoction of roots used to treat horses. (82:34) **Cheyenne** *Ceremonial Medicine* Roots used in ceremonies. *Dermatological Aid* Roots used for sores. *Dietary Aid* Decoction of roots taken to improve the appetite. (69:33) *Gynecological Aid* Infusion of root pieces used by women after childbirth for increased milk flow. (68:8) Infusion of stems taken by pregnant and nursing mothers to increase milk flow. (69:22) **Chippewa** *Gynecological Aid* Decoction of root taken for excessive flowing. (43:358) **Cree, Hudson Bay** *Cathartic* Plant used as a purgative. (as *A. spicata* 78:303) **Cree, Woodlands** *Gynecological Aid* Infusion of small piece of root taken to slow heavy menstrual flow. (91:25) **Eskimo, Arctic** *Poison* Fruits considered poisonous. (106:17) **Ojibwa** *Gastrointestinal Aid* Root eaten by men for stomach troubles. *Gynecological Aid* Infusion of root taken after childbirth "to clear up the system." (130:382) **Ojibwa, South** *Analgesic* and *Gastrointestinal Aid* Decoction of root taken for stomach pain caused by having "swallowed hair." (77:201) **Potawatomi** *Gynecological Aid* Infusion of root given "to purge the patient of afterbirth." (131:74) **Thompson** *Anti-*

rheumatic (*Internal*) Decoction of root taken in a 1-teaspoon dose for arthritis. *Poison* Red and white berried plant considered extremely poisonous. *Pulmonary Aid* Decoction of plant taken for bronchial or lung trouble. (161:245)

Actaea rubra ssp. *arguta*, Red Baneberry
Blackfoot *Cold Remedy* Decoction of root used for colds and coughs. *Cough Medicine* Decoction of root used for coughs and colds. (as *A. arguta* 95:275) **Cheyenne** *Blood Medicine* Infusion of dried roots and stems taken as a blood medicine. (as *A. arguta* 63:174) Infusion of dried, pounded roots and stems used as a blood medicine. (as *A. arguta* 64:174) *Gynecological Aid* Simple or compound decoction of plant taken to increase maternal milk flow. (as *A. arguta* 63:41) Infusion of dried roots and stems taken by women after childbirth. (as *A. arguta* 63:174) Infusion of dried, pounded roots and stems taken after childbirth to make first milk pass off quickly. (as *A. arguta* 64:174) **Okanagon** *Antirheumatic* (*Internal*) Decoction of roots taken for rheumatism. *Dietary Aid* Decoction of roots taken for emaciation. (as *A. arguta* 104:41) **Quileute** *Dermatological Aid* Poultice of chewed leaves applied to boils. **Quinault** *Dermatological Aid* Poultice of chewed leaves applied to wounds. (as *A. arguta* 65:30) **Thompson** *Antirheumatic* (*Internal*) Decoction of roots taken for rheumatism. (as *A. arguta* 104:41) Decoction of root taken for rheumatism. (as *A. arguta* 141:463) *Dietary Aid* Decoction of roots taken for emaciation. (as *A. arguta* 104:41) Decoction of roots taken for emaciation. (as *A. arguta* & *A. eburnea* 141:463) *Poison* Decoction of roots considered poisonous if taken in large quantities. (as *A. arguta* & *A. eburnea* 141:512) *Venereal Aid* Decoction of root taken for syphilis. (as *A. arguta* & *A. eburnea* 141:463)

Actaea rubra ssp. *rubra*, Red Baneberry
Iroquois *Antihemorrhagic* Compound decoction with roots taken for internal hemorrhage. *Antirheumatic* (*External*) Infusion of roots used as a wash for rheumatism. *Psychological Aid* Taken and sprinkled on head to give "young men the right sense." *Veterinary Aid* Infusion of roots given to dogs "when the dog won't hunt anymore." (as *A. spicata* ssp. *rubra* 73:321)

Adenocaulon bicolor, American Trailplant
Cowlitz *Dermatological Aid* Poultice of leaves applied to boils. **Squaxin** *Dermatological Aid* Poultice of leaves applied to scrofula sores. *Tuberculosis Remedy* Poultice of leaves applied to scrofula sores. (65:48)

Adenostoma fasciculatum, Common Chamise
Cahuilla *Antirheumatic* (*External*) and *Disinfectant* Decoction of leaves and branches used to bathe infected, sore, or swollen areas of the body. (11:29) **Coahuilla** *Veterinary Aid* Plant used to make a drink given to sick cows. (9:79)

Adenostoma sparsifolium, Redshank
Cahuilla *Antirheumatic* (*External*) Plant used for arthritis. *Cold Remedy* Leaves used to make a beverage for colds. *Emetic* Infusion of dried leaves taken for stomach ailments by inducing bowel movements or vomiting. *Gastrointestinal Aid* Leaves used to make a beverage for ulcers. Infusion of dried leaves taken for stomach ailments by inducing bowel movements or vomiting. *Laxative* Infusion of dried leaves taken for stomach ailments by inducing bowel movements or vomiting. *Pulmonary Aid* Leaves used to make a beverage for chest ailments. *Veterinary Aid* Poultice of plant and bacon fat applied to saddle sores on horses. (11:30) **Coahuilla** *Analgesic* Infusion of twigs taken for stomach and intestinal pain. *Cathartic* Infusion of twigs used "to produce vomit and bowel relief." *Dermatological Aid* Pulverized twigs mixed with grease and used as a salve. *Emetic* Infusion of twigs used "to produce vomit and bowel relief." *Gastrointestinal Aid* Infusion of twigs taken for stomach and intestinal pain. (9:77, 78) **Diegueño** *Gastrointestinal Aid* Infusion of plant taken for colic. *Toothache Remedy* Infusion of plant used as a mouthwash for toothaches. (74:217)

Adiantum aleuticum, Aleutian Maidenhair
Lummi *Dermatological Aid* Infusion of leaves used as a hair wash. **Makah** *Antihemorrhagic* Leaves chewed for internal hemorrhages from wounds. *Dermatological Aid* Infusion of leaves used as a hair wash. *Gastrointestinal Aid* Leaves chewed for sore chest and stomach troubles. **Skokomish** *Dermatological Aid* Infusion of leaves

used as a hair wash. (as *A. pedatum* var. *aleuticum* 65:14)

Adiantum capillus-veneris, Common Maidenhair
Mahuna *Antirheumatic* (*Internal*) Plant used for rheumatism. (117:60) **Navajo, Kayenta** *Dermatological Aid* Infusion of plant used as a lotion for bumblebee or centipede stings. *Psychological Aid* Plant smoked or infusion of plant used for insanity. (179:14)

Adiantum jordanii, California Maidenhair
Costanoan *Analgesic* Decoction of plant used for "pain below the shoulders." *Blood Medicine* Decoction of plant used to purify the blood. *Gastrointestinal Aid* Decoction of plant used for stomach troubles. *Gynecological Aid* Decoction of plant used to expel the afterbirth and for postparturition. (17:4)

Adiantum pedatum, Northern Maidenhair
Cherokee *Antirheumatic* (*External*) Compound decoction of root applied with warm hands for rheumatism. (66:8) Decoction of roots rubbed on area affected by rheumatism. (152:3) *Antirheumatic* (*Internal*) Infusion taken for rheumatism. *Emetic* Infusion of whole plant given as an emetic "in case of ague and fever." (66:34) Decoction of whole plant used as an emetic in cases of ague and fever. (177:74) *Febrifuge* Infusion of whole plant

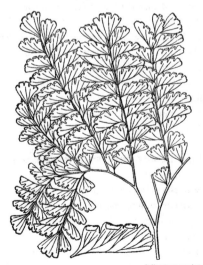

Adiantum pedatum

blown over head and chest of patient for fever. (66:34) Decoction of whole plant used as an emetic in cases of fever. (177:74) *Heart Medicine* Powdered leaves smoked for heart trouble. *Misc. Disease Remedy* Infusion of whole plant given as an emetic "in case of ague and fever." (66:34) Decoction of whole plant used as an emetic in cases of ague. (177:74) *Other* Given for "sudden paralytic attacks as in bad pneumonia of children." *Respiratory Aid* Powdered plant "snuffed" and smoked for asthma. (66:34) **Costanoan** *Blood Medicine* Decoction of plant used to purify the blood. *Gastrointestinal Aid* Decoction of plant used for stomach troubles. (17:5) **Hesquiat** *Respiratory Aid* Infusion of dried fronds burned to ashes, mixed with unknown, and taken for shortness of breath. Green fronds chewed for shortness of breath. *Strengthener* Infusion of dried fronds burned to ashes, mixed with unknown, and taken for strength and endurance. This infusion used especially by dancers in winter. Hesquiat dancers would take nothing but this medicine on day when they were dancing; it made them "light on their feet" and helped them continue dancing for a long time without tiring. Green fronds chewed by dancers in winter for strength and endurance. (159:29) **Makah** *Gastrointestinal Aid* Fronds chewed or eaten for "weak stomach." (55:217) **Menominee** *Antidiarrheal* Compound decoction of root used for dysentery. (44:131) *Gynecological Aid* Blades, stem, and root used for "female maladies." (128:47) **Meskwaki** *Pediatric Aid* Compound containing root and stems used for children who "turn black." (129:237) **Micmac** *Other* Herb used for fits and taken as an "agreeable decoction." (32:54) **Nitinaht** *Ceremonial Medicine* Used by dancers to make them light-footed. (160:61) **Potawatomi** *Gynecological Aid* Infusion of root taken by nursing mothers for caked breast. (131:73)

Adiantum pedatum ssp. *pedatum*, Northern Maidenhair

Iroquois *Analgesic* Decoction of plant used by children for cramps. *Antirheumatic* (*External*) Compound decoction of green roots used as foot soak for rheumatism. *Antirheumatic* (*Internal*) Compound decoction of green roots taken for rheumatism. *Diuretic* Decoction of roots taken for the

cessation of urine due to gall. *Emetic* Infusion of plant induced vomiting as a remedy for love medicine. *Gynecological Aid* Compound decoction or infusion of roots taken for excessive menstruation. Decoction of roots used by "ladies to get period, cleans out" or for abortions. Plant used for abortion pains and pain when about to deliver. *Liver Aid* Decoction of roots taken for the cessation of urine due to gall. (73:258) *Orthopedic Aid* and *Pediatric Aid* Poultice of smashed plant applied to sore back of babies. (73:257) Decoction of plant used by children for cramps. *Snakebite Remedy* Poultice of wet, smashed fronds bound to snakebites. *Venereal Aid* Decoction of plant used as a wash for gonorrhea. Decoction of root taken for venereal disease and used as a wash for sores. (73:258)

Aesculus californica, California Buckeye

Costanoan *Hemorrhoid Remedy* Smashed fruit applied as a salve for hemorrhoids. *Poison* Fruit used as a fish poison. *Toothache Remedy* Decoction of bark used for toothaches and loose teeth. (17:23) **Kawaiisu** *Hemorrhoid Remedy* Broken seeds used as suppositories for piles. *Poison* Raw seeds considered poisonous if eaten. (180:10) **Mendocino Indian** *Poison* Fresh fruit considered poisonous. *Toothache Remedy* Bark placed in cavity of tooth for toothaches. *Veterinary Aid* Fruit given to horses for bot worms and apt to cause an abortion in cows. (33:366) **Pomo** *Poison* Nuts used as poison. (54:14)

Aesculus glabra, Ohio Buckeye

Delaware *Antirheumatic* (*External*) Nuts carried in the pocket for rheumatism. *Ear Medicine* Infusion of ground nuts mixed with sweet oil or mutton tallow and applied for earache. *Poison* Nuts ground and used as fish poison in streams. (151:30) **Delaware, Oklahoma** *Ear Medicine* Poultice of pulverized nuts with sweet oil applied for earache. *Poison* Pulverized nuts used as fish poison called "fish peyote," made the fish dizzy. (150:25, 74) **Mohegan** *Antirheumatic* (*External*) Carried in the pocket for rheumatism pain. (151:78)

Aesculus glabra var. *arguta*, Ohio Buckeye

Kiowa *Emetic* Infusion of the inside of fruit taken as an emetic. (as *A. arguta* 166:41)

Aesculus hippocastanum, Horse Chestnut
Iroquois *Analgesic* Compound of powdered roots used for chest pains. *Pulmonary Aid* Compound of powdered roots used for chest pains. (73:379) **Mohegan** *Antirheumatic* (*External*) Horse chestnut carried in the pocket for rheumatism. **Shinnecock** *Antirheumatic* (*External*) Horse chestnut carried in the pocket for rheumatism. (25:121)

Aesculus pavia, Red Buckeye
Cherokee *Antirheumatic* (*External*) Nut carried in pocket for rheumatism and good luck. *Cancer Treatment* Poultice of pounded nuts used for tumors and infections. *Dermatological Aid* Poultice of pounded nuts used for tumors and infections and as a salve for sores. *Gastrointestinal Aid* Nuts used in various ways for dyspepsia and colic. (66:27) Infusion of roots taken and used as a bath for dyspepsia. (152:39) *Gynecological Aid* Cold, compound infusion given to stop bleeding after delivery. Infusion of bark and cold compound infusion of bark used in delivery. *Hemorrhoid Remedy* Nut carried in pocket for piles. *Orthopedic Aid* Poultice of pounded nuts used for "white swelling" and sprains. *Stimulant* Infusion of ground nutmeat taken to prevent fainting. (66:27)

Agalinis tenuifolia var. ***tenuifolia***, Slenderleaf False Foxglove
Meskwaki *Antidiarrheal* Infusion used for diarrhea. (as *Gerardia tenuifolia* 129:246, 247)

Agastache foeniculum, Blue Giant Hyssop
Cheyenne *Analgesic* Cold infusion of leaves taken for chest pains caused by coughing. (as *A. anethiodora* 63:186) Infusion of leaves used for chest pains from coughing. (as *A. anethiodora* 64:186) *Cold Remedy* Infusion of leaves taken as a cold medicine. *Diaphoretic* Leaves used in a steam bath to induce sweating. *Febrifuge* Powdered leaves rubbed on the body for high fevers. (69:27) *Heart Medicine* Cold infusion of leaves taken for weak heart. (as *A. anethiodora* 63:42, 186) Infusion of leaves used for a weak heart. (as *A. anethiodora* 64:186) Infusion of leaves taken to correct dispirited heart. *Herbal Steam* Leaves used in a steam bath to induce sweating. (69:27) *Pulmonary Aid* Cold infusion of leaves taken for chest pains caused by coughing. (as *A. anethiodora* 63:186)

Cold infusion of leaves taken for chest pain. (as *A. anethiodora* 63:42) *Unspecified* Infusion of leaves taken for its medicinal qualities. (69:27) **Chippewa** *Analgesic* Infusion of root taken for cold and chest pain. (as *A. anethiodora* 43:340) *Burn Dressing* Simple or compound poultice of leaves or stalk applied to burns. (as *A. anethiodora* 43:352) *Cough Medicine* Infusion of root taken for cough of "an internal cold." (as *A. anethiodora* 43:340) **Cree** *Ceremonial Medicine* Flowers frequently included in medicine bundles. (82:51) **Cree, Woodlands** *Antihemorrhagic* Infusion of stem, leaves, and other plants taken for coughing up blood. (91:26)

Agastache nepetoides, Yellow Giant Hyssop
Iroquois *Dermatological Aid* Compound infusion of plants used as wash for poison ivy and itch. (73:422)

Agastache pallidiflora ssp. ***neomexicana*** var. ***neomexicana***, New Mexico Giant Hyssop
Navajo, Ramah *Ceremonial Medicine* Plant used in ceremonial chant lotion. *Cough Medicine* Plant used for bad coughs. *Dermatological Aid* Dried, pulverized root used as dusting powder for sores or cankers. *Disinfectant* Plant used as fumigant for "deer infection." *Febrifuge* Plant used as a fever medicine. *Witchcraft Medicine* Plant used to protect from witches. (as *A. neomexicana* 165:41)

Agastache scrophulariifolia, Purple Giant Hyssop
Meskwaki *Diuretic* Infusion of root used as a diuretic. *Unspecified* Compound of plant heads used medicinally. (129:225)

Agastache urticifolia, Nettleleaf Giant Hyssop
Miwok *Antirheumatic* (*Internal*) Decoction of leaves taken for rheumatism. *Misc. Disease Remedy* Decoction taken for measles. (8:166) **Okanagan-Colville** *Cold Remedy* Infusion of leaves taken as a cold medicine. *Febrifuge* and *Pediatric Aid* Leaves placed in babies' blankets for fevers. (162:109) **Paiute** *Analgesic* Cold infusion of leaves used for stomach pains. *Cold Remedy* Decoction of plant taken for colds. *Dermatological Aid* Poultice of mashed leaves applied to swellings.

Gastrointestinal Aid Cold infusion of leaves used for indigestion and stomach pains. **Shoshoni** *Cathartic* Decoction of plant taken as a physic. (155:33)

Agave sp., Mescal Agave
Hualapai *Dermatological Aid* Used as a facial cream. (169:55)

Ageratina altissima var. **altissima**, White Snakeroot
Cherokee *Antidiarrheal* Taken for diarrhea, gravel, and urinary diseases. *Diuretic* Root used as a diuretic. *Febrifuge* Taken for fever. *Misc. Disease Remedy* Taken for ague. *Stimulant* Root used as a stimulant. *Tonic* Root used as a tonic. *Urinary Aid* Taken for gravel and urinary diseases. (as *Eupatorium rugosum* 66:56) **Iroquois** *Blood Medicine* Decoction of roots taken to separate venereal disease from the blood. (as *Eupatorium rugosum* 73:459) *Cathartic* Decoction of whole plant and roots taken as a physic. (as *Eupatorium rugosum* 73:458) *Diaphoretic* Decoction of roots taken and used as a sweat bath to keep patient cooled. *Gynecological Aid* Decoction or infusion of roots taken for a fallen or inflamed womb. *Panacea* Plant used for anything. *Venereal Aid* Decoction of roots taken to separate venereal disease from the blood. *Veterinary Aid* Infusion of plants given to horses to stop sweating. (as *Eupatorium rugosum* 73:459) *Witchcraft Medicine* Decoction of stems used as a witchcraft medicine. (as *Eupatorium rugosum* 73:458)

Ageratina altissima var. **roanensis**, White Snakeroot
Chickasaw *Toothache Remedy* Roots chewed and held in mouth for toothache. **Choctaw** *Stimulant* and *Tonic* Used as a "warming stimulant and tonic." *Toothache Remedy* Roots chewed and held in mouth for toothache. (as *Eupatorium ageratoides* 23:288) **Meskwaki** *Diaphoretic* Used as a steaming agent in sweat bath. *Stimulant* Smudged and used to revive an unconscious patient. (as *Eupatorium urticaefolium* 129:214)

Ageratina herbacea, Fragrant Snakeroot
Navajo, Ramah *Analgesic* Cold infusion taken and used as lotion for headache. *Febrifuge* Cold infusion taken and used as lotion for fever. (as *Eupatorium herbaceum* 165:51)

Ageratina occidentalis, Western Snakeroot
Zuni *Antirheumatic* (*External*) Ingredient of "schumaakwe cakes" and used externally for rheumatism. *Dermatological Aid* Ingredient of "schumaakwe cakes" and used externally for swelling. (as *Eupatorium occidentale* 143:50)

Agoseris aurantiaca, Orange Agoseris
Navajo, Ramah *Ceremonial Medicine* Plant used as a ceremonial emetic. *Dermatological Aid* Cold infusion taken and used as lotion for arrow or bullet wounds. *Disinfectant* Cold infusion taken and used as lotion for "deer infection." *Emetic* Plant used as a ceremonial emetic. *Orthopedic Aid* Wet leaves rubbed on swollen arms, wrists, or ankles. *Panacea* Root used as a "life medicine." *Witchcraft Medicine* Cold infusion taken and used as lotion for protection from witches. (165:47)

Agoseris glauca var. **dasycephala**, Pale Agoseris
Okanagan-Colville *Dermatological Aid* Infusion of entire plant used to wash sores and rashes. Poultice of latex applied to sores. *Laxative* Infusion of roots taken as a laxative. (162:74) **Thompson** *Dermatological Aid* Milky latex used to remove warts. (161:167)

Agrimonia gryposepala, Tall Hairy Agrimony
Cherokee *Antidiarrheal* Infusion of burs taken to "check bowels." *Blood Medicine* Infusion of root taken to build up blood. *Dermatological Aid* Powdered root compound used for pox. *Dietary Aid* Infusion of root given to satisfy children's hunger. *Febrifuge* Infusion of burs taken for fever. *Gastrointestinal Aid* Cold infusion of pulverized root taken for bowels. *Gynecological Aid* Infusion of burs taken to "check discharge." *Pediatric Aid* Infusion of root given to satisfy children's hunger. (66:22) **Iroquois** *Antidiarrheal* Infusion or decoction used by children for diarrhea, "summer complaint," or vomiting. *Antiemetic* Infusion given to children for diarrhea, "summer complaint," and vomiting. (73:357) *Basket Medicine* Infusion of roots and flowers used on anything to sell, a "basket medicine." *Emetic* Decoction of plants taken

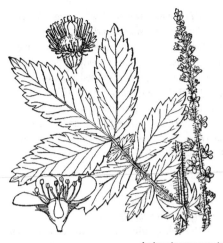

Agrimonia gryposepala

for diarrhea and as emetic for "summer complaint." (73:358) *Other* and *Pediatric Aid* Infusion given to children for diarrhea, "summer complaint," and vomiting. (73:357) **Meskwaki** *Hemostat* Root used as a styptic for nosebleeds. (129: 241) **Ojibwa** *Urinary Aid* Compound containing root used as a medicine for urinary troubles. (130: 383, 384) **Potawatomi** *Hemostat* Plant used as styptic and infusion snuffed for nosebleed by Prairie Potawatomi. (131:76)

Agrimonia parviflora, Harvestlice
Cherokee *Antidiarrheal* Infusion of burs taken to "check bowels." *Blood Medicine* Infusion of root taken to build up blood. *Dermatological Aid* Powdered root compound used for pox. *Dietary Aid* Infusion of root given to satisfy children's hunger. *Febrifuge* Infusion of burs taken for fever. *Gastrointestinal Aid* Cold infusion of pulverized root taken for bowels. *Gynecological Aid* Infusion of burs taken to "check discharge." *Pediatric Aid* Infusion of root given to satisfy children's hunger. (66:22)

Alcea rosea, Hollyhock
Shinnecock *Dermatological Aid* Leaves used to apply infusion of flowers to inflamed areas. (as *Althaea rosea* 25:120)

Alectoria sarmentosa
Nitinaht *Dermatological Aid* Used for wound dressing material and as bandages. (maidenhair moss 160:55)

Aletes acaulis, Stemless Indian Parsley
Keres, Western *Cathartic* Plant used as a cathartic. *Emetic* Plant used as an emetic. (147:25)

Aletris farinosa, White Colicroot
Catawba *Antidiarrheal* Infusion of leaves taken for dysentery. (134:188) Infusion of leaves taken for bloody dysentery. (152:7) *Gastrointestinal Aid* Infusion of leaves taken for colic and stomach disorders. (134:188) Cold infusion of leaves taken for colic and stomach disorders. (152:7) **Cherokee** *Antirheumatic* (*Internal*) Taken for rheumatism. *Carminative* Taken for flatulent colic. *Cough Medicine* Taken for coughs. *Febrifuge* Tonic used for child bed fever. *Gynecological Aid* Tonic used to strengthen womb and root prevented abortion. *Liver Aid* Taken for jaundice. *Pulmonary Aid* Taken for lung diseases. *Tonic* Used for child bed fever and to strengthen womb. *Tuberculosis Remedy* Taken for consumption. *Urinary Aid* Taken for "strangury," a slow, painful urination. (66:57) **Micmac** *Abortifacient* Root used as an emmenagogue. *Gastrointestinal Aid* Root used as a stomachic. *Tonic* Root used as a tonic. (32:54) **Rappahannock** *Gynecological Aid* Infusion of plant given to women and girls for "female troubles." (138:34)

Aleurites moluccana, Indian Walnut
Hawaiian *Abortifacient* Nutshells and gourds burned and the resulting smoke or fumes entered the vagina for swollen wombs. *Dermatological Aid* Baked nutmeats, other plants, and breadfruit milk applied to scrofulous sores, ulcers, and bad sores. *Gastrointestinal Aid* Flowers and other plants pounded and resulting liquid given to infants for stomach or bowel disorders. *Laxative* Nut oil used to make a very strong laxative. *Pediatric Aid* Flowers and other plants pounded and resulting liquid given to infants for stomach or bowel disorders. *Respiratory Aid* Bark and other plants pounded, resulting liquid heated and taken for asthma. *Strengthener* Nutmeats baked, ground, mixed with other plants, and eaten to build up the body. *Tuberculosis Remedy* Baked nutmeats, other plants, and breadfruit milk applied to scrofulous sores. (2:56)

Alisma plantago-aquatica, American Water Plantain

Cree, Woodlands *Gastrointestinal Aid* Dried stem base eaten or grated and taken in water for heart "troubles," including heartburn. Stem base taken for stomachaches, cramps, and stomach flu. *Heart Medicine* Dried stem base eaten or grated and taken in water for heart "troubles," including heartburn. *Laxative* Stem base taken for constipation. *Misc. Disease Remedy* Stem base taken for stomach flu. *Panacea* Powdered stem base and many other herbs used for various ailments. *Stimulant* Stem base given to prevent fainting during childbirth. (91:26) **Iroquois** *Gynecological Aid* Infusion of plant used for "womb troubles." *Kidney Aid* Split roots used for lame back or kidneys. *Orthopedic Aid* Split root used for lame back or kidneys and leaf infusion used as a runner's liniment. *Other* Raw root chewed to strengthen veins. *Tuberculosis Remedy* Decoction of plant or roots or infusion of roots taken for consumption. (73:272)

Alisma subcordatum, American Water Plantain

Cherokee *Dermatological Aid* Used as a poultice on old sores, wounds, bruises, swellings, and ulcers. *Gastrointestinal Aid* Root used for bowel complaints, sores, wounds, and bruises. (66:61)

Allionia incarnata, Trailing Windmills

Navajo, Ramah *Dermatological Aid* Cold infusion of root used as a lotion for swellings. (165:26)

Allium bisceptrum, Twincrest Onion

Mahuna *Dietary Aid* Plant juice used as an appetite restorer. (117:62)

Allium brevistylum, Shortstyle Onion

Cheyenne *Dermatological Aid* Poultice of ground roots and stems applied to carbuncles. (63:171) Poultice of ground roots and stems applied and infusion used as a wash for carbuncles. (64:171)

Allium canadense, Meadow Garlic

Cherokee *Carminative* Used as a carminative. *Cathartic* Used as a mild cathartic. *Diuretic* Used as a diuretic. *Ear Medicine* Used "to remove deafness." *Expectorant* Used as an expectorant. *Kid-*

ney Aid Used for "dropsy." *Misc. Disease Remedy* Used for scurvy. *Pediatric Aid* and *Pulmonary Aid* Tincture used to prevent worms and colic in children and used as a croup remedy. *Respiratory Aid* Used for asthma. *Stimulant* Used as a stimulant. (66:35) **Mahuna** *Dermatological Aid* Plant rubbed on body for protection from insect bites. Plant rubbed on body for protection from lizard, scorpion, and tarantula bites. *Snakebite Remedy* Plant rubbed on body for protection from poisonous snakebites. (117:63)

Allium cepa, Garden Onion

Mohegan *Cold Remedy* Syrup of chopped onions taken for colds. **Shinnecock** *Cold Remedy* Syrup of chopped onions taken for colds. *Disinfectant* Used to destroy germs because of a volatile oil in roots. *Ear Medicine* Heart of onion placed in ear for earache. *Febrifuge* Onion placed in a sick room to draw fever out. *Misc. Disease Remedy* Onion placed in a sick room to draw out flu. (25:120)

Allium cernuum, Nodding Onion

Cherokee *Cold Remedy* Juice taken for colds. *Dermatological Aid* Juice given to children for hives. *Febrifuge* Used as poultice for feet in "nervous fever." *Gastrointestinal Aid* Infusion taken for colic. *Kidney Aid* Juice taken after "horsemint tea" for "gravel and dropsy." *Liver Aid* Juice taken for "liver complaints." *Pediatric Aid* Juice given to children for hives and croup. *Pulmonary Aid* Poultice of fried plant put on chest for croup. Juice given to children for croup. *Respiratory Aid* Juice taken for "phthisic." *Throat Aid* Juice taken for sore throat. *Urinary Aid* Juice taken after "horsemint tea" for "gravel and dropsy." (66:47) **Isleta** *Dermatological Aid* Poultice of onions applied externally for infections. *Throat Aid* Poultice of warm onions applied externally to throat for sore throat. (85:20) **Kwakiutl** *Dermatological Aid* Poultice of soaked bulbs applied to sores and swellings. (157:272) **Makah** *Analgesic* Poultice of chewed plants applied to the chest for pleurisy pains. *Pulmonary Aid* Poultice of chewed plants applied to the chest for pleurisy pains. **Quinault** *Analgesic* Poultice of chewed plants applied to the chest for pleurisy pains. *Pulmonary Aid* Poultice of chewed plants applied to the chest for pleurisy pains. (65:24)

Allium sativum, Cultivated Garlic
Cherokee *Carminative* Used as a carminative.
Cathartic Used as a mild cathartic. *Diuretic* Used
as a diuretic. *Ear Medicine* Used "to remove deafness." *Expectorant* Used as an expectorant. *Kidney Aid* Used for "dropsy." *Misc. Disease Remedy*
Used for scurvy. *Pediatric Aid* and *Pulmonary Aid*
Tincture used to prevent worms and colic in children and used as a croup remedy. *Respiratory Aid*
Used for asthma. *Stimulant* Used as a stimulant.
(66:35)

Allium stellatum, Autumn Onion
Chippewa *Cold Remedy* and *Pediatric Aid* Sweetened decoction of root taken, especially by children, for colds. (43:340)

Allium tricoccum, Wild Leek
Cherokee *Antihemorrhagic* Plant eaten as a
spring tonic. *Cold Remedy* Plant eaten for colds.
Ear Medicine Warm juice used for earache. *Pulmonary Aid* Plant eaten for croup. (66:52) **Chippewa** *Emetic* Decoction of root taken as a quick-
acting emetic. (43:346) **Iroquois** *Anthelmintic*
and *Pediatric Aid* Decoction of plant given to children for worms. *Tonic* Decoction of plant taken as
a spring tonic and "cleans you out." (73:281)

Allium unifolium, Oneleaf Onion
Mendocino Indian *Poison* Plant considered poisonous. (33:323)

Allium vineale, Wild Garlic
Cherokee *Carminative* Used as a carminative.
Cathartic Used as a mild cathartic. *Diuretic* Used
as a diuretic. *Ear Medicine* Used "to remove deafness." *Expectorant* Used as an expectorant. *Kidney Aid* Used for "dropsy." *Misc. Disease Remedy*
Used for scurvy. *Pediatric Aid* and *Pulmonary Aid*
Tincture used to prevent worms and colic in children and used as a croup remedy. *Respiratory Aid*
Used for asthma. *Stimulant* Used as a stimulant.
(66:35) **Mahuna** *Dermatological Aid* Plant
rubbed on body for protection from insect bites.
Plant rubbed on body for protection from lizard,
scorpion, and tarantula bites. *Snakebite Remedy*
Plant rubbed on body for protection from poisonous snakebites. (117:63) **Rappahannock** *Hypotensive* Raw root bulbs chewed for high blood

pressure. *Pulmonary Aid* Raw root bulbs chewed
for shortness of breath. (138:34)

Alnus glutinosa, European Alder
Rappahannock *Panacea* Infusion of bark used
according to diagnosis. (138:31)

Alnus incana, Mountain Alder
Bella Coola *Unspecified* Cones used for medicine.
(158:202) **Blackfoot** *Tuberculosis Remedy* Infusion of bark taken for scrofula. (68:5) **Chippewa**
Blood Medicine Infusion of bark taken for anemia.
(59:128) *Emetic* Compound decoction of scraped
inner bark taken as an emetic. (43:346) *Eye Medicine* Compound decoction of root used as a wash
or compress for sore eyes. (43:360) *Gynecological Aid* Decoction of root with powdered bumble-
bees taken for difficult labor. (43:358) **Cree,
Woodlands** *Eye Medicine* Decoction of inner
bark used as a wash for sore eyes. *Laxative* Bark
removed by scraping downwards used as a laxative. (91:27) **Iroquois** *Analgesic* Infusion of
young plant taken for pain. *Urinary Aid* Decoction
of stems and couch grass rhizomes used for thick
urine. (118:38) **Kutenai** *Abortifacient* Infusion of
bark taken for menstrual regulation. (68:5) **Malecite** *Oral Aid* Bark chewed and used for ulcerated
mouths. (96:245) **Menominee** *Cold Remedy* Infusion of root bark taken to congest loose mucus
during a cold. *Dermatological Aid* Infusion of root
bark used as an astringent, healing wash for sores.
Poultice of inner bark applied to swellings. *Veteri-*

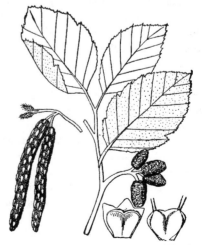

Alnus incana

nary Aid Infusion of root bark used as a wash for horses with saddle gall. (128:26) **Meskwaki** *Antihemorrhagic* and *Pediatric Aid* Decoction of root given to children who pass blood in their stools. (129:206) **Micmac** *Oral Aid* Bark used for ulcerated mouth. (32:54) **Mohegan** *Analgesic* Infusion of twigs used as a liniment for pain of sprains, bruises, backache, and headache. (151:69, 128) *Orthopedic Aid* Infusion of twigs used as a liniment for sprain and backache pains. (151:69, 70) **Ojibwa** *Gastrointestinal Aid* Decoction of root taken as astringent and coagulant after bloody stools. (130:358) **Potawatomi** *Antidiarrheal* Infusion of bark taken for flux. *Dermatological Aid* Juice of inner bark used as a wash for the itch. *Gynecological Aid* Infusion of bark used for "flushing the vagina." *Hemorrhoid Remedy* Infusion of bark injected rectally for piles. (131:43) *Veterinary Aid* Powdered bark used as an astringent for horse galls. (131:116) Powdered inner bark sprinkled on galled spots on ponies. (131:43) **Shuswap** *Dermatological Aid* Decoction of bark used as a wash for sores. *Diaphoretic* Decoction of bark taken to "sweat everything out." *Unspecified* Decoction of bark taken for the body. (102:59)

Alnus incana* ssp. *rugosa, Speckled Alder **Abnaki** *Dermatological Aid* Used for "slight" itches. (as *A. rugosa* 121:155) Decoction of plant, two other plants, and Vaseline used as an ointment for "slight" itches. (as *A. rugosa* var. *americana* 121:165) **Algonquin, Quebec** *Emetic* and *Laxative* Infusion of inner bark taken as an emetic and laxative. *Toothache Remedy* Root bark mixed with molasses and used for toothaches. (as *A. rugosa* 14:153) **Cherokee** *Cathartic* Infusion of roots taken as a cathartic by women during menses. *Emetic* Decoction of inner bark taken to induce vomiting when unable to retain food. Infusion of roots taken as an emetic by women during menses. *Eye Medicine* Infusion of bark rubbed into the eye for eye troubles. *Gastrointestinal Aid* Decoction of inner bark taken to induce vomiting when unable to retain food. *Gynecological Aid* Infusion of roots taken as an emetic and cathartic by women during menses. (as *A. rugosa* 152:14) **Cree, Woodlands** *Eye Medicine* Decoction of inner bark used as a wash for sore eyes. *Laxative* Bark removed by scraping downwards used as a laxative. (as *A.*

rugosa 91:27) **Iroquois** *Antihemorrhagic* Compound decoction with twigs taken for internal hemorrhage. *Cathartic* Decoction of young shoot bark taken as a physic. *Emetic* Decoction of young shoot bark taken as a spring emetic. *Urinary Aid* Infusion of bark or decoction of plant taken for urinating problems. *Venereal Aid* Decoctions used internally or externally for venereal chancres or sores. *Witchcraft Medicine* Decoction used to paint a trap or bow and arrow as a charm to get game. (73:301) **Menominee** *Alterative* Infusion of inner bark used as an alterative. (as *A. rugosa* 128:26)

Alnus incana* ssp. *tenuifolia, Thinleaf Alder **Bella Coola** *Analgesic* Poultice of compound containing buds applied for lung or hip pains. *Antirheumatic (External)* Poultice of compound containing buds applied to lung or hip pain. *Pulmonary Aid* Poultice of compound containing buds applied for lung pains. *Unspecified* Cones used for an "unspecified complaint." (as *A. tenuifolia* 127:55) **Blackfoot** *Tuberculosis Remedy* Infusion of bark taken for scrofula. (as *A. tenuifolia* 82:32) Hot drink made from bark taken for scrofula. (as *A. tenuifolia* 95:275) **Cree, Woodlands** *Eye Medicine* Decoction of inner bark used as a wash for sore eyes. *Laxative* Bark removed by scraping downwards used as a laxative. (as *A. tenuifolia* 91:27) **Gitksan** *Diuretic* Catkins and shavings eaten raw or decoction taken as a diuretic for gonorrhea. *Laxative* Crushed pistillate catkins eaten raw as a laxative. (as *A. tenuifolia* 127:55) *Unspecified* Bark and other plants used to make a salve. (61:152) *Venereal Aid* Catkins and shavings eaten raw or decoction taken as a diuretic for gonorrhea. (as *A. tenuifolia* 127:55) **Keres, Western** *Dermatological Aid* Bark ground into a powder and used on open sores. (as *A. tenuifolia* 147:25) **Okanagan-Colville** *Dietary Aid* Infusion of plant tops given to children with poor appetites. *Gynecological Aid* Decoction of plant tops and leaves taken after childbirth to "clean out." *Pediatric Aid* Infusion of plant tops given to children with poor appetites. *Toothache Remedy* Burnt ashes used to clean the teeth. (as *A. tenuifolia* 162:87) **Sanpoil** *Dermatological Aid* Decoction of bark used as a wash for sores and powder of sapwood used on sores. (as *A. tenuifolia* 109:220)

Alnus rhombifolia, White Alder

Kawaiisu *Unspecified* Plant used as medicine. (180:10) **Mendocino Indian** *Antidiarrheal* Decoction of dried bark taken for diarrhea. *Antihemorrhagic* Decoction of dried bark taken to check hemorrhages for consumption. *Blood Medicine* Decoction of dried bark taken as a blood purifier. *Burn Dressing* Poultice of dried wood applied to burns. *Diaphoretic* Decoction of dried bark taken to perspire. *Emetic* Decoction of dried bark taken as an emetic. *Gastrointestinal Aid* Decoction of dried bark taken for stomachaches. *Gynecological Aid* Decoction of dried bark taken to facilitate childbirth. *Tuberculosis Remedy* Decoction of dried bark taken to check hemorrhages for consumption. (33:332) **Pomo** *Dermatological Aid* and *Pediatric Aid* Decoction of bark used as a wash for babies with skin disease. (54:12) **Pomo, Kashaya** *Dermatological Aid* Decoction of bark used as wash for skin diseases: sores, diaper rash, peeling or itching skin. (60:19)

Alnus rubra, Red Alder

Bella Coola *Cathartic* Decoction of bark taken as a purgative. **Carrier, Northern** *Gastrointestinal Aid* Infusion of ground inner bark injected for biliousness. **Carrier, Southern** *Dermatological Aid* Sap applied to cuts and decoction of bark taken as a purgative. (127:55) **Clallam** *Dermatological Aid* Staminate aments chewed and used for sores. *Gastrointestinal Aid* Pistillate aments chewed and used for the stomach. *Pulmonary Aid* Pistillate aments chewed and used for the lungs. (47:198) **Cowlitz** *Analgesic* and *Orthopedic Aid* Rotten wood rubbed on the body to ease "aching bones." (as *A. oregona* 65:27) **Gitksan** *Analgesic* Infusion of stem bark used as an emetic and purgative for headache and other maladies. (127:55) *Cathartic* Bark used as a purgative. (61:152) Infusion of stem bark used as an emetic and purgative for headache and other maladies. *Cough Medicine* Decoction of bark and root taken in the morning for a cough. *Emetic* Infusion of stem bark used as an emetic and purgative for headache and other maladies. *Unspecified* Infusion of stem bark, not from root, taken for many maladies. (127:55) **Haisla** *Dermatological Aid* Bark used to make a wound dressing and wash. *Tonic* Bark used as a tonic. (61:152) **Hesquiat** *Misc. Disease Remedy* Poul-

Decoction of bark used to make a medicine for internal ailments. *Tuberculosis Remedy* Decoction of bark used to make a medicine for tuberculosis. (159:62) **Hoh** *Unspecified* Infusion of bark used for medicine. (as *A. oregona* 114:61) **Klallam** *Antidiarrheal* Catkins chewed for diarrhea. (as *A. oregona* 65:27) **Kwakiutl** *Analgesic* Poultice of bark applied to sores and aches. *Antihemorrhagic* Bark held in women's mouth for blood-spitting. *Dermatological Aid* Poultice of bark applied or infusion of bark rubbed on sores, aches, and eczema. *Respiratory Aid* Infusion of bark taken for tuberculosis and asthma. *Tuberculosis Remedy* Bark held in women's mouth for tuberculosis. Infusion of bark taken or bark held in women's mouth for tuberculosis. (157:279) **Kwakiutl, Southern** *Analgesic* Poultice of bark, fresh sea wrack, and black twinberry applied for aches and pains. (157:260) **Nitinaht** *Dermatological Aid* Infusion of crushed bark, western hemlock, and grand fir barks taken for bruises. *Internal Medicine* Infusion of bark, western hemlock, and grand fir barks taken for undiagnosed internal injuries. *Orthopedic Aid* Infusion of crushed bark, western hemlock, and grand fir barks taken for broken bones and ribs. *Pulmonary Aid* Infusion of crushed bark, western hemlock, and grand fir barks taken for lung ailments. *Tuberculosis Remedy* Infusion of crushed bark, western hemlock, and grand fir barks taken for tuberculosis. (160:98) *Unspecified* Bark used for medicine. (55:243) **Pomo, Kashaya** *Dermatological Aid* Decoction of bark used as wash for skin diseases: sores, diaper rash, peeling or itching skin. (as *A. oregona* 60:19) **Quileute** *Antidiarrheal* Raw cones eaten for dysentery. (as *A. oregona* 65:27) *Unspecified* Infusion of bark used for medicine. (as *A. oregona* 114:61) **Saanich** *Tonic* Sap used as a tonic. (156:79) **Swinomish** *Cold Remedy* Decoction of bark taken for colds. *Dermatological Aid* Decoction of bark taken for scrofula sores. *Gastrointestinal Aid* Decoction of bark taken for stomach troubles. *Tuberculosis Remedy* Decoction of bark taken for scrofula sores. (as *A. oregona* 65:27) **Thompson** *Dermatological Aid* Infusion of bark used as a wash for scabby skin, eczema, and skin sores. One informant used a concentrated decoction of the bark as a wash for her uncle who had a severe allergic reaction to hops. *Toothache Remedy* Poultice of immature catkins applied to the tooth for toothache. (161:188)

Alnus serrulata, Hazel Alder
Cherokee *Analgesic* Used for childbirth pain and infusion of bark used for various pains. *Blood Medicine* Infusion of bark taken to purify blood and compound infusion used as a blood tonic. *Cathartic* Used as an "emetic and purgative." *Cough Medicine* Infusion of bark taken for cough. *Dermatological Aid* Used for skin eruptions and infusion used to bathe hives. *Emetic* Used as an "emetic and purgative." *Eye Medicine* Infusion of bark "rubbed and blown in eyes for drooping." (66:22) Infusion of bark rubbed into the eye for eye troubles. (152:15) *Febrifuge* Hot infusion of berries taken for fever. *Gastrointestinal Aid* Compound used in steam bath for indigestion, biliousness, and jaundice. *Gynecological Aid* Used for childbirth pain and compound infusion taken for menstrual period. *Heart Medicine* Infusion taken for heart trouble. *Hemorrhoid Remedy* Compound infusion of root taken and used as a bath for piles. *Hypotensive* Cold infusion of bark taken to purify blood or lower blood pressure. *Kidney Aid* Infusion of scraped bark made kidneys act. *Oral Aid* Infusion of bark given to babies for "thrash," a mouth soreness. *Orthopedic Aid* Used for swellings and sprains. *Pediatric Aid* Infusion of bark given to babies for "thrash," a mouth soreness. *Toothache Remedy* Compound infusion of bark held in mouth for toothache. *Urinary Aid* Compound infusion taken to "clear milky urine." (66:22)

Alnus viridis, Sitka Alder
Cree, Hudson Bay *Dermatological Aid* Bark used for the astringent qualities. *Kidney Aid* Bark used for dropsy. (78:303)

Alnus viridis ssp. *crispa*, American Green Alder
Cree, Woodlands *Abortifacient* Decoction of plant used in a steam treatment to bring about menstruation. (as *A. crispa* 91:27) **Eskimo, Alaska** *Dermatological Aid* Poultice of leaves used in the past for infected wounds or sores. The poultice was left in place over the wound until the leaves stuck to it and was then pulled off, removing the "poison" with it. (as *A. crispa* 1:35) **Eskimo,**

Inuktitut *Antirheumatic* (*Internal*) Bark burned as an inhalant for "rheumatism." (as *A. crispa* 176:188) **Okanagan-Colville** *Dietary Aid* Infusion of plant tops given to children with poor appetites. *Gynecological Aid* Decoction of plant tops and leaves taken after childbirth to "clean out." *Pediatric Aid* Infusion of plant tops given to children with poor appetites. *Toothache Remedy* Burnt ashes used to clean the teeth. (as *A. crispa* 162:87) **Tanana, Upper** *Carminative* Decoction of inner bark taken for stomach gas. *Febrifuge* Decoction of inner bark taken for high fevers. *Stimulant* Branches with leaves used for steam bath switches and as a floor covering in the steam bath. (as *A. crispa* 86:5) **Thompson** *Toothache Remedy* Poultice of immature catkins applied to the tooth for toothache. (as *A. crispa* 161:188)

Alnus viridis ssp. *sinuata*, Sitka Alder
Bella Coola *Unspecified* Cones used for an "unspecified complaint." (as *A. sitchensis* 127:55) Cones used for medicine. (as *A. sinuata* 158:202) **Gitksan** *Antihemorrhagic* Pistillate catkins eaten for "throwing blood out." *Cathartic* Pistillate catkins crushed and eaten raw as a physic. (35:225) *Tonic* Bark and other plants used as a tonic. (as *A. crispa* ssp. *sinuata* 61:152) *Venereal Aid* Decoction of pistillate catkins taken for gonorrhea. (35:225)

Alocasia macrorrhizos, Giant Taro
Hawaiian *Analgesic* Plant, other plants, and water taken as a laxative and an appetizer for acute pain in stomach or bowels. *Burn Dressing* Plant made into a salve and used on burns. *Dietary Aid* and *Laxative* Plant, other plants, and water taken as a laxative and an appetizer for acute pain in stomach or bowels. *Love Medicine* Plant used as a stimulant, effecting a constant reminder to the one desired of his or her presence. (2:17)

Aloysia wrightii, Wright's Beebrush
Havasupai *Analgesic* Plant boiled and taken for headaches. *Antirheumatic* (*Internal*) Plant boiled and taken for rheumatism. *Psychological Aid* Plant boiled and taken for slight distempers. **Walapai** *Venereal Aid* Plant used for gonorrhea. (as *Lippia wrightii* 139:285)

Alyxia oliviformis, Maile
Hawaiian *Dermatological Aid* Infusion of
pounded plant and other plants used in a sweat
bath for yellow blotches on the skin. (as *A. clivae-
formis* 2:69)

Amanita muscaria, Amanita
Pomo, Kashaya *Poison* Plant considered poisonous. (60:128)

Amaranthus hybridus, Slim Amaranth
Cherokee *Ceremonial Medicine* Used as an ingredient in a green corn medicine. *Dermatological Aid* Astringent leaves used for profuse menstruation. *Gynecological Aid* Leaves used to
"relieve profuse menstruation." (66:23) **Keres,
Western** *Gastrointestinal Aid* Infusion of plant
used for the stomach. (147:26)

Amaranthus retroflexus, Redroot Amaranth
Cherokee *Ceremonial Medicine* Used as an ingredient in a green corn medicine. *Dermatological
Aid* Astringent leaves used for profuse menstruation. *Gynecological Aid* Leaves used to "relieve
profuse menstruation." (66:23) **Iroquois** *Witchcraft Medicine* Decoction and doll used to "make
a person break out like cancer." (73:316) **Keres,
Western** *Gastrointestinal Aid* Infusion of plant
used for the stomach. (147:26) **Mohegan** *Throat
Aid* Infusion of leaves taken for hoarseness.
(151:70, 128) **Navajo, Ramah** *Antidote* Stem, 3
inches long, made into snake figurine for snake
infection. (165:26)

Amaranthus spinosus, Spiny Amaranth
Cherokee *Ceremonial Medicine* Used as an ingredient in a green corn medicine. *Dermatological
Aid* Astringent leaves used for profuse menstruation. *Gynecological Aid* Leaves used to "relieve
profuse menstruation." (66:23)

Ambrosia acanthicarpa, Flatspine Burr
    Ragweed
Zuni *Abortifacient* Infusion of whole plant taken
and used as wash for "obstructed menstruation."
Toothache Remedy Ground root placed in tooth
for toothache. (as *Gaertneria acanthicarpa*
143:51, 52)

Ambrosia ambrosioides, Ambrosia Leaf Burr
    Ragweed
Pima *Analgesic* and *Antihemorrhagic* Decoction
of crushed roots taken by women for pains and
menstrual hemorrhage. *Cough Medicine* Poultice
of warmed leaves applied to the chest to loosen a
cough. *Gynecological Aid* Decoction of crushed
roots taken by women for pains and menstrual
hemorrhage. (as *Franseria ambrosioides* 38:103)

Ambrosia artemisiifolia, Annual Ragweed
Cherokee *Ceremonial Medicine* Used as an ingredient in green corn medicine. *Dermatological Aid*
Crushed leaves rubbed on insect sting and infusion
of leaf rubbed on hives. *Disinfectant* Juice of wilted
leaves applied to infected toes. *Febrifuge* Infusion
of leaf taken for fever. *Pulmonary Aid* Infusion
taken for pneumonia. (66:52) **Dakota** *Antidiarrheal* Infusion of leaves and plant tops taken for
bloody flux. *Antiemetic* Infusion of leaves and
plant tops taken for vomiting. (57:369) **Delaware**
Blood Medicine Poultice of plant used to prevent
blood poisoning. (151:35) **Delaware, Oklahoma**
Blood Medicine Poultice of plant applied to prevent "blood poison." (150:29) *Dermatological Aid*
Poultice of plant applied to prevent "blood poisoning." (150:29, 74) **Houma** *Gynecological Aid*
Decoction of root taken for menstrual troubles.
(135:65) **Iroquois** *Antidiarrheal* Compound decoction of plants taken for diarrhea with bleeding.
(73:468) *Heart Medicine* Infusion of roots taken

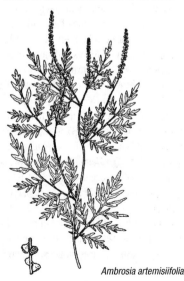

Ambrosia artemisiifolia

for stroke. (73:469) *Orthopedic Aid* Decoction of plants taken for cramps from picking berries. (73: 468) **Lakota** *Antirheumatic* (*External*) Infusion of leaves applied to swellings. (116:35) **Luiseño** *Emetic* Plant used as an emetic. (132:228) **Mahuna** *Dermatological Aid* Infusion of plant used as a wash for minor skin eruptions and scalp diseases. (117:13)

Ambrosia artemisiifolia var. elatior,
Annual Ragweed
Oto *Antiemetic* Bruised leaves laid on scarified abdomen for nausea. (as *A. elatior* 58:132)

Ambrosia chamissonis, Silver Burr Ragweed
Makah *Other* Plant used as medicine for healing. *Strengthener* Plant used as medicine for strength. (55:323)

Ambrosia psilostachya, Cuman Ragweed
Cheyenne *Analgesic* Infusion of leaves and stems taken for bowel pains and bloody stools. (63:188) Infusion of leaves and stem taken for cramps in the bowels. *Antidiarrheal* Infusion of leaves and stem taken for bloody stools. (63:39) *Antihemorrhagic* Infusion of ground leaves and stems taken for bloody stools. (64:188) *Cold Remedy* Infusion of plants taken for colds. (63:188) Infusion of ground leaves and stems taken for colds. (64:188) *Gastrointestinal Aid* Infusion of leaves and stems taken for bowel pains and bloody stools. (63:188) Infusion of leaves and stem taken for bowel cramps. (63:39) Infusion of ground leaves and stems taken for bowel cramps. (64:188) *Laxative* Infusion of ground leaves and stems taken for constipation. (69:18) **Costanoan** *Orthopedic Aid* Poultice of heated leaves applied to aching joints. (17:25) **Diegueño** *Dermatological Aid* Decoction of stems and leaves used after a hair wash as a rinse for dandruff. (70:13) *Gastrointestinal Aid* Infusion of leaves taken for stomach pains. (74: 219) **Gosiute** *Eye Medicine* Poultice of steeped leaves applied to sore eyes. (31:361) **Keres, Western** *Gynecological Aid* Infusion of plant given to women during difficult labor. (147:26) **Kiowa** *Dermatological Aid* Decoction of plant used as a wash for sores. *Veterinary Aid* Decoction of plant used as a wash for sores on horses. (166:55)

Ambrosia tenuifolia, Slimleaf Burr Ragweed
Navajo *Gynecological Aid* Plant used to facilitate delivery of the placenta after childbirth. (as *Franseria tenuifolia* 76:151)

Ambrosia trifida, Great Ragweed
Cherokee *Ceremonial Medicine* Used as an ingredient in green corn medicine. *Dermatological Aid* Crushed leaves rubbed on insect sting and infusion of leaf rubbed on hives. *Disinfectant* Juice of wilted leaves applied to infected toes. *Febrifuge* Infusion of leaf taken for fever. *Pulmonary Aid* Infusion taken for pneumonia. (66:52) **Iroquois** *Antidiarrheal* Compound decoction of plants taken for diarrhea with bleeding. *Blood Medicine* Plant used in a blood medicine. (73:468) **Lakota** *Unspecified* Seeds used medicinally. (116:35) **Meskwaki** *Psychological Aid* Root chewed to drive away fear at night. (129:210)

Amelanchier alnifolia, Saskatoon Serviceberry
Blackfoot *Cathartic* Infusion of plant and chokecherry cambium taken as a purge. (72:68) *Ear Medicine* Decoction of berry juice used for eardrops. *Eye Medicine* Decoction of dried berries or berry juice dripped into the eye and covered with a soft hide piece. (72:80) *Gastrointestinal Aid* Berry juice taken for an upset stomach. *Laxative* Berry juice taken as a mild laxative. (72:65) *Pediatric Aid* Infusion of plant and chokecherry cambium taken by nursing mothers to pass medicinal values to baby. (72:68) **Cheyenne** *Dietary Aid* and *Pediatric Aid* Smashed fruits used to improve loss of appetite in children. (69:34) *Unspecified* Infusion of leaves used for healing. (63:176) Smashed fruits used as an ingredient for medicinal mixtures. (69:34) **Cree, Woodlands** *Cold Remedy* Decoction of sticks taken for bad colds. *Cough Medicine* Decoction of roots taken for coughs. *Diaphoretic* Decoction of stems and snowberry stems taken to cause sweating. *Febrifuge* Decoction of stems and snowberry stems taken for fevers. *Misc. Disease Remedy* Decoction of sticks taken for flu. *Pediatric Aid* Decoction of roots taken for teething sickness. *Pulmonary Aid* Decoction of roots taken for chest pains and lung infections. *Toothache Remedy* Decoction of roots taken for teething sickness. (91:28) **Flathead** *Veterinary*

Aid Sharpened wood used to drain blood and other liquids from horses' swollen ankles. (68:9) **Okanagan-Colville** *Cold Remedy* Decoction of branches taken for colds. *Contraceptive* Decoction of branch ashes and pine branch or bud ashes taken to prevent having children. *Tonic* Decoction of branches taken as a general tonic. (162:120) **Pomo** *Gynecological Aid* Decoction of roots taken for too frequent menstruation. (54:13) **Thompson** *Contraceptive* Decoction of plant and bitter cherry taken as birth control. (161:253) *Gastrointestinal Aid* Decoction of bark taken for stomach troubles. (141:462) *Gynecological Aid* Warm decoction taken and used as a wash after childbirth. (141:471) Warm decoction of stems and twigs taken by women or used as a bath after childbirth. Strong decoction of bark taken by women after childbirth to hasten the dropping of the afterbirth. The decoction was taken immediately after childbirth. The medicine made from the tall variety of saskatoon was said to clean her out and help heal her insides. It was also said to stop her menstrual periods after the baby was born and hence act as a form of birth control. (161:253) *Tonic* Decoction of fresh bark taken as a tonic. (141:471)

***Amelanchier alnifolia* var. *semiintegrifolia*,** Pacific Serviceberry
Bella Coola *Venereal Aid* Compound decoction taken for gonorrhea. (as *A. florida* 127:60)

***Amelanchier arborea*,** Common Serviceberry
Cherokee *Anthelmintic* Compound infusion taken for worms. *Antidiarrheal* Compound infusion taken for diarrhea. *Tonic* Compound infusion taken as a spring tonic. (66:54) **Iroquois** *Venereal Aid* Infusion of bark used for gonorrhea. (73:351)

***Amelanchier arborea* var. *arborea*,** Common Serviceberry
Iroquois *Blood Medicine* Fruits formerly used as a blood remedy. *Gynecological Aid* Fruits, infusion of small branches given to mothers after childbirth for afterpains and hemorrhages. (as *A. oblongifolia* 103:96)

***Amelanchier canadensis*,** Canadian Serviceberry
Cherokee *Anthelmintic* Infusion of bark used as

a bath and given to children with worms. *Pediatric Aid* Infusion of bark used as a bath and given to children with worms. (152:27) **Chippewa** *Antidiarrheal* Compound decoction of root taken for dysentery. (43:344) *Disinfectant* Compound decoction of inner bark used as a disinfectant wash. (43:366) *Gynecological Aid* Compound decoction of bark taken for "female weakness." (43:356) Infusion of root taken to prevent miscarriage after an injury. (43:358) **Iroquois** *Blood Medicine* Fruits formerly used as a blood remedy. *Gynecological Aid* Fruits, infusion of small branches given to mothers after childbirth for afterpains and hemorrhages. (103:96)

***Amelanchier laevis*,** Allegheny Serviceberry
Ojibwa *Gynecological Aid* Infusion of bark taken by expectant mothers. (130:384)

***Amelanchier pallida*,** Pale Serviceberry
Pomo, Kashaya *Gynecological Aid* Decoction of boiled roots taken to check too frequent menstruation. (60:104)

***Amelanchier stolonifera*,** Running Serviceberry
Potawatomi *Tonic* Root bark used to make a tonic. (as *A. spicata* 131:76)

***Amelanchier utahensis*,** Utah Serviceberry
Navajo *Gynecological Aid* Plant used during labor and delivery. (76:148)

***Amelanchier utahensis* ssp. *utahensis*,** Utah Serviceberry
Navajo, Ramah *Ceremonial Medicine* Leaves used as emetics in various ceremonies. *Emetic* Leaves used as a ceremonial emetic. *Panacea* Dried fruit used as a "life medicine." (as *A. mormonica* 165:30)

***Amianthium muscitoxicum*,** Fly Poison
Cherokee *Dermatological Aid* Used for itch. (66:34) Root used as a sure, but severe, cure for itch. (177:74) *Poison* Used to poison crows. (66:34) Root used as a crow poison. (177:74)

***Amorpha canescens*,** Lead Plant
Meskwaki *Anthelmintic* Infusion of leaves used

to kill pinworms or any intestinal worms. *Dermatological Aid* Infusion of leaves used for eczema. (129:227) **Ojibwa, South** *Analgesic* Decoction of root taken for stomach pain. *Gastrointestinal Aid* Decoction of root taken for stomach pain. (77:200) **Omaha** *Analgesic* Moxa of twigs applied for neuralgia. (56:334) Moxa of stems used in cases of neuralgia. (58:93) *Antirheumatic* (*External*) Moxa of twigs applied for rheumatism. (56:334) Moxa of stems used in cases of rheumatism. (58:93) *Dermatological Aid* Powdered, dried leaves blown into cuts and open wounds. (56:334)

Amorpha nana, Dwarf Indigobush
Navajo *Respiratory Aid* Plant used as a snuff for catarrh. (as *A. microphyllus* 45:55)

Ampelopsis cordata, Heartleaf Peppervine
Cherokee *Urinary Aid* Infusion of bark taken for urinary troubles. (152:41)

Amphiachyris dracunculoides, Prairie Broomweed
Comanche *Dermatological Aid* Poultice of boiled flowers used for eczema and skin rashes. (as *Guitierrezia dracunculoides* 84:5)

Amphicarpaea bracteata, American Hogpeanut
Cherokee *Antidiarrheal* Infusion of root taken for diarrhea. *Snakebite Remedy* Infusion of root blown on snakebite wound. (66:38) **Chippewa** *Cathartic* Compound decoction of root taken as a physic. (as *Falcata comosa* 43:346) **Iroquois** *Gastrointestinal Aid* and *Tuberculosis Remedy* Compound decoction of plants taken for a bad stomach caused by consumption. (73:365) **Lakota** *Antirheumatic* (*External*) Poultice of pulverized leaves applied with any salve to swellings. (116:45)

Amsinckia douglasiana, Douglas's Fiddleneck
Costanoan *Unspecified* Plant used for medicinal purposes. (17:13)

Amsonia tomentosa var. *tomentosa*, Woolly Bluestar
Zuni *Snakebite Remedy* Compound poultice of

root applied with much ceremony to rattlesnake bite. (as *A. brevifolia* 54:53)

Anagallis sp., Pimpernel
Mahuna *Venereal Aid* Infusion of plant taken for gonorrhea when the bladder and urinal tract fail. (as *Centunculus* 117:70)

Anaphalis margaritacea, Western Pearly-everlasting
Algonquin, Tête-de-Boule *Burn Dressing* Poultice of boiled leaves applied to burns. (110:119) **Bella Coola** *Tuberculosis Remedy* Plants formerly used for tuberculosis. (158:201) **Cherokee** *Analgesic* Infusion steamed and inhaled for headache. *Cold Remedy* Warm infusion taken for cold and leaves smoked or chewed for colds. *Cough Medicine* Leaves and stems smoked for bronchial cough. *Eye Medicine* Infusion steamed and inhaled for blindness caused by the sun. *Respiratory Aid* Dried leaves smoked for catarrh. *Throat Aid* Used for throat infection. (66:48) **Cheyenne** *Ceremonial Medicine* Powdered flowers chewed and rubbed on body to protect and strengthen warrior. *Disinfectant* Smoke used to purify gift made to the spirits. (63:42) *Unspecified* Plant used as a strong medicine. (63:187) *Veterinary Aid* Plant used in various ways to make horses long-winded. (63:42) Powdered plant rubbed on horse's hoof to make it enduring and untiring. (63:187) Powdered flowers used on the sole of each horse hoof to make it enduring and untiring. (64:187) Powdered flowers put on each hoof and blown between the ears for long-windedness, spirit, and endurance. (82:56) **Chippewa** *Antirheumatic* (*External*) Compound decoction of flowers used as herbal steam for rheumatism and paralysis. *Herbal Steam* and *Orthopedic Aid* Infusion of flower used as herbal steam for rheumatism and paralysis. (43:362) **Delaware, Oklahoma** *Tonic* Compound containing root used as a tonic. (150:74) **Iroquois** *Antidiarrheal* Roots and stalks used for diarrhea and dysentery. *Eye Medicine* Infusion of plants used as wash for sore eyes. *Gastrointestinal Aid* Compound decoction of roots and flowers taken for bruise on back of stomach. (73:465) *Respiratory Aid* Infusion of flowers and roots from another plant used for asthma. (118:63) **Kwakiutl** *Dermatological Aid* Poultice of flowers applied to sores

and swellings. *Internal Medicine* Decoction of flowers taken for internal disorders. (157:278) **Mahuna** *Dermatological Aid* Flowers used for skin ulcers and foot sores. (as *Antennaria margaritacea* 117:11) **Mohegan** *Cold Remedy* Infusion of plant taken for colds. (149:265) Infusion of leaves taken as a cold medicine. (151:70, 128) **Montagnais** *Cough Medicine* Decoction of plant taken for cough. *Tuberculosis Remedy* Decoction of plant taken for consumption. (133:314) **Nitinaht** *Other* Plants rubbed on the hands to soften them for handling or touching sick people. (160:97) **Ojibwa** *Stimulant* Powdered flowers sprinkled on coals and smoke inhaled to revive stroke victim. (130:362, 365) **Okanagan-Colville** *Gastrointestinal Aid* Cooled infusion of roots and shoots taken as a laxative and emetic for a "poison stomach." (162:75) **Potawatomi** *Witchcraft Medicine* Flowers smoked in a pipe or smudged on coals to repel evil spirits. (131:49) **Quileute** *Antirheumatic (Internal)* Whole plant used as a steam bath for rheumatism. (65:48) **Thompson** *Misc. Disease Remedy* Decoction of dried flowers taken for rheumatic fever. (161:167)

Andromeda polifolia, Bog Rosemary
Mahuna *Respiratory Aid* Plant used for catarrh. (117:24)

Andropogon floridanus, Florida Bluestem
Seminole *Analgesic* Roots used with a song or spell as an analgesic. (145:167) Infusion of plant taken for wolf sickness: vomiting, stomach pain, diarrhea, and frequent urination. (145:227) Infusion of roots used for moving sickness: moving pain in the waist region. (145:285) *Antidiarrheal* and *Antiemetic* Infusion of plant taken for wolf sickness: vomiting, stomach pain, diarrhea, and frequent urination. (145:227) *Cough Medicine* Infusion of plant taken and used as bath for gopher-tortoise sickness: cough, dry throat, noisy chest. (145:236) *Gastrointestinal Aid* Infusion of plant taken for wolf sickness: vomiting, stomach pain, diarrhea, and frequent urination. (145:227) *Pulmonary Aid* and *Throat Aid* Infusion of plant taken and used as bath for gopher-tortoise sickness: cough, dry throat, noisy chest. (145:236) *Urinary Aid* Infusion of plant taken for wolf sickness: vom-

iting, stomach pain, diarrhea, and frequent urination. (145:227)

Andropogon gerardii, Big Bluestem
Chippewa *Analgesic* Decoction of root taken for stomach pain. (as *A. furcatus* 43:342) *Diuretic* Simple or compound decoction of root taken as a diuretic. (as *A. furcatus* 43:348) *Gastrointestinal Aid* Decoction of root taken for stomach pain. (as *A. furcatus* 43:342) **Omaha** *Febrifuge* Decoction of blades of grass used as a wash for fevers. *Stimulant* Decoction of blades of grass taken for "general debility and languor." (as *A. furcatus* 58:68, 69)

Andropogon glomeratus, Bushy Bluestem
Catawba *Analgesic* Roots used for backaches. *Orthopedic Aid* Roots used for backaches. (152:5) **Rappahannock** *Dermatological Aid* Infusion of roots taken for the itch and applied to ivy poisoning. *Hemorrhoid Remedy* Compound poultice with roots applied as salve for piles. (138:28)

Andropogon virginicus, Broomsedge Bluestem
Cherokee *Antidiarrheal* Infusion taken to "check bowels." *Ceremonial Medicine* Used as an ingredient in green corn medicine. *Dermatological Aid* Infusion used for frostbite and sores and ooze used to bathe itch. (66:27)

Androsace occidentalis, Western Rockjasmine
Navajo, Ramah *Gynecological Aid* Compound decoction of whole plant used for postpartum hemorrhage. *Pediatric Aid* Compound decoction of whole plant used for birth injury. (165:38)

Androsace septentrionalis, Pygmyflower Rockjasmine
Navajo, Ramah *Analgesic* Cold infusion taken for internal pain. *Panacea* Plant used as "life medicine." *Venereal Aid* Compound decoction of plant taken before sweat bath for venereal disease. (165:38, 39) *Witchcraft Medicine* Plant used as a lotion to give protection from witches. (165:38)

Androsace septentrionalis ssp. ***subulifera***, Pygmyflower Rockjasmine
Navajo, Kayenta *Analgesic* and *Witchcraft Medi-*

cine Plant used for bewitchment and pain from witches' arrows. (179:35)

Anemone canadensis, Canadian Anemone
Chippewa *Dermatological Aid* Poultice of roots applied to wounds and infusion of root used as wash for sores. *Hemostat* Leaves used for nasal hemorrhages, bleeding sores, and wounds. (59:130) **Iroquois** *Anthelmintic* Decoction of roots taken for worms. *Witchcraft Medicine* Compound infusion of plants and liquor used to counteract witch medicine. (73:328) **Meskwaki** *Eye Medicine* Infusion of root used as a wash for crossed eyes, eye twitch, and eye poisoning. (129:238) **Ojibwa** *Ceremonial Medicine* Root eaten to clear throat so one can sing well in medicine lodge ceremony. *Throat Aid* Root eaten to clear throat so one can sing well in ceremonies. (130:382, 383) **Ojibwa, South** *Analgesic* and *Orthopedic Aid* Decoction of root used for pain in the lumbar region. (as *A. pennsylvanicum* 77:201) **Omaha** *Panacea* Highly esteemed medicine taken and applied externally for many illnesses. **Ponca** *Panacea* Highly esteemed medicine taken and applied externally for many illnesses. (58:82)

Anemone cylindrica, Candle Anemone
Meskwaki *Analgesic* Infusion of root taken for headache and dizzy spells. *Burn Dressing* Poultice of leaves applied to bad burns. *Eye Medicine* Decoction of stem and fruit used as a wash for sore eyes. *Psychological Aid* Used as a medicine for "crazy people." *Stimulant* Infusion of root used for headache and dizzy spells. (129:238) **Ojibwa** *Pulmonary Aid* Infusion of root taken for lung congestion and tuberculosis. *Tuberculosis Remedy* Infusion of root used for lung congestion and tuberculosis. (130:383)

Anemone multifida, Pacific Anemone
Blackfoot *Abortifacient* Plant used to cause abortions. (72:60) *Analgesic* Ripe seed head "cotton" burned on hot coals and the smoke inhaled for headaches. (82:35) **Carrier, Southern** *Cold Remedy* Aroma of crushed leaves inhaled for head or lung colds. *Panacea* Decoction of plant, without roots, taken for any sickness. **Gitksan** *Antirheumatic (Internal)* Plant eaten or decoction of plant taken in sweat bath for rheumatism. *Diaphoretic*

Eaten or decoction taken in sweat bath for rheumatism. (127:57) **Okanagon** *Hemostat* Leaves applied to nose for nosebleeds. **Thompson** *Hemostat* Leaves applied to nose for nosebleeds. (104:42) Fresh leaves used to plug nostrils and as an inhalant for nosebleed. (141:474) Wool from seed heads mixed with pitch and used inside the nostril for nosebleeds. *Poison* Plant considered very poisonous. (161:246)

Anemone multifida var. globosa, Hudson's Anemone
Blackfoot *Analgesic* Cottony flower burned on hot coals for headache. (as *A. globosa* 95:274, 275)

Anemone narcissiflora ssp. villosissima, Narcissus Anemone
Aleut *Antihemorrhagic* Decoction of root taken for unspecified hemorrhage. (6:428)

Anemone virginiana, Tall Thimbleweed
Cherokee *Pulmonary Aid* Infusion of root taken for whooping cough. (66:58) **Iroquois** *Antidiarrheal* Cold decoction of roots taken for diarrhea. (73:328) *Emetic* Decoction or infusion of smashed roots or plants taken as an emetic. (73:327) *Love Medicine* Decoction of roots taken as an emetic and used as a wash to cure a love medicine. Infusion of stems and roots used as a love medicine for either sex. *Tuberculosis Remedy* Decoction of roots taken for tuberculosis. (73:328) *Witchcraft Medicine* Compound infusion of smashed plants taken as an emetic to remove bewitchment. Roots placed under the pillow to dream the truth about wife's crookedness. (73:327) Root used as revenge to "kill man who played a trick on man's son." (73:328) **Menominee** *Dermatological Aid* Poultice of root applied to boils. (128:48) **Meskwaki** *Respiratory Aid* Smoke of seeds inhaled for catarrh. *Stimulant* Smoke of seedpod directed up nostril to revive sick and unconscious patient. (129:238)

Anemopsis californica, Yerba Mansa
Cahuilla *Cold Remedy* Infusion of plant used for colds. *Dermatological Aid* Infusion of bark used as a wash for open sores. *Gastrointestinal Aid* Infusion of plant used for stomach ulcers. Decoction of bark taken for ulcers. *Pulmonary Aid* Decoc-

tion of peeled, cut, and squeezed roots taken for pleurisy. *Respiratory Aid* Infusion of plant used for chest congestion. *Veterinary Aid* Infusion of plant used for open sores on cattle. (11:38) **Costanoan** *Analgesic* Decoction of roots used as a general pain remedy. *Dermatological Aid* Dried, powdered plant applied as a disinfectant to wounds. Infusion of plant used as a wash for sores. *Disinfectant* Dried, powdered plant applied as a disinfectant to wounds. *Gynecological Aid* Decoction of roots used for menstrual cramps. (17:8) **Diegueño** *Unspecified* Plant used as medicine. (70:15) **Isleta** *Blood Medicine* Infusion of leaves taken as a blood medicine. *Dermatological Aid* Poultice of damp leaves used on open wounds. *Disinfectant* Infusion of leaves used as a disinfectant on open wounds. *Pulmonary Aid* Infusion of leaves taken for lung hemorrhages. (85:22) **Kawaiisu** *Cold Remedy* Decoction of broken roots taken for colds. *Cough Medicine* Decoction of broken roots taken for coughs. *Dermatological Aid* Leaves used as a salve for cuts and wounds. *Misc. Disease Remedy* Decoction of broken roots taken for diabetes. *Veterinary Aid* Leaves used as a salve for livestock with cuts and wounds. (180:11) **Keres, Western** *Burn Dressing* Poultice of green, chewed leaves applied to burns. *Dermatological Aid* Dried leaves ground into a powder and used on open sores. (147:26) **Mahuna** *Dermatological Aid* Powdered plants used as a disinfectant for knife wounds. *Disinfectant* Powdered plants used as a disinfectant for knife wounds. (117:15) **Paiute** *Laxative* Infusion of roots taken as a laxative. (144:317) *Orthopedic Aid* Decoction of leaves used as a bath for muscular pains and sore feet. (155:33, 34) *Venereal Aid* Infusion of roots taken for gonorrhea. (144:317) **Papago** *Emetic* Decoction of leaves taken as an emetic. (29:65) **Pima** *Cold Remedy* Infusion of dried roots or plant taken for colds. *Cough Medicine* Roots chewed and swallowed or decoction of roots taken for coughs. *Dermatological Aid* Decoction of plant used as a wash and poultice of leaves applied to wounds. *Diaphoretic* Infusion of plant taken for colds and to cause sweating. (38:78) *Emetic* Decoction of crushed root taken as an emetic. (as *Houttuynia californica* 123:80) *Gastrointestinal Aid* Poultice of wet, powdered roots applied for stomachaches. *Other* Infusion of roots taken and used as a wash

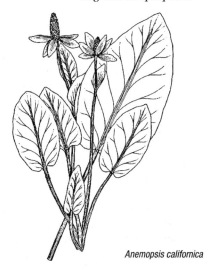

Anemopsis californica

for "bad disease." *Throat Aid* Dry root held in the mouth for sore throats and infusion taken for itchy throat. (38:78) *Tuberculosis Remedy* Decoction of crushed root taken for consumption. (as *Houttuynia californica* 123:80) *Venereal Aid* Infusion of roots used as a wash for syphilis. (38:78) **Shoshoni** *Anticonvulsive* Infusion of whole plant taken for fits. (98:46) *Cold Remedy* Decoction of roots taken as a tonic for general debility following colds. *Dermatological Aid* Poultice of boiled, mashed roots applied to swellings. *Disinfectant* Decoction of roots used as an antiseptic wash. *Gastrointestinal Aid* Decoction of roots taken for stomachaches. *Tonic* Decoction of roots taken as a tonic for general debility following colds. *Venereal Aid* Decoction of plant taken for gonorrhea. (155: 33, 34) **Tubatulabal** *Cold Remedy* Decoction of plant taken for heavy colds. (167:59)

Angadenia berteroi, Pineland Golden Trumpet
Seminole *Dermatological Aid* Decoction of roots taken and used as a wash for sores. (as *Rhabdadenia corallicola* 145:271) *Other* Decoction of roots used by men for menstruation sickness: painful abdominal swelling and impotence. (as *Rhabdadenia corallicola* 145:248) Decoction of roots taken and used as a wash for chronic sickness. (as *Rhabdadenia corallicola* 145:271)

Angelica atropurpurea, Purplestem Angelica
Cherokee *Abortifacient* "Root tonic" taken for obstructed menses. *Carminative* "Root tonic"

taken for flatulent colics. *Cold Remedy* "Root tonic" taken for colds. *Febrifuge* "Root tonic" taken for fever. *Misc. Disease Remedy* "Root tonic" taken for ague. *Oral Aid* "Root tonic" used as gargle for sore mouth. *Sedative* "Root tonic" taken by weakly and nervous females. *Throat Aid* "Root tonic" used as gargle for sore throat. (66:23) **Delaware** *Gastrointestinal Aid* Roots used for stomach disorders. (151:33) **Delaware, Oklahoma** *Gastrointestinal Aid* Root used for stomach disorders. (150:28, 74) **Iroquois** *Analgesic* Compound infusion of plants used as steam bath to sweat out headaches. *Antirheumatic (External)* Plant or root used internally, externally, or in steam bath for rheumatism. (73:400) *Blood Medicine* Dried roots used as blood purifier. *Cold Remedy* Decoction of smashed roots taken for colds. (73:401) *Diaphoretic* Infusion of plants used as steam bath to sweat out rheumatism and headaches. (73:400) *Febrifuge* Decoction of dried roots taken for fevers and chills. *Gynecological Aid* Decoction of roots taken by women for weakness. *Misc. Disease Remedy* Decoction of smashed roots taken for the flu. *Orthopedic Aid* Poultice of roots applied to broken bones. (73:401) *Other* Decoction of roots used as steam bath for frostbite and exposure. (73:400) *Poison* Plant used as poison. *Pulmonary Aid* Infusion of roots used for pneumonia. *Witchcraft Medicine* Plant used to punish evil persons. (73:401) **Menominee** *Analgesic* Poultice of cooked, pounded root applied to painful areas. *Dermatological Aid* Poultice of cooked, pounded root applied to swellings. (128:55)

Angelica breweri, Brewer's Angelica
Miwok *Analgesic* Root chewed for headaches. *Cold Remedy* Root chewed for colds. (8:166) **Paiute** *Cold Remedy* Decoction of roots used for colds or chest ailments. Hot decoction of roots taken for colds. *Cough Medicine* Dried root chewed for sore throats or coughs. *Dermatological Aid* Salve of mashed roots applied to cuts and sores. *Kidney Aid* Decoction of roots taken, instead of drinking water, for kidney ailments. *Throat Aid* Dried root chewed for sore throat and coughs. **Shoshoni** *Adjuvant* Plant used as an adjuvant to improve flavor or amplify effect of medicines. *Analgesic* and *Antirheumatic (External)* Poultice of pulped root applied to rheumatic pains or swellings. *Cold*

Remedy Decoction of roots used for colds or chest ailments. Dried, shaved roots smoked in cigarettes for head colds. Hot decoction of roots and whisky taken for heavy chest colds. *Pediatric Aid* Decoction of split root given to children for whooping cough. *Pulmonary Aid* Decoction of split root in whisky given to children for whooping cough. Poultice of pulped roots applied for pneumonia. *Tonic* Decoction of roots taken in small doses as a tonic. *Tuberculosis Remedy* Decoction of roots taken for tuberculosis. *Venereal Aid* Decoction of roots taken and used as a wash for venereal diseases. *Veterinary Aid* Smoke from root compound inhaled by horses for distemper. **Washo** *Adjuvant* Plant used as an adjuvant to improve flavor or amplify effect of medicines. *Cough Medicine* Dried root chewed for sore throats or coughs. *Misc. Disease Remedy* Infusion of scraped, dried root taken for influenza. *Respiratory Aid* Infusion of scraped, dried root taken for bronchitis. *Throat Aid* Dried root chewed for sore throat or coughs. (155:34, 35)

Angelica dawsonii, Dawson's Angelica
Blackfoot *Antihemorrhagic* Infusion of roots taken for coughing up blood. (72:70) *Antirheumatic (External)* Poultice of chewed roots applied to swellings. (72:75) *Ceremonial Medicine* Roots used as a religious power medicine. (72:40) *Dermatological Aid* Poultice of chewed roots applied to rashes, eczema, and athlete's foot. (72:75) *Dietary Aid* Infusion of roots given to children with malnutrition. *Gastrointestinal Aid* Infusion of roots taken for intestinal ailments. (72:65) *Misc. Disease Remedy* Infusion of roots applied to mumps swellings. *Other* Infusion of roots applied for a disorder characterized by sore groins and underarms. (72:75) *Pediatric Aid* Infusion of roots given to children with malnutrition. (72:65) *Unspecified* Roots used medicinally for unspecified purpose. (72:40) *Veterinary Aid* Root smudge used to fumigate horses with nasal gleet. Infusion of roots given to horses with nasal gleet. Infusion of roots used as a wash for hoof frogs and infections. (72:87)

Angelica genuflexa, Kneeling Angelica
Bella Coola *Cathartic* Decoction of root or raw root taken as a purgative. **Gitksan** *Analgesic* Com-

pound decoction of root taken for headache. *Eye Medicine* Compound decoction of root taken for weak eyes. (127:61)

Angelica lineariloba, Poison Angelica
Paiute, Northern *Antihemorrhagic* Decoction of dried, scraped roots taken for spitting up blood. *Pulmonary Aid* Decoction of dried, scraped roots taken for pneumonia. (49:126)

Angelica lucida, Wild Celery
Aleut *Analgesic* Poultice of leaves applied for internal or external pain. *Cold Remedy* Leaves used to make a tonic for colds. *Throat Aid* Leaves used to make a soothing drink for sore throats. *Tonic* Leaves used to make a tonic for colds. (6:427) **Eskimo** *Panacea* Plant used for most illnesses. *Preventive Medicine* Root eaten as a preventative medicine. *Psychological Aid* Plant used for the feeling of malaise. (126:325) **Eskimo, Inuktitut** *Unspecified* Young stems used medicinally. (176:184) **Eskimo, Kuskokwagmiut** *Disinfectant* Burning stems shaken inside and outside the house for purification. (101:31) **Kwakiutl** *Analgesic* Plant used to prepare sweat bath for localized pains. *Herbal Steam* Plant used to prepare sweat bath for general weakness and localized pains. (as *Coelapleurum gmelini* 16:376) *Hunting Medicine* Plant tied on halibut hooks as a good luck charm. (157:276) *Stimulant* Plant used to prepare sweat bath for general weakness. *Unspecified* Used on

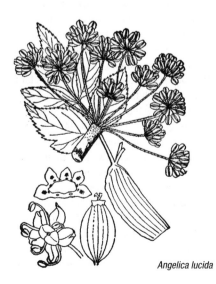

Angelica lucida

heated stones in the steam bath to dry up the patient's disease. (as *Coelapleurum gmelini* 16:376)

Angelica pinnata, Smallleaf Angelica
Gosiute *Unspecified* Root used as medicine. (31:361)

Angelica sylvestris, Woodland Angelica
Micmac *Cold Remedy* Root used for head cold. (32:54) Infusion of roots and spikenard roots used for head colds. (96:259) *Cough Medicine* Root used for cough. (32:54) Infusion of roots and spikenard roots used for coughs. (96:259) *Throat Aid* Root used for sore throat. (32:54) Infusion of roots and spikenard roots used for sore throats. (96:259)

Angelica tomentosa, Woolly Angelica
Pomo, Kashaya *Cold Remedy* Decoction of root used for colds. *Dermatological Aid* Decoction of root used as a strong wash for bathing sores. *Gastrointestinal Aid* Decoction of root used for stomachaches. *Gynecological Aid* Decoction of root used to regulate menses and ease menstrual cramps and discomforts of menopause. *Oral Aid* Root chewed or held in the mouth to prevent bad breath. *Other* Root shavings smoked by the shaman when doctoring. *Throat Aid* Root chewed or held in the mouth to prevent sore throat. Root held in singer's mouth to prevent hoarseness and rawness of throat. (60:20) **Yana** *Analgesic* Decoction of roots taken or poultice of roots applied for headaches. *Antidiarrheal* Decoction of roots taken for diarrhea. *Cold Remedy* Decoction of roots taken for colds. *Panacea* Decoction of roots taken for colds, diarrhea, headaches, and other ailments. (124:253)

Angelica tomentosa var. hendersonii,
   Henderson's Angelica
Mewuk *Antidote* Infusion of plant taken for mussel poisoning. (as *A. hendersoni* 97:366)

Angelica venenosa, Hairy Angelica
Iroquois *Orthopedic Aid* Poultice of plant applied to sprained muscles and twisted joints. *Poison* Roots eaten to commit suicide. (73:400)

Annona reticulata, Custard Apple
Seminole *Kidney Aid* Infusion of flowers taken for kidney disorders. (145:274)

Antennaria anaphaloides, Pearly Pussytoes
Paiute *Dermatological Aid* Plant served as a perfume and placed with clothing or handkerchiefs. (93:116)

Antennaria dioica, Stoloniferous Pussytoes
Gosiute *Eye Medicine* Poultice of steeped plant applied to the eyes for snow-blindness. (31:361)

Antennaria howellii, Howell's Pussytoes
Bella Coola *Analgesic* Decoction of leaves taken for body pain, but not pain in the limbs. (127:65)

Antennaria howellii ssp. neodioica, Field Pussytoes
Ojibwa *Gynecological Aid* Infusion of herb taken after childbirth to purge afterbirth and to heal. (as *A. neodioica* 130:363)

Antennaria parvifolia, Smallleaf Pussytoes
Lakota *Antirheumatic* (*External*) Used for swellings. (116:35) **Navajo, Kayenta** *Blood Medicine* Plant chewed with deer or sheep tallow as a blood purifier. (as *A. aprica* 179:44) **Navajo, Ramah** *Ceremonial Medicine* Plant used ceremonially for mad coyote bite. *Witchcraft Medicine* Cold infusion of root taken for protection from witches. (as *A. aprica* 165:47)

Antennaria plantaginifolia, Woman's Tobacco
Cherokee *Gastrointestinal Aid* Infusion of entire plant given, especially to children, for "bowel complaint." *Gynecological Aid* Infusion taken for excessive discharge in monthly period. *Pediatric Aid* Infusion of entire plant given, especially to children, for "bowel complaint." (66:50) **Iroquois** *Gynecological Aid* Infusion of roots taken for leukorrhea. *Toothache Remedy* Decoction of plant used as a mouthwash for toothaches. (73:464) **Meskwaki** *Gynecological Aid* Infusion of leaves taken after childbirth to prevent sickness. (129:210)

Antennaria rosea, Rosy Pussytoes
Okanagan-Colville *Ceremonial Medicine* Roots dried, powdered, put into hot coals at winter dance, and smoke used to drive away bad spirits and to revive passed-out dancers. *Reproductive Aid* Leaves chewed and swallowed to increase male virility. (162:75)

Antennaria rosulata, Kaibab Pussytoes
Navajo, Ramah *Hunting Medicine* Plants from where deer have slept or browsed used for good luck in hunting. *Pediatric Aid* Compound decoction taken for birth injury. *Witchcraft Medicine* Cold infusion of root taken for protection from witches. (165:47)

Anthemis cotula, Stinking Chamomile
Cherokee *Analgesic* Used as a "sudorific and anodyne for colds." *Anticonvulsive* Used for epilepsy. *Antirheumatic* (*Internal*) Used for rheumatism. *Dermatological Aid* Bruised herb applied externally to "draw blister." *Diaphoretic* Used as a "sudorific and anodyne for colds." *Emetic* Used as an emetic. *Febrifuge* Used for fevers. *Kidney Aid* Used for "dropsy." *Respiratory Aid* Used for asthma. *Sedative* Used for hysterics. *Tonic* Used as a tonic. (66:32) **Iroquois** *Antidiarrheal* Compound decoction of plants, bark, and roots taken for diarrhea. *Antiemetic* Decoction or cold infusion of plants, bark, and roots taken for vomiting. (73:471) *Blood Medicine* Compound decoction of bark, plants, and roots taken as blood purifier. *Emetic* Cold infusion of stalks taken as an emetic when not feeling well and for spring fever. *Febrifuge* Cold infusion of dried roots and stems taken as an emetic for spring fever. (73:472) *Gastrointestinal Aid* Compound decoction of plants taken for too much gall and biliousness. Compound decoction of plants, bark, and roots taken for stomach cramps. (73:471) Cold infusion of stalks taken for ptomaine poisoning. Decoction of plants taken for biliousness. (73:472) *Other* Decoction of plants given to children with "red spots." (73:471) Decoction of plants given to children and adults for "summer complaint." (73:472) *Pediatric Aid* Decoction of plants given to children with "red spots." (73:471) Decoction of plant given to children for "summer complaint" and stomach cramps. (73:472) *Pulmonary Aid* Compound

decoction of plants taken for shortness of breath. (73:471) *Sedative* Cold infusion of dried roots and stems taken as a sedative. (73:472) *Toothache Remedy* Root chewed for toothaches. (73:471) *Venereal Aid* Compound decoction of bark, plants, and roots taken for venereal disease. (73:472) **Karok** *Gynecological Aid* Plant used by pregnant women. (125:390) **Mendocino Indian** *Antirheumatic (External)* Infusion of plants used as a wash for rheumatism. *Cold Remedy* Infusion of plants used as a wash for severe colds. *Eye Medicine* Plant juice used as an eyewash. (33:392) **Mohegan** *Febrifuge* Cold infusion of plant taken for fever. (149:264) Cold infusion of leaves taken for fever. (151:70, 128) *Panacea* Cold infusion of leaves thought to "benefit the entire body." (151:70) **Yuki** *Poison* Plant considered poisonous. (39:94)

Antidesma pulvinatum, Hame
Hawaiian *Antiemetic* Leaves chewed and swallowed for vomiting spells. *Dermatological Aid* Infusion of pounded bark and other plants used as a wash for ulcers and scrofulous sores. *Tuberculosis Remedy* Infusion of pounded bark and other plants used as a wash for scrofulous sores. (2:39)

Apium graveolens, Wild Celery
Houma *Tuberculosis Remedy* Compound decoction of plant with whisky taken for tuberculosis. (135:64)

Aplectrum hyemale, Adam and Eve
Catawba *Analgesic* Pounded, powdered, boiled roots used for head pains. *Dermatological Aid* Pounded, powdered, boiled roots used for boils. (134:188) Poultice of beaten roots applied to boils. (152:10) **Cherokee** *Dietary Aid* Given to endow children with the gift of eloquence and to make them fat. *Pediatric Aid* Given to endow children with the gift of eloquence and to make them fat. (66:51)

Apocynum androsaemifolium, Spreading Dogbane
Cherokee *Veterinary Aid* Used to bathe dogs for mange. (66:32) **Chippewa** *Analgesic* Root used as snuff, herbal steam, poultice or in decoction for headache. *Anticonvulsive* Compound decoction of root taken or sprinkled on chest for convulsions.

(43:336) *Cold Remedy* Weak decoction of root given only to infants for colds. (43:340) *Ear Medicine* Decoction of root poured into ear for soreness. (43:360) *Heart Medicine* Decoction of root taken for heart palpitations. (43:338) *Hemostat* Decoction of root on cotton or mashed root used as a plug in nostril for nosebleed. (43:356) *Pediatric Aid* Weak decoction of root given only to infants for colds. (43:340) *Psychological Aid* Dried, pulverized root used in various ways for insanity. *Vertigo Medicine* Dried, pulverized root used in various ways for dizziness. (43:336) **Cree, Woodlands** *Eye Medicine* Plant used for sore eyes. *Gynecological Aid* Decoction of plant used to increase lactation. (91:28) **Iroquois** *Anthelmintic* Compound infusion of roots taken for worms. *Dermatological Aid* Milk used for warts. *Gastrointestinal Aid* Compound infusion of roots taken for stomach cramps. *Gynecological Aid* Compound infusion of roots taken for evacuation of the placenta. *Liver Aid* Decoction of roots taken as a liver medicine. *Veterinary Aid* Decoction of roots mixed with feed and given to horses with worms. (73:415) **Meskwaki** *Gynecological Aid* Compound containing rind used by a woman with "an injured womb." *Kidney Aid* Root used for dropsy. (129:201) **Montana Indian** *Cathartic* Root, poisonous in large doses, used as a cathartic. *Febrifuge* Root, poisonous in large doses, used as a febrifuge. *Poison* Root poisonous in large doses and poisonous to cattle feeding on it. *Tonic* Root, poisonous in large

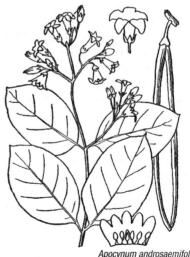

Apocynum androsaemifolium

doses, used as a tonic. (15:6) **Ojibwa** *Analgesic* Root smoke inhaled for headache. *Ceremonial Medicine* Root, considered sacred, eaten during the medicine lodge ceremony. (130:354, 355) Roots eaten during the medicine lodge ceremony. The roots are also chewed to keep the other witch doctors from affecting one with an evil charm. (130:428) *Diuretic* Infusion of root taken as a diuretic during pregnancy. *Gynecological Aid* Infusion of root taken as a diuretic during pregnancy. *Oral Aid* Root used for coated tongue and headache. *Throat Aid* Root eaten for throat trouble. (130:354, 355) **Okanagan-Colville** *Love Medicine* Leaves chewed and the juice and pulp swallowed or dried leaves smoked as an aphrodisiac. (162:72) **Potawatomi** *Diuretic* Root used as a diuretic. *Heart Medicine* Decoction of green berries used as a heart medicine. *Kidney Aid* Decoction of green berries used as a kidney medicine. *Urinary Aid* Root used as a diuretic and urinary medicine. (131:38) **Salish** *Unspecified* Plant used as a medicine. (153:294) **Sanpoil** *Gynecological Aid* Infusion of roots taken about once a week as a contraceptive. (109:219)

Apocynum cannabinum, Indian Hemp
Blackfoot *Dermatological Aid* Decoction of root used as a wash "to prevent hair falling out." *Laxative* Decoction of root taken as a laxative. (95:276) **Cahuilla** *Unspecified* Used for the medicinal properties and as a fibrous material. (11:39) **Cherokee** *Abortifacient* Root used for pox and "uterine obstructions." *Antirheumatic* (*Internal*) Used for rheumatism. *Cough Medicine* Used for coughs. *Dermatological Aid* Root used for pox. *Kidney Aid* Infusion of root taken for "dropsy" and Bright's disease. *Pulmonary Aid* Used for whooping cough. *Respiratory Aid* Used for asthma. (66:38) **Cree, Hudson Bay** *Cathartic* Decoction of chewed leaves and bark taken as a purgative. *Dermatological Aid* Poultice of chewed leaves and bark applied to wounds. *Emetic* Decoction of chewed leaves and bark taken as an emetic. *Unspecified* Plant used as medicine. (as *A. hypericifolium* 78:303) **Iroquois** *Antidiarrheal* Infusion of roots used as a wash for children with diarrhea. *Blood Medicine* Roots used as blood purifier. (73:415) *Emetic* Infusion of roots taken as a spring or summer emetic. *Eye Medicine* Infusion of roots taken

to clear up yellow eyes. (73:416) *Gastrointestinal Aid* Roots used for biliousness. *Laxative* Roots used as a laxative. *Pediatric Aid* Infusion of roots used as a wash for children with diarrhea. (73:415) **Keres, Western** *Gynecological Aid* Crushed leaves rubbed on mothers' breasts to produce more and richer milk. Infusion of plant used by mothers to produce more and richer milk. (as *A. viride* 147:27) **Kutenai** *Veterinary Aid* Tops chewed and used for horses with eyes. (68:12) **Menominee** *Anthelmintic* Decoction of root taken for worms. (as *A. pubescens* 44:131) **Meskwaki** *Kidney Aid, Misc. Disease Remedy,* and *Panacea* Root used as a universal remedy for many things, especially dropsy and ague. (129:201) **Micmac** *Anthelmintic* Root used as a vermifuge. (32:54) **Navajo, Kayenta** *Ceremonial Medicine* Plant used as a Waterway emetic. *Emetic* Plant used as a Waterway emetic. *Other* Plant used for immersion in cold water. (as *A. suksdorfii* var. *angustifolium* 179:36) **Navajo, Ramah** *Analgesic* Decoction of plant taken for persistent stomachache. *Ceremonial Medicine* Leaves used as a ceremonial emetic and cold infusion of leaves used as a ceremonial lotion. *Emetic* Leaves used as a ceremonial emetic. *Gastrointestinal Aid* Decoction of plant taken for persistent stomachache. (as *A. sibiricum* var. *salignum* 165:39) **Okanagan-Colville** *Contraceptive* Decoction of roots taken during monthly periods to become permanently sterile. (162:72) **Penobscot** *Anthelmintic* Infusion of root taken to expel worms. (133:310) **Thompson** *Unspecified* Decoction of root used medicinally. (141:470) *Venereal Aid* Milky stem latex used for venereal disease. (161:159)

Apocynum ×***floribundum***, Intermediate Dogbane
Navajo, Ramah *Ceremonial Medicine* Leaves used as a ceremonial emetic. *Disinfectant* Plant placed on hot rocks and applied to patient's head for "deer infection." *Emetic* Leaves used as a ceremonial emetic. (as *A. medium* 165:39)

Aquilegia canadensis, Red Columbine
Cherokee *Gynecological Aid* Cold infusion used for "flux." *Heart Medicine* Infusion taken for heart trouble. (66:30) **Iroquois** *Dermatological Aid* Compound infusion of plants taken and used as a

wash for poison ivy and itch. *Kidney Aid* Infusion of roots taken before meals for the kidneys. *Witchcraft Medicine* Compound used to detect bewitchment. (73:320) **Meskwaki** *Antidiarrheal* Decoction of root and leaves taken for diarrhea. *Ceremonial Medicine* Decoction of root and leaf used as a "power of persuasion at trade or council." *Gastrointestinal Aid* Root chewed for stomach and bowel troubles. *Love Medicine* Seeds used with love medicine and for smoking. *Urinary Aid* Compound containing root taken "when the contents of the bladder are thick." (129:238, 239) **Ojibwa** *Gastrointestinal Aid* Root considered a good medicine for stomach trouble. (130:383) **Omaha** *Analgesic* Infusion of crushed seeds taken for headache. *Febrifuge* Infusion of crushed seeds taken for fever. *Love Medicine* Pulverized seeds used as a love charm. **Pawnee** *Analgesic* Infusion of crushed seeds taken for headache. *Febrifuge* Infusion of crushed seeds taken for fever. *Love Medicine* Seeds used as a love charm. **Ponca** *Analgesic* Infusion of crushed seeds taken for headache. *Febrifuge* Infusion of crushed seeds taken for fever. *Love Medicine* Pulverized seeds used as a love charm. (58:82, 83)

Aquilegia coerulea, Colorado Blue Columbine **Gosiute** *Analgesic* and *Gastrointestinal Aid* Seed chewed or infusion of roots used for abdominal pains. *Heart Medicine* Plant used as a medicine for the heart. *Panacea* Seed chewed or infusion of roots used when "sick all over." (31:362)

Aquilegia elegantula, Western Red Columbine **Keres, Western** *Blood Medicine* Infusion of plant used as a blood purifier. (147:27)

Aquilegia formosa, Western Columbine **Paiute** *Analgesic* and *Antirheumatic* (*External*) Mashed fresh roots rubbed briskly on aching rheumatic joints. (155:37) *Cold Remedy* Decoction of leaves taken for colds. *Cough Medicine* Leaves chewed for coughs. (87:197) Decoction of roots taken as a cough remedy. (155:37) *Dermatological Aid* Poultice of chewed roots or leaves applied to bee stings. (87:196) Chewed seeds rubbed on body and clothing for perfume, and seeds used in a sachet and stored with clothing. (93:71) *Gastrointestinal Aid* Seeds chewed for stomachaches.

(87:197) *Panacea* Plant used for a variety of maladies. (87:155) *Throat Aid* Leaves chewed for sore throats. (87:197) **Quileute** *Dermatological Aid* Poultice of chewed leaves or milky pulp from scraped roots applied to sores. (65:30) **Shoshoni** *Analgesic* Decoction of roots taken for stomachaches. *Antidiarrheal* Decoction of roots taken for diarrhea. *Dermatological Aid* Mashed ripe seeds rubbed into hair "to discourage head lice." *Emetic* Compound decoction of root taken to induce vomiting. *Gastrointestinal Aid* Decoction of roots and leaves taken for dizziness or biliousness. Decoction of roots taken for stomachaches. *Stimulant* Decoction of roots and leaves taken to counteract dizziness. *Venereal Aid* Decoction of whole plant taken for venereal diseases. (155:37) **Thompson** *Dermatological Aid* Decoction of whole plant used as a wash for the hair and scalp. (141:475) *Love Medicine* Plant used as a charm by women "to gain the affection of men." (141:507) *Strengthener* Root smeared on people's legs to increase stamina before a race. *Veterinary Aid* Root smeared on horse's legs to increase stamina before a race. (161:247)

Aquilegia micrantha, Mancos Columbine **Navajo, Kayenta** *Gynecological Aid* Plant used to deliver placenta. *Hemostat* Plant used as a hemostatic. (179:22)

Aquilegia triternata, Chiricahua Mountain Columbine **Navajo, Kayenta** *Analgesic* and *Ceremonial Medicine* Plant used as a ceremonial fumigant for headaches or other severe pain. (179:22)

Arabis drummondii, Drummond's Rockcress **Okanagon** *Analgesic* Decoction of whole plant taken for pains in the lumbar region. *Kidney Aid* Decoction of whole plant taken for kidney troubles. *Orthopedic Aid* Decoction of whole plant taken for pains in the lumbar region. *Urinary Aid* Decoction of whole plant taken for bladder troubles. (104:41) **Salish** *Venereal Aid* Decoction of plants taken for gonorrhea. (153:294) **Thompson** *Analgesic* Decoction of whole plant taken for pains in the lumbar region. (104:41) Decoction of whole plant taken as a diuretic and for lower back pains. *Dermatological Aid* Poultice of fresh or dried plant applied to sores. *Diuretic* Decoction of whole plant taken as a diuretic. (141:464) *Kidney Aid* Decoction of whole plant taken for kidney troubles. *Orthopedic Aid* Decoction of whole plant taken for pains in the lumbar region. *Urinary Aid* Decoction of whole plant taken for bladder troubles. (104:41) Decoction of whole plant taken as a kidney and bladder medicine. *Venereal Aid* Strong decoction of plant taken for gonorrhea. (141:464)

Arabis fendleri, Fendler's Rockcress
Keres, Western *Gastrointestinal Aid* Infusion of plant used as a stomach medicine. (147:27)
Navajo, Ramah *Panacea* Whole plant used as "life medicine." (165:28)

Arabis glabra, Tower Rockcress
Cheyenne *Cold Remedy* Plant used for colds. (63:174) Infusion of plant taken to check a cold when it first appears. (64:174) *Panacea* Plant used as a general preventive of sickness. (63:174) Infusion of plant taken as a general preventative for sickness. *Pediatric Aid* Infusion of plant given to children as a general preventative for sickness, when sickness is about. (64:174)

Arabis holboellii, Holboell's Rockcress
Thompson *Toothache Remedy* Leaves chewed as a strong medicine for toothache. (161:193)

Arabis perennans, Perennial Rockcress
Navajo, Kayenta *Anticonvulsive* Plant used for hiccups caused by dry throat. *Psychological Aid* Plant used for effects of a bad dream. (179:23)
Navajo, Ramah *Analgesic* Cold infusion taken and used as lotion for general body pain. (165:28)

Arabis puberula, Silver Rockcress
Shoshoni *Antirheumatic (External)* Crushed plant used as a liniment or mustard plaster. (155:37)

Arabis sparsiflora, Sicklepod Rockcress
Okanagan-Colville *Antidiarrheal* Roots chewed and juice swallowed for diarrhea. *Contraceptive* Plant used for birth control. *Eye Medicine* Infusion of whole plant used as an eyewash for sore eyes. *Gastrointestinal Aid* Roots chewed and juice swallowed for heartburn. (162:91)

Aralia californica, California Spikenard
Karok *Antirheumatic (External)* Decoction of roots used as a soak for arthritis. (5:17) **Mendocino Indian** *Cold Remedy* Decoction of dried roots taken for colds. *Febrifuge* Decoction of dried roots taken for fevers. *Gastrointestinal Aid* Decoction of dried roots taken for stomach diseases. *Pulmonary Aid* Decoction of dried roots taken for lung diseases. *Tuberculosis Remedy* Decoction of dried roots taken for consumption. (33:371) **Pomo** *Dermatological Aid* Decoction of roots used as a wash for sores and itching sores. *Panacea* Plant used as a medicine for various ailments. (54:14) **Pomo, Kashaya** *Dermatological Aid* Decoction of root applied externally for open sores and itching. (60:21)

Aralia hispida, Bristly Sarsaparilla
Algonquin, Quebec *Heart Medicine* Infusion of roots taken for heart disease. *Unspecified* Infusion of roots used as a medicinal tea. (14:205) **Potawatomi** *Alterative* Root used as an alterative. *Tonic* Root used as a tonic. (131:40)

Aralia nudicaulis, Wild Sarsaparilla
Abnaki *Blood Medicine* Used as a tonic to strengthen the blood. (121:154) Used to strengthen the blood. (121:170) **Algonquin, Quebec** *Kidney Aid* Infusion of roots given to children for kidney disorders. *Pediatric Aid* Infusion of roots given to children for kidney disorders. (14:205) **Algonquin, Tête-de-Boule** *Ear Medicine* Poultice of chewed roots applied to "sick" ears. (110:119) **Bella Coola** *Analgesic* Decoction of root taken for stomach pain. *Gastrointestinal Aid* Decoction of root taken for stomach pain. (127:61) Decoction of roots taken for stomach pains. (158:201) **Cherokee** *Blood Medicine* Infusion of root taken as a blood tonic. (66:53) **Chippewa** *Abortifacient* Simple or compound decoction of root taken for "stoppage of periods." (43:358) *Blood Medicine* Decoction of root taken for "humor in the blood." (43:340) Mashed root taken as a "remedy for the blood." *Dermatological Aid* Poultice of mashed, fresh root applied to sores. (43:350) *Hemostat* Chewed, fresh root, or dried, powdered root used for nosebleed. (43:356) *Veterinary Aid* Compound infusion of root applied to chest and legs of horse as a stimulant. (43:366) **Cree, Woodlands** *Der-*

matological Aid Poultice of chewed roots applied to wounds to draw out the infection. *Gynecological Aid* Decoction of fruiting stalk used to stimulate lactation. *Oral Aid* Decoction of roots used to wash teething child's infected gums to prevent spread of infection. *Panacea* Powdered roots and many other herbs used for various ailments. *Pediatric Aid* Decoction of roots and other plants taken for teething sickness. Decoction of roots used to wash teething child's infected gums to prevent spread of infection. Decoction of plant, excluding the fruit, used for childhood pneumonia. *Pulmonary Aid* Decoction of plant, excluding the fruit, used for childhood pneumonia. *Toothache Remedy* Decoction of roots and other plants taken for teething sickness. (91:29) **Delaware, Oklahoma** *Tonic* Compound containing root used as a tonic. (150:74) **Iroquois** *Blood Medicine* Infusion of roots taken as a blood medicine and blood purifier. (73:393) *Cancer Treatment* Plant used for cancer. *Cold Remedy* Plant used for colds. (73:394) *Cough Medicine* Compound infusion of roots taken as a consumption cough medicine. *Dermatological Aid* Compound decoction applied as poultice to cuts, sores, and ulcers on legs. Compound infusion of roots applied as salve on venereal disease skin cracks. (73:393) Compound infusion of roots taken for fever sores. Powdered root applied to split skin between the toes. (73:394) *Eye Medicine* Decoction of roots used as a wash for sore eyes. *Gastrointestinal Aid* Infusion of roots taken as a blood medicine or for upset stomach. (73:393) *Misc. Disease Remedy* Plant used for sugar diabetes. *Throat Aid* Compound applied as poultice for sore throat. (73:394) *Tuberculosis Remedy* Compound infusion of roots taken as a consumption cough medicine. *Venereal Aid* Compound infusion of roots applied as salve on venereal disease skin cracks. (73:393) **Kwakiutl** *Antihemorrhagic* Roasted, beaten, broken roots and grease taken for blood-spitting. *Cough Medicine* Roasted, beaten, broken roots and grease taken for coughing. (157:277) **Menominee** *Dermatological Aid* Compound decoction of root used for sores. *Pulmonary Aid* Compound decoction of root taken for "lung trouble." (44:130) **Meskwaki** *Burn Dressing* Poultice of pounded root applied to burns. *Dermatological Aid* Poultice of pounded root applied to sores. *Stimulant* Compound decoction of root

"gives strength to one who is weak." (129:203) **Micmac** *Cough Medicine* Root used as a cough medicine. (32:54) **Mohegan** *Tonic* Complex compound infusion including sarsaparilla root taken as spring tonic. (149:266) Compound decoction of root taken as a spring tonic. (151:70, 128) **Montagnais** *Stimulant* Infusion of root taken for "weakness." *Tonic* Wine made from berries taken as a tonic. (as *A. medicalis* 133:315) **Montana Indian** *Cathartic* Root used as a cathartic. *Tonic* Root used as a tonic. (15:7) **Ojibwa** *Anticonvulsive* Infusion of leaves taken for fits. (112:231) *Blood Medicine* Infusion of plants taken as a blood medicine. (112:237) Infusion of leaves taken as a blood medicine. (112:231) *Dermatological Aid* Poultice of pounded root applied to boils and carbuncles. (130:356) *Hunting Medicine* Roots and sweet flag made into tea and used to soak gill nets before setting out to catch fish at night. (130:428) *Stimulant* Infusion of leaves taken for fainting. (112:231) **Okanagon** *Blood Medicine* Plant used as a blood purifier. *Dermatological Aid* Plant used for pimples. *Tonic* Plant used as a tonic. (104:42) **Penobscot** *Cough Medicine* Compound infusion of powdered root taken for coughs. (133:310) **Potawatomi** *Dermatological Aid* Poultice of pounded root applied to swellings and infections. *Disinfectant* Poultice of root applied to swellings and infections. (131:40, 41) **Thompson** *Blood Medicine* Plant used as a blood purifier. (104:42) Decoction of root taken "for the blood and pimples." (141:471) *Dermatological Aid* Plant used for pimples. (104:42) Decoction of root taken

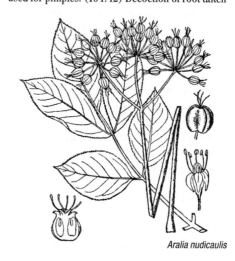

Aralia nudicaulis

"for the blood and pimples." *Stimulant* Decoction of root taken for lassitude and general debility. (141:471) *Tonic* Plant used as a tonic. (104:42) Decoction of root taken as a tonic. (141:471)

Aralia racemosa, American Spikenard
Algonquin, Quebec *Misc. Disease Remedy* Infusion of roots and spurge taken for sugar diabetes. *Tuberculosis Remedy* Infusion of roots taken for tuberculosis. (14:204) **Cherokee** *Burn Dressing* Ooze of beaten roots used as wash for burns. *Cough Medicine* Taken for coughs. *Dermatological Aid* Astringent infusion taken for menstrual problems. Poultice of root ooze used on swellings, fresh wounds, and cuts. *Diaphoretic* Infusion of roots and berries taken as a diaphoretic. *Disinfectant* Infusion of roots and berries taken as an antiseptic. *Expectorant* Taken as an expectorant. *Gynecological Aid* Infusion taken for menstrual problems. *Orthopedic Aid* Taken for weak backs. *Pulmonary Aid* Taken for lung diseases. *Respiratory Aid* Taken for asthma. *Tonic* Infusion of roots and berries taken as a tonic. (66:57) **Chippewa** *Abortifacient* Compound decoction of root taken for "stoppage of periods." (43:358) *Cough Medicine* Decoction of root taken for cough. (43:340) *Dermatological Aid* Poultice of pounded root applied to "draw" and heal boils. (43:350) Poultice of roots applied to boils. (59:137) *Orthopedic Aid* Decoction of root or poultice of root applied to sprain or strained muscles. (43:362) Compound poultice of root or decoction of root applied to fractured bone. (43:366) **Choctaw** *Analgesic* Sweetened decoction of root given to children for "gripes, colic, etc." *Expectorant* Berries and root used as an expectorant. *Eye Medicine* Decoction of root used to steam sore eyes. *Gastrointestinal Aid* Sweetened decoction of root given to children for "gripes, colic, etc." *Pediatric Aid* Berries and root used for many children's complaints. Sweetened decoction of root given to children for "gripes, colic, etc." *Stimulant* Berries and root used as a stimulant. (23:287) **Iroquois** *Abortifacient* Plant used to promote menstruation when stopped by a cold. (73:393) *Anthelmintic* Chewed plant induced tapeworm to pass. (73:392) *Antidiarrheal* Infusion of smashed roots taken for diarrhea. *Antirheumatic (Internal)* Infusion of roots taken at night for rheumatism. (73:391) Compound

used for rheumatism. *Blood Medicine* Compound decoction of roots and bark taken for watery blood and as purifier. *Cough Medicine* Decoction of roots taken for coughs. *Dermatological Aid* Decoction of roots used as wash and applied as poultice to deep cuts. *Gynecological Aid* Decoction of bark taken for prolapse of the uterus or fallen womb. (73:392) Compound decoction of roots taken for miscarriage. (73:393) *Kidney Aid* Compound decoction of roots and bark taken for dropsy or watery blood. *Liver Aid* Compound used for the liver. *Orthopedic Aid* Compound decoction of roots and bark taken for swellings on shins and calves. *Pulmonary Aid* Decoction of roots taken for whooping cough. *Strengthener* Cold infusion of roots taken for more strength. *Tonic* Compound decoction of roots taken by women as a tonic. *Tuberculosis Remedy* Decoction of roots taken for threatening consumption. *Urinary Aid* Compound decoction of bark taken by old men with urinary problems. *Venereal Aid* Compound decoction of roots taken for venereal disease. (73:392) **Malecite** *Analgesic* Roots mixed with red osier dogwood and smoked for headaches. (96:248) Infusion of plant and snakeroot used by women with back and side pain. (96:257) *Cold Remedy* Infusion of roots used for head colds. (96:249) *Kidney Aid* Infusion of plant and snakeroot used for kidney trouble. (96:257) *Strengthener* Infusion of roots used for lassitude in spring. (96:248) *Tuberculosis Remedy* Infusion of roots used for tuberculosis. (96:251) *Venereal Aid* Infusion of plant used for gonorrhea. (96:257) **Menominee** *Analgesic* Root used to make a drink taken for stomachache. *Blood Medicine* Root used in cases of blood poisoning and as a poultice for sores. *Dermatological Aid* Poultice of root applied to sores and used for blood poisoning. *Gastrointestinal Aid* Root used to make a drink said to be good for stomachache. (128:24) **Meskwaki** *Adjuvant* Split root used as a seasoner for other medicines. *Gynecological Aid* Sprayed from the mouth upon women's heads, when they are giving birth. (129:203) **Micmac** *Analgesic* Root used for headaches and female pains. *Antihemorrhagic* Root used for spitting blood. *Cold Remedy* Root used for colds. (32:54, 55) Infusion of roots and angelica roots used for head colds. (96:259) *Cough Medicine* Root used for coughs. (32:54, 55) Infusion of roots and angelica roots used for coughs. (96:259) *Dermatological Aid* Root used for wounds. *Eye Medicine* Root used for sore eyes. *Gynecological Aid* Root used for female pains. *Kidney Aid* Root used for kidney troubles. *Stimulant* Root used for fatigue. *Throat Aid* Root used for sore throats. (32:54, 55) Infusion of roots and angelica roots used for sore throats. (96:259) *Tuberculosis Remedy* Root used for consumption. *Venereal Aid* Root used for gonorrhea. (32:54, 55) **Ojibwa** *Unspecified* Plant used for medicinal purposes. (112:237) **Penobscot** *Antihemorrhagic* Compound infusion of plant taken for "spitting up blood." *Kidney Aid* Compound infusion of plant taken for kidney trouble. *Tonic* Compound infusion of plant taken as a tonic. *Venereal Aid* Compound infusion of plant taken for gonorrhea. (133:311) **Potawatomi** *Dermatological Aid* Hot poultice of pounded root applied to inflammations. (131:41)

Aralia spinosa, Devil's Walking Stick
Cherokee *Antirheumatic* (*Internal*) Used for rheumatism. *Carminative* Used as a carminative for "flatulent colic." *Dermatological Aid* Root used in salve for old sores. *Diaphoretic* Used as a diaphoretic. *Emetic* Infusion of roasted and pounded roots used as strong emetic. (66:31, 32) Decoction of roasted and pounded roots given as a very strong emetic. (177:74) *Orthopedic Aid* Ooze of root used as wash for paralysis. (66:31, 32) *Poison* Green roots considered poisonous. (177:74) *Tonic* Used as a tonic. *Toothache Remedy* Used for rheumatism and "ache of decaying teeth." *Venereal Aid* Used for venereal diseases. (66:31, 32) **Choctaw** *Dermatological Aid* Poultice of mashed, boiled roots applied to boils. *Poultice* Poultice of beaten roots applied to swollen leg veins. **Koasati** *Eye Medicine* Cold infusion of roots used as drops for sore eyes. (152:44) **Rappahannock** *Dermatological Aid* Decoction of root, sugar, and flour or bran used as a salve for boils and sores. *Febrifuge* Decoction of root, sugar, and flour or bran used as a salve for fever. (138:26)

Arbutus menziesii, Pacific Madrone
Cahuilla *Gastrointestinal Aid* Leaves used for stomach ailments. (11:40) **Concow** *Emetic* Plant eaten to cause vomiting. (33:374) **Cowichan** *Burn Dressing* Leaves used for burns. *Dermatological*

Aid Infusion of bark used for cuts and wounds. *Misc. Disease Remedy* Infusion of bark used for diabetes. (156:82) **Karok** *Ceremonial Medicine* Leaves used in the puberty ceremony. (125:387) **Miwok** *Dietary Aid* Cider employed as an appetizer to create appetite. (8:161) *Gastrointestinal Aid* Cider used for stomach trouble. Manzanita cider was dipped with a plume stick from a hawk's tail feather; beverage was sucked from the feathers and was said to create appetite as well as cure stomach troubles. Leaves chewed for stomachache and cramps. (8:161, 162) **Pomo** *Dermatological Aid* Decoction of bark used as a wash for skin sores. (54:14) **Pomo, Kashaya** *Dermatological Aid* Decoction of bark used as a wash for sores and impetigo. Decoction of bark used by women as an astringent to close the pores and make the skin soft. *Love Medicine* Flowers used for love charm poisoning. *Throat Aid* Decoction of bark used as a gargle for sore throat and strep throat. (60:67) **Pomo, Little Lakes** *Cold Remedy* Infusion of leaves taken as a cold medicine. (33:374) **Saanich** *Cold Remedy* Fresh leaves chewed and juice swallowed for bad colds. (156:82) **Salish, Cowichan** *Throat Aid* Leaves chewed and juice swallowed for sore throat. (160:104) **Skokomish** *Cold Remedy* Infusion of leaves taken for colds. *Gastrointestinal Aid* Infusion of leaves taken for ulcerated stomach. *Throat Aid* Infusion of leaves taken for sore throats. (65:44) **Yuki** *Dermatological Aid* Infusion of leaves and bark taken for sores and cuts. (39:47) *Emetic* Plant eaten to cause vomiting. *Gastrointestinal Aid* Infusion of bark taken for stomachaches. (33:374) *Veterinary Aid* Infusion of leaves and bark given to horses with sore backs. (39:47)

Arceuthobium americanum, American Dwarf Mistletoe
Bella Coola *Antihemorrhagic* Decoction taken as a potent medicine for lung hemorrhages. *Pulmonary Aid* Decoction of plant taken as potent medicine for lung hemorrhages. **Carrier, Southern** *Antihemorrhagic* Decoction taken as a potent medicine for mouth hemorrhages. *Dietary Aid* Decoction of plant taken for emaciation and tuberculosis. *Tuberculosis Remedy* Decoction of plant taken for mouth hemorrhages and tuberculosis. (127:56)

Arceuthobium campylopodum, Western
Dwarf Mistletoe
Navajo, Ramah *Ceremonial Medicine* Cold infusion used internally and externally as ceremonial medicine. (165:23)

Arceuthobium occidentale, Digger Pine
Dwarf Mistletoe
Mendocino Indian *Gastrointestinal Aid* Decoction of plant taken for stomachaches. (as *Razoumofskya occidentalis* 33:345)

Arceuthobium vaginatum, Pineland Dwarf
Mistletoe
Navajo, Ramah *Ceremonial Medicine* Decoction of plant used as a ceremonial medicine. (165:23)

Arctium lappa, Greater Burrdock
Cherokee *Antirheumatic* (*Internal*) Used for rheumatism. *Blood Medicine* Infusion of root or seed used to cleanse blood. *Dietary Aid* Used for scurvy. *Gynecological Aid* Used for "weakly females." *Urinary Aid* Used for "gravel." *Venereal Aid* Infusion of root or seed used for venereal diseases. (66:27) **Malecite** *Dermatological Aid* Roots smashed and used with gilead buds for sores. (96:247) *Venereal Aid* Infusion of buds used for chancre. (96:258) **Menominee** *Dermatological Aid* and *Tuberculosis Remedy* Poultice of boiled leaves applied to scrofulous sores on the neck. (44:132) **Micmac** *Dermatological Aid* Buds and roots used for sores. *Venereal Aid* Buds and roots used for chancre. (32:55) **Ojibwa** *Blood Medicine* Roots used as a blood medicine. (112:238)

Arctium minus, Lesser Burrdock
Abnaki *Analgesic* Used for headaches. (121:155) Poultice of leaves applied to the head for headaches. (121:173) *Antirheumatic* (*External*) Used as a medicine for rheumatism. (121:155) *Antirheumatic* (*Internal*) Decoction of roots taken for rheumatism. (121:173) *Febrifuge* Used for trembling fevers. (121:154) Used for trembling fevers. (121:173) *Misc. Disease Remedy* Used for grippe. (121:154) **Cherokee** *Dermatological Aid* Boiled to make "ooze" for leg ulcers and used to bathe swollen legs. (66:27) **Chippewa** *Cough Medicine* Infusion of leaves taken after a coughing spell for a hard, dry cough. (43:340) **Cowlitz** *Pulmonary*

Aid Infusion of roots taken for whooping cough. (65:50) **Delaware** *Antirheumatic* (*Internal*) Infusion of roots used for rheumatism. *Blood Medicine* Infusion of roots used as a blood purifier. *Stimulant* Infusion of roots used as a stimulant. (151:36) **Delaware, Oklahoma** *Antirheumatic* (*Internal*) Infusion of root taken for rheumatism. *Blood Medicine* Infusion of root taken as a blood purifier. *Stimulant* Infusion of root taken as a stimulant. (150:31, 74) **Delaware, Ontario** *Analgesic* Poultice of leaves bound to body for pain. *Blood Medicine* Roots used as a blood purifier. (150:66, 82) **Hoh** *Unspecified* Leaves used to make a rubbing salve. Infusion of leaves and roots used for medicine. (114:70) **Iroquois** *Antirheumatic* (*External*) Poultice of wetted leaves and salt applied to swellings. (118:62) Roots and fruits used for rheumatism. (119:100) *Blood Medicine* Infusion of roots with other roots used to purify the blood. *Dermatological Aid* Poultice of crushed leaves and other leaves applied to blue swellings. (118:62) **Meskwaki** *Analgesic* Compound containing root used by women in labor. *Gynecological Aid* Compound containing root used by women in labor. (129:211) **Micmac** *Dermatological Aid* Roots used for boils and abscesses. (32:55) **Mohegan** *Analgesic* Poultice of leaves applied for rheumatic pains. (151:70) *Antirheumatic* (*External*) Poultice of leaves used for rheumatism. (149:269) Poultice of leaves applied for rheumatic pains. (151:70, 128) *Cold Remedy* Compound infusion of

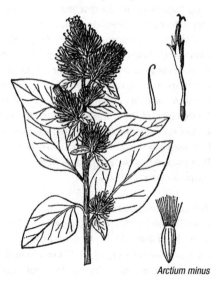

Arctium minus

plants taken for wintertime colds. (149:266) **Nanticoke** *Dermatological Aid* Poultice of leaves applied to boils. (150:57, 84) **Ojibwa** *Analgesic* and *Gastrointestinal Aid* Compound containing root used for stomach pain. *Tonic* Root supposed to have tonic effect. (130:363) **Oto** *Pulmonary Aid* Decoction of root taken for pleurisy. (58:135) **Penobscot** *Dermatological Aid* Poultice of mashed, heated root applied to boils and abscesses. (133:309) **Potawatomi** *Blood Medicine* and *Tonic* Infusion of root taken as a general tonic and blood purifier. (131:49) **Quileute** *Unspecified* Leaves used to make a rubbing salve. Infusion of leaves and roots used for medicine. (114:70)

Arctostaphylos alpina, Alpine Bearberry
Ojibwa *Antirheumatic* (*External*) Infusion of pounded plants used as wash for rheumatism. *Blood Medicine* Decoction of bark taken for internal blood diseases. (112:231) *Ceremonial Medicine* Leaves used for medicine ceremonies. *Narcotic* Leaves smoked to cause intoxication. (112: 238) *Panacea* Infusion of pounded plants used as wash for general illnesses. (112:231) *Unspecified* Leaves used for medicinal purposes. (112:238)

Arctostaphylos columbiana, Hairy
   Manzanita
Pomo *Antidiarrheal* Decoction of bark taken for diarrhea. (54:14) **Pomo, Kashaya** *Antidiarrheal* Decoction of bark used for diarrhea. (60:69)

Arctostaphylos glandulosa, Eastwood's
   Manzanita
Cahuilla *Antidiarrheal* Infusion of leaves used for diarrhea. *Dermatological Aid* Infusion of leaves used for poison oak rash. (11:40) **Pomo** *Unspecified* Plant used as medicine. (54:14) **Pomo, Kashaya** *Antidiarrheal* Decoction of bark taken for diarrhea and bleeding diarrhea. (60:68)

Arctostaphylos glauca, Bigberry Manzanita
Cahuilla *Antidiarrheal* Infusion of leaves used for diarrhea. *Dermatological Aid* Infusion of leaves used for poison oak rash. (11:40)

Arctostaphylos manzanita, Whiteleaf
   Manzanita
Concow *Dermatological Aid* Poultice of chewed

leaves applied to sores. *Veterinary Aid* Plant used for sore backs of horses. **Mendocino Indian** *Poison* Fruit considered poisonous. (33:375) **Miwok** *Dietary Aid* Cider employed as an appetizer to create appetite. *Gastrointestinal Aid* Cider used for stomach trouble. Leaves chewed for stomachache and cramps. (8:161, 162) **Pomo, Calpella** *Cold Remedy* Infusion of leaves taken for severe colds. **Pomo, Little Lakes** *Analgesic* Decoction of leaves used as a wash for headaches. *Antidiarrheal* Leaves used for diarrhea. (33:375)

Arctostaphylos nevadensis, Pine Mat
   Manzanita
Karok *Antidiarrheal* Leaves used for diarrhea. *Antidote* Plant used for poisoning from *Toxicodendron diversiloba*. (5:18)

Arctostaphylos patula, Greenleaf Manzanita
Atsugewi *Burn Dressing* Poultice of leaves applied to burns. Decoction of pounded leaves used for burns. *Dermatological Aid* Decoction of pounded leaves used for cuts. Poultice of leaves applied to cuts. (50:140) **Navajo, Kayenta** *Ceremonial Medicine* and *Emetic* Plant used as a ceremonial emetic. (179:35) **Shoshoni** *Venereal Aid* Decoction of leaves taken for venereal diseases. (155:38)

Arctostaphylos pungens, Pointleaf Manzanita
Cahuilla *Antidiarrheal* Infusion of leaves used for diarrhea. *Dermatological Aid* Infusion of leaves used for poison oak rash. (11:40) **Navajo, Ramah** *Ceremonial Medicine* and *Emetic* Leaves used as a ceremonial emetic. (165:38)

Arctostaphylos tomentosa, Woollyleaf
   Manzanita
Costanoan (Olhonean) *Antihemorrhagic* Infusion of bark powder taken for lung hemorrhages. (97:373) **Miwok** *Dietary Aid* Cider employed as an appetizer to create appetite. *Gastrointestinal Aid* Cider used for stomach trouble. Leaves chewed for stomachache and cramps. (8:161, 162)

Arctostaphylos uva-ursi, Kinnikinnick
Blackfoot *Dermatological Aid* Infusion of plant, mixed with grease and boiled hoof, applied as a salve to itching and peeling scalp, as a salve to

rashes and skin sores, and used as a wash for baby's head. (72:75) *Oral Aid* Infusion of plant used as a mouthwash for cankers and sore gums. (72:66) *Pediatric Aid* Infusion of plant, mixed with grease and boiled hoof, used as a wash for baby's head. (72:75) **Carrier** *Dermatological Aid* Poultice of ground leaves and stems applied to sores. (26:74) Leaves placed on a piece of wood, roasted to a powder, and placed on a cut for rapid healing. Leaves pounded into a paste and applied to boils and pimples. (75:12) **Cherokee** *Kidney Aid* Used for "dropsy." *Urinary Aid* Used for urinary diseases. (66:25) **Cheyenne** *Analgesic* Infusion of stems, leaves, and berries taken for back pain. (63:183) Infusion of stems, leaves, and berries taken for back pain and sprained backs. Poultice of wetted leaves rubbed on the back for pain. (64:183) Infusion of leaves, stems, and berries taken for "persistent" back pain. Leaves wetted and used for pain relief. *Cold Remedy* Berries and other plants used for colds. *Cough Medicine* Berries and other plants used for coughs. (68:40) *Orthopedic Aid* Decoction of plant taken and leaves rubbed on back for painful or sprained back. (63:41) Infusion of stems, leaves, and berries taken for sprained backs. (63:183) Infusion of stems, leaves, and berries taken for sprained backs. (64:183) *Psychological Aid* Leaves burned to drive away bad spirits for people going crazy. *Unspecified* Berries used as an ingredient in medicinal mixtures. (69:25) **Chippewa** *Analgesic* Pulverized, dried leaves compounded and smoked for headache. (43:336) *Hunting Medicine* Roots smoked in pipes as charms to attract game. (43:376) **Cree, Woodlands** *Abortifacient* Infusion of whole plant and velvet leaf blueberry taken to bring menstruation. *Antidiarrheal* Fruit mixed with grease and used for children with diarrhea. *Gynecological Aid* Decoction of stems and blueberry stem taken to prevent miscarriage without causing damage to the baby, and to speed a woman's recovery after childbirth. Roots and several other herbs used to slow excessive menstrual bleeding. *Pediatric Aid* Fruit mixed with grease and used for children with diarrhea. (91:29) **Crow** *Oral Aid* Leaves pulverized and powder used for canker sores of the mouth. **Flathead** *Burn Dressing* Poultice of pulverized leaves used for burns. *Ear Medicine* Smoke from leaves used for earache.

(68:40) **Hoh** *Unspecified* Leaves smoked as medicine. (114:66) **Kwakiutl** *Narcotic* Leaves smoked as a narcotic. (157:282) **Menominee** *Adjuvant* Dried leaves used as a seasoner to make certain female remedies taste good. (128:35) **Navajo, Ramah** *Ceremonial Medicine* and *Emetic* Leaves used as a ceremonial emetic. (165:38) **Ojibwa** *Antirheumatic* (*External*) Infusion of pounded plants used as wash for rheumatism. *Blood Medicine* Decoction of bark taken for internal blood diseases. (112:231) *Ceremonial Medicine* Leaves used for medicine ceremonies. *Narcotic* Leaves smoked to cause intoxication. (112:238) *Panacea* Infusion of pounded plants used as wash for general illnesses. (112:231) *Unspecified* Leaves used for medicinal purposes. (112:238) **Okanagan-Colville** *Antihemorrhagic* Decoction of leaves and stems taken for spitting of blood. *Blood Medicine* Decoction of leaves and stems taken as a blood tonic. *Eye Medicine* Decoction of leaves and stems used as a wash for sore eyes. *Kidney Aid* Decoction of leaves and stems taken as a tonic for the kidneys. *Urinary Aid* Decoction of leaves and stems taken as a tonic for the bladder. (162:101) **Okanagon** *Antihemorrhagic* Decoction of leaves and stems taken for blood-spitting. *Eye Medicine* Decoction of leaves and stems used as a wash for sore eyes. *Kidney Aid* Decoction of leaves and stems taken as a tonic for kidneys. *Tonic* Decoction of leaves and stems taken as a tonic for kidneys and bladder. *Urinary Aid* Decoction of leaves and stems taken as a tonic for bladder. (104:40) **Quileute** *Unspecified* Leaves smoked as medicine. (114:66) **Sanpoil** *Dermatological Aid* Green leaves dried, pulverized, and sprinkled on skin sores. Infusion of entire plant used as hair wash for dandruff and scalp diseases. Infusion of entire plant used as young girls' hair wash to insure growth. *Pediatric Aid* Infusion of entire plant used as young girls' hair wash to insure growth. (109:220) **Tanana, Upper** *Laxative* Raw berries eaten as a laxative. (86:10) **Thompson** *Antihemorrhagic* Decoction of leaves and stems taken for blood-spitting. (104:40) Decoction of root taken for "blood spitting." (141:458) *Dietary Aid* Raw leaves chewed to alleviate thirst. (161:211) *Diuretic* Decoction of leaves and stems taken as a diuretic. *Eye Medicine* Decoction of leaves and stems used as a wash for sore eyes. (141:458) *Kidney Aid*

Decoction of leaves and stems taken as a tonic for kidneys. (104:40) *Oral Aid* Infusion of leaves used as a mouthwash for canker sores and weak gums. *Orthopedic Aid* Infusion of plant taken and used as a wash for broken bones. (161:211) *Tonic* Decoction of leaves and stems taken as a tonic for kidneys and bladder. (104:40) Decoction of leaves and stems taken as a tonic for the kidneys and bladder. (141:458) *Urinary Aid* Decoction of leaves and stems taken as a tonic for bladder. (104:40) Decoction of leaves and stems taken as a tonic for the bladder. (141:458) Infusion of leaves used as a tonic, antiseptic, and astringent for bladder and urinary passage disorders. (161:211)

Arctostaphylos viscida, Sticky Whiteleaf Manzanita
Miwok *Dietary Aid* Cider employed as an appetizer to create appetite. *Gastrointestinal Aid* Cider used for stomach trouble. Leaves chewed for stomachache and cramps. (8:161, 162)

Arenaria aculeata, Prickly Sandwort
Shoshoni *Eye Medicine* Decoction of root used as an eyewash. (155:38)

Arenaria congesta, Ballhead Sandwort
Gosiute *Gastrointestinal Aid* Plant used as bowel medicine. (31:362) **Shoshoni** *Antirheumatic* (*External*) Poultice of steeped leaves applied for swellings. (98:42) *Blood Medicine* Infusion of flower heads and seeds taken as a blood purifier. (100:47) *Dermatological Aid* Poultice of steeped leaves and blossoms used for sun exposure. *Venereal Aid* Poultice of steeped leaves and blossoms used for gonorrheal ulcers. (98:47) **Washo** *Antirheumatic* (*External*) Poultice of steeped leaves applied for swellings. (98:42)

Arenaria eastwoodiae, Eastwood's Sandwort
Hopi *Emetic* Plant used as an emetic for the stomach. (174:34, 75–76)

Arenaria fendleri, Fendler's Sandwort
Navajo, Ramah *Panacea* Root used, only in the summer, as a "life medicine." *Respiratory Aid* Powdered root used as snuff to cause sneezing for "congested nose."

Arenaria lanuginosa ssp. *saxosa*, Spreading Sandwort
Navajo, Ramah *Analgesic* Cold infusion used as lotion on forehead for headache. *Dermatological Aid* Infusion of plant used as lotion for pimples. *Eye Medicine* Infusion of plant used as eye drops. *Febrifuge* Cold infusion used as lotion on forehead for fever. *Respiratory Aid* Infusion of powdered root put in nose to cause sneezing for "congested nose." *Venereal Aid* Strong infusion of plant taken before sweat bath for venereal disease. (as *A. saxosa* 165:26)

Arenaria macradenia, Mojave Sandwort
Kawaiisu *Analgesic* Dried root smoke inhaled for headaches. Poultice of broken roots applied to the head for headaches. Root used as a salve for pain. *Antirheumatic* (*External*) Poultice of broken roots applied to area affected by rheumatism. *Dermatological Aid* Root used as a salve for pimples. *Respiratory Aid* Dried root smoke inhaled to clear the sinuses. (180:12)

Arenaria triflora var. *obtusa*
Gosiute *Cathartic* Plant used as a purgative for babies and adults with intestinal disorders. (31:350) *Gastrointestinal Aid* Plant used as a purgative for babies and adults with intestinal disorders. (31:350) Used as a bowel medicine. (31:362) *Pediatric Aid* Plant used as a purgative for babies and adults with intestinal disorders. (31:350)

Argemone hispida, Rough Pricklypoppy
Paiute *Dermatological Aid* Ground seeds used for sores. (98:44) **Shoshoni** *Cathartic* Infusion of seeds taken as a physic. (98:42)

Argemone munita, Flatbud Pricklypoppy
Kawaiisu *Burn Dressing* Roasted, ripe, and mashed seeds applied as a salve to burns. (180:12)

Argemone polyanthemos, Crested Pricklypoppy
Comanche *Eye Medicine* Sap used for sore eyes. (as *A. intermedia* 24:520) **Paiute** *Burn Dressing* and *Dermatological Aid* Salve of pulverized seeds used on burns, cuts, and sores. **Shoshoni** *Burn Dressing* Salve of pulverized seeds used on burns, sores, or cuts. *Cathartic* Roasted, mashed seeds

taken as powder or pills to serve as a physic. *Dermatological Aid* Poultice of pulverized seed paste applied to bring boils to a head. *Salve* of moistened, pulverized seeds rubbed into hair to kill head lice. *Salve* of pulverized seeds used on burns, cuts, and sores. *Emetic* Roasted, mashed seeds taken as an emetic and physic. *Eye Medicine* Infusion of pulverized seeds used as a wash for sore eyes. *Toothache Remedy* Warmed root used various ways for toothache. (as *A. platyceras* 155:38, 39) **Tubatulabal** *Dermatological Aid* Poultice of pounded, ripe seeds applied to open sores. *Hemorrhoid Remedy* Poultice of pounded, ripe seeds applied to piles. (as *A. platyceras* 167:59) **Washo** *Burn Dressing* Salve of pulverized seeds used on burns, sores, or cuts. *Dermatological Aid* Salve of pulverized seeds used on burns, cuts, and sores. (as *A. platyceras* 155:38, 39)

Argentina anserina, Silverweed Cinquefoil
Blackfoot *Antidiarrheal* Root used for diarrhea. (95:275) *Dermatological Aid* Poultice of chewed roots applied to sores and scrapes. (as *Potentilla anserina* 72:78) *Emetic* Plant soaked in water and the solution taken as an emetic for stomach disorders. (as *Potentilla anserina* 72:68) **Iroquois** *Antidiarrheal* Infusion of plant and another plant given to children for diarrhea. (as *Potentilla anserina* 118:49) *Diuretic* Infusion of leaves used as a diuretic. (as *Potentilla anserina* 119:92) *Pediatric Aid* Infusion of plant and another plant given to children for diarrhea. (as *Potentilla anserina* 118:49) **Kwakiutl** *Analgesic* and *Dermatological Aid* Decoction of root mixed with catfish oil and smeared on painful places. (16:382)

Argentina egedii ssp. egedii, Eged's Pacific Silverweed
Kwakiutl *Dermatological Aid* Poultice of boiled roots and oil applied to sores and swellings. *Eye Medicine* Root juice used as a wash for inflamed eyes. (as *Potentilla pacifica* 157:289) **Tsimshian** *Unspecified* Roots used medicinally for unspecified purpose. (as *Potentilla anserina* ssp. *pacifica* 35:344)

Argyrochosma fendleri, Fendler's Falsecloak Fern
Tewa *Dermatological Aid* Pulverized plant applied

to lips for cold sores. (as *Notholaena fendleri* 115:67, 68)

Argythamnia cyanophylla, Charleston Mountain Silverbush
Navajo *Panacea* Plant used as a "life medicine." (as *Ditaxis cyanophylla* 76:158) **Navajo, Ramah** *Panacea* Root or whole plant used in summer as "the head of the life medicine." (as *Ditaxis cyanophylla* 165:35)

Arisaema dracontium, Greendragon
Menominee *Gynecological Aid* Plant used for "female disorders." (128:23)

Arisaema triphyllum, Jack in the Pulpit
Cherokee *Analgesic* Poultice of root used for headaches and various skin diseases. *Carminative* Used as a carminative. *Cold Remedy* Taken for colds. *Cough Medicine* Taken for dry coughs. *Dermatological Aid* Ointment used for "scald head," ringworm, tetterworm, and "scrofulous sores." Poultice of beaten, boiled roots mixed with meal and used on boils. *Diaphoretic* Used as a diaphoretic. *Expectorant* Used as an expectorant. *Orthopedic Aid* Used as a liniment. *Stimulant* Used as a stimulant. *Throat Aid* Infusion taken for throat irritations. *Tuberculosis Remedy* Given for "consumptions" and ointment used on "scrofulous sores." (66:41) **Chippewa** *Eye Medicine* Decoction of root used as a wash for sore eyes. (43:360) **Iroquois** *Analgesic* Compound snuff used for headaches. Decoction or infusion of roots taken for pains. *Antidiarrheal* Decoction of plant given to children for diarrhea. *Blood Medicine* Cold infusion of roots taken "for nonconception caused by cold blood." *Dermatological Aid* Plant used for face sores and hot poultice of plant applied to bruises. (73:276) *Eye Medicine* Steam from decoction of plant used for sore eyes. (73:277) *Febrifuge* Compound decoction steam used "when a person has cold sweats, not very sick." *Gynecological Aid* Cold infusion of roots taken "for nonconception caused by cold blood." (73:276) *Nose Medicine* Steam from decoction of plant used to "make you sneeze." (73:277) *Orthopedic Aid* Compound infusion of powdered plants taken for cramps. Hot poultice of plant applied to bruises and for lameness. (73:276) Compound of pow-

dered plant and alcohol used as a liniment for sore joints. (73:277) *Pediatric Aid* Decoction of plant given to children for diarrhea. Infusion of roots used as a wash for listless babies. *Respiratory Aid* Compound of chopped root and whisky taken for bronchial colds. Compound snuff used for catarrh. *Stimulant* Infusion of roots used as a wash for listless babies. *Tuberculosis Remedy* Compound decoction used as poultice for infected and swollen tubercular glands. (73:276) *Veterinary Aid* Ground plant added to mare's feed to induce pregnancy and reduce listlessness. (73:275) **Malecite** *Dermatological Aid* Poultice of dried, pounded plants used for abscesses and boils. (96:247) **Menominee** *Eye Medicine* Poultice of pulverized root applied to sore eyes. (128:23) *Witchcraft Medicine* Compounded pulverized root used in lip incision to counteract "witchery" to face. (44:129) **Meskwaki** *Ceremonial Medicine* Seed used as a magical diagnostic medicine to predict recovery or death. *Poison* Finely chopped root put in meat for enemies, to cause pain and death. (129:202) Root cooked with meat used in abandoned vessels to poison enemy during war. (129:272) *Sedative* Compound used in very small doses for insomnia. *Snakebite Remedy* Root used for rattlesnake bite swellings. (129:202) **Micmac** *Dermatological Aid* Parts of plant used for boils and abscesses. *Orthopedic Aid* Parts of plant used as a liniment used for external use. (32:55) **Mohegan** *Analgesic* and *Antirheumatic* (*External*) Infusion of dried root used as a liniment for pain. (151:70, 128) *Orthopedic Aid* Infusion of plant

used as a liniment. *Poison* Infusion of plant poisonous when taken internally. (149:269) Infusion of root, poisonous if swallowed, gargled for sore throat. (151:70) *Throat Aid* Infusion of root taken for sore throat. (149:269) Dilute infusion of root gargled for sore throat. (151:70, 128) **Ojibwa** *Eye Medicine* Root used for sore eyes. (130:356) *Unspecified* Plant used for medicinal purposes. (112:246) **Pawnee** *Analgesic* Crushed corm sprinkled on head and temples for headache and general pain. *Antirheumatic* (*External*) Poultice of pulverized corm applied as counterirritant for rheumatism. (58:69) **Penobscot** *Orthopedic Aid* Infusion of plant used as a liniment "for general external use." *Poison* Infusion of plant considered poisonous. (133:310) **Rappahannock** *Dermatological Aid* Compound dried root meal poultice applied for swelling and boils. (138:32)

Arisaema triphyllum ssp. *quinatum*, Jack in the Pulpit
Choctaw *Blood Medicine* Decoction of root taken "to make blood." (as *A. quinatum* 20:23) Decoction of plant taken to make blood. (as *A. quinatum* 152:6)

Arisaema triphyllum ssp. *triphyllum*, Jack in the Pulpit
Iroquois *Contraceptive* Infusion of rhizomes used by women for temporary sterility. (as *A. atrorubens* 118:69)

Aristida divaricata, Poverty Threeawn
Keres, Western *Burn Dressing* Grass ashes rubbed on burns. (147:27)

Aristolochia californica, California Dutchman's Pipe
Miwok *Cold Remedy* Decoction taken for colds. (8:167)

Aristolochia macrophylla, Pipevine
Cherokee *Dermatological Aid* Decoction of root applied externally for "swelling of feet and legs." *Urinary Aid* Compound infusion of "stalk chips" taken for "yellowish urine." (66:32)

Aristolochia serpentaria, Virginia Snakeroot
Cherokee *Abortifacient* Infusion taken for

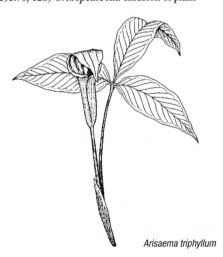
Arisaema triphyllum

obstructions. *Analgesic* Infusion taken for sharp darting pains and used as an anodyne. Taken for sharp pains in the breast and used as a wash for headache. (66:55) Infusion of roots taken for breast pains. (152:20) *Antirheumatic* (*Internal*) Infusion taken for rheumatism. *Cold Remedy* Infusion taken or root chewed for colds and cold infusion of plant used for pain. *Cough Medicine* Taken for coughs. *Disinfectant* Used as an antiseptic. *Diuretic* Used as a diuretic. *Febrifuge* Taken for fever. *Gastrointestinal Aid* Used to "stop mortification and prevent putrefaction in the bowels," dyspepsia. *Misc. Disease Remedy* Used as a tonic for typhus fevers and taken for ague. Used for "black-yellow" diseases. *Nose Medicine* Used as a poultice for "nose made sore by constant blowing." *Pulmonary Aid* Infusion taken for pleurisy. *Snakebite Remedy* Root chewed and saliva spit on snakebite. *Stimulant* Used by "persons of weak, phlegmatic habits" and for dizziness or fainting. *Throat Aid* Used as a gargle for sore throat. *Tonic* Used as a tonic for typhus fevers. *Toothache Remedy* Poultice of bruised root applied to tooth for toothache. (66:55) **Choctaw** *Analgesic* Infusion of root taken for stomach pain. (20:24) Cold infusion of roots taken for stomach pains. (152:20) *Gastrointestinal Aid* Infusion of root taken for stomach pains. (20:24) Cold infusion of roots taken for stomach pains. (152:20) **Delaware** *Tonic* Used singly or combined with wintergreen to make a tonic. (151:39) **Delaware, Oklahoma** *Tonic* Root used alone or with wintergreen as a tonic. (150:32, 74) **Micmac** *Anticonvulsive* Root used for fits. (32:55) **Mohegan** *Snakebite Remedy* Poultice of plant applied to snakebites. (149:266) Poultice of pounded root applied to snakebite. (151:70, 128) **Nanticoke** *Anthelmintic* Infusion of plant taken for intestinal worms. (150:57, 84) **Natchez** *Febrifuge* Warm decoction of plant taken for fevers. (148:667) Decoction of plant taken for fevers. (152:20) **Penobscot** *Anticonvulsive* Infusion of root used for "fits." (133:310) **Rappahannock** *Dermatological Aid* Compound poultice with mashed roots used as salve for spider bites. *Febrifuge* Infusion of leaves taken for chills. *Snakebite Remedy* Compound poultice with mashed roots used as salve for snakebites. (138:27)

Armoracia rusticana, Horseradish
Cherokee *Abortifacient* Used for "obstructed menses." *Antirheumatic* (*Internal*) Used for rheumatism. *Cold Remedy* Used for colds. *Dietary Aid* Used to increase the appetite. *Diuretic* Used as a diuretic. *Gastrointestinal Aid* Used to aid digestion. *Oral Aid* Roots chewed for tongue and mouth diseases. *Respiratory Aid* Used for asthma. *Throat Aid* Infusion gargled for sore throat. *Tonic* Used as a tonic. *Urinary Aid* Used for "gravel." (66:39) **Delaware, Ontario** *Analgesic* Poultice of leaves applied for neuralgia. (as *Rorippa armoracia* 150: 66, 82) **Iroquois** *Blood Medicine* Infusion of smashed roots taken for the blood. *Misc. Disease Remedy* Plant used for sugar diabetes. (as *A. lapathifolia* 73:342) **Mohegan** *Toothache Remedy* Poultice of leaves, with midrib removed, bound to cheeks for toothache. (as *Roripa amoracia* 149:266) Poultice of leaf bound to the face for toothaches. (as *Rorippa amoracia* 151:75, 132)

Arnica acaulis, Common Leopardbane
Catawba *Analgesic* Infusion of roots taken for back pain. *Orthopedic Aid* Infusion of roots taken for back pain. (134:189)

Arnica cordifolia, Heartleaf Arnica
Okanagan-Colville *Love Medicine* Roots used as a love medicine. Roots were mixed with a robin's heart and tongue and with ocher paint. The mixture was dried and powdered. The user went into the water and faced east, recited certain words, mentioned the name of the person he desired, and marked his face with the powdered arnica mixture. (162:75) **Shuswap** *Eye Medicine* Plant used for sore eyes. (102:58) **Thompson** *Antirheumatic* (*External*) Poultice of mashed plant used for swellings. *Dermatological Aid* Poultice of mashed plant used for bruises and cuts. *Tuberculosis Remedy* Infusion of plant taken for tuberculosis. (161:169)

Arnica latifolia, Broadleaf Arnica
Okanagan-Colville *Love Medicine* Roots used as a love medicine. (162:75) **Thompson** *Unspecified* Plant used medicinally for unspecified purpose. (141:473)

Arnoglossum atriplicifolium, Armoglossum
Cherokee *Cancer Treatment* Poultice used for

cancer and to draw out blood or poisonous matter. *Dermatological Aid* Poultice used for cuts and bruises. (as *Cacalia atriplicifolia* 66:58)

Aronia melanocarpa, Black Chokeberry
Potawatomi *Cold Remedy* Infusion of berry used for colds. (as *Pyrus melanocarpa* 131:76)

Artemisia absinthium, Absinth Sagewort
Chippewa *Orthopedic Aid* Boiled plant top used as warm compress for sprain or strained muscles. (43:362) **Mohegan** *Anthelmintic* Infusion of leaves taken as a vermifuge. (151:70, 128) **Okanagan-Colville** *Cold Remedy* Decoction or infusion of twigs taken for head colds. Poultice of pounded leaves applied for chest colds. *Gastrointestinal Aid* Infusion of split roots taken for stomach ailments. *Gynecological Aid* Plant used as a sanitary napkin to "heal the mother's insides" after a baby's birth. *Misc. Disease Remedy* Poultice of pounded leaves applied for flu. *Orthopedic Aid* Poultice of mashed, boiled plant applied or decoction of plant used as a wash for broken limbs. *Tuberculosis Remedy* Decoction or infusion of twigs taken for tuberculosis. *Venereal Aid* Decoction or infusion of twigs taken for venereal disease. (162:75)

Artemisia alaskana, Alaska Sagebrush
Tanana, Upper *Cancer Treatment* Decoction taken for cancers. *Cold Remedy* Decoction taken for colds. *Cough Medicine* Decoction taken for coughs. *Eye Medicine* Cooled decoction used as a wash for eyes. *Misc. Disease Remedy* Decoction taken for diabetes. (86:17)

Artemisia arctica, Boreal Sagebrush
Tanana, Upper *Cancer Treatment* Decoction taken for cancer. *Cold Remedy* Decoction taken for colds. *Cough Medicine* Decoction taken for coughs. *Eye Medicine* Cooled decoction used as a wash for eyes. *Misc. Disease Remedy* Decoction taken for diabetes. (86:17)

Artemisia australis, Oahu Wormwood
Hawaiian *Febrifuge* Decoction of pounded leaves, trunk, and roots used as a steam bath and wash for high fevers. *Pulmonary Aid* Leaves used as an ingredient in a medicine for lung troubles. *Repro-*

ductive Aid Leaves used as an ingredient for asthma medicine. (2:7)

Artemisia biennis, Biennial Wormwood
Cherokee *Analgesic* Used for cramps and painful menstruation. *Anthelmintic* Poultice applied to stomach for worms and seeds in molasses taken for worms. *Dermatological Aid* Used for sores and wounds. *Gastrointestinal Aid* Used for cramps and colic. *Gynecological Aid* Used for painful menstruation. (66:62)

Artemisia californica, California Sagebrush
Cahuilla *Cold Remedy* Leaves used for colds. *Gynecological Aid* Decoction of plant taken to start menstrual activity, for easy childbirth, and postnatal recovery, and to prevent dysmenorrhea and ease menopause trauma. *Pediatric Aid* Decoction of plant given to newborn babies 1 day after birth to flush out their system. *Unspecified* Plant used in the sweat houses for various cures. (11:42) **Costanoan** *Analgesic* Poultice of leaves applied to the tooth for pain. *Antirheumatic (External)* Decoction of plant used as a bath for rheumatism. *Cold Remedy* Decoction of plant used as a bath for colds. *Cough Medicine* Decoction of plant used as a bath for coughs. *Dermatological Aid* Poultice of leaves applied to wounds. *Respiratory Aid* Poultice of plant applied to the back or decoction of plant taken for asthma. *Toothache Remedy* Poultice of leaves applied to the tooth for pain. (17:25) **Mahuna** *Gynecological Aid* Infusion of plants taken for vaginal troubles. (117:14)

Artemisia campestris, Field Sagewort
Blackfoot *Abortifacient* Decoction of leaves taken to abort difficult pregnancies. (72:60) *Antirheumatic (External)* Chewed leaf spittle applied to rheumatic parts. (72:78) *Cough Medicine* Infusion of dried leaves taken for coughs. (72:71) *Dermatological Aid* Infusion of roots used, especially for children, as a hair tonic. Infusion of roots cleansed and used for scalp infections. (72:123) Infusion of leaves applied to eczema. (72:75) *Eye Medicine* Poultice of chewed leaves applied to sore eyes. (72:80) *Gastrointestinal Aid* Fresh leaves chewed for stomach troubles. (72:66) *Oral Aid* Leaves chewed by runners for the mentholating properties. (72:101) *Pediatric Aid* Infusion of

roots used, especially for children, as a hair tonic. (72:123) *Veterinary Aid* Infusion of roots used for back sores on horses. (72:87) **Lakota** *Diuretic* Infusion of roots used to cause urination. *Gastrointestinal Aid* Infusion of roots used to cause bowel movements. *Gynecological Aid* Infusion of roots used by women for difficult births. *Sedative* Pulverized roots put on sleeping man's face so his horses could be stolen. (116:35) **Shuswap** *Cold Remedy* Decoction of plants taken for colds. *Cough Medicine* Decoction of plants taken for coughs. *Dermatological Aid* Poultice of steamed branches applied to bruises and sores. *Panacea* Decoction of plants taken as a medicine for everything. *Tuberculosis Remedy* Decoction of plants taken for tuberculosis. (102:58)

Artemisia campestris ssp. *borealis* var. *borealis*, Pacific Wormwood

Menominee *Abortifacient* Compound infusion of leaf taken to restore menstrual flow. (as *A. canadensis* 128:29) **Meskwaki** *Burn Dressing* Poultice of leaves applied to bad burns. (as *A. canadensis* 129:211) **Okanagon** *Antidiarrheal* Decoction of whole plant used for diarrhea. *Gynecological Aid* Decoction of fresh or dried leaves taken by women after childbirth. **Thompson** *Antidiarrheal* Decoction of whole plant used for diarrhea. (as *A. canadensis* 104:41) Decoction of plant taken for diarrhea. (as *A. canadensis* 141:470) *Gynecological Aid* Decoction of fresh or dried leaves taken by women after childbirth. (as *A. canadensis* 104:41) Decoction of fresh or dried leaves taken postpartum to hasten recovery. *Unspecified* Decoction of root used medicinally. (as *A. canadensis* 141:470)

Artemisia campestris ssp. *caudata*, Field Wormwood

Tewa *Antiemetic* Leaves and stems chewed and juice swallowed when one was "sick at the stomach." *Febrifuge* Infusion of leaves and stems taken for "chills." (as *A. forwoodii* 115:53)

Artemisia campestris ssp. *pacifica*, Pacific Wormwood

Havasupai *Unspecified* Sprays used in the sweat baths or infusion of leaves taken for sicknesses. (as *A. pacifica* 171:245) **Navajo, Kayenta** *Ceremonial Medicine* Plant used as a ceremonial fumigant ingredient. *Disinfectant* Plant used as a ceremonial fumigant ingredient. (as *A. pacifica* 179:45)

Artemisia cana, Silver Sagebrush

Lakota *Unspecified* Used as a medicine. (116:35) **Montana Indian** *Dermatological Aid* Decoction of leaves used as a hair restorer. *Dietary Aid* Leaves chewed to allay thirst. *Tonic* Decoction of leaves used as a general tonic. *Unspecified* Decoction of leaves used for various complaints. (15:7)

Artemisia carruthii, Carruth's Sagewort

Navajo, Ramah *Cough Medicine* Infusion of leaves taken for cough. *Dermatological Aid* Cold infusion used as lotion for sores. *Diaphoretic* Leaves used in sweat bath medicine. *Febrifuge* Infusion of leaves taken for fever. *Misc. Disease Remedy* Cold infusion of leaves taken for fever, influenza, and cough. *Panacea* Root used as a "life medicine." *Veterinary Aid* Cold infusion of leaves used as lotion for sheep's sore back. (165:48) **Zuni** *Analgesic* Seeds placed on coals and used as a sweat bath for body pains from a serious cold. (as *A. wrightii* 143:42, 43)

Artemisia douglasiana, Douglas's Sagewort

Costanoan *Analgesic* and *Antirheumatic* (*External*) Decoction of plant used as a compress for rheumatism pain. *Dermatological Aid* Decoction of plant used as a compress for wounds. *Ear Medicine* Poultice of heated leaves applied to the ear for earaches. *Respiratory Aid* Decoction of plant used for asthma. *Urinary Aid* Decoction of plant used for urinary problems. (17:25) **Karok** *Antirheumatic* (*External*) Poultice of leaves applied for rheumatism and arthritis. (5:18) **Kawaiisu** *Abortifacient* Infusion of plant used when the menstrual flow had stopped. *Dermatological Aid* Infusion of plant used as a hair wash to prevent the hair from falling out. *Other* Infusion of plant used as a bath for mother and father after childbirth. *Pediatric Aid* Infusion of plant used to "prevent a girl from aging prematurely." (180:12) **Miwok** *Analgesic* Leaves worn in nostrils for headaches. *Antirheumatic* (*Internal*) Decoction of leaves taken for rheumatism. *Ceremonial Medicine* Leaves worn in nostrils by mourners when crying, the pungent odor clearing the head. *Witchcraft Medi-*

cine Leaves rubbed on body to keep ghosts away. Plant worn on a necklace to prevent dreaming of the dead. Poisoned leaves carried to avoid personal injury. Leaves rubbed on corpse handlers to ward off ghosts of the deceased. (as *A. vulgaris* var. *heterophylla* 8:167) **Paiute** *Analgesic* Poultice of crushed, green leaves used as a compress for headaches. *Misc. Disease Remedy* Burning plant used as an inhalant for grippe. (155:39) **Paiute, Northern** *Cold Remedy* Branches put over a bed of ashes and slept on for colds. *Febrifuge* Branches put over a bed of ashes and slept on for fevers. (49:125) **Pomo, Kashaya** *Analgesic* Decoction or infusion of leaves taken for stomachache and cramps associated with diarrhea. *Dermatological Aid* Poultice of warmed leaves used on baby's severed umbilical cord. Decoction or infusion of leaves used for washing itching sores. *Gastrointestinal Aid* Decoction or infusion of leaves taken for stomachache and cramps associated with diarrhea. *Gynecological Aid* Decoction or infusion of leaves taken to stop excessive menstruation or to ease cramps. (60:119) **Tolowa** *Anthelmintic* Infusion of fresh leaves taken by children for "pin worms." *Antirheumatic* (*External*) Poultice of fresh leaves used for arthritis. Fresh leaves used as a liniment. *Orthopedic Aid* Fresh leaves used as a steamed herb for fractures. *Pediatric Aid* Infusion of fresh leaves taken by children for "pin worms." (5:18) **Washo** *Analgesic* Decoction of leaves used as a wash for headaches. *Antirheumatic* (*External*) Decoction of leaves used as a liniment for rheumatism. (155:39) **Yuki** *Analgesic* Decoction of leaves taken for pains or "troubles inside." Poultice of pounded leaves applied for rheumatism, arthritic or back pains. *Antidiarrheal* Decoction of leaves taken for dysentery. *Antirheumatic* (*External*) Poultice of pounded leaves applied for rheumatism or arthritic pains. *Dermatological Aid* Infusion used as wash and poultice of plant applied to cuts, bruises, and sores. Poultice of chewed leaves applied to spot affected by hunting accident. *Gynecological Aid* Infusion of plant used as a steam bath for difficulties attending childbirth. *Orthopedic Aid* Poultice of pounded plant applied for back pains. *Veterinary Aid* Infusion of plant given to injured animals. (39:45) **Yurok** *Anthelmintic* Infusion of fresh leaves taken by children for "pin worms." *Antirheumatic* (*Exter-*

nal) Poultice of fresh leaves used for arthritis. Fresh leaves used as a liniment. *Orthopedic Aid* Fresh leaves used as a steamed herb for fractures. *Pediatric Aid* Infusion of fresh leaves taken by children for "pin worms." (5:18)

Artemisia dracunculus, Wormwood
Costanoan *Antidiarrheal* Decoction of roots used for dysentery. *Gastrointestinal Aid* Decoction of roots used for infants with colic. *Pediatric Aid* Decoction of roots used for infants with colic. *Urinary Aid* Decoction of roots used for urinary problems. (17:26) **Crow** *Eye Medicine* Infusion of stems and leaves used as an eyewash for snowblindness. Poultice of leaves used for the eyes. **Flathead** *Antirheumatic* (*External*) Infusion of foliage used lukewarm for swollen feet and legs. *Dermatological Aid* Foliage dried, powdered, and used for open sores. (68:45) **Kawaiisu** *Antirheumatic* (*External*) Infusion of leaves used as a wash for rheumatism. (180:13) **Luiseño** *Unspecified* Plant used for medicinal purposes. (132:228) **Okanagan-Colville** *Analgesic* Poultice of mashed, dampened leaves applied to the forehead for headaches. *Antirheumatic* (*External*) Leaves used in a steam bath for rheumatic or arthritic pain. *Dermatological Aid* Leaves used in diapers or used as a diaper for diaper rash and skin rawness. *Gynecological Aid* Leaves used as sanitary napkins. *Pediatric Aid* Leaves used in diapers or used as a diaper for diaper rash and skin rawness.

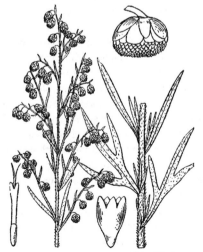

Artemisia dracunculus

Tonic Infusion of roots and yarrow roots taken as a general tonic. (162:76) **Sanpoil** *Cold Remedy* Cold infusion of root used for colds. (109:217) **Shuswap** *Gynecological Aid* Plant used by women at childbirth. *Stimulant* Decoction of leaves and roots used as a bath for tiredness. *Witchcraft Medicine* Plant used to keep away sickness and germs. (102:58) **Thompson** *Antirheumatic* (*External*) Decoction of plant used as a "liniment" for arthritis. *Cold Remedy* Plant used as a wash for colds. *Dermatological Aid* Infusion or decoction of plant used as a bathing solution for swelling and discoloration of bruises. *Pediatric Aid* Plant used as a wash for colds, especially for babies and for chickenpox, to help the itching. *Veterinary Aid* Decoction of plant used after injuries to wash horses' legs every day until healed. (161:169)

Artemisia dracunculus ssp. *dracunculus*, Wormwood

Chippewa *Abortifacient* Decoction of root taken for "stoppage of periods." Infusion or decoction of root or leaf and stalk used for "stoppage of periods." (as *A. dracunculoides* 43:356) *Antidiarrheal* Infusion of dried leaves and tops taken for chronic dysentery. (as *A. dracunculoides* 43:344) *Dermatological Aid* Poultice of chewed, fresh, or dried leaves and flowers applied to wounds. (as *A. dracunculoides* 43:356) Compound decoction of root used as wash to strengthen hair and make it grow. (as *A. dracunculoides* 43:350) *Gynecological Aid* Decoction of root taken for "excessive flowing." Decoction of whole plant taken to aid in difficult labor. (as *A. dracunculoides* 43:356) *Heart Medicine* Infusion of leaf and flower taken or fresh leaf chewed for heart palpitations. (as *A. dracunculoides* 43:338) *Herbal Steam* Strong decoction of root used "for steaming old people to make them stronger." *Pediatric Aid* Strong decoction of root used as a strengthening bath for children. *Strengthener* Decoction of root used as strengthening bath for child and herbal steam for elderly. (as *A. dracunculoides* 43:362) **Navajo, Ramah** *Dermatological Aid* Cold infusion used as lotion for cuts. Used as hair rinse to make hair long and soft. (165:48) **Okanagan** *Analgesic* Infusion of whole plant used as a head wash for headaches. *Antirheumatic* (*External*) Plant used in the sweat house for rheumatism. *Diaphoretic*

Plant used in the sweat house for rheumatism and stiff joints. *Gynecological Aid* Infusion of whole plant used as a bath for women after childbirth. *Orthopedic Aid* Plant used in the sweat house for stiff joints. (104:41) **Omaha** *Abortifacient* Decoction of plant taken for irregular menstruation. *Love Medicine* Chewed root put on clothes as a love charm. *Unspecified* Plant used in the smoke treatment of unspecified illnesses. (58:134) **Paiute** *Antirheumatic* (*External*) Hot decoction of branches used as a wash for rheumatism. Hot poultice of plant tops applied to sprains, swellings, or rheumatism. *Dermatological Aid* Poultice of plant tops applied for swellings. *Gynecological Aid* Decoction of whole plant taken as a tonic after childbirth. *Orthopedic Aid* Poultice of plant tops applied for sprains. *Tonic* Decoction of whole plant taken as a tonic after childbirth. (155:39, 40) **Pawnee** *Antirheumatic* (*External*) Decoction of tops used as a wash for rheumatism. *Unspecified* Plant used in the smoke treatment of unspecified illnesses. **Ponca** *Unspecified* Plant used in the smoke treatment of unspecified illnesses. (58:134) **Shoshoni** *Cathartic* Hot decoction of branches taken as a physic. *Cold Remedy* Hot decoction of branches taken for colds. *Dermatological Aid* Decoction of whole plant used as a wash for nettle stings. *Eye Medicine* Steam from boiling plant used for eye trouble. *Herbal Steam* Steam from boiling plant used for eye trouble. *Throat Aid* Poultice of pulped, green plant applied to sore throat or neck glands. *Venereal Aid* Decoction of whole plant taken or used as a wash for venereal diseases. (155:39, 40) **Thompson** *Analgesic* Infusion of whole plant used as a head wash for headaches. (104:41) Decoction of plant used to wash the head and temples for headache. Fresh plants used as a bed in the sweat bath for aching bones or muscles. (141:463) *Antirheumatic* (*External*) Plant used in the sweat house for rheumatism. (104:41) Fresh plants used as a bed in the sweat bath for rheumatism. (141:463) *Diaphoretic* Plant used in the sweat house for rheumatism and stiff joints. (104:41) Whole plant steamed to cause sweating for rheumatism and other aches. (141:463) *Gynecological Aid* Infusion of whole plant used as a bath for women after childbirth. (104:41) Decoction of plant used as a wash for women after childbirth. (141:463) *Orthopedic Aid* Plant used in the sweat house for stiff joints. (104:41) Plants used in sweat bath for sprains, stiff or aching joints, or muscles. (141:463) *Poison* Plant considered poisonous "if it enters the blood." (141:512) **Winnebago** *Febrifuge* Infusion of plant top sprinkled on the body for fevers. *Love Medicine* Chewed root put on clothes as a love charm. *Unspecified* Plant used in the smoke treatment of unspecified illnesses. (58:134)

Artemisia dracunculus ssp. *glauca*, Dragon Wormwood

Ponca *Burn Dressing* Decoction of plant taken and used as a wash for burns. (as *A. glauca* 80:152)

Artemisia filifolia, Sand Sagebrush

Comanche *Gynecological Aid* Padding of plants placed over hot coals as a bed after childbirth. (24:520) **Hopi** *Dermatological Aid* Plant used for boils. (34:288) Plant used for boils. (174:32, 94) *Gastrointestinal Aid* Infusion of plant and juniper branches taken for indigestion. (34:288) Simple or compound decoction of plant taken for indigestion. (174:33, 94) **Navajo, Ramah** *Snakebite Remedy* Strong infusion taken in large amounts and used as lotion for snakebites. (165:48) **Tewa** *Carminative* Plant chewed or decoction taken for indigestion and flatulence. (115:44) *Dermatological Aid* Plant used for boils. *Gastrointestinal Aid* Infusion of plant and juniper branches taken for indigestion. (34:288) Leaves chewed or decoction taken for indigestion or biliousness. Poultice of plant steeped in boiling water applied to stomach. (115:44)

Artemisia frigida, Fringed Sagewort

Arapaho *Cough Medicine* Infusion of leaves taken as a cough medicine. (98:38) **Blackfoot** *Cold Remedy* Infusion of leaves taken for colds. *Cough Medicine* Infusion of leaves taken for coughs. (82:56) *Dermatological Aid* Poultice of chewed leaves applied to wounds to lessen the swelling. (72:83) *Febrifuge* Decoction of roots or tops taken for "mountain fever." (95:275) *Gastrointestinal Aid* Plant tops chewed and liquid swallowed for heartburn. (82:56) Plant chewed for heartburn. (95:275) *Gynecological Aid* Pad of the plant worn by women during menses to reduce skin irritation.

(72:79) Infusion of plant taken by women during menses. (82:56) *Hemostat* Soft leaves used to stuff a bleeding nostril. (72:83) *Misc. Disease Remedy* Decoction of roots and tops taken for mountain fever. (82:56) *Stimulant* Crushed leaves used to revive gophers after children clubbed them while playing a game. (72:109) *Veterinary Aid* Horses rolled in patches of the plant to treat their wounds. Infusion of plant given to horses for coughing, sneezing, and to clean the sinuses. (72:87) **Cheyenne** *Ceremonial Medicine* Plant used in the Sun Dance ceremony. (69:18) *Gynecological Aid* Infusion of plant taken by women during menses. (82:56) *Hemostat* Plant braid tied around the head for nosebleed. (69:18) **Chippewa** *Anticonvulsive* Compound infusion or decoction of root taken for "fits." (41:63, 64) Compound decoction of root taken for convulsions. (43:336) *Disinfectant* Dried leaves burned to disinfect room of contagious patient. (43:366) *Gastrointestinal Aid* Infusion of leaves taken or leaf smoke inhaled for biliousness. (43:364) *Hemostat* Compound infusion or decoction of root used on bleeding wounds. (41:63, 64) Compound decoction of root used on bleeding wounds. (43:336) *Stimulant* Compound infusion or decoction of root taken or used externally as stimulant. (41:63, 64) Compound decoction of root taken as a stimulant. *Tonic* Compound infusion or decoction of root taken as a tonic. (43:364) **Cree, Woodlands** *Analgesic* Leaves used for headaches associated with fevers. *Febrifuge* Decoction of leaves taken for fevers. (91:30) **Dakota** *Abortifacient* Decoction of plant taken and used as wash for irregular menstruation. (58:134) **Delaware, Oklahoma** *Ceremonial Medicine* Leaves chewed as "ceremonial" medicine. (150:74) **Great Basin Indian** *Antihemorrhagic* Leaves used for stopping a hemorrhage. (100:50) **Isleta** *Gastrointestinal Aid* Infusion of plant used as a stomach medicine. (85:22) **Montana Indian** *Pulmonary Aid* Decoction used for lung troubles. *Tuberculosis Remedy* Decoction used for consumption. (15:7) **Navajo, Ramah** *Cough Medicine* Decoction of leaves taken for cough. *Panacea* Root used as a "life medicine." *Toothache Remedy* Hot poultice of leaves applied for toothache. (165:48) **Okanagan-Colville** *Cold Remedy* Infusion of leaves and branches taken for colds. *Misc. Disease Remedy* Infusion of leaves and branches taken for flu. (162:

76) **Omaha** *Abortifacient* Decoction of plant taken and used as wash for irregular menstruation. **Pawnee** *Abortifacient* Decoction of plant taken and used as wash for irregular menstruation. **Ponca** *Abortifacient* Decoction of plant taken and used as wash for irregular menstruation. (58:134) **Potawatomi** *Stimulant* Leaves and flowers fumed on live coals to revive comatose patient. (131:49) **Sioux** *Abortifacient* Decoction used for menstrual irregularity. (68:45) **Tanana, Upper** *Cancer Treatment* Decoction taken for cancer. *Cold Remedy* Decoction taken for colds. *Cough Medicine* Decoction taken for coughs. *Eye Medicine* Cooled decoction used as a wash for eyes. *Misc. Disease Remedy* Decoction taken for diabetes. (86:17) **Tewa** *Carminative* Leaves chewed or decoction taken for indigestion or flatulence. *Gastrointestinal Aid* Leaves chewed or decoction taken for indigestion or biliousness. Poultice of plant steeped in boiling water applied to stomach for gastritis. (115:54) **Thompson** *Unspecified* Plant used medicinally for unspecified purpose. (141:465) *Venereal Aid* Decoction of plant taken as medicine, possibly for venereal disease. (161:170) **Zuni** *Cold Remedy* Infusion of whole plant taken as a cold remedy. (143:42)

Artemisia furcata var. heterophylla,
Forked Sagewort

Luiseño *Unspecified* Plant used for medicinal purposes. (as *A. heterophylla* 132:228) **Mendocino Indian** *Analgesic* Decoction of leaves taken for headaches. *Antidiarrheal* Decoction of leaves taken for diarrhea. *Antidote* Juice used as an antidote for effects of poison oak. *Antirheumatic (External)* Poultice of leaves applied or leaves used in sweat bath for rheumatism. *Cold Remedy* Decoction of leaves taken or bruised leaves placed in nostril for colds. *Eye Medicine* Decoction of leaves used as a wash for sore eyes. *Febrifuge* Decoction of leaves taken for fevers. *Gastrointestinal Aid* Decoction of leaves taken for colic and stomachaches. *Gynecological Aid* Poultice of leaves applied after childbirth to promote blood circulation. *Herbal Steam* Poultice of leaves applied or leaves used in sweat bath for rheumatism. *Respiratory Aid* Decoction of leaves taken for bronchitis. (as *A. heterophylla* 33:392) **Paiute** *Febrifuge* and *Pedi-*

atric Aid Steeped leaves put next to a baby's skin for fever. (as *A. heterophylla* 98:40)

Artemisia ludoviciana, Louisiana Sagewort

Blackfoot *Dermatological Aid* Leaves put into moccasins as a foot deodorant. (72:124) Poultice of leaves applied to blisters and burst boils. (72:75) *Pediatric Aid* Leaves chewed, especially by children, during the sweat for respiratory disorders. *Pulmonary Aid* Infusion of leaves taken for chest constrictions. *Respiratory Aid* Leaves chewed, especially by children, during the sweat for respiratory disorders. *Throat Aid* Infusion of leaves taken for throat constrictions. (72:71) *Veterinary Aid* Infusion of plant given to horses for coughing, sneezing, and to clean the sinuses. (72:87) **Cheyenne** *Analgesic* Snuff of crushed leaves used for headache. (68:44) Crushed leaves used as snuff for headaches. *Ceremonial Medicine* Plant used in ceremonies. *Hemostat* Crushed leaves used as snuff for nosebleeds. (69:18) *Nose Medicine* Leaves crushed and used as a snuff for nosebleeds. *Respiratory Aid* Leaves crushed and used as a snuff for sinuses. (68:44) Crushed leaves used as snuff for sinus attacks. (69:18) *Unspecified* Plants rubbed on the body for immunity to sickness. (68:44) **Comanche** *Dermatological Aid* Leaves chewed and used for insect and spider bites. (84:7) **Crow** *Dermatological Aid* Salve of plants and neck fat used for sores. Infusion used as an astringent for eczema, and for underarm and foot

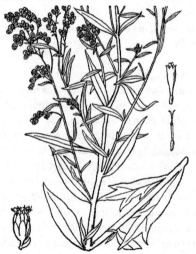

Artemisia ludoviciana

perspiration and odor. **Flathead** *Cold Remedy* Infusion used for colds. *Dermatological Aid* Infusion used for bruises and itching. **Gros Ventre** *Febrifuge* Infusion used for high fevers. (68:44) **Havasupai** *Unspecified* Sprays used in the sweat baths or infusion of leaves taken for sicknesses. (171:245) **Kutenai** *Dermatological Aid* Decoction of plants used for sores. (68:44) **Lakota** *Antidiarrheal* Infusion used for diarrhea. *Cold Remedy* Infusion used for colds. *Throat Aid* Infusion used for sore throats. (88:46) **Meskwaki** *Dermatological Aid* Poultice of leaves applied to old sores. Tincture of leaves used for old sores, especially scrofulous sores. *Throat Aid* Infusion of leaves taken for tonsillitis and sore throat. *Tuberculosis Remedy* Tincture of leaves used for old sores, especially scrofulous sores. *Veterinary Aid* Smudge of leaves used to "smoke ponies when they have the distemper." (129:211) **Mewuk** *Cathartic* Infusion of plant used as a mild cathartic. *Dermatological Aid* Poultice of bruised leaves applied to cuts and sores. (97:366) *Disinfectant* Infusion of plant used as a disinfectant to wash the bodies of the mourners after funerals. (97:353) *Gastrointestinal Aid* Infusion of plant used for indigestion. (97:366) *Other* Plant worn around the neck by orphans after parents death to keep the ghost away and prevent sickness. (97:353) *Panacea* Small bundles of plant made into necklaces to keep disease away. (97:336) *Unspecified* Plant used as a medicine. (as *A. lucoviciana* 97:338) Infusion of plant taken, used as a wash, or poultice applied as medicine. (97:353) *Veterinary Aid* Used for horses with sore backs. (97:366) **Navajo** *Unspecified* Used by the medicine men. (45:81) **Navajo, Ramah** *Panacea* Root used as a "life medicine." (165:48) **Ojibwa** *Veterinary Aid* Plant used as a horse medicine. (130:363) **Okanagan-Colville** *Carminative* Infusion of plant taken and splashed on the body during sweat bathing to "clear his wind." *Strengthener* Infusion of plant taken and splashed on body during sweat bathing by hunters, to walk long distances. (162:78) **Poliklah** *Eye Medicine* Poultice of plant applied to sore eyes. (97:173) **Thompson** *Antirheumatic* (*External*) Decoction of plant used as a "liniment" for arthritis. *Cold Remedy* Decoction of plant used as a wash for colds. Hot decoction of plant taken, especially by the elderly, for colds. *Disinfectant* Plant

used as incense to disinfect the house. *Gastrointestinal Aid* Plant used for overeating or indigestion. *Misc. Disease Remedy* Hot decoction of plant taken, especially by the elderly, for influenza. *Orthopedic Aid* Poultice of plant boiled with "any kind of weeds" and used on injured areas as a bone setter. (161:170) **Yokut** *Unspecified* Used as medicine. (as *A. lucoviciana* 97:437) **Yurok, South Coast (Nererner)** *Dermatological Aid* Infusion of plant used for itching skin and as a lotion for sores. *Eye Medicine* Infusion of plant used for sore eyes. (97:169)

Artemisia ludoviciana ssp. *incompta*, Mountain Sagewort

Bella Coola *Unspecified* Used as a medicine. **Carrier, Northern** *Analgesic* Hot infusion of plant taken for headache. **Carrier, Southern** *Dermatological Aid* Poultice of chewed plant applied to sprains and swellings. *Orthopedic Aid* Poultice of chewed leaves applied to sprains. (as *A. discolor* 127:65)

Artemisia ludoviciana ssp. *ludoviciana*, Foothill Sagewort

Cheyenne *Ceremonial Medicine* Plant used in ceremonies. *Psychological Aid* Plant used to drive away bad or ominous dreams. (as *A. gnaphalodes* 63:190) **Chippewa** *Antidote* Dried flowers placed on coals and the fumes used as an antidote to "bad medicine." (as *A. gnaphalodes* 43:376) Smoke of burned flowers inhaled as antidote for "bad medicine." (as *A. gnaphalodes* 43:366) **Keres, Western** *Antirheumatic* (*External*) Crushed plant rubbed on body as a liniment for soreness or stiffness. *Diaphoretic* Plant used as an ingredient in the sweat bath. *Other* Plant placed in shoes to keep feet from sweating. (as *A. gnaphaloides* 147:28) **Kiowa** *Gastrointestinal Aid* Infusion of plants taken for stomach troubles. *Pulmonary Aid* Infusion of plants taken for the lungs or to cut phlegm. (as *A. gnaphalodes* 166:56) **Omaha** *Ceremonial Medicine* Plant used in rites of lustration for humans or beasts. (as *A. gnaphaloides* 56:321) *Febrifuge* Decoction of leaves used as a bath for fevers. *Hemostat* Dried, powdered leaves applied to nostrils for nasal hemorrhage. (as *A. gnaphalodes* 56:334) **Paiute** *Analgesic* Decoction of plant used as a soaking bath for aching feet. Hot or cold decoction of whole plant or young growth taken for stomachaches. Poultice of steamed plants or bruised leaves used for rheumatism or other aches. Poultice of steeped leaves used as a compress for headaches. *Antidiarrheal* Decoction of plant taken for diarrhea. *Antirheumatic* (*External*) Branches used in a sweat bath for rheumatism. Poultice of steamed plants or bruised leaves used for rheumatism or other aches. *Dermatological Aid* Decoction of plant used as a wash for rashes, itching, or skin eruptions. Poultice of leaves or stems and leaves applied to swellings, boils, and sores. *Disinfectant* Branches used as a bed in a sweat bath to steam out infection of influenza. *Eye Medicine* Decoction of leaves used as an eyewash. *Febrifuge* Poultice of steeped leaves used, especially for babies, as a compress for fevers. *Gastrointestinal Aid* Decoction of whole plant or shoots taken for stomachaches. *Gynecological Aid* Decoction of root or entire plant taken as a tonic after childbirth. Infusion of leaves used as a regulator of menstrual disorders. *Herbal Steam* and *Misc. Disease Remedy* Branches used as a bed in a sweat bath to steam out infection of influenza. *Orthopedic Aid* Decoction of plant used as a soaking bath for aching feet. *Pediatric Aid* Poultice of steeped leaves used, especially for babies, as a compress for fevers. *Tonic* Decoction of root or entire plant taken as a tonic after childbirth. *Venereal Aid* Decoction of plant tops taken for venereal diseases. (as *A. gnaphalodes* 155:40–42) **Sanpoil** *Analgesic* Leaves placed in the nostrils for an hour for a headache. *Cold Remedy* Leaves placed in the nostrils for an hour for a cold. *Dermatological Aid* Pulverized leaves sprinkled on sores "to hasten their healing." (as *A. vulgaris* var. *ludoviciana* 109:217) **Shoshoni** *Analgesic* Decoction of leaves taken for headaches. Hot or cold decoction of whole plant or young growth taken for stomachaches. Poultice of steeped leaves used, especially for babies, as a compress for fevers. *Antidiarrheal* Decoction of plant tops taken for diarrhea. *Cathartic* Decoction of whole plant or shoots taken as a physic. *Cold Remedy* Compound decoction of plant tops taken for colds. Compound decoction of whole plant taken for heavy colds. Decoction of branches taken in small doses for colds. Decoction of leaves taken for colds. Decoction of tops alone, or sometimes with roots, taken for colds.

Cough Medicine Compound decoction of plant tops taken for coughs. Compound decoction of whole plant or plant tops taken for coughs. Compound decoction of whole plant taken for coughs. Decoction of branches taken in small doses for coughs. Simple or compound decoction of leaves taken for coughs. *Dermatological Aid* Decoction of plant used as a wash for rashes, itching, or skin eruptions. *Disinfectant* Decoction of plant tops taken for severe infections. *Eye Medicine* Infusion of leaves used as an eyewash. *Febrifuge* Compound decoction of whole plant taken for fevers. Poultice of steeped leaves used, especially for babies, as a compress for fevers. *Gastrointestinal Aid* Decoction of whole plant or shoots taken for stomachaches. *Gynecological Aid* Infusion of leaves used as a regulator of menstrual disorders. *Misc. Disease Remedy* Decoction of branches taken for influenza. *Pediatric Aid* Poultice of steeped leaves used, especially for babies, as a compress for fevers. **Washo** *Analgesic* Decoction of leaves taken and used as a cooling, aromatic wash for headaches. *Cold Remedy* Decoction of leaves taken for "heavy colds" and head colds. *Cough Medicine* Decoction of leaves taken for colds, coughs, and headaches. (as *A. gnaphalodes* 155:40–42)

***Artemisia ludoviciana* ssp. *mexicana*,** Mexican White Sagebrush
Kiowa *Dermatological Aid* Poultice of chewed leaves applied to sores. *Herbal Steam* Plant used as a purifying agent in the sweat house. *Throat Aid* Leaves chewed for sore throats. (as *A. mexicana* 166:56)

***Artemisia nova*,** Black Sagebrush
Shoshoni *Cold Remedy* Decoction of leaves taken for colds. *Cough Medicine* Decoction of leaves taken for coughs. (155:43)

***Artemisia spinescens*,** Bud Sagebrush
Paiute *Analgesic* Decoction of branches taken for chronic stomach troubles and cramps. *Antirheumatic* (*External*) Decoction of stems and leaves used as a wash for rheumatism. *Cold Remedy* Decoction of root taken for colds. *Cough Medicine* Decoction of root taken for coughs. *Dermatological Aid* Green leaves rubbed on bed patients to prevent bedsores. Mashed, green leaves mixed

with tobacco and used as a salve for sores or bruises. Poultice of mashed, green leaves applied to "draw out boils." Poultice of mashed green leaves or young branches applied to swellings. *Diuretic* Decoction of flowers and leaves taken for "stoppage of the bladder." *Gastrointestinal Aid* Decoction of branches taken for stomach trouble, cramps, or indigestion. *Pulmonary Aid* Decoction of root taken for chest congestion, coughs, or colds. Strained decoction of leaves and flowers taken for tubercular hemorrhage. (155:43, 44) *Urinary Aid* Plant juice heated and taken for bladder trouble. (98:41) **Shoshoni** *Dermatological Aid* Crushed, moistened leaves rubbed onto the skin for irritations and rashes. Poultice of whole plant, either fresh or boiled, applied to rash or itch. *Hemostat* Decoction of leaves sniffed for nosebleed. *Misc. Disease Remedy* Decoction of whole plant taken and used as a wash for influenza. *Pulmonary Aid* Decoction of branches taken for tubercular hemorrhage. (155:43, 44)

Artemisia tilesii, Tilesius's Wormwood
Eskimo *Cancer Treatment* Plant used as an antitumor agent. *Disinfectant* Plant used as an infection inhibitor. *Febrifuge* Plant used as a fever medicine. (126:326) **Eskimo, Alaska** *Antirheumatic* (*External*) Infusion of fresh or dried leaves used for arthritic-like ailments. Infusion of stems used for discomfort of swollen areas. *Hemostat* Poultice of leaves used to stop bleeding. *Laxative* Infusion of seed heads and plant tops used as a laxative. *Respiratory Aid* Plant boiled and the vapors inhaled for congestion. *Tonic* Infusion of plant taken daily as a tonic. (1:38) **Eskimo, Inuktitut** *Dermatological Aid* Poultice of plant applied to skin infections. (176:186) **Eskimo, Kuskokwagmiut** *Dermatological Aid* Poultice of dried, shredded plant applied to skin infections. *Orthopedic Aid* Plant used as switch during steam bath for a sprained or sore limb. (101:33) **Eskimo, Western** *Gastrointestinal Aid* Decoction of plant taken for stomachache. (90:13) *Orthopedic Aid* Poultice of heated leaves applied to painful joint and used internally. (90:5, 13) **Tanaina** *Antirheumatic* (*Internal*) Plant used for diseases from rheumatism to tuberculosis. *Misc. Disease Remedy* Plant used for diseases from rheumatism to tuberculosis. *Tuberculosis Remedy* Plant used for diseases from

rheumatism to tuberculosis. (126:329) **Tanana, Upper** *Antirheumatic* (*External*) Decoction of above-the-ground part of the plant used as a body wash for aches and pains. Poultice of leaves applied or decoction of leaves used as a wash for swellings and body aches. *Blood Medicine* Poultice of leaves applied or decoction of leaves used as a wash for blood poisoning. *Cough Medicine* Leaves chewed for coughs. *Dermatological Aid* Poultice of leaves applied or decoction of leaves used as a wash for skin rashes and cuts. *Disinfectant* Poultice of leaves applied or decoction of leaves used as a wash for infections. *Eye Medicine* Decoction of above-the-ground part of the plant used as an eyewash. *Oral Aid* Decoction of above-the-ground part of the plant taken for mouth sores. (86:17)

Artemisia tridentata, Big Sagebrush
Cahuilla *Disinfectant* Dried leaves and stems burned, in the homes and sweat houses, as a disinfectant. *Respiratory Aid* Dried leaves and stems burned, in the homes and sweat houses, as an air purifier. (11:43) **Coahuilla** *Gastrointestinal Aid* Decoction of leaves taken for stomach complaints. (9:78) **Diegueño** *Cold Remedy*, *Cough Medicine*, and *Respiratory Aid* Infusion of fresh or dried leaves taken for a bad cold with coughing and bronchitis. (74:220) **Flathead** *Cold Remedy* Infusion taken for colds. *Pulmonary Aid* Infusion taken for pneumonia. (68:45) **Gosiute** *Antirheumatic* (*External*) and *Antirheumatic* (*Internal*) Plant

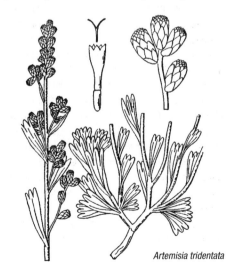

Artemisia tridentata

used externally and internally for rheumatism. *Cold Remedy* Plant used for colds. *Cough Medicine* Plant used for coughs. *Febrifuge* Plant used for fevers. (31:351) Infusion of leaves used for febrile conditions. (31:363) *Panacea* Plant used as a panacea. (31:351) **Havasupai** *Cold Remedy* Stems and leaves used for colds. *Cough Medicine* Stems and leaves used for coughs. *Dermatological Aid* Decoction of leafy stems and leaves used as a wash for sores or pimples. *Gastrointestinal Aid* Stems and leaves used for intestinal upset. *Nose Medicine* Stems and leaves used for runny noses. *Throat Aid* Stems and leaves used for sore throats. (171:246) **Hopi** *Gastrointestinal Aid* Plant used for digestive disorders. (174:34, 94) *Orthopedic Aid* Infusion of leaves taken for ailing ilium. (46:17) **Kawaiisu** *Analgesic* Decoction of plant fumes inhaled for headaches. *Cold Remedy* Decoction of plant fumes inhaled for head colds and chest colds. Decoction or infusion of leaves taken for bad colds. *Cough Medicine* Infusion of leaves taken for colds and coughs. *Herbal Steam* Decoction of plant fumes inhaled for head colds, chest colds, and headaches. *Misc. Disease Remedy* Decoction of leaves taken for influenza or bad colds. (180:13) **Klamath** *Antidiarrheal* Decoction of herbage used internally for diarrhea. (37:105) Decoction of herbs taken for diarrhea. (140:131) *Antirheumatic (External)* Poultice of herbage used as a substitute for liniment. *Eye Medicine* Decoction of herbage used as an eyewash. (37:105) Decoction of herbs used as an eyewash. *Orthopedic Aid* Smashed herbs used as substitute for liniment. (140:131) **Lakota** *Unspecified* Used as a medicine. (116:36) **Montana Indian** *Antidiarrheal* Decoction of herb taken for diarrhea. *Eye Medicine* Decoction of herb used externally as an eyewash. *Orthopedic Aid* Mashed herbs used as a substitute for liniment and as a poultice. (15:7) **Navajo** *Analgesic* Compound of plants used for headaches. (45:81) *Ceremonial Medicine* Plant used for religious and medicinal ceremonies. (76:158) *Cold Remedy* Plant used for colds. *Febrifuge* Plant used for fevers. *Gastrointestinal Aid* Decoction of plants taken for stomachaches. *Gynecological Aid* Infusion of plants taken by women as an aid for deliverance. *Sports Medicine* Plant taken before long hikes and athletic contests to rid the body of lingering, undesirable things. (45:81) **Navajo, Kayenta** *Laxative* Plant used for constipation. *Snakebite Remedy* Infusion of plant taken and used as a lotion for water snake bites. (179:45) **Navajo, Ramah** *Analgesic* Decoction of leaves taken for postpartum pain. *Cough Medicine* Decoction of leaves taken for "big cough." *Dermatological Aid* Poultice of wet leaves applied to swellings. *Diaphoretic* Plant used in a sweat bath medicine. *Gynecological Aid* Decoction of leaves taken for postpartum pain. *Veterinary Aid* Cold infusion of leaves used as lotion for cuts on sheep. (165:48) **Okanagan-Colville** *Cold Remedy* Decoction of leaves and branches taken for colds. Infusion of roots taken for colds. *Diaphoretic* Decoction of leaves and branches taken to cause sweating during a cold. *Oral Aid* Decoction of leaves and branches taken for tonsillitis. *Throat Aid* Decoction of leaves and branches taken for sore throats. Infusion of roots taken for sore throats. (162:78) **Paiute** *Analgesic* Burning plant used as an inhalant for headache. Decoction of branches taken for headache. Decoction of branches taken for stomachaches, especially children's. (155:44–47) *Ceremonial Medicine* Sagebrush used by dancers to pat themselves to be made spiritually clean, curing ceremonies. (93:119) *Cold Remedy* Plant chewed for colds. (144:317) Burning branches used as an inhalant for head colds. Compound decoction of plant tops taken for colds. Decoction of leaves taken or raw leaves eaten for colds. Poultice of mashed, green leaves applied for chest colds. (155:44–47) *Dermatological Aid* Poultice of mashed leaves applied to burns and sores. Infusion of leaves applied to the scalp as a hair tonic. (93:119) Decoction of leaves used as an antiseptic wash for cuts, wounds, or sores. Poultice of wet, steeped leaves applied to bullet wounds. Pulverized leaves used as a talcum powder for babies. (155:44–47) *Diaphoretic* Infusion of leaves taken to produce sweating during a fever. (144:317) *Disinfectant* Decoction of leaves used as an antiseptic wash for cuts, wounds, or sores. (155:44–47) *Emetic* Infusion of leaves taken as an emetic for respiratory diseases. (93:119) *Febrifuge* Infusion of leaves taken to produce sweating during a fever. (144:317) Decoction of leaves taken for malarial fever. (155:44–47) *Gastrointestinal Aid* Leaves chewed for indigestion. (98:45) Plant chewed for stomach disorders. (144:317) Decoction of branches used for stomachaches, especially children's. Raw leaves chewed for indigestion. *Gynecological Aid* Decoction of plant taken as a general tonic, especially after childbirth. *Misc. Disease Remedy* Decoction of leaves taken for malarial fever. *Orthopedic Aid* Decoction of branches used as liniment for lumbago, muscular cramps and sore feet. *Pediatric Aid* Decoction of branches used for stomachaches, especially children's. Finely pulverized dried leaves used as a baby powder. *Pulmonary Aid* Compound decoction of leaves taken and poultice of decoction used for pneumonia. Poultice of mashed, green leaves applied for chest colds. (155:44–47) *Respiratory Aid* Infusion of leaves taken as an emetic for respiratory diseases. (93:119) *Tonic* Decoction of plant taken as a general tonic, especially after childbirth. (155:44–47) **Paiute, Northern** *Analgesic* Small plant pieces stuffed into the nostrils for headaches. Decoction of leaves taken for headaches. *Antidiarrheal* Decoction of leaves taken for diarrhea. *Antirheumatic* (*External*) Poultice of ground leaves and tobacco applied to swellings on adults or children. *Cold Remedy* Decoction of leaves taken for colds. Small plant pieces stuffed into the nostrils for colds. (49:128) Branches put over a bed of ashes and slept on for colds. (49:125) *Emetic* Decoction of leaves taken as an emetic. *Febrifuge* Poultice of ground leaves and cold water applied to the body for fevers. Poultice of ground leaves and tobacco applied to children for fevers. (49:128) Branches put over a bed of ashes and slept on for fevers. (49:125) *Pediatric Aid* Poultice of ground leaves and tobacco applied to children for fevers. Poultice of ground leaves and tobacco applied to swellings on adults or children. *Stimulant* Blossoms dipped in water and the blossomed branch used to comb the hair for fainting spells. (49:128) **Salish** *Cold Remedy* Plant used for colds. (153:294) **Sanpoil** *Cold Remedy* Infusion of pulverized leaves and stems taken for colds. *Diaphoretic* Infusion of stem tips and seedpods taken as a diaphoretic. *Gastrointestinal Aid* Infusion of stem tips and seedpods taken for indigestion and biliousness. *Laxative* Various infusions of leaves, stems, and seedpods taken as laxatives. *Misc. Disease Remedy* Infusion of pulverized leaves and stems taken for "la grippe." *Tuberculosis Remedy* Infusion of stem tips and seedpods taken for indigestion and tuberculosis. (109:217)

Shoshoni *Analgesic* Decoction of branches taken for stomach cramps. Decoction of leaves used as a wash for headaches. Hot poultice of branches applied for various aches and pains. Poultice of crushed, moistened, green leaves applied to forehead for headache. *Antidote* Decoction of leaves taken or leaf chewed as an antidote for any poisoning. *Antirheumatic* (*External*) Poultice of boiled branches applied for aches and pains, especially rheumatism. *Cold Remedy* Compound decoction of plant tops taken for colds. Decoction of leaves taken or raw leaves eaten for colds. *Cough Medicine* Decoction of branches with salt taken for coughs. Decoction of leaves and salt taken for pneumonia coughs. *Dermatological Aid* Decoction of branches used for red ant bites. Decoction of leaves used as an antiseptic wash for cuts, wounds, or sores. Poultice of leaf decoction or powdered branches used for sores, cuts, or wounds. *Diaphoretic* Decoction of leaves taken to cause sweating and break a fever. *Disinfectant* Decoction of leaves used as an antiseptic wash for cuts, wounds, or sores. Warm decoction of leaves used as an antiseptic bath for newborns. *Emetic* Decoction of plant tops taken for colds and an overdose acts as an emetic. *Eye Medicine* Poultice of steeped leaves applied to inflamed eyes. *Febrifuge* Decoction of leaves taken to cause sweating and break a fever. (155:44–47) *Gastrointestinal Aid* Leaves chewed for indigestion. (98:45) Hot decoction of branches taken for stomach cramps. Raw leaves chewed for indigestion. *Gynecological Aid* Decoction of plant taken as a general tonic, especially after childbirth. *Orthopedic Aid* Decoction of branches used as a wash or liniment for lumbago or muscular cramps. *Pediatric Aid* Decoction of leaves used as a warm antiseptic bath for newborn babies. *Pulmonary Aid* Decoction of leaves with salt taken for cough of pneumonia. *Throat Aid* Strained decoction of leaves gargled for sore throat. *Tonic* Decoction of plant taken as a general tonic, especially after childbirth. *Toothache Remedy* Poultice of mashed leaves applied to cheek for toothache. (155:44–47) **Shuswap** *Cold Remedy* Decoction of plants inhaled for a bad cold. *Disinfectant* Plant used to fumigate the house and keep germs off. *Witchcraft Medicine* Plant used to fumigate the house and keep germs off. (102:58) **Tewa** *Carminative* Leaves eaten as a carminative. *Cough Medi-*

cine Leaves eaten as a cough remedy and expectorant. *Expectorant* Leaves chewed and swallowed as an expectorant. *Gastrointestinal Aid* Leaves eaten for indigestion. (115:45) **Thompson** *Antirheumatic* (*External*) Decoction of plant used as a bath to "rest your bones" and relax you. Decoction of plant used as a bath for muscular ailments. (161:172) *Cold Remedy* Decoction of leaves taken and poultice or plugs of leaves used in nostrils for colds. (141:459) Decoction of leafless twigs taken for colds. Decoction of branches taken for colds. One informant's mother said that this sage was too strong and powerful to drink. She said, "you wouldn't have any more kids. No children." She said that seems to close something up in one's system, that it is just too powerful. Weak decoction of plant used as a wash for colds. *Panacea* Dried branch smoke used to fumigate the house, to protect the inhabitants against sickness. (161:172) *Stimulant* Bruised leaves used as an inhalant to revive a patient. (141:459) *Throat Aid* Decoction of leafless twigs taken for laryngitis. (161:172) *Tuberculosis Remedy* Decoction of stems and leaves taken for consumption and colds. (141:459) **Ute** *Unspecified* Decoction of leaves used as a medicine. (30:32) **Washo** *Cold Remedy* Decoction of leaves taken for colds. *Disinfectant* Branches burned as fumigant for sickroom or for utensils used for childbirth. *Tonic* Decoction of plant taken as a general tonic. (155:44–47) **Zuni** *Antirheumatic* (*External*) Infusion of leaves used for body aches. *Cold Remedy* Infusion of leaves taken as a cold medicine. *Dermatological Aid* Leaves in shoes used for athlete's foot infection, fissures between toes, and foot deodorant. (22:374)

Artemisia tripartita, Threetip Sagebrush
Okanagan-Colville *Cold Remedy* Infusion of roots taken for colds. Decoction of leaves and branches taken for colds. *Diaphoretic* Decoction of leaves and branches taken to cause sweating during a cold. *Oral Aid* Decoction of leaves and branches taken for tonsillitis. *Throat Aid* Infusion of roots taken for sore throats. Decoction of leaves and branches taken for sore throats. (162:79)

Artemisia tripartita ssp. ***tripartita***, Idaho Threetip Sagebrush
Navajo *Analgesic* Plant used for headaches. (as *A.*

trifida 45:97) *Ceremonial Medicine* Plant burned to charcoal and given to patient to blacken legs and forearms in Mountain Chant Ceremony. *Dermatological Aid* Infusion of plant used as a wash for wounds caused by removed corns. (as *A. trifida* 45:82)

Artemisia vulgaris, Common Wormwood
Karok *Analgesic* Infusion of plant taken by women for the pains of afterbirth. *Cold Remedy* Poultice of branches applied for colds. *Gynecological Aid* Infusion of plant taken by women for the pains of afterbirth. *Panacea* Poultice of branches applied for any kind of sickness. (125:390) **Kiowa** *Anthelmintic* Plant used as a "worm" medicine. (166:57) **Miwok** *Analgesic* Leaves worn in nostrils for headaches. *Antirheumatic* (*Internal*) Decoction of leaves taken for rheumatism. *Ceremonial Medicine* Leaves worn in nostrils by mourners when crying, the pungent odor clearing the head. *Witchcraft Medicine* Leaves rubbed on body to keep ghosts away. Plant worn on a necklace to prevent dreaming of the dead. Poisoned leaves carried to avoid personal injury. Leaves rubbed on corpse handlers to ward off ghosts of the deceased. (8:167) **Paiute** *Cold Remedy* Poultice of crushed leaves applied to the chest for colds. (87:197) *Dermatological Aid* Decoction of tops applied to gonorrheal sores. *Orthopedic Aid* Plant used for female backache and knee-ache. *Venereal Aid* Decoction of tops applied to gonorrheal sores. (144:317) **Pomo** *Dermatological Aid* Poultice of heated leaves applied to newborn baby's navel. *Gynecological Aid* Decoction of leaves taken to stop excessive menstruation. Plant used in childbirth. *Pediatric Aid* Poultice of heated leaves applied to newborn baby's navel. (54:15) **Tlingit** *Herbal Steam* and *Pulmonary Aid* Plant taken or used in steam bath for pleurisy. (89:283)

Artemisia vulgaris var. ***kamtschatica***,
    Kamtschat's Wormwood
Aleut *Antirheumatic* (*External*) Heated plant used externally as a "switch" for rheumatism. (as *A. unalaskensis* 6:426) *Dermatological Aid* Poultice of heated leaves applied to minor cuts. *Orthopedic Aid* Poultice of heated leaves applied to sore muscles. (as *A. unalaskensis* 6:425) *Tonic* Decoc-

tion of leaves taken as a tonic, especially good "for dying persons." (as *A. unalaskensis* 6:427)

Artocarpus altilis, Breadfruit
Hawaiian *Dermatological Aid* Milk and other plants used for skin diseases, boils, cuts, and cracked skin. *Oral Aid* Milk and other plants used for mouth sores. (as *A. incisa* 2:38)

Aruncus dioicus, Bride's Feathers
Cherokee *Dermatological Aid* Beaten root applied to bee stings on the face. *Eye Medicine* Beaten root applied to bee stings on the eye. *Gynecological Aid* Infusion of root used to prevent excessive bleeding at childbirth. *Orthopedic Aid* Infusion of root used to bathe swollen feet. *Urinary Aid* Infusion taken for excessive urination. (66:36) **Haihais** *Unspecified* Roots used medicinally for unspecified purpose. **Kitasoo** *Unspecified* Roots used medicinally for unspecified purpose. (35:342) **Thompson** *Gastrointestinal Aid* Decoction of washed roots taken for internal ailments. Infusion of plant taken for internal wounds and stomach problems. *Misc. Disease Remedy* Decoction of washed roots taken for influenza. It was said that too much of the decoction should not be taken because it would make you sick. (161:257)

Aruncus dioicus* var. *acuminatus, Bride's Feathers
Thompson *Cold Remedy* Decoction of root taken for colds and influenza. *Dermatological Aid* Decoction of root taken for "swellings" and stalk ashes and grease used as a salve. *Gastrointestinal Aid* Decoction of root taken for indigestion and general stomach disorders. *Misc. Disease Remedy* Decoction of roots taken for colds and influenza. *Orthopedic Aid* Salve of stalk ashes and grease used for paralysis. (as *A. acuminatus* 141:457)

Aruncus dioicus* var. *vulgaris, Bride's Feathers
Bella Coola *Analgesic* Decoction of root taken for stomach pain. (as *A. sylvester* 127:59) *Antidiarrheal* Infusion of roots used for diarrhea. (as *A. sylvester* 158:208) *Diuretic* Decoction of root taken as a diuretic and for gonorrhea. *Gastrointestinal Aid* Decoction of root taken for stomach pain. (as *A. sylvester* 127:59) Infusion of roots used for

stomach pain. (as *A. sylvester* 158:208) *Misc. Disease Remedy* Decoction of root in grease of mountain goat taken for smallpox. *Venereal Aid* Decoction of root taken for gonorrhea and stomach pain. (as *A. sylvester* 127:59) **Klallam** *Dermatological Aid* Salve of root ashes rubbed on sores. (as *A. sylvester* 65:33) **Kwakiutl** *Cough Medicine* Scraped roots held in the mouth for coughs. Dried root held in mouth for cough. (as *A. aruncus* 16:381) Dried, soaked root held in the mouth for coughing. *Love Medicine* Root used as a love charm. (as *A. sylvester* 157:288) **Lummi** *Dermatological Aid* Plant used for sores. *Misc. Disease Remedy* Raw leaves chewed for smallpox. (as *A. sylvester* 65:33) **Makah** *Antirheumatic (External)* Infusion of roots used for rheumatism. (as *A. sylvester* 55:261) *Dermatological Aid* Plant used for sores. (as *A. sylvester* 65:33) *Internal Medicine* Root juice taken for internal healing. (as *A. sylvester* 55:261) *Kidney Aid* Infusion of roots taken for kidney trouble. (as *A. sylvester* 65:33) Mixture of pounded roots taken for kidney pain. (as *A. sylvester* 160:116) *Unspecified* Used for medicine. Roots used to make a very good medicine. (as *A. sylvester* 55:261) *Venereal Aid* Infusion of roots taken for gonorrhea. (as *A. sylvester* 65:33) **Nitinaht** *Febrifuge* Infusion of pounded roots taken for bad fevers. *Misc. Disease Remedy* Infusion of pounded roots taken for measles-like illnesses. (as *A. sylvester* 160:116) **Quileute** *Dermatological Aid* Poultice of scraped roots applied to sores. *Tonic* Infusion of pounded roots taken as a general tonic. **Quinault** *Dermatological Aid* Plant used for sores. **Skagit** *Cold Remedy* Infusion of roots taken for colds. *Dermatological Aid* Plant used for sores. *Throat Aid* Infusion of roots taken for sore throats. Poultice of twig and root ashes with bear grease applied to throat swellings. (as *A. sylvester* 65:33) **Tlingit** *Blood Medicine* Infusion of root used for "diseases of the blood." (as *Spiraea aruncus* 89:283)

Arundinaria gigantea, Giant Cane
Houma *Kidney Aid* and *Stimulant* Decoction of root taken to stimulate the kidneys and "renew strength." (as *A. macrosperma* 135:61) **Seminole** *Cathartic* Decoction of root used as a cathartic. (145:275)

Arundinaria gigantea ssp. tecta, Switch Cane
Choctaw *Analgesic* Decoction of roots taken for breast pain. (as *A. tecta* 152:6) **Houma** *Kidney Aid* and *Stimulant* Decoction of root taken to stimulate the kidneys and "renew strength." (as *A. tecta* 135:61)

Arundo donax, Giant Reed
Cahuilla *Orthopedic Aid* Used as a splint for broken limbs. (11:102)

Asarum canadense, Canadian Wildginger
Abnaki *Cold Remedy* Decoction of plant and another plant used for colds. (121:166) *Cough Medicine* Used for coughs. (121:154) **Algonquin, Quebec** *Anticonvulsive* Infusion of roots given to infants for convulsions. *Febrifuge* Infusion of roots taken for fevers. *Pediatric Aid* Infusion of roots given to infants for convulsions. (14:159) **Cherokee** *Abortifacient* Used for "scant or painful menstruation" and infusion taken "to start periods." (66:35, 36) *Analgesic* Decoction of plant taken to cause vomiting for stomach pain. (152:21) *Anthelmintic* Root used as powerful stimulant and for worms. *Antidiarrheal* Infusion taken for "flux." *Blood Medicine* Compound infusion of root used "for blood." (66:35, 36) *Breast Treatment* Infusion of whole plant used as a wash for swollen breasts. (152:21) *Cold Remedy* Root used for colds. *Cough Medicine* Root used for coughs. *Dermatological Aid* Fresh leaves applied to wounds and liquid or salve used on sores. (66:35, 36)

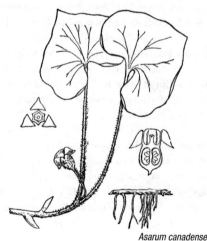
Asarum canadense

Emetic Infusion of plant taken as an emetic for swollen breasts and stomach pain. (152:21) *Eye Medicine* Snuff of dried leaves used for head and eyes. *Febrifuge* Taken for typhus fever, "ague and fever." *Gastrointestinal Aid* Compound infusion used for poor digestion. (66:35, 36) Decoction of plant taken to cause vomiting for stomach pain. (152:21) *Gynecological Aid* Used for "scant or painful menstruation" and infusion taken to start periods. *Heart Medicine* Compound infusion used for poor digestion and infusion of root used "for heart trouble." *Misc. Disease Remedy* Taken for typhus fever, "ague and fever." *Sedative* Leaves, roots, or blossoms used for hysterical or nervous debility. *Stimulant* Root used as powerful stimulant. (66:35, 36) **Chippewa** *Adjuvant* Root combined with other herbs to strengthen their action. (43:342) *Dermatological Aid* Compound poultice of chopped root applied to inflammations. (43:348) Roots used for bruises and contusions. (59:129) *Gastrointestinal Aid* Root cooked with foods to aid digestion. (43:342) *Orthopedic Aid* Compound poultice of root applied to fractured bones. (43:366) **Iroquois** *Adjuvant* "Plant may be added to all kinds of medicine to make them stronger." (73:309) *Analgesic* Cold infusion of roots given to children with headaches and fevers. (73:308) Infusion of plant taken for long-lasting headaches. (73:309) *Anticonvulsive* Compound decoction given to children with convulsions. (73:308) Plant and other plants given to children with convulsions and fevers. (118:41) *Antiemetic* Compound decoction taken for heaves. *Blood Medicine* Complex compound decoction taken as blood purifier. (73:310) *Cathartic* Infusion of root taken as a spring tonic by the old and works as a physic. (73:309) *Cold Remedy* Decoction of roots taken for scarlet fever, colds, and "peevies." Infusion of roots taken for colds and typhoid fever. (73:310) *Cough Medicine* Decoction of root taken for coughs and measles. (73:309) Compound decoction taken for coughs. (73:310) *Dermatological Aid* Compound used for boils. (73:311) *Diaphoretic* Cold infusion or decoction of roots taken for any kind of fever and sweating. *Dietary Aid* Decoction taken to become fit to visit the sick and for the lack of appetite. *Disinfectant* Infusion or decoction used as hand and face wash for ghost contamination. (73:309) *Febrifuge* Plant used several ways for adults and children with fevers. (73:308) Plant and other plants given to children with convulsions and fevers. (118:41) *Misc. Disease Remedy* Compound decoction of roots taken for typhoid, measles, and scarlet fever. *Pediatric Aid* Compound infusion given "when babies cry until they hold their breath." Infusion of roots given to children with headaches, fevers, or convulsions. (73:308) Plant and other plants given to children with convulsions and fevers. (118:41) *Psychological Aid* Infusion taken to prevent bad dreams caused by the dead. (73:308) *Pulmonary Aid* Infusion taken and used as a wash for fever and chest congestion, then vomit. *Respiratory Aid* Infusion of root taken for asthma. *Stimulant* Decoction of roots taken for fevers, colds, and as a stimulant. (73:310) Compound used for laziness. (73:311) *Throat Aid* Poultice used for sore throat. (73:310) *Tonic* Infusion of root taken as a spring tonic by the old and works as a physic. (73:309) Compound infusion taken for fevers and as a general tonic. (73:311) *Tuberculosis Remedy* Compound infusion of roots taken for tuberculosis. (73:310) *Urinary Aid* Decoction of roots taken for urinary disorders and urine stoppage. (73:309) *Venereal Aid* Complex compound decoction taken for venereal disease. *Veterinary Aid* Compound decoction given to horses for coughs or heaves. (73:310) Decoction with whisky given to horses that are sick from not being used. (73:311) *Witchcraft Medicine* Plant used several ways to detect or protect people from witchcraft. (73:308) Decoction or infusion used internally or externally before visiting the sick. (73:309) **Malecite** *Gastrointestinal Aid* and *Pediatric Aid* Infusion of small roots used by children with cramps. (96:255) **Menominee** *Gastrointestinal Aid* Decoction of root used for indigestion. (44:130) Fresh or dried root used as a mild stomachic. Root eaten to protect "weak stomach" so that desired food may be eaten. (128:24, 25) **Meskwaki** *Adjuvant* Used as a seasoner and for sore throats. *Analgesic* Compound used for stomach cramps. *Antidote* Root cooked with spoiled meat to prevent ptomaine poisoning. *Ear Medicine* Cooked root placed in ear for earache or sore ears. *Gastrointestinal Aid* Compound used for stomach cramps. *Hunting Medicine* Root chewed and spittle put on bait to enable fisherman to catch catfish. *Pulmonary Aid* Compound used for lung

trouble. *Throat Aid* Used for sore throat and as a medicine used as a seasoning. (129:204) **Micmac** *Analgesic* and *Gastrointestinal Aid* Root used for cramps and as a stomachic. *Tonic* Root used for cramps and as a stomachic. (32:55) **Montagnais** *Panacea* Plant had "general medicinal properties." (133:314) **Ojibwa** *Dietary Aid* Root chewed by sick person as an appetite stimulant. (130:357) *Gastrointestinal Aid* Roots chewed or infusion of roots taken for stomach pain. (4:2250) **Potawatomi** *Antiemetic* Root used to help the appetite of persons who could not keep anything in their stomachs. (131:96)

Asarum caudatum, British Columbia
Wildginger

Bella Coola *Analgesic* Decoction of plant used externally for headache, intestinal pain, and knee pain. *Antirheumatic (External)* Decoction of plant used externally for knee pain. *Gastrointestinal Aid* Decoction of plant used externally for intestinal pain. Decoction of plant taken for stomach pain. (127:56) Decoction of roots taken for stomach pains. (158:201) **Okanagan-Colville** *Cold Remedy* Infusion of roots taken for colds. *Laxative* Infusion of roots taken as a laxative. (162:74) **Okanagon** *Gastrointestinal Aid* Decoction of rhizomes taken for stomach troubles, indigestion, and colic. (104:40) **Pomo** *Dermatological Aid* Poultice of heated leaves applied to boils. (54:13) **Pomo, Kashaya** *Dermatological Aid* Poultice of fresh, warmed leaves used to bring boils to a head. Decoction of leaves used to wash sores. *Toothache Remedy* Poultice of fresh, warmed leaves used for toothaches. (60:50) **Skagit** *Dietary Aid* Leaves eaten to increase appetite. *Tonic* Decoction of leaves taken as a tonic. *Tuberculosis Remedy* Dried leaves used for tuberculosis. (65:28) **Thompson** *Dermatological Aid* Dried, powdered leaves rubbed on the hands as a deodorant. (161:165) *Gastrointestinal Aid* Decoction of rhizomes taken for stomach troubles, indigestion, and colic. (104:40) Decoction of rhizome taken as a stomach tonic and for indigestion and colic. (141:460) *Pediatric Aid* and *Sedative* Whole plant or stems put in infant's bed to quiet baby and for illness. (141:508) *Tonic* Decoction of rhizomes taken as a tonic for the stomach. (141:460) *Unspecified* Fresh or dried leaves used as a medicine. (161:165) **Tolowa** *Dis-*

infectant Poultice of leaves applied for any infections. **Yurok** *Dermatological Aid* and *Pediatric Aid* Leaves used to keep a newborn baby's navel from becoming infected. (5:19)

Asclepias asperula ssp. capricornu,
Antelope Horns

Navajo, Kayenta *Respiratory Aid* Plant used as a snuff for catarrh. (as *Asclepiodora decumbens* 179:37) **Navajo, Ramah** *Ceremonial Medicine* Plant used as ceremonial emetic. *Emetic* Plant used as ceremonial emetic. *Veterinary Aid* Infusion taken and used as lotion for mad dog or mad coyote bite on humans or animals. (as *Asclepiodora decumbens* 165:39)

Asclepias auriculata, Eared Milkweed
Navajo, Kayenta *Respiratory Aid* Plant used for nasal congestion from a cold. (as *Acerates auriculata* 179:36)

Asclepias californica, California Milkweed
Kawaiisu *Dermatological Aid* Dried, powdered plant applied to spider bites. (180:13)

Asclepias cordifolia, Heartleaf Milkweed
Miwok *Unspecified* Root used as a medicine. (8:167)

Asclepias cryptoceras, Pallid Milkweed
Paiute *Analgesic* Decoction of root used as a wash for headaches. *Dermatological Aid* Latex used for ringworm. (155:47) **Paiute, Northern** *Dermatological Aid* Poultice of dried, powdered roots applied to sores. (49:125) **Shoshoni** *Veterinary Aid* Juice of plant used for horse with sore back. (98:49)

Asclepias eriocarpa, Woollypod Milkweed
Costanoan *Cold Remedy* Decoction of plant and plant salve used for colds. *Dermatological Aid* Milky juice used to reduce corns. *Other* Powdered, dried roots inhaled to cause sneezing. *Respiratory Aid* Burning dried plant smoke inhaled for asthma. (17:12) **Mendocino Indian** *Dermatological Aid* Plant juice applied to cuts, sores, and warts. (33:379)

Asclepias exaltata, Poke Milkweed
Omaha *Gastrointestinal Aid* Raw root eaten for stomach trouble. **Ponca** *Gastrointestinal Aid* Root eaten raw for stomach trouble. (58:110)

Asclepias fascicularis, Mexican Whorled Milkweed
California Indian *Snakebite Remedy* Poultice of fresh leaves used for snakebite. (as *A. mexicana* 98:47) **Mendocino Indian** *Poison* Flowers considered poisonous. (as *A. mexicana* 33:380)

Asclepias hallii, Hall's Milkweed
Navajo *Gynecological Aid* Infusion of plant used as tonic after deliverance. (45:69) **Navajo, Kayenta** *Veterinary Aid* Plant poisonous to livestock. (179:36)

Asclepias incarnata, Swamp Milkweed
Chippewa *Pediatric Aid* Infusion of root used as a strengthening bath for children. *Strengthener* Infusion of root used as a strengthening bath for children and adults. (43:364) **Iroquois** *Dermatological Aid* Cold infusion of roots applied to heal baby's navel. *Diuretic* Decoction of plants taken for too little urine. *Kidney Aid* Decoction of plants taken for the kidneys. *Orthopedic Aid* Decoction of plants taken for lame backs. (73:418) *Other* Compound decoction of roots taken and used as wash for stricture. (73:417) *Pediatric Aid* Cold infusion of roots applied to heal baby's navel. *Strengthener* Infusion of roots taken and used as wash to give

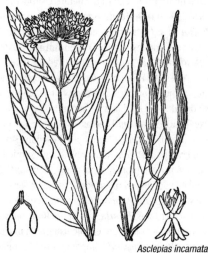

Asclepias incarnata

strength. *Toothache Remedy* Dried stems made into cord and used for tooth extraction. *Urinary Aid* Decoction of plants taken for too much urine. *Witchcraft Medicine* Decoction of plant used to increase one's strength to be able to physically punish a witch. (73:418) **Meskwaki** *Anthelmintic* Infusion of root used to drive the tapeworms from a person in 1 hour. *Carminative* Root used as a carminative. *Cathartic* Root used as a cathartic. *Diuretic* Root used as a diuretic. *Emetic* Root used as an emetic. (129:205)

Asclepias involucrata, Dwarf Milkweed
Keres, Western *Gastrointestinal Aid* Infusion of plant used as a stomach medicine. (147:30) **Navajo, Kayenta** *Toothache Remedy* Poultice of heated roots applied for toothaches. (179:36) **Zuni** *Unspecified* Dry powdered root and saliva used for unspecified illness. (22:373)

Asclepias latifolia, Broadleaf Milkweed
Isleta *Respiratory Aid* Ground leaf and stem powder inhaled for catarrh. (85:23)

Asclepias nyctaginifolia, Mojave Milkweed
Navajo, Kayenta *Antidiarrheal* and *Pediatric Aid* Infusion of plant given to infants with diarrhea. (179:37)

Asclepias perennis, Aquatic Milkweed
Cherokee *Analgesic* Infusion of root taken with root of "virgin's bower" for backache. *Dermatological Aid* Rubbed on warts to remove them. *Kidney Aid* Plant taken for "dropsy." *Laxative* Plant taken as a laxative. *Urinary Aid* Plant taken for "gravel." *Venereal Aid* Infusion of root taken for venereal diseases. *Veterinary Aid* Infusion given for "milksick (mastitis)." (66:44)

Asclepias pumila, Plains Milkweed
Lakota *Antidiarrheal* Infusion of leaves taken for diarrhea. *Pediatric Aid* Infusion of leaves taken by children with diarrhea. (116:34)

Asclepias quadrifolia, Fourleaf Milkweed
Cherokee *Analgesic* Infusion of root taken with root of "virgin's bower" for backache. *Dermatological Aid* Rubbed on warts to remove them. *Kidney Aid* Plant taken for "dropsy." *Laxative* Plant

taken for as a laxative. *Urinary Aid* Plant taken for "gravel." *Venereal Aid* Infusion of root taken for venereal diseases. *Veterinary Aid* Infusion given for "milksick (mastitis)." (66:44)

Asclepias speciosa, Showy Milkweed
Cheyenne *Eye Medicine* Decoction of plant tops strained and used as an eye medicine. (68:66) Decoction of plant tops used as an eyewash for blindness or snow-blindness. (69:14) **Flathead** *Gastrointestinal Aid* Fresh roots chewed or dried, pulverized, and boiled and used for stomachache. (68:66) **Lakota** *Unspecified* Used as a medicine. (116:34) **Miwok** *Dermatological Aid* Milk of plant applied to warts. *Venereal Aid* Decoction of root taken in small doses for venereal diseases. (8:167) **Navajo, Kayenta** *Ceremonial Medicine* and *Emetic* Plant used as an Eagleway, Female Shootingway, Beautyway, and Beadway emetic. (179:37) **Okanagan-Colville** *Antirheumatic* (*External*) Poultice of mashed roots applied for rheumatism. *Dermatological Aid* Latex rubbed on skin sores. (162:74) **Okanagon** *Analgesic* Decoction of roots taken for headaches and general debility. (104:42) **Paiute** *Antirheumatic* (*External*) Decoction of root used as a wash for rheumatism. *Cough Medicine* Decoction of root taken for cough, especially from tuberculosis. *Dermatological Aid* Latex or pulverized seeds used as an antiseptic and healing agent on sores. *Misc. Disease Remedy* Hot decoction of root taken to "bring out the rash of measles." *Snakebite Remedy* Decoction of seeds used to draw poison from snakebites. *Tuberculosis Remedy* Decoction of root taken for cough, especially from tuberculosis. **Shoshoni** *Antidiarrheal* Decoction of root taken for "bloody diarrhea." *Dermatological Aid* Latex applied to remove corns and calluses. Latex used as an antiseptic and healing agent on sores, cuts, and ringworm. Poultice of mashed root applied to swellings. *Venereal Aid* Latex used as an antiseptic and healing agent on syphilitic sores. (155:48) **Thompson** *Analgesic* Decoction of roots taken for headaches and general debility. (104:42) *Dermatological Aid* Milky juice from stem used as face cream. *Dietary Aid* Decoction of root taken for "general out-of-sorts feeling and emaciation." (141:470) *Poison* Root poisonous in large amounts. (141:513) *Tonic*

Decoction of root taken for "general out-of-sorts feeling and emaciation." (141:470)

Asclepias stenophylla, Slimleaf Milkweed **Lakota** *Dietary Aid* Root given to children to increase the appetite. (116:34)

Asclepias subulata, Rush Milkweed **Pima** *Cathartic* Plant used as a physic. *Emetic* Plant used as an emetic. *Eye Medicine* Plant used for sore eyes. *Gastrointestinal Aid* Plant used for stomach disorders. *Panacea* Plant used for many ailments. *Poison* Plant considered poisonous. (38:81)

Asclepias subverticillata, Whorled Milkweed **Hopi** *Gynecological Aid* Used by the mother to produce a flow of milk. (as *A. galioides* 164:164) Plant used to increase mother's milk flow. (as *A. galioides* 174:36, 87) **Keres, Western** *Gynecological Aid* Crushed leaves rubbed on mothers' breasts to produce more and richer milk. Infusion of plant used by mothers for more and richer milk. (as *A. galioides* 147:30)

Asclepias syriaca, Common Milkweed **Cherokee** *Analgesic* Infusion of root taken with root of "virgin's bower" for backache. *Dermatological Aid* Rubbed on warts to remove them. *Kidney Aid* Plant taken for "dropsy." *Laxative* Plant taken as a laxative. *Urinary Aid* Plant taken for "gravel." *Venereal Aid* Infusion of root taken for venereal diseases. *Veterinary Aid* Infusion given for "milksick (mastitis)." (66:44) **Chippewa** *Gynecological Aid* Cold decoction of root added to food to produce postpartum milk flow. (43:360) **Iroquois** *Antirheumatic (External)* Stalks cooked as greens and used for rheumatism. (103:93) *Contraceptive* Infusion of dried, pulverized roots and rhizomes taken by women for temporary sterility. (118:59) *Dermatological Aid* Milk used for warts, bee stings, and cuts. *Gastrointestinal Aid* Infusion of leaves taken as a stomach medicine. *Gynecological Aid* Compound decoction of plants taken to prevent hemorrhage after childbirth. *Kidney Aid* Compound used for dropsy. (73:417) *Other* Compound decoction of roots taken for stricture. (73:416) *Unspecified* Poultice of cotton applied to sick parts. (118:59) **Menominee** *Pul-*

monary Aid Buds eaten or decoction of root used for chest discomfort. (44:130) **Ojibwa** *Gynecological Aid* Root used as a female remedy for unspecified ailment. (130:357) **Potawatomi** *Unspecified* Root used for unspecified ailments. (131:42) **Rappahannock** *Dermatological Aid* Milk of fresh plant applied to warts and ringworm. (138:32)

Asclepias tuberosa, Butterfly Milkweed **Cherokee** *Analgesic* Used for breast, stomach, and intestinal pains. *Antidiarrheal* Seeds boiled in "new milk" and used for diarrhea. *Expectorant* Used as an expectorant and taken for pleurisy. *Gynecological Aid* Infusion used for "bloody flux." *Heart Medicine* Infusion of root used for heart trouble. *Laxative* Seeds or root used as gentle laxative. *Pulmonary Aid* Used as an expectorant and taken for pleurisy and lung inflammations. (66:27) **Delaware** *Antirheumatic (External)* Roots used for rheumatism. *Gynecological Aid* Roots administered to women following childbirth. *Pulmonary Aid* Roots used for pleurisy. (151:37) **Delaware, Oklahoma** *Antirheumatic (Internal)* Root used for rheumatism. *Gynecological Aid* Root used to make a drink taken by women after childbirth. *Pulmonary Aid* Root used for pleurisy. (150:31, 74) **Iroquois** *Other* Infusion of roots used as a wash for arms, shoulders, and body for lifting. *Sports Medicine* Poultice of smashed roots applied to legs, and running shoes dampened or washed for running strength. (73:416) **Menominee** *Dermatological Aid* Poultice of root used or decoction taken for bruises and swellings. (44:132) Simple or compound poultice of pulverized root used on cuts, wounds, and bruises. (128:25) *Orthopedic Aid* Poultice of root used or decoction taken for lameness. *Tonic* Decoction of pounded root taken as a tonic. (44:132) **Mohegan** *Pulmonary Aid* Dried root used for pleurisy. (151:70, 128) **Navajo, Ramah** *Ceremonial Medicine* Plant used in ceremonial chant lotion. *Dermatological Aid* Decoction or infusion of various plant parts used for dog or coyote bites. *Misc. Disease Remedy* Plant used for influenza. (165:39) **Omaha** *Ceremonial Medicine* Ceremony connected with the obtaining and distribution of this prized root. *Dermatological Aid* Fresh and dried root used in several ways on wounds and sores. *Pulmonary Aid* and *Respiratory Aid* Root eaten raw for bronchial and pulmonary trouble. **Ponca** *Pulmonary Aid* Root eaten raw for pulmonary trouble. *Respiratory Aid* Root eaten raw for bronchial trouble. (58:109) **Rappahannock** *Snakebite Remedy* Poultice of bruised leaves bound to snakebites. (138:30)

Asclepias verticillata, Whorled Milkweed **Choctaw** *Diaphoretic* Root used as a sudorific. *Snakebite Remedy* Root chewed, saliva swallowed, and strong decoction taken for snakebite. *Stimulant* Root used as a stimulant. (23:287) **Hopi** *Gynecological Aid* Infusion of entire plant taken by nursing mother with scanty flow of milk. (46:18) **Lakota** *Gynecological Aid* Used by mothers to increase their milk. (116:34) **Navajo** *Nose Medicine* Plant used for nose troubles. *Throat Aid* Plant used for throat troubles. (45:96)

Asclepias viridiflora, Green Milkweed **Blackfoot** *Antirheumatic* (*External*) Poultice of chewed roots applied to swellings. *Dermatological Aid* Poultice of chewed roots applied to rashes. Poultice of chewed roots applied to diarrhea rash. (72:75) *Eye Medicine* Poultice of chewed roots applied to sore eyes. (as *A. viridis flora* 72:80) *Oral Aid* Poultice of chewed roots applied to nursing baby's sore gums. *Pediatric Aid* Poultice of chewed roots applied to diarrhea rash and nursing baby's sore gums. (72:75) *Throat Aid* Root chewed for sore throats. (72:71) **Lakota** *Antidiarrheal* Pulverized roots given to children with diarrhea. *Gynecological Aid* Infusion of whole plant taken by mothers to increase their milk. *Pediatric Aid* Pulverized roots given to children with diarrhea. (116:34)

Asparagus officinalis, Garden Asparagus **Cherokee** *Dietary Aid* Infusion of plant taken for rickets. (66:24) **Iroquois** *Antirheumatic* (*External*) Compound decoction with roots used as a foot soak for rheumatism. (73:282) Stalks cooked as greens and used for rheumatism. (103:93) *Blood Medicine* Compound decoction with bark taken before meals for the blood. (73:282)

Asplenium horridum, Lacy Spleenwort **Hawaiian** *Blood Medicine* Infusion of plant, other ingredients, and coconut milk taken for impure blood. *Oral Aid* Buds and burnt potato peel chewed

for sore mouths. *Stimulant* Scraped wood, other ingredients, and water taken and used as wash for fainting spells and muscle stiffness. (2:14)

Asplenium nidus, Birdnest Fern **Hawaiian** *Dermatological Aid* Leaves and other plants pounded, squeezed, and resulting liquid used for ulcers or scrofulous sores. *Oral Aid* Shoots and other plants pounded, squeezed, and resulting liquid used for children with mouth sores. *Pediatric Aid* Shoots and other plants pounded, squeezed, and resulting liquid given to children for general weakness, and used for children with mouth sores. *Strengthener* Shoots and other plants pounded, squeezed, and resulting liquid given to children for general weakness, and taken for general body weakness. *Tuberculosis Remedy* Leaves and other plants pounded, squeezed, and resulting liquid used for scrofulous sores. (2:22)

Asplenium pseudofalcatum, Iwaiwa **Hawaiian** *Dermatological Aid* Leaf ashes, nut juice, and fruit milk mixed and used on sores. Infusion of leaves used as a bath to beautify children. *Oral Aid* Leaf ashes, nut juice, and fruit milk mixed and used on sores about the mouth. (2:29)

Asplenium rhizophyllum, Walking Fern **Cherokee** *Breast Treatment* Compound used for swollen breasts. (66:61) Decoction of whole plant rubbed on swollen breast. *Emetic* Decoction of whole plant taken to induce vomiting for swollen breasts. (as *Camptosorus rhizophyllus* 152:3)

Asplenium trichomanes, Maidenhair Spleenwort **Cherokee** *Abortifacient* Taken for irregular menses. *Breast Treatment* Infusion taken for "breast diseases" and "acrid humors." *Cough Medicine* Infusion taken for coughs. *Liver Aid* Taken for "liver complaints." (66:34)

Aster carolinianus, Climbing Aster **Seminole** *Dermatological Aid* Plant used for snake sickness: itchy skin. (145:166) Decoction of leaves taken and used as a body steam for snake sickness: itchy skin. (145:239)

Aster conspicuus, Showy Aster
Okanagan-Colville *Dermatological Aid* Roots
soaked in hot or cold water and used as a wash for
sores, boils, wounds, and infections. Poultice of
leaves applied to boils. *Hemorrhoid Remedy* Roots
soaked in hot or cold water and used as a wash for
hemorrhoids. Poultice of leaves applied to hemorrhoids. *Toothache Remedy* Roots applied to the
tooth for toothaches. *Unspecified* Roots soaked
in hot or cold water and taken for gonorrhea and
other ailments. *Venereal Aid* Roots soaked in hot
or cold water and taken for gonorrhea. *Veterinary
Aid* Roots used for cuts with maggots on horses.
(162:79)

Aster cordifolius, Common Blue Wood Aster
Ojibwa *Hunting Medicine* Root used to make a
smoke or incense to attract deer near enough to
shoot it with a bow and arrow. A number of the
composites as well as plants from other families
are used in the hunting charms. The deer carries
its scent or spoor in between its toes, and wher-
ever the foot is impressed into the ground, other
animals can detect its presence. This allows dogs
to track them. It is a peculiar scent and the Ojibwa
tries successfully to counterfeit it with roots and
herbs. The root of this aster is but one of 19 that
can be used. They say that the white man drives
the deer away when he smokes cigarettes or ci-
gars, but the Indian brings them closer. (130:428)

Aster cusickii, Cusick's Aster
Cheyenne *Ear Medicine* Infusion of dried stems
used as drops for earaches. (63:187) Infusion of
dried stems used as ear drops for earaches.
(64:187)

Aster ericoides var. **ericoides**, Heath Aster
Meskwaki *Herbal Steam* Used in the sweat bath.
Stimulant Used to revive an unconscious patient.
(as *A. multiflorus* 129:212)

Aster falcatus var. **commutatus**, Cluster
    Aster
Zuni *Dermatological Aid* Ground blossoms mixed
with yucca suds and used to wash newborn infants
and make their hair grow. *Pediatric Aid* Ground
blossoms mixed with yucca suds and used to wash
newborn infants. This medicine was said to make

the hair grow on the head and to give strength to
the body. *Strengthener* Ground blossoms mixed
with yucca suds and used as a strengthening wash
for newborn infants. (as *A. incanopilosus* 143:84)

Aster falcatus var. **crassulus**, Rough White
    Prairie Aster
Navajo, Ramah *Snakebite Remedy* Compound
decoction of plant taken and used as lotion for
snakebite. (as *A. commutatus* var. *crassulus*
165:48)

Aster foliaceus, Alpine Leafybract Aster
Okanagan-Colville *Veterinary Aid* Decoction
of whole plant used as wash for sores on a horse's
back. (162:80) **Okanagon** *Dietary Aid* Decoction
of roots taken for loss of appetite. *Gastrointestinal
Aid* Decoction of roots taken for stomach swelling,
dyspepsia, and indigestion. **Thompson** *Dietary
Aid* Decoction of roots taken for loss of appetite.
(104:41) Decoction of roots used to stimulate appetite. (141:461) *Gastrointestinal Aid* Decoction
of roots taken for stomach swelling, dyspepsia,
and indigestion. (104:41) Decoction of root taken
for various stomach discomforts. *Venereal Aid*
Strong decoction of root mixed with salmon oil
and taken for syphilis. (141:461)

Aster furcatus, Forked Aster
Potawatomi *Analgesic* Infusion of leaves rubbed
on head for severe headache. (131:49, 50)

Aster laevis, Smooth Aster
Meskwaki *Herbal Steam* Entire plant used to fur-
nish smoke in sweat bath. *Stimulant* Smoke forced
into nostrils of unconscious patient to revive him.
(129:211, 212)

Aster lanceolatus ssp. **hesperius**, Siskiyou
    Aster
Zuni *Dermatological Aid* Decoction of plant used
to dress arrow or bullet wounds. Dried, pulverized
plant used for abrasions made by ceremonial
mask. *Hemostat* Smoke from crushed blossoms
inhaled for nosebleed. (as *A. hesperius* 143:43)

Aster lanceolatus ssp. *lanceolatus* var.
  lanceolatus, White Panicle Aster
Iroquois *Febrifuge* Infusion of plant and another
plant used for fevers. (as *A. paniculatus* 118:65)

Aster lateriflorus, Calico Aster
Meskwaki *Herbal Steam* Entire plant used as a
smoke or steam in sweat bath. *Psychological Aid*
Blossoms smudged "to cure a crazy person who
has lost his mind." (129:212)

Aster linariifolius, Ionactis
Cherokee *Analgesic* Poultice of roots used for
pain. *Antidiarrheal* Infusion of root taken for diarrhea. *Febrifuge* Infusion taken for fever. *Respiratory Aid* Ooze of roots sniffed for catarrh. (66:24)

Aster macrophyllus, Bigleaf Aster
Iroquois *Blood Medicine* Roots used as a blood
medicine. *Laxative* and *Venereal Aid* Compound
decoction of roots taken to loosen the bowels for
venereal disease. (73:462) **Ojibwa** *Analgesic* Infusion of root used to bathe the head for headache.
Hunting Medicine Plant used as a charm in hunting. (130:363) Plant smoked as one of the hunting
charms to attract deer. (130:429) *Unspecified*
Young and tender leaves eaten and act as a medicine at the same time that they are food. (130:398)

Aster nemoralis, Bog Aster
Chippewa *Ear Medicine* Decoction of root used
as drops or on a compress for sore ear. (43:360)

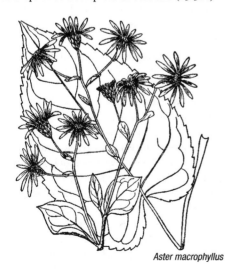
Aster macrophyllus

Aster novae-angliae, New England Aster
Cherokee *Analgesic* Poultice of roots used for
pain. *Antidiarrheal* Infusion of root taken for diarrhea. *Febrifuge* Infusion taken for fever. *Respiratory Aid* Ooze of roots sniffed for catarrh. (66:24)
Chippewa *Hunting Medicine* Roots smoked in
pipes as a charm to attract game. (43:376) **Iroquois** *Dermatological Aid* Decoction of plants
used for weak skin. *Febrifuge* Decoction of roots
and leaves taken for all kinds of fevers. (73:463)
Infusion of whole plant and rhizomes from another
plant taken by mothers with intestinal fevers. (118:
65) *Love Medicine* Plant used as a love medicine.
(73:462) **Meskwaki** *Stimulant* Smudged and
used to revive an unconscious patient. (129:212)
Potawatomi *Stimulant* Plant used as a fumigating
reviver by the Prairie Potawatomi. (131:50)

Aster oblongifolius, Aromatic Aster
Navajo, Ramah *Witchcraft Medicine* Decoction
used as lotion for protection from witches.
(165:48)

Aster praealtus var. *coerulescens*, Willowleaf Aster
Navajo, Ramah *Ceremonial Medicine* Decoction
used ceremonially for snakebite. *Eye Medicine*
Cold infusion of whole plant used as a ceremonial
eyewash. *Gastrointestinal Aid* Cold infusion of
whole plant used for stomachache. *Hunting Medicine* Dried leaves smoked for good luck in hunting.
Internal Medicine Cold infusion of whole plant
used for internal injury. *Snakebite Remedy* Decoction used ceremonially for snakebite. (as *A. coerulescens* 165:48)

Aster praealtus var. *praealtus*, Willowleaf
  Aster
Meskwaki *Stimulant* Used to revive an uncon-
scious patient. (as *A. salicifolius* 129:212)

Aster prenanthoides, Crookedstem Aster
Iroquois *Cold Remedy* Compound decoction of
roots taken for colds. *Febrifuge* Decoction of roots
given to babies with fevers. *Kidney Aid* Compound
decoction of roots taken for the kidneys. *Pediatric
Aid* Decoction of roots given to babies with fevers.
(73:463)

Aster puniceus, Purplestem Aster
Chippewa *Hunting Medicine* Root tendrils smoked with tobacco as a charm to attract game. (43:376) **Cree, Woodlands** *Abortifacient* Decoction of roots taken for failure to menstruate. *Diaphoretic* Decoction of roots taken to cause sweating and reduce a fever. *Febrifuge* Decoction of roots taken to cause sweating and reduce a fever. *Gynecological Aid* Decoction of roots taken to make a woman well after childbirth. *Orthopedic Aid* Roots used for facial paralysis. *Pediatric Aid* and *Toothache Remedy* Decoction of roots taken for teething sickness. Chewed root applied to tooth for toothache. (91:31) **Iroquois** *Cold Remedy* Infusion of roots taken for colds. *Febrifuge* Infusion of roots taken for fevers. *Misc. Disease Remedy* Infusion of roots taken for typhoid. *Pulmonary Aid* Infusion of roots taken for pneumonia. *Tuberculosis Remedy* Infusion of roots taken for consumption. (73:463)

Aster shortii, Short's Aster
Potawatomi *Unspecified* Infusion of flowering tops used for unspecified ailments. (131:50)

Aster simmondsii, Simmonds's Aster
Seminole *Other* Infusion of plant used for sunstroke. (145:303)

Aster subulatus* var. *ligulatus, Annual Saltmarsh Aster
Kawaiisu *Analgesic* Decoction of roots used as a wash for headaches. *Toothache Remedy* Mashed roots applied to the tooth for toothache. (as *A. exilis* 180:14)

Aster umbellatus, Parasol Aster
Mohegan *Gastrointestinal Aid* Infusion of leaves said to be good for the stomach. (151:70, 128) **Potawatomi** *Witchcraft Medicine* Flowers smudged to repel evil spirits from sickroom. (131:50)

Astragalus adsurgens* var. *robustior, Prairie Milkvetch
Cheyenne *Dermatological Aid* Ground leaf and stem sprinkled on skin in cases of poison ivy. (as *A. nitidus* 63:40) Ground leaves and stems applied to skin affected by poison ivy. (as *A. nitidus*

63:179) Ground leaves and stems sprinkled on watery poison ivy rash. (as *A. nitidus* 64:179)

Astragalus allochrous, Halfmoon Milkvetch
Navajo, Ramah *Ceremonial Medicine* Leaves used as a ceremonial emetic. *Emetic* Leaves used as a ceremonial emetic. (165:31, 32)

Astragalus americanus, American Milkvetch
Cree, Woodlands *Gastrointestinal Aid* Roots chewed for stomachaches, cramps, or stomach flu. *Misc. Disease Remedy* Roots chewed for stomach flu. (91:31)

Astragalus amphioxys, Crescent Milkvetch
Zuni *Snakebite Remedy* Fresh or dried root chewed by medicine man before sucking snakebite and poultice applied to wound. (22:376)

Astragalus bisulcatus* var. *haydenianus, Hayden's Milkvetch
Navajo, Ramah *Ceremonial Medicine* and *Emetic* Fruit used as ceremonial emetic. *Eye Medicine* Infusion of plant used as an eyewash. *Toothache Remedy* Poultice of chewed leaves applied for toothache. (as *A. haydenianus* 165:32)

Astragalus calycosus* var. *scaposus, Torrey's Milkvetch
Navajo, Kayenta *Dermatological Aid* Plant used as a lotion and poultice applied to injuries from hailstones. *Other* Plant used as a lotion for illness from exposure. *Poultice* Plant used as a lotion and poultice applied to injuries from water. (as *A. scaposus* 179:27) **Shoshoni** *Venereal Aid* Decoction of scraped roots taken for venereal disease. (as *A. scaposus* 155:49)

Astragalus canadensis, Canadian Milkvetch
Blackfoot *Antihemorrhagic* Roots chewed or infusion of root taken for spitting up blood. (72:71) *Dermatological Aid* Poultice of chewed roots applied to cuts. (72:83) *Pediatric Aid* and *Pulmonary Aid* Root boiled and the steam used to bathe a child's aching chest. (72:71) **Dakota** *Febrifuge* and *Pediatric Aid* Infusion of roots given to children with fevers. (57:365) **Lakota** *Analgesic* Roots pulverized and chewed for chest and back pains. *Antihemorrhagic* Roots and wild licorice roots

used for spitting of blood. *Cough Medicine* Infusion of roots taken for coughs. *Pulmonary Aid* Roots pulverized and chewed for chest pains. (116:45)

Astragalus canadensis var. canadensis, Canadian Milkvetch
Dakota *Febrifuge* and *Pediatric Aid* Decoction of root used as a febrifuge for children. (as *A. caroliniana* 58:91)

Astragalus convallarius var. convallarius, Timber Milkvetch
Gosiute *Veterinary Aid* Plant used as a horse medicine. (as *A. junceus* 31:363)

Astragalus crassicarpus, Groundplum Milkvetch
Chippewa *Anticonvulsive* Compound infusion or decoction of root taken for "fits." (41:63, 64) Compound decoction of root taken for convulsions. (43:336) *Hemostat* Compound infusion or decoction of root used on bleeding wounds. (41:63, 64) Compound decoction of root used on bleeding wounds. (43:336) *Stimulant* Compound infusion or decoction of root taken or used externally as stimulant. (41:63, 64) Compound decoction of root taken as a stimulant. *Tonic* Compound decoction of root taken as a tonic. (43:364) **Lakota** *Veterinary Aid* Used as medicine for horses. (116:46)

Astragalus gracilis, Slender Milkvetch
Lakota *Gynecological Aid* Roots chewed by mothers with no milk. (116:46)

Astragalus humistratus var. sonorae, Groundcover Milkvetch
Navajo, Ramah *Ceremonial Medicine* Plant used as a ceremonial chant lotion. *Dermatological Aid* Dried plant used as a dusting powder for sores. *Panacea* Leaves or whole plant used as "life medicine." (165:32)

Astragalus kentrophyta var. elatus, Tall Spiny Milkvetch
Navajo, Ramah *Ceremonial Medicine* Cold infusion of whole plant used as a ceremonial chant lotion. *Panacea* Root used as a "life medicine." (as *A. impensus* 165:32)

Astragalus kentrophyta var. kentrophyta, Spiny Milkvetch
Navajo *Misc. Disease Remedy* Plant used for rabies. (as *Kentrophyta montana* 45:56)

Astragalus lonchocarpus, Rushy Milkvetch
Navajo, Kayenta *Emetic* Plant used as an emetic. *Poultice* Poultice of plant applied to goiter. (179:27)

Astragalus mollissimus, Woolly Milkvetch
Mahuna *Poison* Plant considered poisonous. (117:36)

Astragalus mollissimus var. matthewsii, Matthews's Woolly Milkvetch
Navajo, Ramah *Ceremonial Medicine* and *Emetic* Leaves used as a ceremonial emetic. (as *A. matthewsii* 165:32)

Astragalus pachypus, Thickpod Milkvetch
Kawaiisu *Analgesic* Decoction of roots taken for menstrual pains. *Gynecological Aid* Decoction of roots taken for menstrual pains. (180:14)

Astragalus pattersonii, Patterson's Milkvetch
Navajo, Kayenta *Ear Medicine* Plant used for any disease of the ears. *Emetic* Plant used as an emetic. *Eye Medicine* Plant used for any disease of the eyes. *Misc. Disease Remedy* Plant used for mumps. *Other* Plant used for sore throats or swollen neck. *Throat Aid* Plant used for any disease of the throat. (179:27)

Astragalus praelongus, Stinking Milkvetch
Navajo, Ramah *Ceremonial Medicine* and *Emetic* Leaves used as a ceremonial emetic. (165:32)

Astragalus purshii, Woollypod Milkvetch
Thompson *Dermatological Aid* Decoction of whole plant used as a wash for the head, hair, and whole body. (141:473, 474) *Disinfectant* Decoction of roots taken and poured on head in sweat house for purification. (141:504) *Hunting Medicine* Decoction of plant poured onto hunting equipment which had "lost its luck." (141:507)

Astragalus purshii var. tinctus, Woollypod Milkvetch
Kawaiisu *Analgesic* and *Gynecological Aid* Decoction of roots taken for menstrual pains. (180:15)

Astragalus racemosus, Alkali Poisonvetch
Lakota *Poison* Plant poisonous to livestock. (116:46)

Astragalus sesquiflorus, Sandstone Milkvetch
Navajo, Kayenta *Ceremonial Medicine* Plant used as a ceremonial emetic. *Dermatological Aid* Plant used as a lotion and poultice of plant applied to ringworm. *Emetic* Plant used as a ceremonial emetic. (179:28)

Athyrium filix-femina, Common Ladyfern
Chippewa *Diuretic* Compound decoction of root taken for "stoppage of urine." (43:348) **Cowlitz** *Analgesic* Infusion of stems taken for body pains. (65:14) **Hesquiat** *Cancer Treatment* Young, unfurling fronds eaten for internal ailments, such as cancer of the womb. (159:29) **Makah** *Gynecological Aid* Decoction of pounded stems taken by women to ease labor. (65:14) **Meskwaki** *Analgesic* and *Gynecological Aid* Decoction of root taken by women for bosom pains caused by childbirth. (as *Asplenium filix-femina* 129:237) **Ojibwa** *Dermatological Aid* Grated dried root used as healing powder for sores. *Gynecological Aid* Infusion of root induced milk flow in patients with caked breast. (as *Asplenium filis-femina* 130:381) **Pota-**

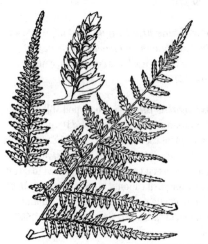

Athyrium filix-femina

watomi *Gynecological Aid* Infusion of root taken for caked breasts and other female disorders. (as *Asplenium filix-femina* 131:73) **Thompson** *Antihemorrhagic* Infusion of plant used for vomiting blood. (161:88)

Athyrium filix-femina ssp. angustum, Subarctic Ladyfern
Iroquois *Febrifuge* Infusion of rhizomes and whole New England aster plant taken by mothers with intestinal fevers. *Reproductive Aid* Infusion of plant, vinegar bark, and flower stalks taken to prevent women's water from breaking. *Venereal Aid* Infusion of rhizomes and sensitive fern used by men with venereal diseases. (as *A. angustum* 118:34)

Athyrium filix-femina ssp. cyclosorum, Subarctic Ladyfern
Bella Coola *Eye Medicine* Simple or compound decoction of root used as a wash for sore eyes. (as *Asplenium cyclosorum* 127:48)

Atriplex argentea, Silverscale Saltbush
Navajo, Ramah *Analgesic* Leaves used as a fumigant for pain. *Dermatological Aid* Poultice of leaves applied to spider bites. *Other* Cold infusion used for sickness from drinking bad water and to purify water. (165:24) **Zuni** *Dermatological Aid* Poultice of chewed root applied to sores and rashes. *Gastrointestinal Aid* Infusion of root taken for stomachache. (22:374)

Atriplex canescens, Fourwing Saltbush
Havasupai *Dermatological Aid* Leaves made into a soapy lather and used to wash the hair. *Misc. Disease Remedy* Leaves made into a soapy lather and used for itches or rashes, such as chickenpox or measles. (171:217) **Hopi** *Ceremonial Medicine* Plant used for kiva fires. (46:21) **Isleta** *Poison* Infectious wood used to make poison arrowheads for war purposes. (85:24) **Jemez** *Dermatological Aid* Poultice of crushed leaves applied to ant bites, probably to reduce the swelling and pain. *Stimulant* Leaves put unto a fire and smoke used to revive badly hurt, weak, and faint person. (36:20) **Navajo** *Dermatological Aid* Plant used for ant bites. (76:148) **Navajo, Kayenta** *Emetic* Plant used as an emetic. *Gastrointestinal Aid* Plant used for stomach disease. (179:20) **Navajo, Ramah**

Analgesic Decoction of tops or roots taken as an emetic for gastric pain. *Ceremonial Medicine* Whole plant used as a ceremonial emetic. *Cough Medicine* Decoction of leaves or roots taken for bad cough. *Dermatological Aid* Poultice of leaves applied to ant bites. Leaf and stem ash rubbed on the scalp as a hair tonic. *Emetic* Whole plant used as a ceremonial emetic. *Gastrointestinal Aid* Decoction of tops or roots taken as an emetic for gastric pain. *Nose Medicine* Leaves used as snuff for nose trouble. *Toothache Remedy* Poultice of warm, pulverized root applied for toothache. *Veterinary Aid* Compound decoction given to sheep for bloating from overeating. (165:24) **Shoshoni** *Cathartic* Decoction of fresh roots with salt taken as a physic. (155:50) **Zuni** *Dermatological Aid* Poultice of fresh or dried flower used for ant bites. (22:374) Infusion of dried root and blossoms or poultice of blossoms used for ant bites. (143:44) *Hunting Medicine* Twigs attached to prayer plumes and sacrificed to the cottontail rabbit to ensure good hunting. (143:88)

Atriplex confertifolia, Shadscale Saltbush
Hopi *Anticonvulsive* Plant burned and smoke inhaled for epileptic medicine. (as *A. jonesii* 34:293) **Navajo** *Veterinary Aid* Plant rubbed on horses to repel gnats. (76:149) **Paiute, Northern** *Antirheumatic* (*External*) Leaves boiled and used as a liniment for sore muscles and aches. *Cold Remedy* Poultice of mashed leaves applied to the chest and decoction of leaves taken for colds. (49:125)

Atriplex lentiformis, Big Saltbush
Cahuilla *Cold Remedy* Dried leaves smoked for head colds. Fresh leaves chewed for head colds. *Nose Medicine* Crushed flowers, stems, and leaves steamed and inhaled for nasal congestion. (11:45) **Pima** *Dermatological Aid* Poultice of powdered roots applied to sores. (38:66) Poultice of powdered root applied to sores. (123:80)

Atriplex obovata, Mound Saltbush
Hopi *Anticonvulsive* Plant burned and smoke inhaled for epileptic medicine. (34:293)

Atriplex polycarpa, Cattle Saltbush
Maricopa *Antirheumatic* (*External*) Moxa of dried galls burned on the affected area for rheuma-

tism. **Pima** *Antirheumatic* (*External*) Moxa of galls placed on area affected by rheumatism. (38:67)

Aureolaria flava, Smooth Yellow False Foxglove
Cherokee *Antidiarrheal* Compound decoction taken for dysentery. *Other* Infusion taken while fasting for 4 days for apoplexy. (66:35)

Aureolaria laevigata, Entireleaf Yellow False Foxglove
Cherokee *Antidiarrheal* Compound decoction taken for dysentery. *Other* Infusion taken while fasting for 4 days for apoplexy. (66:35)

Aureolaria pedicularia, Fernleaf Yellow False Foxglove
Cherokee *Antidiarrheal* Compound decoction taken for dysentery. *Other* Infusion taken while fasting for 4 days for apoplexy. (66:35)

Aureolaria pedicularia* var. *pedicularia, Fernleaf Yellow False Foxglove
Chickasaw *Emetic* Plant used as an emetic. *Misc. Disease Remedy* Plant used as an antiscorbutic. (as *Dasystoma pedicularia* 23:289)

Aureolaria virginica, Downy Yellow False Foxglove
Cherokee *Antidiarrheal* Decoction of plants taken for dysentery. (as *Gerardia virginica* 152:57)

Baccharis douglasii, Saltmarsh Baccharis
Costanoan *Dermatological Aid* Decoction of plant used as a wash for wounds. Dried, powdered stems applied as a disinfectant to wounds. Poultice of heated leaves and animal fat applied to boils. *Disinfectant* Dried, powdered stems applied as a disinfectant to wounds. *Kidney Aid* Infusion of plant taken for kidney ailments. (17:26) **Luiseño** *Dermatological Aid* Decoction of leaves used as a bath for sores and wounds. (132:228)

Baccharis pilularis, Coyotebrush
Costanoan *Panacea* Infusion of plant used as a general remedy. (17:26)

Baccharis pteronioides, Yerba de Pasmo
Yavapai *Antirheumatic* (*External*) Decoction
of leaves and roots used as wash for rheumatism.
Venereal Aid Decoction of leaves and roots used as
wash for gonorrhea. (53:261)

Baccharis salicifolia, Mule's Fat
Cahuilla *Dermatological Aid* Leaves used in a hair
wash solution to prevent baldness. *Gynecological
Aid* Decoction of leaves and stems used as a female
hygienic agent. (as *B. viminea* 11:46) **Coahuilla**
Eye Medicine Infusion of leaves used as an eyewash. (as *B. glutinosa* 9:78) **Costanoan** *Dermatological Aid* Infusion of leaves and twigs used as
wash for scalp and hair to encourage growth. (as
B. viminea 17:26) **Diegueño** *Dermatological Aid*
Infusion of leaves used as a wash or poultice of
leaves applied to bruises, wounds, or insect stings.
(as *B. glutinosa* 74:220) **Navajo, Kayenta** *Febrifuge* Compound infusion of plants used as a lotion
for chills from immersion. (as *B. glutinosa* 179:45)

Baccharis sarothroides, Desert Broom
Diegueño *Cough Medicine* Infusion of plant taken
for coughs. *Gastrointestinal Aid* Infusion of plant
taken for stomachaches. (74:220)

Baccharis wrightii, Wright's Baccharis
Navajo, Ramah *Ceremonial Medicine* and *Emetic*
Plant used as a ceremonial emetic. *Venereal Aid*
Strong decoction of plant taken in large amounts
for sexual infection. (165:49)

Bacopa caroliniana, Blue Waterhyssop
Seminole *Cough Medicine* Plant used for turtle
sickness: trembling, short breath, and cough. (as
Hydrotrida caroliniana 145:237) *Other* Complex
infusion of leaves taken for chronic conditions. (as
Hydrotrida caroliniana 145:272) *Respiratory Aid*
and *Sedative* Plant used for turtle sickness: trembling, short breath, and cough. (as *Hydrotrida
caroliniana* 145:237)

Bahia dissecta, Ragleaf Bahia
Keres, Western *Cathartic* Infusion of plant used
as a cathartic. *Emetic* Infusion of plant used as an
emetic. (147:32) **Navajo, Ramah** *Analgesic* Compound decoction taken for menstrual pain. *Antirheumatic* (*Internal*) Compound decoction of

plant taken for arthritis. *Contraceptive* Compound
decoction of plant taken as contraceptive. *Gynecological Aid* Compound decoction of plant taken for
menstrual pain. (165:49) **Zuni** *Analgesic* Powdered plant rubbed on affected parts for headache. *Antirheumatic* (*External*) Powdered plant
rubbed on affected parts for rheumatism. (as *Villa-
nova dissecta* 143:62)

Baileya multiradiata, Desert Marigold
Keres, Western *Dermatological Aid* Plant
rubbed under arms as deodorant. (147:32)

Balsamita major, Costmary
Iroquois *Ear Medicine* Infusion of one smashed
leaf used as drops for earaches. (as *Chrysanthemum balsamita* var. *tanacetoides* 73:472)

Balsamorhiza deltoidea, Deltoid Balsamroot
Kawaiisu *Cold Remedy* Decoction of split roots
taken for colds. *Cough Medicine* Decoction of split
roots taken for coughing. (180:15)

Balsamorhiza hookeri var. ***hirsuta***, Hairy
  Balsamroot
Paiute *Gastrointestinal Aid* Decoction of root
considered good for severe stomach. *Urinary Aid*
Decoction of root considered good for bladder
troubles. **Washo** *Gynecological Aid* Decoction of
root taken for female complaints. (as *B. hirsuta*
155:50)

Balsamorhiza incana, Hoary Balsamroot
Cheyenne *Analgesic* Infusion of leaves, roots,
and stems taken for stomach pains and headaches.
(63:189) Decoction of leaves, roots, and stems
taken for stomach pains. Decoction of leaves,
roots, and stems used as a steam bath for headaches. (64:189) *Cold Remedy* Plant used for colds.
(63:189) Plant used for colds. (64:189) Infusion
of leaves, stems, and roots taken for colds. (69:20)
Gastrointestinal Aid Infusion of leaves, roots, and
stems taken for stomach pains. (63:189) Decoction of leaves, roots and stems taken for stomach
pains. (64:189) Infusion of leaves, stems, and
roots taken for stomach pains. (69:20)

Balsamorhiza sagittata, Arrowleaf Balsamroot
Blackfoot *Antirheumatic (Internal)* Root smudge
smoke inhaled for body aches. (72:78) *Dermatological Aid* Poultice of chewed roots applied to blisters and sores. (72:75) **Cheyenne** *Analgesic* Infusion of leaves, roots, and stems taken for stomach
pains and headaches. (63:189) Steam of decoction
of plant inhaled for headache and used as wash on
head. (63:38) Decoction of leaves, roots, and
stems taken for stomach pains. (63:38, 39) *Cold
Remedy* Plant used for colds. (63:189) Infusion of
leaves, stems, and roots taken for colds. (69:20)
Febrifuge Infusion of root taken for fever. (63:38)
Gastrointestinal Aid Infusion of leaves, roots, and
stems taken for stomach pains. (63:189) Decoction of leaves, roots, and stems taken for stomach
pain. (63:38) Infusion of leaves, stems, and roots
taken for stomach pains. (69:20) *Gynecological
Aid* Decoction of root taken when labor begins, to
insure easy delivery. (63:38) *Oral Aid* Root chewed
and saliva allowed to run down throat for sore
mouth and throat. *Panacea* Root chewed and
rubbed over the body for any sickness. (63:38, 39)
Throat Aid Root chewed and saliva allowed to run
down throat for sore throat. *Toothache Remedy*
Root chewed for toothaches. (63:38) **Flathead**
Burn Dressing Poultice of coarse, large leaves
used for burns. *Cathartic* Infusion of roots taken
as a cathartic. *Pulmonary Aid* Infusion of roots
taken for whooping cough. *Tuberculosis Remedy*
Infusion of roots taken for tuberculosis. *Urinary
Aid* Infusion of roots taken to increase urine.
(68:20) **Gosiute** *Dermatological Aid* Poultice of
pounded or chewed root paste applied to arrow
or gunshot wounds. (31:348) Chewed roots or
pounded root salve applied to fresh wounds.
(31:363) *Hemostat* Poultice of plant applied to
arrow or gunshot wound hemorrhages. (31:348)
Kutenai *Dermatological Aid* Poultice of root infusion used for wounds, cuts, and bruises. (68:20)
Miwok *Analgesic* Decoction of ground root
cooled and taken for headaches. *Antirheumatic
(Internal)* Decoction of ground root cooled and
taken for rheumatism. *Diaphoretic* Decoction of
root taken to produce profuse perspiration for
rheumatism. (8:167) **Okanagan-Colville** *Burn
Dressing* Poultice of dried, powdered leaves applied to severe skin burns. *Diaphoretic* Leaves

placed on glowing coals and laid on to cause profuse sweating. (162:80) **Paiute** *Analgesic* Decoction of root taken for stomachaches. *Dermatological Aid* Poultice of mashed root applied to insect
bites or swellings. Powdered, dried root applied
to syphilitic sores. *Disinfectant* Root burned as a
fumigant in the sickroom. *Gastrointestinal Aid*
Decoction of root taken for stomachaches. *Tuberculosis Remedy* Root sap taken for consumption.
Venereal Aid Decoction of root taken over a long
period of time for venereal disease. Poultice of
dry, powdered root applied to syphilitic sores.
(155:50, 51) **Sanpoil** *Analgesic* Poultice of root
prepared in various ways and applied to painful
areas. *Dermatological Aid* Infusion of root rubbed
into hair and scalp to help hair grow. Poultice of
root prepared in various ways and applied to
bruised areas. Pulverized root sprinkled on sores
and boils. (109:219) **Shoshoni** *Dermatological
Aid* Poultice of mashed root applied to insect bites
or swellings, and to syphilitic sores. *Eye Medicine*
Decoction of root used as an eyewash. *Venereal
Aid* Poultice of mashed root applied to syphilitic
sores. (155:50, 51) **Shuswap** *Dermatological Aid*
Infusion of leaves used as a wash for poison ivy
and running sores. (102:59) **Thompson** *Antidiarrheal* Seeds eaten for dysentery. (161:175)
Dietary Aid Root sucked and chewed for hunger.
(141:493) *Sedative* Young shoots, when eaten in
great quantities, caused sleepiness like sleeping
pills. (161:175) **Washo** *Disinfectant* Root burned
as a fumigant in the sickroom. (155:50, 51)

Baptisia alba var. ***macrophylla***, Largeleaf
Wild Indigo
Choctaw *Dermatological Aid* Poultice of roots
and leaves applied to swellings. **Koasati** *Antirheumatic (Internal)* Decoction of roots taken for
rheumatism. (as *B. leucantha* 152:31) **Meskwaki**
Dermatological Aid Root used for old sores and
compound used on knife or ax wounds. *Hemorrhoid Remedy* Compound containing root used for
piles. *Kidney Aid* Compound infusion taken for
dropsy. *Respiratory Aid* Decoction of root used for
catarrh. *Snakebite Remedy* Compound containing
root used for rattlesnake bite. (as *B. leucantha*
129:228)

Baptisia australis, Blue Wild Indigo
Cherokee *Antiemetic* Cold infusion used for vomiting. *Cathartic* Used as a purgative. *Emetic* Used as an emetic. *Gynecological Aid* Poultice used "to allay inflammation and stop mortification." *Toothache Remedy* Hot infusion of root or beaten root held against tooth for toothache. (66:40)

Baptisia bracteata, Longbract Wild Indigo
Pawnee *Gastrointestinal Aid* Pulverized seeds mixed with buffalo fat and applied to abdomen for colic. (58:90)

Baptisia tinctoria, Horseflyweed
Cherokee *Antiemetic* Cold infusion used for vomiting. *Cathartic* Used as a purgative. *Emetic* Used as an emetic. *Gynecological Aid* Poultice used "to allay inflammation and stop mortification." *Toothache Remedy* Hot infusion of root or beaten root held against tooth for toothache. (66:40) **Delaware** *Dermatological Aid* Infusion of roots used to clean cuts and ulcers. *Gynecological Aid* Infusion of roots used as a douche. (151:37) **Delaware, Oklahoma** *Dermatological Aid* Infusion of root used as a wash to clean cuts and ulcers. (150:31, 74) *Gynecological Aid* Infusion of root used as a douche. (150:31) **Iroquois** *Antirheumatic (Internal)* Compound used for rheumatism. *Gastrointestinal Aid* Decoction of roots rubbed on the stomach for cramps. *Liver Aid* Infusion of plant taken to concentrate bile. *Orthopedic Aid* Decoction of roots rubbed on the arms and legs

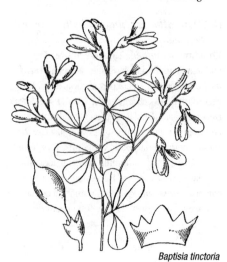

Baptisia tinctoria

for cramps. (73:363) **Micmac** *Antihemorrhagic* Root used for spitting blood. *Kidney Aid* Root used for kidney trouble. *Venereal Aid* Root used for gonorrhea. (32:55) **Mohegan** *Dermatological Aid* Infusion of plant used as wash for cuts and wounds. (149:266) Infusion of root used as a healing lotion for cuts or bruises. (151:70, 128) **Nanticoke** *Orthopedic Aid* Compound containing plant used as a lotion on sprains. (150:56, 84) **Ojibwa** *Unspecified* Plant used for medicinal purposes. (112:235) **Penobscot** *Antihemorrhagic* Compound infusion of plant taken for "spitting up blood." *Kidney Aid* Compound infusion of plant taken for kidney trouble. *Tonic* Compound infusion of plant taken as a tonic. *Venereal Aid* Compound infusion of plant taken for gonorrhea. (133:311)

Barbarea vulgaris, Garden Yellowrocket
Cherokee *Blood Medicine* Cooked salad eaten to purify blood. (66:31) **Mohegan** *Cough Medicine* Infusion of leaves taken every half hour for coughs. **Shinnecock** *Cough Medicine* Infusion of leaves taken every half hour for coughs. (25:118)

Barbula unguiculata, Moss
Seminole *Antirheumatic (External)* and *Febrifuge* Plant used for fire sickness: fever and body aches. (145:203)

Bellis perennis, Lawndaisy
Iroquois *Gastrointestinal Aid* Decoction of plant clusters taken for bad stomach. (73:461)

Berberis canadensis, American Barberry
Cherokee *Antidiarrheal* Infusion of scraped bark taken for diarrhea. (66:48)

Berberis vulgaris, Common Barberry
Micmac *Oral Aid* Bark and root used for ulcerated gums. *Throat Aid* Bark and root used for sore throat. (32:55) **Mohegan** *Febrifuge* Cold, compound decoction of berries taken for fever. (149:269) Juice of berries mixed with water and used for fever. (151:70, 128) *Throat Aid* Berries used for sore throat and fever. (151:128) **Penobscot** *Oral Aid* Poultice of pounded root or bark applied to ulcerated gums. *Throat Aid* Pounded root or bark used for sore throat. (133:309) **Shinnecock** *Liver*

Aid Decoction of leaves taken three times a day for jaundice. (25:119)

Berchemia scandens, Alabama Supplejack
Choctaw *Blood Medicine* Plant used for the blood. (152:40) **Houma** *Reproductive Aid* Decoction of leaf and bark taken for "impotency in male or female." Decoction of leaves and bark taken by males or females for impotency. (135:57) **Koasati** *Cough Medicine* Cold infusion of burned stems taken as a cough medicine. (152:40) **Seminole** *Other* Complex infusion of stems taken for chronic conditions. (145:272)

Berlandiera lyrata, Lyreleaf Greeneyes
Keres, Western *Psychological Aid* Dried roots burned, ground, and tossed on hot coals or smoke inhaled to give courage. *Sedative* Dried roots burned, ground, and tossed on hot coals or smoke inhaled for nervousness. (147:33)

Berula erecta, Cutleaf Waterparsnip
Apache, White Mountain *Unspecified* Leaves and blossoms used for medicinal purposes. (113:155) **Zuni** *Antirheumatic* (*External*) Ingredient of "schumaakwe cakes" and used externally for rheumatism. (143:44) *Dermatological Aid* Infusion of whole plant used as wash for rashes and athlete's foot infection. (22:379) Ingredient of "schumaakwe cakes" and used externally for swelling. (143:44)

Besseya plantaginea, White River Coraldrops
Navajo, Ramah *Ceremonial Medicine* Plant used as ceremonial emetic. *Dermatological Aid* Dried root or leaf used as dusting powder on skin sores or infant's sore navel. *Diuretic* Cold infusion of plant taken by hunters for anuria. *Emetic* Plant used as ceremonial emetic. *Hunting Medicine* Lotion from plant applied to body for protection while hunting and in war. *Panacea* Root used as a "life medicine." *Pediatric Aid* Cold infusion of root used for birth injuries. Dried root or leaves used as dusting powder for skin sores or infant's sore navel. *Witchcraft Medicine* Lotion from plant applied to body for protection from witches. (165:43)

Betula alleghaniensis, Yellow Birch
Ojibwa, South *Diuretic* Compound decoction of inner bark taken as a diuretic. (as *B. excelsa* 77:199)

Betula alleghaniensis var. ***alleghaniensis***, Yellow Birch
Delaware, Oklahoma *Cathartic* Decoction of bark taken as a cathartic. *Emetic* Decoction of bark taken as an emetic. (as *B. lutea* 150:25, 74) *Gastrointestinal Aid* and *Liver Aid* Decoction of bark taken "to remove bile from the intestines." (as *B. lutea* 150:25) **Iroquois** *Blood Medicine* Complex compound used as a blood purifier. *Dermatological Aid* Complex compound decoction used as wash for affected parts of "Italian itch." (as *B. lutea* 73:300) *Gynecological Aid* Decoction of plant used for lactation. (as *B. lutea* 73:301) **Micmac** *Other* Wood used as a hot-water bottle. (as *B. lutea* 32:55) **Ojibwa** *Blood Medicine* Decoction of bark taken for internal blood diseases. (as *B. lutea* 112:231) **Potawatomi** *Adjuvant* Infusion of twigs used as a seasoner for medicines. (as *B. lutea* 131:44)

Betula lenta, Sweet Birch
Algonquin, Quebec *Unspecified* Infusion of plant used for many medicinal purposes. (14:151) **Cherokee** *Antidiarrheal* Leaves chewed or infusion taken for dysentery. *Cold Remedy* Infusion taken for colds. *Gastrointestinal Aid* Infusion of bark taken for the stomach. *Urinary Aid* Infusion of bark taken for "milky urine." (66:25) **Chippewa** *Antidiarrheal* Decoction of bark taken for diarrhea. *Pulmonary Aid* Bark used for pulmonary troubles and decoction of bark taken for pneumonia. (59:128) **Iroquois** *Blood Medicine* Compound decoction taken when the "blood gets bad and cold." *Cold Remedy* Compound infusion taken by women "when they catch cold with the menses." *Febrifuge* Compound decoction taken for fever. *Gynecological Aid* Compound decoction taken by women who have gonorrhea and are pregnant. *Orthopedic Aid* Compound decoction taken for soreness. *Stimulant* Compound decoction taken "when a person tires." *Unspecified* "Highly valued medicine because it sustains the deer, the mainstay of life." (73:300) **Mohegan** *Tonic* Complex compound infusion including black birch bark taken as spring tonic. (149:266) Inner bark used to make a tonic. (151:70, 128)

Betula nana, Bog Birch
Eskimo, Western *Analgesic* and *Gastrointestinal Aid* Compound decoction of leaves taken for stomachache and intestinal discomfort. (as *B. exilis* 90:5)

Betula nigra, River Birch
Cherokee *Antidiarrheal* Leaves chewed or infusion taken for dysentery. *Cold Remedy* Infusion taken for colds. *Gastrointestinal Aid* Infusion of bark taken for the stomach. *Urinary Aid* Infusion of bark taken for "milky urine." (66:25) Decoction of inner bark taken for difficult urination with discharge. (152:15) **Chippewa** *Analgesic* and *Gastrointestinal Aid* Decoction of bark taken for stomach pain. (43:342)

Betula occidentalis, Water Birch
Blackfoot *Abortifacient* Flowers and leaves included in two separate bundles and used for conception. Decoction of flowers and leaves taken when bundle to stop conception fails. (72:60)

Betula papyrifera, Paper Birch
Algonquin, Quebec *Dermatological Aid* and *Pediatric Aid* Bark powder used for diaper rash and other skin rashes. (14:152) **Chippewa** *Cathartic* Infusion of inner bark used as an enema. (43:364) **Cree, Woodlands** *Burn Dressing* Poultice of outer bark used to bandage a burn. *Dermatological Aid* Dried, finely powdered rotten wood used as baby powder to prevent rashes. Dried inner bark ground, added to pitch and grease, and used as ointment for persistent scabs and rashes. Decoction of inner bark used as a wash for skin rashes and other skin sores. *Diaphoretic* Decoction of wood taken to cause sweating. *Gynecological Aid* Decoction of wood taken to ensure an adequate supply of milk for breast feeding. Decoction of wood and inner bark used for "women's troubles." *Orthopedic Aid* Decoction of wood taken for back pain. *Pediatric Aid* Dried, finely powdered rotten wood used as baby powder to prevent rashes. Decoction of stems or branches taken for teething sickness. *Toothache Remedy* Decoction of stems or branches taken for teething sickness. *Venereal Aid* Wood mixed with other materials and used for gonorrhea. (91:32) **Iroquois** *Gynecological Aid* Burned bark ashes used to "shrivel the womb."

(73:300) **Koyukon** *Unspecified* Plant spirit used by the shaman to heal sick people. (99:53) **Menominee** *Antidiarrheal* Decoction of inner bark used for dysentery. *Tonic* Decoction of branch tips used as a tonic. (44:131) **Ojibwa** *Adjuvant* Root used as a seasoner for medicines. *Analgesic* Root bark cooked with maple sugar as syrup for stomach cramps. (as *B. alba* var. *papyrifera* 130:358) *Blood Medicine* Decoction of bark taken for internal blood diseases. (112:231) *Gastrointestinal Aid* Compound decoction of root bark taken to alleviate stomach cramps. (as *B. alba* var. *papyrifera* 130:358) **Potawatomi** *Adjuvant* Infusion of twigs used as a seasoner for medicines. (as *B. alba* var. *papyrifera* 131:43, 44) **Shuswap** *Analgesic* Plant used for pain. (102:60) **Tanana, Upper** *Orthopedic Aid* Bark used as casts for broken limbs. A soft material such as a cloth was placed next to the skin on the broken limb over which birch bark was wrapped and tied. The birch bark was then heated until it shrank to fit the limb. (86:5) **Thompson** *Cold Remedy* Sap tapped from trees in early spring and taken for colds. *Contraceptive* Bark used for contraception. One informant recalled a case in which a woman in childbirth did not want any more children. An old woman told her to take the afterbirth, stick it with an old bone awl, wrap it in fish net and then in a piece of birch bark, and place it high up on a particular kind of tree. The patient was then given an infusion of bitter cherry or saskatoon wood and after that had no more children *Cough Medicine* Sap tapped from trees in early spring and taken for coughs. (161:189)

Betula populifolia, Gray Birch
Iroquois *Hemorrhoid Remedy* Decoction of bark taken for bleeding piles. (73:300) **Malecite** *Dermatological Aid* Inner bark scrapings used for swelling in infected cuts. (96:245) **Micmac** *Dermatological Aid* Inner bark used for infected cuts. *Emetic* Inner bark used as an emetic. (32:55)

Betula pubescens ssp. pubescens, Downy Birch
Cree, Hudson Bay *Dermatological Aid* Boiled, powdered wood applied to chafed skin. (as *B. alba* 78:303)

Betula pumila* var. *glandulifera, Glandulose Birch
Ojibwa *Gynecological Aid* Infusion of cones taken during menses and for strength after childbirth. *Respiratory Aid* Smoke of cones inhaled for catarrh. (130:358)

Bidens bipinnata, Spanish Needles
Cherokee *Anthelmintic* Infusion taken for worms. *Throat Aid* Leaves chewed for sore throat. (66:57)

Bidens coronata, Crowned Beggarticks
Seminole *Analgesic* and *Antidiarrheal* Infusion of roots taken for sun sickness: eye disease, headache, high fever, and diarrhea. (145:206) *Antirheumatic (External)* Plant used for fire sickness: fever and body aches. (145:204) *Eye Medicine* Infusion of roots taken for sun sickness: eye disease, headache, high fever, and diarrhea. (145:206) Infusion of whole plant taken and used as a bath for mist sickness: eye disease, fever, and chills. (145:209) *Febrifuge* Plant used for fire sickness: fever and body aches. (145:204) Infusion of roots taken for sun sickness: eye disease, headache, high fever, and diarrhea. (145:206) Infusion of whole plant taken and used as a bath for mist sickness: eye disease, fever, and chills. (145:209)

Bignonia capreolata, Cross Vine
Cherokee *Blood Medicine* Infusion of leaf taken to purify blood. (as *Anisostichus capreolata* 66:31) Infusion of leaves used to cleanse the blood. (177:74) **Choctaw** *Kidney Aid* Decoction of mashed bark used as a steam bath for dropsy. (152:57) **Creek** *Unspecified* Plant used medicinally for unspecified purpose. (as *B. crucigera* 148:670) **Houma** *Misc. Disease Remedy* Infusion of mashed root used as a gargle for diphtheria. (135:65) **Koasati** *Analgesic* Decoction of bark used as a bath and taken for headaches. *Antirheumatic (Internal)* Decoction of leaves taken for rheumatism. (152:57)

Blechnum spicant, Deer Fern
Hesquiat *Cancer Treatment* Leaflets chewed for internal cancer. *Dermatological Aid* Fronds used as a good medicine for skin sores. This medicine was first learned about from watching the deer,

who rub their antler stubs on this plant when their antlers break off. (159:29) **Kwakiutl** *Antidiarrheal* Compound decoction of root taken or root held in mouth for diarrhea. (as *Struthiopteris spicant* 16:381) Compound decoction of roots taken for diarrhea. (157:266) **Makah** *Gastrointestinal Aid* Green leaves chewed for stomach distress. *Pulmonary Aid* Green leaves chewed for lung trouble. **Quileute** *Orthopedic Aid* Poultice of fresh leaves applied to paralyzed parts of the body. *Panacea* Decoction of leaves taken for general ill health. **Quinault** *Gastrointestinal Aid* Raw leaves chewed for colic. (as *Struthiopteris spicant* 65:15)

Blephilia ciliata, Downy Pagodaplant
Cherokee *Analgesic* Poultice of leaves used for headache. (66:45)

***Bobea* sp.**, Ahakea
Hawaiian *Blood Medicine* Bark used as a blood purifier. *Dermatological Aid* Bark used for skin ulcers. (2:5)

Boschniakia glabra
Tlingit *Dermatological Aid* Compound containing root used for sores. (89:284)

Boschniakia hookeri, Vancouver Groundcone
Hesquiat *Cough Medicine* Roots used for coughs. (159:70)

Bothriochloa saccharoides, Silver Bluestem
Kiowa *Oral Aid* Stem used as a toothpick. Stem used as a toothpick. (166:13)

Botrychium virginianum, Rattlesnake Fern
Abnaki *Other* Used as a demulcent. (121:155) *Pediatric Aid* and *Unspecified* Decoction of plant given to children with illness. (121:162) **Cherokee** *Emetic* Decoction of roots taken to cause vomiting. (152:4) *Snakebite Remedy* Decoction of root "boiled down to syrup" and rubbed on snakebite. (66:34) **Chickasaw** *Diaphoretic* Plant used as a diaphoretic. (23:288, 289) *Emetic* Decoction of root used as an emetic. (23:288, 289) *Expectorant* Decoction of root used as an emetic and plant used as an expectorant. (23:288, 289) **Chippewa** *Snakebite Remedy* Poultice of mashed, fresh root applied to snakebite and used as repel-

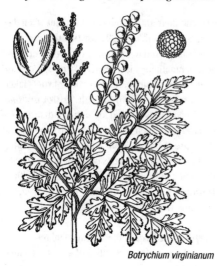

Botrychium virginianum

lent. (43:352) **Ojibwa** *Pulmonary Aid* Plant said to be good for lung trouble. *Tuberculosis Remedy* Plant said to be good for consumption. (130:377) **Ojibwa, South** *Dermatological Aid* Poultice of bruised root applied to cuts. (77:201) **Potawatomi** *Unspecified* Compound containing root used medicinally. (131:67)

Botrychium virginianum ssp. *virginianum*, Rattlesnake Fern
Iroquois *Cough Medicine* and *Tuberculosis Remedy* Cold infusion of root and liquor taken for the cough of consumption. (73:261)

Bouteloua gracilis, Blue Grama
Navajo, Ramah *Antidote* Compound decoction of plant taken to counteract overdose of "life medicine." *Dermatological Aid* Roots chewed and blown on cuts. *Gynecological Aid* Decoction of whole plant taken as a postpartum medicine. *Panacea* Cold, compound infusion of root used internally and externally as "life medicine." *Veterinary Aid* Roots chewed and blown on incisions of castrated colts. (165:15, 16)

Bouteloua simplex, Matted Grama
Navajo, Ramah *Dermatological Aid* Ashes applied to sores. *Throat Aid* Cold infusion used internally and externally for sore throat. (165:16)

Bovista pila, Puffball
Haisla & Hanaksiala *Poison* Spores dangerous, especially harmful to the eyes. (35:134)

Bovista plumbea, Puffball
Haisla & Hanaksiala *Poison* Spores dangerous, especially harmful to the eyes. (35:134)

Bovistella sp., Puffball
Haisla & Hanaksiala *Poison* Spores dangerous, especially harmful to the eyes. (35:134)

Boykinia jamesii, James's Telesonix
Cheyenne *Antihemorrhagic* and *Pulmonary Aid* Infusion of dried plant taken for lung hemorrhages. (as *Saxifraga jamesi* 63:175) Infusion of finely powered plant taken for lung hemorrhage. (as *Saxifraga jamesi* 64:175)

Boykinia occidentalis, Coastal Brookfoam
Quileute *Tuberculosis Remedy* Raw leaves eaten for tuberculosis. (as *B. elata* 65:31) **Yuki** *Unspecified* Roots used medicinally for unspecified purpose. (as *Therofon elatum* 33:353)

Brachyactis frondosa, Leafy Rayless Aster
Paiute *Antirheumatic* (*External*) Infusion of stems and flowers used as a wash for rheumatism. *Blood Medicine* and *Tonic* Infusion of dried stems taken as a general blood tonic. (as *A. frondosus* 155:48, 49)

Brassica juncea, India Mustard
Navajo, Ramah *Gastrointestinal Aid* Plant used as a stomach medicine. (165:28)

Brassica napus, Rape
Cherokee *Dietary Aid* Taken to increase the appetite. *Febrifuge* Taken for fever and "nervous fever." *Kidney Aid* Taken for "dropsy." *Misc. Disease Remedy* Taken for "ague." *Orthopedic Aid* Taken for palsy. *Pulmonary Aid* Used as a poultice for croup. *Respiratory Aid* Given for "phthisic" or asthma. *Stimulant* Taken as a stimulant. *Tonic* Taken as a tonic. (66:46) **Iroquois** *Dermatological Aid* Poultice of hot, dried leaves applied to sores and boils. (73:341) **Micmac** *Cold Remedy* Bark used for colds. *Cough Medicine* Bark used

for coughs. *Misc. Disease Remedy* Bark used for grippe and smallpox. (32:55)

Brassica nigra, Black Mustard

Cherokee *Dietary Aid* Taken to increase appetite. *Febrifuge* Taken for fever and "nervous fever." *Kidney Aid* Taken for "dropsy." *Misc. Disease Remedy* Taken for "ague." *Orthopedic Aid* Taken for palsy. *Pulmonary Aid* Used as a poultice for croup. *Respiratory Aid* Given for "phthisic" or asthma. *Stimulant* Taken as a stimulant. *Tonic* Taken as a tonic. (66:46) **Hoh** *Unspecified* Plants used for medicine. (114:61) **Meskwaki** *Cold Remedy* Snuff of ground seeds used for head colds. (129:219) **Mohegan** *Analgesic* Poultice of mustard applied to body pains. Poultice of wilted leaves applied to the skin for headache. (25:120) Poultice of leaves bound to the skin for headache. (149:264) Poultice of fresh leaves applied to headaches. (151:71, 128) *Toothache Remedy* Poultice of wilted leaves applied to the skin for toothache. (25:120) Poultice of leaves bound to the skin for toothache. (149:264) Poultice of fresh leaves applied to toothaches. (151:71, 128) **Quileute** *Unspecified* Plants used for medicine. (114:61) **Shinnecock** *Analgesic* Poultice of mustard applied to body pains. Poultice of wilted leaves applied to the skin for headache. *Emetic* Mustard mixed with flour and water and taken to make "insides come up." *Toothache Remedy* Poultice of wilted leaves applied to the skin for toothache. (25:120)

Brassica oleracea, Cabbage

Cherokee *Dermatological Aid* Poultice of wilted leaf used for boils. (66:28) **Rappahannock** *Analgesic* Poultice of green leaves bound to head for headache. (138:25)

Brassica rapa var. *rapa*, Birdrape

Ojibwa *Unspecified* Plant used for medicinal purposes. (as *B. campestris* 112:232)

Brickellia ambigens

Keres, Western *Antirheumatic (External)* Dried, ground leaves mixed with water and used as a salve. *Carminative* and *Dietary Aid* Infusion of plant taken for flatulence and overeating. *Liver Aid* Infusion of plant used as liver medicine. (147:33)

Brickellia brachyphylla, Plumed Brickellbush

Navajo, Ramah *Disinfectant* and *Pediatric Aid* Root used with "lizard figurine" for prenatal "lizard infection." (165:49)

Brickellia californica, California Brickellbush

Diegueño *Febrifuge* Infusion of leaves taken for fevers. (74:220) **Navajo, Kayenta** *Ceremonial Medicine* Plant used as a ceremonial emetic following clan incest. *Dermatological Aid* Plant used as a lotion on infant sores caused by prenatal infection. *Emetic* Plant used as a ceremonial emetic following clan incest. *Pediatric Aid* Plant used as a lotion on infant sores caused by prenatal infection. (179:45) **Navajo, Ramah** *Cough Medicine* Cold infusion of leaves taken and used as lotion for cough or fever. *Febrifuge* Infusion of leaves taken and used as lotion for cough or fever. (165:49)

Brickellia eupatorioides var. *eupatorioides*, False Boneset

Navajo, Ramah *Cough Medicine* and *Other* Decoction of root taken for old injury or cough. (as *Kuhnia rosmarinifolia* 165:52)

Brickellia grandiflora, Tasselflower Brickellbush

Gosiute *Poison* Seeds had poisonous effects. *Unspecified* Root used as medicine. (31:364) **Keres, Western** *Antirheumatic (External)* Dried, ground leaves mixed with water and used as a

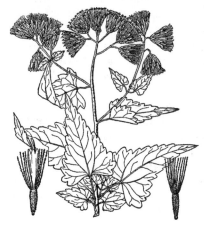

Brickellia grandiflora

salve. *Carminative* Infusion of plant taken for flatulence. *Dietary Aid* Infusion of plant taken for
overeating. *Liver Aid* Infusion of plant used as a
liver medicine. (147:33) **Navajo, Ramah** *Analgesic* Cold infusion of dried leaves taken for headache. *Ceremonial Medicine* and *Emetic* Plant used
as a ceremonial emetic. *Misc. Disease Remedy*
Cold infusion of dried leaves taken for influenza.
(165:49)

Brickellia oblongifolia var. **linifolia**,
Narrowleaf Brickellbush
Navajo, Kayenta *Dermatological Aid* and *Pediatric Aid* Plant lotion used on infant ear and finger
sores caused by prenatal infection. (179:46) **Shoshoni** *Gastrointestinal Aid* Decoction of stems
and leaves taken as a stomach medicine. (155:52)

Brodiaea sp., Grass Nut
Mahuna *Dermatological Aid* Plant used as a
shampoo for the hair. (117:40)

Bromus carinatus, California Brome
Hesquiat *Poison* Long, sharp-awned fruit were
said to be very dangerous if swallowed. (159:56)

Bromus tectorum, Cheat Grass
Navajo, Kayenta *Ceremonial Medicine* Infusion
of plant used as a face wash for God-Imperson-
ators. (179:15)

Broussaisia arguta, Kanawao
Hawaiian *Pediatric Aid* Fruits eaten from conception until the child feeds itself to increase the
child's survival rate. *Reproductive Aid* Fruits eaten
with baked eggs to bring about conception by barren women. *Strengthener* Fruits eaten from conception until the child feeds itself to increase the child's
survival rate. (as *Broussaisa pelluoida* 2:48)

Broussonetia papyrifera, Paper Mulberry
Apache, Chiricahua & Mescalero *Narcotic*
Plant used as a narcotic. (as *B. secundiflora* 28:54)

Bryum capillare, Moss
Seminole *Antirheumatic* (*External*) and *Febrifuge* Plant used for fire sickness: fever and body
aches. (145:203)

Buchloe dactyloides, Buffalo Grass
Keres, Western *Dermatological Aid* Stolons
crushed with yucca root or soaked in water and
used as a head bath to make the hair grow. (as
Bulbilis dactyloides 147:34)

Bursera microphylla, Elephant Tree
Cahuilla *Dermatological Aid* Sap used for skin
diseases. *Panacea* Sap used for almost any disease. (11:48)

Butomus umbellatus, Flowering Rush
Iroquois *Veterinary Aid* Decoction of whole plant
and bark from another plant added to cow and
horse feed for worms. (118:66)

Caesalpinia bonduc, Yellow
Nicker
Hawaiian *Blood Medicine* Beans
and other plants pounded, squeezed
and the resulting liquid taken to purify the blood.
Laxative and *Pediatric Aid* Beans ground and
taken as a laxative by infants, children and adults.
Pulmonary Aid Beans and other plants pounded,
squeezed, and resulting liquid taken to clear the
chest of tough phlegm. (2:47)

Caesalpinia jamesii, James's Holdback
Zuni *Veterinary Aid* Infusion of plant given to
sheep to make them "prolific." (as *Hoffmanseggia
jamesii* 143:54)

Caesalpinia kavaiensis, Uhiuhi
Hawaiian *Blood Medicine* Bark, young leaves,
and other plants pounded, squeezed, and resulting
liquid taken to purify the blood. (as *Mezoneurum
kauaiense* 2:38)

Calamagrostis rubescens, Pine Grass
Thompson *Gynecological Aid* Dried grass rubbed
until soft and used as sanitary napkins. (161:140)

Calla palustris, Water Arum
Cree, Woodlands *Orthopedic Aid* Aerial stems
used for sore legs. *Poison* Plant poisonous to touch
and eat. (91:33) **Gitksan** *Antihemorrhagic* Decoction of root taken for hemorrhage. *Eye Medicine*
Decoction of root taken for "cleaning the eyes of

the blind." *Misc. Disease Remedy* Decoction of roots taken for influenza and hemorrhage. *Respiratory Aid* Decoction of root taken for shortness of breath. (127:53) *Tonic* Plant used in a spiritual spring tonic. (62:26) **Iroquois** *Snakebite Remedy* Compound decoction of roots and stems used as poultice on snakebites. (73:278) **Potawatomi** *Dermatological Aid* Poultice of pounded root applied to swellings. (131:40)

Calliandra eriophylla, Fairyduster
Yavapai *Gynecological Aid* Decoction of leaves and stems taken after childbirth. (53:261)

Calliandra humilis, Dwarf Stickpea
Navajo, Ramah *Panacea* Plant used as "life medicine." (165:32) **Zuni** *Dermatological Aid* Powdered root used three times a day for rashes. (22:376)

Callicarpa americana, American Beautyberry
Alabama *Antirheumatic* (*External*) Decoction of roots and branches used in sweat bath for rheumatism. *Diaphoretic* Decoction of root and branch used in sweat bath for malarial fever and rheumatism. *Febrifuge* Decoction of roots and branches used in sweat bath for malarial fevers. (148:663) Decoction of roots and leaves used as sweat bath for malarial fever. *Herbal Steam* and Decoction of roots and leaves used as sweat bath for malarial fever. **Choctaw** *Antidiarrheal* Decoction of roots taken for dysentery. (152:52) *Gastrointestinal Aid* Decoction of roots and berries taken for colic. (20:24) Decoction of roots and berries taken for colic. *Other* Decoction of roots taken during attacks of dizziness. **Koasati** *Gastrointestinal Aid* Decoction of roots taken for stomachaches. (152:52) **Seminole** *Dermatological Aid* Plant used for snake sickness: itchy skin. (145:166) Roots or stem bark used for snake sickness: itchy skin. (145:239) *Urinary Aid* Decoction of root bark taken for urine retention. (145:274)

Callirhoe involucrata, Purple Poppymallow
Dakota *Analgesic* Decoction of root taken for internal pains. Smoke of dried root used to bathe aching body parts. *Cold Remedy* Root smoke inhaled for head cold. (58:103)

Calocedrus decurrens, Incense Cedar
Klamath *Herbal Steam* Branches and twigs used in administering a sweat bath. (as *Libocedrus decurrens* 37:88) **Mendocino Indian** *Gastrointestinal Aid* Decoction of leaves taken for stomach troubles. (as *Libocedrus decurrens* 33:306) **Paiute** *Cold Remedy* Infusion of leaves steam inhaled for colds. (as *Libocedrus decurrens* 93:46)

Calochortus aureus, Golden Mariposa Lily
Hopi *Ceremonial Medicine* Plant used in the Flute ceremony. (46:18) **Navajo, Ramah** *Panacea* Bulb used as "life medicine." (as *C. nuttallii* var. *aureus* 165:20)

Calochortus gunnisonii, Gunnison's Mariposa Lily
Cheyenne *Unspecified* Dried, chopped bulbs used as an ingredient for a medicinal mixture. *Veterinary Aid* Root put into a horse's mouth before running the animal in a race. (69:12) **Keres, Western** *Antirheumatic* (*Internal*) Infusion of plant taken for swellings. (147:34) **Navajo, Ramah** *Ceremonial Medicine* Plant used as a ceremonial medicine. *Dermatological Aid* Juice of leaf applied to pimples. *Gynecological Aid* Decoction of whole plant taken to ease delivery of placenta. *Panacea* Bulb used as "life medicine." (165:20)

Calochortus macrocarpus, Sagebrush Mariposa Lily
Okanagan-Colville *Dermatological Aid* Poultice of mashed bulbs applied to the skin for poison ivy. (162:41) **Thompson** *Eye Medicine* Mashed bulbs placed in cheesecloth and used for the eyes. (161:119)

Caltha leptosepala ssp. *leptosepala* var. *leptosepala*, White Marshmarigold
Okanagon *Dermatological Aid* Poultice of chewed plant applied to inflamed wounds. **Thompson** *Dermatological Aid* Poultice of chewed plant applied to inflamed wounds. (as *C. rotundifolia* 104:42) Fresh plant chewed and spit on wounds and poultice of crushed plant used. (as *C. rotundifolia* 141:467)

Caltha palustris, Yellow Marshmarigold
Abnaki *Poison* Plant considered poisonous. (121:
155) **Alaska Native** *Poison* Raw leaves considered
poisonous. (71:19) **Chippewa** *Cold Remedy* Decoction of root taken as diaphoretic, expectorant,
and emetic for colds. (43:340) *Dermatological
Aid* Poultice of boiled and mashed roots applied
to sores. (59:130) *Diaphoretic* Decoction of root
taken as a diaphoretic and emetic for colds.
(43:340) *Diuretic* Compound decoction of leaves
and stalks taken as a diuretic. (43:348) *Emetic*
Decoction of root taken as a diaphoretic and
emetic for colds. (43:340) *Gynecological Aid*
Compound decoction of root taken during "confinement." (43:360) *Tuberculosis Remedy* Poultice of mashed or powdered root applied to scrofula sores. (43:354) **Eskimo, Inupiat** *Poison*
Young shoots poisonous, if not boiled. (83:143)
Eskimo, Western *Laxative* Infusion of leaves
taken for constipation. (90:14) **Iroquois** *Emetic*
and *Love Medicine* Infusion of smashed roots
taken to vomit against a love charm. (73:323)

Calvatia sp.
Haisla & Hanaksiala *Poison* Spores dangerous,
especially harmful to the eyes. (35:134)

Calycadenia fremontii, Frémont's Western
   Rosinweed
Yana *Febrifuge* Cooked, dried, pounded seeds
eaten for chills. (as *Hemizonia multiglandulosa*
124:252)

Calycanthus floridus, Eastern Sweetshrub
Cherokee *Dermatological Aid* Bark ooze used
on children's sores and infusion used for hives.
Emetic Roots used as a strong emetic. (66:58)
Roots used as very strong emetics. (177:74) *Eye
Medicine* Cold infusion of bark used as eye drops
for persons losing eyesight. *Pediatric Aid* Bark
ooze used on children's sores and infusion used
for hives. (66:58) *Poison* Seeds used to poison
wolves. (177:74) *Urinary Aid* Roots used for urinary and bladder complaints. (66:58)

Calycanthus floridus var. glaucus, Eastern
   Sweetshrub
Cherokee *Urinary Aid* Infusion of bark taken for
urinary troubles. (as *C. fertilis* 152:23)

Calycanthus occidentalis, Western Sweetshrub
Pomo *Cold Remedy* Decoction of scraped bark
taken for severe colds. (54:13) **Pomo, Kashaya**
Cold Remedy Infusion of dried or fresh, peeled
bark used for chest colds. *Expectorant* Infusion of
dried or fresh, peeled bark used to cough up the
phlegm in the chest. *Gastrointestinal Aid* Infusion
of dried or fresh, peeled bark used for stomach
problems. *Throat Aid* Infusion of dried or fresh,
peeled bark used for sore throat. (60:109)

Calylophus hartwegii ssp. **fendleri**,
   Hartweg's Sundrops
Navajo, Ramah *Panacea* Plant used as "life medicine," especially for internal bleeding. (as *Oenothera hartwegii* var. *fendleri* 165:38)

Calypso bulbosa, Fairyslipper Orchid
Thompson *Anticonvulsive* Bulbs chewed or flowers sucked for mild epilepsy. (161:135)

Calypso bulbosa var. americana, Fairyslipper Orchid
Thompson *Unspecified* Plants used as charms for
unspecified purpose. (as *Cytherea bulbosa*
141:506)

Calystegia longipes, Paiute False Bindweed
Kawaiisu *Venereal Aid* Decoction of roots taken
for gonorrhea. (180:17)

Calystegia occidentalis ssp. **fulcrata**,
   Chaparral False Bindweed
Karok *Love Medicine* Plant used as a love medi-
cine. (as *Convolvulus fulcratus* 125:388)

Camassia quamash, Small Camas
Blackfoot *Gynecological Aid* Decoction of roots
taken to induce labor. Infusion of grass taken for
vaginal bleeding after birth and to help expel the
afterbirth. (72:60)

Camassia scilloides, Atlantic Camas
Creek *Unspecified* Plant used medicinally for unspecified purpose. (as *C. esculenta* 148:667)

Camellia sinensis, Tea
Makah *Hemostat* Poultice of leaves applied to
stop bleeding. (55:287)

Camissonia multijuga, Froststem Suncup
Navajo, Kayenta *Other* Infusion of plant used for
injuries by water or hail or dreaming of it. (as
Oenothera multijuga 179:33)

Camissonia tanacetifolia ssp. **tanacetifolia**, Tansyleaf Eveningprimrose
Navajo *Dermatological Aid* Plant rubbed on as a
liniment for boils. (as *Oenothera tanacetifolia*
45:67)

Campanula aparinoides, Marsh Bellflower
Iroquois *Gynecological Aid* Decoction of stems
taken by young women to induce childbirth.
(73:451)

Campanula divaricata, Small Bonny Bellflower
Cherokee *Antidiarrheal* Infusion of root taken for
diarrhea. (66:37)

Campanula parryi, Parry's Bellflower
Navajo, Kayenta *Gynecological Aid* Plant taken
by pregnant woman when female baby was desired.
(179:44) **Navajo, Ramah** *Dermatological Aid*
Dry plant used as a dusting powder for sores.
(165:47) **Zuni** *Dermatological Aid* Blossoms
chewed and saliva applied to skin as a depilatory.
Poultice of chewed root applied to bruises.
(143:44)

Campanula rotundifolia, Bluebell Bellflower
Chippewa *Ear Medicine* Infusion of root used as
drops for sore ear. (43:362) **Cree, Woodlands**
Heart Medicine Root chewed for heart ailments.
(91:34) **Navajo, Ramah** *Analgesic* Plant used as
ceremonial fumigant for head trouble. *Ceremonial
Medicine* Plant used as ceremonial fumigant for
various ailments. *Disinfectant* Plant used as ceremonial fumigant for deer infection. *Eye Medicine*
Plant used as ceremonial fumigant for eye. *Hunting Medicine* Plant rubbed on body for protection
while hunting. *Witchcraft Medicine* Plant rubbed
on body for protection from witches. (165:47)
Ojibwa *Pulmonary Aid* Compound containing

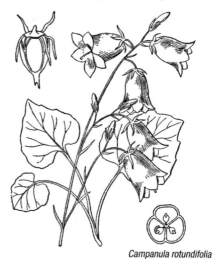

Campanula rotundifolia

root used for lung troubles. (130:360) **Thompson**
Eye Medicine Decoction of plant taken or used as
a wash for sore eyes. (161:196)

Campanulastrum americanum, American
Bellflower
Iroquois *Pulmonary Aid* Infusion of smashed
roots taken for whooping cough. (73:451)
Meskwaki *Cough Medicine* Leaves used for
coughs. *Tuberculosis Remedy* Leaves used for
consumption. (129:206)

Canavalia galeata, 'Awikiwiki
Hawaiian *Dermatological Aid* Infusion of leaves,
shoots, bark, and other plants used as a bath for
itch, ringworm, and skin diseases. (2:21)

Cannabis sativa, Marijuana
Iroquois *Psychological Aid* Used after patient gets
well but does not think that he has recovered.
Stimulant "This plant will get you going."
(73:306)

Capsella bursa-pastoris, Shepherd's Purse
Cheyenne *Analgesic* Cold infusion of leaves and
stems taken for head pains. (as *Bursa bursa-
pastoris* 63:174) Infusion of powdered leaves and
stems taken or small quantities of powder eaten
for head pains. (as *Bursa bursa-pastoris* 64:174)
Chippewa *Analgesic* Decoction of entire plant
taken for dysentery cramps. *Antidiarrheal* Decoction of whole plant taken for dysentery and cramps.

Gastrointestinal Aid Decoction of whole plant taken for stomach cramps and dysentery. (as *Bursa bursa-pastoris* 43:344) **Costanoan** *Antidiarrheal* Infusion of plant used for dysentery. (17:9) **Mahuna** *Antidiarrheal* Infusion of plants taken for dysentery and diarrhea. (117:7) **Menominee** *Dermatological Aid* Infusion of whole plant used as a wash for poison ivy. (as *Bursa bursa-pastoris* 44:134) Infusion of plant used as a wash for poison ivy. (128:33) **Meskwaki** *Unspecified* Used as a medicine. (129:219) **Mohegan** *Analgesic* Infusion of seedpods taken for stomach pains. (151:71) *Anthelmintic* Infusion of seedpods taken for stomach, the pungency killed internal worms. (as *Bursa bursa-pastoris* 149:265) Infusion of seedpods taken as a vermifuge. (151:71, 128) *Gastrointestinal Aid* Infusion of seedpods taken for stomach, the pungency killed internal worms. (as *Bursa bursa-pastoris* 149:265) Infusion of seedpods taken for stomach pains. (151:71)

Capsicum annuum var. *frutescens*,
Cayenne Pepper

Cherokee *Cold Remedy* Plant used for colds. *Febrifuge* Poultice applied to soles of feet "in nervous or low fevers." *Gastrointestinal Aid* Plant used for colics. *Poultice* Poultice used for gangrene and poultice applied to feet for fevers. *Stimulant* Plant used as a powerful stimulant. (as *C. frutescens* 66:48) **Navajo, Ramah** *Gynecological Aid* and *Pediatric Aid* Powdered chili pepper rubbed on breast to wean nursing child. (as *C. frutescens* var. *longum* 165:42)

Cardamine concatenata, Cutleaf Toothwort
Iroquois *Analgesic* Poultice of smashed roots applied to the head for headaches. *Cold Remedy* Used for colds. *Dietary Aid* Used to stimulate appetite and regulate stomach. *Gastrointestinal Aid* Plant used for colds, to stimulate appetite, and to regulate the stomach. (73:340) *Hallucinogen* Plant used to mesmerize. (73:339) *Heart Medicine* Roots used several ways for heart palpitations or other heart diseases. (73:340) *Hunting Medicine* Roots rubbed on guns, traps, fishing lines or hooks, a "hunting medicine." *Love Medicine* Roots or plant placed in pocket or mouth to attract women, a "love medicine." *Panacea* Compound infu-

sion taken or placed on injured part, a "Little Water Medicine." (73:339)

Cardamine diphylla, Crinkle Root
Algonquin, Quebec *Febrifuge* Infusion of plant given to children for fevers. *Heart Medicine* Infusion of plant and sweet flag root taken for heart disease. *Pediatric Aid* Infusion of plant given to children for fevers. (as *Dentaria diphylla* 14:173) **Cherokee** *Analgesic* Poultice of root used for headache. *Cold Remedy* Root chewed for colds. *Throat Aid* Infusion gargled for sore throat and root chewed for colds. (66:59) **Delaware** *Gastrointestinal Aid* Roots used as a stomach medicine. (as *Dentaria diphylla* 151:37) *Venereal Aid* Infusion of roots combined with other plants and used for scrofula and venereal disease. (as *Dentaria diphylla* 151:34) **Delaware, Oklahoma** *Gastrointestinal Aid* Compound containing root used as a stomach remedy. *Tuberculosis Remedy* Compound containing root used for "scrofula." *Venereal Aid* Compound containing root used for venereal disease. (as *Dentaria diphylla* 150:31, 76) **Iroquois** *Breast Treatment* Infusion of whole plant taken to strengthen the breasts. (as *Dentaria diphylla* 118:45) *Carminative* Raw root chewed for stomach gas. *Dermatological Aid* Poultice of roots applied to swellings. *Febrifuge* Cold infusion of plant taken for fever. *Love Medicine* Infusion of roots taken when "love medicine is too strong." *Other* Cold infusion of plant taken for "summer complaint." *Psychological Aid* Infusion of roots taken when the "heart jumps and the head goes wrong." *Pulmonary Aid* Compound used for chest pains. (73:341) *Tuberculosis Remedy* Infusion of plant taken at the beginning of tuberculosis. (as *Dentaria diphylla* 118:45) **Malecite** *Pediatric Aid* Infusion of roots used as a tonic for children. (as *Dentaria diphylla* 96:252) *Throat Aid* Green or dried roots chewed and used for hoarseness. (as *Dentaria diphylla* 96:247) Green or dry roots chewed and used to clear the throat. *Tonic* Infusion of roots used as a tonic. (as *Dentaria diphylla* 96:252) **Micmac** *Sedative* Root used as a sedative. *Throat Aid* Root used to clear the throat and for hoarseness. *Tonic* Root used as a tonic. (as *Dentaria diphylla* 32:56)

Cardamine douglassii, Limestone Bittercress
Iroquois *Antidote* Infusion of smashed roots used
to counteract any kind of poison. *Witchcraft Medicine* Infusion of smashed roots used to divine the
perpetrator of witchcraft. (73:340)

Cardamine maxima, Large Toothwort
Menominee *Gastrointestinal Aid* Good medicine
for the stomach. (as *Dentaria maxima* 128:65)
Ojibwa *Gastrointestinal Aid* Roots used as a good
medicine for the stomach. (as *Dentaria maxima*
130:399)

Cardamine rhomboidea, Bulbous Bittercress
Iroquois *Poison* Roots used as a poison to kill.
(as *C. bulbosa* 73:340)

Carex brevior, Fescue Sedge
Iroquois *Gynecological Aid* Compound infusion
of plant taken for evacuation of the placenta.
(73:275)

Carex inops ssp. **heliophila**, Sun Sedge
Navajo, Ramah *Disinfectant* Cold infusion of
plant used as lotion for "eagle infections." *Gastrointestinal Aid* Cold infusion of plant taken to relieve discomfort from overeating. (as *C. pensylvanica* var. *digyna* 165:19)

Carex microptera, Smallwing Sedge
Navajo, Ramah *Ceremonial Medicine* and *Emetic*
Plant used as a ceremonial emetic. (as *C. festivella*
165:19)

Carex nebrascensis, Nebraska Sedge
Cheyenne *Ceremonial Medicine* Plant used in the
Sun Dance and Massaum ceremonies. (69:7)

Carex oligosperma, Fewseed Sedge
Iroquois *Emetic* Compound decoction taken as
an emetic before running or playing lacrosse.
(73:275)

Carex plantaginea, Plantainleaf Sedge
Menominee *Snakebite Remedy* Root used as a
charm to prevent snakebite and spittle from
chewed root used on snakebite. (128:34)

Carex platyphylla, Broadleaf Sedge
Iroquois *Other* Used several ways to "wash the
snowsnake," a snowsnake medicine. (73:274)

Carex prasina, Drooping Sedge
Iroquois *Emetic* Decoction taken as an emetic.
Gastrointestinal Aid Decoction taken "when stomach is bad from an unknown cause." *Veterinary
Aid* Decoction given to hunting dogs "when stomach is bad from an unknown cause." (73:275)

Carex vulpinoidea, Fox Sedge
Iroquois *Other* Compound decoction of roots
used as a "rooster fighting medicine." (73:275)

Carica papaya, Papaya
Hawaiian *Breast Treatment* Infusion of fruit
taken by mothers for dry breasts. *Dermatological
Aid* Milk and other plants mixed and applied to
deep cuts. (2:43)

Carnegia gigantea, Saguaro
Pima *Gynecological Aid* Plant used to make the
milk flow after childbirth. *Orthopedic Aid* Dead
ribs used as splints for broken bones. (38:53)

Carpinus caroliniana, American Hornbeam
Cherokee *Antidiarrheal* Compound infusion
taken for flux. *Dermatological Aid* Compound infusion taken for "navel yellowness." Compound
infusion of astringent inner bark taken for flux.
Urinary Aid Compound infusion taken for cloudy
urine. (66:39) Decoction of inner bark taken for

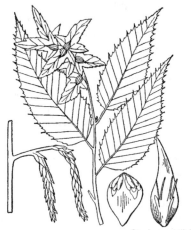

Carpinus caroliniana

difficult urination with discharge. (152:15) **Delaware, Ontario** *Gynecological Aid* Compound infusion of root or bark taken for "diseases peculiar to women." *Tonic* Compound infusion of root or bark taken for "general debility." (150:68) **Iroquois** *Antidiarrheal* Decoction used as a wash or infusion of vine given to babies with diarrhea. *Dermatological Aid* Complex compound decoction used as wash for affected parts of "Italian itch." *Gynecological Aid* Compound decoction taken to facilitate childbirth and for parturition. *Other* Compound used for "big injuries." *Pediatric Aid* Decoction used as a wash or infusion of vine given to babies with diarrhea. *Tuberculosis Remedy* Compound decoction of bark chips taken for consumption. (73:299)

Carum carvi, Caraway
Abnaki *Analgesic* Used as an analgesic. (121:155) **Cree, Woodlands** *Pediatric Aid* and *Sedative* Seed given to a crying child to quiet him or her. (91:34) **Iroquois** *Veterinary Aid* Rhizomes given to pigs to make them stronger. (118:55)

Carya alba, Mockernut Hickory
Cherokee *Abortifacient* Used for female obstructions. *Analgesic* Used for poliomyelitis pain. *Cold Remedy* Used for colds. *Dermatological Aid* Bark used as a dressing for cuts. Astringent and detergent inner bark used as dressing for cuts. *Diaphoretic* Used as a diaphoretic. *Emetic* Used as an emetic. *Gastrointestinal Aid* Used to invigorate the stomach. *Liver Aid* Used for bile. *Misc. Disease Remedy* Used for poliomyelitis pain. *Oral Aid* Bark chewed for sore mouth. (as *C. tomentosa* 66:38) Chewed inner bark used for sore mouth. (as *C. tomentosa* 152:14) *Orthopedic Aid* Infusion of bark taken by ballplayers to make limbs supple. (as *C. tomentosa* 66:38) **Delaware, Ontario** *Gynecological Aid* Compound infusion of bark taken for "female disorder." *Tonic* Compound infusion of bark taken as a tonic for general debility. (150:82)

Carya cordiformis, Bitternut Hickory
Iroquois *Dermatological Aid* Nutmeat oil formerly used for the hair, either alone or mixed with bear grease. (170:123) **Meskwaki** *Diuretic* Infusion of bark taken "to make the urine free." *Laxative* Infusion of bark taken "to make the bowels

loose." *Panacea* Infusion of bark taken for "simple sicknesses." (129:224)

Carya illinoinensis, Pecan
Comanche *Dermatological Aid* Pulverized leaves rubbed on affected part for ringworm. (24:520) **Kiowa** *Tuberculosis Remedy* Decoction of bark taken for tuberculosis. (as *C. pecan* 166:20)

Carya laciniosa, Shellbark Hickory
Cherokee *Abortifacient* Used for female obstructions. *Analgesic* Used for poliomyelitis pain. *Cold Remedy* Used for colds. *Dermatological Aid* Bark used as a dressing for cuts. Astringent and detergent inner bark used as dressing for cuts. *Diaphoretic* Used as a diaphoretic. *Emetic* Used as an emetic. *Gastrointestinal Aid* Used to invigorate the stomach. *Liver Aid* Used for bile. *Misc. Disease Remedy* Used for poliomyelitis pain. *Oral Aid* Bark chewed for sore mouth. *Orthopedic Aid* Infusion of bark taken by ballplayers to make limbs supple. (66:38)

Carya ovata, Shagbark Hickory
Chippewa *Analgesic* Fresh, small shoots steamed as inhalant for headache. *Herbal Steam* Fresh small shoots placed on hot stones as herbal steam for headache. (as *Hicoria alba* 43:338) **Delaware, Ontario** *Gynecological Aid* Compound infusion of bark taken for "diseases peculiar to women." *Tonic* Compound infusion of bark taken for "general debility." (150:68) **Iroquois** *Anthelmintic* Compound decoction with white from inside bark taken by adults for worms. *Antirheumatic (External)* Decoction of bark applied as a poultice for arthritis. *Antirheumatic (Internal)* Decoction of bark taken for arthritis. (73:297) *Dermatological Aid* Nutmeat oil formerly used for the hair, either alone or mixed with bear grease. (170:123)

Carya pallida, Sand Hickory
Cherokee *Abortifacient* Used for female obstructions. *Analgesic* Used for poliomyelitis pain. *Cold Remedy* Used for colds. *Dermatological Aid* Bark used as a dressing for cuts. Astringent and detergent inner bark used as dressing for cuts. *Diaphoretic* Used as a diaphoretic. *Emetic* Used as an emetic. *Gastrointestinal Aid* Used to invigorate the stomach. *Liver Aid* Used for bile. *Misc. Disease

Remedy Used for poliomyelitis pain. *Oral Aid* Bark chewed for sore mouth. *Orthopedic Aid* Infusion of bark taken by ballplayers to make limbs supple. (66:38)

Cassiope mertensiana, Western Moss Heather
Thompson *Tuberculosis Remedy* Decoction of plant taken over a period of time for tuberculosis and spitting up blood. (161:215)

Cassytha filiformis, Devil's Gut
Hawaiian *Gynecological Aid* Plant pounded, water added, and taken by women to remove blood from the womb while giving birth. *Respiratory Aid* Plant and other plants pounded, water added, and taken to remove phlegm causing congestion in the chest. (2:46)

Castanea dentata, American Chestnut
Cherokee *Cough Medicine* Compound decoction of leaves used as cough syrup. *Dermatological Aid* Leaves from young sprouts dipped in hot water and put on sores. *Gastrointestinal Aid* Infusion given for the stomach. *Gynecological Aid* Cold, compound infusion of bark used to stop bleeding after childbirth. *Heart Medicine* Infusion of year-old leaves taken for heart trouble. *Misc. Disease Remedy* Infusion given for typhoid. *Pediatric Aid* Warmed galls applied to make infant's navel recede. (66:29) **Iroquois** *Dermatological Aid* Compound decoction used as wash for parts affected by "Italian itch." Compound wood powder used for chafed babies. (73:302) Nutmeat oil formerly used for the hair, either alone or mixed with bear grease. (170:123) *Pediatric Aid* Compound wood powder used for chafed babies. *Veterinary Aid* Bark mixed into young dog's food for worms. (73:302) **Mohegan** *Antirheumatic* (*Internal*) Leaves used for rheumatism. *Cold Remedy* Leaves used for colds. (151:128) *Pulmonary Aid* Infusion of leaves used for whooping cough. (149:265) Infusion of leaves taken for whooping cough. (151:71, 128)

Castanea pumila, Allegheny Chinkapin
Cherokee *Analgesic* Brittle leaves heated and blown on patient for headaches. *Dermatological Aid* Used for fever blisters. *Febrifuge* Used for "chills and cold sweats." (66:29) Infusion of dried

leaves used as a wash for fevers, chills, and cold sweats. **Koasati** *Gastrointestinal Aid* Decoction of roots taken for stomach troubles. (152:16)

Castela emoryi, Thorn of Christ
Yavapai *Dermatological Aid* Milky fluid of pulverized buds rubbed on face to stop pimples. (as *Holocantha emoryi* 53:261)

Castilleja affinis, Indian Paintbrush
Costanoan *Dermatological Aid* and *Disinfectant* Decoction of plant used as a wash or powdered plant applied to infected sores. (17:15)

Castilleja angustifolia, Northwestern Indian Paintbrush
Navajo *Gastrointestinal Aid* Plant used for stomach troubles. (45:96) **Quileute** *Abortifacient* Infusion of whole plant taken to regulate menstruation. (65:46) **Shuswap** *Eye Medicine* Decoction of roots, stems, and leaves used for weak or sore eyes. (102:69)

Castilleja angustifolia* var. *dubia, Northwestern Indian Paintbrush
Navajo, Kayenta *Dermatological Aid* Plant used for spider bites. (as *C. chromosa* 179:41)

Castilleja coccinea, Scarlet Indian Paintbrush
Cherokee *Poison* Infusion used "to destroy your enemies." (66:40) **Chippewa** *Cold Remedy* Infusion of flower taken for colds. *Orthopedic Aid* Simple or compound decoction of flowers used for paralysis. (43:362) **Menominee** *Love Medicine* Herb secreted onto the person who is the object of the enamor, a love charm. (128:81)

Castilleja hispida, Harsh Indian Paintbrush
Okanagan-Colville *Dermatological Aid* Plant pounded up and put into moccasins for "sweaty feet." (162:138)

Castilleja integra, Wholeleaf Indian Paintbrush
Navajo *Burn Dressing* Plant used for burns. (76:159) *Gastrointestinal Aid* Infusion of crushed leaves taken for stomach troubles. (45:76) **Navajo, Ramah** *Blood Medicine* Compound decoction of root used to "clean out the blood" after internal injury. *Burn Dressing* Poultice of leaves applied to

burns. *Gynecological Aid* Decoction of leaf taken
during pregnancy to keep baby small, for easy
labor. (165:43, 44)

Castilleja linariifolia, Wyoming Indian Paintbrush
Hopi *Contraceptive* Decoction of plant used to
prevent conception. (34:297) Decoction of plant
used as a contraceptive. (174:35, 91) *Gynecological Aid* Decoction of plant used for excessive menstrual discharge. (34:297) Decoction of plant used
to ease menstrual difficulties. (174:35, 91) **Navajo,
Ramah** *Analgesic* Plant used for stomachaches.
Gastrointestinal Aid Plant used for stomachache.
Gynecological Aid Decoction of leaf taken during
pregnancy to keep baby small, for easy labor.
(165:44) **Shoshoni** *Blood Medicine* Decoction
of root taken as a blood purifier. *Cathartic* Decoction of root taken as a physic. *Emetic* Decoction of
root taken as an emetic. *Venereal Aid* Decoction
of root taken over a long period of time for venereal disease. (155:53) **Tewa** *Contraceptive* Decoction of plant used to prevent conception. *Gynecological Aid* Decoction of plant used for excessive
menstrual discharge. (34:297)

Castilleja lineata, Marshmeadow Indian
  Paintbrush
Navajo *Gastrointestinal Aid* Infusion of crushed,
dried leaves taken for stomach troubles. (45:76)

Castilleja miniata, Scarlet Indian Paintbrush
Gitksan *Antihemorrhagic* Decoction of entire
plant taken for bleeding, stiff lungs. *Cathartic* Decoction of entire plant taken as a purgative. *Cough
Medicine* Decoction of seeds taken for coughs.
Diuretic Decoction of entire plant taken as a diuretic. *Eye Medicine* Decoction of entire plant taken
for sore eyes. *Kidney Aid* Decoction of entire plant
taken for lame back, perhaps from kidney trouble.
Orthopedic Aid Decoction of entire plant taken for
lame back, stiff lungs, and sore eyes. *Pulmonary
Aid* Decoction of entire plant taken for bleeding,
stiff lungs. (127:63) **Navajo, Ramah** *Hunting
Medicine* Plant used with any witchcraft plant to
protect hunters. *Witchcraft Medicine* Plant used
in a drink and lotion as protection from witches.
(165:44) **Thompson** *Unspecified* Broken plant

parts used in the house for decoration or for medicine. (161:284)

Castilleja parviflora, Mountain Indian Paintbrush
Ute *Gastrointestinal Aid* Roots used for bowel
troubles. (30:33)

Castilleja sessiliflora, Downy Paintedcup
Menominee *Dermatological Aid* Flowers and
leaves macerated in bear grease and used as invig-
orating hair oil. (128:53)

Castilleja stenantha, Largeflower Indian
  Paintbrush
Kawaiisu *Dermatological Aid* Decoction of leaves
used as a wash for sores. (180:17)

Castilleja thompsonii, Thompson's Indian
  Paintbrush
Okanagan-Colville *Dermatological Aid* Plant
tops dried, powdered, and placed on open cuts to
draw out the germs. (162:138)

Catabrosa aquatica, Water Whorlgrass
Crow *Ceremonial Medicine* Burned as incense
during certain ceremonies. **Montana Indian**
Ceremonial Medicine Burned as incense during
certain ceremonies. (as *Glyceria aquatica* 15:12)
Shoshoni *Stimulant* Decoction of plant taken as
a stimulant. *Tonic* Decoction of plant taken as a
tonic. (155:53)

Catharanthus roseus, Madagascar Periwinkle
Hawaiian *Blood Medicine* Bark and other plants
pounded, the resulting liquid heated and taken to
purify the blood. (as *Lochnera rosea* 2:51)

Caulanthus crassicaulis, Thickstem Wild
  Cabbage
Shoshoni *Blood Medicine* Infusion of root taken
as a blood tonic. (155:53)

Caulophyllum thalictroides, Blue Cohosh
Cherokee *Anticonvulsive* Syrup or decoction of
root given for "fits and hysterics." *Antirheumatic*
(*Internal*) Root used for rheumatism. *Dermatological Aid* Leaves rubbed on "oak-poison." *Gastrointestinal Aid* Taken for "colics and nerves" or

root ooze held in mouth for toothache. *Gynecological Aid* Plant promoted childbirth and used for womb inflammation. *Sedative* Syrup or decoction of root given for "fits and hysterics." *Toothache Remedy* Root ooze held in mouth for toothache. (66:30) **Chippewa** *Analgesic* Compound decoction of root taken for cramps. (43:344) *Antihemorrhagic* Infusion of scraped root taken for lung hemorrhages. *Emetic* Infusion of scraped root taken as an emetic. (43:346) *Gastrointestinal Aid* Compound infusion of root taken for indigestion. (43:342) Compound decoction of root taken for stomach cramps. (43:344) Infusion of scraped root taken for biliousness. (43:346) *Pulmonary Aid* Decoction of root taken for lung trouble. (43:340) **Iroquois** *Antirheumatic* (*External*) Infusion of roots used as a foot and leg bath for rheumatism. *Antirheumatic* (*Internal*) Compound decoction taken for rheumatism. *Emetic* Infusion of smashed roots taken to vomit for gallstones. *Febrifuge* Decoction of roots taken for any kind of fever. *Liver Aid* Infusion of smashed roots taken to vomit for gallstones. *Tonic* Roots used as a tonic. (73:333) **Menominee** *Gynecological Aid* Decoction of root taken to suppress profuse menstruation. (128:25) **Meskwaki** *Gynecological Aid* Decoction of root taken for profuse menstruation. *Urinary Aid* Decoction of root taken by men as a genitourinary remedy. (129:205) **Mohegan** *Kidney Aid* Root, "very rare," used for kidney disorders. (151:71, 128) **Ojibwa** *Analgesic* Root used for stomach cramps accompanying painful menstruation. *Emetic* Decoction of root taken as an emetic. *Gynecological Aid* Root used for stomach cramps accompanying painful menstruation. (130:358) **Omaha** *Febrifuge* Plant used as a fever medicine. (56:335) Decoction of root, considered highly effective, given for fevers. **Ponca** *Febrifuge* Decoction of root given for fevers. (58:83) **Potawatomi** *Gynecological Aid* Infusion of root taken to suppress profuse menstruation and aid in childbirth. (131:43)

Ceanothus americanus, New Jersey Tea
Alabama *Orthopedic Aid* Decoction of root used as a wash for injured legs or feet. (148:664) Decoction of roots used as a bath for injured feet and legs. (152:40) **Cherokee** *Gastrointestinal Aid* Infusion of root taken for "bowel complaint." *Tooth-*

ache Remedy Infusion of root held on aching tooth. (66:46) **Chippewa** *Gastrointestinal Aid* Infusion of roots taken for constipation with bloating and shortness of breath. *Laxative* Infusion of roots taken for constipation with bloating and shortness of breath. *Pulmonary Aid* Infusion of roots taken for pulmonary troubles. *Respiratory Aid* Infusion of roots taken for constipation with bloating and shortness of breath. (59:136) **Iroquois** *Abortifacient* Decoction of roots taken for suppressed menses from catching cold. Decoction taken as an abortifacient when fetus is hurt within 2 or 3 months. (73:381) *Antidiarrheal* Compound decoction of plants taken for diarrhea. *Blood Medicine* Infusion of roots taken for the blood. *Cold Remedy* Infusion of roots taken for colds. (73:382) *Dermatological Aid* Powdered bark applied to open sores caused by venereal disease. (73:381) *Misc. Disease Remedy* Compound decoction of plants taken for sugar diabetes. *Oral Aid* Decoction of bark used as a wash for sore roof of the mouth. *Other* and *Pediatric Aid* Compound decoction of dried roots given to children with "summer complaint." (73:382) *Urinary Aid* Decoction of roots taken by women with urinating problems caused by colds. *Venereal Aid* Decoction of roots taken for venereal disease. (73:381) **Menominee** *Cough Medicine* Decoction of root taken for cough with a "tendency to consumption." (44:130) *Gastrointestinal Aid* Infusion of roots used as a cure-all for stomach troubles. (128:49) **Meskwaki** *Antidiarrheal* Boiled root chewed as main remedy for flux. *Dermatological Aid* Root and bark were strongly astringent. *Gastrointestinal Aid* Root, strongly astringent with great powers, used for bowel troubles. *Snakebite Remedy* Root used for snakebite. (129:240, 241)

Ceanothus fendleri, Fendler's Ceanothus
Keres, Western *Oral Aid* Leaves chewed for sore mouth. (147:35) **Navajo** *Sedative* Compound infusion taken and poultice of plants applied for nervousness. (45:62) **Navajo, Kayenta** *Ceremonial Medicine* and *Emetic* Plant used as a Plumeway emetic. (179:31) **Navajo, Ramah** *Ceremonial Medicine* and *Emetic* Leaves and stems used as an emetic in various ceremonies. (165:36)

Ceanothus herbaceus, Jersey Tea
Chippewa *Cough Medicine* Decoction of root
taken as a cough remedy. (as *C. ovatus* 43:340)

Ceanothus integerrimus, Deerbrush
Karok *Gynecological Aid* Plant used by women
who have suffered an injury in childbirth.
(125:386)

Ceanothus leucodermis, Chaparral White-
thorn
Diegueño *Dermatological Aid* Leaves picked
when only the leaves were out, boiled, and used as
a wash for itch. Leaves and cascara leaves boiled
and used for poison oak. Decoction of berries,
whole branch with berries or leaves used as bath
for itch, sores, or impetigo. Blossom, leaf, or berry
sap used by rubbing area affected by itch, sores, or
impetigo. (70:15)

Ceanothus sanguineus, Redstem Ceanothus
Okanagan-Colville *Burn Dressing* Poultice of
dried, powdered bark applied to burns. (162:119)
Sanpoil *Dermatological Aid* Poultice of "sap
wood" sprinkled on grease or oil applied to sores
or wounds. (109:217)

Ceanothus thyrsiflorus, Blueblossom
Ceanothus
Poliklah *Pediatric Aid* Decoction of leaves and
twigs used to wash newborn babies. (97:173)

Ceanothus velutinus, Snowbrush Ceanothus
Great Basin Indian *Other* Infusion of leaves taken
for diagnosis and certain results mean certain
things. (100:49) **Karok** *Dermatological Aid*
Leaves used as a deodorant. (125:386) **Modesse**
Cough Medicine Infusion of leaves taken for
coughs. *Febrifuge* Infusion of leaves taken for fevers. (97:223) **Okanagan-Colville** *Ceremonial
Medicine* Decoction of plant tops with leaves used
as a cleansing solution in the sweat house. *Dermatological Aid* Decoction of plant tops with leaves
used as a hair wash for dandruff, used to bathe
babies to prevent diaper rash, and used to "condition" adult skin. Infusion of branches used to wash
sores and eczema. Poultice of dried, powdered
leaves applied or mixed with pitch and used as a
salve for sores. Poultice of dried, powdered leaves

used as a "baby powder." *Orthopedic Aid* Infusion
of leaves taken for broken bones. *Pediatric Aid*
Decoction of plant tops with leaves used to bathe
babies to prevent diaper rash. Poultice of dried,
powdered leaves used as a "baby powder." (162:
120) **Okanagon** *Analgesic* Decoction of stems
and leaves used internally and externally for dull
pains. (104:40) **Oregon Indian, Warm Springs**
Unspecified Infusion of leaves taken for puzzling
illnesses. (98:40) **Shuswap** *Misc. Disease Remedy* Decoction of plants taken for the flu. (102:65)
Thompson *Analgesic* Decoction of stems and
leaves used internally and externally for dull
pains. (104:40) Decoction of stem and leaf taken
and used as a wash for dull, body pains. (141:457)
Antidiarrheal Infusion of leaves and twigs used for
diarrhea. *Antirheumatic (External)* Decoction of
branches used as a wash for rheumatism. Decoction of leaves used as a bath or leaves used in a
steam bath for rheumatism or arthritis. Infusion of
leaves and twigs used for arthritis. *Antirheumatic
(Internal)* Decoction of plant taken for arthritis.
Cancer Treatment Decoction of plant used for
cancer. *Dietary Aid* Decoction of branches taken
for weight loss. *Orthopedic Aid* Infusion of leaves
and twigs with Indian hellebore used for broken
limbs. *Panacea* Decoction of branches taken for
general illness. *Unspecified* Decoction of branches
taken for an unspecified ailment. Plant used in
sweat bath for an unspecified illness. (161:252)
Venereal Aid Compound decoction of branches
taken for mild forms of gonorrhea. (141:457)

Celastrus scandens, American Bittersweet
Cherokee *Analgesic* Strong compound infusion
used for pain of childbirth. *Antirheumatic (External)* Thorny branch used to scratch rheumatism.
Cough Medicine Root chewed for cough. *Dermatological Aid* Decoction of highly astringent leaves
taken for bowel complaint. Used as wash for "foul
ulcers." *Gastrointestinal Aid* Infusion of bark
used to settle stomach and decoction given for
bowel complaint. *Gynecological Aid* Strong infusion combined with red raspberry leaves and used
for childbirth pains. (66:25) **Chippewa** *Cancer
Treatment* Boiled roots used as an ointment for
cancer. (59:135) *Cathartic* Decoction of root
used, especially for babies, as a physic. (43:344)
Dermatological Aid Decoction of stalk applied to

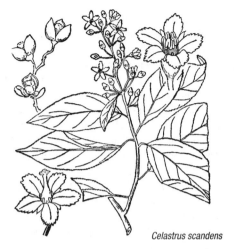

Celastrus scandens

skin "eruptions." (43:350) Boiled roots used as an ointment for any obstinate sore. (59:135) *Diuretic* Decoction of root taken for "stoppage of urine." (43:348) *Pediatric Aid* Decoction of root used, especially for babies, as a physic. (43:344) **Creek** *Analgesic, Gynecological Aid*, and *Orthopedic Aid* Plant used by women with urinary trouble or pain in small of back. *Urinary Aid* Plant used by women with urinary trouble. (148:661) **Delaware** *Dermatological Aid* Poultice or salve of roots used for skin eruptions. *Liver Aid* Infusion of roots used to clear up liver spots. (151:37) **Delaware, Ontario** *Tuberculosis Remedy* Root taken for consumption. (150:66, 82) **Iroquois** *Abortifacient* Decoction of roots taken by young girls who catch cold and do not menstruate. Infusion of leaves and stems taken as a regulator by women. *Blood Medicine* Compound decoction of plants taken to make blood or for watery blood. (73:376) Infusion of root bark with another plant and wine taken for anemia. (118:54) *Cold Remedy* Decoction of roots taken by young girls who catch cold and do not menstruate. *Diuretic* Infusion of leaves and stems taken as a diuretic. *Febrifuge* Infusion of leaves and stems taken for fever and soreness from pregnancy. *Gynecological Aid* Infusion of leaves and stems taken for fever and soreness from pregnancy. *Kidney Aid* Compound decoction of roots and bark taken for dropsy or watery blood. Infusion of roots taken for kidney trouble following childbirth. *Other* Decoction of roots used as a wash on lips of bad children. *Pediatric Aid* Decoction of roots used as wash on lips or gums of bad or teething

children. *Poison* Berries considered poisonous. *Toothache Remedy* Decoction of roots used as a wash on lips and gums of teething child. *Urinary Aid* Infusion of leaves and stems taken for urine stoppage. (73:376) **Meskwaki** *Analgesic* and *Gynecological Aid* Compound containing root used for "the relief of women in labor." (129:208, 209) **Oglala** *Poison* Plant considered poisonous. (58:102) **Ojibwa** *Gastrointestinal Aid* Berries used for stomach trouble. (130:362) *Unspecified* Plant used for medicinal purposes. (112:233)

Celtis laevigata, Sugarberry
Houma *Throat Aid* Decoction of bark taken for sore throat. *Venereal Aid* Compound decoction of bark with powdered shells taken for venereal disease. (135:57)

Celtis laevigata var. *reticulata*, Netleaf Hackberry
Navajo, Kayenta *Gastrointestinal Aid* Plant used for indigestion. (as *C. reticulata* 179:18)

Celtis occidentalis, Common Hackberry
Houma *Throat Aid* Decoction of bark taken for sore throat. *Venereal Aid* Compound decoction of bark with powdered shells taken for venereal disease. (135:57) **Iroquois** *Abortifacient* Decoction taken "for suppressed menses in girls, cause: working in the sun." *Cold Remedy* Compound decoction taken by "women when they catch cold with the menses." *Gynecological Aid* Decoction of bark used as "woman's medicine" and regulated menses. (73:306) **Meskwaki** *Veterinary Aid* Inner bark fed to ponies as a conditioner. (129:250)

Cenchrus calyculatus, Ka-mano-mano
Hawaiian *Dermatological Aid* Shoots, leaves, roots, and other plants pounded and resulting liquid used on fresh, deep cuts. *Tuberculosis Remedy* Shoots, leaves, roots, and other plants pounded and resulting liquid used on scrofulous sores. (2:48)

Centaurea americana, American Star Thistle
Kiowa *Dermatological Aid* Poultice of leaves applied to skin sores. (166:58)

Centaurea melitensis, Maltese Star Thistle
Mahuna *Kidney Aid* Plant used for the kidneys.
(117:69)

Centaurium exaltatum, Desert Centaury
Miwok *Analgesic* Decoction of stems and leaves
taken for internal pains. *Gastrointestinal Aid*
Decoction of stems and leaves taken for stomachache. *Toothache Remedy* Decoction of stems and
leaves taken for toothaches. *Tuberculosis Remedy*
Decoction of stems and leaves taken for consumption. (8:168)

Centaurium muehlenbergii, Muhlenberg's
    Centaury
Mahuna *Febrifuge, Gastrointestinal Aid*, and
Laxative Infusion of plants taken for constipation
caused by stomach fevers. (as *Erythaea muehlenbergii* 117:8)

Centaurium venustum, Charming Centaury
Luiseño *Febrifuge* Infusion of plant taken for
fevers. (as *Erythraea venusta* 132:230) **Miwok**
Febrifuge Decoction of flowers and leaves taken
for fever. *Misc. Disease Remedy* Decoction of flowers and leaves taken for ague. *Pulmonary Aid*
Decoction of flowers, leaves, and brandy taken for
pneumonia. (8:168)

Cephalanthus occidentalis, Common Button-
    bush
Chickasaw *Eye Medicine* Poultice of warmed
roots applied to the head for eye troubles.
(152:58) **Choctaw** *Antidiarrheal* Strong decoction
of tree bark taken as a favorite medicine for dysentery. (23:287) *Eye Medicine* Decoction of bark
used as wash for sore eyes. (20:24) Decoction of
bark used as a bath for sore eyes. (152:58) *Febrifuge* Root bark and bark used as a febrifuge. *Tonic*
Root bark and bark used as a tonic. (23:287)
Toothache Remedy Bark chewed for toothache.
(20:24) Bark chewed for toothaches. (152:58)
Kiowa *Antihemorrhagic* Decoction of roots taken
for hemorrhages. (166:51) **Koasati** *Antirheumatic*
(*Internal*) Decoction of leaves taken for rheumatism. *Orthopedic Aid* Decoction of roots taken for
enlarged muscles. (152:58) **Meskwaki** *Emetic*
Inner bark, very important medicine, used as an
emetic. (129:243) **Seminole** *Analgesic* Decoction

of bark taken for headaches. (145:283) *Antidiarrheal* Decoction of plant taken for wolf ghost sickness: diarrhea and painful defecation. (145:228)
Antiemetic Decoction of roots or berries used for
horse sickness: nausea, constipation, and blocked
urination. (145:189) *Blood Medicine* Decoction of
roots taken for menstruation sickness: yellow eyes
and skin, weakness, and shaking head. (145:247)
Cathartic Decoction of plant taken for wolf ghost
sickness: diarrhea and painful defecation. (145:
228) *Febrifuge* Decoction of bark taken for fevers.
Gastrointestinal Aid Decoction of bark taken for
stomachaches. (145:283) *Laxative* Decoction of
roots or berries used for horse sickness: nausea,
constipation, and blocked urination. (145:189)
Other and *Strengthener* Decoction of roots taken
for menstruation sickness: yellow eyes and skin,
weakness, and shaking head. (145:247) *Unspecified* Plant used for medicinal purposes. (145:162)
Urinary Aid Decoction of roots or berries used for
horse sickness: nausea, constipation, and blocked
urination. (145:189) Plant taken for urine retention. (145:273)

Cerastium arvense, Field Chickweed
Iroquois *Dermatological Aid* Decoction of plant
used as an astringent. *Gynecological Aid* Decoction of plant taken for injuries and miscarriage.
Decoction taken to "stop bleeding and stops child
from passing through uterus." (73:317)

Cerastium beeringianum, Bering Chickweed
Navajo, Ramah *Veterinary Aid* Cold infusion of
plant used for sheep or horses with eye troubles.
(165:26)

Cerastium fontanum ssp. ***vulgare***, Big
    Chickweed
Cherokee *Anthelmintic* and *Pediatric Aid* Compound infusion of stem and root given to children
for worms. (as *C. holosteoides* 66:29)

Cercis canadensis, Eastern Redbud
Alabama *Febrifuge* Cold infusion of roots and inner bark taken for fever. (152:31) *Pulmonary Aid*
Infusion of root and inner bark taken for congestion. (148:665) *Respiratory Aid* Cold infusion of
roots and inner bark taken for congestion. (152:31)
Cherokee *Pulmonary Aid* Infusion of bark given

for whooping cough. (66:52) **Delaware** *Antiemetic* Infusion of bark used as a cold drink for vomiting. *Febrifuge* Infusion of bark used as a cold drink for fever. (151:30) **Delaware, Oklahoma** *Antiemetic* Infusion of bark taken for vomiting. *Febrifuge* Infusion of bark taken for fever. (150:25, 74)

Cercis canadensis* var. *texensis, California Redbud
Mendocino Indian *Febrifuge* Bark used for chills and fever. (as *C. occidentalis* 33:356)

Cercocarpus ledifolius, Curlleaf Mountain Mahogany
Gosiute *Burn Dressing* Poultice of powdered green wood applied to burns. (31:350) Charred wood powder applied to burns. (31:365) **Kawaiisu** *Ear Medicine* Dried, powdered plant exudation applied for earaches. Dried exudation ground into a powder and applied to earaches. *Gynecological Aid* Decoction of bark and leaves taken for "women's disease." *Venereal Aid* Decoction of bark taken for gonorrhea. (180:18) **Paiute** *Analgesic* Decoction of bark taken for stomachaches. *Antidiarrheal* Compound infusion of scraped bark given to children for diarrhea. Decoction of bark taken for diarrhea. *Blood Medicine* Cold decoction of bark taken as a blood tonic. *Burn Dressing* Powder or paste of bark or wood applied to burns. (155:53–55) *Cold Remedy* Infusion of bark taken for colds. (98:38) Decoction or infusion of dried bark or leaves taken for colds and coughs. *Cough Medicine* Decoction of bark or infusion of bark or leaves taken for coughs and colds. *Dermatological Aid* Powder or paste of bark or wood applied to sores, cuts, or wounds. *Gastrointestinal Aid* Decoction of bark taken for stomachaches and stomach ulcers. *Heart Medicine* Decoction of leaves or bark taken for heart disorders. *Pediatric Aid* Compound infusion of scraped bark given to children for diarrhea. *Pulmonary Aid* Decoction of bark taken for pneumonia. *Tuberculosis Remedy* Simple or compound decoction of dried bark used for tuberculosis. *Venereal Aid* Decoction of bark taken for venereal diseases. Pulverized wood sprinkled on syphilitic sores. (155:53–55) **Paiute, Northern** *Antihemorrhagic* Decoction of dried bark taken for spitting up blood. *Tuberculosis Remedy* Decoc-

tion of dried bark taken for tuberculosis. (49:129) **Shoshoni** *Antidiarrheal* Compound infusion of scraped bark given to children for diarrhea. *Blood Medicine* Cold decoction of bark taken as a blood tonic. *Burn Dressing* Powder or paste of bark or wood applied to burns. *Cold Remedy* Decoction of bark taken for colds. *Cough Medicine* Decoction of bark taken for coughs. *Dermatological Aid* Poultice of pulverized leaves and bark applied to swellings. Powder or paste of bark or wood applied to sores, cuts, or wounds. *Eye Medicine* Strained decoction of inner bark used as a wash for eye diseases. *Heart Medicine* Decoction of leaves or bark taken for heart disorders. *Misc. Disease Remedy* Infusion of inner bark taken for diphtheria. *Pediatric Aid* Compound infusion of scraped bark given to children for diarrhea. (155:53–55) *Tuberculosis Remedy* Compound decoction of bark taken for tuberculosis. (155:122) *Unspecified* Decoction of soft inner bark taken for unspecified purpose. *Venereal Aid* Compound decoction of bark taken as an "unfailing cure for syphilis." (155:53–55)

Cercocarpus montanus, True Mountain Mahogany
Keres, Western *Strengthener* Infusion of leaves used as a strengthener. (147:35) **Navajo** *Gastrointestinal Aid* Roots and bark used for stomach troubles. (45:53) **Navajo, Ramah** *Gastrointestinal Aid* Compound decoction of leaves taken and used as lotion for sickness from overeating. *Gynecological Aid* Decoction of plant used to hasten postpartum recovery. *Hunting Medicine* Leaves from shrubs browsed by deer chewed by hunter for good luck in hunting. *Panacea* Root used as a "life medicine." (165:30) **Tewa** *Laxative* Cold infusion of plant or leaves taken as a laxative. (115:45)

Cercocarpus montanus* var. *glaber, Birchleaf Mountain Mahogany
Apache, White Mountain *Burn Dressing* Wood burned, the charcoal powdered and applied to burns. (as *C. parvifolius* 113:156) **Kawaiisu** *Cough Medicine* Decoction of roots used for coughing. *Internal Medicine* Decoction of roots used for internal ills. (as *C. betuloides* 180:18) **Mahuna** *Venereal Aid* Infusion of bark and roots taken for venereal disease or gonorrhea gleet (urethral discharge). (as *C. betulaefolius* 117:70)

Chaenactis douglasii, Douglas's Dustymaiden
Gosiute *Analgesic* and *Orthopedic Aid* Mashed
plant rubbed on limbs for soreness or aching.
(31:365) **Great Basin Indian** *Heart Medicine*
and *Pediatric Aid* Infusion of whole plant given to
children to slow their heartbeats. (100:50) **Okanagon** *Dermatological Aid* Infusion used as wash
for chapped hands, pimples, boils, tumors, and
swellings. *Snakebite Remedy* Infusion of plant
used as wash for insect and snake bites. (104:42)
Paiute *Analgesic* Infusion of young leaves taken
or put on the hair for headaches. (93:118) *Cold
Remedy* Decoction of plant or leaves taken for
colds. *Cough Medicine* Decoction of plant or leaves
taken for coughs. (155:55, 56) *Dermatological Aid*
Poultice of crushed leaves applied to swellings.
(87:196) Poultice of crushed, fresh plants or
leaves applied to swellings. *Heart Medicine* Infusion of plant used as a heart depressant. (155:55,
56) *Orthopedic Aid* Poultice of crushed leaves applied to sprains. (87:196) *Snakebite Remedy* Poultice of pulped leaves and stems applied to rattlesnake bites. (155:55, 56) **Sanpoil** *Cathartic*
Decoction of roots taken by family of dead one
as a purge to avoid illness. *Tuberculosis Remedy*
Decoction of roots taken by family of dead one to
avoid taking consumption. (109:221) **Shoshoni**
Dermatological Aid Poultice of crushed fresh
plants or leaves applied to swellings. *Emetic* Decoction of plant taken as an emetic for indigestion.
Gastrointestinal Aid Decoction of plant taken as
an emetic for indigestion or sour stomach. *Kidney
Aid* Decoction of plants used as a bath for swollen
limbs or dropsical conditions. (155:55, 56)
Thompson *Dermatological Aid* Infusion of plant
used as wash for chapped hands, pimples, boils,
and tumors. Infusion of whole plant taken for
swellings. (104:42) Decoction of plant used on
various skin conditions and insect bites. Decoction
of whole plant taken for any kind of swellings. *Gastrointestinal Aid* Mild decoction taken as a tonic
for the stomach. (141:473) *Snakebite Remedy* Infusion of plant used as wash for insect and snake
bites. (104:42) Strong decoction of entire plant
applied to insect and snake bites. *Stimulant* Mild
decoction of entire plant taken as a tonic for the
stomach and lassitude. *Tonic* Mild decoction taken
as a tonic for the stomach and lassitude. (141:473)

Unspecified Plant considered a good medicine.
(161:178)

Chaenactis douglasii* var. *douglasii,
    Douglas's Dustymaiden
Okanagan-Colville *Eye Medicine* Infusion of
roots used as an eyewash. (162:82)

Chaenactis santolinoides, Santolina Pin-
    cushion
Kawaiisu *Analgesic* and *Orthopedic Aid* Decoction of roots taken for sore chest, sore shoulders,
and internal soreness. (180:19)

Chaenactis stevioides, Steve's Dustymaiden
Nevada Indian *Heart Medicine* and *Pediatric Aid*
Infusion of plant used to slow down heartbeats of
children with fevers. (98:40)

Chaerophyllum procumbens, Spreading
    Chervil
Chickasaw *Emetic* and *Poison* Poisonous root
used as an emetic. (23:289)

Chaetopappa ericoides, Rose Heath
Havasupai *Gastrointestinal Aid* Decoction of
whole plant or roots taken or used as a wash for
digestive troubles. *Pediatric Aid* Decoction of
whole plant or roots given or used as a wash for
children with digestive troubles. (as *Leucelene
ericoides* 171:248) **Hopi** *Nose Medicine* Infusion
of root used to "aid a sore nose." (as *Aster leuce-*

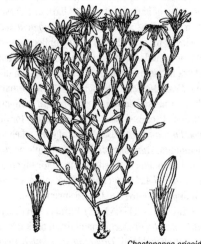

Chaetopappa ericoides

lene 174:34, 95) *Panacea* Root used as a universal panacea. *Pediatric Aid* Infusion of herb used to "quiet the baby." (as *Aster leucelene* 174:95) *Reproductive Aid* Plant used to determine the sex of a child. This is quite an ambiguous reference. The text says this: "This plant is used by the Hopi Indians as genetic factor among the Indian clans. Genetic factor refers to the choice of a small (female) or large (male) plant to assist in determining the sex of a child." It is, therefore, unclear if the plant is used to detect whether the fetus is male or female, or to cause the child to be one or the other. Elsewhere, this author tells us that the Hopi make a decoction of the leaves of juniper "which is said to be a laxative and is taken by women who desire a female child." This suggests that the second possibility may be the correct one, with administration of large plants if you want a son and small ones if you want a daughter. (as *Aster arenosus* 34:290) *Sedative* Infusion of root used to "quiet the baby." (as *Aster leucelene* 174:36, 95) *Stimulant* Plant used as a stimulant. (as *Aster leucelene* 174:31) **Keres, Western** *Antirheumatic* (*External*) Poultice or infusion of plant used for swellings. (as *Leucelene ericoides* 147:52) **Navajo, Kayenta** *Kidney Aid* Infusion of plant with sumac berries taken for kidney disease. *Urinary Aid* Infusion of plant with sumac berries taken for bladder disease. (as *Aster ericaefolius* 179:45) **Navajo, Ramah** *Nose Medicine* Dried pulverized plant used as snuff or cold infusion used as drops for "nose trouble." *Snakebite Remedy* Poultice of chewed leaves applied and infusion taken for snakebite. *Toothache Remedy* Leaves chewed for toothache. (as *Aster arenosus* 165:48) **Zuni** *Analgesic* Infusion of pulverized plant applied for pain from cold or rheumatism. *Antirheumatic* (*External*) Infusion of whole plant rubbed on body for swelling and rheumatic pain. *Cold Remedy* Infusion of whole plant rubbed on body for pain from a cold. *Dermatological Aid* Infusion of pulverized plant rubbed over body for swellings. *Gynecological Aid* Warm infusion of plant taken to "hasten parturition." (as *Leucelene ericoides* 143:55)

Chamaebatia foliolosa, Sierran Mountain Misery
Miwok *Antirheumatic* (*Internal*) Infusion of leaves taken for rheumatism. *Cold Remedy* Decoc-tion of leaves taken for colds. *Cough Medicine* Decoction of leaves taken for coughs. *Misc. Disease Remedy* Infusion of leaves taken for chickenpox, measles, and smallpox. *Venereal Aid* Leaves used as ingredient in medicines for venereal diseases. (8:168)

Chamaebatiaria millefolium, Fernbush
Gosiute *Venereal Aid* Plant used for gonorrhea. (31:365) Poultice of plant applied or plant used as wash for venereal diseases. (as *Spiraea mille-folium* 31:351) **Navajo, Ramah** *Hunting Medicine* Leaves rolled in corn husk smoked for good luck in hunting. (165:30) **Paiute** *Orthopedic Aid* Compound decoction of young shoots taken for lumbago. **Shoshoni** *Analgesic* and *Gastrointestinal Aid* Decoction of fresh or dried leaves taken for stomachaches or cramps. (155:56, 57)

Chamaecrista fasciculata, Sleepingplant
Cherokee *Sports Medicine* Root medicine used to keep ballplayers from tiring. *Stimulant* Compound infusion given for fainting spells. (as *Cassia fasci-culata* 66:54) **Seminole** *Antiemetic* Cold decoction of plant used for nausea. (as *Chamaecrista brachista* 145:276)

Chamaecrista nictitans ssp. *nictitans* var. *nictitans*, Partridge Pea
Cherokee *Sports Medicine* Root medicine used to keep ballplayers from tiring. *Stimulant* Compound infusion given for fainting spells. (as *Cassia nicti-tans* 66:54)

Chamaecyparis nootkatensis, Alaska Cedar
Bella Coola *Adjuvant* Soft bark used as cover for poultices of *Trautvetteria grandis* and *Ranun-culus acris*. (127:49) **Kwakiutl** *Antirheumatic* (*External*) Plant used in sweat baths for arthritis and rheumatism. *Dermatological Aid* Infusion of branch tips used as a wash for sores and swellings. Poultice of chewed leaves applied to sores. Sharp boughs rubbed on sores and swellings until skin was broken. *Herbal Steam* Plant used in sweat baths for arthritis and rheumatism. *Kidney Aid* Compound decoction of leaves applied to swelling on woman's kidney. *Panacea* Infusion of branch tips taken for general illness. *Strengthener* Bark ash and oil used as a lotion to give strength to the

very ill. (157:266) **Kwakiutl, Southern** *Anti-rheumatic* (*External*) Branches placed on top of burning sea wrack as part of a steam treatment for rheumatism. *Strengthener* Branches placed on top of burning sea wrack as part of a steam treatment for general sickness. (157:261)

Chamaecyparis thyoides, Atlantic White Cedar
Ojibwa, South *Analgesic* Decoction of leaves used as herbal steam for headache and backache. Poultice of crushed leaves and bark applied for headache. (as *Cupressus thyoides* 77:198)

Chamaedaphne calyculata, Leather Leaf
Potawatomi *Dermatological Aid* Poultice of leaves applied to inflammations. *Febrifuge* Infusion of leaves used for fevers. (131:56)

Chamaemelum nobile, Garden Dogfennel
Cherokee *Abortifacient* Infusion of flower or herb used for "female obstructions." *Antiemetic* Used for vomiting. *Dermatological Aid* Used as poultice for ulcers and "hard swellings." *Gastrointestinal Aid* Used for colic and bowel complaints. *Sedative* Infusion of flower or herb used for "hysterical affections." (as *Anthemis nobilis* 66:28) **Mahuna** *Gastrointestinal Aid* Plant used to regulate unsettled stomachs or for babies suffering from colic. *Pediatric Aid* Plant used for babies suffering from colic. (as *Anthemis nobilis* 117:7)

Chamaesaracha coronopus, Greenleaf Five Eyes
Navajo, Kayenta *Dermatological Aid* Plant used for swellings. *Other* Compound containing plant used in cases of drowning. (179:41)

Chamaesyce albomarginata, Whitemargin Sandmat
Diegueño *Dermatological Aid* Decoction of plant used to wash sores. (as *Euphorbia albinomarginata* 70:21) **Kawaiisu** *Snakebite Remedy* Ground leaves and flowers used as a salve for rattlesnake bites. *Veterinary Aid* Poultice applied or decoction of leaves given to animals with snakebites. (as *Euphorbia albomarginata* 180:31) **Keres, Western** *Eye Medicine* Crushed plant rubbed on sore eyes. *Gynecological Aid* Leaves rubbed on mothers' breasts to produce more and richer milk. (as *Eu-*

phorbia albomarginata 147:44) **Navajo, Ramah** *Analgesic* Cold infusion used for stomachache. *Gastrointestinal Aid* Cold infusion of plant taken for stomachache. *Hemostat* Poultice of plant used as a hemostatic. (as *Euphorbia albomarginata* 165:35) **Shoshoni** *Snakebite Remedy* Poultice of crushed, whole plant applied to snakebites. *Tonic* Decoction of plant taken as a tonic for general debility. (as *Euphorbia albomarginata* 155:73, 74) **Zuni** *Gynecological Aid* Leaves and roots eaten to promote lactation. (as *Euphorbia albomarginata* 22:376)

Chamaesyce fendleri, Fendler's Sandmat
Hopi *Dietary Aid* Young roots fed to sick baby whose mother's milk was failing. (174:84) *Oral Aid* Dried, ground plant used as soothing lip balm. (174:33, 83–84) *Pediatric Aid* Young roots fed to sick baby whose mother's milk was failing. (174:84)

Chamaesyce fendleri var. *fendleri*, Fendler's Sandmat
Navajo *Gastrointestinal Aid* Infusion of plant taken for stomachache. (as *Euphorbia fendleri* 76:151) **Navajo, Ramah** *Analgesic* Cold infusion or decoction used for stomachache and diarrhea. *Antidiarrheal* Cold infusion or decoction of plant taken for diarrhea. *Ceremonial Medicine* Plant used as a ceremonial medicine. *Dermatological Aid* Plant used topically for warts and poison ivy. *Gastrointestinal Aid* Cold infusion or decoction of plant taken for stomachache. *Gynecological Aid* Pulverized plant used topically as a galactagogue and for breast injuries. *Hemostat* Poultice of chewed plant applied to cuts as a hemostatic. *Toothache Remedy* Hot poultice of plant applied for toothache. *Veterinary Aid* Milky juice applied to snakebite in livestock. (as *Euphorbia fendleri* 165:35)

Chamaesyce geyeri, Geyer's Sandmat
Lakota *Preventive Medicine* Used as a medicine as protection for the head. (as *Euphorbia geyeri* 116:45)

Chamaesyce glyptosperma, Ribseed Sandmat
Iroquois *Gland Medicine* Compound decoction of stems taken and used as a wash for goiter. *Gyne-*

cological Aid Plant used to stimulate lactation. (as *Euphorbia glyptosperma* 73:369) **Thompson** *Snakebite Remedy* Fresh plant rubbed on all snakebites, but especially rattlesnake bites. (as *Euphorbia glyptosperma* 141:462)

Chamaesyce hypericifolia, Graceful Sandmat
Cherokee *Urinary Aid* Infusion of bruised roots taken for yellow urine. (as *Euphorbia hypericifolia* 152:35)

Chamaesyce lata, Hoary Sandmat
Navajo *Cathartic* Plant used as a purge. *Gastrointestinal Aid* Plant used for upset stomachs. (as *Euphorbia lata* 76:151)

Chamaesyce maculata, Spotted Sandmat
Cherokee *Cancer Treatment* Decoction prepared with herbs and taken for cancer. *Cathartic* Taken as a purgative. *Dermatological Aid* "Juice rubbed on skin eruptions, especially on children's heads." Juice used as ointment for "sores and sore nipples." *Gynecological Aid* Infusion taken for bleeding after childbirth. *Pediatric Aid* "Juice rubbed on skin eruptions, especially on children's heads." *Toothache Remedy* Root used for toothache. *Urinary Aid* Infusion of bruised root taken for urinary diseases. *Venereal Aid* Decoction taken for gonorrhea and "similar diseases." (as *Euphorbia maculata* 66:45) **Costanoan** *Blood Medicine* Infusion of plant taken to purify the blood. *Dermatological Aid* Decoction of plant used as a wash for cuts. Milky juice applied to pimples and infusion of foliage used as a hair wash. *Eye Medicine* Decoction of plant used as a wash for eyes. (as *Euphorbia maculata* 17:9)

Chamaesyce melanadenia, Squaw Sandmat
Cahuilla *Dermatological Aid* Sap used for bee stings and sores. *Ear Medicine* Sap used for earaches. (as *Euphorbia melanadenia* 11:73)

Chamaesyce multiformis var. ***multiformis***, Variable Sandmat
Hawaiian *Breast Treatment* Plant milk and other ingredients taken for dry breasts. *Dietary Aid* Buds or leaves chewed by the mother for the benefit of the nursing baby. Buds or leaves chewed by nursing mothers to stimulate the appetite, helpful in milk production. *Laxative* Buds or leaves chewed by nursing mothers as a laxative. *Pediatric Aid* Buds chewed by the mother and given to babies till the age of 6 months. Buds or leaves chewed by the mother for the benefit of the nursing baby. *Reproductive Aid* Buds, leaves, and other plants pounded and resulting liquid taken for female reproductive organ weakness. *Strengthener* Buds and leaves used for general debility of the body. *Tuberculosis Remedy* Poultice of plant milk and other ingredients applied to scrofulous sores. *Unspecified* Buds chewed by the mother and given to babies till the age of 6 months. (as *Euphorbia multiformis* 2:11)

Chamaesyce nutans, Eyebane
Houma *Dermatological Aid* Milk from stem rubbed on skin for itching and eczema. Poultice of crushed leaves applied to bad sores. (as *Euphorbia nutans* 135:65, 66) *Gastrointestinal Aid* Cool decoction of plant in milk given to babies for sickness from bad milk. (as *Euphorbia nutans* 135:65) *Pediatric Aid* Cool decoction of plant in milk given to babies for sickness from bad milk. (as *Euphorbia nutans* 135:65, 66)

Chamaesyce ocellata ssp. ***arenicola***, Contura Creek Sandmat
Paiute *Dermatological Aid* Poultice of mashed plant applied to swellings. (as *Euphorbia arenicola* 155:74) *Eye Medicine* Infusion of whole plant used as an eyewash. (as *Euphorbia arenicola* 98:39) Decoction of leaves used as an eyewash. (as *Euphorbia arenicola* 155:74)

Chamaesyce ocellata ssp. ***ocellata***, Contura Creek Sandmat
Miwok *Blood Medicine* Decoction of leaves taken as a blood purifier. *Snakebite Remedy* Mashed leaves rubbed into snakebite to prevent swelling. (as *Euphorbia ocellata* 8:169)

Chamaesyce polycarpa var. ***polycarpa***, Smallseed Sandmat
Luiseño *Snakebite Remedy* Plant used for rattlesnake bites. (as *Euphorbia polycarpa* 132:231) **Pima** *Dermatological Aid* Poultice of plant applied to scorpion and snakebites. *Diaphoretic* Plant chewed to cause vomiting and sweating for

snakebites. *Emetic* Roots chewed to vomit for
stomach troubles, snakebites, and constipation.
Gastrointestinal Aid Roots chewed to vomit and
loosen bowels for stomach troubles. *Laxative*
Roots chewed to loosen bowels for stomach troubles and constipation. *Poison* Plant considered
poisonous. *Snakebite Remedy* Plant chewed to
cause vomiting and sweating for snakebites. Plant
juice used as wash and poultice of plant applied to
snakebites. (as *Euphorbia polycarpa* 38:99) **Shoshoni** *Eye Medicine* Infusion of plant used as an
eyewash. *Tonic* Infusion of plant taken as a tonic
"for any general, indisposed feeling." (as *Euphorbia polycarpa* 155:74) **Zuni** *Gynecological Aid*
Warm gruel made with plant and white cornmeal
taken to promote milk flow. (as *Euphorbia polycarpa* 143:51)

Chamaesyce revoluta, Threadstem Sandmat
Navajo, Kayenta *Dermatological Aid* Plant used
as a lotion for chafing and sores. (as *Euphorbia
revoluta* 179:30)

Chamaesyce serpyllifolia, Thymeleaf Sandmat
Omaha *Antidiarrheal* Dried leaves rubbed into
abdominal scratches for children's dysentery.
Gastrointestinal Aid Dried leaves rubbed into abdominal scratches for children's bloating. **Ponca**
Gynecological Aid Decoction of plant taken to encourage milk flow in nursing mothers. (58:99)
Decoction of plant taken by young mothers for
scanty or lack of milk. (80:151)

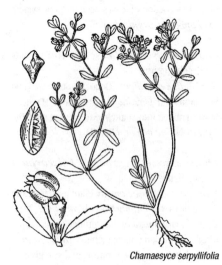

Chamaesyce serpyllifolia

Chamaesyce serpyllifolia ssp. *serpyllifolia*, Thymeleaf Sandmat
Apache, White Mountain *Oral Aid* Plant chewed
to sweeten the saliva. (as *Euphorbia serpyllifolia*
113:158) **Miwok** *Dermatological Aid* Decoction of
leaves used as wash for running sores. *Snakebite
Remedy* Poultice of plant applied, must be done
immediately, to rattlesnake bites. (as *Euphorbia
serpyllifolia* 8:170) **Navajo, Ramah** *Analgesic*
Cold infusion or decoction of plant taken for stomachache. *Antidiarrheal* Cold infusion or decoction
of plant taken for diarrhea. *Ceremonial Medicine*
Plant used as a ceremonial medicine. *Dermatological Aid* Plant used topically for warts and poison
ivy. *Gastrointestinal Aid* Cold infusion or decoction of plant taken for stomachache. *Gynecological Aid* Pulverized plant used topically as a galactagogue and for breast injuries. *Hemostat* Poultice
of chewed plant applied to cuts as a hemostatic.
Toothache Remedy Hot poultice of plant applied
for toothache. *Veterinary Aid* Milky juice applied
to snakebite in livestock. (as *Euphorbia serpyllifolia* 165:35) **Zuni** *Cathartic* Plant used as a cathartic. *Emetic* Plant used as an emetic. *Gynecological Aid* Plant used to increase the flow of milk
in nursing mother. (as *Euphorbia serpyllifolia*
143:51)

Chaptalia tomentosa, Woolly Sunbonnets
Seminole *Antirheumatic* (*External*) Decoction
of leaves rubbed on body and body steamed for
deer sickness: numb, painful limbs and joints.
(145:192) *Urinary Aid* Decoction of roots taken
for urine retention. (145:274)

Cheilanthes fendleri, Fendler's Lipfern
Keres, Western *Gynecological Aid* Infusion of
plant used as a douche after childbirth. (147:36)

Cheilanthes wootonii, Beaded Lipfern
Navajo, Ramah *Dermatological Aid* Cold infu-
sion of plant used as a lotion for gunshot wounds.
Panacea Plant used as "life medicine." (165:11)

Cheirodendron gaudicchaudii, Olapa
Hawaiian *Respiratory Aid* Root bark and other
plants pounded, squeezed, and the resulting liquid
taken for asthma. (as *C. caudicchaudii* 2:33)

Chelidonium majus, Greater Celandine
Iroquois *Veterinary Aid* Infusion of whole plant, another plant, and milk given to pigs that drool and have sudden movements. (118:45)

Chelone glabra, White Turtlehead
Algonquin, Quebec *Unspecified* Infusion of roots and cedar bark used as a medicinal tea. (14:230) **Cherokee** *Anthelmintic* Infusion of blooms taken for worms. *Dermatological Aid* Used for sores or skin eruptions. *Dietary Aid* Taken to increase appetite. *Febrifuge* Infusion of blooms taken for fevers. *Laxative* Infusion of blooms taken as a laxative. (66:59) **Iroquois** *Liver Aid* Compound decoction of roots taken for too much gall. *Witchcraft Medicine* Infusion of smashed roots taken as an anti-witchcraft medicine. (73:434) **Malecite** *Contraceptive* Infusion of plants used to prevent pregnancy. (96:258) **Micmac** *Contraceptive* Herb used to prevent pregnancy. (32:55)

Chenopodium album, Lamb's Quarters
Carrier *Blood Medicine* Decoction of plant taken to improve the blood. (26:86) **Cherokee** *Dietary Aid* Cooked salad greens eaten to "keep healthy." (66:42) **Cree, Woodlands** *Antirheumatic (External)* Decoction of plant used as wash for painful limbs. *Antirheumatic (Internal)* Decoction of plant taken for painful limbs. (91:35) **Eskimo, Inupiat** *Carminative* Leaves and stems cooked with beans to reduce the intestinal gas from eating the beans. (83:64) **Iroquois** *Antidiarrheal* Cold infusion of whole plant taken for diarrhea. (73:315) *Burn Dressing* Compound used as salve on burns. (73:316) *Gynecological Aid* Compound decoction used as wash and applied as poultice when bothered by milk flow. (73:315) **Mendocino Indian** *Gastrointestinal Aid* Leaves used for stomachaches. (33:346) **Meskwaki** *Dermatological Aid* Infusion of root used for urethral itching. (129:209) **Navajo** *Dietary Aid* Plant used as a nutrient. (76:149) **Navajo, Kayenta** *Burn Dressing* Poultice of plant applied to burns. (179:20) **Navajo, Ramah** *Antidote* Stem, 3 inches long, made into snake figurine for snake infection. (165:24) **Paiute** *Emetic* Leaf chewed as an emetic. (as *C. alba* 144:317) **Potawatomi** *Misc. Disease Remedy* Plant considered a medicinal food used to prevent

or cure scurvy. (131:47) Leaves included in the diet for scurvy or to prevent it. (131:98)

Chenopodium ambrosioides, Mexican Tea
Creek *Febrifuge* Unspecified plant part used "in cases of fever." (148:657) Plant used as a fever medicine. (152:22) *Panacea* Plant used for "a great many ailments." *Tonic* Plant used as "a sort of spring tonic." (148:657) Plant used as a spring tonic. (152:22) **Houma** *Analgesic* Poultice of crushed leaves applied for headaches. *Anthelmintic* and *Pediatric Aid* Decoction of leaves in milk given to children for worms. (135:63) **Koasati** *Anthelmintic* Decoction of leaves taken for worms. (152:22) **Mahuna** *Abortifacient* Roots used for delayed menstrual period. (117:14) **Miwok** *Antirheumatic (External)* Plant used as wash for rheumatic parts. *Dermatological Aid* Poultice of boiled or raw plant applied to swellings. *Toothache Remedy* Plant used for toothache or an ulcerated tooth. *Venereal Aid* Plant used as wash for gonorrhea and injected into affected parts. (8:168) **Natchez** *Anthelmintic* Plant given to children for worms. *Febrifuge* Plant used as a fever medicine. *Pediatric Aid* Plant given to children for worms. (152:22) **Rappahannock** *Anthelmintic* Stewed seeds taken for worms. *Tonic* Stewed seeds taken as a tonic. (138:30) **Seminole** *Blood Medicine* Decoction of whole plant taken for worm sickness: pale skin and laziness. (145:241) *Gastrointestinal Aid* Infusion of root bark taken for stomach troubles. (145:276) *Pulmonary Aid* and *Sedative* Plant taken and rubbed on the body for lion disease: chest cramps, nervousness, and walking continually. (145:233) *Stimulant* Decoction of whole plant taken for worm sickness: pale skin and laziness. (145:241)

Chenopodium botrys, Jerusalem Oak Goosefoot
Cherokee *Analgesic* Cold infusion taken orally and used to moisten head for headache. *Anthelmintic* Decoction of any part of plant in sweet milk given for worms. *Cold Remedy* Cold infusion taken orally and used to moisten head for colds. *Misc. Disease Remedy* Warm infusion of root taken in winter for "fever diseases." (66:41)

Chenopodium californicum, California Goosefoot

Cahuilla *Gastrointestinal Aid* Decoction of entire plant used for stomach disorders. (11:52) **Costanoan** *Orthopedic Aid* Decoction of root applied as a poultice for numb or paralyzed limbs. (17:11) **Kawaiisu** *Dermatological Aid* Plant used as a hair wash. *Emetic* Decoction of leaves and stems taken as an emetic. *Poison* Plant considered poisonous. (180:19)

Chenopodium capitatum, Blite Goosefoot

Navajo, Kayenta *Dermatological Aid* Plant used as a lotion for head bruises. *Eye Medicine* Plant used as a lotion for black eyes. (179:21) **Potawatomi** *Pulmonary Aid* Juice of seeds and infusion of plant used for lung congestion. (131:47)

Chenopodium graveolens, Fetid Goosefoot

Keres, Western *Emetic* Plant used as an emetic. (as *C. cornutum* 147:36) **Zuni** *Analgesic* and *Herbal Steam* Plant steeped in water and vapor inhaled for headache. (as *C. cornutum* 143:45)

Chenopodium incanum, Mealy Goosefoot

Navajo, Ramah *Antidote* Stem, 3 inches long, made into snake figurine for snake infection. (165:25)

Chenopodium oahuense, Alaweo

Hawaiian *Dermatological Aid* Plant used for beautifying the skin. Bark mixture eaten by nursing mother to beautify the skin of the child during growth and development. *Dietary Aid* Bark chewed by nursing mother to benefit the child. Juice mixed with other plants and given to children to fatten or add weight. *Pediatric Aid* Buds chewed by children with general weakness. Bark chewed by nursing mother to benefit the child. Bark mixture eaten by nursing mother to beautify the skin of the child during growth and development. Juice mixed with other plants and given to children to fatten or add weight. *Strengthener* Buds chewed by children with general weakness. (as *Chenepodium sandwicheum* 2:20)

Chimaphila maculata, Striped Prince's Pine

Cherokee *Analgesic* Poultice of root used for pain. *Antirheumatic (Internal)* Tops and roots used for rheumatism. *Cancer Treatment* Used as a wash for cancer and ulcers. *Cold Remedy* Infusion of leaves used for colds. *Dermatological Aid* Decoction used for tetter and ringworm. *Emetic* Infusion given to make baby vomit and poultice of root used for pain. *Febrifuge* Infusion of leaves used for fevers. *Pediatric Aid* Infusion given to make baby vomit and poultice of root used for pain. *Poison* Infusion used to kill rats. *Tuberculosis Remedy* Used as a wash for scrofula. *Urinary Aid* Tops and roots used for urinary problems. *Veterinary Aid* Infusion given for "milksick." (66:62) **Nanticoke** *Misc. Disease Remedy* Plant used for ague. (150:84)

Chimaphila menziesii, Little Prince's Pine

Karok *Gynecological Aid* Decoction of leaves taken for female troubles. *Kidney Aid* and *Urinary Aid* Decoction of leaves taken for kidney and bladder troubles. (5:23)

Chimaphila umbellata, Pipsissewa

Abnaki *Cold Remedy* Used for head colds. (121:154) *Nose Medicine* Powdered leaves mixed with bark from another plant and used as snuff for nasal inflammation. (121:170) **Catawba** *Analgesic* and *Orthopedic Aid* Plant used for backache. (152:47) **Chippewa** *Eye Medicine* Decoction of root used as drops for sore eyes. (43:360) *Venereal Aid* Plant used for gonorrhea. (59:138) **Cree, Woodlands** *Antihemorrhagic* Infusion or decoction of plant with other species used for coughing

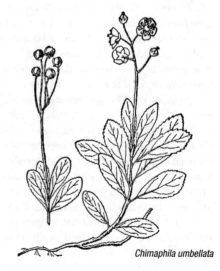

Chimaphila umbellata

up blood. Decoction of plant taken for coughing up blood. *Heart Medicine* Used for pain and fever caused by chest ailments due to heart conditions such as angina pectoris. *Orthopedic Aid* Decoction of plant used for backaches. *Pulmonary Aid* Decoction of plant used for stabbing pain in the chest. (91:35) **Delaware** *Blood Medicine* Infusion of plant, mallow root, elder flowers, and dwarf elder bark used as a blood purifier. *Dermatological Aid* Infusion of plant used for blisters. *Pulmonary Aid* Infusion of plant, mallow root, elder flowers, and dwarf elder bark used to remove lung mucus. *Urinary Aid* Infusion of plant, mallow root, elder flowers, and dwarf elder bark used for bladder inflammation. *Venereal Aid* Infusion of plant, mallow root, elder flowers, and dwarf elder bark used for scrofula. (151:35) **Delaware, Oklahoma** *Blood Medicine* Compound containing plant taken as a blood purifier. *Dermatological Aid* Infusion of plant applied to blisters. *Expectorant* Compound containing plant taken to help remove mucus from the lungs. *Tuberculosis Remedy* Compound containing plant taken for "scrofula." *Urinary Aid* Compound containing plant used for bladder inflammation. (150:29, 74) **Flathead** *Eye Medicine* Solution of plant used as eye medicine. (68:34) **Karok** *Orthopedic Aid* Poultice of plant applied or infusion of leaves taken for backaches. (125:387) **Kutenai** *Eye Medicine* Solution of plant used as eye medicine. *Kidney Aid* Infusion of plant used for kidney trouble. (68:34) **Malecite** *Blood Medicine* Infusion of plants used as a blood purifier. (96:253) *Tuberculosis Remedy* Infusion of plants and juniper roots used for consumption. (96:251) **Menominee** *Adjuvant* Plant used as a seasoner to make female remedies taste good. (128:35) *Blood Medicine* Decoction of leaves taken to "clear the blood." (44:129) *Gynecological Aid* Compound decoction of root taken after childbirth to aid internal healing. (44:133) **Micmac** *Antirheumatic (Internal)* Herb used for rheumatism. *Blood Medicine* Herb used as a blood purifier. *Dermatological Aid* Herb used for blisters. *Gastrointestinal Aid* Herb used for stomach trouble. *Kidney Aid* Herb used for kidney trouble. (32:56) Used for kidney pains. (122:57) *Misc. Disease Remedy* Herb used for smallpox. *Tuberculosis Remedy* Herb used for consumption. *Urinary Aid* Herb used for "cold in bladder." (32:56) Infusion of roots, hemlock,

parsley, and curled dock used for colds in the bladder. (96:259) **Mohegan** *Dermatological Aid* Infusion of plant applied to blisters. (149:265) Infusion of leaves applied to blisters. (151:71, 128) **Montagnais** *Diaphoretic* Decoction of plant taken to induce sweating. (133:316) **Montana Indian** *Febrifuge* Decoction of the herb or root used as a febrifuge for fevers. (15:9) Infusion taken for fever. (68:34) **Nanticoke** *Misc. Disease Remedy* Infusion of plant taken for ague. (150:56) **Ojibwa** *Gastrointestinal Aid* Infusion of plant used for stomach troubles. (130:368) **Okanagan-Colville** *Blood Medicine* Infusion of roots and leaves taken as a blood purifier. Decoction of whole plant taken as a blood purifier. *Cold Remedy* Infusion of roots and leaves taken for long-lasting colds. *Dietary Aid* Decoction of whole plant taken as an appetizer. *Kidney Aid* Infusion of roots and leaves taken to "clean out" the kidneys. *Tuberculosis Remedy* Infusion of roots and leaves taken for tuberculosis. (162:101) **Okanagon** *Dermatological Aid* Poultice of crushed plant applied to leg and foot swellings. *Gynecological Aid* Plant chewed or infusion of leaves taken by women before and after childbirth. (104:42) **Penobscot** *Dermatological Aid* Infusion of plant applied to blisters. (133:309) **Rappahannock** *Blood Medicine* Infusion of roots taken to benefit blood. *Dietary Aid* Infusion of dried roots in brandy taken or chewed for the appetite. *Gastrointestinal Aid* Infusion of dried roots in brandy taken or chewed for the stomach. *Tonic* Infusion of dried roots in brandy used as a tonic for feeling low. *Veterinary Aid* Crushed and dried leaves mixed with the feed of mules to remove "bot worms." (138:26) **Saanich** *Antirheumatic (External)* Leaves put in bath water of sprinters and canoers as a liniment for sore muscles. (156:83) **Thompson** *Dermatological Aid* Poultice of crushed plant applied to leg and foot swellings. (104:42) *Gynecological Aid* Plant chewed or infusion of leaves taken by women before and after childbirth. (104:41) Plant chewed at childbirth to ease confinement. (141:462) Warm decoction of leaves taken before and after childbirth. *Orthopedic Aid* Poultice of crushed, fresh plant applied to leg and foot swellings. *Tonic* Decoction of leaves taken as a tonic for general indisposition. (141:477)

Chimaphila umbellata ssp. *cisatlantica*, Pipsissewa

Iroquois *Adjuvant* Plant mixed, as a medicine strengthener, with any medicine. (73:408) *Analgesic* Compound decoction of roots taken for urinating pain. *Anthelmintic* Infusion of plants given to babies with worms. (73:407) *Antirheumatic (Internal)* Compound decoction of plants taken for rheumatism. (73:408) *Blood Medicine* Decoction of roots or stems taken to purify bad blood or for blood chills. *Cancer Treatment* Decoction of stalks and roots taken for stomach cancer. *Dermatological Aid* Infusion of dried roots taken for pimples and sores on the face and neck. *Diuretic* Leaves and stems used as a diuretic. *Febrifuge* Infusion of plants taken by feverish and drowsy pregnant women. *Gynecological Aid* Compound decoction of bark and roots taken to induce pregnancy. Compound infusion of leaves and bark taken for miscarriage. Infusion of plants taken by feverish and drowsy pregnant women. (73:407) *Kidney Aid* Compound decoction of roots taken for the kidneys and dropsy. (73:408) *Laxative* Compound decoction of roots taken as a laxative. *Pediatric Aid* Infusion of plants given to babies with worms. *Stimulant* Infusion of plants taken by feverish and drowsy pregnant women. (73:407) *Tonic* Compound decoction of roots and bark taken as a tonic. (73:408) *Urinary Aid* Compound decoction of roots taken for urinating pain. *Venereal Aid* Compound decoction taken as blood purifier and for venereal disease. (73:407)

Chimaphila umbellata ssp. *occidentalis*, Pipsissewa

Yurok *Antirheumatic (External)* Leaves used for various aches and pains and to relax the muscles. *Kidney Aid* Leaves used for kidney ailments. (5:23)

Chionanthus virginicus, White Fringetree

Choctaw *Dermatological Aid* Decoction of bark used as wash or poultice as dressing for cuts or bruises. (20:23) Decoction of roots or bark used as a wash for infected sores and wounds. Poultice of beaten bark applied to cuts and bruises. *Disinfectant* Decoction of roots used as a wash for infected sores. **Koasati** *Dermatological Aid* Decoction of bark used as a wash for cuts. (152:50)

Chlorogalum pomeridianum, Wavyleaf Soapplant

Cahuilla *Dermatological Aid* Saponaceous material used as a dandruff shampoo. (11:54) **Costanoan** *Dermatological Aid* Pounded stalks used as a wash for dandruff. *Poison* Bulb used as a fish poison. (17:28) **Mendocino Indian** *Dermatological Aid* Plant used as a hair wash for dandruff. *Poison* Root considered poisonous. (33:319) **Mewuk** *Poison* Plant considered poisonous. (97:336) **Pomo** *Dermatological Aid* Plant juice rubbed on area affected by poison oak. (33:319) Bulb used as a soap for washing the hair and to prevent lice. (54:12) **Pomo, Kashaya** *Dermatological Aid* Bulb used as soap for washing body, hair, and utensils. (60:107) **Wailaki** *Analgesic* Bulb rubbed on body for cramps. *Antirheumatic (External)* Bulb rubbed on body for rheumatism. *Carminative* Decoction of bulbs taken for gas. *Dermatological Aid* Poultice of roasted bulbs used antiseptically for sores. *Disinfectant* Poultice of roasted bulbs used antiseptically for sores. *Diuretic* Decoction of bulbs taken as a diuretic. *Gastrointestinal Aid* Decoction of bulbs taken for stomachaches. *Laxative* Decoction of bulbs taken as a laxative. (33:319)

Chorizanthe staticoides, Turkish Rugging

Tubatulabal *Dermatological Aid* Infusion of entire plant used as lotion for pimples. (167:59)

Chrysobalanus icaco, Icaco Coco Plum

Seminole *Love Medicine* Decoction of wood ashes placed on the tongue to cleanse the body and strengthen the marriage. (145:250)

Chrysophyllum oliviforme, Satinleaf

Seminole *Love Medicine* Decoction of wood ashes placed on the tongue to cleanse the body and strengthen the marriage. (145:250)

Chrysopsis mariana, Maryland Goldenaster

Delaware *Pediatric Aid* Infusion of roots used to quiet infants. Infusion of roots used as a tonic for sickly children. *Sedative* Infusion of roots used to quiet infants. *Tonic* Infusion of roots used as a tonic for sickly children. (151:33) **Delaware, Oklahoma** *Sedative* Infusion of root given to infants to quiet them. *Tonic* Infusion of root used as a tonic for "sickly children." (150:28, 74)

Chrysothamnus depressus, Longflower Rabbitbrush

Navajo, Ramah *Gynecological Aid* Decoction of plant used to facilitate labor and delivery of placenta. (165:49)

Chrysothamnus greenei, Greene's Rabbitbrush

Navajo *Dermatological Aid* and *Misc. Disease Remedy* Infusion of plant tops used as a wash for chickenpox and measles eruptions. (45:83)

Chrysothamnus nauseosus, Rubber Rabbitbrush

Cahuilla *Toothache Remedy* Decoction of twigs taken for toothaches. (11:54) **Cheyenne** *Cold Remedy* Infusion of flower parts taken or burning plant smoke inhaled for colds. *Cough Medicine* Infusion of flower parts taken for coughs. (69:20) *Dermatological Aid* Decoction of leaves and stem used as wash and taken for sores, especially smallpox. (as *C. nauseosa* 63:39, 40) Infusion of leaves and stems used as a wash to heal eruptions or sores. (63:187) Infusion of leaves and stems used as a wash or taken for eruptions or body sores. (64:187) Infusion of leaves and stems used for sores and skin eruptions. (69:20) *Misc. Disease Remedy* Decoction of leaves and stem taken for smallpox. (as *C. nauseosa* 63:39, 40) Infusion of leaves and stems taken for smallpox. (63:187) Infusion of leaves and stems taken for smallpox. (64:187) *Psychological Aid* Burning leaf and branch smoke used to drive away the cause of nightmares. *Tuberculosis Remedy* Infusion of flower parts taken for tuberculosis. (69:20) **Coahuilla** *Analgesic* Infusion of twigs taken for chest pain. *Cough Medicine* Infusion of twigs taken for coughs. (as *Bigilovia graveolens* 9:79) **Klamath** *Dermatological Aid* Poultice of herbage used to raise blisters. (as *Chondrophora nauseosa* 37:106) Poultice of smashed herbs applied to blisters. (as *Chondrophora nauseosa* 140:131) **Okanagan-Colville** *Gynecological Aid* Leaves used as a sanitary napkin. Leaves used as a sanitary napkin particularly after childbirth, to "heal the insides."

(162:83) **Thompson** *Antidiarrheal* Decoction of plant taken for diarrhea. *Cold Remedy* Decoction of plant taken for colds. *Gastrointestinal Aid* Decoction of plant taken for stomach cramps. *Other* Plant used as a medicine for "drinking and bathing." *Panacea* Decoction of plant taken for "all diseases." *Tuberculosis Remedy* Decoction of plant taken for tuberculosis. *Urinary Aid* Decoction of plant taken for colds, venereal diseases, bladder trouble, and tuberculosis. *Venereal Aid* Decoction of plant taken for venereal disease. (161:178)

Chrysothamnus nauseosus ssp. *albicaulis*, Rubber Rabbitbrush

Sanpoil *Veterinary Aid* Container of brush lighted and held under horse's nostrils for distemper. Salve of branches and leaves used on horses to keep horseflies and gnats away. (109:217) **Shoshoni** *Antidiarrheal* Decoction of roots and tops taken for bloody diarrhea. *Cold Remedy* Compound decoction of stems taken for colds. Infusion of leaves taken as a cold medicine. *Cough Medicine* Compound decoction of stems taken for coughs. Decoction of stems and leaves taken for coughs. *Gastrointestinal Aid* Infusion of leaves taken for stomach disorders. *Tonic* Infusion of dried leaves and flowers taken as a general tonic. (155:57)

Chrysothamnus nauseosus ssp. *bigelovii*, Rubber Rabbitbrush

Navajo, Kayenta *Ceremonial Medicine* and *Emetic* Plant used as a ceremonial emetic. (179:46) **Navajo, Ramah** *Analgesic* Leaves made into a lotion and used for headache and decoction of root used for menstrual pain. *Cathartic* Compound decoction of leaves used as a cathartic. (165:49, 50) *Ceremonial Medicine* Leaves used as a ceremonial emetic. (165:49) *Cold Remedy* Strong decoction of root taken for colds. *Cough Medicine* Strong decoction of root taken for cough. *Emetic* Leaves used as an emetic for several ceremonies. *Febrifuge* Strong decoction of root taken for fever. *Gynecological Aid* Strong decoction of root taken for menstrual pain. (165:49, 50) **Tewa** *Oral Aid* and *Pediatric Aid* White galls from plants hung around babies' necks to stop dribbling. (as *C. bigelovii* 115:45)

Chrysothamnus nauseosus* ssp. *latisqua-meus, Rubber Rabbitbrush
Isleta *Poison* Wood used to make poisonous war arrows. (as *C. latisquameus* 85:26)

Chrysothamnus parryi* ssp. *howardii,
Howard's Rabbitbrush
Hopi *Ceremonial Medicine* Plant used in initiatory ceremonials. (as *Bigelovia howardii* 46:20)

Chrysothamnus viscidiflorus, Green Rabbitbrush
Hopi *Dermatological Aid* Poultice of chewed plant tips applied to boils. (as *Bigelovia douglasii* 46:20) **Paiute** *Cold Remedy* Infusion of crushed leaves taken or used as a wash for colds. (87:197) Infusion of crushed leaves taken for colds. *Cough Medicine* Decoction of young growth taken for coughs. *Diaphoretic* Branches used as a bed in the sweat bath for rheumatism. **Shoshoni** *Antirheumatic (External)* Poultice of moistened, crushed stems and leaves applied for rheumatism. *Misc. Disease Remedy* Hot compound decoction of plant taken for influenza. *Toothache Remedy* Finely mashed leaves inserted in tooth cavities for toothaches. (155:57, 58)

Chrysothamnus viscidiflorus* ssp. *viscidiflorus* var. *stenophyllus, Green Rabbitbrush

Chrysothamnus viscidiflorus* ssp. *viscidiflorus* var. *viscidiflorus, Green Rabbitbrush
Navajo *Emetic* Plant used to make a sick person vomit. (45:84)

Cibotium chamissoi, Chamisso's Manfern
Hawaiian *Analgesic* Infusion of powdered bark and other plants taken for chest pains. *Antirheumatic (External)* Very fine, downy hairs burned and the heat applied to hardened muscles and tired limbs. *Blood Medicine* Infusion of powdered bark and other plants taken to purify the blood. *Dietary Aid* Infusion of powdered bark and other plants taken to stimulate the appetite, and taken for weight loss. *Sedative* Very fine, downy hairs burned and the heat applied for nervousness. (as *Cibatium whamissoi* 2:43)

Cichorium intybus, Chicory
Cherokee *Tonic* Infusion of root used as a tonic for nerves. (66:29) **Iroquois** *Dermatological Aid* Decoction of roots used as a wash and poultice applied to chancres and fever sores. (73:476)

Cicuta douglasii, Western Water Hemlock
Alaska Native *Poison* Roots considered poisonous. (71:153) **Bella Coola** *Cathartic* Roots used as a purgative. (127:61) *Emetic* Infusion of grated tubers taken as an emetic to "clean out the bile in the stomach." (158:200) **Haisla & Hanaksiala** *Poison* Roots considered poisonous. (35:212) **Kawaiisu** *Analgesic* and *Orthopedic Aid* "Mashed root put on a hot stone and sore limbs laid directly over it." *Poison* Plant considered poisonous. (180:20) **Kutenai** *Dermatological Aid* Roots pounded and used for sores. *Emetic* Infusion of roots taken with large amounts of warm water as an emetic. This remedy was used cautiously because of the poisonous effects of larger doses of water hemlocks. (68:71) **Kwakiutl** *Antidiarrheal* Cold, compound infusion of burned, pulverized bark taken for diarrhea. (157:270) *Cathartic* Poultice of soaked roots applied to the stomach as a purgative. *Dermatological Aid* Poultice of roots applied to draw out thorns and splinters. *Emetic* Root extract and grease taken to induce vomiting. *Misc. Disease Remedy* Roots smashed, steamed, peeled, powdered, mixed with oil, and taken for any serious disease. *Poison* Plant considered highly poisonous. (157:276) **Montana Indian** *Analgesic* Roots used for headaches. *Snakebite Remedy* Poultice of

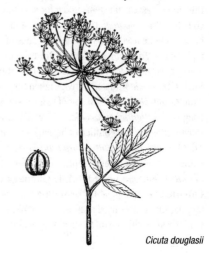

Cicuta douglasii

split roots used for rattlesnake bites. (68:71) **Okanagan-Colville** *Poison* Plant considered a very bad poison. (162:60) **Paiute** *Antirheumatic* (*External*) Decoction of mashed roots used as a soothing solution for "rheumatism" and tired and aching feet. (93:96) **Salish, Coast** *Cathartic* Used with caution as a purgative. *Emetic* Used with caution to induce vomiting. (156:89) **Shuswap** *Poison* Plant considered poisonous. (102:56) **Thompson** *Analgesic* Poultice of root used for severe pain in the legs and back. Decoction of plant used as a wash for aching bones. *Orthopedic Aid* Boiled, roots used by bedridden patients, or poultice of roots used for broken hips. The bedridden patient's back was splashed with water and the boiled, mashed roots placed on the back to help the patient recover. The informant warned that the poultice should not be left on for more than half an hour and that because of its toxicity it should never be taken internally. Decoction of plant used as a wash for broken bones. (161:150) *Panacea* Root eaten to protect against disease and give feeling of "perfect wellness." (as *Cicuta vagans* 141:476) *Poison* Roots known to be poisonous to both humans and animals. (as *Cicuta vagans* 141:513) Considered one of the most toxic plants in North America for people, horses, cattle, and sheep. (161:150) *Veterinary Aid* Roots known to be poisonous to animals. (as *Cicuta vagans* 141:513)

Cicuta maculata, Spotted Water Hemlock
Alaska Native *Poison* Roots considered poisonous. (71:153) **Cherokee** *Ceremonial Medicine* Root chewed, if dizziness occurred person would die soon, if not, long life. *Contraceptive* Roots eaten for four consecutive days "to become sterile forever." (66:31) Roots chewed and swallowed by women as form of contraception and become sterile. (152:45) **Cree, Woodlands** *Antirheumatic* (*External*) Dried roots powdered, made into a liniment, and applied externally. (91:35) **Iroquois** *Dermatological Aid* Poultice of smashed roots applied for lameness, running sores, or cuts. *Disinfectant* Handling plants caused fits and decoction used as floor wash to prevent disease. *Orthopedic Aid* Decoction of plants used on bruises, sprains, sore joints, or broken bones. *Poison* Roots chewed to commit suicide. *Veterinary Aid* Poultice of smashed roots applied to horses for lameness or running sores. (73:398) **Klamath** *Poison* Poisonous roots mixed with rattlesnake poison or decomposed animal liver and used to poison arrows. (37:101) **Lakota** *Poison* Plant poisonous to humans. (116:33) **Ojibwa** *Hunting Medicine* Root used in hunting medicine smoked to attract the buck deer near enough to shoot with bow and arrow. (130:432) *Unspecified* Root used medicinally. (130:390)

Cicuta maculata* var. *angustifolia, Spotted Water Hemlock
Montana Indian *Poison* Fleshy roots known as a virulent poison and sometimes used for suicide. (as *Cicuta occidentalis* 15:10) **Paiute** *Analgesic* Poultice of roasted roots applied to "deaden muscular pain." *Antirheumatic* (*External*) Poultice of roasted roots applied to rheumatic joints. *Dermatological Aid* Poultice of roasted roots applied for ordinary swellings. *Orthopedic Aid* Poultice of roasted roots applied to "deaden muscular pain." *Snakebite Remedy* Poultice of pulped root applied to rattlesnake bites for the swelling. **Shoshoni** *Eye Medicine* Cool decoction of root used as a wash for sore eyes or granulated lids. *Orthopedic Aid* Poultice of roots applied to "deaden muscular pain." *Poison* Root pulp considered poisonous for open wounds. (as *Cicuta occidentalis* 155:58, 59)

Cicuta maculata* var. *maculata, Spotted Water Hemlock
Seminole *Febrifuge* Decoction of leaves, roots, and stems used as a bath for high fevers. (as *Cicuta curtissii* 145:282)

Cicuta virosa, Mackenzie's Water Hemlock
Alaska Native *Poison* Roots considered poisonous. (as *Cicuta mackenziana* 71:153) **Eskimo, Inupiat** *Poison* Whole plant considered poisonous. (as *Cicuta mackenziana* 83:137) **Eskimo, Kuskokwagmiut** *Poison* Root "considered to be poisonous to people." (as *Cicuta mackenziana* 101:21) **Eskimo, Western** *Poison* Roots considered poisonous. (as *Cicuta mackenziana* 90:17) **Haisla & Hanaksiala** *Poison* Roots considered poisonous. (as *Cicuta mackenzieana* 35:212)

Cimicifuga racemosa, Black Bugbane
Cherokee *Abortifacient* Used to stimulate men-

struation. *Analgesic* Used as an anodyne. (66:30) Infusion of root "in spirits" used for rheumatic pains. (177:73, 74) *Antirheumatic (Internal)* Infusion of roots in alcoholic spirits used for rheumatism. (66:30) Infusion of root "in spirits" used for rheumatic pains. (177:73, 74) *Cold Remedy* Infusion taken for colds. *Cough Medicine* Infusion taken for coughs. *Dermatological Aid* Given for hives. Infusion of slightly astringent plant taken for rheumatism. *Diuretic* Used as a diuretic. *Laxative* Infusion taken for constipation. *Pediatric Aid* and *Sedative* Given to make babies sleep. *Stimulant* Given for fatigue. *Tonic* Used as a tonic. *Tuberculosis Remedy* Infusion taken for colds, coughs, "consumption," and constipation. (66:30) **Delaware** *Tonic* Used with elecampane and stone root to make a tonic. (151:33) Combined with elecampane and stone roots to make a tonic. (151:39) **Delaware, Oklahoma** *Tonic* Compound containing root used as a tonic. (150:32, 74) **Iroquois** *Antirheumatic (External)* Decoction of roots or plants used as a soak and steam bath for rheumatism. (73:320) *Blood Medicine* Root used as a blood purifier. (73:321) *Gynecological Aid* Infusion of roots taken to "promote the flow of milk in women." *Orthopedic Aid* and *Pediatric Aid* Poultice of smashed leaves applied to babies with sore backs. (73:320) **Micmac** *Kidney Aid* Root used for kidney trouble. (32:56) **Penobscot** *Kidney Aid* Root used to make a medicine and taken for kidney trouble. (133:310, 311)

Cinchona calisaya, Quinine
Cherokee *Reproductive Aid* Infusion of plant taken for impotence. *Tonic* Used to make a tonic. (as *C. ledgeriana* 66:49)

Cinna arundinacea, Sweet Woodreed
Iroquois *Misc. Disease Remedy* Compound decoction of plants taken for sugar diabetes. (73:274)

Circaea lutetiana ssp. *canadensis*, Broadleaf Enchanter's Nightshade
Iroquois *Dermatological Aid* Plant used on wounds. *Other* Compound infusion taken and used as wash on injured part, a "Little Water Medicine." (73:391)

Cirsium altissimum, Tall Thistle
Cherokee *Analgesic* Infusion of leaves taken for neuralgia. *Gastrointestinal Aid* Warm infusion of roots taken to help person who overeats. *Poultice* Roots used as poultice and decoction of bruised plant used to poultice sore jaw. (as *Carduus altissimus* 66:58)

Cirsium arvense, Canadian Thistle
Abnaki *Anthelmintic* Used as a vermifuge. (121:155) Decoction of roots used by children for worms. *Pediatric Aid* Decoction of roots used by children for worms. (121:173) **Iroquois** *Oral Aid* Infusion of roots used for mouth sickness. (118:63) **Mohegan** *Oral Aid* and *Pediatric Aid* Infusion of leaves used as a mouthwash for infants. (151:71, 128) *Pulmonary Aid* Plant used for lung trouble. (151:128) *Tuberculosis Remedy* Decoction of plant taken for consumption. (149:269) **Montagnais** *Tuberculosis Remedy* Decoction of plant used for consumption. (133:314) Decoction of plant taken for consumption. (149:269) **Ojibwa** *Gastrointestinal Aid* Plant used as a "bowel tonic." (130:364)

Cirsium calcareum, Cainville Thistle
Hopi *Anthelmintic* Plant used as a worm remedy. (as *C. pulchellum* 174:34, 95, 96) *Dermatological Aid* Plant used for itching. (as *C. pulchellum* 174:32, 95, 96) *Laxative* Plant used as a laxative. *Throat Aid* Decoction of plant used for tickling throat caused by a cold. (as *C. pulchellum* 174:34, 95–96) **Navajo, Ramah** *Eye Medicine* Cold infusion of root used as a wash for sore eyes. (165:50)

Cirsium discolor, Field Thistle
Cree *Dermatological Aid* Poultice of root paste applied to linen cloths and bound to the wound. (12:490) **Iroquois** *Dermatological Aid* Compound decoction of roots taken or poultice of roots applied to boils. *Hemorrhoid Remedy* Compound decoction of plants taken for piles. (73:475) **Meskwaki** *Analgesic* Infusion of root used for stomachaches. *Gastrointestinal Aid* Infusion of root taken for stomachache. (129:213)

Cirsium eatonii, Eaton's Thistle
Gosiute *Dermatological Aid* Plant used for

wounds, cuts, or sores. (as *Cnicus eatoni* 31:349, 366)

Cirsium horridulum, Yellow Thistle
Houma *Dermatological Aid* Infusion of leaves and root in whisky recognized as a strong astringent. *Expectorant* Infusion of leaf and root in whisky taken to clear phlegm from lungs and throat. *Throat Aid* Infusion of leaves and root in whisky taken to clear throat and lungs of phlegm. (135:57)

Cirsium neomexicanum, New Mexico Thistle
Navajo *Febrifuge* Plant used for chills and fevers. (45:96) **Navajo, Ramah** *Eye Medicine* Cold infusion of root used as a wash for eye diseases. *Panacea* Root used as a "life medicine." Cold infusion of plant taken when one "feels bad all over." *Veterinary Aid* Cold infusion of root used as a wash for livestock with eye diseases. (165:50)

Cirsium ochrocentrum, Yellowspine Thistle
Kiowa *Burn Dressing* Decoction of blossoms used as wash for burns. *Dermatological Aid* Decoction of blossoms used as wash for sores. (166:58) **Zuni** *Contraceptive* Infusion of root taken by both partners as a contraceptive. (22:374) *Diaphoretic* Infusion of whole plant taken as a diaphoretic for syphilis. *Diuretic* Infusion of whole plant taken as a diuretic for syphilis. *Emetic* Infusion of whole plant taken as an emetic for syphilis. (as *Carduus ochrocentrus* 143:44, 45) *Misc. Disease Remedy* Infusion of fresh or dried root taken three times a day for diabetes. *Venereal Aid* Infusion of whole plant taken for syphilis. (22:374) Infusion of whole plant taken for syphilis. (as *Carduus ochrocentrus* 143:44, 45)

Cirsium pallidum, Pale Thistle
Keres, Western *Diuretic* Roots used as a diuretic. (147:37)

Cirsium remotifolium, Fewleaf Thistle
Kwakiutl *Oral Aid* Root skins dried, soaked in water, and used as a wash for mouth rashes and cankers. Infusion of root used to wipe out child's mouth for rash and cankers. Root held in mouth for rash or cankers in mouth and infusion used for children. *Pediatric Aid* Infusion of root used to

wipe out child's mouth for rash and cankers. (as *Carduus remaliflorus* 16:383)

Cirsium rothrockii, Rothrock's Thistle
Navajo, Kayenta *Febrifuge* Plant used for fevers caused by injuries. *Misc. Disease Remedy* Roots used as a lotion or eaten raw for smallpox. *Panacea* Plant used as a life medicine. (179:46)

Cirsium undulatum, Wavyleaf Thistle
Comanche *Venereal Aid* Decoction of root used for gonorrhea. (24:521) **Navajo, Ramah** *Eye Medicine* Cold infusion of root used as a wash for eye diseases. *Panacea* Root used as a "life medicine." Cold infusion of plant taken when one "feels bad all over." *Veterinary Aid* Cold infusion of root used as a wash for livestock with eye diseases. (165:50) **Shuswap** *Gastrointestinal Aid* Root used for the stomach and body. (102:59)

Cirsium vulgare, Bull Thistle
Cherokee *Analgesic* Infusion of leaves taken for neuralgia. *Gastrointestinal Aid* Warm infusion of roots taken to help person who overeats. *Poultice* Roots used as poultice and decoction of bruised plant used to poultice sore jaw. (as *Carduus lanceolatus* 66:58) **Delaware** *Antirheumatic (External)* Hot infusion of roots or twigs used as a steam treatment for muscular swellings and stiff joints. (as *Cirsium lanceolatum* 151:36) **Delaware, Oklahoma** *Antirheumatic (External)* Infusion of whole plant used as herbal steam for rheumatism. (as *C. lanceolatum* 150:30, 74) *Herbal Steam* Infusion of roots or twigs used as herbal steam for rheumatism. (as *C. lanceolatum* 150:30) **Iroquois** *Cancer Treatment* Plant used for cancer. *Hemorrhoid Remedy* Plant used for bleeding piles. (as *C. lanceolatum* 73:475) Decoction of whole plant taken and poultice of plant and wool applied to hemorrhoids. (as *C. lanceolatum* 118:63) *Hemostat* Plant used for bleeding piles. (as *C. lanceolatum* 73:475) **Meskwaki** *Adjuvant* Root used as a seasoner for medicines. (as *C. lanceolatum* 129:213) **Navajo** *Emetic* Decoction of plant taken to induce vomiting. (as *C. lanceolatum* 45:84) **Ojibwa** *Analgesic* and *Gastrointestinal Aid* Root used by men and women for stomach cramps. (as *C. lanceolatum* 130:364) **Potawatomi** *Adjuvant*

Fresh flower centers chewed to mask unpleasant flavors in medicines. (as *C. lanceolatum* 131:51)

Citrullus lanatus* var. *lanatus, Watermelon
Cherokee *Kidney Aid* Infusion of seeds taken for kidney trouble. *Pediatric Aid* and *Urinary Aid* Seeds chewed for bed-wetting. (as *C. vulgaris* 66:61) **Cheyenne** *Diuretic* Decoction of seeds taken as a diuretic. (as *C. vulgaris* 69:24) **Chickasaw** *Urinary Aid* Decoction of mashed seeds taken for blood in the urine. (as *C. vulgaris* 152:59) **Iroquois** *Urinary Aid* Compound decoction of roots and seeds taken for urine stoppage. (as *C. vulgaris* 73:451) **Kiowa** *Poison* Unripened plant considered poisonous. (as *C. vulgaris* 166:53) **Rappahannock** *Kidney Aid* Infusion of seeds taken for gravel (kidney stones). *Veterinary Aid* Infusion of seeds given to horses for gravel (kidney stones). (as *C. vulgaris* 138:30)

Clarkia purpurea* ssp. *quadrivulnera, Winecup Fairyfan
Mendocino Indian *Eye Medicine* Decoction of leaves used as a wash for sore eyes. (as *Godetia albescens* 33:370)

Claytonia perfoliata, Miner's Lettuce
Shoshoni *Analgesic* Poultice of mashed plants applied for rheumatic pains. *Antirheumatic (External)* Poultice of plants applied as a counterirritant for rheumatic pains. (155:59) **Thompson** *Eye Medicine* Plant used for sore eyes and for "helping someone to see the right." (161:241)

Claytonia perfoliata* ssp. *perfoliata* var. *perfoliata, Miner's Lettuce
Mahuna *Dietary Aid* Plant juice used as an appetite restorer. (as *Montia perfoliata* 117:62)

Claytonia sibirica, Siberian Springbeauty
Cowlitz *Dermatological Aid* Cold infusion of stems used as a hair wash. **Quileute** *Dermatological Aid* Cold infusion of stems used as a hair wash for dandruff. *Eye Medicine* Juice from stems used as a wash for eyes. *Urinary Aid* Infusion of plants taken as an urinative. **Quinault** *Gynecological Aid* Whole plant chewed by women during pregnancy. **Skagit** *Throat Aid* Infusion of plants taken for sore throats. *Tonic* Infusion of plants taken as

a general tonic. (65:29) **Skagit, Upper** *Throat Aid* Infusion of plant used as a general tonic for sore throats. (154:42) **Skokomish** *Dermatological Aid* Cold infusion of stems used as a hair wash. **Snohomish** *Dermatological Aid* Cold infusion of stems used as a hair wash. (65:29) **Tlingit** *Venereal Aid* Compound poultice of leaves applied for syphilis. (as *C. alsinoides* 89:284)

Claytonia sibirica* var. *sibirica, Siberian Springbeauty
Hesquiat *Dermatological Aid* Poultice of chewed leaves used on cuts and sores. *Eye Medicine* Stem juice squeezed into the eye for sore, red eyes. (as *Montia sibirica* 159:71)

Claytonia virginica, Virginia Springbeauty
Iroquois *Anticonvulsive* Cold infusion or decoction of powdered roots given to child with convulsions. (73:317) *Contraceptive* Eating raw plants permanently prevented conception. (73:318) *Pediatric Aid* Cold infusion or decoction of powdered roots given to child with convulsions. (73:317)

Clematis baldwinii* var. *baldwinii, Baldwin's Clematis
Seminole *Other* Infusion of plant used for sunstroke. (as *Viorna baldwinii* 145:303)

Clematis columbiana, Rock Clematis
Okanagan-Colville *Dermatological Aid* Infusion of leaves alone or the stems and leaves used as a hair wash to prevent gray hair. Poultice of pounded, dampened leaves applied to the feet for sweaty feet. (162:117) **Thompson** *Dermatological Aid* Plant used as a head wash and for scabs and eczema. (141:459)

Clematis columbiana* var. *columbiana, Rock Clematis
Navajo, Ramah *Orthopedic Aid* Cold infusion of plant used as a lotion for swollen knee or ankle. (as *C. pseudoalpina* 165:27)

Clematis hirsutissima, Hairy Clematis
Montana Indian *Analgesic* Decoction of leaves used for headaches. *Veterinary Aid* Scraped root held in nostril of fallen horse and acted as a stimulant to animal. (as *C. douglasii* 15:10) **Navajo,**

Ramah *Analgesic* and *Respiratory Aid* Root used for congested nose pain. *Witchcraft Medicine* Cold infusion of plant or root taken and used as a lotion to protect from witches. (as *C. eriophora* 165:27)

Clematis lasiantha, Pipestem Clematis
Miwok *Burn Dressing* Pulverized plant charcoal dusted onto burns. *Dermatological Aid* Pulverized plant charcoal dusted onto running sores. (8:168) **Shasta** *Cold Remedy* Decoction of pounded, whole stem or bark used as a steam bath for colds. Roots burned or chewed for colds. *Herbal Steam* Decoction of pounded, whole stem or bark used as a steam bath for colds. (79:340)

Clematis ligusticifolia, Western White Clematis
Costanoan *Analgesic* Poultice of foliage applied for chest pains. (17:7) **Dakota** *Veterinary Aid* Plant used as a horse medicine. (82:35) **Gosiute** *Unspecified* Plant used as a medicine. (31:366) **Great Basin Indian** *Dermatological Aid* Roots used to make a shampoo. (100:47) **Lakota** *Analgesic* Infusion of roots taken for headaches. (116:55) **Mahuna** *Dermatological Aid* Infusion of plant used as a wash for skin eruptions. (117:17) **Mendocino Indian** *Cold Remedy* Stems and leaves chewed for colds. *Throat Aid* Stems and leaves chewed for sore throats. (33:347) **Montana Indian** *Cold Remedy* Chewed for colds. *Throat Aid* Chewed for sore throats. (15:10) **Navajo** *Analgesic* Plant used for pain. *Gynecological Aid* Plant used

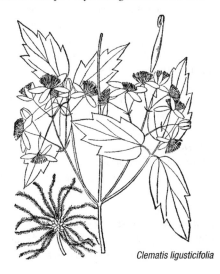
Clematis ligusticifolia

as tonic after deliverance. *Tonic* Plant used as tonic after deliverance. (45:47) **Navajo, Kayenta** *Dermatological Aid* Plant used for spider or sand cricket bites. (179:22) **Navajo, Ramah** *Analgesic* Cold infusion of plant used as lotion for backache. *Orthopedic Aid* Cold infusion of plant used as lotion for backache or swollen legs or arms. *Witchcraft Medicine* Cold infusion of plant or root taken and used as a lotion to protect against witches. (165:27) **Nevada Indian** *Dermatological Aid* Dried, powdered root used for shampoo. (98:57) **Nez Perce** *Veterinary Aid* Plant used as a horse medicine. (82:35) **Okanagan-Colville** *Contraceptive* Stalk and roots used to make a women's contraceptive. *Dermatological Aid* Decoction of mashed leaves and branches rubbed into the scalp as a shampoo to kill hair root "germs." (162:117) **Okanagon** *Tonic* Decoction of plants taken as a tonic for general or out-of-sorts feeling. (104:40) **Oregon Indian** *Dermatological Aid* Leaves and bark used as shampoo. (98:57) *Febrifuge* Infusion of white portion of bark used for fever. (98:40) **Paiute** *Kidney Aid* Decoction of leaves used as a wash or tub bath for dropsical conditions. (155:59, 60) **Sanpoil** *Dermatological Aid* Lather of leaves and water applied to sores or boils. *Veterinary Aid* Lather of leaves and water applied to animals for sores or boils. (as *C. lingusticifolia* 109:220) **Shoshoni** *Analgesic* Branches used to whip sore or painful areas as a counterirritant. Crushed dried leaves used as snuff or fresh leaves smelled for headaches. Decoction of roots taken for stomachaches or cramps. Poultice of mashed leaves applied for rheumatic pains. *Antirheumatic (External)* Poultice of mashed leaves applied for rheumatic pains. *Burn Dressing* Poultice of mashed, moistened seeds applied to severe burns. *Dermatological Aid* Simple or compound poultice of leaf for used swellings, bruises, wounds, or boils. *Gastrointestinal Aid* Decoction of leaves or roots taken for stomachaches or cramps. *Kidney Aid* Decoction of leaves used as a wash or tub bath for dropsical conditions. *Orthopedic Aid* Decoction of leaves used as a bath for tired feet. *Venereal Aid* Powdered leaves or decoction applied as a healing agent for syphilitic sores. (155:59, 60) **Thompson** *Dermatological Aid* Plant used as a head wash and for scabs and eczema. (141:459) Sap used for boils. *Other* Decoction of plant used to bathe babies if they seemed to take after animals or deceased people. *Pediatric Aid* Decoction of plant given to children who habitually wet their beds. Decoction of plant used to bathe babies if they seemed to take after animals or deceased people. (161:247) *Tonic* Decoction of plants taken as a tonic for general or out-of-sorts feeling. (104:40) Mild decoction of plant taken as a tonic or "remedy for general disorder." (141:459) *Toothache Remedy* Poultice of cut stem pieces applied to the tooth for toothache. *Urinary Aid* Decoction of plant given to children who habitually wet their beds. (161:247) **Yavapai** *Gastrointestinal Aid* Decoction of pulverized root taken for stomachaches. (53:261)

Clematis occidentalis var. *occidentalis*,
   Western Blue Virginsbower
Blackfoot *Veterinary Aid* Infusion of plant given to horses as a diuretic. (as *C. verticellaris* 72:88)

Clematis viorna, Vasevine
Meskwaki *Panacea* Root used to make a drink taken for "any kind of common sickness." (129:239)

Clematis virginiana, Devil's Darning Needles
Cherokee *Analgesic* Infusion with milkweed used for backache. *Ceremonial Medicine* Used as an ingredient in green corn medicine. *Gastrointestinal Aid* Infusion of root taken for stomach trouble and infusion taken for nerves. *Kidney Aid* Infusion of root taken for kidneys. *Orthopedic Aid* Infusion with milkweed used for backache. (66:60) **Iroquois** *Dermatological Aid* Root powder and infusion of roots used on venereal disease sores. *Hallucinogen* Decoction of stems used as a wash to induce strange dreams. *Kidney Aid* Taken for burning kidney troubles. *Urinary Aid* Taken for burning kidney troubles. *Venereal Aid* Root powder and infusion of roots used on venereal disease sores. (73:330)

Cleome lutea, Yellow Spiderflower
Navajo, Kayenta *Ceremonial Medicine* Plant used with ceremonial tobacco in some chants. *Dermatological Aid* Plant used for ant bites. (179:25)

Cleome serrulata, Rocky Mountain Beeplant
Gosiute *Eye Medicine* Poultice of pounded, soaked leaves applied to sore eyes. (as *C. integrifolia* 31:366) **Navajo, Ramah** *Blood Medicine* Decoction of seeds used ceremonially to give "good blood." *Ceremonial Medicine* Decoction of seeds used ceremonially to improve voice and give "good blood." *Dermatological Aid* Cold infusion of leaves used as a body and shoe deodorant. *Throat Aid* Decoction of seeds used ceremonially to improve voice. (165:29) **Oregon Indian** *Febrifuge* Infusion of whole plant taken for fever. (98:40) **Tewa** *Gastrointestinal Aid* Infusion of plant taken for stomach disorders and poultice of plant used on abdomen. (as *Peritoma serrulatum* 115:58, 59)

Clermontia arborescens, 'Oha Wai Nui
Hawaiian *Breast Treatment* Milk and other plants mixed, poured into a sweet potato, and eaten for restoring or producing milk. *Dermatological Aid* Milk, breadfruit milk, and a finely ground plant mixed and put into bad and deep cuts. *Respiratory Aid* Fruits with other plants pounded, squeezed, and the resulting liquid taken for asthma. (2:30)

Clethra acuminata, Mountain Sweetpepperbush
Cherokee *Antiemetic* Decoction of bark scrapings taken for vomiting bile. (152:47) *Emetic* Inner bark used to make a drink taken to induce vomiting of "disordered bile." (66:22) Decoction of inner bark taken to cause vomiting when unable to retain food. (152:47) *Febrifuge* Decoction of bark and "wild cherry" bark taken to break high fever. *Gastrointestinal Aid* Hot infusion of bark taken for "bowel complaint." (66:22) Decoction of inner bark taken to cause vomiting when unable to retain food. *Liver Aid* Decoction of bark scrapings taken for vomiting bile. (152:47)

Clintonia andrewsiana, Western Bluebeadlily
Pomo *Poison* Plant considered poisonous. (54:12)
Pomo, Kashaya *Poison* Plant considered poisonous. (60:34)

Clintonia borealis, Yellow Bluebeadlily
Algonquin, Quebec *Dermatological Aid* Poultice of leaves applied to open wounds. *Disinfectant*

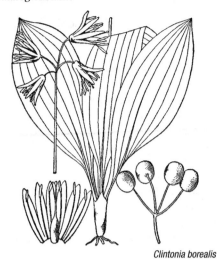

Clintonia borealis

Poultice of leaves applied to infections. (14:138) **Algonquin, Tête-de-Boule** *Dermatological Aid* Poultice of leaves applied to wounds and ulcers. (110:126) **Chippewa** *Burn Dressing* Poultice of fresh leaf applied to burns. *Dermatological Aid* Decoction of leaves applied externally to scrofulous sores. (43:354) **Iroquois** *Heart Medicine* Decoction of plant taken for the heart. *Misc. Disease Remedy* Compound decoction of smashed whole plants taken for sugar diabetes. (73:283) **Menominee** *Antidote* Plant put on bite of dog which has eaten plant, to draw out the poison. (128:40, 41) **Ojibwa** *Antidote* Root applied to draw poison from bite made by dog which has eaten the plant. (130:373) *Dermatological Aid* Poultice of roots used on wound caused by dog's northern clintonia-poisoned teeth. (130:430) *Gynecological Aid* Infusion of root used to aid parturition. (130:373) *Poison* Roots chewed by dogs to poison their teeth and kill animals they bite. (130:430) **Potawatomi** *Unspecified* Plant used as a medicine for unspecified ailments. (131:62)

Clintonia umbellulata, White Bluebeadlily
Iroquois *Basket Medicine* Decoction of whole plant "makes people buy baskets," a basket medicine. *Febrifuge* Infusion of whole plant taken for chills. (73:283)

Clintonia uniflora, Bride's Bonnet
Bella Coola *Dermatological Aid* Decoction of plant used as a wash for the body. Poultice of

toasted leaf applied to wounds. *Eye Medicine* Poultice of toasted leaf applied to eyes. (127:53) **Cowlitz** *Dermatological Aid* Juice from smashed plants used as a wash for cuts. *Eye Medicine* Juice from smashed plants used as a wash for sore eyes. (65:25) **Haisla & Hanaksiala** *Dermatological Aid* Poultice of plant applied to wounds and decoction of plant used to wash the body. *Eye Medicine* Poultice of plant applied to the eyes. (35:194) **Micmac** *Urinary Aid* Root juice taken with water for gravel. (as *Smilacrina borealis* 133:317)

Clitoria mariana, Atlantic Pigeonwings
Cherokee *Oral Aid* Infusion held in mouth for 10 to 20 minutes for thrush. (66:47)

Cneoridium dumosum, Bush Rue
Luiseño *Unspecified* Plant used for medicinal purposes. (132:231)

Cocculus carolinus, Carolina Coralbead
Houma *Blood Medicine* Root used to make a drink taken as a blood clarifier. (135:63)

Cocos nucifera, Coconut Palm
Hawaiian *Abortifacient* Fruit shells burned and the smoke used for swollen wombs. *Dermatological Aid* Young shoots used for deep cuts. *Other* Young meat applied as a rub for the brain. *Strengthener* Dried meat ash used for general debility of the body. *Unspecified* Oil used as a good rub. (2:73)

Coeloglossum viride* var. *virescens, Longbract Frog Orchid
Iroquois *Gynecological Aid* Compound decoction with plant taken to bring away placenta after childbirth. (as *Habenaria viridis* ssp. *bracteata* 73: 289) **Ojibwa** *Love Medicine* Root smuggled into another's food as an aphrodisiac. (as *Habenaria bracteata* 130:377) Plant used as a sort of love charm and often put to bad use. (as *Habenaria bracteata* 130:431)

Coix lacryma-jobi, Job's Tears
Cherokee *Pediatric Aid* Seeds strung around baby's neck for teething. *Toothache Remedy* Seeds strung around baby's neck for teething. *Unspeci-*

fied Long strands of seeds used for various unspecified medicinal purposes. (66:41)

Coleogyne ramosissima, Blackbrush
Kawaiisu *Venereal Aid* Decoction of bark taken
for gonorrhea. (180:21)

Collinsia parviflora, Smallflower Blue Eyed
  Mary
Navajo, Kayenta *Veterinary Aid* Plant used to
make a horse run fast. (179:42) **Ute** *Dermatological Aid* Plant used externally for sore flesh.
(30:33)

Collinsia violacea, Violet Blue Eyed Mary
Creek *Tuberculosis Remedy* Infusion of root
taken for colds, coughs, consumption, and whooping cough. **Natchez** *Cold Remedy* Infusion of root
taken for colds. *Cough Medicine* Infusion of root
taken for coughs. (148:667) Infusion of roots taken
for coughs. (152:56) *Pulmonary Aid* Infusion of
root taken for consumption and whooping cough.
(148:667) *Tuberculosis Remedy* Infusion of roots
taken for consumption. (152:56)

Collinsonia canadensis, Rich Weed
Cherokee *Breast Treatment* Compound used for
swollen breasts. (66:52) Decoction of plant applied
for swollen breasts. (152:53) *Dermatological Aid*
Mashed flowers and leaves used as a deodorant.
(66:52) *Emetic* Decoction of plant taken to cause
vomiting. (152:53) *Veterinary Aid* Infusion used as
a drench for horses with colic. (66:52) **Iroquois**
Analgesic Poultice of powdered leaves applied to
the forehead for headaches. *Antidiarrheal* Compound decoction of roots taken for diarrhea with
blood. *Antirheumatic* (*External*) Decoction of
roots taken and used as foot, back, and leg soak
for rheumatism. *Antirheumatic* (*Internal*) Compound decoction of roots taken and used as foot
soak for rheumatism. *Blood Medicine* Roots used
as a blood medicine. *Dermatological Aid* Roots
used for boils. *Heart Medicine* Decoction of roots
taken for heart trouble. *Kidney Aid* Decoction of
roots taken for kidney trouble. *Panacea* Decoction
of roots taken for any ailment. *Pediatric Aid* Infusion of smashed roots given to strengthen listless
children. *Stimulant* Infusion of smashed roots giv-
en to children for listlessness. (73:429) *Strength-*

ener Infusion of smashed roots used as a wash for
babies to give them strength. (73:428)

Collomia grandiflora, Largeflower Mountain-
  trumpet
Okanagan-Colville *Febrifuge* Infusion of roots
taken for high fevers. *Laxative* Infusion of leaves
and stalks taken for constipation and to "clean out
your system." Infusion of roots taken as a laxative.
(162:111)

Collomia linearis, Narrowleaf Mountain-
  trumpet
Gosiute *Dermatological Aid* Poultice of mashed
plant applied to wounds and bruises. (as *Gilia
linearis* 31:370)

Colocasia esculenta, Coco Yam
Hawaiian *Laxative* Flesh and other plants
pounded, squeezed, and resulting liquid taken as
a laxative. (as *Coloccasia antiquorum* 2:47) *Unspecified* Plant used to make a draft and given to
the sick. (as *Arum esculentum* 94:67)

Comandra umbellata, Bastard Toadflax
Cherokee *Dermatological Aid* Juice applied to
cut or sore. *Kidney Aid* Compound infusion used
for kidneys. (66:24) **Meskwaki** *Analgesic* Infusion of leaf taken for lung pains. *Cold Remedy*
Medicine licked to ease labored breathing caused
by a cold or other illness. *Pulmonary Aid* Infusion
of leaf taken for lung pains. *Respiratory Aid* Medicine of immature florets licked to ease labored
breathing from cold, etc. (129:246)

Comandra umbellata ssp. pallida, Pale
  Bastard Toadflax
Navajo *Dermatological Aid* Decoction of plant
used as a foot bath for corns. (as *C. pallida* 76:
150) **Navajo, Kayenta** *Eye Medicine* Plant used
for sore eyes. *Narcotic* Plant used as a narcotic.
Oral Aid Plant used as a mouthwash for canker
sores. (as *Commandra pallida* 179:18) **Thompson** *Dermatological Aid* Decoction of plant used
as a wash for sores. (161:281) *Eye Medicine* Fresh
roots mixed with woman's milk and used as a
wash for sore or inflamed eyes. (as *Comandra
pallida* 141:459) **Ute** *Analgesic* Roots used for
headaches. (as *Commandra pallida* 30:33)

Comarum palustre, Purple Marshlocks
Chippewa *Antidiarrheal* Decoction of root taken for dysentery. (as *Potentilla palustris* 43:344) **Ojibwa** *Analgesic* Plant used alone for stomach cramps. *Gastrointestinal Aid* Plant used for stomach cramps. (as *Potentilla palustris* 130:384, 385)

Commelina dianthifolia, Birdbill Dayflower
Keres, Western *Tuberculosis Remedy* Infusion of plant used as a strengthener for weakened tuberculosis patients. (147:38) **Navajo, Ramah** *Veterinary Aid* Cold simple or compound infusion given to livestock as an aphrodisiac. (165:19)

Commelina erecta* var. *angustifolia,
Whitemouth Dayflower
Seminole *Other* Mucilaginous sap used to soothe irritations. (as *C. angustifolia* 145:303)

Comptonia peregrina, Sweet Fern
Algonquin, Quebec *Analgesic* Infusion of leaves taken or crushed leaf perfume inhaled for headaches. (14:149) **Cherokee** *Anthelmintic* Infusion taken for roundworms. (66:58) **Chippewa** *Ceremonial Medicine* Burned, dried leaves used as incense in religious ceremonies. *Febrifuge* Infusion of leaves taken for fevers. *Unspecified* Leaves used for medicine. (as *Myrica asplenifolia* 59:127) **Delaware** *Blood Medicine* Infusion of plant, mallow root, elder flowers, and dwarf elder used as a blood purifier. *Dermatological Aid* Infusion of plant used for blisters. *Pulmonary Aid* Infusion of

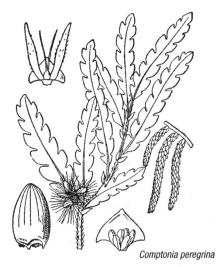

Comptonia peregrina

plant, mallow root, elder flowers, and dwarf elder used to remove mucus from the lungs. *Urinary Aid* Infusion of plant, mallow root, elder flowers, and dwarf elder used for bladder inflammation. *Venereal Aid* Infusion of plant, mallow root, elder flowers, and dwarf elder used for scrofula. (as *Myrica asplenifolia* 151:35) **Delaware, Oklahoma** *Blood Medicine* Infusion of plant taken as a blood purifier. *Dermatological Aid* Infusion of plant applied to blisters and leaves used for poison ivy rash. *Expectorant* Infusion of plant taken to help remove mucus from the lungs. *Tuberculosis Remedy* Plant used for scrofula. *Urinary Aid* Complex compound containing plant used for bladder inflammation. (as *Myrica asplenifolia* 150:29, 76) **Malecite** *Dermatological Aid* Infusion of plant and yarrow used as a liniment for swelling. (as *Myrica asplenifolia* 96:245) *Respiratory Aid* Plants smoked and used for catarrh. (as *Myrica asplenifolia* 96:248) **Menominee** *Adjuvant* Plant used as a seasoner and potent medicine in childbirth. *Gynecological Aid* Decoction of plants used as a potent medicine in childbirth. *Poison* Compound containing leaves sprinkled on medicine to kill a hated person. (as *Myrica asplenifolia* 128:42) *Tonic* Compound decoction of root taken as a mild tonic. (44:133) **Micmac** *Analgesic* Root used for headache and inflammation. *Dermatological Aid* Leaves used for sprains, swellings, poison ivy, and inflammation. (32:56) Leaves used for swellings and poison ivy. (as *Myrica asplenifolia* 32:58) *Orthopedic Aid* Leaves used for sprains. (32:56) Leaves used for sprains, swellings, and poison ivy. (as *Myrica asplenifolia* 32:58) *Respiratory Aid* Leaves used for catarrh. (32:56) Leaves used for catarrh and poison ivy. (as *Myrica asplenifolia* 32:58) *Stimulant* Berries, bark, and leaves used as an "exhilarant" and beverage. (32:56) **Mohegan** *Dermatological Aid* Infusion of leaves used as a wash for poison ivy. (as *Myrica asplenifolia* 149:264) Infusion of leaves used as poison ivy lotion. (as *Myrica asplenifolia* 151:74, 130) **Ojibwa** *Analgesic* Infusion of leaves taken for flux and stomach cramps. *Antidiarrheal* Infusion of leaves taken for stomach cramps and flux. *Gastrointestinal Aid* Decoction of leaves taken for stomach cramps and flux. (as *Myrica asplenifolia* 130:375) **Penobscot** *Dermatological Aid* Infusion of leaves rubbed on skin for poison ivy. (as *Myrica aspleni-*

folia 133:309) **Potawatomi** *Dermatological Aid* Infusion of leaves used for itch. (as *Myrica aspleni-folia* 131:65) **Shinnecock** *Dermatological Aid* Infusion of leaves rubbed on the skin for itch. (25:119)

Conioselinum chinense, Chinese Hemlock-parsley
Micmac *Urinary Aid* Infusion of roots, hemlock, prince's pine, and curled dock used for colds in the bladder. (96:259)

Conioselinum gmelinii, Pacific Hemlock-parsley
Aleut *Cold Remedy* Leaves used to make a tonic for colds. *Throat Aid* Leaves used to make a soothing drink for sore throats. (6:427) **Kwakiutl** *Antirheumatic* (*External*) and *Herbal Steam* Plant used in sweat baths for arthritis and rheumatism. (as *C. pacificum* 157:266) Plant used in steam bath for general weakness. *Stimulant* Plant used in steam bath for general weakness. (as *C. pacificum* 157:276)

Conioselinum scopulorum, Rocky Mountain Hemlockparsley
Navajo, Kayenta *Blood Medicine* Plant used as a postpartum blood purifier. *Gynecological Aid* Plant used as a postpartum blood purifier. *Respiratory Aid* Plant smoked for catarrh. *Snakebite Remedy* Infusion of plant used as a snake repellent. (179:34)

Conium maculatum, Poison Hemlock
Klallam *Love Medicine* Roots rubbed on woman's body to attract the attention of a man. *Poison* Roots considered poisonous. (65:42) **Lakota** *Poison* All plant parts very poisonous. (116:33) **Snohomish** *Poison* Roots considered poisonous. (65:42)

Conocephalum conicum, Cone Headed Liverwort
Haisla & Hanaksiala *Burn Dressing* Plant pulverized, mixed with mountain goat fat, and used for sunburns. (as *C. conicum* 35:145) **Nitinaht** *Eye Medicine* Plant used as an eye medicine and for cataracts. *Kidney Aid* Plant formerly used for kidney troubles. *Psychological Aid* Plant eaten to

stop recurring dreams of having sex with the deceased. (as *C. conicum* 160:58)

Conopholis alpina var. **mexicana**, Mexican Squawroot
Keres, Western *Tuberculosis Remedy* Infusion of plant used as a strengthener for weakened tuberculosis patients. (as *C. mexicana* 147:38)

Consolida ajacis, Doubtful Knight's Spur
Cherokee *Heart Medicine* Infusion taken "for heart." *Poison* Root "makes cows drunk and kills them." (as *Delphinium ajacis* 66:42)

Convolvulus arvensis, Field Bindweed
Navajo, Ramah *Dermatological Aid* Cold infusion of plant taken and used as a lotion for spider bites. *Gastrointestinal Aid* Cold infusion taken with food after swallowing a spider. (165:39) **Pomo** *Gynecological Aid* Decoction of plant taken for excessive menstruation. (54:15) **Pomo, Kashaya** *Gynecological Aid* Decoction of stem with leaves taken for excessive menstruation. (60:73)

Conyza canadensis, Canadian Horseweed
Cahuilla *Antidiarrheal* Infusion of leaves used for diarrhea. (11:56)

Conyza canadensis var. **canadensis**, Canadian Horseweed
Blackfoot *Antidiarrheal* Plant used for chronic diarrhea. *Antihemorrhagic* Plant used for childbirth hemorrhage. (as *Erigeron canadensis* 82:56) **Chippewa** *Analgesic* Decoction of root and leaves taken for stomach pain. *Gastrointestinal Aid* Decoction of root and leaves taken for stomach pain. (as *Erigeron canadensis* 43:342) *Gynecological Aid* Infusion of whole plant taken for "female weakness." (as *Erigeron canadensis* 43:356) **Cree, Hudson Bay** *Antidiarrheal* Plant used as a diarrhea medicine. (as *Erigeron canadensis* 78:303) **Hawaiian** *Antirheumatic* (*External*) Leaves and other plant parts pounded and resulting liquid applied to sore joints. *Orthopedic Aid* Leaves and other plant parts pounded and resulting liquid applied to sprains and backaches. Leaves, shoots, and other plants pounded and resulting liquid used for injuries caused by accidents. (as *Erigen canadense* 2:25) **Hopi** *Analgesic* Poul-

tice of rubbed plant applied to temples for head-ache. (as *Erigeron canadensis* 174:33, 96) **Houma** *Gynecological Aid* Hot infusion of root taken for leukorrhea. (as *Erigeron canadense* 135:64) **Iroquois** *Anticonvulsive, Febrifuge,* and *Pediatric Aid* Infusion of whole plant and roots from another plant used for children with convulsions and fevers. (as *Erigeron canadensis* 118:65) **Keres, Western** *Burn Dressing* Crushed plant rubbed on sunburns. *Dermatological Aid* Plant beaten into a paste and rubbed on the skin for blotches or liver spots. (as *Leptilon canadense* 147:51) **Meskwaki** *Diaphoretic* Used as a steaming agent in sweat bath. (as *Erigeron canadensis* 129:213) **Navajo, Kayenta** *Dermatological Aid* Plant used as a lotion for pimples. *Disinfectant* Hot poultice of plant applied to infants with prenatal infection. *Ear Medicine* Hot poultice of plant applied for earaches. *Gastrointestinal Aid* Plant used for stomachaches. *Pediatric Aid* Hot poultice of plant applied to infants with prenatal infection. (as *Erigeron canadensis* 179:47) **Navajo, Ramah** *Dermatological Aid* Poultice of crushed leaves or cold infusion of leaves used as a lotion for pimples. *Snakebite Remedy* Cold infusion taken or used as lotion for snakebite. (as *Erigeron canadensis* 165:50) **Ojibwa** *Hunting Medicine* Disk florets smoked as one of the hunting charms. (as *Erigeron canadensis* 130:429) **Potawatomi** *Veterinary Aid* Plant used as a medicine for horses. (as *Erigeron canadensis* 131:51, 52) **Seminole** *Cold Remedy* Infusion of leaves and bark taken and steam inhaled for runny nose, stuffy head, and sore throat. *Cough Medicine* Infusion of leaves and bark taken and steam inhaled for coughs. (as *Leptilon canadense* 145:279) *Love Medicine* Plant rubbed on the body by a doctor to rid himself of his wife. (as *Leptilon canadense* 145:401) *Respiratory Aid* Infusion of leaves and bark taken and steam inhaled for asthma. (as *Leptilon canadense* 145:279) **Zuni** *Respiratory Aid* Crushed flowers inserted in nostrils to cause sneezing, relieving "rhinitis." (as *Leptilon canadense* 143:55)

***Coprosma* sp.**, Maile-kaluhea
Hawaiian *Dermatological Aid* Infusion of pounded vines, roots, and other plants strained and used as a wash for skin ulcers, and for skin diseases. *Tuberculosis Remedy* Infusion of pounded vines, roots, and other plants strained and used as a wash for scrofulous sores. (2:69) *Unspecified* Whole plant dried, stored, and used under the direction of a medicine man. (2:72)

Coptis macrosepala, Goldthread
Tlingit *Pulmonary Aid* Compound infusion of plant used for lung inflammations. (89:283)

Coptis trifolia, Threeleaf Goldthread
Iroquois *Anthelmintic* Compound decoction or infusion of roots taken for stomach cramps and worms. *Antiemetic* Infusion or decoction of roots taken, especially for babies, for vomiting. *Blood Medicine* Complex compound decoction taken as a blood purifier and blood remedy. *Emetic* Decoction of roots taken to vomit for jaundice, for the eyeballs, and dizziness. *Eye Medicine* Infusion or decoction of roots taken or used as drops for sore eyes. *Gastrointestinal Aid* Compound decoction of roots taken for stomach cramps and worms. Infusion of roots taken for vomiting, biliousness, and jaundice. *Oral Aid* Infusion of roots used for sore mouths of children and trench mouth. *Pediatric Aid* Decoction of roots given to "little babies when they throw up often." Infusion of roots used as a wash or poultice applied to sore mouths of children. (73:322) Decoction of plant given to babies with sickness caused by bad blood from mother. (73:323) *Throat Aid* Cold, compound infusion with plant taken for trench mouth and raw throat. (73:322) *Unspecified* Decoction of plant given to

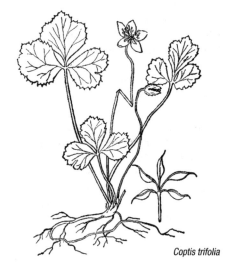

Coptis trifolia

babies with sickness caused by bad blood from mother. (73:323) *Venereal Aid* Complex compound decoction taken as a blood purifier and for venereal disease. (73:322) **Malecite** *Oral Aid* and *Pediatric Aid* Infusion of plant used for children with sore mouths. (96:245) **Menominee** *Oral Aid* Astringent root used as a wash for oral cankers and babies' teething pains. *Pediatric Aid* Root yielded astringent mouthwash for sore throat and teething babies. *Throat Aid* Roots used in astringent mouthwash for babies with sore throats. *Toothache Remedy* Roots used in astringent mouthwash for teething babies. (128:48) **Micmac** *Oral Aid* Herb used for sore and diseased mouth. (32:56) **Mohegan** *Oral Aid* Infusion of plant used as a mouthwash for babies. (149:265) Infusion of leaves used as a mouthwash for infants. (151:72, 128) *Pediatric Aid* Infusion of plant used as a mouthwash for babies. (149:265) Infusion of leaves used as a mouthwash for infants. (151:72, 128) **Ojibwa** *Oral Aid* Decoction of root used as a wash for sore mouth and to soothe mouth of teething baby. *Pediatric Aid* Decoction of root used to soothe mouth of teething baby. (130:383) **Penobscot** *Oral Aid* Stems chewed for mouth sores and mouths irritated by tobacco smoking. (133:309) **Potawatomi** *Analgesic* Root used for babies with teething pains. *Oral Aid* Roots used for sore gums and especially for pain of teething babies. *Pediatric Aid* Roots used especially for pain of teething babies. (131:74)

Coptis trifolia ssp. **groenlandica**, Threeleaf Goldthread

Abnaki *Cold Remedy* Decoction of plant and another plant used for colds. (as *C. groenlandica* 121:167) *Cough Medicine* Used for coughs. (as *C. groenlandica* 121:154) **Algonquin, Quebec** *Antidiarrheal* Infusion of rhizomes taken for diarrhea. *Eye Medicine* Infusion of rhizomes used as an eyewash. *Heart Medicine* Infusion of rhizomes taken for heart disease. *Toothache Remedy* Infusion of rhizomes taken for toothaches. (as *C. groenlandica* 14:167) **Algonquin, Tête-de-Boule** *Cold Remedy* Boiled roots used for serious colds. *Respiratory Aid* Boiled roots used for respiratory troubles. (as *C. groenlandica* 110:126) **Iroquois** *Ear Medicine* Infusion of plant, with another plant, used as ear drops for earaches. *Gastrointestinal Aid* Infusion of roots taken to ease digestion. (as

C. groenlandica 118:42) *Oral Aid* Roots chewed for mouth pains. (as *C. groenlandica* 119:87) **Malecite** *Unspecified* Used for medicines. (as *C. groenlandica* 137:6) **Micmac** *Unspecified* Roots chewed for medicinal use. (as *C. groenlandica* 136:258)

Corallorrhiza maculata, Summer Coralroot

Navajo, Kayenta *Dermatological Aid* Infusion of plant used as a lotion for ringworm or skin disease. (179:17) **Nevada Indian** *Cold Remedy* Infusion of dried, whole plant bits taken for colds. (98:37) **Paiute** *Blood Medicine* Decoction of stalks used to "build up the blood" of pneumonia patients. *Pulmonary Aid* Infusion of dried stalks taken to "build up the blood" of pneumonia patients. **Shoshoni** *Blood Medicine* Decoction of stalks used to "build up the blood" of pneumonia patients. *Pulmonary Aid* Infusion of dried stalks taken to "build up the blood" of pneumonia patients. (155:60)

Corallorrhiza maculata ssp. **maculata**, Summer Coralroot

Iroquois *Basket Medicine* Infusion of pounded root used as a basket medicine. (73:290) *Hunting Medicine* Root placed in a half cup of water and used to wash guns and clothes as a hunting medicine. *Love Medicine* Infusion of pounded roots used as a love medicine. *Tuberculosis Remedy* Compound infusion of roots taken for tuberculosis. (73:291) *Veterinary Aid* Infusion of whole plant added to horse's grain for heaves. *Witchcraft Medicine* Infusion of pounded roots used as an anti-witch medicine. (73:290)

Cordylanthus ramosus, Bushy Bird's Beak

Navajo *Emetic* Infusion of plant taken to induce vomiting. *Gynecological Aid* Infusion of plant taken by menstruating women to stop menses. *Hemostat* Infusion of plant used by men for nosebleeds. (45:76) *Orthopedic Aid* Plant used to prevent broken ribs. (45:96) *Venereal Aid* Infusion of plant taken for syphilis. (45:76) **Shoshoni** *Venereal Aid* Decoction of plant taken for venereal disease, or "bad disease." (155:60)

Cordylanthus wrightii, Wright's Bird's Beak

Navajo *Venereal Aid* Decoction of plant used for

syphilis. (45:76) **Navajo, Kayenta** *Ceremonial Medicine* Plant used for ceremonial purposes. *Gynecological Aid* Plant used for prolapse of the uterus. (179:42) **Navajo, Ramah** *Analgesic* Decoction of plant taken for menstrual pain and by men for leg or body aches. *Gynecological Aid* Decoction of plant taken for menstrual pain. (165:44)

Cordyline fruticosa, Tiplant
Hawaiian *Febrifuge* Leaves applied to the head, chest, and abdomen for dry fevers. *Nose Medicine* Flowers and other plants pounded and resulting liquid fumes inhaled for nose growths. *Pulmonary Aid* Leaves, shoots, and other plants mixed with water and taken for chest congestion from tough phlegm. *Respiratory Aid* Flowers and other plants pounded, resulting liquid mixed with potato or poi and eaten for asthma. *Sedative* Leaves made into a wreath and worn to provide a restful condition of the nerves and body. (as *C. terminalis* 2:49)

Coreopsis leavenworthii, Leavenworth's Tickseed
Seminole *Other* Infusion of plant used for heat prostration. (145:303)

Coreopsis palmata, Stiff Tickseed
Meskwaki *Orthopedic Aid* Decoction of seeds used internally and as a poultice for one who is crippled. (129:213)

Coreopsis tinctoria, Golden Tickseed
Cherokee *Antidiarrheal* Infusion of root taken for flux. (66:59)

Coreopsis tinctoria var. *tinctoria*, Golden Tickseed
Navajo, Ramah *Ceremonial Medicine* Plant used in ceremonial chant lotion. *Disinfectant* Cold infusion of dried plant taken with salt for "lightning infection." *Panacea* Root used as a "life medicine." *Venereal Aid* Plant used as fumigant for sexual infection. (as *C. cardaminefolia* 165:50) **Zuni** *Reproductive Aid* Infusion of whole plant, except for the root, taken by women desiring female babies. (as *C. cardaminefolia* 143:84)

Coreopsis tripteris, Tall Tickseed
Meskwaki *Analgesic* Decoction of stems taken for internal pains. *Antihemorrhagic* Decoction of stems taken for internal bleeding. (129:213)

Corethrogyne filaginifolia, Common Sandaster
Kawaiisu *Cold Remedy, Diaphoretic,* and *Herbal Steam* Infusion of twigs and leaves used as steam bath to induce sweating for colds. (180:22)

Cornus alternifolia, Alternateleaf Dogwood
Cherokee *Analgesic* Bark chewed for headache. *Anthelmintic* Compound infusion of bark and root used for childhood diseases like worms and measles. *Antidiarrheal* Compound infusion taken for diarrhea. *Antidote* Infusion of beaten bark used for bathing after "poisons of any kind." *Blood Medicine* Infusion taken "for blood." *Dermatological Aid* Root bark astringent and compound infusion taken for diarrhea. Root bark used for unspecified poultices and poultice of bark ooze applied to ulcers. *Diaphoretic* Infusion of flower taken "to sweat off flu." *Disinfectant* Root bark used as an antiseptic and astringent. *Febrifuge* Root bark used as a febrifuge. *Gastrointestinal Aid* Infusion of flower taken for colic. *Gynecological Aid* Infusion of bark used by women for backache. *Misc. Disease Remedy* Compound infusion of bark and root used for childhood diseases like worms and measles. Infusion of flower taken "to sweat off flu." *Pediatric Aid* Compound infusion of bark and root

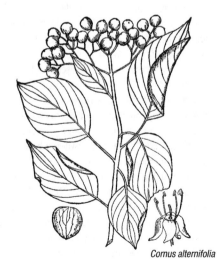

Cornus alternifolia

used for childhood diseases like worms and measles. *Stimulant* Root bark used as a stimulant. *Throat Aid* Infusion of inner bark taken for "lost voice." *Tonic* Root bark used as a tonic. (66:32) **Chippewa** *Cough Medicine* Inner bark used as a cough remedy. (59:138) *Eye Medicine* Compound decoction of root used as a wash or compress for sore eyes. Infusion of scraped root used as a wash or on a compress for sore eyes. (43:360) *Hunting Medicine* Roots used as a charm on muskrat traps. (43:376) **Iroquois** *Cold Remedy* Compound decoction of bark taken for colds. *Cough Medicine* Compound decoction of bark taken for coughing. (73:407) *Dermatological Aid* Poultice of powdered bark applied to heal the navel and blisters. (73:406) Infusion of bark applied as poultice to swollen areas. *Emetic* Compound decoction of bark taken as an emetic, especially for coughs. (73:407) *Eye Medicine* Plant used in a wash for eyes. *Gynecological Aid* Compound decoction of bark taken by pregnant women who have had gonorrhea. *Pediatric Aid* Poultice of powdered bark applied to heal navel. *Respiratory Aid* Decoction of bark taken to vomit for coughs or bronchial coughs. (73:406) *Tuberculosis Remedy* Compound decoction of bark taken for tuberculosis. (73:407) *Venereal Aid* Compound infusion used as wash on parts affected by venereal disease. (73:406) **Menominee** *Antidiarrheal* Bark liquid injected rectally and poultice of bark applied to anus for diarrhea. *Cancer Treatment* One reported case: poultice of bark plus something else cured facial cancer. *Hemorrhoid Remedy* Bark used to make a liquid and injected rectally for piles. (128:32, 33) **Ojibwa** *Emetic* Inner bark used as an emetic. (130:366) **Potawatomi** *Eye Medicine* Infusion of bark used as a wash for granulation of the eyelids. (131:54)

Cornus amomum, Silky Dogwood
Iroquois *Analgesic* Compound decoction of roots taken for urinating pain. *Dermatological Aid* Infusion of bark used as wash or powdered bark applied to gonorrhea sores. (73:402) Complex compound decoction used as wash for affected parts of "Italian itch." *Emetic* Decoction of bark taken as an emetic. (73:403) *Laxative* Compound decoction of roots taken as a laxative. *Pediatric Aid* Infusion of bark used as wash to make babies sleep. (73:402) *Poultice* Poultice of smashed bark ap-

plied for goiter. *Pulmonary Aid* Infusion of bark taken for chest congestion. (73:403) *Sedative* Infusion of bark used as wash to make babies sleep. *Urinary Aid* Compound decoction of roots taken for urinating pain. *Venereal Aid* Infusion of bark used as wash or powdered bark applied to gonorrhea sores. (73:402) **Menominee** *Antidiarrheal* Plant known as maimakwukwa and infusion of bark injected rectally for diarrhea. *Ceremonial Medicine* Plant known as kinnikinnick and bark smoked ceremonially. (128:32)

Cornus amomum ssp. *obliqua*, Silky Dogwood
Iroquois *Gastrointestinal Aid* Infusion of bark taken for dyspepsia. (as *C. obliqua* 118:54)

Cornus canadensis, Bunchberry Dogwood
Abnaki *Analgesic* Used for side pains. (121:155) Decoction of whole plant taken for side pains. (121:170) **Algonquin, Quebec** *Cathartic* Infusion of leaves used as a cathartic tea. (14:211) **Algonquin, Tête-de-Boule** *Cold Remedy* Decoction of plant and other plants used for colds. *Gynecological Aid* Plant mixed with other plants and used by women for stomachaches. (110:128) **Carrier, Northern** *Unspecified* Used as a medicine for unspecified malady. **Carrier, Southern** *Eye Medicine* Strong decoction of plant, without berries, used as an eyewash. (127:62) **Delaware** *Analgesic* Bark used for body pains. (151:31) **Delaware, Oklahoma** *Analgesic* Compound containing bark used for body pain. (150:26, 74) **Hoh** *Tonic* Infusion of bitter bark used as a tonic. (114:66) **Iroquois** *Cold Remedy* Decoction of whole plant taken for coughs. *Febrifuge* Decoction of whole plant taken for fevers. *Tuberculosis Remedy* Decoction of whole plant taken for tuberculosis. (73:402) **Malecite** *Anticonvulsive* Infusion of roots, leaves, and berries used for fits. (96:256) **Micmac** *Anticonvulsive* Berries, roots, and leaves used for fits. (32:56) **Montagnais** *Orthopedic Aid* Infusion of plant used as a medicine for paralysis. (133:315) **Ojibwa** *Gastrointestinal Aid* Infusion of root used for infant colic. *Pediatric Aid* Infusion of root used for infant colic. (130:366, 367) **Paiute** *Eye Medicine* Mashed roots strained through a clean cloth and used as an eyewash for the removal of foreign objects. Mashed roots strained through

a clean cloth and used as an eyewash for eye soreness. (93:98) **Quileute** *Tonic* Infusion of bitter bark used as a tonic. (114:66) **Thompson** *Dermatological Aid* Leaf ash or powdered, toasted leaves sprinkled on sores. (141:458)

Cornus drummondii, Roughleaf Dogwood
Iroquois *Venereal Aid* Infusion of switches taken for gonorrhea. (73:403)

Cornus florida, Flowering Dogwood
Cherokee *Analgesic* Bark chewed for headache. *Anthelmintic* Compound infusion of bark and root used for childhood diseases like worms and measles. (66:32) Infusion of bark used as a bath and given to children with worms. (152:46) *Antidiarrheal* Compound infusion taken for diarrhea. *Antidote* Infusion of beaten bark used for bathing after "poisons of any kind." *Blood Medicine* Compound infusion taken for "for blood." *Dermatological Aid* Root bark astringent and compound infusion taken for diarrhea. Root bark used for unspecified poultices and poultice of bark ooze applied to ulcers. (66:32) Root bark used for wounds. (177:74) *Diaphoretic* Infusion of flower taken "to sweat off flu." *Disinfectant* Root bark used as an antiseptic and astringent. *Febrifuge* Root bark used as a febrifuge. *Gastrointestinal Aid* Infusion of flower taken for colic. *Gynecological Aid* Infusion of bark used by women for backache. *Misc. Disease Remedy* Compound infusion of bark and root used for childhood diseases like worms and measles. Infusion of flower taken "to sweat off flu." *Pediatric Aid* Compound infusion of bark and root used for childhood diseases like worms and measles. (66:32) Infusion of bark used as a bath and given to children with worms. (152:46) *Poultice* Root bark used in poultices. (177:74) *Stimulant* Root bark used as a stimulant. *Throat Aid* Infusion of inner bark taken for "lost voice." (66:32) Decoction of inner bark taken to loosen phlegm for hoarseness. (152:46) *Tonic* Root bark used as a tonic. (66:32) **Delaware** *Tonic* Roots used as a tonic. (151:31) **Delaware, Oklahoma** *Tonic* Compound containing root used as a tonic. (150:26, 74) **Houma** *Febrifuge* Decoction of root or bark scrapings taken for fever. *Misc. Disease Remedy* Decoction of root or bark scrapings taken for malaria. (135:55) **Iroquois** *Blood Medicine* Compound decoction of

stems and roots taken for blood chills. (73:402) **Rappahannock** *Antidiarrheal* Infusion of root bark taken for diarrhea. *Blood Medicine* Decoction of dried bark from roots used to purify the blood. *Tonic* Decoction of dried bark from roots used as a tonic. (138:33)

Cornus foemina, Stiff Dogwood
Cherokee *Throat Aid* Infusion used for "lost voice." (as *C. stricta* 66:30, 31) **Houma** *Febrifuge* Decoction of root or bark scrapings taken for fever. *Misc. Disease Remedy* Decoction of root or bark scrapings taken for malaria. (as *C. stricta* 135:55)

Cornus nuttallii, Pacific Dogwood
Green River Group *Cathartic* Plant used as a physic. *Emetic* Plant used as an emetic. (65:42) **Hoh** *Tonic* Infusion of bitter bark used as a tonic. (114:66) **Karok** *Herbal Steam* Boughs used in the fire of the sweat house. (125:387) **Lummi** *Laxative* Decoction of bark taken as a laxative. (65:42) **Quileute** *Tonic* Infusion of bitter bark used as a tonic. (114:66) **Thompson** *Blood Medicine* Decoction of two bark strips and two cascara bark strips taken as a "blood purifier." (161:204) *Gastrointestinal Aid* Decoction of wood or bark taken for stomach trouble. (141:461) Decoction of two bark strips and two cascara bark strips taken for ulcers. *Psychological Aid* Strained decoction of flower heads used to wash the skin for "seven year itch." *Pulmonary Aid* Decoction of two bark strips and two cascara bark strips taken to improve hunters lungs before hiking. (161:204)

Cornus racemosa, Gray Dogwood
Iroquois *Dermatological Aid* Decoction of bark applied as poultice to cuts. (as *C. paniculata* 73:405) *Gastrointestinal Aid* Compound decoction taken, used as wash, and poultice applied to swollen abdomen. *Orthopedic Aid* Compound poultice of bark applied to swollen legs after the birth of a baby. *Venereal Aid* Compound powder poultice "put in bag, place penis in bag and tie around waist." (as *C. paniculata* 73:406) *Veterinary Aid* Decoction of bark applied as poultice to cuts on horses. (as *C. paniculata* 73:405) **Meskwaki** *Analgesic* Infusion of bark held in mouth for neuralgia. *Antidiarrheal* Infusion of bark used, espe-

cially for children, as an enema for flux. *Oral Aid* Infusion of bark held in mouth for toothache. *Pediatric Aid* Infusion of bark given, often to children, as an enema for flux. *Stimulant* Smudged bark used to revive an unconscious patient. *Tuberculosis Remedy* Infusion of root used for consumption. (as *C. paniculata* 129:218, 219) **Ojibwa** *Antidiarrheal* Infusion of bark used for flux. *Hemorrhoid Remedy* Bark forced into the anus for piles. (as *C. paniculata* 130:367)

Cornus rugosa, Roundleaf Dogwood
Iroquois *Cathartic* Bark taken as a general cathartic or emetic. *Emetic* Decoction of bark taken as an emetic. *Kidney Aid* Compound decoction of roots taken for the kidneys. *Tuberculosis Remedy* Compound infusion of smashed roots taken for tuberculosis. (73:405)

Cornus sericea, Red Osier Dogwood
Cree, Hudson Bay *Cold Remedy* Decoction of bark taken as an emetic for colds. *Cough Medicine* Decoction of bark taken as an emetic for coughs. *Emetic* Decoction of bark taken as an emetic for coughs, colds, and fevers. *Febrifuge* Decoction of bark taken as an emetic for fevers. (78:303) **Ojibwa** *Ceremonial Medicine* Bark smoked for various ceremonies. *Unspecified* Bark used for medicinal purposes. (112:237) **Thompson** *Anthelmintic* Fruit considered a good "tonic," especially for intestinal worms. *Antidiarrheal* Decoction of branches, wild rose, and chokecherry branches taken for diarrhea. *Antiemetic* Decoction of branches, wild rose, and chokecherry branches taken for vomiting. *Cold Remedy* Decoction of branches taken for colds. *Panacea* Plant used as a medicine for anything by the elderly. *Pediatric Aid* Decoction of plant, squaw currant, branches, and fir or tamarack used as a baby bath. *Poison* Sap used on arrowheads for the poisonous effect upon animals. *Strengthener* Decoction of plant, squaw currant branches, and fir or tamarack used as a baby bath. (161:204)

Cornus sericea* ssp. *occidentalis, Western Dogwood
Hoh *Tonic* Infusion of bitter bark used as a tonic. **Quileute** *Tonic* Infusion of bitter bark used as a tonic. (as *C. occidentalis* 114:66) **Snohomish**

Eye Medicine Infusion of bark used for sore eyes. (as *C. pubescens* 65:42) **Thompson** *Gynecological Aid* Compound decoction of twigs taken by women after childbirth. (as *C. pubescens* 141:461) Simple or compound decoction of various plant parts taken after childbirth. (as *C. pubescens* 141:475)

Cornus sericea* ssp. *sericea, Red Osier Dogwood
Abnaki *Eye Medicine* Used for sore eyes. (as *C. stolonifera* 121:155) Decoction of bark and bark from two other plants used for eye pain. (as *C. stolonifera* 121:170) **Algonquin, Quebec** *Cold Remedy* Infusion of bark shavings taken for colds. *Hemorrhoid Remedy* Bark shavings used to stop bleeding. (as *C. stolonifera* 14:211) **Apache, White Mountain** *Ceremonial Medicine* Plant used in medicine ceremonies. (as *Svida stolonifera* 113:161) **Bella Coola** *Eye Medicine* Infusion of inner bark used for sties and other eye infections. (as *C. stolonifera* 158:203) **Blackfoot** *Cold Remedy* Infusion of bark taken for chest colds. (as *C. stolonifera* 72:71) *Liver Aid* Infusion of cambium taken for liver troubles and related disorders. (as *C. stolonifera* 72:66) *Poison* Chewed berry spittle used on arrow points and musket balls to cause infections in the wound. (as *C. stolonifera* 72:84) **Carrier** *Analgesic* Poultice of water-soaked, inner bark applied with warmed ashes as a painkiller. *Pulmonary Aid* Bark scraped, mixed with tobacco, and smoked for lung sickness. (as *C. stolonifera*

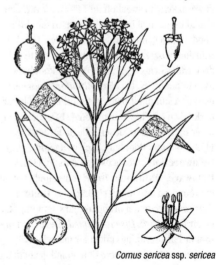

Cornus sericea ssp. *sericea*

26:71) **Carrier, Northern** *Dermatological Aid* Compound decoction of bark taken for body sores. *Orthopedic Aid* Compound decoction of bark taken for weakness or paralysis. *Stimulant* Compound decoction of bark taken for constitutional weakness. (as *C. stolonifora* 127:62) **Chippewa** *Antidiarrheal* Infusion of bark taken for diarrhea. *Dermatological Aid* Infusion of bark taken for eruptions caused by poison ivy. (as *C. stolonifera* 59:138) *Eye Medicine* Compound decoction of root used as a wash or compress for sore eyes. (as *C. stolonifera* 43:360) **Costanoan** *Febrifuge* Decoction of inner bark used for fevers. (as *C. californica* 17:24) **Cree, Woodlands** *Eye Medicine* Fruit or pith used to make a wash for snow-blindness. Pith used for cataracts. (as *C. stolonifera* 91:36) **Gosiute** *Narcotic* Plant used for the similar effect to opium. (as *C. stolonifera* 31:366) **Iroquois** *Analgesic* Infusion of bark taken for headaches. (as *C. alba* ssp. *stolonifera* 73:403) *Cold Remedy* Plant used for colds. (as *C. alba* ssp. *stolonifera* 73:405) *Cough Medicine* Infusion of bark taken for coughs. *Emetic* Decoction or infusion of bark taken as an emetic, especially for consumption. (as *C. alba* ssp. *stolonifera* 73:403) *Eye Medicine* Plant used in a wash for eyes. (as *C. alba* ssp. *stolonifera* 73:405) *Hemostat* Infusion of bark taken for nose or mouth hemorrhages. *Oral Aid* Infusion of bark taken for nose or mouth hemorrhages. (as *C. alba* ssp. *stolonifera* 73:403) *Panacea* Bark smoked for every ailment. *Psychological Aid* Compound decoction of bark taken for craziness. (as *C. alba* ssp. *stolonifera* 73:404) *Pulmonary Aid* Compound infusion of bark taken for pain or congestion of the chest. (as *C. alba* ssp. *stolonifera* 73:405) *Sports Medicine* Decoction of bark taken by lacrosse players and runners to vomit. (as *C. alba* ssp. *stolonifera* 73:404) *Tuberculosis Remedy* Compound decoction taken to vomit during the initial stages of consumption. (as *C. alba* ssp. *stolonifera* 73:403) *Witchcraft Medicine* Compound of plant and dried snake's blood used as a "witching medicine." (as *C. alba* ssp. *stolonifera* 73:405) **Malecite** *Analgesic* Plants mixed with spikenard roots and smoked for headaches. *Eye Medicine* Plants chewed or soaked in warm water and used for sore eyes. *Respiratory Aid* Plants smoked and used for catarrh. *Throat Aid* Infusion of plants used as a gargle for sore throats. (as *C.*

stolonifera 96:248) **Micmac** *Analgesic* Herb used for headache. *Eye Medicine* Herb used for sore eyes. *Respiratory Aid* Herb used for catarrh. *Throat Aid* Herb used for sore throat. (as *C. stolonifera* 32:56) **Montana Indian** *Dermatological Aid* Decoction of bark used as a wash for ulcers. (as *C. stolonifera* 15:11) **Navajo, Kayenta** *Ceremonial Medicine* and *Emetic* Plant used as a Mountaintop-way emetic. (as *C. stolonifera* 179:35) **Navajo, Ramah** *Ceremonial Medicine* and *Emetic* Plant used as a ceremonial emetic. (as *C. stolonifera* 165:38) **Ojibwa** *Ceremonial Medicine* Bark smoked for various ceremonies. (as *C. stolonifera* 112:237) **Okanagan-Colville** *Blood Medicine* Decoction of inner bark and chokecherry bark or alder bark taken to clear the blood, taken to help circulation, and taken for the blood after childbirth. *Cold Remedy* Inner bark dried, mixed with kinnikinnick or tobacco, and smoked for colds. Poultice of inner bark alone or mixed with goose oil applied to babies for a chest cold. *Contraceptive* Decoction of inner bark and other bark taken after childbirth to prevent frequent pregnancies. *Dermatological Aid* Decoction of sticks taken for poison ivy rashes. Decoction of inner bark and chokecherry bark or alder bark taken for sores and rashes. Decoction of wood and bark used to wash skin, hair, and scalp for dandruff, falling hair, and itchy scalp. Decoction of wood, bark, cow parsnip roots, and chokecherry wood and bark used for sores and scabs. Berries rubbed into the scalp to prevent graying hair. *Gastrointestinal Aid* Decoction of sticks taken in the sweat house to cause vomiting for an upset stomach condition. *Gynecological Aid* Decoction of inner bark and chokecherry or alder bark taken to clean out the womb after childbirth. Poultice of inner bark applied to the back and belly to "heal a woman's insides" after childbirth. *Heart Medicine* Infusion of inner cambium taken for "heart conditions." *Other* Decoction of inner bark and chokecherry bark or alder bark taken to heal the body. *Panacea* Decoction of inner bark and chokecherry bark or alder bark taken for any kind of sickness. *Pediatric Aid* Poultice of inner bark alone or mixed with goose oil applied to babies for a chest cold. *Unspecified* Decoction of bark or entire branch used as a medicine. (as *C. stolonifera* 162:96) **Okanagon** *Gynecological Aid* Decoction of bark or leaves taken by women soon after childbirth. (as *C. stolonifera* 104:42) **Potawatomi** *Antidiarrheal* Root bark used for diarrhea and flux, "the most efficacious remedy." (as *C. stolonifera* 131:55) **Saanich** *Gastrointestinal Aid* Bark soaked in warm water and taken to induce vomiting to clean out the stomach. *Respiratory Aid* Bark soaked in warm water and taken to induce vomiting for improved breathing. (as *C. stolonifera* 156:81) **Shuswap** *Kidney Aid* Plant used for weak kidneys. *Pediatric Aid* and *Urinary Aid* Plant used for children for bed-wetting. (as *C. stolonifera* 102:61) **Thompson** *Gynecological Aid* Decoction of bark or leaves taken by women soon after childbirth. (as *C. stolonifera* 104:42) Simple or compound decoction of various plant parts taken after childbirth. (as *C. stolonifera* 141:475) **Wet'suwet'en** *Dermatological Aid* Bark used to make a skin wash. *Febrifuge* Bark used for fevers. *Hemorrhoid Remedy* Bark used for postpartum hemorrhaging. (as *C. stolonifera* 61:152)

Coronilla varia, Purple Crownvetch
Cherokee *Antirheumatic* (*External*) Plant crushed and rubbed on rheumatism. *Emetic* Used as an emetic. (66:60) Decoction of bark taken as an emetic. (152:31) *Orthopedic Aid* Plant crushed and rubbed on cramps. (66:60)

Corydalis aurea, Scrambledeggs
Navajo, Kayenta *Antidiarrheal* Plant used for diarrhea. *Dermatological Aid* Plant used for hand sores. *Disinfectant* and *Gynecological Aid* Plant used for puerperal infection. *Veterinary Aid* Plant sprinkled on livestock for snakebites. (179:23) **Ojibwa** *Stimulant* Root smoke inhaled to clear the head and revive the patient. (130:370)

Corydalis aurea* ssp. *occidentalis,
    Scrambledeggs
Navajo *Antirheumatic* (*Internal*) Plant used as a rheumatic remedy. (as *C. montana* 45:96) **Navajo, Ramah** *Analgesic* Cold infusion taken for stomachache and used as lotion for backache. *Gastrointestinal Aid* Cold infusion of plant taken for stomachache. *Gynecological Aid* Compound decoction of plant used for menstrual difficulties. *Orthopedic Aid* Cold infusion of plant used as a lotion for backache. *Other* Plant used for injuries.

Throat Aid Cold infusion of plant taken and used as a lotion for sore throat. (165:28)

Corydalis sempervirens, Rock Harlequin
Iroquois *Hemorrhoid Remedy* Compound decoction of plants taken and used as a wash for piles. (73:339)

Corylus americana, American Hazelnut
Cherokee *Dermatological Aid* Infusion of scraped bark taken for hives. *Emetic* Compound of inner bark taken "to vomit bile." (66:37) Decoction of inner bark taken to induce vomiting when unable to retain food. (152:16) **Chippewa** *Analgesic* Compound containing charcoal pricked into temples with needles for headache. (43:338) **Iroquois** *Antidiarrheal* and *Antiemetic* Compound decoction taken for "summer disease—vomiting, diarrhea and cramps." *Antihemorrhagic* Raw nuts taken for hay fever, childbirth hemorrhage, and prenatal strength. (73:297) *Blood Medicine* Compound infusion taken as a blood purifier and for prenatal strength. (73:298) *Dermatological Aid* Nutmeat oil formerly used for the hair, either alone or mixed with bear grease. (170:123) *Gastrointestinal Aid* Compound decoction taken for summer disease: vomiting, diarrhea, and cramps. *Gynecological Aid* Decoction or raw nuts taken for childbirth hemorrhage and prenatal strength. *Pediatric Aid* Compound decoction of roots given when "baby's teeth are coming in." (73:297) Compound infusion taken or raw nuts eaten for prenatal strength. *Respiratory Aid* Compound decoction of buds taken for hay fever. (73:298) *Toothache Remedy* Compound decoction of roots given when "baby's teeth are coming in." (73:297) **Menominee** *Adjuvant* Inner bark used "with other herbs as a binder to cement the virtues of all." (128:26) **Ojibwa** *Dermatological Aid* Poultice of boiled bark applied to help close and heal cuts. (130:359)

Corylus cornuta, Beaked Hazelnut
Abnaki *Eye Medicine* Used for sore eyes. (121:155) Decoction of bark and bark from two other plants used for eye pain. (121:165) **Algonquin, Quebec** *Gastrointestinal Aid* Infusion of branches and leaves used for intestinal disorders. *Heart Medicine* Infusion of branches and leaves used for heart troubles. (14:151) **Algonquin,**

Tête-de-Boule *Heart Medicine* Infusion of branch tips taken for heart problems. (110:128) **Iroquois** *Antirheumatic (External)* Poultice of branches applied for rheumatism. (119:85) *Emetic* Compound decoction of bark taken to vomit. *Pediatric Aid* Decoction of bark given to children for teething. (73:298) Infusion of stems and other plant stems made into a necklace used by children for teething pain. (118:38) *Psychological Aid* Compound decoction of bark used as a wash for loneliness. *Toothache Remedy* Decoction of bark given to children for teething. (73:298) Infusion of stems and other plant stems made into a necklace used by children for teething pain. (118:38) **Thompson** *Throat Aid* Buds chewed to become a good singer. (161:190)

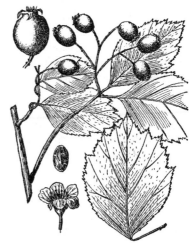
Crataegus douglasii

Corylus cornuta **var.** *cornuta*, Beaked Hazelnut
Ojibwa *Anthelmintic* Hairs of husk used as a medicine to expel worms. *Dermatological Aid* Poultice of boiled bark applied to help close and heal cuts. (as *C. rostrata* 130:359) **Potawatomi** *Dermatological Aid* Inner bark used as an astringent. (as *C. rostrata* 131:44)

Cosmos parviflorus, Southwestern Cosmos
Navajo, Ramah *Ceremonial Medicine* Cold infusion of dried leaves used as ceremonial chant lotion. (165:50)

Crataegus calpodendron, Pear Hawthorn
Meskwaki *Analgesic* Infusion of twigs used for a pain in the side and bladder trouble. *Stimulant* Infusion of root bark used in cases of "general debility." *Urinary Aid* Fruit used for bladder ailments. (as *C. tomentosa* 129:241)

Crataegus chrysocarpa, Fireberry Hawthorn
Blackfoot *Laxative* Decoction of dried berries taken during the winter as a mild laxative. (72:66) **Ojibwa, South** *Antidiarrheal* Compound decoction of root taken for diarrhea. (as *C. coccinea* 77:200) **Potawatomi** *Gastrointestinal Aid* Fruit used for stomach complaints. (as *C. rotundifolia* var. *bicknellii* 131:76)

Crataegus douglasii, Black Hawthorn
Kwakiutl *Dermatological Aid* Poultice of chewed leaves applied to swellings. (157:288) **Okanagan-Colville** *Antidiarrheal* Infusion of shoots given to children for diarrhea. *Antirheumatic (External)* Thorn used to pierce areas affected by arthritic pain. The upper end of the thorn was ignited and burned down to the point buried into the skin. This treatment was very painful, but after a scab had formed and disappeared, the arthritic pain also disappeared. *Oral Aid* Infusion of new shoots used to wash a baby's mouth for mouth sores. *Pediatric Aid* Infusion of new shoots used to wash a baby's mouth for mouth sores. Infusion of shoots given to children for diarrhea. (162:124) **Okanagon** *Dermatological Aid* Spines used as probes for boils and ulcers. *Gastrointestinal Aid* Decoction of sapwood, bark, and roots taken as a stomach medicine. (as *C. brevispina* 104:40) **Thompson** *Antidiarrheal* Fruit considered a good health food for diarrhea. Infusion of bark taken for diarrhea and dysentery. (161:258) *Dermatological Aid* Spines used as probes for boils and ulcers. (as *C. brevispina* 104:40) Spines used as probes "for ripe boils and ulcers." (141:457) *Gastrointestinal Aid* Decoction of sapwood, bark, and roots taken as a stomach medicine. (as *C. brevispina* 104:40) Decoction of sap, bark, wood, or root taken as stomach medicine. (141:457) *Panacea* Fruit considered a good health food for general sickness. (161:258)

Crataegus punctata, Dotted Hawthorn
Iroquois *Gastrointestinal Aid* Infusion of little

branches without leaves and other plants taken for large stomachs. (118:46) *Gynecological Aid* Compound decoction of shoots and bark taken to stop menstrual flow. *Witchcraft Medicine* Decoction taken to prevent "breaking out like cancer" caused by witchcraft. (73:351)

Crataegus rivularis, River Hawthorn
Mendocino Indian *Poison* Thorns considered poisonous. (33:355)

Crataegus spathulata, Littlehip Hawthorn
Cherokee *Dietary Aid* Berries eaten "for appetite." *Heart Medicine* Infusion of bark taken for good circulation. *Preventive Medicine* Infusion of bark taken "to prevent current spasms." (66:37)

Crataegus submollis, Quebec Hawthorn
Iroquois *Witchcraft Medicine* Decoction and doll used to "make a person break out like cancer." (73:351)

Crepis acuminata, Longleaf Hawksbeard
Shoshoni *Analgesic* Poultice of seeds or plant applied to sore breasts after childbirth. *Eye Medicine* Pulverized root sprinkled in eye to dislodge object and clear inflammation. *Gynecological Aid* Poultice of seeds or whole plant applied to sore breasts to induce milk flow. (155:62)

Crepis atribarba, Slender Hawksbeard
Okanagan-Colville *Orthopedic Aid* Infusion of pounded green tops used in a foot bath for a "sweaty feet" condition. (162:83)

Crepis modocensis, Siskiyou Hawksbeard
Paiute *Dermatological Aid* Latex applied to bee stings or insect bites. **Shoshoni** *Eye Medicine* Decoction of root used as a wash for sore eyes. *Gynecological Aid* Poultice of mashed plant applied to women's caked breasts. (as *C. scopulorum* 155:62)

Crepis runcinata, Fiddleleaf Hawksbeard
Meskwaki *Cancer Treatment* and *Dermatological Aid* Poultice of whole plant applied "to open up a carbuncle or cancer." (129:213)

Crepis runcinata ssp. *glauca*, Fiddleleaf Hawksbeard
Keres, Western *Psychological Aid* Infusion of young plants drunk for homesickness and lonesomeness. (as *C. glauca* 147:40)

Crotalaria rotundifolia, Rabbitbells
Seminole *Throat Aid* Infusion of pods used for sore throats. (as *C. maritima* 145:281)

Crotalaria sagittalis, Arrowhead Rattlebox
Delaware *Narcotic* Roots used as a strong narcotic. *Venereal Aid* Roots used for venereal disease. (151:34) **Delaware, Oklahoma** *Narcotic* Root considered to be a very strong narcotic. *Venereal Aid* Root used for venereal disease. (150:29, 74) **Mohegan** *Blood Medicine* Root taken as a blood purifier. (151:72, 128)

Croton californicus, California Croton
Cahuilla *Ear Medicine* and *Pediatric Aid* Warm decoction of mashed stems and leaves placed in the child's ear for earaches. *Poison* Toxic plant used only in small dosages for illnesses. *Respiratory Aid* Hot decoction of mashed stems and leaves taken for congestion caused by colds. (11:56) **Diegueño** *Cough Medicine* Decoction of whole plant taken for coughs. (74:218) **Luiseño** *Abortifacient* Plant used for abortions. (132:231)

Croton pottsii var. *pottsii*, Potts's Leatherweed
Mahuna *Kidney Aid* Infusion of plant taken for kidney infections. (as *C. corymbosus* 117:68)

Croton setigerus, Croton
Concow *Analgesic* Poultice of fresh, bruised leaves applied to chest for internal pains. *Febrifuge* Decoction of plant used as a bath or decoction taken for chills and fevers. *Misc. Disease Remedy* Decoction of plant used as a bath for typhoid and other fevers. (33:363) **Costanoan** *Antidiarrheal* Decoction of roots used for dysentery. (as *Eremocarpus setigerus*, turkey mullein 17:8) **Diegueño** *Veterinary Aid* Mashed stems and leaves placed in wormy, open wounds on horses to kill the worms and heal the sores. (as *Eremocarpus setigerus*, turkey mullein 70:20) **Kawaiisu** *Analgesic* Decoction of plant used as a wash or

taken for headaches. *Heart Medicine* Infusion of plant taken for heart palpitations. (as *Eremocarpus setigerus*, turkey mullein 180:28) **Modesse** *Kidney Aid* Plant dried for a year to take on great power and used for dropsy. (as *Eremocarpus setigerus*, turkey mullein 97:224) **Neeshenam** *Misc. Disease Remedy* Decoction of plants taken for ague. (as *Eremocarpus setigerus*, turkey mullein 107:376) **Pomo** *Antidiarrheal* Decoction of smashed plant used for bleeding diarrhea. *Poison* Plant considered poisonous. (as *Eremocarpus setigerus*, turkey mullein 54:13) **Pomo, Kashaya** *Antidiarrheal* Decoction of mashed, boiled root taken for bleeding diarrhea. (as *Eremocarpus setigerus*, turkey mullein 60:75)

Croton texensis, Texas Croton
Apache, White Mountain *Cathartic* Infusion of plant taken as a purgative. *Gastrointestinal Aid* Infusion of plant taken for stomach troubles. (113:156) **Hopi** *Emetic* Plant used as an emetic to "relieve the stomach." (174:34, 84) *Eye Medicine* Plant used in a very strong eyewash. (174:33, 84) **Isleta** *Ear Medicine* Seeds used in ears as a hearing aid in cases of partial deafness. *Laxative* Infusion of leaves taken or fresh leaves eaten as a laxative. (85:27) **Jemez** *Analgesic* Decoction of ground whole plant, roots, and salt taken for headaches. *Antirheumatic* (*Internal*) Decoction of ground whole plant, roots, and salt taken for body aches. *Misc. Disease Remedy* Decoction of ground whole plant, roots, and salt taken for grippe. (36:22) **Keres, Western** *Cathartic* Infusion of plant used as a cathartic. *Dermatological Aid* Ground seed powder used on open sores. *Hemorrhoid Remedy* Crushed roots used as a salve for piles. (147:40) **Lakota** *Gastrointestinal Aid* Infusion of leaves taken for stomach pains. (116:45) **Pawnee** *Pediatric Aid* Decoction of leaves used to bathe sick babies. (58:99) **Zuni** *Antiemetic* Decoction of plant taken for "sick stomach." *Cathartic* Decoction of plant taken as a purgative. *Diuretic* Decoction of plant taken as a diuretic. (143:45) *Gastrointestinal Aid* Infusion of leaves taken for stomachaches. (22:375) *Snakebite Remedy* Fresh or dried root chewed by medicine man before sucking snakebite and poultice applied to wound. (22:376) *Venereal Aid* Infusion of leaves taken for

gonorrhea. Infusion of leaves taken for syphilis. (22:375)

Cryptantha cinerea var. ***cinerea***, James's Catseye
Navajo, Kayenta *Disinfectant* and *Pediatric Aid* Plant given to newborn infant for prenatal snake or toad infection. *Snakebite Remedy* Poultice of plant applied or plant used as lotion for snakebites. *Veterinary Aid* Poultice of plant applied or plant used as lotion for livestock with snakebites. (as *C. jamesii* var. *multicaulis* 179:40) **Navajo, Ramah** *Ceremonial Medicine* Root used as ceremonial medicine. *Dermatological Aid* Poultice of root or powdered root applied to sores. *Panacea* Cold infusion of root used as "life medicine." *Pediatric Aid* Cold infusion of whole plant used for birth injury. (as *C. jamesii* var. *multicaulis* 165:40)

Cryptantha cinerea var. ***jamesii***, James's Catseye
Hopi *Analgesic* Poultice of pounded plant applied for body pains. (as *Cryptanthe jamesii* 174:32, 88) **Zuni** *Dermatological Aid* Powdered root used for a sore anus. (as *Cryptantha jamesii* 22:374)

Cryptantha crassisepala, Thicksepal Catseye
Hopi *Dermatological Aid* Plant used for boils or any swelling. (174:32, 33, 38) **Keres, Western** *Poison* Plant considered a bad, poisonous weed. (147:40) **Navajo, Kayenta** *Dermatological Aid* Plant used as a lotion for itching. (179:39) **Zuni** *Stimulant* Hot infusion of pulverized plant applied to limbs for fatigue. (143:45)

Cryptantha fendleri, Sanddune Catseye
Navajo, Ramah *Cough Medicine* Decoction of plant taken for coughs. (165:40)

Cryptantha flava, Brenda's Yellow Catseye
Hopi *Cancer Treatment* Plant used for the cancer and growth in the throat. (34:301) **Navajo, Kayenta** *Eye Medicine* Plant used as a dusting powder for sore eyes. *Gastrointestinal Aid* Plant used for intestinal inflammation. *Gynecological Aid* Plant used for postpartum purification. (179:39)

Cryptantha fulvocanescens, Tawny Catseye
Navajo *Gynecological Aid* Decoction of plants

taken at childbirth. (76:150) **Navajo, Ramah** *Snakebite Remedy* Cold infusion used as lotion for snakebite. *Toothache Remedy* Poultice of leaves applied for toothache. (165:40)

Cryptantha fulvocanescens var. *fulvocanescens*, Tawny Catseye
Navajo *Analgesic* Plant used for pain from a fall. *Cold Remedy* Plant chewed for colds. *Cough Medicine* Plant chewed for coughs. (as *Oreocarya fulvocanescens* 45:72)

Cryptantha sericea, Silky Catseye
Ute *Gastrointestinal Aid* Roots used as a stomach medicine. (as *Krynitzkia sericea* 30:35)

Cryptogramma sitchensis, Sitka Rockbrake
Thompson *Eye Medicine* Infusion of washed, strained fronds used as an eyewash. *Liver Aid* Infusion of washed, strained fronds taken for gallstones. (as *C. crispa* 161:88)

Cucurbita foetidissima, Missouri Gourd
Apache, Western *Veterinary Aid* Poultice of mashed stems, leaves, and roots soaked in hot water and applied to sores on horses' backs. (21:192) **Cahuilla** *Cathartic* Decoction of dried roots used as a physic. *Dermatological Aid* Ground fruit shell used as a hair shampoo. Macerated roots applied to ulcers. Pulp used for open sores. *Emetic* Decoction of dried roots used as an emetic. *Other* Dried gourds used to make ladles, syringes for feminine hygiene, and rattles. *Veterinary Aid* Poultice of

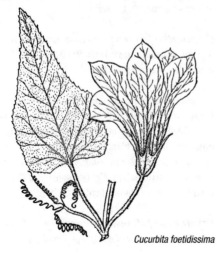

Cucurbita foetidissima

crushed pulp applied to saddle sores on horses. (11:57) **Coahuilla** *Veterinary Aid* Poultice of crushed root and sugar applied to saddle sores on horses. (as *Cucerbita perennis*, mock orange 9:80) **Dakota** *Panacea* Root used for any ailment, according to the doctrine of signatures. (as *Pepo foetidissima* 58:116, 117) **Isleta** *Pulmonary Aid* Decoction of roots used for chest pains. (85:27) **Keres, Western** *Dermatological Aid* Poultice of crushed roots applied to boils or other sores. (147:40) **Kiowa** *Emetic* Decoction of peeled roots taken as an emetic. (166:53) **Omaha** *Analgesic* Pulverized root mixed with water and taken for pains. (as *Cucurbita perennis* 48:584) *Dietary Aid* Plant used as an appetizer. (56:335) *Gynecological Aid* Root used in cases of protracted labor. (as *C. perennis* 48:585) *Panacea* Root used for any ailment, according to the doctrine of signatures. (as *Pepo foetidissima* 58:116, 117) *Tonic* Plant used as a tonic. (56:335) **Paiute** *Cathartic* Decoction of root taken as a physic for venereal disease. *Dermatological Aid* Decoction of root used to kill maggots in wounds. *Emetic* Decoction of root taken as an emetic for venereal disease. *Venereal Aid* Decoction of root taken as an emetic and physic for venereal diseases. Pulverized seeds sprinkled on venereal sores. (155:62, 63) **Pawnee** *Panacea* Root used for any ailment, according to the doctrine of signatures. **Ponca** *Panacea* Root used for any ailment, according to the doctrine of signatures. (as *Pepo foetidissima* 58:116, 117) **Shoshoni** *Cathartic* Decoction of root taken as a physic for venereal disease. *Emetic* Decoction of root taken as an emetic for venereal disease. (155:62, 63) *Venereal Aid* Infusion of plant taken for gonorrhea and syphilis. (98:47) Decoction of root taken as an emetic and physic for venereal diseases. (155:62, 63) *Veterinary Aid* Infusion of plant given to horses for bloat or worms. (98:48) **Tewa** *Laxative* Infusion of pulverized root taken as a laxative. (115:63) **Winnebago** *Panacea* Root used for any ailment, according to the doctrine of signatures. (as *Pepo foetidissima* 58:116, 117) **Zuni** *Antirheumatic* (*External*) Poultice of powdered seeds, flowers, and saliva applied to swellings. (22:375)

Cucurbita maxima, Winter Squash
Hawaiian *Dermatological Aid* Fruit meat and

water taken for bad skin blotches. *Gynecological Aid* Fruits and shoots or buds with other plants pounded, mixed with water, and used for fallen wombs. *Laxative* Fruits mixed with water and used for internal cleaning of the bowels. *Psychological Aid* Leaves and young shoots eaten for partial insanity due to lack of sleep. (2:28) **Ojibwa** *Diuretic* Infusion of seeds taken as a diuretic. (130:367)

Cucurbita pepo, Field Pumpkin
Cherokee *Anthelmintic* Seeds eaten for worms. *Ceremonial Medicine* Used as an ingredient in green corn medicine. *Diuretic* Taken as a diuretic. *Kidney Aid* Taken for "dropsy." *Urinary Aid* Browned seeds eaten for bed-wetting. Taken for "gravel," "scalding of the urine," and spasms of urinary passage. (66:51) **Iroquois** *Diuretic* and *Pediatric Aid* Infusion of seeds given to children with reduced urination. (118:61) **Menominee** *Diuretic* Pulverized seeds taken in water "to facilitate the passage of urine." (128:33) **Meskwaki** *Gynecological Aid* Decoction of stem used for "female ills." (129:220) **Navajo** *Gastrointestinal Aid* Leaves used for upset stomachs. (76:150) **Pima** *Dermatological Aid* Ground seed paste used to cleanse and soften the skin. (38:72) **Zuni** *Antirheumatic* (*External*) and *Dermatological Aid* Ingredient of "schumaakwe cakes" and used externally for rheumatism and swelling. Poultice of seeds and blossoms applied to cactus scratches. (143:45, 46)

Cuminum cyminum, Cumin
Apalachee *Unspecified* Plant water used for medicinal purposes. (as *C. cymium* 67:98)

Cunila marina, Common Dittany
Cherokee *Analgesic* Infusion taken for headache. *Cold Remedy* Infusion taken for colds. *Diaphoretic* Infusion taken to increase perspiration. *Febrifuge* Infusion taken for fever. *Gynecological Aid* Strong infusion taken to increase labor pains and aid in childbirth. *Snakebite Remedy* Used as a snakebite remedy. *Stimulant* Used as a stimulant. *Tonic* Used as a tonic. (as *C. origanoides* 66:32)

Cupressus macrocarpa, Monterey Cypress
Costanoan *Antirheumatic* (*Internal*) Decoction of foliage used for rheumatism. (17:6)

Cupressus nevadensis, Paiute Cypress
Kawaiisu *Analgesic* Decoction of dried seeds taken for sore chest. *Cold Remedy* Decoction of dried seeds taken for colds. *Cough Medicine* Decoction of dried seeds taken for coughing. *Gynecological Aid* Hot or cold infusion of cones taken for menstruation problems. *Kidney Aid* Hot or cold infusion of cones taken for kidney problems. *Orthopedic Aid* Hot or cold infusion of cones taken for backaches. (180:22)

Curcuma longa, Common Turmeric
Hawaiian *Blood Medicine* Bulbs, shoots, and other plants pounded, squeezed, and resulting liquid taken to cleanse the blood. *Nose Medicine* Bulbs and other plants pounded, squeezed, and the resulting liquid fumes inhaled for nose growths or odors. *Oral Aid* Bark and other plants pounded, squeezed, and the resulting liquid used to gargle. (as *C. louza* 2:33)

Cuscuta californica, Chaparral Dodder
Diegueño *Antidote* Infusion of plant, picked from buckwheat plants, taken for black widow spider bites. (70:17) **Kawaiisu** *Hemostat* Chewed stem juice or powdered plant snuffed up the nose for nosebleeds. (180:23)

Cuscuta compacta, Compact Dodder
Pawnee *Love Medicine* Vine used by girls to divine sincerity of suitors. (as *C. paradoxa* 58:110)

Cuscuta gronovii, Scaldweed
Cherokee *Dermatological Aid* Used as poultice for bruises. (66:32)

Cuscuta megalocarpa, Bigfruit Dodder
Navajo, Ramah *Ceremonial Medicine* Plant used as ceremonial emetic. *Emetic* Plant used as ceremonial emetic. (as *C. curta* 165:39)

Cycloloma atriplicifolium, Winged Pigweed
Hopi *Analgesic* Plant used for headache. (174:33, 74) *Antirheumatic* (*Internal*) Plant used for rheumatism. *Febrifuge* Plant used for fever. (174:32, 74)

Cymopterus bulbosus, Bulbous Springparsley
Keres, Western *Gastrointestinal Aid* Plant eaten as a stomach medicine. (as *Phellopterus bulbosus*

147:59) **Navajo, Ramah** *Panacea* Plant used as "life medicine." (165:38)

Cymopterus newberryi, Sweetroot Springparsley
Navajo, Kayenta *Dermatological Aid* Infusion of plant taken and used as a lotion for wounds. (179:34)

Cymopterus purpurascens, Widewing Springparsley
Navajo, Kayenta *Analgesic* Plant used for backache. *Antiemetic* and *Gastrointestinal Aid* Plant used to settle stomach after vomiting from swallowing a fly. *Orthopedic Aid* Plant used for backache. (179:34)

Cynodon dactylon var. *dactylon*, Bermuda Grass
Keres, Western *Veterinary Aid* Infusion of diseased grass used as a wash in castrating domestic animals. (as *Capriola dactylon* 147:35)

Cynoglossum grande, Pacific Hound's Tongue
Concow *Burn Dressing* Grated roots used for inflamed burns and scalds. **Pomo, Potter Valley** *Gastrointestinal Aid* Grated roots used for stomachaches. *Venereal Aid* Root used for venereal diseases. (33:382)

Cynoglossum officinale, Gypsyflower
Iroquois *Antihemorrhagic* Compound infusion of plants taken for consumption with hemorrhage. (73:420) *Cancer Treatment* Decoction of plant used as a wash and applied as poultice to leg cancer. *Dermatological Aid* Compound infusion used as wash and applied as poultice to running sores. *Kidney Aid* Compound infusion used as wash and applied as poultice for dropsy. (73:421) *Tuberculosis Remedy* Compound infusion of plants taken for consumption with hemorrhage. (73:420) *Venereal Aid* Decoction of roots taken and used as a wash for internal venereal disease. (73:421)

Cynoglossum virginianum, Wild Comfrey
Cherokee *Cancer Treatment* Root used for cancer. *Ceremonial Medicine* Used as an ingredient in green corn medicine. *Dermatological Aid* Compound decoction of roots given for itch. (as *Gyno-*

glossom virginianum 66:30) Decoction of roots used as a bath and taken for itching genitals. (152:52) *Psychological Aid* Compound decoction taken every 4 days for "bad memory." *Urinary Aid* Root syrup taken for milky urine and compound decoction used for bad memory. (as *Gynoglossom virginianum* 66:30)

Cynoglossum virginianum var. *boreale*, Wild Comfrey
Ojibwa *Analgesic* Plant burned on live coals and fumes inhaled for headaches. (as *C. boreale* 130:359, 360)

Cyperus esculentus, Chufa Flatsedge
Navajo, Ramah *Ceremonial Medicine* and *Emetic* Plant used as a ceremonial emetic. (165:19) **Pima** *Cold Remedy* Roots chewed for colds. *Cough Medicine* Roots chewed for coughs. *Snakebite Remedy* Poultice of chewed roots applied to snakebites. *Veterinary Aid* Chewed roots placed in horse's nostrils as a stimulant. (38:98)

Cyperus laevigatus, Smooth Flatsedge
Hawaiian *Cold Remedy* Stalks crushed into fine particles and used as a snuff for hard head colds. *Dermatological Aid* Stalks crushed into fine particles and used for deep cuts, boils, skin ulcers, and other skin diseases. *Strengthener* Flower and stalk ashes and kukui nut juice mixed and rubbed on the tongue for general debility. *Venereal Aid* Stalks crushed into fine particles, mixed with water and clay, and taken for penis burning disease. (2:9)

Cypripedium acaule, Pink Lady's Slipper
Algonquin, Quebec *Gynecological Aid* Roots used for menstrual disorders. *Venereal Aid* Roots used for venereal disease. (14:143) **Algonquin, Tête-de-Boule** *Gastrointestinal Aid* Infusion of roots used for stomachaches. *Kidney Aid* and *Pediatric Aid* Infusion of roots used by children for kidney troubles. *Urinary Aid* Infusion of roots used for urinary tract problems. (110:128) **Cherokee** *Analgesic* Root used for neuralgia and other pain and infusion taken for "rupture pains." *Anthelmintic* Infusion of root given for worms. *Anticonvulsive* Roots used for "spasms" and "fits." *Cold Remedy* Infusion of root taken for colds and hot infusion of root taken for flu. *Gastrointestinal Aid* Compound

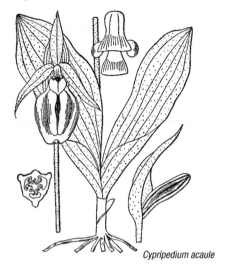
Cypripedium acaule

infusion taken for stomach cramps. *Gynecological Aid* Infusion taken for "female trouble." *Kidney Aid* Compound infusion taken for kidney trouble. *Misc. Disease Remedy* Infusion taken for diabetes and hot infusion of root taken for flu. *Sedative* Roots used for "fits" and "hysterical affections." (66:42) **Iroquois** *Analgesic* Decoction taken for pains all over the skin and body, caused by bad blood. *Dermatological Aid* Poultice of smashed leaves bound to bite of mad dog. (73:289) **Menominee** *Urinary Aid* Root used in "male disorders." (128:44) **Meskwaki** *Love Medicine* Compound containing root used as a love medicine. (129:233, 234) **Micmac** *Sedative* Root used for nervousness. (32:56) **Penobscot** *Sedative* Infusion of plant taken for "nervousness." (133:310) **Rappahannock** *Panacea* Compound of dried roots and whisky taken for general ailments. (138:32)

Cypripedium arietinum, Ramhead Lady's Slipper

Iroquois *Analgesic* Decoction of whole plant taken for intestinal trouble with inflation and pains. *Gastrointestinal Aid* Decoction of whole plant taken for intestinal trouble with inflation and pains. (73:288)

Cypripedium montanum, Mountain Lady's Slipper

Okanagan-Colville *Reproductive Aid* Infusion of leaves and stalks taken by a pregnant woman to have a small baby. (162:52)

Cypripedium parviflorum, Lesser Yellow Lady's Slipper

Cherokee *Analgesic* Root used for neuralgia and other pain and infusion taken for "rupture pains." *Anthelmintic* Infusion of root given for worms. *Anticonvulsive* Roots used for "spasms" and "fits." *Cold Remedy* Infusion of root taken for colds and hot infusion of root taken for flu. *Gastrointestinal Aid* Compound infusion taken for stomach cramps. *Gynecological Aid* Infusion taken for "female trouble." *Kidney Aid* Compound infusion taken for kidney trouble. *Misc. Disease Remedy* Infusion taken for diabetes and hot infusion of root taken for flu. *Sedative* Roots used for "fits" and "hysterical affections." (as *C. calceolus* 66:42) **Iroquois** *Blood Medicine* Compound decoction taken as blood medicine when "blood is bad from scrofula." (as *C. calceolus* ssp. *parviflorum* 73:289) *Febrifuge* Compound decoction taken for fever. *Orthopedic Aid* Compound decoction for soreness. (as *C. calceolus* ssp. *parviflorum* 73:288) *Sedative* Used as a nerve medicine. Infusion of root taken for nervousness or lack of energy. *Stimulant* Root decoction or infusion taken for nervousness, tiredness, and lack of energy. *Tuberculosis Remedy* Compound decoction taken as blood medicine when "blood is bad from scrofula." (as *C. calceolus* ssp. *parviflorum* 73:289)

Cypripedium pubescens, Greater Yellow Lady's Slipper

Cherokee *Anthelmintic* Decoction of roots taken for worms. (as *C. calceolus* var. *pubescens* 152:11) **Chippewa** *Dermatological Aid* Poultice of chopped, moistened root applied to inflammations. (as *C. hirsutum* 43:348) *Gastrointestinal Aid* Infusion of root taken in small doses for indigestion. *Toothache Remedy* Dried, powdered root moistened and applied to decayed teeth for toothache. (as *C. hirsutum* 43:342) **Iroquois** *Analgesic* Roots used with another plant for lower back pain. *Pulmonary Aid* Infusion of roots used for "too much wind in the chest." *Tuberculosis Remedy* Roots used with another plant for tuberculosis. (as *C. calceolus* var. *pubescens* 118:69) **Menominee** *Gynecological Aid* Plant used in "female disorders." *Hallucinogen* Plant used in sacred bundles to induce dreams of the supernatural. (as *C. parviflorum* pubescens 128:44) **Ojibwa** *Gyneco-*

logical Aid Root used for all female troubles. (as *C. parviflorum* var. *pubescens* 130:377)

Cyrtandra sp., Kanawao-keokeo
Hawaiian *Pediatric Aid* Fruits eaten from conception until the child feeds itself to increase the child's survival rate. Fruits eaten by infants for a weak physical constitution. *Reproductive Aid* Fruits eaten with baked eggs to bring about conception by barren women. *Strengthener* Fruits eaten from conception until the child feeds itself to increase the child's survival rate. Fruits eaten by infants for a weak physical constitution. (2:49)

Cystopteris fragilis, Brittle Bladderfern
Navajo, Ramah *Dermatological Aid* Cold, compound infusion of plant taken and used as lotion for injury. (165:11)

Cystopteris protrusa, Lowland Bladderfern
Cherokee *Febrifuge* Compound infusion given for chills. (66:33)

Dalea aurea, Golden Prairieclover
Dakota *Antidiarrheal* Infusion of leaves taken for dysentery. (as *Parosela aurea* 57:366) Decoction of leaves used for dysentery. (as *Parosela aurea* 58:94) *Gastrointestinal Aid* Infusion of leaves taken for stomachaches. (as *Parosela aurea* 57:366) Decoction of leaves used for colic. (as *Parosela aurea* 58:94)

Dalea candida var. **candida**, White Prairie-clover
Navajo *Analgesic* Compound of plants used for abdomen pain caused by colds and loose bowels. Roots chewed for pain. *Gastrointestinal Aid* Compound of plants used for abdomen pain caused by colds and loose bowels. *Toothache Remedy* Plant used as toothache medicine. (as *Petalostemon candidus* 45:57) **Navajo, Ramah** *Analgesic* Plant used for stomachache. *Disinfectant* Compound decoction used for "snake infection." Decoction of plant used for "snake infection." *Febrifuge* and *Gastrointestinal Aid* Plant used for stomachache. *Panacea* Plant used as "life medicine," especially for fever. *Veterinary Aid* Compound decoction used for "snake infection" in sheep. (as *Petaloste-*

mum candidum 165:33) **Pawnee** *Panacea* Infusion of root taken as a prophylactic to keep away disease. (as *Petalostemum candidum* 58:94)

Dalea candida var. **oligophylla**, White Prairieclover
Hopi *Emetic* Plant recognized as a strong emetic. (as *Petalostemon oligophyllum* 174:34, 80) **Keres, Western** *Dermatological Aid* Infusion of roots used as a hair wash to keep it from falling. (as *Petalostemon cliogophyllus* 147:58) **Navajo, Kayenta** *Dermatological Aid* Poultice of plant applied to arrow wounds. *Panacea* Plant used as a life medicine. *Veterinary Aid* Plant used for sheep with constipation. (as *Petalostemum oligophyllum* 179:29)

Dalea compacta, Compact Prairieclover
Zuni *Dermatological Aid* Poultice of root applied to sores and rashes. *Gastrointestinal Aid* Infusion of root taken for stomachache. (22:376)

Dalea enneandra, Nineanther Prairieclover
Dakota *Poison* Root considered poisonous. (as *Parosela enneandra* 57:366)

Dalea formosa, Featherplume
Jemez *Cathartic* Decoction of leaves taken as a cathartic. (as *Parosela formosa* 36:25) **Keres, Western** *Emetic* Infusion of leaves used as an emetic before breakfast. *Strengthener* Infusion of leaves used by runners to increase endurance and long wind. (as *Parosela formosa* 147:57)

Dalea lanata var. **lanata**, Woolly Prairie-clover
Navajo, Kayenta *Dermatological Aid* Poultice of plant applied to centipede bites. (as *Parosela lanata* 179:28)

Dalea nana var. **nana**, Dwarf Prairieclover
Keres, Western *Pediatric Aid* and *Strengthener* Infusion of plant used as a tonic for weak children. (as *Parosela nana* 147:57)

Dalea purpurea, Purple Prairieclover
Montana Indian *Dermatological Aid* Poultice of steeped, bruised leaves applied to fresh wounds. (as *Petalostemon violaceus* 15:17)

Dalea purpurea* var. *purpurea, Violet
Prairieclover
Chippewa *Heart Medicine* Decoction of leaves
and blossoms taken for heart trouble. (as *Petalostemon purpureus* 43:338) **Meskwaki** *Antidiarrheal* Compound containing florets used for diarrhea. *Misc. Disease Remedy* Infusion of root taken
for measles. (as *Petalostemum purpureum* 129:
229) **Navajo** *Pulmonary Aid* Plant used for pneumonia. (as *Petalostemum purpureum* 76:154)
Pawnee *Panacea* Infusion of root taken as a prophylactic to keep away disease. (as *Petalostemum
purpureum* 58:94)

Dalea villosa* var. *villosa, Silky Prairieclover
Lakota *Cathartic* Roots used as a purge. *Throat
Aid* Leaves and blossoms eaten for swellings inside
the throat. (as *Petalostemon villosum* 116:47)

Dalibarda repens, Robin Runaway
Iroquois *Blood Medicine* Complex compound
decoction of powdered plants taken as a blood
purifier. *Venereal Aid* Complex compound decoction of powdered plants taken for venereal disease.
(73:357)

Daphne mezereum, Paradise Plant
Cherokee *Analgesic* Root bark used for nocturnal
venereal disease pains. Root bark used for venereal
disease pains. *Diaphoretic* Used as a diaphoretic.
Stimulant Used as a stimulant. *Venereal Aid* Root
bark used for venereal disease pains. (66:32)

Darmera peltata, Indian Rhubarb
Karok *Gynecological Aid* Infusion of roots taken
by women to prevent fetus from getting too large.
(as *Peltiphyllum peltatum* 125:384)

Dasylirion durangensis
Tarahumara *Ceremonial Medicine* Used in the
annual ceremonial curing of animals and fields
from sickness and lightning. (13:60)

Datisca glomerata, Durango Root
Costanoan *Throat Aid* Decoction of plant used for
sore throat and swollen tonsils. (17:9) **Miwok**
Antirheumatic (*External*) Decoction of pulverized
root used as a wash for rheumatism. *Dermatologi-

cal Aid Decoction of pulverized root used as a
wash for sores. (8:168)

Datura discolor, Desert Thornapple
Pima *Analgesic* Infusion of leaves taken to mitigate the pains of childbirth. *Dermatological Aid*
Poultice of pounded leaves applied to sores or to
draw pus from a boil. *Ear Medicine* Poultice of
heated flowers applied to ears for earaches. *Eye
Medicine* Plant juice used as a wash for sore eyes.
Gastrointestinal Aid Plant used for ulcers. *Gynecological Aid* Infusion of leaves taken to mitigate
the pains of childbirth. *Hemorrhoid Remedy* Plant
used for hemorrhoids. *Other* Roots chewed to become crazy for "bad disease." (38:85)

Datura ferox, Chinese Thornapple
Keres, Western *Psychological Aid* Roots eaten to
see into the future. (as *D. quercifolia* 147:41)

Datura stramonium, Jimson Weed
Cherokee *Dermatological Aid* Poultice of wilted
leaves used on boils. *Respiratory Aid* Smoked for
asthma. (66:41) **Delaware** *Dermatological Aid*
Poultice of crushed leaves applied to fresh wounds.
Hemorrhoid Remedy Seeds pounded, mixed with
tallow and salve, and used for piles. (151:37)
Delaware, Oklahoma *Dermatological Aid* Poultice of seeds and leaves applied to wounds. *Hemorrhoid Remedy* Crushed seeds and tallow used as
a salve for piles. (150:31, 74) **Iroquois** *Poison*
Seeds considered poisonous. (118:56) **Mohegan**

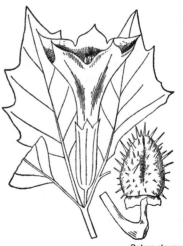

Datura stramonium

Dermatological Aid Poultice of crushed leaves, considered a "powerful plant," applied to cuts. (151:72, 128) **Rappahannock** *Dermatological Aid* Decoction of green or parched leaves used as salve on wounds. (138:27) Decoction of leaves applied to parts affected with inflammation. (138:28) *Febrifuge* Poultice of parched leaves bound to fevered part. (138:27) Decoction of leaves applied to parts affected with fever. *Poison* Seeds and leaves poisonous. *Pulmonary Aid* Poultice of decoction of leaves mash applied to the chest for pneumonia. (138:28) *Throat Aid* Compound poultice with crushed seeds rubbed on sore throat. (138:27)

Datura wrightii, Sacred Thornapple
Apache, White Mountain *Ceremonial Medicine* Powdered roots used in the religious-medicine ceremonies. *Disinfectant* Plant juice or ground flowers and roots used as a disinfectant. *Narcotic* Powdered roots used as a narcotic. (as *D. meteloides* 113:156) **Cahuilla** *Analgesic* Powdered leaves made into an ointment and applied as a painkiller in setting bones, and applied for pain in specific areas of the body. *Antidote* Plant paste used for poisonous tarantula, snake, spider, and insect bites. *Antirheumatic* (*External*) Powdered leaves made into an ointment and applied to swellings. *Hallucinogen* Most universally used hallucinogenic and medicinal plant known to humans. Used by the shaman to transcend reality and enter other worlds. *Datura* offered the shaman not only a means to transcend reality and come into contact with specific guardian spirits, it also enabled him to go on magical flights to other worlds or transform himself into other life forms such as the mountain lion or eagle. Such magical flights were a necessary and routine activity for Cahuilla shaman. A shaman might use the drug to visit the land of the dead, returning to the profane world with information useful to his people, or he might pursue a falling star to recapture a lost soul and return it to its owner. *Hunting Medicine* Used by hunters on long treks to increase strength, allay hunger, and gain power to capture game. *Other* Plant used to diagnose ailments and permitted the shamans to "see" the pain or disease. Plant used to divine cures for diseases. *Poison* An extremely poisonous plant. *Respiratory Aid* Leaves steamed

and vapor inhaled for severe bronchial or nasal congestion. *Snakebite Remedy* Plant paste used for poisonous tarantula, snake, spider, and insect bites. *Sports Medicine* Used to enhance mental perception when playing "peon," the gambling game. *Toothache Remedy* Powdered leaves made into an ointment and applied for toothache pain. *Unspecified* Crushed leaves and roots, with other parts, mixed into a medicinal paste. Most universally used hallucinogenic and medicinal plant known to humans. *Veterinary Aid* Plant paste used for saddle sores on horses. **Chumash** *Hallucinogen* and *Unspecified* Most universally used hallucinogenic and medicinal plant known to humans. (as *D. meteloides* 11:60) **Coahuilla** *Hallucinogen* Plant used as a "delirient," but with extreme danger, as it can cause death. (as *D. meteloides* 9:80) *Poison* Pulverized plant given with water to cause death and now almost wholly avoided. (as *D. meteloides* 9:75) *Veterinary Aid* Crushed plant mixed with water and rubbed into saddle sores on horses. (as *D. meteloides* 9:80) **Costanoan** *Analgesic* Poultice of heated leaves applied for chest pains. *Cathartic* Dried leaves smoked as a purgative. *Dermatological Aid* Ground leaves used as a salve for boils. *Eye Medicine* Flower dew used as an eyewash. *Hallucinogen* Dried leaves smoked as a hallucinogen. *Love Medicine* Seeds and tobacco smoked as an aphrodisiac. *Respiratory Aid* Poultice of heated leaves applied for respiratory problems. (as *D. meteloides* 17:14) **Diegueño** *Hallucinogen* Most universally used hallucinogenic and medicinal plant known to humans. (as *D. meteloides* 11:60) Well known as a hallucinogenic plant used in rites marking boys' initiation into the toloache cult. *Poison* Plant considered poisonous. (as *D. meteloides* 70:17) *Unspecified* Most universally used hallucinogenic and medicinal plant known to humans. **Gabrielino** *Hallucinogen* and *Unspecified* Most universally used hallucinogenic and medicinal plant known to humans. (as *D. meteloides* 11:60) **Havasupai** *Dermatological Aid* Leaf folded several times and rubbed onto red ant bite. *Narcotic* Leaves or seeds, when eaten, made a person intoxicated for a day or more. (as *D. meteloides* 171:239) **Hopi** *Hallucinogen* Root chewed to induce visions by medicine man while making a diagnosis. (as *D. meteloides* 34:306) Roots chewed by doctor to induce visions while making diagnosis. (as *D. meteloides* 174:31, 89) *Narcotic* Plant used as a narcotic. (as *D. meteloides* 34:306) Plant well known for the narcotic properties. (as *D. meteloides* 174:89) *Other* Used to cure meanness. (as *D. meteloides* 174:37) *Poison* Plant sometimes fatal and given to a person "who is mean" to cure "meanness." (as *D. meteloides* 174:89) *Psychological Aid* Plant used as a cure for "meanness." (as *D. meteloides* 34:306) *Stimulant* Plant rarely used as a stimulant as it was sometimes fatal. (as *D. meteloides* 174:31, 89) **Kawaiisu** *Analgesic* Infusion of mashed roots taken for the pain of broken bones. Plant used for pain and swellings. *Antirheumatic (External)* Infusion of mashed roots used as a bath for rheumatic and arthritic limbs. *Ceremonial Medicine* Plant used for the puberty ceremony. *Dermatological Aid* Plant used for swellings and as a wash for cuts. *Hallucinogen* Plant used as a hallucinogen to induce dreams and visions. *Orthopedic Aid* Infusion of mashed roots taken for the mending of broken bones. *Pediatric Aid* Plant used for the puberty ceremony. *Poison* Plant considered poisonous. (180:23) **Keres, Western** *Dermatological Aid* Poultice of crushed leaves or roots used for boils. Poultice of burned, ground leaves used for boils. *Poison* Root killed any humans or other animals if eaten. (as *D. metefoides* 147:41) **Luiseño** *Ceremonial Medicine* Root juice used in boys' puberty ceremony to induce stupefaction. (as *D. meteloides* 132:229) *Hallucinogen* Most universally used hallucinogenic and medicinal plant known to humans. (as *D. meteloides* 11:60) *Narcotic* Root juice used in boys' puberty ceremony to induce stupefaction. (as *D. meteloides* 132:229) *Unspecified* Most universally used hallucinogenic and medicinal plant known to humans. (as *D. meteloides* 11:60) **Mahuna** *Dermatological Aid* Plant used as an antivenin for tarantula bites. *Narcotic* Smoked leaves or infusion of leaves taken as a narcotic. *Poison* Plant considered poisonous. *Snakebite Remedy* Plant used as an antivenin for rattlesnake bites. (as *D. meteloides* 117:43) **Miwok** *Hallucinogen* Root eaten to induce delirium which achieved supernatural power. Decoction of plant taken to induce delirium which achieved supernatural power. (as *D. meteloides* 8:169) **Navajo** *Veterinary Aid* Infusion of leaf used as wash for wounds of sheep after castration. (as *D. meteloides* 76:160)

Navajo, Kayenta *Narcotic* Plant used as a narcotic. *Orthopedic Aid* Poultice of plant applied for sprains and fractures. (as *D. meteloides* 179:41) **Navajo, Ramah** *Analgesic* Cold infusion of root taken and used as a lotion for injury pain, a narcotic. *Ceremonial Medicine* Plant used as a ceremonial medicine. *Hallucinogen* Plant caused hallucinations and made "you drunk like from whisky." *Hunting Medicine* Plant mixed with pollen and smoked by hunters to make deer tame. *Narcotic* Cold infusion of root taken and used as a lotion for injury pain, a narcotic. *Veterinary Aid* Cold infusion of flower used as an eyewash for blindness in horses and lotion used for sores. *Witchcraft Medicine* Plant used by witches, but cannot harm one who knows how to use it. (as *D. meteloides* 165:42) **Paiute** *Blood Medicine* Decoction of ground, soaked roots taken for blood poisoning in the foot. *Hallucinogen* Decoction of ground, soaked roots taken to have visions, especially visitations from the dead. Seeds eaten to see dead relatives. (as *D. meteloides* 144:318) *Narcotic* Roots used to make a narcotic tea and not used medicinally. (as *D. meteloides* 155:66, 67) *Other* Plant enabled one to ascertain one's life span and those "whose days were numbered." Plant taken to find lost objects and remember where things were hidden. (as *D. meteloides* 144:318) **Paiute, Northern** *Hallucinogen* Roots eaten to discover things or see things that could not be seen with ordinary powers. *Poison* Plant poisonous if used incorrectly. (as *D. meteloides* 49:126) **Shoshoni** *Hallucinogen* Decoction of root taken to become unconscious and have visions. (as *D. meteloides* 98:50) *Narcotic* Roots used to make a narcotic tea and not used medicinally. (as *D. meteloides* 155:66, 67) **Tubatulabal** *Antirheumatic (Internal)* Infusion of plant taken for rheumatism. *Dermatological Aid* Plant used for wounds. Poultice of dried, pounded root applied to inflamed sores. *Gastrointestinal Aid* Plant used for bloat. *Laxative* Plant used for constipation. *Sedative* Cold infusion of plant taken to fall into a stupor. (as *D. meteloides* 167:59) **Ute** *Narcotic* Used as a narcotic. (as *D. meteloides* 29:26) **Yavapai** *Hunting Medicine* Decoction of leaves taken or leaves eaten for success in deer hunt. (as *D. meteloides* 53:261) **Yokut** *Ceremonial Medicine* Decoction of roots used as a ceremonial narcotic. *Gastrointestinal*

Aid Decoction of roots taken for inflammation of the bowels (appendicitis). *Other* Decoction of roots taken for many different diseases. (as *D. meteloides* 97:423) **Yuma** *Narcotic* Used as a narcotic. (as *D. meteloides* 29:26) **Zuni** *Anesthetic* Powdered root given as an anesthetic for surgery. *Dermatological Aid* Poultice of root and flower meal applied to wounds to promote healing. (as *D. meteloides* 143:46, 48) *Narcotic* Used as a narcotic. (as *D. meteloides* 29:26) Powdered root given as a narcotic for surgery. (as *D. meteloides* 143:46, 48)

Daucus carota, Queen Anne's Lace
Cherokee *Dermatological Aid* Infusion used as a wash for swelling. (66:51) **Delaware** *Misc. Disease Remedy* Infusion of full-blooming blossoms used for diabetes. (151:35) **Delaware, Oklahoma** *Misc. Disease Remedy* Infusion of fresh blossoms taken for diabetes. (150:29, 76) **Iroquois** *Blood Medicine* Decoction of roots taken by men for a blood disorder. *Dermatological Aid* Decoction of roots taken by men for pimples and paleness. *Dietary Aid* Decoction of roots taken by men with no appetite. *Diuretic* Decoction of roots taken for urine stoppage. (73:402) *Gynecological Aid* Plant used for fallen womb. (73:401) **Micmac** *Cathartic* Leaves used as a purgative. (32:56) **Mohegan** *Misc. Disease Remedy* Infusion of blossoms, must be full bloom, taken for diabetes. (149:269) Infusion of blossoms, must be in full bloom, taken for diabetes. (151:72, 130)

Daucus pusillus, American Wild Carrot
Costanoan *Blood Medicine* Decoction of plant taken to clean the blood. *Cold Remedy* Decoction of plant taken for colds. *Dermatological Aid* Decoction of plant taken for itching. *Febrifuge* Decoction of plant taken for fevers. *Snakebite Remedy* Decoction of plant taken for snakebites. (17:23) **Miwok** *Snakebite Remedy* Poultice of chewed plant applied to snakebite. (8:169)

Delphinium bicolor, Little Larkspur
Blackfoot *Antidiarrheal* Infusion of plant given to children with diarrhea. (72:82) *Dermatological Aid* Infusion of plant used by women to shine and straighten their hair. (72:124) *Oral Aid* Infusion of plant given to children with frothy mouth. *Pediat-*

ric Aid Infusion of plant given to children with diarrhea, frothy mouth, and fainting spells. *Stimulant* Infusion of plant given to children with fainting spells. (72:82) **Gosiute** *Poison* Plant considered poisonous. (31:367)

Delphinium carolinianum ssp. ***virescens***, Carolina Larkspur
Lakota *Poison* Plant poisonous to cattle. (as *D. virescens* 116:55)

Delphinium geraniifolium, Clark Valley Larkspur
Hopi *Ceremonial Medicine* Plant taken as an emetic in the Po-wa-mu ceremony. *Gynecological Aid* Decoction of plant and juniper used to bathe mother during the lying-in period. (34:307)

Delphinium hesperium, Foothill Larkspur
Mendocino Indian *Poison* Plant poisonous to cattle. (33:347)

Delphinium menziesii, Menzies's Larkspur
Chehalis *Dermatological Aid* Poultice of stalks and roots applied to sores. *Poison* Whole plant considered poisonous. (65:30) **Navajo** *Unspecified* Powdered petals sometimes used by the medicine man instead of larkspur petals. (45:47) **Thompson** *Love Medicine* Plant used as a charm by women "to help them obtain & hold affection of men." (141:506)

Delphinium nudicaule, Red Larkspur
Mendocino Indian *Narcotic* Plant had narcotic properties. (33:347)

Delphinium parryi, San Bernardino Larkspur
Kawaiisu *Orthopedic Aid* Dried, ground root used as a salve for swollen limbs. (180:25)

Delphinium scaposum, Tall Mountain Larkspur
Hopi *Ceremonial Medicine* Plant taken as an emetic in Po-wa-mu ceremony. (34:308) Plant used as a ceremonial emetic. (174:76) *Emetic* Plant used as a ceremonial emetic. (174:34, 76) *Gynecological Aid* Decoction of plant and juniper used to bathe mother during the lying-in period. (34:308) Compound decoction of plant used as a

wash for mother after childbirth. (174:36, 76)
Navajo *Unspecified* Powdered petals used by the
medicine man. (45:47) **Navajo, Kayenta** *Gynecological Aid* Plant eaten by women to become prolific. *Veterinary Aid* Plant eaten by goats to become
prolific. (179:22)

Delphinium tricorne, Dwarf Larkspur
Cherokee *Heart Medicine* Infusion taken "for
heart." *Poison* Root "makes cows drunk and kills
them." (66:42)

Dennstaedtia punctilobula, Eastern Hay-
scented Fern
Cherokee *Febrifuge* Compound infusion taken
for chills. (66:33, 34) **Mahuna** *Antihemorrhagic*
Plant used for lung hemorrhages. (117:19)

Descurainia incana ssp. ***incisa***, Mountain
Tansymustard
Gitksan *Dermatological Aid* Mashed and applied
to bad cuts. (as *Sisymbrium incisum* 127:57)
Navajo, Kayenta *Dermatological Aid* Plant used
as a lotion for frozen body parts. *Throat Aid* Plant
used as a lotion for sore throats. (as *D. incisa*
179:23)

Descurainia pinnata, Western Tansymustard
Cahuilla *Gastrointestinal Aid* Ground seeds used
for stomach ailments. (11:66) **Navajo, Ramah**
Toothache Remedy Poultice of plant applied for
toothache. (165:28)

Descurainia pinnata ssp. ***pinnata***, Western
Tansymustard
Pima *Dermatological Aid* Infusion of leaves used
for sores. (as *Sophia pinnata* 123:77) **Ute** *Unspecified* Used as medicine. (as *Sisymbrium canescens* 30:36)

Descurainia sophia, Herb Sophia
Navajo, Ramah *Toothache Remedy* Poultice of
plant applied for toothache. (165:28) **Paiute** *Dermatological Aid* Poultice of ground seeds applied
to burns and sores, including sores on horses. *Veterinary Aid* Poultice of ground seeds applied to
sores on horses. (93:74)

Desmanthus illinoensis, Prairie Bundle-
flower
Paiute *Eye Medicine* Five seeds placed in eye at
night for trachoma and washed out in morning.
(155:67) **Pawnee** *Dermatological Aid* Decoction
of leaves used as a wash for itch. (as *Acuan illinoensis* 58:89)

Desmodium canadense, Showy Ticktrefoil
Iroquois *Gastrointestinal Aid* Decoction of root
taken for biliousness. (73:364)

Desmodium glutinosum, Pointedleaf
Ticktrefoil
Iroquois *Basket Medicine* Cold infusion of
smashed roots used as a "basket medicine."
(73:364)

Desmodium illinoense, Illinois Ticktrefoil
Meskwaki *Adjuvant* Plant in combination with
others used as a powerful medicine. (129:228)

Desmodium incanum var. ***incanum***, Zarza-
bacoa Comun
Seminole *Analgesic* Plant used for adult's sickness caused by adultery: headache, body pains,
and crossed fingers. (as *D. supina* 145:256) Decoction of leaves taken for headaches. *Febrifuge*
Decoction of leaves taken for fevers. *Gastrointestinal Aid* Decoction of leaves taken for stomachaches. (as *D. supinum* 145:282)

Desmodium nudiflorum, Nakedflower
Ticktrefoil
Cherokee *Analgesic* Infusion of root used as a
wash for cramps. *Oral Aid* Roots chewed for sore
gums and mouth, including pyorrhea. (66:59)

Desmodium paniculatum, Panicledleaf
Ticktrefoil
Houma *Analgesic* and *Stimulant* Infusion of root
in whisky taken for weakness or cramps. (135:63)

Desmodium perplexum, Perplexed Ticktrefoil
Cherokee *Analgesic* Infusion of root used as a
wash for cramps. *Oral Aid* Roots chewed for sore
gums and mouth, including pyorrhea. (66:59)

Desmodium sandwicense, Hawaii Ticktrefoil
Hawaiian *Cold Remedy* Leaves sun dried, crushed
into a powder, mixed with tea, and taken for head
colds. *Respiratory Aid* Leaves sun dried, crushed,
and smoked in a pipe for asthma. *Strengthener*
Leaves sun dried, crushed into a powder, mixed
with tea, and taken for general debility. *Tuberculosis Remedy* Decoction of whole plant and other
plants used as a wash for scrofulous sores. (as *D.
uncinatum* 2:51)

Dicentra chrysantha, Golden Eardrops
Kawaiisu *Analgesic* and *Heart Medicine* Dried,
mashed roots placed in heated bag and applied to
the heart for heart pains. (180:26)

Dicentra cucullaria, Dutchman's Breeches
Iroquois *Sports Medicine* Compound infusion of
leaves used as liniment by runners to strengthen
limbs. (73:339) **Menominee** *Love Medicine*
Plant, most important love charm, thrown by
young swain at his intended to hit her with it. Root
chewed by young swain and breath attracts girl,
even against her will. (128:81)

Dicentra formosa, Pacific Bleedinghearts
Skagit *Anthelmintic* Decoction of pounded roots
taken as a worm medicine. *Dermatological Aid*
Infusion of crushed plants used as a wash to make
hair grow. *Toothache Remedy* Raw roots chewed
for toothaches. (65:31) **Thompson** *Unspecified*
Root used as some kind of medicine. (161:225)

Dichanthelium laxiflorum, Openflower
 Rosette Grass
Seminole *Analgesic* Infusion of leaves rubbed on
the abdomen for labor pains. (as *Panicum xalapense* 145:323) *Antirheumatic* (*External*) Whole
plant used for rabbit sickness: muscular cramps.
(as *Panicum xalapense* 145:194) *Cough Medicine*, *Pulmonary Aid*, and *Throat Aid* Infusion of
plant taken and used as bath for gopher-tortoise
sickness: cough, dry throat, noisy chest. (as *Panicum xalapense* 145:236)

Dichanthelium oligosanthes* var. *oligosanthes, Heller's Rosette Grass
Lakota *Poison* Plant poisonous to horses. (as
Panicum oligosanthes 116:30)

Dichanthelium oligosanthes* var. *scribnerianum, Scribner's Rosette Grass
Navajo, Ramah *Ceremonial Medicine* and *Disinfectant* Decoction of plant used ceremonially for
"snake infection." (as *Panicum seribnerianum*
165:17)

Dichanthelium strigosum* var. *glabrescens, Roughhair Rosette Grass
Seminole *Analgesic* Infusion of leaves rubbed on
the abdomen for labor pains. (as *Panicum polycaulon* 145:323) *Antirheumatic* (*External*) Whole
plant used for rabbit sickness: muscular cramps.
(as *Panicum polycaulon* 145:194) *Cough Medicine*, *Pulmonary Aid*, and *Throat Aid* Infusion of
plant taken and used as bath for gopher-tortoise
sickness: cough, dry throat, noisy chest. (as *Panicum polycaulon* 145:236)

Diervilla lonicera, Northern Bush Honeysuckle
Algonquin, Tête-de-Boule *Diuretic* Leaves used
as a diuretic. (110:128) **Chippewa** *Analgesic*
Compound decoction of leaves taken for stomach
pain. (43:342) *Eye Medicine* Infusion of bark used
as an eyewash. (59:141) *Gastrointestinal Aid*
Compound decoction of leaves taken for stomach
pain. (43:342) *Laxative* Infusion of bark taken for
constipation. (59:141) **Cree, Woodlands** *Eye
Medicine* Cooled infusion or decoction of roots or
stems put into the eyes for soreness. *Gynecological Aid* Infusion of roots taken to ensure a good
supply of breast milk. (91:37) **Iroquois** *Blood*

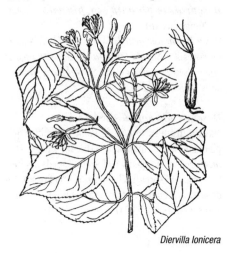

Diervilla lonicera

Medicine Decoction of plant or roots taken as a blood medicine. *Gynecological Aid* Compound decoction of bark and plants taken for prolapse of the uterus. *Pediatric Aid* Decoction of plant or roots given to "spoiled babies with adulterous mother." *Urinary Aid* Compound decoction of bark and plants taken by old men who cannot retain urine. *Venereal Aid* Compound decoction of roots taken for gonorrhea. (73:442) **Menominee** *Blood Medicine* Compound decoction of stalk used to "clear the blood." (44:129) *Diuretic* Infusion of root taken as a mild diuretic. *Psychological Aid* Infusion of root used for senility and as a mild diuretic. (128:27) **Meskwaki** *Urinary Aid* Infusion of root taken by "one who is urinating blood." *Venereal Aid* Compound decoction of root taken for gonorrhea. (129:206, 207) **Ojibwa** *Urinary Aid* Compound containing root used as a valued urinary remedy. (130:360) **Potawatomi** *Diuretic* Simple or compound infusion of root taken as a diuretic. *Other* Compound infusion of twigs used for vertigo. *Venereal Aid* Infusion of root taken for gonorrhea. (131:45)

Digitaria setigera, East Indian Crabgrass
Hawaiian *Antihemorrhagic* Grass pounded, mixed with water, strained, and taken for stomach and bowel hemorrhage. *Eye Medicine* Shoots chewed into a thick liquid and blown into the eye for cataracts. *Laxative* Leaves chewed by mothers and fed to children as a laxative. Shoot chewed and swallowed as a laxative. *Pediatric Aid* Shoots chewed by mothers and given to infants for run-down condition. Leaves chewed by mothers and fed to children as a laxative. *Strengthener* Shoots chewed by mothers and given to infants for run-down condition. Shoots chewed for run-down condition. (as *Panicum pruricus* 2:55)

Dimorphocarpa wislizeni, Touristplant
Apache, White Mountain *Ceremonial Medicine* Infusion of plant taken at medicine ceremonies. *Dermatological Aid* Infusion of plant used as wash for swellings. *Throat Aid* Infusion of plant used as wash for throat troubles. (as *Dithyraea wislizeni* 113:157) **Hopi** *Dermatological Aid* Pods ground and sprinkled on wounds. (as *Dithyrea wislizeni* 34:311) Dried, powdered leaves sprinkled on abrasions. (as *Biscutella wislizeni* 46:15) Ground

stalk used as a salve for all kinds of sores. (as *Dithyraea wislizenii* 164:163) Powdered plant sprinkled on wounds. (as *Dithyrea wislizeni* 174: 32, 77) **Keres, Western** *Nose Medicine* Crushed seeds and leaves inhaled for catarrh or sore nose. (as *Dithyraea wislizeni* 147:41) **Navajo, Kayenta** *Dermatological Aid* Infusion of plant taken and used as lotion for centipede or sand cricket bites. *Hemorrhoid Remedy* Poultice of plant applied to hemorrhoids. *Pediatric Aid* and *Toothache Remedy* Plant chewed by children to strengthen teeth. (as *Dithyraea wislizeni* 179:24) **Navajo, Ramah** *Dermatological Aid* Cold infusion of plant used as a lotion for itch. Poultice of leaves used to remove scabs. (as *Dithyrea wizlizenii* 165:28) **Zuni** *Dermatological Aid* Warm infusion of pulverized plant applied to swelling, especially the throat. (as *Dithyraea wislizeni* 143:48, 49) *Emetic* Flower and fruit eaten as an emetic for stomachaches. (as *Dithyraea wislizeni* 22:375) *Psychological Aid* Decoction of entire plant given for delirium. (as *Dithyraea wislizeni* 143:48, 49) Infusion of plant taken by men to "loosen their tongues so they may talk like fools & drunken men." It was said that this infusion should never be given to women because they "should not be made to talk too much." (as *Dithyraea wislizeni* 143:91)

Dioscorea villosa, Wild Yam
Meskwaki *Analgesic* Root used by women for pain at childbirth. *Gynecological Aid* Root used by women for pain at childbirth. (129:220)

Diospyros virginiana, Common Persimmon
Cherokee *Antidiarrheal* Syrup taken for bloody discharge from bowels. *Dermatological Aid* Astringent plant used for sore throat and mouth. *Gastrointestinal Aid* Bark chewed for heartburn. Compound used in steam bath for indigestion or biliousness. *Hemorrhoid Remedy* Used as a wash for piles. *Liver Aid* Cold infusion of bark taken for bile and liver. *Oral Aid* Syrup used for thrush. *Throat Aid* Syrup used for sore throat. *Toothache Remedy* Compound infusion used for toothache. *Venereal Aid* Used for venereal diseases. (66:49) **Rappahannock** *Oral Aid* Infusion of inner bark used as a wash for thrash. *Throat Aid* Infusion of north side bark taken for sore throat. (138:25)

Diphylleia cymosa, American Umbrellaleaf
Cherokee *Diaphoretic* Infusion taken as a diaphoretic. *Disinfectant* Used as an antiseptic. *Diuretic* Taken as a diuretic. *Misc. Disease Remedy*
Infusion taken for smallpox. (66:59, 60)

Diplacus aurantiacus, Orange Bush Monkeyflower
Tubatulabal *Gastrointestinal Aid* Decoction of
leaves and flowers taken for stomachaches.
(167:59)

Diplacus aurantiacus* ssp. *aurantiacus,
Orange Bush Monkeyflower
Costanoan *Kidney Aid* Decoction of plant used
for kidney problems. *Urinary Aid* Decoction of
plant used for bladder problems. (as *Mimulus aurantiacus* 17:15) **Mahuna** *Antidiarrheal* Infusion
of leaves, flowers, and stems taken for diarrhea.
(as *Dipsacus glutinosus* 117:6) **Pomo, Kashaya**
Eye Medicine Strained decoction of flower, stem,
and leaves used as an eyewash for sore eyes. (as
Mimulus aurantiacus 60:72)

Diplacus longiflorus, Southern Bush Monkeyflower
Tubatulabal *Gastrointestinal Aid* Decoction of
leaves and flowers taken for stomachaches.
(167:59)

Diplazium meyenianum, Meyen's Twinsorus
Fern
Hawaiian *Dermatological Aid* Young shoots powdered, mixed with milk and nuts, and applied to
boils. (as *Dilazium arnottii* 2:44)

Dipsacus fullonum, Fuller's Teasel
Iroquois *Dermatological Aid* Infusion of leaves
used as a wash for acne or "worms in the face."
Poison Powdered roots considered poisonous. (as
D. sylvestris 73:450)

Dirca palustris, Eastern Leatherwood
Algonquin, Quebec *Laxative* Infusion of inner
bark taken as a laxative tea. (14:202) **Chippewa**
Cathartic Infusion of stalk taken or green stalk
chewed as a physic. (43:346) *Dermatological Aid*
Compound decoction of root used as wash to
strengthen hair and make it grow. (43:350) *Pul-*

monary Aid Infusion of roots taken for pulmonary
troubles. (59:137) **Iroquois** *Analgesic* Compound
infusion of bark and roots taken for back pains.
Blood Medicine Compound decoction or infusion
of roots taken to purify the blood. (73:388) *Cathartic* Bark and wood used as a strong purgative.
(118:50) *Dermatological Aid* Decoction of
branches applied as poultice to swellings on the
leg or limbs. (73:387) Compound infusion taken
for dark circles and puffiness around the eyes.
Compound used for neck sores. (73:388) *Emetic*
Infusion of bark and wood used as an emetic to
remove yellow from the stomach. The yellow in the
stomach was a sickness brought by the Europeans.
As they introduced tea, butter, and tobacco, the
yellow accumulated in the stomach and could not
be evacuated. (118:50) *Eye Medicine* Compound
infusion taken for dark circles and puffiness
around the eyes. *Gynecological Aid* Compound
decoction of bark and roots taken to induce pregnancy. *Internal Medicine* Root used for internal
inflammation. *Kidney Aid* Compound infusion of
bark and roots taken for kidney troubles. *Laxative*
Decoction or infusion of smashed roots or bark
taken as a laxative. (73:388) *Love Medicine* Decoction of stems used as an aphrodisiac. (73:389)
Misc. Disease Remedy Infusion of smashed roots
taken for typhoid fever. (73:388) *Orthopedic Aid*
Infusion of roots taken for a strained back or back
pains. (73:387) *Strengthener* Decoction of stems
used to increase strength. (73:389) *Tonic* Compound decoction of roots taken as a blood medicine or tonic. *Tuberculosis Remedy* Whole plant

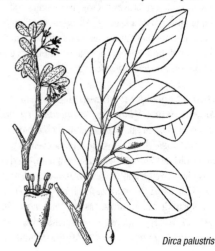

Dirca palustris

used for consumption. *Urinary Aid* Compound infusion of roots taken for kidneys or for male urination problems. *Venereal Aid* Compound infusion of powdered roots taken for gonorrhea and syphilis. Decoction of roots taken to remove venereal germs from the blood. (73:388) **Menominee** *Diuretic* Infusion of roots taken as a diuretic. *Kidney Aid* Infusion of root taken as a diuretic for kidney troubles. (128:54) **Ojibwa** *Diuretic* Infusion of bark taken as a diuretic. (130:390) *Urinary Aid* Infusion of twigs taken for urinary infections. (4:2306) **Potawatomi** *Diuretic* Infusion of inner bark taken as a diuretic. (131:85)

Disporum hookeri, Drops of Gold
Costanoan *Kidney Aid* Fruit used for the kidneys. (17:28)

Disporum hookeri* var. *oreganum, Oregon Drops of Gold
Klallam *Poison* Plant considered poisonous. **Makah** *Love Medicine* Plant used as a love medicine. (as *D. oreganum* 65:25)

Disporum smithii, Largeflower Fairybells
Makah *Love Medicine* Plant used as a love medicine. (65:25)

Disporum trachycarpum, Roughfruit Fairybells
Blackfoot *Eye Medicine* Fresh seed used to clear matter from the eye. A fresh seed was inserted and the closed eye rubbed until the seed was watered out with the matter clinging to it. Seeds placed in the eye overnight and infusion of bark used as an eyewash for snow-blindness. (72:80) **Okanagan-Colville** *Dermatological Aid* Infusion of leaves used as a wash for wounds. *Hemostat* Poultice of dampened, bruised leaves applied to bleeding wounds. *Unspecified* Berries used to make medicine. (162:44)

Distichlis spicata, Inland Saltgrass
Kawaiisu *Dermatological Aid* Decoction of plant taken for doodlebug bites that cause pimples. *Heart Medicine* Infusion of plant taken "when the heart beats fast." *Laxative* Infusion of plant taken as a laxative. *Venereal Aid* Cold infusion of plant taken for gonorrhea. (180:26) **Yokut** *Cold Remedy* Decoction of salt cooked into a gum, placed in the mouth, and allowed to melt for bad colds. *Dietary Aid* Decoction of salt cooked into a gum, placed in the mouth, and allowed to melt for loss of appetite. (97:423)

Dodecatheon hendersonii, Mosquito Bills
Pomo, Kashaya *Sedative* Flowers hung on baby baskets to make the baby sleepy. (as *D. henersonii* 60:105)

Dodecatheon jeffreyi, Tall Mountain Shootingstar
Thompson *Love Medicine* Flowers used by women "to obtain the love of men and to help them control men." (141:506)

Dodecatheon pulchellum* ssp. *pauciflorum, Pride of Ohio
Okanagan-Colville *Eye Medicine* Infusion of roots used as a wash for sore eyes. (as *D. pauciflorum* 162:117)

Dodecatheon pulchellum* ssp. *pulchellum, Darkthroat Shootingstar
Blackfoot *Eye Medicine* Cooled infusion of leaves used for eye drops. (as *D. radicatum* 72:81) *Oral Aid* and *Pediatric Aid* Infusion of leaves gargled, especially by children, for cankers. (as *D. radicatum* 72:76)

Dodonaea viscosa, Florida Hopbush
Hawaiian *Ceremonial Medicine* Infusion of leaves and other plants used as a wash to keep evil influences away. *Dermatological Aid* Infusion of leaves and other plants used as a wash for rash and itch. *Misc. Disease Remedy* Infusion of leaves and other plants used as a wash for contagious diseases. (2:3)

Draba helleriana, Heller's Whitlowgrass
Keres, Western *Other* Plant made into a drink and taken when not feeling well. (147:42) **Navajo, Ramah** *Ceremonial Medicine* Plant used in various ways as a ceremonial medicine. *Cough Medicine* Decoction of leaves taken for bad cough, sore kidney, or gonorrhea. *Emetic* Whole plant used as a ceremonial emetic. *Eye Medicine* Cold infusion of leaves used as ceremonial eyewash. *Kidney Aid*

Decoction of leaves taken for sore kidney, bad cough, or gonorrhea. *Panacea* Root used as a "life medicine." *Venereal Aid* Decoction of leaves taken for gonorrhea, sore kidney, or bad cough. *Witchcraft Medicine* Cold infusion of plant taken and used as a lotion to protect against witches. (165:28)

Draba incerta, Yellowstone Whitlowgrass
Blackfoot *Abortifacient* Plant used to cause abortions. (72:60) *Nose Medicine* Infusion of roots taken for nosebleeds. (72:71)

Draba rectifructa, Mountain Whitlowgrass
Navajo *Diuretic* Infusion of plants taken as a diuretic. (as *D. montana* 45:49)

Draba reptans, Carolina Whitlowgrass
Navajo, Ramah *Dermatological Aid* Poultice of crushed leaves applied to sores. (165:28)

Dracocephalum parviflorum, American Dragonhead
Navajo, Kayenta *Antidiarrheal* Plant used for infants with diarrhea. *Panacea* Plant used as a life medicine. *Pediatric Aid* Plant used for infants with diarrhea. (as *Moldavica parviflora* 179:40) **Navajo, Ramah** *Analgesic* Cold, compound infusion of leaves taken for headache. *Eye Medicine* Cold infusion of leaves used as an eyewash. *Febrifuge* Cold, compound infusion of leaves taken for fever. (as *Moldavica parviflora* 165:41)

Drosera capillaris, Pink Sundew
Seminole *Dermatological Aid* Sticky, plant glands rubbed on ringworm sores. (145:211)

Drosera rotundifolia, Roundleaf Sundew
Kwakiutl *Dermatological Aid* Plant used for corns, warts, and bunions. *Love Medicine* Plant used as a "medicine to make women love-crazy," a love charm. (157:281)

Drymaria glandulosa, Fendler's Drymary
Navajo, Ramah *Dermatological Aid* Poultice of chewed plant applied to mouse bite. (as *D. fendleri* 165:26)

Dryopteris arguta, Coastal Woodfern
Costanoan *Dermatological Aid* Infusion of fronds used as a hair wash. (17:5) **Mewuk** *Antiemetic* Decoction of roots taken for vomiting. *Antihemorrhagic* Decoction of roots taken for spitting blood and other internal bleeding. (as *D. rigida arguta* 97:366)

Dryopteris campyloptera, Mountain Woodfern
Eskimo, Western *Analgesic* and *Gastrointestinal Aid* Compound decoction of leaves taken for stomachache and intestinal discomfort. (as *D. austriaca* 90:5) **Hesquiat** *Cancer Treatment* Young shoots used cancer of the womb. (as *D. austriaca* 159:29)

Dryopteris carthusiana, Spinulose Woodfern
Bella Coola *Antidote* Root eaten as an antidote for poison from eating shellfish in early summer. (as *Aspidium spinulosum* 127:48)

Dryopteris cristata, Crested Woodfern
Ojibwa *Gastrointestinal Aid* Infusion of root used for stomach trouble. (as *Aspidium cristatum* 130:381)

Dryopteris expansa, Spreading Woodfern
Klallam *Dermatological Aid* Poultice of pounded roots applied to cuts. **Snohomish** *Dermatological Aid* Infusion of leaves used as a hair wash. (as *D. dilatata* 65:14)

Dryopteris filix-mas, Male Fern
Bella Coola *Antidote* Rhizomes eaten raw to neutralize plant and shellfish poisoning. (158:197) **Cherokee** *Anthelmintic* Infusion of root taken for worms. (66:34)

Dryopteris marginalis, Marginal Woodfern
Cherokee *Antirheumatic* (*Internal*) Infusion of root used alone or in a compound for rheumatism. *Emetic* Infusion of root taken as an emetic. *Toothache Remedy* Warm infusion held in mouth for toothache. (66:34)

Dudleya pulverulenta, Chalk Liveforever
Diegueño *Dermatological Aid* Fleshy leaves used to remove corns and calluses. Three descriptions

of its use, essentially the same but differing in detail, were given by the three consultants: (1) Prick the leaf all over with a pin or needle, put it on the stove, and bake it on one side, then the other. Place the leaf over the corn or callus and leave it there to remove the growth. (2) Heat the leaf over the fire, peel the skin off one side, place the leaf over the corn or callus—peeled side down—and leave it there to remove the corn or callus. (3) Cook the leaf over a flame, peel one side, and prick the peeled side with a needle and bind the leaf over the corn or callus to remove it. *Respiratory Aid* Decoction of roots taken for asthma. (70:19)

Dugaldia hoopesii, Owlsclaws

Great Basin Indian *Analgesic* Snuff of crushed blossoms and string plant leaves inhaled for headaches. *Respiratory Aid* Snuff of crushed blossoms inhaled for hay fever. (as *Helenium hoopesii* 100:50) **Navajo** *Antiemetic* Plant used to inhibit vomiting. (as *Helenium hoopesii* 45:87)

Dyssodia papposa, Fetid Marigold

Dakota *Veterinary Aid* Plant given to horses for coughs. (as *Boebera papposa* 57:369) Compound decoction of plant used for horses with coughs. (as *Boebera papposa* 58:132, 133) **Keres, Western** *Febrifuge* Infusion of fresh or dried plants taken or used as a rub for fever. *Other* Plant smoked for epileptic fits. (as *Boebera papposa* 147:33) **Lakota** *Analgesic* Plant breathed in for headaches. *Antihemorrhagic* Decoction of plant and gumweed blossoms taken for the spitting of blood. *Reproductive Aid* Pulverized leaves used for breathing difficulties. (116:37) **Navajo, Ramah** *Dermatological Aid* Poultice of chewed leaves applied to ant bites. *Gastrointestinal Aid* Cold infusion of plant taken after swallowing a red ant. (165:50) **Omaha** *Analgesic* Leaves stuffed up nostrils to cause nosebleed for headache. (as *Boebera papposa* 58:132, 133)

Echeandia flavescens, Torrey's Craglily

Navajo, Ramah *Gynecological Aid* Cold infusion of root taken to ease delivery of placenta. *Veterinary Aid* Cold infusion of root used as a lotion on sheep's swollen leg. Cold simple or compound infusion given to livestock as an aphrodisiac. (as *Anthericum torreyi* 165:20)

Echinacea angustifolia, Blacksamson Echinacea

Blackfoot *Toothache Remedy* Roots chewed to cause mouth numbness for toothaches. (82:56) **Cheyenne** *Analgesic* Infusion of leaves and roots rubbed on painful necks. (63:188) Infusion of powdered leaves and roots used as a wash for sore and painful necks. (64:188) *Oral Aid* Infusion of leaves and roots taken for sore mouth or gums. (63:188) Infusion of powdered leaves and roots taken or root chewed for sore mouth or gums. Root used to stimulate the flow of saliva. (64:188) *Orthopedic Aid* Infusion of leaves and roots rubbed on painful necks. (63:188) Infusion of powdered leaves and roots used as a wash for sore and painful necks. (64:188) *Throat Aid* Infusion of leaves and roots taken for sore throat. (63:188) Infusion of powdered leaves and roots taken or root chewed for sore throat. (64:188) *Toothache Remedy* Root juice used for toothaches. (63:188) Infusion of powdered leaves and roots used for toothaches. (64:188) **Dakota** *Analgesic* Juice used as wash for pain from burns. Plant used in smoke treatment for headache. *Antidote* Plant used as an antidote for many poisonous conditions. *Burn Dressing* Juice used as wash for pain from burns. Juice used by jugglers as wash for arms, to protect against boiling water. *Misc. Disease Remedy* Poultice of plant applied to enlarged glands, as in mumps. *Other* Plant used in the steam bath to "render the great heat endurable." *Snakebite Remedy* Plant used for snake and other venomous bites and stings in unspecified ways. *Toothache Remedy* Plant applied to tooth for toothache. *Veterinary Aid* Plant used in smoke treatment for horses with distemper. (58:131) **Lakota** *Antirheumatic (External)* Poultice of chewed roots applied to swellings. (116:37) *Dermatological Aid* Poultice used for wounds and sores. (88:47) *Gastrointestinal Aid* Plant chewed for stomachaches. *Oral Aid*

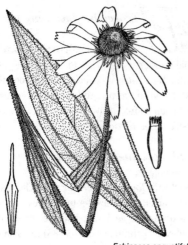

Echinacea angustifolia

distemper. **Pawnee** *Analgesic* Juice used as wash for pain from burns. Plant used in smoke treatment for headache. *Antidote* Plant used as an antidote for many poisonous conditions. *Burn Dressing* Juice used as wash for pain from burns. Juice used by jugglers as wash for arms, to protect against boiling water. *Misc. Disease Remedy* Poultice of plant applied to enlarged glands, as in mumps. *Other* Plant used in the steam bath to "render the great heat endurable." *Snakebite Remedy* Plant used for snake and other venomous bites and stings in unspecified ways. *Toothache Remedy* Plant applied to tooth for toothache. *Veterinary Aid* Plant used in smoke treatment for horses with distemper. **Ponca** *Analgesic* Juice used as wash for pain from burns. Plant used in smoke treatment for headache. *Antidote* Plant used as an antidote for many poisonous conditions. *Burn Dressing* Juice used as wash for pain from burns. Juice used by jugglers as wash for arms, to protect against boiling water. *Misc. Disease Remedy* Poultice of plant applied to enlarged glands, as in mumps. *Other* Plant used in the steam bath to "render the great heat endurable." *Snakebite Remedy* Plant used for snake and other venomous bites and stings in unspecified ways. *Toothache Remedy* Plant applied to tooth for toothache. *Veterinary Aid* Plant used in smoke treatment for horses with distemper. (58:131) **Sioux**, **Teton** *Analgesic* Root used for bowel pain. *Gastrointestinal Aid* Root used for bowel pain. *Throat Aid* Root used for tonsillitis. *Toothache Remedy* Root used as toothache remedy. (42:270) **Winnebago** *Analgesic* Juice used as wash for pain from burns. Plant used in smoke treatment for headache. *Antidote* Plant used as an antidote for many poisonous conditions. *Burn Dressing* Juice used as wash for pain from burns. Juice used by jugglers as wash for arms, to protect against boiling water. Plant used to make mouth insensitive to hot coals put in mouth for show. *Misc. Disease Remedy* Poultice of plant applied to enlarged glands, as in mumps. *Other* Plant used in the steam bath to "render the great heat endurable." *Snakebite Remedy* Plant used for snake and other venomous bites and stings in unspecified ways. *Toothache Remedy* Plant applied to tooth for toothache. *Veterinary Aid* Plant used in smoke treatment for horses with distemper. (58:131)

Plant chewed when thirsty. *Other* Plant chewed for overperspiring. (116:37) *Throat Aid* Roots chewed for tonsillitis. *Toothache Remedy* Roots chewed or powdered and used for toothache. (88:47) Plant chewed for toothaches. (116:37) **Montana Indian** *Oral Aid* Dried root with "smarting, acrid taste" caused a profuse flow of saliva. *Snakebite Remedy* Root used as an antidote for rattlesnake bites. (15:11) **Omaha** *Analgesic* Juice used as wash for pain from burns. Plant used in smoke treatment for headache. (58:131) *Anesthetic* Poultice of smashed roots applied as an anesthetic to arms and hands. *Antidote* Poultice of smashed roots applied to septic diseases. (56:333) Plant used as an antidote for many poisonous conditions. (58:131) *Blood Medicine* Poultice of smashed roots applied to septic diseases. (56:333) *Burn Dressing* Juice used as wash for pain from burns. Juice used by jugglers as wash for arms, to protect against boiling water. (58:131) *Dermatological Aid* Poultice of smashed roots applied to stings and septic diseases. (56:333) *Eye Medicine* Plant used for sore eyes and roots used for eye troubles. (56:335) *Misc. Disease Remedy* Poultice of plant applied to enlarged glands, as in mumps. *Other* Plant used in the steam bath to "render the great heat endurable." (58:131) *Snakebite Remedy* Poultice of smashed roots applied to snakebites. (56:333) Plant used for snake and other venomous bites and stings in unspecified ways. *Toothache Remedy* Plant applied to tooth for toothache. *Veterinary Aid* Plant used in smoke treatment for horses with

***Echinacea angustifolia* var. *angustifolia*,**
Blacksamson Echinacea
Kiowa *Cough Medicine* Ground root chewed for coughs. *Throat Aid* Ground root chewed for sore throats. (as *Brauneria angustifolia* 166:57) **Meskwaki** *Analgesic* Root used for stomach cramps and fits. *Anticonvulsive* Compound containing root used for stomach cramps and fits. *Gastrointestinal Aid* Root used for stomach cramps and fits. (as *Brauneria angustifolia* 129:212)

***Echinacea pallida*, Pale Purple Coneflower**
Cheyenne *Antirheumatic* (*Internal*) Decoction of roots and leaves taken for rheumatism and arthritis. (68:38) Decoction of roots taken for rheumatism and arthritis. (69:20) *Burn Dressing* Decoction of roots used for burns. (68:38) Decoction of roots used as a wash for burns. *Cold Remedy* Root chewed for colds. (69:20) *Dermatological Aid* Roots mixed with puffball mushroom spores and skunk oil and used for boils. (68:38) Roots used for boils. *Dietary Aid* Root chewed to increase the flow of saliva and prevent thirst. *Febrifuge* Decoction of roots used as a wash for fevers. (69:20) *Misc. Disease Remedy* Decoction of roots and leaves taken for mumps and measles. (68:38) Decoction of roots taken for smallpox, mumps, and measles. (69:20) *Oral Aid* Infusion of powdered roots and leaves taken for sore mouth and gums. *Throat Aid* Infusion of powdered roots and leaves taken for sore throat. *Toothache Remedy* Roots chewed for toothache. (68:38) Root chewed for toothaches, especially cavities. (69:20) **Crow** *Cold Remedy* Roots chewed and used for colds. *Gastrointestinal Aid* Infusion of roots taken for colic. *Toothache Remedy* Roots chewed for toothache. (68:38) **Dakota** *Anthelmintic* Decoction of roots taken as a vermifuge. (as *Brauneria pallida* 57:361) *Dermatological Aid* Poultice of roots applied to inflammation to relieve the burning sensation. (as *Brauneria pallida* 57:368) *Eye Medicine* Decoction of roots used for sore eyes. (as *Brauneria pallida* 57:367) *Snakebite Remedy* Plant used as an antidote for snakebites. (as *Brauneria pallida* 57:368) **Sioux** *Analgesic* Plant used in the smoke treatment for headache. *Antidote* Used as an antidote for rattlesnake and other venomous bites, stings, and poisonous conditions. *Burn Dressing* Decoction of roots used for burns.

Toothache Remedy Roots chewed for toothache. *Veterinary Aid* Plant used in the smoke treatment for horses with distemper. (68:38)

***Echinacea purpurea*, Eastern Purple Coneflower**
Choctaw *Cough Medicine* Root chewed, saliva swallowed, and tincture of root used for cough. *Gastrointestinal Aid* Root chewed, saliva swallowed, and tincture of root used for dyspepsia. (23:288) **Delaware** *Venereal Aid* Roots combined with staghorn sumac roots and used for venereal disease. (as *Brauneria purpurea* 151:33) Infusion of roots used for advanced cases of venereal disease. (as *Brauneria purpurea* 151:35) **Delaware, Oklahoma** *Venereal Aid* Simple or compound infusion of root, highly effective, taken for gonorrhea. (as *Brauneria purpurea* 150:29, 74)

***Echinocactus williamsii*, Mescal**
Omaha *Other* Plant used for alcohol addiction. (56:318)

***Echinocereus coccineus*, Scarlet Hedgehog Cactus**
Navajo *Heart Medicine* Plant used as a heart stimulant. *Poison* Plant considered poisonous. (45:64)

***Echinochloa crus-pavonis* var. *macera*,**
Gulf Cockspur Grass
Navajo, Ramah *Ceremonial Medicine* and *Emetic* Plant used as a ceremonial emetic. (as *E. crusgalli* var. *zelayensis* 165:16)

Echinocystis brandegei
Tubatulabal *Dermatological Aid* Burned, ripe seeds rubbed on pimples and newborn baby's navel. *Pediatric Aid* Burned, ripe seeds rubbed on newborn baby's navel. (167:59)

***Echinocystis lobata*, Wild Cucumber**
Cherokee *Abortifacient* Taken for "obstructed menses." *Antirheumatic* (*Internal*) Infusion taken for rheumatism. *Febrifuge* Taken for chills and fevers. *Kidney Aid* Infusion taken for kidneys. (66:40) **Menominee** *Analgesic* Poultice of pulverized root used for headache. *Love Medicine* Root used in love potions. *Panacea* Plant considered to be "the greatest of all medicines" and always use-

ful. *Tonic* Decoction of root taken as a bitter tonic. (128:33, 34) **Meskwaki** *Analgesic* Poultice of pounded root applied for headache. *Panacea* Compound containing root used as a universal remedy for all sicknesses. (129:220) **Ojibwa** *Gastrointestinal Aid* Infusion of root used as a bitter medicine for stomach troubles. *Tonic* Infusion of root used as a tonic. (130:367, 368)

Echium vulgare, Common Vipersbugloss
Cherokee *Urinary Aid* Compound taken for milky urine. (66:60) **Iroquois** *Gynecological Aid* Compound infusion of roots taken for the evacuation of the placenta. (73:421) **Mohegan** *Kidney Aid* Infusion of root taken for the kidneys. (149:266) Leaves or root, "a rare plant," used for kidney disorders. (151:72, 130)

Elaeagnus commutata, Silverberry
Blackfoot *Dermatological Aid* and *Pediatric Aid* Strong decoction of bark and grease used as a salve for children with frostbite. (72:85) **Thompson** *Venereal Aid* Decoction of roots and sumac roots taken for syphilis. This medicine was considered very poisonous and had to be taken with fish head soup to counteract the poison. One informant who was treated with this medicine recovered from syphilis but, afterwards, could never have children. (161:207)

Eleocharis geniculata, Canada Spikesedge
Seminole *Analgesic* Infusion of leaves taken as an emetic for rainbow sickness: fever, stiff neck, and backache. (as *E. caribaea* 145:210) Infusion of leaves taken as an emetic for thunder sickness: fever, dizziness, headache, and diarrhea. *Antidiarrheal* Infusion of leaves taken as an emetic for thunder sickness: fever, dizziness, headache, and diarrhea. (as *E. caribaea* 145:213) *Antirheumatic* (*External*) Plant used for fire sickness: fever and body aches. (as *E. caribaea* 145:203) *Emetic* Infusion of leaves taken as an emetic for rainbow sickness: fever, stiff neck, and backache. (as *E. caribaea* 145:210) Infusion of leaves taken as an emetic for thunder sickness: fever, dizziness, headache, and diarrhea. (as *E. caribaea* 145:213) *Febrifuge* Plant used for fire sickness: fever and body aches. (as *E. caribaea* 145:203) Infusion of leaves taken as an emetic for rainbow sickness: fever, stiff

neck, and backache. (as *E. caribaea* 145:210) Infusion of leaves taken as an emetic for thunder sickness: fever, dizziness, headache, and diarrhea. (as *E. caribaea* 145:213) *Unspecified* Plant used for medicinal purposes. (as *E. caribaea* 145:162) *Urinary Aid* Decoction of plant taken for urine retention. (as *E. caribaea* 145:274) *Vertigo Medicine* Infusion of leaves taken as an emetic for thunder sickness: fever, dizziness, headache, and diarrhea. (as *E. caribaea* 145:213)

Eleocharis montevidensis, Sand Spikerush
Navajo, Ramah *Ceremonial Medicine* and *Emetic* Plant used as a ceremonial emetic. (165:19)

Eleocharis rostellata, Beaked Spikerush
Navajo, Ramah *Ceremonial Medicine* and *Emetic* Plant used as a ceremonial emetic. (165:19)

Elliottia pyroliflorus, Copperbush
Kitasoo *Dietary Aid* Decoction of plant used as an appetite stimulant. (as *Cladothamnus pyroliflorus* 35:332)

Elodea canadensis, Canadian Waterweed
Iroquois *Emetic* Infusion of plant taken as a strong emetic. (as *Anacharis canadensis* 118:66)

Elymus canadensis, Canada Wildrye
Iroquois *Ceremonial Medicine* Decoction of plant with other plants used as medicine to soak corn seeds before planting. (170:19) *Kidney Aid* Compound decoction of roots taken for the kidneys. *Other* Compound decoction of plants taken for stricture. (73:274)

Elymus glaucus, Blue Wildrye
Karok *Other* Plant used as a medicine to settle quarrels between families or individuals. (125:380)

Elymus hystrix var. ***hystrix***, Eastern Bottlebrush Grass
Iroquois *Ceremonial Medicine* Decoction of leaves and reed grass rootstocks used as medicine to soak corn seeds before planting. (as *Hystrix patula* 170:18)

***Elymus trachycaulus* ssp. *trachycaulus*,**
Slender Wheatgrass
Navajo, Ramah *Veterinary Aid* Leaves eaten by
dogs, causing emesis. (as *Agropyron trachycaulum* 165:15)

***Elytrigia repens* var. *repens*,** Quack Grass
Cherokee *Orthopedic Aid* Decoction used to wash
swollen legs and infusion taken for "gravel." *Urinary Aid* Infusion taken for "gravel" and "[in] continence and bedwetting." (as *Agropyron repens*
66:31) **Iroquois** *Anthelmintic* Used as a worm
remedy. (as *Agropyron repens* 73:274) *Urinary
Aid* Infusion of rhizomes and stems from another
plant used for thick urine. (as *Agropyron repens*
118:67)

***Empetrum nigrum*,** Black Crowberry
Bella Coola *Cathartic* Decoction of green leaves
taken as a purgative. (127:60) **Cree, Woodlands**
Diuretic and *Pediatric Aid* Leafy branches used,
especially for children with a fever, as a diuretic.
(91:38) **Tanana, Upper** *Antidiarrheal* Decoction
or infusion of stems taken for diarrhea. Berries
cooked and eaten for diarrhea. *Cold Remedy* Decoction of leaves, stems, Hudson bay tea, and
young spruce tree tip used for colds. *Eye Medicine*
Cooled decoction of roots used as an eyewash to
remove a growth. *Kidney Aid* Decoction of leaves
and stems taken for kidney troubles. (86:12)

***Encelia farinosa*,** Goldenhills
Cahuilla *Toothache Remedy* Decoction of blos-

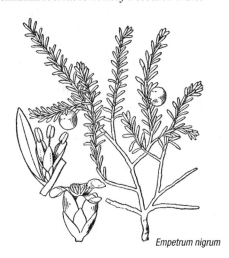
Empetrum nigrum

soms, leaves, and stems held in the mouth for
toothaches. (11:69) **Pima** *Analgesic* Poultice of
plant applied for pain. (38:102)

***Encelia frutescens* var. *resinosa*,** Button
Brittlebush
Navajo, Kayenta *Dermatological Aid* Plant used
for shingles. (179:47)

***Encelia virginensis* var. *actonii*,** Acton's
Brittlebush
Kawaiisu *Analgesic* and *Antirheumatic* (*External*) Decoction of leaves and flowers used as a wash
for rheumatic pains. *Veterinary Aid* Decoction of
leaves used as a wash for horses with cuts and
bruises. (180:27) **Tubatulabal** *Antirheumatic*
(*External*) Compound decoction of roots used as
a wash for rheumatism. (as *E. actoni* 167:59)

***Enceliopsis nudicaulis*,** Nakedstem Sunray
Shoshoni *Antidiarrheal* Decoction of root taken
for bloody diarrhea. *Cough Medicine* Decoction of
leaves taken for coughs. *Venereal Aid* Decoction
of root taken for venereal disease. (155:67, 68)

***Ephedra antisyphilitica*,** Clapweed
Pima *Venereal Aid* Plant used for syphilis.
(123:80) **Tewa** *Antidiarrheal* Leaves and stems
chewed or decoction taken for diarrhea. (115:46)

***Ephedra californica*,** California Jointfir
Diegueño *Blood Medicine* Infusion of branches
taken to purify the blood. *Dietary Aid* Infusion of
branches taken to improve the appetite. (70:19)
Gastrointestinal Aid Infusion of plant taken for
stomachaches caused by eating too much food or
eating bad food. (74:216) *Kidney Aid* Infusion of
branches taken for the kidneys. (70:19)

***Ephedra fasciculata*,** Arizona Jointfir
Pima *Dermatological Aid* Poultice of dried, powdered roots applied to sores. *Venereal Aid* Poultice
of dried, powdered roots applied for syphilis.
(38:76)

***Ephedra nevadensis*,** Nevada Jointfir
Apache, White Mountain *Venereal Aid* Infusion
of stems and leaves taken for gonorrhea or first
stages of syphilis. (113:157) **Cahuilla** *Blood Medi-*

cine Decoction of fresh or dried twigs used to purify the blood. *Other* Decoction of fresh or dried twigs used to "clear the system." (11:70) **Coahuilla** *Unspecified* Plant used for unspecified medicinal purposes. (9:73, 74) **Navajo** *Kidney Aid* Infusion of stems and leaves taken for kidney troubles. *Venereal Aid* Infusion of stems and leaves taken for venereal troubles. (113:157) **Paiute** *Adjuvant* Twigs used in medicines "to lessen disagreeable flavors." *Burn Dressing* Compound decoction of plant used as a salve for burns. *Venereal Aid* Decoction of twigs and branches taken for venereal diseases. **Shoshoni** *Dermatological Aid* Poultice of powdered twigs and branches applied to sores. *Diuretic* Decoction of twigs and branches taken to stimulate urination. *Venereal Aid* Decoction of twigs and branches taken for venereal diseases. (155:68) **Zuni** *Venereal Aid* Infusion of stems and leaves taken for venereal troubles. (113:157) Infusion of whole plant, except root, taken for syphilis. (143:49)

Ephedra torreyana, Torrey's Jointfir
Hopi *Venereal Aid* Plant used for syphilis. (174:35, 63) **Isleta** *Dermatological Aid* Decoction of leaves and stems used to make a lotion for itching skin. (85:28) **Keres**, **Western** *Cough Medicine* Infusion of stems used as a cough medicine. *Diaphoretic* Stems used as an ingredient in the sweat bath. *Kidney Aid* Infusion of stems taken or stems chewed for kidney trouble. *Urinary Aid* Infusion of stems taken or stems chewed for bladder trouble. (147:42) **Navajo**, **Ramah** *Cough Medicine* Decoction of whole plant taken for bad cough. *Gastrointestinal Aid* Decoction of whole plant taken for stomachache. (165:14)

Ephedra trifurca, Longleaf Jointfir
Cocopa *Dermatological Aid* Poultice of pulverized or boiled stems and leaves applied to sores. (52: 268) **Navajo** *Gastrointestinal Aid* Infusion of dried plants taken for stomach troubles. *Kidney Aid* Infusion of dried plants taken for kidney affections. *Venereal Aid* Infusion of dried plants taken for venereal disease. Wood burned for venereal disease. Wood burned with charcoal, buffalo hair, wood rat hair, and bat hair in a hole in the middle of the hogan. The person with venereal disease sits over the hole and the smudge covers his exposed

parts and cures him. (45:24) **Pima** *Dermatological Aid* Moxa used to burn the boils caused by "bad disease." Poultice of plant applied to bleeding sores caused by venereal disease. *Other* Plant used as an "antileuretic." *Venereal Aid* Poultice of plant applied to bleeding sores caused by venereal disease. (38:76)

Ephedra viridis, Mormon Tea
Havasupai *Emetic* Used to make a draft and taken to vomit for bowel complaints. *Laxative* Used to make a draft and taken to clear the bowels. (139:285) **Hopi** *Tonic* Dried flowers and stems taken as a tonic. *Venereal Aid* Plant used for syphilis. (34:312) Plant used for syphilis. (174:64) **Kawaiisu** *Blood Medicine* Infusion of stems taken for anemia. *Orthopedic Aid* Infusion of stems taken for backaches. (180:27) **Navajo** *Cough Medicine* Decoction of plant tops taken as a cough medicine. (45:24) *Venereal Aid* Strong infusion of plant used for syphilis. (92:19) **Paiute** *Antidiarrheal* Compound infusion of plant given to children for diarrhea. *Antirheumatic (Internal)* Infusion or decoction of twigs or branches taken for rheumatism. *Blood Medicine* Infusion or decoction of twigs or branches taken as a blood purifier. *Cold Remedy* Infusion or decoction of twigs or branches taken for colds. *Dermatological Aid* Dried, powdered stems applied to sores. *Gastrointestinal Aid* Infusion or decoction of twigs or branches used for stomach ulcers and disorders. *Kidney Aid* Infusion or decoction of twigs or branches taken as a kidney regulator. *Pediatric Aid* Compound infusion of plant given to children for diarrhea. *Tonic* Infusion or decoction of twigs or branches taken as a tonic. *Urinary Aid* Infusion or decoction of twigs or branches used as a kidney regulator and for bladder. *Venereal Aid* Decoction of twigs taken for syphilis or gonorrhea. (155:68– 70) **Paiute**, **Northern** *Dermatological Aid* Poultice of dried, powdered stems applied to sores. (49:128) **Shoshoni** *Antidiarrheal* Compound infusion of plant given to children for diarrhea. *Blood Medicine* Infusion or decoction of twigs or branches taken as a blood purifier. *Burn Dressing* Poultice of moistened, powdered stems applied to burns. *Cathartic* Decoction of root or salted decoction of stems taken as a physic. *Cold Remedy* Infusion or decoction of twigs or branches taken for

colds. *Dermatological Aid* Dried, powdered stems alone or mixed with pitch and used as a salve for sores. *Gastrointestinal Aid* Infusion or decoction of twigs or branches taken for stomach disorders. *Kidney Aid* Infusion or decoction of twigs or branches taken as a kidney regulator. *Pediatric Aid* Compound infusion of plant given to children for diarrhea. *Tonic* Infusion or decoction of twigs or branches taken as a tonic. *Urinary Aid* Infusion or decoction of twigs or branches used as a kidney regulator and for bladder. *Venereal Aid* Simple or compound decoctions of plant parts taken for syphilis or gonorrhea. (155:68–70) **Tewa** *Tonic* Dried flowers and stems taken as a tonic. *Venereal Aid* Plant used for syphilis. (34:312) **Tubatulabal** *Blood Medicine* Decoction of stalks and leaves used for the blood. *Venereal Aid* Decoction of stalks and leaves used for syphilis. (167:59) **Washo** *Gynecological Aid* Infusion or decoction of twigs or branch used for delayed or difficult menstruation. (155:68–70)

Epifagus virginiana, Beech Drops
Iroquois *Antidiarrheal* Infusion of plants taken for diarrhea caused by menstruating women. (73:437)

Epigaea repens, Trailing Arbutus
Algonquin, Quebec *Kidney Aid* Infusion of leaves used for kidney disorders. (14:216) **Cherokee** *Analgesic* Decoction of plant taken to cause vomiting for abdominal pains. *Antidiarrheal* Infusion of plant given to children with diarrhea. *Emetic* Decoction of plant taken to cause vomiting for abdominal pains. (152:48) *Gastrointestinal Aid* Compound infusion taken for indigestion. (66:23) Decoction of plant taken to cause vomiting for abdominal pains. (152:48) *Kidney Aid* Infusion taken for kidneys and "chest ailment." (66:23) *Pediatric Aid* Infusion of plant given to children with diarrhea. (152:48) *Pulmonary Aid* Infusion used for "chest ailment." (66:23) **Iroquois** *Analgesic* Compound used for labor pains in parturition. *Antirheumatic (Internal)* Compound decoction of plant taken for rheumatism. *Gastrointestinal Aid* Decoction of leaves taken to aid digestion. *Gynecological Aid* Compound used for labor pains in parturition. *Kidney Aid* Decoction of whole plant or

roots, stalks, and leaves taken for the kidneys. (73:410)

Epilobium angustifolium, Fireweed
Abnaki *Cough Medicine* Roots used for coughs. (121:154) **Algonquin, Tête-de-Boule** *Dermatological Aid* Poultice of boiled roots applied to "sick" skin. (110:128) **Bella Coola** *Dermatological Aid* Poultice of roasted and mashed root applied to boils. (127:60) Poultice of roasted and mashed roots applied to boils. (158:207) **Blackfoot** *Dermatological Aid* Powdered inner cortex rubbed on the hands and face to protect them from the cold during the winter. (72:112) *Laxative* and *Pediatric Aid* Infusion of roots and inner cortex given to babies as an enema for constipation. (72:66) **Chippewa** *Dermatological Aid* Poultice of moistened fresh or dried leaf used for bruises or to remove a sliver. (43:352) **Cree, Woodlands** *Dermatological Aid* Poultice of barked, macerated roots applied to boils, abscesses, or wounds to draw out the infection. Poultice of leaves applied to bruises. Poultice of barked, chewed roots applied to cuts and wounds. (91:38) **Eskimo, Alaska** *Laxative* Infusion of old, dry leaves used as a laxative. (1:36) **Eskimo, Western** *Analgesic* and *Gastrointestinal Aid* Compound decoction of leaves taken for stomachache and intestinal discomfort. (90:5) **Iroquois** *Analgesic* Infusion of bark applied as poultice for pain anywhere in the body. *Basket Medicine* Infusion of plant used as a "basket medicine." *Internal Medicine* Decoction of roots taken for internal injuries from lifting.

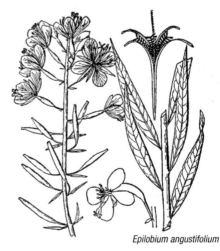

Epilobium angustifolium

(73:389) *Kidney Aid* Compound infusion of roots taken for kidneys or for male urination problems. *Orthopedic Aid* Poultice of smashed roots applied to swollen knees. (73:390) *Panacea* Compound infusion of twigs and roots taken as a panacea for pain. *Tuberculosis Remedy* Compound decoction of roots taken for consumption. *Urinary Aid* Infusion of roots taken for burning urination and other urination problems. *Witchcraft Medicine* Compound decoction of plants and a doll used for black magic. (73:389) **Kwakiutl** *Cancer Treatment* Poultice of seeds, down, and oil applied to wound after cutting open the tumor. *Dermatological Aid* Poultice of seeds, down, and oil applied to wound after cutting open the tumor. (157:287) **Menominee** *Dermatological Aid* Root used to make a wash for swellings. (128:43) **Navajo, Kayenta** *Gastrointestinal Aid* Plant used for gastritis. (179:32) **Ojibwa** *Dermatological Aid* Poultice of pounded root applied to boils and carbuncles. (130:376) **Potawatomi** *Unspecified* Plant used as a medicine for unspecified ailments. (131:66) **Skokomish** *Tuberculosis Remedy* Infusion of roots taken for tuberculosis. **Snohomish** *Throat Aid* Infusion of roots taken for sore throats. **Swinomish** *Other* Decoction of whole plants used as a bath for invalids. *Poison* Infusion of plant considered poisonous. (65:41) **Thompson** *Dermatological Aid* Decoction of plant used as a wash for sores. (161:235)

Epilobium angustifolium ssp. *angustifolium*, Fireweed

Cheyenne *Antihemorrhagic* Infusion of dried leaves or dried roots taken for bowel hemorrhages. (as *Chamoenerion angustifolium* 63:181) Infusion of dried, pulverized leaves taken for bowel hemorrhage. (as *Chamaenerion angustifolium* 64:181) *Gastrointestinal Aid* Infusion of dried leaves or dried roots taken for bowel hemorrhages. (as *Chamoenerion angustifolium* 63:181)

Epilobium brachycarpum, Autumn Willowweed

Okanagan-Colville *Dermatological Aid* Infusion of plant tops applied to the hair as a conditioner for dandruff and hair manageability. (as *E. paniculatum* 162:111)

Epilobium canum ssp. *angustifolium*, Hummingbird Trumpet

Costanoan *Dermatological Aid* Decoction of plant used for infected sores. *Disinfectant* Decoction of plant used for infected sores. *Febrifuge* Decoction of plant used for infant's fever. *Panacea* Decoction of plant used as a general remedy. *Pediatric Aid* Decoction of plant used for infant's fever. *Urinary Aid* Decoction of plant used for urinary problems. (as *Zauschneria californica* 17:22) **Miwok** *Antihemorrhagic* Used by women after parturition for hemorrhages. *Cathartic* Decoction of leaves taken as a cathartic. *Gynecological Aid* Used by women after parturition for hemorrhages. *Kidney Aid* Decoction of leaves taken for kidney trouble. *Tuberculosis Remedy* Decoction of leaves taken for tuberculosis. *Urinary Aid* Decoction of leaves taken for bladder trouble. *Venereal Aid* Used for syphilis. (as *Zauschneria californica* 8:174)

Epilobium ciliatum ssp. *ciliatum*, Coast Willowweed

Hopi *Analgesic* Plant used for leg pains. (as *E. adenocaulon* 174:33, 86) **Navajo, Kayenta** *Orthopedic Aid* Infusion used as lotion and poultice of roots applied to muscular cramps. (as *E. adenocaulon* 179:32) **Potawatomi** *Antidiarrheal* Infusion of root used "to check diarrhea." (as *E. adenocaulon* 131:66)

Epilobium latifolium, Dwarf Fireweed

Eskimo, Inupiat *Dermatological Aid* Leaves, rich in vitamins A and C, eaten for healthy, beautiful skin. *Eye Medicine* Leaves, rich in vitamins A and C, eaten for healthy, beautiful eyes. (83:26)

Epilobium minutum, Small Willowweed

Okanagan-Colville *Antidiarrheal* and *Pediatric Aid* Infusion of roots and stems given to children for diarrhea. (162:111)

Epipactis gigantea, Giant Helleborine

Navajo, Kayenta *Ceremonial Medicine* Plant used in girl's puberty rite. *Other* Plant used for general body disease. *Pediatric Aid* Plant used to purify a newborn infant and plant used in girl's puberty rite. (179:17)

Epixiphium wislizeni, Balloonbush
Keres, **Western** *Antirheumatic* (*External*)
Leaves heated with stones and rubbed on swellings. *Snakebite Remedy* Leaves heated with stones and rubbed onto snakebites. (as *Maurandia wislizeni* 147:53)

Equisetum arvense, Field Horsetail
Blackfoot *Dermatological Aid* Poultice of stem pieces applied to rash under the arm and in the groin. (72:76) *Diuretic* Infusion of fertile stem roots used as a powerful diuretic. (72:69) *Orthopedic Aid* Powdered stems put in moccasins to avoid foot cramps when traveling long distances. (72:112) *Veterinary Aid* Infusion of fertile stem roots given to horses as a diuretic. Infusion of fertile stem roots rubbed on the groins of horses. Powdered stems and water given to perk a horse up. (72:88) **Cherokee** *Kidney Aid* Infusion taken for kidneys. *Laxative* Strong infusion taken for constipation. (66:39) **Cheyenne** *Veterinary Aid* Infusion of stems and leaves given to horses for coughs. (63:169) Infusion of leaves and stems given to horses with a hard cough. (64:169) **Chippewa** *Urinary Aid* Decoction of stems taken for dysuria. (59:122) **Iroquois** *Analgesic* Used for headaches and pains. *Antirheumatic* (*Internal*) Used for rheumatism. *Orthopedic Aid* Used for joint aches. *Pediatric Aid* Raw stems chewed by teething babies. (73:261) Infusion of rhizomes and hazel stems given to children for teething. (118:33) *Toothache Remedy* Raw stems chewed by teething babies. (73:261) Infusion of rhizomes and hazel stems given to children for teething. (118:33) **Kwakiutl** *Dermatological Aid* Poultice of rough leaves and stems applied to cuts and sores. (157: 263) **Ojibwa** *Kidney Aid* Infusion of whole plant used for dropsy. (130:368) **Okanagan-Colville** *Antirheumatic* (*Internal*) Infusion of stems taken for lumbago. *Dermatological Aid* Plant pounded, mixed with water, and used to wash areas of the body affected by poison ivy. *Diuretic* Infusion of stems taken as a diuretic to stimulate the kidneys. *Orthopedic Aid* Infusion of stems taken for backaches. *Stimulant* Infusion of stems taken for sluggishness due to a cold. *Venereal Aid* Decoction of plant and false box taken or used as a bath for syphilis and gonorrhea. *Veterinary Aid* Given to thin, old horses with diarrhea after eating fresh

grass in spring. (162:17) **Pomo**, **Kashaya** *Dermatological Aid* Decoction of plant used as a wash for itching or open sores. (60:58) **Potawatomi** *Analgesic* Infusion of whole plant used for lumbago. *Kidney Aid* Infusion of plant used for kidney trouble. *Orthopedic Aid* Infusion of plant used for lumbago. *Urinary Aid* Infusion of plant used for bladder trouble. (131:55, 56) **Saanich** *Blood Medicine* Tender, young shoots eaten raw or boiled and thought to be "good for the blood." (156:68) **Thompson** *Dermatological Aid* Decoction or infusion of stems used after childbirth to expel the afterbirth more quickly. *Urinary Aid* Decoction of new plant tops taken for "stoppage of urine." (161:86)

Equisetum hyemale, Scouringrush Horsetail
Blackfoot *Veterinary Aid* Infusion used as a drench for horse medicine. (68:58) Decoction of foliage used in horse medicine as a drench. (82:16) Decoction of plant used as a horse medicine. (95:276) **Carrier** *Kidney Aid* Decoction of plant taken for kidney problems. *Urinary Aid* Decoction of plant taken for the inability to pass water. (26:84) **Cherokee** *Kidney Aid* Infusion taken for kidneys. *Laxative* Strong infusion taken for constipation. (66:39) **Cheyenne** *Veterinary Aid* Plant used as a medicine for horses. (69:4) **Chippewa** *Disinfectant* Leaves burned as a disinfectant. (43: 366) **Cree** *Abortifacient* Used for irregular menstruation. (68:58) Decoction of plant and two unknown roots used to correct menstrual irregulari-

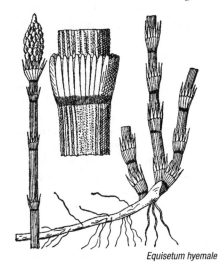

Equisetum hyemale

ties. (82:16) **Crow** *Analgesic* Poultice used for bladder and prostate pains. *Diuretic* Infusion of stems used as a diuretic. **Flathead** *Diuretic* Infusion of stems used as a diuretic. (68:58) **Hoh** *Ceremonial Medicine* Rootstocks eaten during medicinal ceremonies. (114:57) **Iroquois** *Urinary Aid* Infusion of rhizomes taken by old people "when the urine is too red." (118:33) **Karok** *Ceremonial Medicine* Plant used in ceremonial cleansing for the priests in First Salmon ceremony. *Eye Medicine* Decoction of plant used as a wash or poultice of stalks applied for sore eyes. (125:378) **Mahuna** *Urinary Aid* Infusion of dried plants taken for prostate gland troubles. (117:21) **Makah** *Antidiarrheal* Raw shoots chewed for diarrhea. (65:15) **Menominee** *Gynecological Aid* Decoction of rushes taken after childbirth "to clear up the system." *Kidney Aid* Decoction of rushes taken for kidney troubles. (128:34) **Meskwaki** *Venereal Aid* Infusion of whole plant taken by both men and women for gonorrhea. (129:220) **Ojibwa** *Unspecified* Plant used as a medicine. (130:418) **Okanagan-Colville** *Antirheumatic* (*Internal*) Infusion of stems taken for lumbago. *Dermatological Aid* Decoction of stems used as a wash on children for skin sores. Plant pounded, mixed with water, and used to wash areas of the body affected by poison ivy. *Diuretic* Infusion of stems taken as a diuretic to stimulate the kidneys. *Eye Medicine* Stem fluid used as an eyewash. *Orthopedic Aid* Infusion of stems taken for backaches. *Pediatric Aid* Decoction of stems used as a wash on children for skin sores. *Stimulant* Infusion of stems taken for sluggishness due to a cold. *Venereal Aid* Decoction of plant and false box taken or used as a bath for syphilis and gonorrhea. *Veterinary Aid* Given to thin, old horses with diarrhea after eating fresh grass in spring. (162:17) **Quileute** *Ceremonial Medicine* Rootstocks eaten during medicinal ceremonies. (114:57) *Sports Medicine* Plant rubbed on swimmers to make them feel strong. **Quinault** *Abortifacient* Decoction taken to regulate menses, informant insisted not an abortive. *Eye Medicine* Infusion of roots or root juice used as a wash for sore eyes. (65:15) **Sanpoil** *Adjuvant* Used as a drinking tube for medicine and used for giving medicine to infants. *Pediatric Aid* Used as a drinking tube for medicine and used for giving medicine to infants. (109:218) **Thompson** *Eye Medicine*

Stem liquid used for sore eyes or decoction of stems used for sore, itchy eyes or cataracts. *Gynecological Aid* Decoction of roots taken during difficult childbirth, to accelerate it. Decoction or infusion of stems taken after childbirth to expel the afterbirth more quickly. *Urinary Aid* Decoction of new growths taken for bladder trouble. (161:86)

Equisetum hyemale var. *affine*, Scouringrush Horsetail

Iroquois *Diuretic* Decoction of plant taken for urinating too infrequently. *Eye Medicine* Infusion of whole plant used as an eyewash for white spot on the eye. *Kidney Aid* Decoction of plant taken for kidney trouble. *Other* Decoction of plant taken for backache or "summer complaint." *Urinary Aid* Decoction of plant taken for urinating too much. Decoction used by women with excessive urination who are ruptured. *Venereal Aid* Compound decoction of roots taken for gonorrhea. (73:262)

Equisetum laevigatum, Smooth Horsetail

Costanoan *Abortifacient* Decoction of plant used for retarded menstruation. *Contraceptive* Decoction of plant used as a contraceptive. *Dermatological Aid* Decoction of stalks used as a hair wash. *Urinary Aid* Decoction of plant used for bladder ailments. (17:4) **Diegueño** *Hypotensive* Infusion of stems taken for high blood pressure. (70:19) **Hoh** *Ceremonial Medicine* Rootstocks eaten during medicinal ceremonies. (114:57) **Hopi** *Ceremonial Medicine* Dried, ground plant used for ceremonial bread. (46:17) **Keres, Western** *Hemorrhoid Remedy* Plant chewed before meals for piles. (147:42) **Navajo, Kayenta** *Analgesic* and *Orthopedic Aid* Infusion of plant taken or cold infusion used as a lotion for backaches. (as *E. kansanum* 179:15) **Navajo, Ramah** *Disinfectant* Compound decoction of plant used for "lightning infection." (165:11) **Okanagan-Colville** *Antirheumatic* (*Internal*) Infusion of stems taken for lumbago. *Cold Remedy* Decoction of plant and chokecherry twigs given to children for colds. *Dermatological Aid* Plant pounded, mixed with water, and used to wash areas of the body affected by poison ivy. *Diuretic* Infusion of stems taken as a diuretic to stimulate the kidneys. *Orthopedic Aid* Infusion of stems taken for backaches. *Pediatric Aid* Decoction of plant and chokecherry twigs given to children for colds. *Stimulant* Infusion of stems taken for sluggishness due to a cold. *Venereal Aid* Decoction of plant and false box taken or used as a bath for syphilis and gonorrhea. *Veterinary Aid* Given to thin, old horses with diarrhea after eating fresh grass in spring. (162:17) **Okanagon** *Burn Dressing* Poultice of plant ash and grease applied to burns. (104:41) **Pomo, Kashaya** *Kidney Aid* Decoction of whole plant taken for kidney trouble and associated back trouble. (as *E. funstoni* 60:59) **Quileute** *Ceremonial Medicine* Rootstocks eaten during medicinal ceremonies. (114:57) **Thompson** *Burn Dressing* Poultice of plant ash and grease applied to burns. (104:41) *Eye Medicine* Stem liquid used for sore eyes or decoction of stems used for sore, itchy eyes or blindness. *Gynecological Aid* Decoction of roots taken to accelerate a difficult childbirth. Decoction or infusion of stems taken after childbirth to expel the afterbirth more quickly. *Urinary Aid* Decoction of new growths taken for bladder trouble. (161:86)

Equisetum palustre, Marsh Horsetail
Ojibwa *Gastrointestinal Aid* Infusion or decoction of plants taken for stomach or bowel troubles. *Laxative* Decoction of plants taken for sick stomach, bowels, or for constipation. (112:231)

Equisetum sylvaticum, Woodland Horsetail
Eskimo, Alaska *Antihemorrhagic* Infusion of branches and stems used for internal bleeding. Green plants could be used, but a stronger medicine could be made from plants collected in autumn. The plant was also dried for future use, but only the stems and branches were used. The tea from this plant was strong and bitter. (1:33) **Menominee** *Hemostat* Poultice of pulverized stem applied to stop bleeding. *Kidney Aid* Infusion of stems used for dropsy. (128:35) **Ojibwa** *Kidney Aid* Infusion of plant used for kidney trouble and dropsy. (130:368)

Equisetum telmateia, Giant Horsetail
Kwakiutl *Dermatological Aid* Poultice of rough leaves and stems applied to cuts and sores. (157:263) **Saanich** *Blood Medicine* Tender, young shoots eaten raw or boiled and thought to be "good for the blood." (156:68) **Thompson** *Urinary Aid* Decoction of new plant tops used for

"stoppage of urine." (161:86) **Yuki** *Diuretic* Decoction of plant taken as a diuretic. (39:47)

Equisetum telmateia* var. *braunii, Giant Horsetail
Pomo, Kashaya *Gynecological Aid* Decoction of stem taken for menstrual cramps. (60:58) **Tolowa** *Oral Aid* and *Pediatric Aid* Stem rubbed on child's teeth to keep them from gritting their teeth. (5:29)

Equisetum variegatum, Variegated Scouring-rush
Yuki *Eye Medicine* Plant used for sore eyes. (33:304)

Eremocrinum albomarginatum, Lonely Lily
Navajo, Kayenta *Snakebite Remedy* Plant used for snakebites. (179:17)

Eriastrum densifolium, Giant Woolstar
Kawaiisu *Dermatological Aid* and *Venereal Aid* Dried, pounded flowers and roots used as a salve for venereal sores. (180:28)

Eriastrum eremicum, Desert Woolstar
Paiute *Antidiarrheal* Decoction of plant taken for diarrhea. *Gastrointestinal Aid* Decoction of plant taken as a stomach medicine. *Pediatric Aid* Infusion of plant used for children with tuberculosis. *Tuberculosis Remedy* Infusion of plant used for children with tuberculosis. (as *Gilia eremica* var. *arizonica* 155:80)

Eriastrum filifolium, Lavender Woolstar
Paiute *Cathartic* Decoction of plant taken as a physic. *Emetic* Decoction of plant taken as an emetic. **Shoshoni** *Analgesic* and *Antirheumatic* (*External*) Decoction of plant used as a bath for rheumatic pains. *Cathartic* Decoction of plant taken as a physic. *Emetic* Decoction of plant taken as an emetic. *Venereal Aid* Decoction of plant taken for venereal disease. (as *Gilia filifolia* var. *sparsiflora* 155:80, 81)

Eriastrum sparsiflorum, Great Basin Woolstar
Paiute, Northern *Gastrointestinal Aid* Decoction of stalks taken as an emetic for stomach troubles. (49:128)

Eriastrum virgatum, Wand Woolstar
Paiute *Throat Aid* Decoction of entire plant used as a gargle for sore throats. (as *Hugelia virgata* 144:317)

Ericameria arborescens, Goldenfleece
Miwok *Antirheumatic* (*External*) Decoction of leaves used for rheumatism. Poultice of twigs and leaves applied to rheumatic parts. *Dermatological Aid* Poultice of leaves applied to bring boils to a head. *Gastrointestinal Aid* Decoction of leaves taken for stomach trouble. *Gynecological Aid* Decoction of leaves taken during menstruation and after parturition for pain. *Orthopedic Aid* Poultice of leaves applied to foot sores. (as *Haplopappus aborescens* 8:170)

Ericameria bloomeri, Rabbitbush Heathgoldenrod
Klamath *Dermatological Aid* Poultice of leaves used to draw blisters. (as *Chrysothamnus bloomeri* 37:106) Poultice of smashed leaves applied to blisters. (as *Chrysothamnus bloomeri* 140:131)

Ericameria brachylepis, Chaparral Heathgoldenrod
Diegueño *Dermatological Aid* Decoction of fresh or dried, entire plant used as a wash for wounds. *Misc. Disease Remedy* Decoction of fresh or dried, entire plant taken for "pasmo," a malady with chills. (as *Aplopappus propinquus* 74:219)

Ericameria cooperi, Cooper's Heathgoldenrod
Tubatulabal *Antirheumatic* (*External*) Compound decoction of stalks and flowers used as a wash for rheumatism. (as *E. monactis* 167:59)

Ericameria cuneata var. **cuneata**, Cliff Heathgoldenrod
Miwok *Cold Remedy* Decoction of stems taken for colds. (as *Haplopappus cuneatus* 8:170)

Ericameria linearifolia, Narrowleaf Heathgoldenrod
Kawaiisu *Antirheumatic* (*External*) Decoction of leaves and flowers applied to limbs for rheumatism. *Dermatological Aid* Decoction of leaves and flowers applied to soreness, bruises, and cuts.

Decoction of roots used as a hair wash to make the hair grow. *Orthopedic Aid* Decoction of roots used as a wash for tired feet. *Veterinary Aid* Decoction of leaves and flowers applied to sore backs of horses. (as *Haplopappus linearifolius* var. *interior* 180:33) **Tubatulabal** *Antirheumatic* (*External*) Compound decoction of leaves and flowers used as a wash for rheumatism. (as *Stenotopsis linearifolius* 167:59)

Ericameria nana, Dwarf Heathgoldenrod
Paiute *Antidiarrheal* Decoction of plant taken for diarrhea. *Cold Remedy* Decoction of flowering heads and stems or stems alone used for colds. *Cough Medicine* Decoction of flowering heads and stems used for coughs and colds. *Eye Medicine* Decoction of roots used as a wash for sore eyes. *Febrifuge* Decoction of whole plant taken for high fevers. *Gastrointestinal Aid* Decoction of whole plant taken for stomach troubles. *Misc. Disease Remedy* Decoction of whole plant taken for grippe and high fever. **Shoshoni** *Analgesic* Decoction of flowering tops taken for stomachaches or stomach cramps. *Cold Remedy* Decoction of flowering heads and stems or whole plant used for colds. *Cough Medicine* Decoction of flowering heads and stems used for coughs and colds. *Eye Medicine* Decoction of roots used as a wash for sore eyes. *Gastrointestinal Aid* Decoction of flowering tops taken for stomachaches or cramps. (as *Aplopappus nanus* 155:36)

Ericameria palmeri var. **palmeri**, Palmer's Heathgoldenrod
Cahuilla *Dermatological Aid* Poultice of boiled leaves applied to sores. *Throat Aid* Leaves soaked in a pan of boiling water and steam inhaled for sore throats. (as *Haplopappus palmeri* 11:75) **Coahuilla** *Analgesic* Poultice of leaves and twigs applied to feet for swelling and pain. *Orthopedic Aid* Hot poultice of leaves and twigs bound to feet for swelling and pain. (as *Aplopappus palmeri* 9:78)

Ericameria parishii, Parish's Heathgoldenrod
Luiseño *Unspecified* Plant used for medicinal purposes. (as *Bigelovia parishii* 132:228)

Erigenia bulbosa, Harbinger of Spring
Cherokee *Toothache Remedy* Chewed for toothache. (66:48)

Erigeron aphanactis var. **aphanactis**,
  Rayless Shaggy Fleabane
Paiute *Analgesic* Decoction of whole plant taken for stomachaches and cramps. *Cathartic* Decoction of whole plant, a violent remedy, taken as a physic. *Emetic* Decoction of whole plant, a violent remedy, taken as an emetic. *Gastrointestinal Aid* Decoction of plant taken for stomachaches and cramps. **Shoshoni** *Analgesic* Decoction of whole plant taken for stomachaches and cramps. *Eye Medicine* Decoction of plant used as an eyewash. *Gastrointestinal Aid* Decoction of plant taken for stomachaches and cramps. (as *E. concinnus* var. *aphanactis* 155:70, 71)

Erigeron bellidiastrum, Western Daisy
  Fleabane
Navajo, **Ramah** *Ceremonial Medicine* Cold infusion of dried leaves used as ceremonial chant lotion. (165:50)

Erigeron caespitosus, Tufted Fleabane
Paiute *Antidiarrheal* Strong decoction of root taken for diarrhea. *Eye Medicine* Cool decoction of root used as an eyewash. (155:70)

Erigeron canus, Hoary Fleabane
Navajo, **Ramah** *Ceremonial Medicine* Plant used in ceremonial chant lotion. *Disinfectant* Plant used for "deer infection." (165:50)

Erigeron compositus, Cutleaf Daisy
Thompson *Dermatological Aid* Plant chewed, possibly taken internally, and spit on sores. (141:465) *Orthopedic Aid* Decoction of plant and any kind of "weeds" used for broken bones. (161:180)

Erigeron concinnus, Navajo Fleabane
Navajo, **Ramah** *Analgesic* Cold infusion taken and used as lotion for general body pain. *Disinfectant* Plant used for "antelope infection." (165:50) **Shoshoni** *Venereal Aid* Infusion of whole plant taken for gonorrhea. (98:47)

Erigeron concinnus var. **condensatus**,
  Navajo Fleabane
Navajo, **Kayenta** *Analgesic* Plant used as a lotion for headaches. *Gynecological Aid* Plant used for difficult labor. (179:47)

Erigeron divergens, Spreading Fleabane
Navajo *Gynecological Aid* Infusion of plant taken by women as an aid for deliverance. (45:85)
Navajo, **Kayenta** *Analgesic* Plant used as a snuff for headaches. (179:47) **Navajo**, **Ramah** *Ceremonial Medicine* Plant used ceremonially in several ways. *Disinfectant* Cold infusion of plant taken and used as a lotion for "lightning infection." *Eye Medicine* Cold, compound infusion of plant used as an eyewash. *Panacea* Root used as a "life medicine." *Snakebite Remedy* Compound used for snakebites. (165:50)

Erigeron eximius, Sprucefir Fleabane
Navajo, **Ramah** *Ceremonial Medicine* Cold infusion of plant taken and used ceremonially as a lotion for various ills. *Cough Medicine* Cold infusion of plant taken and used as a lotion for cough. *Febrifuge* Cold infusion of plant taken and used as a lotion for fever. *Hunting Medicine* Infusion of plant used internally and externally for protection in warfare or hunting. *Misc. Disease Remedy* Cold infusion of plant taken and used as a lotion for influenza. *Witchcraft Medicine* Cold infusion of plant taken and used as a lotion for protection from witches. (as *E. superbus* 165:51)

Erigeron filifolius, Threadleaf Fleabane
Thompson *Dermatological Aid* Toasted, powdered stems and leaves sprinkled on sores, cuts, and wounds. (141:473) Plant chewed, possibly taken internally, and spit on sores. (141:465) *Unspecified* Decoction of plant and any kind of "weeds" used for broken bones. (161:180)

Erigeron flagellaris, Trailing Fleabane
Navajo, **Ramah** *Ceremonial Medicine* Cold infusion of leaves used ceremonially as a medicine and as a fumigant. (as *E. nudiflorus* 165:50, 51) *Dermatological Aid* Poultice of chewed leaves applied to spider bites and used as a hemostat. (165:50) *Disinfectant* Cold infusion of leaves used ceremonially for "lightning infection." (as *E. nudiflorus*

165:50, 51) *Hemostat* Poultice of chewed leaves applied as a hemostatic. *Snakebite Remedy* Compound poultice of plant applied to snakebite. *Veterinary Aid* Cold infusion of leaves used as eyewash for livestock. (as *E. nudiflorus* 165:50, 51)

Erigeron foliosus var. stenophyllus, Leafy
   Fleabane
Kawaiisu *Analgesic* Infusion of roots used as a wash for headaches. *Toothache Remedy* Root held between the teeth for toothache. (180:28) **Miwok** *Dermatological Aid* Decoction of root and vinegar weed used as a bath for pustules and skin eruptions from smallpox. (8:173, 174) *Febrifuge* Decoction of washed and pounded root taken for fever. *Misc. Disease Remedy* Decoction of washed and pounded root taken for ague. *Toothache Remedy* Root chewed and placed in cavity. (8:169)

Erigeron formosissimus, Beautiful Fleabane
Navajo, Ramah *Hunting Medicine* Cold, compound infusion taken and used as lotion for good luck in hunting. (165:50)

Erigeron grandiflorus, Largeflower Fleabane
Gosiute *Poison* Roots used for arrow poison. (31:368)

Erigeron linearis, Desert Yellow Fleabane
Okanagan-Colville *Tuberculosis Remedy* Decoction of whole plant taken for tuberculosis. (162:83)

Erigeron neomexicanus, New Mexico
   Fleabane
Navajo, Kayenta *Dermatological Aid* Powdered plant applied to dog or bear bite sores. *Gastrointestinal Aid* Plant used for stomachaches caused by eating unripe fruit. (179:47)

Erigeron peregrinus ssp. callianthemus,
   Subalpine Fleabane
Cheyenne *Analgesic* and *Orthopedic Aid* Infusion of roots, stems, and flowers used as steam bath for backaches. (as *E. salsuginosus* 63:187) Infusion of dried, pulverized roots, stems, and flowers used as a steam bath or taken for backaches. *Other* Infusion of dried, pulverized roots, stems, and flowers used as a steam bath or taken for dizziness. (as *E. salsuginosus* 64:187) *Stimulant* Infusion of roots,

stems and flowers used as steam bath when dizzy and drowsy. (as *E. salsuginosus* 63:187) Infusion of dried, pulverized roots, stems, and flowers used as a steam bath or taken for drowsiness. (as *E. salsuginosus* 64:187)

Erigeron philadelphicus, Philadelphia
   Fleabane
Blackfoot *Antidiarrheal* Plant used for chronic diarrhea. *Antihemorrhagic* Plant used for childbirth hemorrhage. (82:56) **Cherokee** *Abortifacient* Taken for "suppressed menstruation." *Analgesic* Used as a poultice for headache. *Anticonvulsive* and *Antihemorrhagic* Used for hemorrhages, "spitting of blood," and epilepsy. *Cold Remedy* Cold infusion of root taken and root chewed for colds. *Cough Medicine* Taken for coughs. *Dermatological Aid* Astringent plant boiled, mixed with tallow, and used on sores. Boiled plant mixed with tallow and used on sores. *Diaphoretic* Used as a sudorific. *Diuretic* Used as a diuretic. *Eye Medicine* Taken for "dimness of sight." *Kidney Aid* Taken for gout and infusion taken "for kidneys." (66:35) **Houma** *Gynecological Aid* Decoction of root taken for "menstruation troubles." (135:62) **Iroquois** *Dermatological Aid* Compound infusion of plants used as wash for poison ivy and itch. Poultice of plants applied to running sores. *Pulmonary Aid* Decoction of whole plant taken to open the lungs. (73:464) **Meskwaki** *Analgesic* Snuff of powdered florets used for sick headaches. (129:213, 21) *Cold Remedy* Powdered disk florets used

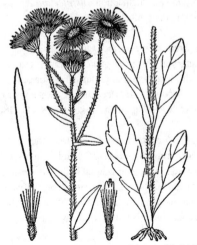

Erigeron philadelphicus

as snuff to make one sneeze for cold or catarrh. (129:213) *Respiratory Aid* Snuff of powdered florets used to make patient sneeze for catarrh. (129:213, 214) **Ojibwa** *Cold Remedy* Smoke of dried flowers inhaled for head cold. Snuff of pulverized flowers used to cause sneezing to loosen head colds. *Febrifuge* Infusion of flowers used to break fevers. (130:364) **Okanagan-Colville** *Analgesic* Infusion of leaves and blossoms taken for headaches. (162:83)

Erigeron pulchellus, Robin's Plantain
Cherokee *Abortifacient* Taken for "suppressed menstruation." *Analgesic* Used as a poultice for headache. *Anticonvulsive* and *Antihemorrhagic* Used for hemorrhages, "spitting of blood," and epilepsy. *Cold Remedy* Cold infusion of root taken and root chewed for colds. *Cough Medicine* Taken for coughs. *Dermatological Aid* Astringent plant boiled, mixed with tallow, and used on sores. Boiled plant mixed with tallow and used on sores. *Diaphoretic* Used as a sudorific. *Diuretic* Used as a diuretic. *Eye Medicine* Taken for "dimness of sight." *Kidney Aid* Taken for gout and infusion taken "for kidneys." (66:35) **Iroquois** *Cold Remedy* Decoction of roots taken for colds. *Cough Medicine* Decoction of roots taken for coughs. *Tuberculosis Remedy* Decoction of plants and flowers taken for consumption. (73:464)

Erigeron pumilus, Shaggy Fleabane
Okanagan-Colville *Eye Medicine* Infusion of roots used to wash the eyes as an "eye tonic." (162:84)

Erigeron speciosus var. ***macranthus***, Aspen Fleabane
Navajo, Ramah *Analgesic* Compound decoction taken for menstrual pain and as a contraceptive. *Contraceptive* Compound decoction of plant used as a contraceptive. *Gynecological Aid* Compound decoction of plant used for menstrual pain. (as *E. macranthus* 165:50)

Erigeron strigosus var. ***strigosus***, Prairie Fleabane
Catawba *Heart Medicine* Infusion of roots taken for heart troubles. (as *E. ramosus* 134:191) Infusion of roots taken for heart troubles. (as *E. ramo-*

sus 152:61) **Ojibwa** *Analgesic* Plant used for sick headache. (as *E. ramosus* 130:364)

Eriodictyon angustifolium, Narrowleaf Yerbasanta
Hualapai *Dermatological Aid* Decoction of leaves used as a wash for cuts. *Gastrointestinal Aid* Decoction of leaves taken for indigestion. *Laxative* Decoction of leaves taken as a laxative. *Orthopedic Aid* Decoction of leaves used as a wash for tired feet. (169:48) **Paiute** *Antidiarrheal* Decoction of leaves taken for diarrhea. *Antiemetic* Decoction of leaves taken for vomiting. *Cold Remedy* Decoction of leaves or shoots taken for colds. *Cough Medicine* Decoction of leaves or shoots taken for coughs. *Expectorant* Decoction of leaves or plant tops used as an expectorant for lungs or tuberculosis. *Pulmonary Aid* Infusion of leaves or tops taken as an expectorant for pulmonary troubles. *Tuberculosis Remedy* Decoction of leaves or plant tops used as an expectorant for lungs or tuberculosis. **Shoshoni** *Analgesic* Infusion of leaves taken for stomachaches. Poultice of decoction of stems, leaves, and flowers applied for rheumatic pains. *Antirheumatic* (*External*) Decoction of plant used in hot compresses for rheumatic pains. *Cold Remedy* Decoction of leaves or shoots taken for colds. *Cough Medicine* Decoction of leaves or shoots taken for coughs. *Expectorant* Decoction of leaves or plant tops used as an expectorant for lungs or tuberculosis. *Gastrointestinal Aid* Decoction of leaves taken for stomachaches. *Pulmonary Aid* Infusion of leaves or tops taken as an expectorant for pulmonary troubles. *Tuberculosis Remedy* Decoction of leaves or plant tops used as an expectorant for lungs or tuberculosis. *Venereal Aid* Decoction of leaves taken for venereal disease. (155:71, 72)

Eriodictyon californicum, California Yerbasanta
Atsugewi *Antirheumatic* (*External*) Branches and leaves used in a steam bath for rheumatism. Steam of burned branches and leaves used for rheumatism. *Cold Remedy* Juice of chewed plant used for colds. Plant chewed and juice swallowed for colds. *Herbal Steam* Branches and leaves used in a steam bath for rheumatism. *Pulmonary Aid* Plant chewed and juice swallowed for whooping

cough. Juice of chewed plant used for whooping cough. (50:140) **Coahuilla** *Analgesic* Decoction of leaves used as a wash for "sore parts" or painful, fatigued limbs. *Dermatological Aid* Poultice of leaves applied to men and animals with sores. *Orthopedic Aid* Decoction of leaves used as a wash for painful or fatigued limbs. *Veterinary Aid* Poultice of leaves applied to men and animals with sores. (9:78) **Costanoan** *Analgesic* Poultice of heated leaves applied to the forehead for headaches. *Antirheumatic (External)* Decoction of plant used for rheumatism. *Blood Medicine* Decoction of plant used to purify the blood. *Cold Remedy* Infusion of plant used for colds. *Dermatological Aid* and *Disinfectant* Plant combined with other herbs and used for infected sores. *Eye Medicine* Infusion of plant used as an eyewash. *Respiratory Aid* Decoction of plant used or leaves chewed or smoked for asthma. *Tuberculosis Remedy* Decoction of plant used for tuberculosis. (17:13) **Karok** *Cold Remedy* Decoction of leaves taken for colds. *Pulmonary Aid* Decoction of leaves taken for pleurisy. *Tuberculosis Remedy* Decoction of leaves taken for tuberculosis. (125:388) **Kawaiisu** *Cold Remedy* Infusion of leaves taken as a cold medicine. *Gastrointestinal Aid* Infusion of leaves used for stomach problems. *Venereal Aid* Infusion of leaves taken for gonorrhea. (180:29) **Mahuna** *Antirheumatic (Internal)* Plant used for rheumatism. *Cough Medicine* Plant used for coughs. *Pulmonary Aid* Plant used for pneumonia. *Respiratory Aid* Plant used for asthma. (117:19) **Mendocino Indian** *Cold Remedy* Leaves used for colds and asthma. *Respiratory Aid* Leaves used for inflammation of the bronchial tubes or asthma. (33:381) **Miwok** *Antirheumatic (External)* Poultice of leaves used as plasters on aching or sore spots. *Antirheumatic (Internal)* Infusion of leaves and flowers taken for rheumatism. Leaves chewed for rheumatism. *Cold Remedy* Infusion of leaves and flowers taken for colds. Leaves chewed for colds. Leaves smoked in form of cigarette for colds. *Cough Medicine* Infusion of leaves and flowers taken for coughs. Leaves chewed for coughs. Leaves smoked in form of cigarette for coughs. *Dermatological Aid* Poultice of mashed leaves applied to cuts, wounds, and abrasions. *Gastrointestinal Aid* Infusion of leaves and flowers taken for stomachaches. Leaves chewed for stomachache.

Orthopedic Aid Poultice of mashed leaves applied to fractured bones in order to keep down the swelling, aid the knitting, and for pain. (8:169) **Pomo** *Expectorant* Infusion of gummy leaf taken as an expectorant. (98:38) **Pomo, Kashaya** *Blood Medicine* Decoction of leaves used as a blood purifier. *Cough Medicine* Decoction of leaves used as a cough medicine. *Dermatological Aid* Decoction of leaves used to make a wash for sores. *Febrifuge* Decoction of leaves used to bring down the fever of a cold. (60:74) **Round Valley Indian** *Antirheumatic (Internal)* Infusion of leaves taken for rheumatism. *Blood Medicine* Infusion of leaves taken as a blood purifier. *Febrifuge* Infusion of leaves used as a wash for fevers. *Misc. Disease Remedy* Leaves used for grippe. *Respiratory Aid* Infusion of leaves taken or used as wash for catarrh. *Tuberculosis Remedy* Infusion of leaves taken or used as wash for consumption. (33:381) **Yokut** *Diaphoretic* Infusion of plant taken and used as a steam for sweating. (yerba santa 97:437) **Yuki** *Cough Medicine* Plant used in cough syrup. *Dermatological Aid* Poultice of leaves applied to scabby sores. (39:47) **Yurok** *Cold Remedy* Infusion of leaves taken for colds. *Cough Medicine* Infusion of leaves taken for coughs. (5:30)

Eriodictyon crassifolium, Thickleaf Yerbasanta
Luiseño *Unspecified* Plant used for medicinal purposes. (132:230)

Eriodictyon lanatum, San Diego Yerbasanta
Diegueño *Cold Remedy* Decoction of leaves, with or without honey, taken for colds. *Cough Medicine* Decoction of leaves, with or without honey, taken for coughs. (as *E. trichocalyx* ssp. *lanatum* 70:21) Decoction of leaves taken for coughs. (74:219)

Eriodictyon tomentosum, Woolly Yerbasanta
Luiseño *Unspecified* Plant used for medicinal purposes. (132:230)

Eriodictyon trichocalyx, Hairy Yerbasanta
Cahuilla *Antirheumatic (External)* Poultice of fresh, pounded leaves applied to sore or fatigued limbs for rheumatism. *Antirheumatic (Internal)* Decoction of leaves taken for rheumatism. *Blood Medicine* Decoction of leaves used as a blood

purifier. *Cold Remedy* Decoction of leaves used for colds. *Cough Medicine* Decoction of leaves used for coughs. Decoction of three leaves and ½ teaspoon of sugar taken for coughs, 1 teaspoon every 4 hours. *Febrifuge* Decoction of leaves applied as a liniment for fevers. *Oral Aid* Fresh leaves chewed as a thirst quencher. *Respiratory Aid* Decoction of leaves used for asthma and catarrh. *Throat Aid* Decoction of leaves used for sore throats. *Tuberculosis Remedy* Decoction of leaves used for tuberculosis. (11:71)

Eriogonum abertianum var. abertianum, Abert's Buckwheat
Navajo, Ramah *Dermatological Aid* Decoction of plant used as lotion for skin cuts. *Veterinary Aid* Decoction of plant used as lotion for skin cuts on horses. (165:23)

Eriogonum alatum, Winged Buckwheat
Navajo *Analgesic* Plant used for pain. (45:42) **Navajo, Kayenta** *Dermatological Aid* Plant used as a lotion for rashes. *Panacea* Plant used as a life medicine. (179:19) **Navajo, Ramah** *Antidiarrheal* Cold infusion of root used for diarrhea. *Ceremonial Medicine* Cold infusion of root used as a ceremonial medicine. *Cough Medicine* Cold infusion of root used for bad cough. *Dermatological Aid* Powdered root mixed with tallow and used as ointment for infant's sore navel. *Oral Aid* Cold infusion of root used as a mouthwash for sore gums. *Panacea* Cold infusion of root used as an important "life medicine." *Pediatric Aid* Powdered root mixed with tallow and used as ointment for infant's sore navel. (165:23) **Zuni** *Emetic* Root eaten as an emetic for stomachaches. (22:378) *Other* Infusion of powdered root taken after a fall and relieve general misery. (143:49)

Eriogonum androsaceum, Rockjasmine Buckwheat
Thompson *Analgesic* Decoction of plant taken for internal pains, especially stomach pain. Plants used in steam bath for rheumatism, stiff and aching joints and muscles. *Antirheumatic (External)* Plants used in steam bath for aching and rheumatic joints. Plants steamed in sweat bath for rheumatism and various aches and stiffness. *Dermatological Aid* Salve of dry leaves or leaf ash mixed with

grease used for swellings. *Gastrointestinal Aid* Decoction of plant taken for stomach pain. *Herbal Steam* Plants steamed in sweat bath for rheumatism and various aches and stiffness. *Orthopedic Aid* Plants used in steam bath for sprains, stiff and aching joints and muscles. *Other* Mild or medium decoction taken for general indisposition. *Venereal Aid* Strong decoction of plant used for syphilis. (141:470)

Eriogonum annuum, Annual Buckwheat
Lakota *Diuretic* Infusion of plant used for urination problems. *Oral Aid* and *Pediatric Aid* Infusion of plant used for children with sore mouths. (116:54) **Navajo, Ramah** *Ceremonial Medicine* Plant used as a ceremonial medicine. *Dermatological Aid* Cold infusion taken or used as lotion for red ant bite. *Disinfectant* Cold infusion taken for "lightning infection." *Other* Cold infusion taken or used as lotion for sickness from swallowing an ant. *Panacea* Plant used as a "life medicine," "the boss of all medicines." *Witchcraft Medicine* Cold infusion used for protection against witches. (165:23)

Eriogonum baileyi, Bailey's Buckwheat
Tubatulabal *Dermatological Aid* Infusion of entire plant used as lotion for pimples. (167:59)

Eriogonum cernuum, Nodding Buckwheat
Navajo, Kayenta *Dermatological Aid* Plant used for rashes. *Kidney Aid* Infusion of plant used for kidney disease. (179:19) **Navajo, Ramah** *Dermatological Aid* Poultice of chewed leaves applied to red ant bite. (165:23)

Eriogonum compositum, Arrowleaf Buckwheat
Okanagan-Colville *Cold Remedy* Decoction of roots and stems taken for colds. *Dermatological Aid* Decoction of roots and stems used to wash infected cuts. Poultice of mashed leaves applied to cuts or infusion of leaves used as a wash for cuts and sores. (162:112) **Sanpoil** *Antidiarrheal* Decoction of root taken for diarrhea. (109:218)

Eriogonum corymbosum, Crispleaf Buckwheat
Havasupai *Analgesic* Decoction of leaves taken three times a day for headaches. (171:216)

Eriogonum divaricatum, Divergent Buckwheat

Navajo, Kayenta *Ceremonial Medicine* Plant used for "Big Snake chant." *Orthopedic Aid* Poultice of plant applied to back for leg paralysis. *Snakebite Remedy* Plant smoked for snakebites. (179:19)

Eriogonum elatum, Tall Woolly Buckwheat
Mahuna *Cathartic* Branch chewed or infusion of plant taken as a physic. (117:20)

Eriogonum elongatum, Longstem Buckwheat
Mahuna *Blood Medicine* Plant used as a blood tonic. *Hypotensive* Plant used for high blood pressure and hardening of arteries. (117:22)

Eriogonum fasciculatum, Eastern Mojave Buckwheat
Coahuilla *Analgesic* Decoction of leaves taken for headache and stomach pain. *Eye Medicine* Infusion of flower used as an eyewash. *Gastrointestinal Aid* Decoction of leaves taken for stomach pain and headache. (9:78) **Costanoan** *Urinary Aid* Decoction of plant used for urinary problems. (17:11) **Diegueño** *Antidiarrheal* Decoction of flowers given to babies for diarrhea. *Emetic* Decoction of flowers taken to "throw up badness in the stomach." (70:21) *Heart Medicine* Decoction of dried flowers or dried roots taken for a healthy heart. (74:216) *Pediatric Aid* Decoction of flowers given to babies for diarrhea. (70:21) **Navajo** *Witchcraft Medicine* Decoction of plants used as an antiwitchcraft medicine. (45:42) **Omaha** *Dermatological Aid* Poultice of powdered root applied to wounds. (48:49) **Zuni** *Dermatological Aid* Poultice of powdered root applied to cuts and arrow or bullet wounds. *Gynecological Aid* Decoction of root taken after parturition to heal lacerations. *Throat Aid* Decoction of root taken for hoarseness and colds involving the throat. (143:49)

Eriogonum fasciculatum* var. *polifolium, Eastern Mojave Buckwheat
Tubatulabal *Antidiarrheal* Decoction of dried flowers given to children for bloody flux. Infusion of dried heads taken for diarrhea. *Gastrointestinal Aid* Infusion of dried heads taken for stomach-

aches. *Pediatric Aid* Decoction of dried flowers given to children for bloody flux. (167:59)

Eriogonum gracillimum, Rose and White Buckwheat
Tubatulabal *Dermatological Aid* Infusion of entire plant used as lotion for pimples. (167:59)

Eriogonum heracleoides, Parsnipflower Buckwheat
Okanagan-Colville *Cold Remedy* Decoction of roots and stems taken for colds. *Dermatological Aid* Decoction of roots and stems used to wash infected cuts. Poultice of mashed leaves applied to cuts or infusion of leaves used as a wash for cuts and sores. (162:112) **Sanpoil** *Antidiarrheal* Decoction of root taken for diarrhea. (109:218) **Thompson** *Analgesic* Decoction of plant taken for internal pains, especially stomach pain. Plants used in steam bath for rheumatism, stiff and aching joints and muscles. *Antirheumatic (External)* Plants used in steam bath for aching and rheumatic joints. Plants steamed in sweat bath for rheumatism and various aches and stiffness. (141:470) *Ceremonial Medicine* Decoction of whole plant used as a purifying ceremonial wash in the sweat house. (141:505) *Dermatological Aid* Salve of dry leaves or leaf ash mixed with grease used for swellings. (141:470) Infusion of plant used as a wash for sores. (161:237) *Disinfectant* Decoction of whole plant used as a purifying ceremonial wash in the sweat house. (141:505) *Eye Medicine* Decoction of leaves used as a wash for sore eyes. (161:237) *Gastrointestinal Aid* Decoction of plant taken for stomach pain. *Herbal Steam* Plants steamed in sweat bath for rheumatism and various aches and stiffness. *Orthopedic Aid* Plants used in steam bath for sprains, stiff and aching joints and muscles. *Other* Mild or medium decoction taken for general indisposition. (141:470) *Pulmonary Aid* Decoction of washed, clean plant taken for sickness on the lung. *Tuberculosis Remedy* Decoction of washed, clean plant taken for tuberculosis. Infusion of plant taken in large quantities for tuberculosis. *Unspecified* Decoction of plant taken or used as a wash for an unspecified illness. (161:237) *Venereal Aid* Strong decoction of plant used for syphilis. (141:470)

Eriogonum inflatum, Native American
Pipeweed
Navajo, Kayenta *Dermatological Aid* Plant used
as a lotion for bear or dog bite. (179:19)

Eriogonum jamesii, James's Buckwheat
Apache, White Mountain *Ceremonial Medicine*
Plant used in medicine ceremonies. *Oral Aid* Plant
chewed to sweeten the saliva. *Unspecified* Plant
used for medicinal purposes. (113:157) **Keres,
Western** *Heart Medicine* Roots chewed for a heart
medicine. *Psychological Aid* Infusion of roots used
for despondency. (147:43) **Navajo, Kayenta** *Psychological Aid* Plant smoked when disturbed by
dreaming of tobacco worms. (179:19) **Navajo,
Ramah** *Analgesic* Decoction of whole plant taken
to ease labor pains. *Contraceptive* Root used as a
contraceptive. *Gastrointestinal Aid* Cold infusion
of whole plant taken to kill a swallowed red ant.
Gynecological Aid Decoction of whole plant taken
to ease labor pains. *Panacea* Root used as a "life
medicine." (165:23) **Zuni** *Eye Medicine* Root
soaked in water and used as a wash for sore eyes.
Gastrointestinal Aid Fresh or dried root eaten for
stomachaches. (22:378) *Oral Aid* Root carried in
mouth for sore tongue, then buried in river bottom.
(143:50)

Eriogonum latifolium, Seaside Buckwheat
Costanoan *Cold Remedy* Decoction of root, stalk,
and leaves taken for colds. *Cough Medicine* Decoction of root, stalk, and leaves taken for coughs.
(17:11) **Round Valley Indian** *Analgesic* Decoction of leaves, stems, and roots taken for stomach
pains and headaches. *Eye Medicine* Decoction of
roots used for sore eyes. *Gastrointestinal Aid* Decoction of leaves, stems, and roots taken for stomach pains. *Gynecological Aid* Decoction of leaves,
stems, and roots taken for female complaints.
(33:345)

Eriogonum leptophyllum, Slenderleaf Buckwheat
Navajo, Ramah *Analgesic* Decoction of whole
plant used for postpartum pain. *Gynecological Aid*
Decoction of whole plant used for postpartum
pain and to aid in placenta delivery. *Panacea* Decoction of whole plant used as a "life medicine."

Snakebite Remedy Decoction of whole plant used
internally and externally for snakebite. (165:23)

Eriogonum longifolium, Longleaf Buckwheat
Comanche *Gastrointestinal Aid* Infusion of root
taken for stomach trouble. (24:521)

Eriogonum microthecum, Slender Buckwheat
Paiute *Tuberculosis Remedy* Decoction of roots
or tops used for tuberculosis. *Urinary Aid* Decoction of stems and leaves used for bladder trouble.
Shoshoni *Antirheumatic (External)* Decoction
of plant used in hot compresses or as a wash for
lameness or rheumatism. *Cough Medicine* Decoction of roots and sometimes tops taken for tubercular cough. *Orthopedic Aid* Decoction of whole
plant used as a wash or as a compress for lameness. *Tuberculosis Remedy* Decoction of roots or
tops used for tuberculosis. (155:72)

Eriogonum niveum, Snow Buckwheat
Okanagan-Colville *Cold Remedy* Decoction of
roots and stems taken for colds. *Dermatological
Aid* Decoction of roots and stems used to wash infected cuts. Poultice of mashed leaves applied to
cuts or infusion of leaves used as a wash for cuts
and sores. (162:112)

Eriogonum nudum* var. *oblongifolium,
Naked Buckwheat
Karok *Gastrointestinal Aid* Roots used for abdominal ailments. (5:30)

Eriogonum nudum* var. *pauciflorum,
Naked Buckwheat
Kawaiisu *Cold Remedy* Infusion of roots taken
for colds. *Cough Medicine* Infusion of roots taken
for coughs. (180:30)

Eriogonum ovalifolium, Cushion Buckwheat
Gosiute *Eye Medicine* Plant used as an eye medicine. *Gastrointestinal Aid* Plant used for stomachaches. (31:369) *Venereal Aid* Poultice of plant applied or plant used as wash for venereal diseases.
(31:351) **Paiute** *Cold Remedy* Decoction of root
taken as a cold remedy. **Shoshoni** *Cold Remedy*
Decoction of root taken as a cold remedy. (155:72)
Ute *Unspecified* Used as medicine. (30:34)

Eriogonum racemosum, Redroot Buckwheat
Navajo, **Kayenta** *Analgesic* Plant used for back-aches and side aches. *Orthopedic Aid* Plant used for backaches and side aches. (179:19) **Navajo**, **Ramah** *Blood Medicine* Cold infusion of whole plant taken for blood poisoning or internal injuries. (165:23)

Eriogonum roseum, Wand Buckwheat
Tubatulabal *Dermatological Aid* Infusion of entire plant used as lotion for pimples. (as *E. virgatum* 167:59)

Eriogonum rotundifolium, Roundleaf Buck-wheat
Keres, **Western** *Emetic* Infusion of roots used as an emetic to eliminate the ozone in cases of lightning shock. *Psychological Aid* Plant eaten by children to become good looking. *Sedative* Infusion of roots used for lightning shock. (147:43) **Navajo** *Emetic* Plant taken to vomit after swallowing ants. (45:42) *Throat Aid* Leaves used for sore throats. *Unspecified* Roots used as medicine. (76:150)

Eriogonum sphaerocephalum, Rock Buck-wheat
Paiute *Antidiarrheal* Decoction of root taken for diarrhea. *Cold Remedy* Decoction of root taken for colds. **Shoshoni** *Antidiarrheal* Decoction of root taken for diarrhea. (155:73)

Eriogonum tenellum, Tall Buckwheat
Keres, **Western** *Febrifuge* Hot infusion of plant given to mothers after childbirth for fever. *Gynecological Aid* Infusion of roots or raw roots given to women during difficult labor. Infusion of plant used as a douche after childbirth. (147:43)

Eriogonum umbellatum, Sulphur Wild-buckwheat
Kawaiisu *Dermatological Aid* and *Venereal Aid* Mashed flowers used as a salve for gonorrheal sores. (180:30) **Mahuna** *Gastrointestinal Aid* Infusion of blossoms taken for ptomaine poisoning. (117:49) **Navajo**, **Kayenta** *Disinfectant* Plant used as a fumigant for biliousness. *Emetic* Plant used as an emetic for biliousness. *Gastrointestinal Aid* Plant used as a fumigant or emetic for biliousness. (179:20) **Nevada Indian** *Cold Remedy* Infu-sion of roots taken for colds. (98:37) **Paiute** *Analgesic* Decoction of roots taken for stomachaches. *Antirheumatic* (*External*) Poultice of mashed leaves, often with roots, used for lameness or rheumatism. (155:73) *Cold Remedy* Infusion of roots taken for colds. (144:317) Hot decoction of roots taken for colds. *Gastrointestinal Aid* Decoction of root taken for stomachaches. *Orthopedic Aid* Poultice of leaves, and sometimes roots, applied for lameness or rheumatism. **Shoshoni** *Antirheumatic* (*External*) Poultice of mashed leaves, often with roots, used for lameness or rheumatism. *Cold Remedy* Hot decoction of roots taken for colds. *Orthopedic Aid* Poultice of leaves, and sometimes roots, applied for lameness or rheumatism. (155:73)

Eriogonum umbellatum* var. *majus, Sulphurflower Buckwheat
Cheyenne *Gynecological Aid* Infusion of pow-dered stems and flowers taken for constant menses. (as *E. subalpinum* 63:172) Infusion of powdered stems and flowers taken for lengthy menses. (as *E. subalpinum* 64:172) Stems and flowers powdered, made into a tea, and used for menses that ran too long. (69:32)

Eriogonum umbellatum* var. *stellatum, Sulphurflower Buckwheat
Klamath *Burn Dressing* Leaves placed on burns to soothe the pain. (as *E. stellatum* 37:95) Poul-tice of leaves applied to burns. (as *E. stellatum* 140:131)

Eriogonum wrightii, Bastardsage
Navajo, **Kayenta** *Emetic* Plant used as an emetic. (179:20)

Erioneuron pulchellum, Low Woollygrass
Havasupai *Laxative* Decoction of blades taken as a laxative. (as *Tridens pulchellus* 171:210)

Eriophorum angustifolium, Tall Cottongrass
Eskimo, **Kuskokwagmiut** *Panacea* Raw stems eaten to restore good health to persons in gener-ally poor health. (101:27)

Eriophorum angustifolium ssp. *subarcticum*, Tall Cottongrass
Eskimo, Inuktitut *Unspecified* "Female" stems used medicinally. (176:184)

Eriophorum callitrix, Arctic Cottongrass
Ojibwa *Hemostat* Matted fuzz used as a "hemostatic." (130:368)

Eriophorum russeolum, Red Cottongrass
Eskimo, Western *Dermatological Aid* Poultice of "cotton" from plant applied to boils to absorb the pus. (90:17) *Eye Medicine* "Cotton" from plant put in corner of eye to absorb fluid from "watery eyes." (90:22)

Eriophorum scheuchzeri, White Cottongrass
Eskimo, Western *Dermatological Aid* Poultice of "cotton" from plant applied to boils to absorb the pus. (90:17)

Eriophyllum lanatum, Woolly Eriophyllum
Chehalis *Love Medicine* Dried flowers used as a love charm. **Skagit** *Dermatological Aid* Leaves rubbed on the face to prevent chapping. (65:49)

Eriophyllum lanatum var. *leucophyllum*, Common Woollysunflower
Miwok *Antirheumatic* (*External*) Poultice of leaves bound on body over aching parts. (as *E. caespitosum* 8:169)

Erodium cicutarium, Redstem Stork's Bill
Costanoan *Misc. Disease Remedy* Infusion of leaves used for typhoid fever. (17:8) **Jemez** *Gynecological Aid* Plant and roots eaten by women to produce more milk for the nursing children. (36:22) **Navajo, Kayenta** *Dermatological Aid* Plant used for wildcat, bobcat, or mountain lion bites. *Disinfectant* Plant used for infections. (179:29) **Zuni** *Dermatological Aid* Poultice of chewed root applied to sores and rashes. *Gastrointestinal Aid* Infusion of root taken for stomachache. (22:376)

Eryngium alismifolium, Modoc Eryngo
Paiute *Antidiarrheal* Infusion of whole plant used for diarrhea. (98:42) Infusion of plant taken for diarrhea. (155:73)

Eryngium aquaticum, Rattlesnakemaster
Alabama *Emetic* Infusion of plant taken as an emetic. **Cherokee** *Emetic* and *Gastrointestinal Aid* Infusion of plant taken to cause vomiting for nausea. (152:45) **Choctaw** *Antidote* Root used as an "anti-poison"; especially good for snakebite. *Diuretic* Root used as a powerful diuretic. *Expectorant* Root used as a powerful expectorant. *Snakebite Remedy* Root used as an "anti-poison"; especially good for snakebite. *Stimulant* Root used as a powerful stimulant. *Venereal Aid* Plant used for gonorrhea. (23:287) **Delaware** *Anthelmintic* Used for intestinal tape and "pin" worms. (151:35) **Delaware, Oklahoma** *Anthelmintic* Root used for tapeworms and pinworms. *Venereal Aid* Root used alone and in compound for venereal disease. (150:29, 76) **Koasati** *Emetic* Decoction of roots taken as an emetic. (152:45)

Eryngium yuccifolium, Button Eryngo
Cherokee *Pulmonary Aid* Decoction used to prevent whooping cough. *Snakebite Remedy* Used as snakebite remedy. *Toothache Remedy* Infusion held in mouth for toothaches. (66:27) **Creek** *Analgesic* Cold infusion of root taken for neuralgia and kidney troubles. (148:655, 656) Cold infusion of pounded roots taken for neuralgia. (152:45) *Antirheumatic* (*Internal*) Plant used with "deer potato" for rheumatism. *Blood Medicine* Infusion of root taken "to cleanse the system and purify the blood." (148:655, 656) Plant used to cleanse the system and purify the blood. (152:45) *Cathartic* Plant used as a physic called "the war physic."

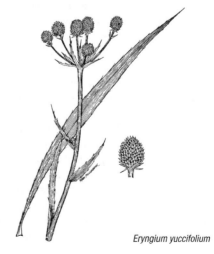

Eryngium yuccifolium

Gastrointestinal Aid Plant used for diseases of the spleen. *Kidney Aid* Cold infusion of root taken for kidney troubles and neuralgia. (148:655, 656) Cold infusion of pounded roots taken for kidney troubles. (152:45) *Panacea* Infusion of root used to produce "an access of health." *Sedative* Plant used to produce a feeling of peace and tranquility. *Snakebite Remedy* Infusion of root used for snakebite. (148:655, 656) Plant used for snakebites. (152:45) *Venereal Aid* Compound infusion of root taken for "the clap." (148:655, 656) **Meskwaki** *Antidote* Root used as an antidote for poisons and for bladder trouble. *Ceremonial Medicine* Leaves and fruit formerly introduced into rattlesnake medicine song and dance. *Snakebite Remedy* Root used for rattlesnake bites and bladder trouble. *Urinary Aid* Root used for bladder trouble and as an antidote for poisons. (129:248) **Natchez** *Antidiarrheal* Infusion of parched leaves taken for dysentery. *Hemostat* Stem and leaves chewed for nosebleeds. (152:45)

Eryngium yuccifolium var. *synchaetum*, Button Eryngo

Seminole *Analgesic* Plant used for pains. (as *E. synchaetum* 145:161) Decoction of roots used for cow sickness: lower chest pain, digestive disturbances, and diarrhea. (as *E. synchaetum* 145:191) Infusion of plant taken by men for menstruation sickness: stomachache, headache, and body soreness. (as *E. synchaetum* 145:248) Decoction of plant taken for dead people's sickness. (as *E. synchaetum* 145:257) *Antidiarrheal* Decoction of roots used for cow sickness: lower chest pain, digestive disturbances, and diarrhea. (as *E. synchaetum* 145:191) Infusion of plant taken for otter sickness: severe diarrhea, bloody stools, and severe stomachache. *Antihemorrhagic* Infusion of plant taken for otter sickness: severe diarrhea, bloody stools, and severe stomachache. (as *E. synchaetum* 145:223) *Antirheumatic* (*External*) Cold infusion of plant used as a bath for body aches. (as *E. synchaetum* 145:215) *Antirheumatic* (*Internal*) Infusion of plant taken by men for menstruation sickness: stomachache, headache, and body soreness. (as *E. synchaetum* 145:248) *Ceremonial Medicine* Plant used as a ceremonial emetic. (as *E. synchaetum* 145:161) Roots used as an emetic in purification after funerals, at doctor's school, and after death of patient. (as *E. synchaetum* 145:167) Plant used to make a medicine taken by students in medical training. (as *E. synchaetum* 145:95) *Dermatological Aid* Plant used for sores. (as *E. synchaetum* 145:161) Plant used for snake sickness: itchy skin. (as *E. synchaetum* 145:166) Decoction of plant taken and used as a body steam for snake sickness: itchy skin. (as *E. synchaetum* 145:238) *Dietary Aid* Decoction of plant taken for dead people's sickness. (as *E. synchaetum* 145:257) *Emetic* Decoction of plant and other plants taken as an emetic by doctors to strengthen his internal medicine. (as *E. synchaetum* 145:145) Roots used as an emetic to "clean the insides." (as *E. synchaetum* 145:167) Plant used as an emetic by the doctor to prevent the next patient from getting worse. (as *E. synchaetum* 145:184) Infusion of roots taken as an emetic during religious ceremonies. (as *E. synchaetum* 145:408) *Febrifuge* Decoction of plant taken for dead people's sickness. (as *E. synchaetum* 145:257) *Gastrointestinal Aid* Decoction of roots used for cow sickness: lower chest pain, digestive disturbances, and diarrhea. (as *E. synchaetum* 145:191) Infusion of plant taken for otter sickness: severe diarrhea, bloody stools, and severe stomachache. (as *E. synchaetum* 145:223) Infusion of plant taken by men for menstruation sickness: stomachache, headache, and body soreness. (as *E. synchaetum* 145:248) Decoction of plant taken and root chewed for stomachaches. (as *E. synchaetum* 145:276) *Heart Medicine* Roots eaten as a heart medicine. (as *E. synchaetum* 145:304) *Orthopedic Aid* Decoction of plant taken for dead people's sickness. (as *E. synchaetum* 145:257) Decoction of roots applied to foot swellings. (as *E. synchaetum* 145:288) *Panacea* Plant used medicinally for everything. (as *E. synchaetum* 145:161) *Respiratory Aid* Decoction of plant taken for dead people's sickness. (as *E. synchaetum* 145:257) *Snakebite Remedy* Plant used for snakebites. (as *E. synchaetum* 145:295) *Stimulant* Decoction of plant taken for dead people's sickness. (as *E. synchaetum* 145:257) *Unspecified* Plant used for medicinal purposes. (as *E. synchaetum* 145:161) Plant used medicinally. (as *E. synchaetum* 145:164)

Erysimum asperum, Plains Wallflower

Okanagan-Colville *Dermatological Aid* Poultice

of pounded, whole plant applied to open, fresh wounds. (162:92) **Sioux, Teton** *Analgesic* Infusion of crushed seed taken and used externally for stomach or bowel cramps. *Gastrointestinal Aid* Infusion of crushed seeds used for stomach or bowel cramps. (as *Cheirinia aspera* 42:269)

Erysimum capitatum, Sanddune Wallflower
Hopi *Tuberculosis Remedy* Plant used for advanced cases of tuberculosis. (34:315) **Navajo, Ramah** *Analgesic* Crushed leaves "smelled" for headache. *Ceremonial Medicine* and *Emetic* Whole plant used as a ceremonial emetic. *Gynecological Aid* Whole plant chewed and blown over patient to aid in difficult labor. *Respiratory Aid* Pulverized pods snuffed to cause sneezing for "congested nose." *Toothache Remedy* Poultice of warmed root applied for toothache. (165:28, 29) **Zuni** *Antirheumatic* (*External*) Infusion of whole plant used for muscle aches. *Emetic* Flower and fruit eaten as an emetic for stomachaches. (22:375)

Erysimum capitatum var. *capitatum*, Sanddune Wallflower
Keres, Western *Antirheumatic* (*External*) Poultice of chewed leaves applied to swellings. (as *E. wheeleri* 147:43)

Erysimum cheiranthoides, Wormseed Wallflower
Chippewa *Dermatological Aid* Decoction of root applied to skin eruptions. (43:350)

Erysimum inconspicuum, Shy Wallflower
Hopi *Tuberculosis Remedy* Plant used for tuberculosis. (34:316)

Erythrina herbacea, Redcardinal
Alabama *Gastrointestinal Aid* Cold infusion of root taken by women for bowel pain. (148:666) **Choctaw** *Tonic* Decoction of leaves taken as a general tonic. (20:23) **Creek** *Analgesic* Cold infusion of root taken by women for bowel pain. (148:666) **Seminole** *Antiemetic* Decoction of roots or berries used for horse sickness: nausea, constipation, and blocked urination. (145:188) *Antirheumatic* (*External*) Decoction of "beans" or inner bark used as a body rub and steam for deer sickness: numb, painful limbs and joints. (145:192) *Laxa-*

tive and *Urinary Aid* Decoction of roots or berries used for horse sickness: nausea, constipation, and blocked urination. (145:188)

Erythrina sandwicensis, Wili Wili
Hawaiian *Venereal Aid* Flowers used for venereal diseases. Infusion of pounded bark taken for sexual organ diseases. (as *E. monosperma* 2:74)

Erythronium americanum, American Troutlily
Cherokee *Dermatological Aid* Warmed leaves crushed and juice poured over "wound that won't heal." *Febrifuge* Infusion of root given for fever. *Hunting Medicine* Root chewed and spit into river to make fish bite. *Stimulant* Compound infusion given for fainting. (66:43) **Iroquois** *Contraceptive* Raw plants, except the roots, taken by young girls to prevent conception. *Dermatological Aid* Poultice of smashed roots used for swellings and removing slivers. (73:282)

Erythronium grandiflorum, Dogtooth Lily
Montana Indian *Dermatological Aid* Poultice of crushed bulb-like roots applied to boils. (15:11) **Okanagan-Colville** *Cold Remedy* Corms used for bad colds. (162:45)

Erythronium oregonum ssp. *oregonum*, Oregon Fawnlily
Wailaki *Dermatological Aid* Poultice of crushed plant applied to boils. (as *E. giganteum* 33:320)

Eschscholzia californica, California Poppy
California Indian *Toothache Remedy* Leaves used for toothache. (as *Escholtzia californica* 98:45) **Costanoan** *Pediatric Aid* Flowers laid underneath bed to put child to sleep. *Poison* "Plant avoided by pregnant or lactating women as smell may be poisonous." *Sedative* Flowers laid underneath bed to put child to sleep. (17:9) **Mahuna** *Poison* Plant considered poisonous. (117:34) **Mendocino Indian** *Analgesic* Root juice used as a wash for headaches. *Dermatological Aid* Root juice used as a wash for suppurating sores. *Emetic* Root juice taken as an emetic. *Gastrointestinal Aid* Root juice taken for stomachaches. *Gynecological Aid* Root juice used as a wash by women to stop the secretion of milk. *Narcotic* Root used for

the stupefying effect. *Toothache Remedy* Root placed in cavity of tooth for toothaches. *Tuberculosis Remedy* Root juice taken for consumption. (as *Eschscholtzia douglasii* 33:351) **Pomo, Kashaya** *Gynecological Aid* Mashed seedpod rubbed on a nursing mother's breast to dry up her milk. Decoction of mashed seedpod rubbed on a nursing mother's breast to dry up her milk. (60:94)

Eschscholzia parishii, Parish's Goldenpoppy **Kawaiisu** *Dermatological Aid* Poultice of dried, ground roots applied to venereal sores. *Venereal Aid* Root used for gonorrhea and syphilis. (180:31)

Escobaria vivipara var. *vivipara*, Spinystar **Blackfoot** *Antidiarrheal* Fruit eaten in small amounts for diarrhea. (as *Mamillaria vivipara* 72:67) *Eye Medicine* Seed inserted into the eye to remove matter. (as *Mammilaria vivpara* 72:81)

Eucalyptus sp., Eucalyptus, Nuholani **Cahuilla** *Cold Remedy* Leaves used in steam treatments for colds. The leaves were boiled in water and the patient held his head over the bowl. A blanket was then placed over the patient, who inhaled the steam to relieve sinus congestion. (11:73) **Hawaiian** *Analgesic* Oil used for rubbing over backaches and rheumatic pain. *Antirheumatic (External)* Oil used for rubbing over rheumatic pain. *Dermatological Aid* Oil used for rubbing over sores and cuts. *Febrifuge* Leaves used in sweat baths for fevers. *Orthopedic Aid* Oil used for rubbing over sprains. (2:73)

Euonymus americana, American Strawberry-bush **Cherokee** *Analgesic* Infusion taken for stomach-ache. *Antihemorrhagic* Taken for "breast complaints" or "spitting blood." *Dermatological Aid* Astringent infusion of bark sniffed for sinus. Used for "white swelling." *Disinfectant* Used as an antiseptic. *Expectorant* Used as an expectorant. *Gynecological Aid* Infusion of root used for "falling of the womb." *Orthopedic Aid* Infusion of bark rubbed on cramps in veins. *Other* Compound infusion taken for "bad disease." *Respiratory Aid* Infusion sniffed for sinus. *Tonic* Used as a tonic. *Urinary Aid* Compound decoction used for "irregular urination." (66:38) Infusion of bark taken for urinary

troubles. (152:38) *Venereal Aid* Infusion of root used for "claps." (66:38) **Iroquois** *Abortifacient* Decoction of plants taken for suppressed menses. Decoction taken to stimulate suppressed menses, not taken when pregnant. *Gynecological Aid* Decoction of vine taken for excessive menstrual flow. *Urinary Aid* Compound decoction of plant taken for difficult urination due to excess gall. (73:375)

Euonymus atropurpurea, Eastern Wahoo **Meskwaki** *Dermatological Aid* Poultice of pounded, fresh trunk bark applied to old facial sores. *Eye Medicine* Infusion or decoction of bark used as a wash for weak or sore eyes. (as *Evonymus atropurpurea* 129:209) **Mohegan** *Cathartic* Infusion of plant used as a physic. (as *Evonymus atropurpurea* 149:265) Infusion of leaves taken as a physic. (151:72, 130) **Winnebago** *Gynecological Aid* Decoction of inner bark taken for uterine trouble. (58:102)

Euonymus europaea, European Spindletree **Iroquois** *Anthelmintic* Compound decoction of plant taken to remove worms caused by solid food taboo. Decoction of bark given to children with worms. *Cathartic* Infusion of roots taken as a physic. *Dietary Aid* Infusion of roots taken to stimulate the appetite. *Pediatric Aid* Decoction of bark given to children with worms. *Urinary Aid* Decoction of roots taken for bloody urine. (73:374)

Euonymus obovata, Running Strawberrybush **Iroquois** *Other* Compound decoction of plants taken for stricture caused by bad blood. (73:375) *Urinary Aid* Decoction of vines taken for difficult urination. (73:376) *Witchcraft Medicine* Compound infusion of plants taken by people who are bewitched. (73:375)

Eupatorium maculatum, Spotted Joepyeweed **Algonquin, Quebec** *Gynecological Aid* Used for menstrual disorders and to facilitate the recovery of women after childbirth. *Venereal Aid* White flowered plant used for males and pink flowered plant used for females for venereal disease. (14:238) **Cherokee** *Adjuvant* Section of stem used to blow or spray medicine. *Antirheumatic (Internal)* Root used for rheumatism. *Diuretic* Root used as a diuretic. *Gynecological Aid* Root used for "female problems." *Kidney Aid* Root used for "dropsy" and infusion taken for kidney trouble. *Misc. Disease Remedy* Root used for gout and "dropsy." *Other* Infusion of root used as a wash "after becoming sick from odor of corpse." *Tonic* Infusion of root used as a tonic during pregnancy. *Urinary Aid* Compound decoction of root taken for "difficult urination." (66:41, 42) **Chippewa** *Antirheumatic* (*External*) Decoction of root used as a wash for joint inflammations. (43:348) *Pediatric Aid* and *Sedative* Decoction of root used as a quieting bath for fretful child. (43:364) **Iroquois** *Antidiarrheal* Compound decoction of smashed plants taken for diarrhea. *Antirheumatic* (*External*) Compound plants used for the liver and rheumatism. *Carminative* Compound decoction of plants taken for stomach gas. *Cold Remedy* Infusion of roots taken for colds. *Febrifuge* Infusion of roots taken for chills and fever. *Gastrointestinal Aid* Decoction of dried roots taken for dried stomach. (73:456) *Gynecological Aid* Infusion of roots taken for soreness of womb and abdomen after childbirth. *Kidney Aid* Infusion of roots taken for kidney trouble. (73:455) *Liver Aid* Compound infusion of roots taken for liver sickness. *Love Medicine* Compound decoction of roots used as a wash for anti-love medicine. *Tuberculosis Remedy* Decoction of dried roots taken for consumption. *Venereal Aid* Decoction of roots taken for gonorrhea. (73:456)

Eupatorium perfoliatum, Common Boneset
Abnaki *Orthopedic Aid* Used to mend bones. (121:154) **Cherokee** *Cathartic* Used as a purgative. *Cold Remedy* Infusion taken for colds. *Diaphoretic* Used as a sudorific. *Disinfectant* and *Diuretic* Used as a tonic, sudorific, stimulant, emetic, and diuretic. *Emetic* Used as an emetic. *Febrifuge* Taken for fever. *Gastrointestinal Aid* Taken for the "biliary system." *Misc. Disease Remedy* Infusion taken for "ague," colds and flu. *Stimulant* Used as a stimulant. *Throat Aid* Infusion taken for sore throat. *Tonic* Used as a tonic. (66:26) **Chippewa** *Abortifacient* Root used to correct irregular menses. *Antirheumatic* (*External*) Poultice of boiled plant tops applied for rheumatism. (59:142) *Hunting Medicine* Root fibers applied to whistles and used as a charm to attract deer. (43:376) *Snakebite Remedy* Poultice of chewed plants applied to rattlesnake bites.

(59:142) **Delaware** *Febrifuge* Infusion of roots and occasionally the leaves used for chills and fever. (151:33) **Delaware**, **Oklahoma** *Febrifuge* Infusion of root, sometimes with leaves, used for chills and fever. (150:28, 76) **Delaware**, **Ontario** *Gastrointestinal Aid* Infusion of leaves, considered a powerful herb, taken as a stomach medicine. (150:67, 82) **Iroquois** *Analgesic* Infusion of roots taken for pains in the stomach and on the left side. Poultice of smashed plants applied for headaches. (73:457) *Cold Remedy* Compound decoction of roots taken for colds. Infusion of stems with leaves taken during the onset of a cold. (73:458) *Dermatological Aid* Infusion of roots used as a wash and applied as poultice to syphilitic chancres. (73:456) *Febrifuge* Infusion of whole plant, plant tops, or roots taken for fevers. *Gastrointestinal Aid* Infusion of roots taken for pains in the stomach. (73:457) *Hemorrhoid Remedy* Plant used for piles. *Kidney Aid* Compound decoction of roots taken for the kidneys. (73:458) *Laxative* Compound decoction of flowers and leaves taken as a laxative. (73:456) *Misc. Disease Remedy* Decoction of smashed plants and roots taken for typhoid. (73:458) *Orthopedic Aid* Cold, compound infusion of leaves applied as poultice to broken bones. *Other* Decoction of roots taken for stricture caused by menstruating girls. *Poison* Plant put in enemy's liquor flask to kill him. *Psychological Aid* Decoction of smashed roots taken to stop the liquor habit. (73:457) *Pulmonary Aid* Decoction of roots taken for pneumonia and pleurisy. (73:458) *Venereal Aid* Infusion of roots used as a wash and applied as poultice to syphilitic chancres.

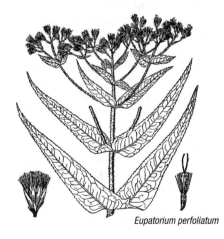

Eupatorium perfoliatum

(73:456) *Veterinary Aid* Infusion of whole plant given to horses with fevers. *Witchcraft Medicine* Plant used for sorcery. (73:457) **Koasati** *Emetic* Decoction of leaves taken as an emetic. *Urinary Aid* Decoction of roots taken for urinary troubles. (152:61) **Menominee** *Febrifuge* Infusion of whole plant used for fever. (128:30) **Meskwaki** *Anthelmintic* Infusion of leaves and blossoms used to expel worms. *Snakebite Remedy* Root used for snakebite. (129:214) **Micmac** *Kidney Aid* Parts of plant used for kidney trouble. *Venereal Aid* Parts of plant used for persons spitting blood and gonorrhea. (32:56) **Mohegan** *Cold Remedy* Bitter infusion taken for colds. (25:118) Infusion taken for colds. (149:265) Simple or compound infusion of leaves taken in small doses for colds. (151:72, 130) *Febrifuge* Bitter infusion taken for fever. (25:118) Infusion taken for fevers. (149:265) Infusion of leaves taken in small doses for colds and fever. (151:72, 130) *Gastrointestinal Aid* Leaves used for stomach trouble and colds. (151:130) *Panacea* Infusion taken for many ailments and general illness. (149:265) Infusion of leaves taken in small doses for "general debility." (151:72, 130) *Tonic* Complex compound infusion including boneset taken as spring tonic. (149:266) **Nanticoke** *Febrifuge* Compound infusion of whole plant taken for chills and fever. (150:56, 84) **Penobscot** *Antihemorrhagic* Compound infusion of plant taken for "spitting up blood." *Kidney Aid* Compound infusion of plant taken for kidney trouble. *Tonic* Compound infusion of plant taken as a tonic. *Venereal Aid* Compound infusion of plant taken for gonorrhea. (133:311) **Rappahannock** *Tonic* Infusion of dried leaves, picked before flowers matured, taken as a tonic. (138:34) **Seminole** *Emetic* Decoction of plant used as a gentle emetic. *Febrifuge* Plant used as a fever medicine. (145:283) **Shinnecock** *Cold Remedy* Bitter infusion taken for colds. *Diaphoretic* Infusion taken cold, then a hot cup before bed to cause perspiring. *Febrifuge* Bitter infusion taken for fever. (25:118)

Eupatorium pilosum, Rough Boneset

Cherokee *Breast Treatment* Used for "breast complaints." *Cold Remedy* Used for colds. *Laxative* Used as a laxative. *Respiratory Aid* Used for "phthisic." *Tonic* Used as a tonic. *Urinary Aid* Taken to increase urination. (66:38)

Eupatorium purpureum, Sweetscented Joepyeweed

Cherokee *Adjuvant* Section of stem used to blow or spray medicine. *Antirheumatic (Internal)* Root used for rheumatism. *Diuretic* Root used as a diuretic. *Gynecological Aid* Root used for "female problems" and infusion of root used as a tonic during pregnancy. *Kidney Aid* Root used for "dropsy" and infusion taken for kidney trouble. *Misc. Disease Remedy* Root used for gout and "dropsy." *Other* Infusion of root used as a wash "after becoming sick from odor of corpse." *Tonic* Root used for "female problems" and infusion of root used as a tonic during pregnancy. *Urinary Aid* Compound decoction of root taken for "difficult urination." (66:41, 42) **Chippewa** *Cold Remedy* Vapors from infusion of plant tops inhaled for colds. *Gynecological Aid* Plant used to counteract the bad effects of a miscarriage. (59:142) **Mahuna** *Laxative* Infusion of roots taken as a laxative. (117:18) **Menominee** *Gynecological Aid* Compound decoction of root taken after childbirth "for internal healing." (44:133) *Urinary Aid* Plant used for diseases of the genitourinary canal. (128:30) **Meskwaki** *Love Medicine* Root kept in mouth and nibbled when wooing women. (129:214) **Navajo** *Antidote* Plant used as an antidote for poison. *Dermatological Aid* Decoction of plant taken for arrow wounds. (45:85) **Ojibwa** *Pediatric Aid* Strong solution of root used as strengthening wash for infants. (130:364) **Potawatomi** *Burn Dressing* Poultice of fresh leaves applied to burns. *Gynecological Aid* Root used "to clear up afterbirth." (131:52) **Rappahannock** *Blood Medicine* An ingredient of a blood medicine. (138:31)

Eupatorium purpureum var. **purpureum**, Sweetscented Joepyeweed

Iroquois *Other* Compound infusion used as wash on injured parts, a "Little Water Medicine." (as *E. falcatum* 73:455)

Eupatorium serotinum, Lateflowering Thoroughwort

Houma *Febrifuge* Decoction of flowers taken for typhoid fever. *Misc. Disease Remedy* Decoction of flowers taken for typhoid fever. (135:64)

Euphorbia corollata, Flowering Spurge
Cherokee *Cancer Treatment* Decoction prepared with herbs and taken for cancer. *Cathartic* Taken as a purgative. *Dermatological Aid* "Juice rubbed on skin eruptions, especially on children's heads." Juice used as an ointment for "sores and sore nipples." *Gynecological Aid* Infusion taken for bleeding after childbirth. *Pediatric Aid* "Juice rubbed on skin eruptions, especially on children's heads." *Toothache Remedy* Root used for toothache. *Urinary Aid* Infusion of bruised root taken for urinary diseases. (66:45) Infusion of bruised roots taken for yellow urine. (152:35) *Venereal Aid* Decoction taken for gonorrhea and "similar diseases." (66:45) **Meskwaki** *Anthelmintic* Compound infusion of root used to expel pinworms. *Antirheumatic* (*Internal*) Decoction of root taken for rheumatism. *Cathartic* Decoction of root or compound taken before breakfast as a physic. (129: 220, 221) **Micmac** *Emetic* Root used as an emetic. (32:56) **Ojibwa** *Cathartic* Infusion of pounded root taken before eating as a physic. (130:369)

Euphorbia dentata, Toothed Spurge
Keres, **Western** *Gynecological Aid* Plant eaten by mothers to produce more milk. (as *Poinsettia dentata* 147:62)

Euphorbia helioscopia, Madwoman's Milk
Iroquois *Gastrointestinal Aid* and *Pediatric Aid* Infusion of plant given to babies with stomachaches. (118:41)

Euphorbia incisa, Mojave Spurge
Navajo, **Kayenta** *Gynecological Aid* Plant used to increase fertility. *Veterinary Aid* Plant used to increase fertility in livestock. (179:30)

Euphorbia ipecacuanhae, American Ipecac
Cherokee *Diaphoretic* Used as a diaphoretic. *Emetic* Used as an emetic. *Expectorant* Used as an expectorant. *Gynecological Aid* and *Pulmonary Aid* "Stops violent hemorrhaging from lungs and womb when given in small doses." (as *Cephaelis ipecacuanha* 66:40)

Euphorbia lurida, San Francisco Mountain
Spurge
Navajo, **Ramah** *Gynecological Aid* Poultice of root applied to hard areas of "caked breast." (165:35)

Euphorbia marginata, Snow on the Mountain
Lakota *Antirheumatic* (*External*) Infusion of crushed leaves used as a liniment for swellings. *Gynecological Aid* Infusion of plant used by mothers without milk. (116:45) **Pawnee** *Poison* Plant considered poisonous. (as *Dichrophyllum marginatum* 58:99)

Euphorbia robusta, Rocky Mountain Spurge
Navajo *Cathartic* Compound infusion of plants taken for purging. *Dermatological Aid* Plant rubbed as a liniment or poultice of plant applied to boils and pimples. *Gynecological Aid* Compound infusion of plants taken for confinement. (as *E. montana* 45:60) **Navajo**, **Kayenta** *Analgesic* Plant used for injuries and pain. *Witchcraft Medicine* Plant used for bewitchment. (179:30)

Euthamia graminifolia, Flattop Goldentop
Chippewa *Analgesic* Decoction of root taken for chest pain. *Pulmonary Aid* Decoction of root taken for lung trouble, especially chest pain. (43:340)

Euthamia graminifolia var. **graminifolia**,
Flattop Goldentop
Ojibwa *Analgesic* Infusion of flowers taken for chest pain. *Hunting Medicine* Plant used in a hunting medicine. (as *Solidago graminifolia* 130:366) Flowers used in the hunting medicine and smoked to simulate the odor of a deer's hoof. (as *Solidago graminifolia* 130:429) **Potawatomi** *Febrifuge* Infusion of blossoms used for some kinds of fevers. (as *Solidago graminifolia* 131:53)

Evernia vulpina
Blackfoot *Dermatological Aid* Plant blackened in a fire and rubbed on rashes, eczema, and wart sores. *Gastrointestinal Aid* Infusion of plant and marrow taken for stomach disorders like ulcers. (72:76) **Wailaki** *Dermatological Aid* Used for drying running sores. **Yuki** *Dermatological Aid* Used for drying running sores. (98:44)

***Evolvulus nuttallianus*,** Shaggy Dwarf
  Morningglory
Navajo, Kayenta *Nose Medicine* Plant used as a
snuff for itching in the nose and sneezing. (as *E.
pilosus* 179:37)

***Fagopyrum esculentum*,**
Fagopyrum
Iroquois *Pediatric Aid* Decoction
of plant given when "baby is sick
because of mother's adultery."
Witchcraft Medicine Decoction
taken by the mother "who is running around,
making baby sick." (73:313)

***Fagus grandifolia*,** American Beech
Cherokee *Anthelmintic* Nuts chewed for worms.
(66:25) **Chippewa** *Pulmonary Aid* Bark used for
pulmonary troubles. (59:128) **Iroquois** *Abortifacient* Bark used for abortions, only when mother
was suffering. *Blood Medicine* Complex compound
used as a blood purifier. *Burn Dressing* Compound decoction of leaves applied as poultice to
burns or scalds. *Dermatological Aid* Compound
decoction taken when "skin becomes thin."
(73:302) Nutmeat oil formerly used for the hair,
either alone or mixed with bear grease. (170:123)
Liver Aid Compound decoction taken for yellow
skin and gall. *Tuberculosis Remedy* Compound
decoction of bark taken for consumption. (73:302)
Malecite *Dermatological Aid* Leaves used for
sores. (96:246) **Menominee** *Unspecified* Inner
bark of the trunk and root used in medicinal compounds. (128:36) **Micmac** *Venereal Aid* Leaves
used for chancre. (32:56) **Potawatomi** *Burn
Dressing* Decoction of leaves used for burned or
scalded wounds. *Dermatological Aid* Decoction
of leaves used to restore frostbitten extremities.
(131:58) **Rappahannock** *Dermatological Aid*
Compound infusion of north side bark used as a
wash for poison ivy. (138:34)

***Fallugia paradoxa*,** Apache Plume
Navajo, Kayenta *Witchcraft Medicine* Plant used
as witchcraft to cause insanity. (179:26) **Navajo,
Ramah** *Ceremonial Medicine* Cold infusion of
leaves used as a ceremonial lotion and leaves used
as a ceremonial emetic. *Emetic* Leaves used as an

emetic in various ceremonies. (165:30, 31) **Tewa**
Dermatological Aid Infusion of leaves used as
shampoo, to promote growth of hair. (115:46, 47)

***Fendlera rupicola*,** Cliff Fendlerbush
Navajo *Gastrointestinal Aid* Infusion of inner bark
taken for swallowed ants. (45:51) **Navajo, Kayenta**
Cathartic Plant used as a cathartic. *Ceremonial
Medicine* Plant used for Plumeway, Nightway, Male
Shootingway, and Windway ceremonies. (179:25)

***Festuca subverticillata*,** Nodding Fescue
Iroquois *Heart Medicine* Decoction of smashed
roots taken for heart disease. *Other* Compound
used as a "corn medicine." (as *F. obtusa* 73:273)

***Ficus aurea*,** Florida Strangler Fig
Seminole *Dermatological Aid* Poultice of mashed
bark applied to cuts and sores. (145:300)

***Filipendula rubra*,** Queen of the Prairie
Meskwaki *Heart Medicine* Root used as an important medicine for various heart troubles. *Love
Medicine* Compound containing root used as a
love medicine. (129:241, 242)

***Foeniculum vulgare*,** Sweet Fennel
Cherokee *Carminative* Used for colic and given
to children for flatulent colic. *Cold Remedy* Used
as a tonic and given for colds and to children for
flatulence. *Gastrointestinal Aid* Used for colic and
given to children for flatulent colic. *Gynecological
Aid* Used as a tonic and given to women in labor.
Pediatric Aid Used for colic and given to children
for flatulent colic. *Tonic* Used as a tonic. (66:33)
Pomo, Kashaya *Eye Medicine* Strained decoction
of seeds used as an eyewash. *Gastrointestinal Aid*
Seeds chewed for upset stomach, indigestion, and
heartburn. (60:44)

***Fomes igniarius*,** Shelf Fungus
Eskimo, Inuktitut *Laxative* Infusion of plant
taken as a laxative. (176:187)

Fomitopsis officinalis
Haisla & Hanaksiala *Tuberculosis Remedy*
Decoction of ground plant taken for tuberculosis.
(35:138)

Forestiera acuminata, Eastern Swampprivet
Houma *Panacea* Decoction of roots and bark
taken as a "health beverage." (135:63)

Forestiera pubescens var. ***pubescens***,
   Stretchberry
Navajo, **Ramah** *Ceremonial Medicine* Leaves
used as a ceremonial emetic. *Disinfectant* Plant
used for "bear infection." *Emetic* Leaves used as a
ceremonial emetic. (as *F. neomexicana* 165:39)

Fouquieria splendens, Ocotillo
Mahuna *Blood Medicine* Plant used as a blood
specific, purifier, and tonic. (117:28)

Fragaria chiloensis, Beach Strawberry
Quileute *Burn Dressing* Poultice of chewed leaves
applied to burns. (65:36)

Fragaria vesca, Woodland Strawberry
Okanagan-Colville *Dermatological Aid* Poultice
of leaf powder and deer fat applied to sores. *Disinfectant* Leaf powder applied to any open sore as a
disinfectant. *Oral Aid* and *Pediatric Aid* Leaf powder dusted into baby's sore mouth. (162:125)
Potawatomi *Gastrointestinal Aid* Root used for
stomach complaints. (131:76, 77) **Thompson** *Antidiarrheal* Infusion of roots or whole plant taken
for diarrhea or dysentery. Decoction of leaves
taken for diarrhea. *Pediatric Aid* Infusion of roots
or whole plant bottle fed to babies for diarrhea or
dysentery. Decoction of leaves given to children for
diarrhea. (161:259)

Fragaria vesca ssp. ***californica***, California
   Strawberry
Diegueño *Antidiarrheal* Decoction of leaves taken
for diarrhea. (70:21) **Navajo**, **Ramah** *Panacea*
Whole plant used as "life medicine." (as *F. califor-
nica* 165:31)

Fragaria virginiana, Virginia Strawberry
Blackfoot *Antidiarrheal* Decoction of roots used
for diarrhea. (82:38) **Cherokee** *Antidiarrheal* Infusion taken for dysentery. *Gastrointestinal Aid*
Taken for visceral obstructions. *Kidney Aid* Taken
for disease of the kidneys. *Liver Aid* Taken for jaundice. *Misc. Disease Remedy* Taken for scurvy. *Psychological Aid* Kept in home to insure happiness.

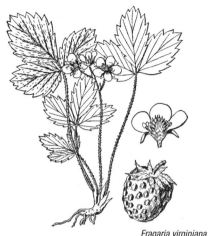

Fragaria virginiana

Sedative Infusion taken to calm nerves. *Toothache
Remedy* Fruit held in mouth to remove tartar from
teeth. *Urinary Aid* Taken for disease of the bladder.
(66:57) **Chippewa** *Misc. Disease Remedy* and
Pediatric Aid Infusion of root given for "cholera
infantum." (43:346) **Iroquois** *Unspecified* Fruits
eaten as a spring medicine. (103:96) **Malecite**
Abortifacient Infusion of plant and dwarf raspberry used for irregular menstruation. (96:258)
Micmac *Abortifacient* Parts of plant used for irregular menstruation. (32:56) **Ojibwa** *Analgesic*
Infusion taken for stomachaches. *Gastrointestinal
Aid* and *Pediatric Aid* Infusion of root used, especially for babies, for stomachache. (130:384)
Okanagan-Colville *Dermatological Aid* Poultice
of leaf powder and deer fat applied to sores. *Disinfectant* Leaf powder applied to any open sore as
a disinfectant. *Oral Aid* and *Pediatric Aid* Leaf
powder dusted into baby's sore mouth. (162:125)
Thompson *Antidiarrheal* Infusion of roots or
whole plant taken for diarrhea or dysentery. Decoction of leaves taken for diarrhea. *Dermatological Aid* Berries used as deodorant. *Pediatric Aid*
Infusion of roots or whole plant bottle fed to babies
for diarrhea or dysentery. Decoction of leaves given
to children for diarrhea. (161:259)

Frangula betulifolia ssp. ***betulifolia***,
   Beechleaf Frangula
Navajo, **Kayenta** *Ceremonial Medicine* Plant used
in a hoop for the emetic ceremony of Mountain-top-
way. *Emetic* Plant used in a hoop for the emetic

ceremony of Mountain-top-way. (as *Rhamnus betulaefolia* 179:31)

Frangula californica, California Buckthorn **Neeshenam** *Toothache Remedy* Heated root held in the mouth for toothaches. (107:376)

Frangula californica ssp. **californica**,
California Buckthorn
Costanoan *Cathartic* Decoction of inner bark used as a purgative. *Dermatological Aid* Decoction of leaves used for poison oak dermatitis. *Laxative* Dried, ground inner bark used as a laxative. (as *Rhamnus californica* 17:22) **Kawaiisu** *Antidote* Crushed berries used to counteract poisoning. *Burn Dressing* Crushed leaves and berries rubbed into burns. *Dermatological Aid* Crushed berries applied to infected sores. Crushed leaves and berries used for wounds. *Disinfectant* Crushed berries applied to infected sores. *Hemostat* Crushed berries used to stop the flow of blood. *Laxative* Ripe berries eaten as a laxative. *Unspecified* Roots or dried seeds used as medicine. (as *Rhamnus californica* ssp. *tomentella* 180:58) **Mahuna** *Cathartic* Powdered bark used as a cathartic for constipation. (as *Rhamnus californica* 117:21) **Mendocino Indian** *Cathartic* Bark used as a cathartic. *Kidney Aid* Bark used for kidney troubles. *Misc. Disease Remedy* Bark used for grippe. *Psychological Aid* Decoction of bark taken for mania. (as *Rhamnus californica* 33:368) **Mewuk** *Cathartic* Infusion of bark and leaves used as a cathartic. (as *Rhamnus californica* 97:366) **Modesse** *Antirheumatic* (*External*) Used as a medicine for rheumatism. *Cathartic* Used as a cathartic. (as *Rhamnus californica* 97:224) **Pomo** *Laxative* Decoction of bark taken for constipation. *Poison* Berries considered poisonous. (as *Rhamnus californica* 54:14) **Pomo, Kashaya** *Laxative* Decoction of bark stored for a whole year and taken for constipation. Fresh berries eaten as a laxative. (as *Rhamnus californica* 60:39) **Yokia** *Misc. Disease Remedy* Decoction of bark taken for grippe. (as *Rhamnus californica* 33:368)

Frangula californica ssp. **occidentalis**,
California Buckthorn
Cahuilla *Laxative* Infusion of berries taken as a laxative. Dried, ground bark used for constipation.

Tonic Infusion of berries taken as a tonic. (as *Rhamnus californica* ssp. *occidentalis* 11:131)

Frangula californica ssp. **tomentella**,
California Buckthorn
Diegueño *Cathartic* Decoction of bark used as a physic. *Dermatological Aid* Decoction of bark and salt used as a bath for poison oak. (as *Rhamnus californica* ssp. *tomentella* 70:37)

Frangula caroliniana, Carolina Buckthorn **Creek** *Liver Aid* Infusion of wood taken for jaundice. (as *Rhamnus caroliniana* 148:667) **Delaware, Oklahoma** *Cathartic* Decoction of bark taken as a cathartic. *Emetic* Decoction of bark taken as an emetic. (as *Rhamnus caroliniana* 150:25, 78) *Gastrointestinal Aid* and *Liver Aid* Decoction of bark taken "to remove bile from the intestines." (as *Rhamnus caroliniana* 150:25)

Frangula purshiana, Pursh's Buckthorn **Bella Coola** *Laxative* Infusion of bark taken as a strong laxative. (as *Rhamnus purshiana* 158:208) **Clallam** *Dermatological Aid* Poultice of bark used for wounds. (as *Rhamnus purshiana* 47:201) **Cowlitz** *Laxative* Bark used as a laxative. (as *Rhamnus purshiana* 65:40) **Flathead** *Cathartic* Infusion of bark used as a purgative. (as *Rhamnus purshiana* 68:56) *Poison* Fruit considered poisonous. (as *Rhamnus purshiana* 15:21) **Green River Group** *Laxative* Bark used as a laxative. (as *Rhamnus purshiana* 65:40) **Haisla & Hanaksiala** *Laxative* Infusion of bark used as a laxative. (as *Rhamnus purshianus* 35:262) **Hesquiat** *Anthelmintic* Decoction of bark, infusion of bark or chewed bark used by children for worms. *Gastrointestinal Aid* Decoction of bark, infusion of bark or chewed bark used for general stomach upset. *Laxative* Decoction of bark, infusion of bark or chewed bark used as a laxative. It was believed that the bigger the tree, the stronger the medicine. Thick bark from the larger trees was used if a very strong dose was required; thin bark from young trees was used for a mild dose. (as *Rhamnus purshiana* 159:71) **Karok** *Cathartic* Infusion of bark taken as a physic. (as *Rhamnus purshiana* 125: 385) **Klallam** *Laxative* Bark used as a laxative. (as *Rhamnus purshiana* 65:40) **Klamath** *Emetic* Infusion of foliage, twigs, and bark taken as an emetic. Berries used as an emetic. (as *Rhamnus purshiana* 37:100) Infusion of leaves, twigs, bark, and berries taken as an emetic. (as *Rhamnus purshiana* 140:131) **Kutenai** *Cathartic* Infusion of bark used as a purgative. (as *Rhamnus purshiana* 68:56) **Kwakiutl** *Gastrointestinal Aid* Decoction of dried bark taken for biliousness. *Laxative* Decoction of dried bark taken as a laxative. (as *Rhamnus purshiana* 157:288) **Lummi** *Laxative* Bark used as a laxative. (as *Rhamnus purshiana* 65:40) **Makah** *Adjuvant* Bark mixed with crab apple bark to prevent the crab apple from constipating the user. *Laxative* Used as a laxative. (as *Rhamnus purshiana* 55:286) Bark used as a laxative. (as *Rhamnus purshiana* 65:40) **Montana Indian** *Emetic* Decoction of leaves, bark, and fruit used as an emetic. *Unspecified* Bark used as a source of medicine. (as *Rhamnus purshiana* 15:21) **Nitinaht** *Disinfectant* Infusion of spring or early summer bark used as a disinfectant for cuts, wounds, and sores. *Gastrointestinal Aid* Infusion of spring or early summer bark taken as a tonic for bowel regularity. *Laxative* Infusion of spring or early summer bark taken as a mild but effective laxative. (as *Rhamnus purshiana* 160:115) **Okanagan-Colville** *Antirheumatic* (*Internal*) Infusion of bark taken for rheumatism and arthritis. *Blood Medicine* Infusion of bark taken as a blood purifier. *Laxative* Infusion of bark taken as a mild laxative. (as *Rhamnus purshiana* 162:120) **Paiute** *Gastrointestinal Aid* Decoction of bark taken for "any trouble in the stomach." (as *Rhamnus purshiana* 93:89) **Quileute** *Laxative* Bark used as a laxative. (as *Rhamnus purshiana* 65:40) *Panacea* Infusion of bark used for "any sort of disease." *Venereal Aid* Infusion of bark taken for gonorrhea. (as *Rhamnus purshiana* 114:65) **Quinault** *Laxative* Bark used as a laxative. (as *Rhamnus purshiana* 65:40) **Salish, Coast** *Tonic* Bark soaked in cold water and used as an excellent tonic. (as *Rhamnus purshiana* 156:86) **Sanpoil** *Cathartic* Decoction of bark used as a cathartic. (as *Rhamnus purshiana* 109:221) **Shuswap** *Laxative* Decoction of bark taken as a laxative. (as *Rhamnus purshiana* 102:65) **Skagit** *Antidiarrheal* Decoction of inner bark taken for dysentery. *Dermatological Aid* Salve of bark ashes and grease rubbed on swellings. *Laxative* Bark used as a laxative. (as *Rhamnus purshiana* 65:40) **Skagit,**

Upper *Laxative* Decoction of bark used as a laxative. (as *Rhamnus purshiana* 154:42) **Squaxin** *Dermatological Aid* Poultice of chewed bark applied or infusion of bark used as a wash for sores. *Laxative* Bark used as a laxative. **Swinomish** *Laxative* Bark used as a laxative. (as *Rhamnus purshiana* 65:40) **Thompson** *Analgesic* Decoction of four bark strips used as a skin wash for sciatica. (as *Rhamnus purshiana* 161:253) *Cathartic* Strong decoction of bark or wood used as a physic. (as *Rhamnus purshiana* 141:473) Strong or mild decoction of bark and sometimes wood used as a physic. *Gastrointestinal Aid* Decoction of two bark strips and flowering dogwood bark taken for ulcers. (as *Rhamnus purshiana* 161:253) *Laxative* Mild decoction of bark or wood used as a laxative. (as *Rhamnus purshiana* 141:473) *Liver Aid* Infusion of bark and red elderberry roots taken for liver diseases. (as *Rhamnus purshiana* 161:253) **Tolowa** *Laxative* Bark used as a laxative. (as *Rhamnus purshiana* 5:50) **West Coast Indian** *Cathartic* Infusion of root bark or bark taken as a cathartic. *Panacea* Infusion of root bark or bark taken for most any sort of disease. *Poison* Infusion of root bark or bark taken in large doses caused death. *Venereal Aid* Infusion of root bark or bark taken for gonorrhea. (as *Rhamus purshiana* 111:133) **Yurok** *Laxative* Decoction of bark or bark chewed as a laxative. (as *Rhamnus purshiana* 5:50) **Yurok, South Coast (Nererner)** *Cathartic* Decoction of bark used as a cathartic medicine. (as *Rhamnus purshiana* 97:169)

Frangula rubra **ssp.** *rubra*, Red Buckthorn
Miwok *Cathartic* Decoction of bark taken as a cathartic. (as *Rhamnus rubra* 8:172)

Frasera albomarginata, Desert Elkweed
Navajo, Kayenta *Dermatological Aid* Poultice of plant applied to gunshot wounds. (179:36)

Frasera albomarginata **var.** *induta*, Desert
Elkweed
Shoshoni *Eye Medicine* Decoction of root used as an eyewash. (155:75)

Frasera caroliniensis, American Columbo
Cherokee *Antidiarrheal* Root used as tonic and taken for dysentery. *Antiemetic* Used to "check

vomiting." *Dietary Aid* Taken for dysentery and given for "want of appetite." *Disinfectant* Used as an antiseptic. *Gastrointestinal Aid* Root used for indigestion, colics, and cramps. *Tonic* Root used as tonic. (as *Swertia caroliniensis* 66:30)

Frasera montana, White Elkweed
Okanagan-Colville *Tuberculosis Remedy* Infusion of roots taken for tuberculosis. (162:106)

Frasera speciosa, Showy Frasera
Apache *Unspecified* Root used to make a medicine. (100:49) **Cheyenne** *Antidiarrheal* Infusion of dried leaves taken for diarrhea. (63:184) Infusion of dried, pulverized leaves or roots taken for diarrhea. (64:184) **Havasupai** *Cold Remedy* Cooled decoction of roots taken for colds and similar troubles. *Gastrointestinal Aid* Cooled decoction of roots taken for digestive upsets and similar troubles. *Venereal Aid* Cooled decoction of roots used in conjunction with the sweat bath for gonorrhea. (as *Swertia radiata* 171:236) **Isleta** *Analgesic* Poultice of large, salted leaves applied to the head for headaches. *Pulmonary Aid* Decoction of large, fleshy root used as a lung medicine for asthma. *Throat Aid* Decoction of large, fleshy root used as a throat medicine for asthma. (85:29) **Navajo** *Sedative* Plant used for alarm and nervousness. (as *Swertia radiata* 45:97) **Navajo, Kayenta** *Panacea* Plant used as a life medicine. *Veterinary Aid* Ground plant sprinkled on incision when castrating livestock. (179:36) **Navajo, Ramah** *Psychological Aid* Dried leaves mixed with mountain tobacco and smoked to "clear the mind if lost." *Strengthener* Cold, compound infusion rubbed on hunters to strengthen them. *Veterinary Aid* Cold, compound infusion rubbed on hunters' horses to strengthen them. (165:39) **Shoshoni** *Panacea* Decoction of roots taken as a tonic for any general weakness or illness. *Tonic* Decoction of root taken as a tonic for any general weakness or illness. (155:76)

Fraxinus americana, White Ash
Abnaki *Abortifacient* Used as an emmenagogue. (121:154) Infusion of bark taken by women to provoke menses. (121:172) **Cherokee** *Gastrointestinal Aid* Tonic of inner bark taken for liver and stomach. *Gynecological Aid* Infusion of bark used to "check discharge." (66:23) **Delaware, Okla-**

homa *Cathartic* Decoction of bark taken as a cathartic. *Emetic* Decoction of bark taken as an emetic. (150:25, 76) *Gastrointestinal Aid* and *Liver Aid* Decoction of bark taken "to remove bile from the intestines." (150:25) **Iroquois** *Blood Medicine* Compound used for bad blood. (73:412) *Cathartic* Decoction of bark taken as a physic. (73:411) *Dermatological Aid* Compound infusion of bark taken and applied as poultice to syphilitic lumps. Compound used for neck sores. (73:412) *Ear Medicine* Infusion of plant, with another plant, used as ear drops for earaches. Branch sap used for earaches. (118:60) *Emetic* Bark chewed to cause vomiting and clean out the insides, as a hunting medicine for deer. *Gastrointestinal Aid* Compound decoction of bark taken for stomach cramps. *Hunting Medicine* Bark chewed to cause vomiting and clean out the insides, as a hunting medicine for deer. *Laxative* Compound decoction of bark taken as a laxative. (73:412) *Reproductive Aid* Compound decoction of roots and bark taken to induce pregnancy. *Snakebite Remedy* Decoction of roots taken and applied as poultice to snakebites. (73:411) *Venereal Aid* Compound infusion of bark taken and applied as poultice to syphilitic lumps. *Veterinary Aid* Compound decoction of plants mixed with feed as a laxative for horses. (73:412) **Meskwaki** *Dermatological Aid* Infusion of bark used for sores, itch, and vermin on the scalp. *Snakebite Remedy* Decoction of flowers taken as an antidote for a bite, probably a snakebite. (129:233) **Micmac** *Gynecological Aid* Leaves used for cleansing after childbirth. (32:56) **Ojibwa**

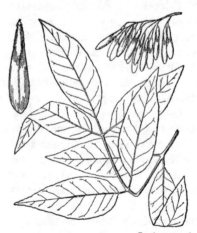

Fraxinus americana

Unspecified Root bark used for medicinal purposes. (112:245) **Penobscot** *Gynecological Aid* Strong decoction of leaves taken after childbirth for cleansing. (133:310)

Fraxinus latifolia, Oregon Ash
Costanoan *Febrifuge* Cold infusion of twigs used for fevers. *Snakebite Remedy* Leaves placed in sandals as a snake repellent. (17:12) **Cowlitz** *Anthelmintic* Infusion of bark taken for worms. (as *F. oregana* 65:45) **Karok** *Preventive Medicine* Bark used to prevent bad effect on medicine by ceremonially impure person. (as *F. oregona* 125:388) **Yokia** *Dermatological Aid* Mashed roots used for wounds. (as *F. oregana* 33:378)

Fraxinus nigra, Black Ash
Cherokee *Gastrointestinal Aid* Tonic of inner bark taken for liver and stomach. *Gynecological Aid* Infusion of bark used to "check discharge." (66:23) **Iroquois** *Analgesic* Infusion of bark taken for painful urination. *Antirheumatic (External)* Compound infusion of roots and bark used as foot soak for rheumatism. (73:412) *Ear Medicine* Compound infusion of roots used as drops for earaches. *Laxative* Compound decoction of bark taken as a laxative. *Other* Compound decoction of bark taken for stricture. *Reproductive Aid* Compound decoction of roots and bark taken to induce pregnancy. (73:413) *Urinary Aid* Infusion of bark taken for painful urination. (73:412) *Veterinary Aid* Compound decoction of plants mixed with feed given to horses as a laxative. (73:413) **Menominee** *Adjuvant* Inner bark used as a seasoner for medicines. (128:43) **Meskwaki** *Laxative* Compound infusion of wood used to loosen the bowels. *Panacea* Inner bark of trunk considered a remedy for any internal ailments. (129:233) **Ojibwa, South** *Eye Medicine* Infusion of inner bark applied to sore eyes. (as *F. sambucifolia* 77:200)

Fraxinus pennsylvanica, Green Ash
Algonquin, Tête-de-Boule *Psychological Aid* Infusion of inner bark taken for depression. *Stimulant* Infusion of inner bark taken for fatigue. (110:128) **Ojibwa** *Tonic* Compound containing inner bark used as a tonic. (130:376) **Omaha** *Ceremonial Medicine* Plant used in various rituals. (as *F. viridis* 56:322)

Fremontodendron californicum, California Flannelbush
Kawaiisu *Cathartic* Infusion of inner bark taken as a physic. (180:32)

Freycinetia arborea, 'Ie'ie
Hawaiian *Analgesic* Shoots and leaves laid over the sheets in bed for severe body pain. *Gynecological Aid* Stems and other plants pounded, squeezed, and resulting juice taken for excessive menses. *Pediatric Aid* Shoots and other plants pounded, squeezed, and the resulting juice given to children with general debility. *Strengthener* Shoots and other plants pounded, squeezed, and the resulting juice given to children with general debility, or taken for general debility. (as *F. arnotti* 2:22)

Fritillaria atropurpurea, Spotted Missionbells
Lakota *Cancer Treatment* Plant pulverized into a salve and applied to scrofulous swellings. (116:27) **Ute** *Poison* Decoction of bulbs and roots in large quantities regarded dangerously poisonous. *Unspecified* Decoction of bulbs and roots used as medicine. (30:34)

Fucus gardneri, Sea Wrack
Kwakiutl, Southern *Analgesic* Poultice applied for aches and pains. *Antirheumatic (External)* and *Strengthener* Plants used to make a steam bath for general sickness. *Venereal Aid* Fresh plants rubbed on legs and feet for locomotor ataxia. (157:260)

Gaillardia aristata, Common Gaillardia
Blackfoot *Breast Treatment* Infusion of plant rubbed on nursing mother's sore nipples. *Dermatological Aid* Poultice of chewed, powdered roots applied to skin disorders. (72:76) *Eye Medicine* Infusion of plant used as an eyewash. (72:81) *Gastrointestinal Aid* Infusion of roots taken for gastroenteritis. (72:66) *Nose Medicine* Infusion of plant used as nose drops. (72:71) *Orthopedic Aid* Infusion of flower heads used as a foot wash. (72:124) *Veterinary Aid* Infusion of roots rubbed on saddle sores and places where the hair was falling out. Infusion of

roots used for horses as an eyewash for minor lacerations. (72:88) **Okanagan-Colville** *Analgesic* Flowers used to "paint" the body for pain. *Kidney Aid* Decoction of plant taken for kidney problems. *Orthopedic Aid* Poultice of mashed plant applied for backaches. *Venereal Aid* Infusion or decoction of whole plant used as a bath for venereal disease. (162:84) **Thompson** *Analgesic* Decoction of plant taken for headache and general indisposition. (141:469) *Cancer Treatment* Infusion of whole plant used for cancer. *Misc. Disease Remedy* Poultice of lightly toasted, pounded plant mixed with bear grease and used for "mumps." *Tuberculosis Remedy* Decoction of plant taken for tuberculosis. (161:181)

Gaillardia pinnatifida, Red Dome Blanket-
 flower
Hopi *Analgesic* Plant used as a diuretic for painful urination. (174:96) *Diuretic* Taken as a diuretic. (34:320) Plant used as a diuretic for painful urination. (174:35, 96) **Keres**, **Western** *Gynecological Aid* Plant rubbed on mothers' breasts to wean infant. *Psychological Aid* Infusion of plant used to become good drummers. (147:44) **Navajo** *Misc. Disease Remedy* Infusion of leaves taken and poultice of leaves applied for gout. (45:86) **Navajo**, **Kayenta** *Other* Plant used for the effects of immersion. *Witchcraft Medicine* Plant used for bewitchment. (179:48) **Navajo**, **Ramah** *Antiemetic* Two cupfuls of decoction taken for heartburn and nausea. *Gastrointestinal Aid* Decoction of plant taken for heartburn and nausea. *Respiratory Aid* Plant used as snuff for "congested nose." (165:51)

Gaillardia pulchella var. *pulchella*, Fire-
 wheel
Keres, **Western** *Gynecological Aid* Plant rubbed on mothers' breasts to wean infant. *Psychological Aid* Infusion of plant used to become good drummers. (as *G. neo-mexicana* 147:44)

Galactia volubilis, Downy Milkpea
Seminole *Analgesic* Roots used for baby sickness caused by adultery: appetite loss, fever, headache, and diarrhea. (145:253) Roots used for adult's sickness caused by adultery: headache, body pains and crossed fingers. (145:256) *Antidiarrheal* Roots used for baby sickness caused by adultery:

appetite loss, fever, headache, and diarrhea. (145:253) Cold infusion of roots taken for baby's sickness: vomiting, diarrhea, and grogginess. *Antiemetic* Cold infusion of roots taken for baby's sickness: vomiting, diarrhea, and grogginess. (145:306) *Dietary Aid* Roots used for baby sickness caused by adultery: appetite loss, fever, headache, and diarrhea. (145:253) Roots and mother's milk or canned milk used for baby's sickness: refusal to suckle. (145:255) *Febrifuge* and *Pediatric Aid* Roots used for baby sickness caused by adultery: appetite loss, fever, headache, and diarrhea. (145:253) Roots and mother's milk or canned milk used for baby's sickness: refusal to suckle. (145:255) Cold infusion of roots taken for baby's sickness: vomiting, diarrhea, and grogginess. (145:306) *Reproductive Aid* Infusion of roots taken and rubbed on the body for protracted labor. (145:323) *Stimulant* Cold infusion of roots taken for baby's sickness: vomiting, diarrhea, and grogginess. (145:306) *Unspecified* Plant used for medicinal purposes. (145:162)

Galax urceolata, Beetleweed
Cherokee *Kidney Aid* Infusion of root taken for kidneys. *Sedative* Infusion taken for "nerves." (as *G. aphylla* 66:35)

Galeopsis tetrahit, Brittlestem Hempnettle
Iroquois *Emetic* and *Witchcraft Medicine* Infusion of roots taken to vomit as a cure for bewitching. (73:425) **Potawatomi** *Pulmonary Aid* Infusion of plant used for pulmonary troubles. (131:61)

Galium aparine, Stickywilly
Cherokee *Laxative* Infusion taken to "move bowels." (66:36) **Chippewa** *Dermatological Aid* Cold infusion of stems rubbed on skin troubles. (59:141) **Cowlitz** *Love Medicine* Infusion of plant used as a bath by women to be successful in love. *Poison* Plant considered poisonous. (65:46) **Gosiute** *Veterinary Aid* Plant used as a horse medicine. (31:370) **Iroquois** *Dermatological Aid* Compound infusion of plants used as wash for poison ivy and itch. (73:439) **Meskwaki** *Emetic* Decoction of whole plant taken as an emetic. (129:243) **Micmac** *Antihemorrhagic* Parts of plant used for persons spitting blood and gonor-

rhea. *Kidney Aid* Parts of plant used for kidney trouble. *Venereal Aid* Parts of plant used for gonorrhea. (32:56) **Nitinaht** *Dermatological Aid* Plant good for the hair, making it grow long. (55:316) **Ojibwa** *Diuretic* Infusion of whole plant used as a diuretic. *Kidney Aid* Infusion of whole plant used for kidney trouble. *Urinary Aid* Infusion of whole plant used for gravel, urine stoppage, and allied ailments. (130:386) **Penobscot** *Antihemorrhagic* Compound infusion of plant taken for "spitting up blood." *Kidney Aid* Compound infusion of plant taken for kidney trouble. *Tonic* Compound infusion of plant taken as a tonic. *Venereal Aid* Compound infusion of plant taken for gonorrhea. (133:311)

Galium asprellum, Rough Bedstraw
Choctaw *Diaphoretic* Whole plant used as a diaphoretic. *Diuretic* Whole plant used as a diuretic. *Misc. Disease Remedy* Whole plant used for measles. (23:287)

Galium boreale, Northern Bedstraw
Choctaw *Abortifacient* Decoction of whole plant used as a "deobstruent." *Contraceptive* Decoction of whole plant used to prevent pregnancy. *Diaphoretic* Whole plant used as a diaphoretic. *Diuretic* Whole plant used as a diuretic. (23:287) **Cree, Hudson Bay** *Diuretic* Leaves used as a diuretic. (78:303) **Shuswap** *Poison* Plant considered poisonous. (102:68)

Galium circaezans, Licorice Bedstraw
Cherokee *Cough Medicine* Taken for coughs. *Expectorant* Used as an expectorant. *Respiratory Aid* Taken for asthma. *Throat Aid* Taken for hoarseness. (66:43)

Galium concinnum, Shining Bedstraw
Meskwaki *Kidney Aid* Infusion of whole plant used for kidney trouble. *Misc. Disease Remedy* Infusion of whole plant used for ague. *Urinary Aid* Infusion of whole plant used for bladder trouble. (129:244)

Galium fendleri, Fendler's Bedstraw
Navajo, Ramah *Analgesic* Infusion of plant taken and used as lotion for headache. *Ceremonial Medicine* and *Emetic* Plant used as a ceremonial

emetic. *Misc. Disease Remedy* Infusion of plant taken and used as lotion for influenza. (165:45)

Galium tinctorium, Stiff Marsh Bedstraw
Ojibwa *Pulmonary Aid* Infusion of whole plant used for "beneficial effect upon the respiratory organs." (130:386, 387)

Galium trifidum, Threepetal Bedstraw
Ojibwa *Dermatological Aid* Infusion of plant used for skin diseases like eczema and ringworm. *Tuberculosis Remedy* Infusion of plant used for skin diseases like scrofula. (130:387)

Galium triflorum, Fragrant Bedstraw
Cherokee *Gastrointestinal Aid* Infusion taken for gallstones. (66:25) **Iroquois** *Love Medicine* Compound used as love medicine. *Orthopedic Aid* and *Pediatric Aid* Poultice of whole plant applied to babies for backaches. *Urinary Aid* Compound decoction taken and poultice applied to swollen testicles or ruptures. (73:440) **Karok** *Love Medicine* Plant placed in women's bed as a love medicine. (125:389) **Klallam** *Dermatological Aid* Poultice of smashed plants applied to the hair to make it grow. (65:46) **Kwakiutl** *Analgesic* Nettles or vines and then hellebore used to rub the chest for chest pains. (16:379) Plant rubbed on the skin for chest pains. (157:291) **Makah** *Dermatological Aid* Poultice of smashed plants applied to the hair to make it grow. (65:46) **Menominee** *Kidney Aid* Infusion of herb used "to clear up kidney troubles." (128:51) **Miwok** *Kidney Aid* Decoction of plant taken as a tea for dropsy. (8:170) **Quileute** *Love Medicine* Plant used by women to attract men. **Quinault** *Dermatological Aid* Poultice of smashed plants applied to the hair to make it grow. (65:46)

Galium uniflorum, Oneflower Bedstraw
Choctaw *Dermatological Aid* Whole plant used as an astringent. *Diaphoretic* Whole plant used as an diaphoretic. *Diuretic* Whole plant used as an diuretic. (23:287)

Gamochaeta purpurea, Spoonleaf Purple Everlasting
Houma *Cold Remedy* Decoction of dried plant taken for colds. *Misc. Disease Remedy* Decoction

of dried plant taken for grippe. (as *Gnaphalium purpureum* 135:64)

Garrya elliptica, Wavyleaf Silktassel
Pomo, **Kashaya** *Abortifacient* Infusion of leaves taken to bring on a woman's period. (60:106)

Garrya flavescens* ssp. *pallida, Pallid Silktassel
Kawaiisu *Cold Remedy* Decoction of plant taken for colds. *Gastrointestinal Aid* Infusion of leaves taken for stomachaches. *Laxative* Infusion of leaves taken as a laxative. *Venereal Aid* Infusion of leaves taken for gonorrhea. (180:32)

Gaultheria hispidula, Creeping Snowberry
Algonquin, **Quebec** *Gastrointestinal Aid* Infusion of leaves used as a tonic for overeating. (14:216) **Anticosti** *Sedative* Used to facilitate sleeping. (as *Chiogenes hispidula* 120:68) **Micmac** *Unspecified* Decoction of leaves or whole plant taken for unspecified purpose. (as *Vaccinium hispidotum* 133:317)

Gaultheria procumbens, Eastern Teaberry
Algonquin, **Quebec** *Analgesic* Infusion of plant used for headaches and general discomforts. *Cold Remedy* Infusion of plant used for colds. (14:216) *Unspecified* Used to make tea and medicinal tea. (14:116) Infusion of plant used as a medicinal tea. (14:216) **Algonquin**, **Tête-de-Boule** *Cold Remedy* Poultice of whole plant applied to the chest for

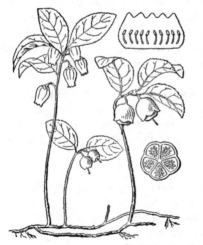

Gaultheria procumbens

colds. Infusion of leaves used for colds. *Gastrointestinal Aid* Infusion of leaves used for stomachaches. *Misc. Disease Remedy* Infusion of leaves used for grippe. (110:129) **Cherokee** *Antidiarrheal* Leaves chewed for dysentery. *Cold Remedy* Infusion taken for colds. *Gastrointestinal Aid* Infusion of root taken with trailing arbutus for chronic indigestion. *Oral Aid* Leaves chewed for tender gums. (66:61) **Chippewa** *Blood Medicine* Decoction of plants taken as spring and fall tonic to keep blood in good order. *Cold Remedy* Plant used for colds. *Tonic* Decoction of plants taken as spring and fall tonic to keep blood in good order. (59:138) **Delaware** *Antirheumatic* (*External*) Plants used with poke root, mullein leaves, wild cherry, and black cohosh barks for rheumatism. (151:33) *Kidney Aid* Infusion of plant used for kidney disorders. (151:36) *Tonic* Plants used with poke root, mullein leaves, wild cherry, and black cohosh barks as a tonic. (151:33) **Delaware**, **Oklahoma** *Antirheumatic* (*Internal*) Complex compound containing entire plant taken for rheumatism. *Tonic* Complex compound containing entire plant taken as a tonic. (150:28, 76) **Iroquois** *Anthelmintic* Compound infusion of roots taken as blood remedy and for tapeworms. *Antirheumatic* (*Internal*) Plant used for rheumatism and arthritis. (73:410) *Blood Medicine* Compound decoction or infusion taken as blood purifier or blood remedy. *Cold Remedy* Decoction of leaves taken for colds. (73:409) *Kidney Aid* Compound decoction of plants taken for the kidneys. (73:410) *Venereal Aid* Compound decoction taken as blood purifier and for venereal disease. (73:409) **Menominee** *Antirheumatic* (*Internal*) Infusion of leaf and berry taken for rheumatism. (128:35) **Mohegan** *Kidney Aid* Infusion taken for kidney trouble. (25:121) Infusion of leaves taken as a kidney medicine. (151:72, 130) **Ojibwa** *Antirheumatic* (*Internal*) Infusion of leaves taken for rheumatism and "to make one feel good." (130:369) Young, tender leaves used as a beverage tea and rheumatic medicine. (130:400) **Potawatomi** *Analgesic* Infusion of leaves used for lumbago and rheumatism. *Antirheumatic* (*Internal*) Infusion of leaves taken for rheumatism and lumbago. *Febrifuge* Infusion of leaves used for fevers. (131:56, 57) **Shinnecock** *Kidney Aid* Infusion taken for kidney trouble. (25:121)

Gaultheria shallon, Salal
Bella Coola *Dermatological Aid* Poultice of toasted, pulverized leaves applied to cuts. (127:63) **Klallam** *Burn Dressing* Poultice of chewed leaves applied to burns. (65:43) **Makah** *Oral Aid* Leaves used to dry the mouth. **Nitinaht** *Gastrointestinal Aid* Infusion of leaves used as a stomach tonic. (55:299) *Reproductive Aid* Large leaves eaten by both newly wed husband and wife for a firstborn baby boy. (160:104) **Quileute** *Dermatological Aid* Poultice of chewed leaves applied to sores. **Quinault** *Antidiarrheal* Decoction of leaves taken for diarrhea. *Gastrointestinal Aid* Leaves chewed for heartburn and colic. **Samish** *Cough Medicine* Infusion of leaves taken for coughs. *Tuberculosis Remedy* Infusion of leaves taken for tuberculosis. **Skagit** *Tonic* Infusion of leaves taken as a convalescent tonic. (65:43) **Skagit, Upper** *Other* Infusion of leaves taken as a convalescent tea. (154:38) **Swinomish** *Cough Medicine* Infusion of leaves taken for coughs. *Tuberculosis Remedy* Infusion of leaves taken for tuberculosis. (65:43)

Gaura coccinea, Scarlet Beeblossom
Navajo, Ramah *Antiemetic* Cold infusion given to settle child's stomach after vomiting. *Panacea* Plant used as "life medicine," especially for serious internal injury. *Pediatric Aid* Cold infusion given to settle child's stomach after vomiting. (165:37)

Gaura hexandra ssp. gracilis, Harlequin-bush
Navajo, Ramah *Gastrointestinal Aid* Infusion of plant taken for stomachache. (as *G. gracilis* 165:37)

Gaura parviflora, Velvetweed
Hopi *Snakebite Remedy* Decoction of root taken for snakebite. (174:86) **Isleta** *Dermatological Aid* Fresh, soft leaves worn as a headband for their cooling effect in hot weather. (85:30) **Keres, Western** *Febrifuge* Leaves used for fever and the cooling effect. *Sedative* Fresh leaves used in pillows to overcome insomnia. (147:44) **Navajo** *Burn Dressing* Infusion of plant used for burns. *Dermatological Aid* Infusion of plant used for inflammation. (45:66) **Navajo, Kayenta** *Disinfectant* Plant used as a fumigant. *Gynecological Aid* Poultice of plant applied for postpartum sore

breast. (179:33) **Zuni** *Snakebite Remedy* Fresh or dried root chewed by medicine man before sucking snakebite and poultice applied to wound. (22:377)

Gaylussacia baccata, Black Huckleberry
Cherokee *Antidiarrheal* Infusion of leaves and infusion of bark taken for dysentery. *Kidney Aid* Infusion of leaves taken for Bright's disease and dysentery. (66:39) **Iroquois** *Blood Medicine* Berries considered "good" for the blood. (103:96) *Ceremonial Medicine* Berries used ceremonially by those desiring health and prosperity for the coming season. (170:142) *Liver Aid* Berries considered "good" for the liver. (103:96)

Gayophytum ramosissimum, Pinyon Groundsmoke
Navajo, Kayenta *Dermatological Aid* Plant used as a lotion for cuts. *Psychological Aid* Plant used for the effects of a dream of a spider bite. (179:33) **Navajo, Ramah** *Hemostat* Poultice applied to cuts as a hemostatic. (165:37)

Geastrum sp., Earth Star
Isleta *Dermatological Aid* Spores used as baby powder similar to talcum. (85:30) **Keres, Western** *Ear Medicine* Spores used in the ear for running ear. (147:45)

Gelsemium sempervirens, Evening Trumpet-flower
Delaware *Blood Medicine* Roots used as a blood purifier. (151:33) **Delaware, Oklahoma** *Blood Medicine* Root used as a blood purifier. *Dermatological Aid* Compound containing root used as a salve. (150:28, 76)

Gentiana affinis, Pleated Gentian
Navajo *Analgesic* Plant used as a snuff for headaches. *Stimulant* Plant used for fainting. *Witchcraft Medicine* Plant used as an antidote for witchcraft. (45:69)

Gentiana alba, Plain Gentian
Potawatomi *Alterative* Infusion of root taken as an alterative. (as *G. flavida* 131:58, 59)

Gentiana andrewsii, Closed Bottle Gentian
Iroquois *Analgesic* Infusion of roots used as a

wash and taken for pain and headaches. *Eye Medicine* Infusion of roots used as drops for sore eyes. (73:413) *Febrifuge* Infusion of roots taken for chills. *Liver Aid* Compound used as a liver medicine. *Orthopedic Aid* Poultice of roots applied for muscular soreness. *Psychological Aid* Compound infusion of roots taken and used as wash for lonesomeness and craziness. *Witchcraft Medicine* Dried root hung in house as an anti-witch charm. Infusion of dried roots taken for headaches and to cure jealous witchcraft. (73:414) **Meskwaki** *Gynecological Aid* Root used for "caked breast." *Snakebite Remedy* Root used for snakebite. (129:222)

Gentiana saponaria, Harvestbells
Dakota *Tonic* Simple or compound decoction of root taken as a tonic. **Winnebago** *Tonic* Simple or compound decoction of root taken as a tonic. (as *Dasystephana puberula* 58:109)

Gentianella propinqua, Fourpart Dwarf-gentian
Tanana, Upper *Cold Remedy* Decoction of leaves, stems, and flowers taken for colds. *Cough Medicine* Decoction of leaves, stems, and flowers taken for coughs. (86:17)

Gentianella quinquefolia, Agueweed
Cherokee *Cathartic* Root used as a cathartic. *Gastrointestinal Aid* Used for "dyspepsy," "weak stomach and hysterical affections." *Laxative* Root used as a laxative. *Sedative* Used for "weak stomach and hysterical affections." *Stimulant* Root used as a stimulant. *Tonic* Root used as a tonic. (66:35) **Iroquois** *Anthelmintic* Plant used for worms. *Antidiarrheal* Infusion of plants taken for diarrhea. *Gastrointestinal Aid* Plant used for stomachaches. *Pulmonary Aid* Infusion of plants taken for sore chest. (73:414) **Meskwaki** *Hemostat* Liquid from root used for hemorrhages. (129:222)

Gentianopsis crinita, Greater Fringedgentian
Delaware *Blood Medicine* Infusion of roots used as a blood purifier. *Gastrointestinal Aid* Infusion of roots used as a stomach strengthener. (151:39) **Delaware, Oklahoma** *Blood Medicine* Infusion of root taken as a blood purifier. *Gastrointestinal Aid* Infusion of root taken as a "stomach strength-ener." (150:32, 76) **Rappahannock** *Blood Medicine* An ingredient of a blood medicine. (138:31)

Geocaulon lividum, False Toadflax
Cree, Hudson Bay *Cathartic* Decoction of chewed leaves and bark taken as a purgative. *Dermatological Aid* Poultice of chewed leaves and bark applied to wounds. *Emetic* Decoction of chewed leaves and bark taken as an emetic. *Unspecified* Plant used as medicine. (as *Comandra livida* 78:303)

Geranium atropurpureum, Western Purple Cranesbill
Navajo, Kayenta *Other* Plant used for overexertion. (179:29) **Navajo, Ramah** *Panacea* Plant used as "life medicine." (165:34)

Geranium caespitosum, Pineywoods Geranium
Keres, Western *Dermatological Aid* Roots bruised into a paste for sores. (147:45)

Geranium caespitosum var. fremontii, Frémont's Geranium
Gosiute *Antidiarrheal* Decoction of roots used for diarrhea. *Dermatological Aid* Plant used as an astringent. (as *G. fremontii* 31:370)

Geranium erianthum, Woolly Geranium
Aleut *Throat Aid* Leaves used in a gargle for sore throat. (6:428)

Geranium lentum, Mogollon Geranium
Navajo, Ramah *Dermatological Aid* Poultice of moist leaves and root applied to injuries, a "life medicine." *Panacea* Decoction of plant taken for internal injury, a "life medicine." (165:34)

Geranium maculatum, Spotted Geranium
Cherokee *Dermatological Aid* Astringent, compound decoction used as a wash for thrush in child's mouth. Used for open wounds and to remove canker sores. *Hemostat* Used as a styptic. *Oral Aid* and *Pediatric Aid* Decoction and fox grapes used to wash children's mouths for "thrush." (66:35) **Chippewa** *Antidiarrheal* Infusion of roots taken for diarrhea. (59:134) *Oral Aid* Dried, pulverized root put in mouth, especially by children, for sores. *Pediatric Aid* Dried, powdered

root placed in mouth, especially by children, for soreness. (43:342) **Choctaw** *Dermatological Aid* Root used as powerful astringent. *Venereal Aid* Root used for "the venereal." (23:287) **Iroquois** *Antidiarrheal* Infusion of plant taken for diarrhea. (73:367) *Dermatological Aid* Decoction of roots used as a wash for face sores or parts infected with itch. Poultice of powdered or chewed roots applied to unhealed navel of babies. (73:366) *Emetic* Decoction of roots taken as an emetic. *Heart Medicine* Decoction of roots taken for heart trouble. *Laxative* Infusion of plant used to "clean out the innards." *Love Medicine* Root placed in victim's tea to counteract a love medicine. (73:367) *Oral Aid* Roots used several ways for sore mouth, trench mouth, and chancre sores. *Pediatric Aid* Decoction of roots given to child with sore mouth, trench mouth, or chancre sores. (73:366) Poultice of chewed or powdered roots applied to severed umbilical cord. *Throat Aid* Decoction of smashed roots used as a wash for sore throats. (73:367) *Venereal Aid* Compound infusion of root used as wash on parts affected by venereal disease. Decoction of roots taken for venereal disease. (73:366) **Menominee** *Antidiarrheal* Root used for "flux and like troubles." (128:36, 37) **Meskwaki** *Analgesic* Infusion of root used for neuralgia and toothache. *Antidiarrheal* Compound containing root used for diarrhea. *Burn Dressing* Poultice of decoction of root applied to burns and infusion used for toothache. *Hemorrhoid Remedy* Poultice of pounded root bound on the anus to cause piles to recede. *Oral Aid* Infusion of root used for pyor-

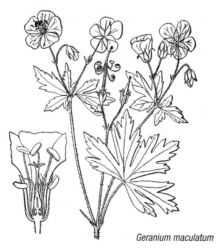
Geranium maculatum

rhea, sore gums, and toothache. *Toothache Remedy* Infusion of root used for aching teeth and sore gums. (129:222, 223) **Ojibwa** *Antidiarrheal* Root used for flux and sore mouth. *Oral Aid* Root used for sore mouths and flux. (130:370, 371)

Geranium oreganum, Oregon Geranium
Miwok *Antirheumatic* (*External*) Decoction of root rubbed on aching joints. (as *G. incisum* 8:170) **Montana Indian** *Antidiarrheal* Root used for diarrhea. *Dermatological Aid* Root used as an astringent. (as *G. incisum* 15:12) **Salish** *Oral Aid* Leaf held between lips for sore lips. (as *G. incisum* 153:293)

Geranium richardsonii, Richardson's Geranium
Cheyenne *Hemostat* Infusion of dried roots taken or powdered leaves used as snuff for nosebleed. (63:179) *Nose Medicine* Pulverized leaf rubbed on the nose and powder snuffed up the nostrils for nosebleeds. Infusion of powdered roots taken for nosebleeds. (64:179) **Navajo, Ramah** *Panacea* Plant used as "life medicine." (165:34) **Thompson** *Unspecified* Plant used medicinally for unspecified purpose. (141:461)

Geranium viscosissimum, Sticky Geranium
Blackfoot *Cold Remedy* Infusion of leaves and simple sweat bath taken for colds. (72:72) *Eye Medicine* Infusion of leaves used for sore eyes. (72:81) *Other* Infusion of leaves applied to the head and eaten for large head, from dropsy or severe malnutrition. Two cases were described of a young girl and a woman whose heads became abnormally large, as with dropsy or severe malnutrition. An infusion of the leaves was applied to the head and consumed, effecting temporary recovery, but both lost their hair and died later. (72:82) **Okanagan-Colville** *Unspecified* Poultice of pounded, heated roots applied medicinally. (162:106) **Sanpoil** *Dermatological Aid* Poultice of crushed leaves applied to sores. *Eye Medicine* Decoction of roots used as a wash for sore eyes. (109:219) **Thompson** *Gynecological Aid* Plant used as a medicine for women. *Love Medicine* Plant used as a love charm or love potion. (161:225) *Unspecified* Plant used medicinally for unspecified purpose. (141:461) Roots used for medi-

cine. *Witchcraft Medicine* Flowers possibly used for witchcraft. (161:225)

Geum aleppicum, Yellow Avens
Cree, Woodlands *Diaphoretic* Decoction of root and other herbs used to make a person sweat. *Panacea* Powdered roots used in a many herb remedy for various ailments. *Pediatric Aid* Decoction of root alone or with other herbs used for teething sickness. *Throat Aid* Decoction of root used for sore throats. *Toothache Remedy* Decoction of root alone or with other herbs used for teething sickness. Decoction of root used for sore teeth. (91:39) **Iroquois** *Anticonvulsive* Decoction of roots taken for convulsions. *Antidiarrheal* Compound infusion or decoction of roots taken for diarrhea. *Emetic* Compound decoction of roots taken to vomit as cure for love medicine. *Febrifuge* Decoction of roots taken for high fevers. *Love Medicine* Compound decoction of roots taken to vomit as cure for love medicine. *Veterinary Aid* Compound decoction mixed with horse feed and used as nose drops for cramps. (73:353) **Malecite** *Cough Medicine* Infusion of one root used by children with coughs. *Pediatric Aid* Infusion of one root used by children with croup. Infusion of one root used by children with coughs. *Pulmonary Aid* Infusion of one root used by children with croup. (as *G. strictum* 96:249) **Micmac** *Cough Medicine* Roots used for coughs and croup. *Pulmonary Aid* Root used for coughs and croup. (as *G. strictum* 32:57) **Ojibwa, South** *Analgesic* Weak decoction of root taken for chest soreness. *Cough Medicine* Weak decoction of root taken for cough. *Pulmonary Aid* Weak decoction of root taken for chest soreness. (as *G. strictum* 77:200)

Geum calthifolium, Calthaleaf Avens
Aleut *Cold Remedy* Decoction of root taken as a tonic for colds and sore throat. *Dermatological Aid* Poultice of plant applied to sores "that refused to heal." *Throat Aid* Decoction of root taken as a tonic for colds and sore throats. *Tonic* Decoction of root taken as a tonic. (6:427)

Geum canadense, White Avens
Chippewa *Gynecological Aid* Root used for "female weakness." (43:356) **Iroquois** *Love Medicine* Decoction of whole plant used as a love medi-

cine. *Panacea* Compound infusion taken or placed on injured part, a "Little Water Medicine." (73:353)

Geum macrophyllum, Largeleaf Avens
Bella Coola *Analgesic* Decoction of root taken for stomach pain. *Dermatological Aid* Poultice of chewed or bruised leaves applied to boils. *Gastrointestinal Aid* Decoction of root taken for stomach pain. **Carrier, Southern** *Dermatological Aid* Poultice of boiled leaves applied to bruises. *Panacea* Decoction of leaves taken for any sickness. (127:59) **Chehalis** *Contraceptive* Infusion of leaves taken to avoid conception. (65:37) **Clallam** *Dermatological Aid* Leaves used for boils. (47:202) **Gosiute** *Unspecified* Decoction of roots used as a medicine. (31:370) **Hesquiat** *Gastrointestinal Aid* Entire plant, including the roots, eaten as a medicine for stomach pains or excess acid. *Gynecological Aid* Young, small leaves chewed after childbirth to heal the womb. (159:72) **Klallam** *Gynecological Aid* Raw leaves chewed during labor. (65:37) **Ojibwa** *Gynecological Aid* Plant used as a female remedy. (130:384) **Okanagan-Colville** *Gynecological Aid* Infusion of roots taken by women after childbirth. (162:126) **Quileute** *Dermatological Aid* Poultice of leaves applied to boils. **Quinault** *Dermatological Aid* Poultice of smashed leaves applied to cuts. *Gynecological Aid* Raw leaves chewed during labor. (65:37) *Panacea* Leaves chewed as a universal remedy, "good for everything." (175:276) **Snohomish** *Dermatological Aid* Poultice of leaves applied to boils. (65:37)

Geum macrophyllum var. **perincisum**, Largeleaf Avens
Cree, Woodlands *Pediatric Aid* and *Toothache Remedy* Decoction of root with other herbs used for teething sickness. (91:39)

Geum rivale, Purple Avens
Algonquin, Tête-de-Boule *Antihemorrhagic* Decoction of roots boiled four times and used for the spitting of blood. (110:129) **Iroquois** *Antidiarrheal* Infusion of roots taken for diarrhea. *Febrifuge* Infusion of roots taken for fevers. (73:354) **Malecite** *Antidiarrheal* and *Pediatric Aid* Infusion of one root used by children with diarrhea. (96:255) **Micmac** *Antidiarrheal* Root used for

diarrhea or dysentery. (32:57) Decoction of root taken, especially by children, for dysentery. *Cold Remedy* Decoction of root taken, especially by children, for colds. *Cough Medicine* Decoction of root taken, especially by children, for coughs. *Pediatric Aid* Decoction of root taken, especially by children, for dysentery, coughs, and colds. (as *G. nivale* 133:316)

Geum triflorum, Prairie Smoke
Blackfoot *Cough Medicine* Infusion of plant taken as a general tonic for severe coughs. (72:72) *Dermatological Aid* Infusion of roots and grease applied as a salve to sores, rashes, blisters, and flesh wounds. (72:76) Infusion of roots applied to wounds. (72:84) *Eye Medicine* Decoction of roots used for sore or swollen eyes. (82:38) *Oral Aid* Infusion of roots used as a mouthwash for cankers. (72:66) *Respiratory Aid* Scraped roots mixed with tobacco and smoked to "clear the head." (72:79) *Throat Aid* Infusion of roots used as a mouthwash for sore throats. (72:66) *Tonic* Leaves dried, crushed, mixed with other medicines, and used as a tonic. (82:38) *Veterinary Aid* Infusion of roots used for bleeding and promoted rapid healing on horse boils and castration wounds. (72:88) **Okanagan-Colville** *Cold Remedy* Infusion of roots taken for colds. *Dietary Aid* Infusion of roots taken for the lack of appetite due to "poor blood." *Febrifuge* Infusion of roots taken for fevers. *Gynecological Aid* Infusion of roots taken by women to "heal her insides" from a vaginal yeast infection. *Love Medicine* Infusion of roots taken as a love potion by a woman who wanted to win back the affections of a man. *Misc. Disease Remedy* Infusion of roots taken for flu. (162:126) **Thompson** *Analgesic* Decoction of root used as a wash for pain. Plants used in the sweat bath for aching joints and sore, stiff muscles. *Antirheumatic (External)* Plants used in the sweat bath for rheumatism and stiff joints and muscles. (141:466) *Disinfectant* Decoction of whole plant used as a wash after the purifying sweat bath. (141:504) *Herbal Steam* Plants used in the sweat bath for rheumatism and stiff joints and muscles. Plants steamed in the sweat bath for rheumatism and joint and muscle stiffness. *Orthopedic Aid* Decoction of root used as a wash for body stiffness. Plants used in the sweat bath for sprains, aching and stiff joints

and muscles. *Tonic* Decoction of root taken as a tonic. (141:466)

Geum triflorum* var. *ciliatum, Old Man's Whiskers
Blackfoot *Blood Medicine* Infusion of roots taken to build the blood. (as *Sieversia ciliata* 100:48) *Eye Medicine* Decoction of plant used as a wash for sore and inflamed eyes. (as *Sieversia ciliata* 95:275) Decoction of root applied to eyes. (as *Sieversia ciliata* 98:39) Infusion of roots taken for sore eyes. (as *Sieversia ciliata* 100:48) **Chippewa** *Gastrointestinal Aid* Compound decoction of root taken for indigestion. (as *Sieversia ciliata* 43:342) *Stimulant* Dried root chewed as strong stimulant before feats of endurance. (as *Sieversia ciliata* 43:364) *Veterinary Aid* Dried, powdered root added to horse's feed as a stimulant before a race. (as *Sieversia ciliata* 43:366) **Paiute** *Veterinary Aid* Decoction of roots given to stimulate tired horses. (as *G. ciliatum* 93:81)

Gilia inconspicua, Shy Gilia
Navajo, Ramah *Febrifuge* Cold, compound infusion of plant taken and used as lotion for fever. (165:40)

Gilia leptomeria, Sand Gilia
Navajo, Kayenta *Dermatological Aid* Poultice of plant applied to scorpion stings or worm bites. *Sedative* Plant used as a soporific. *Tonic* Infusion of plant taken or plant smoked as a tonic. (179:38)

Gilia rigidula* ssp. *acerosa, Bluebowls
Keres, Western *Antirheumatic (External)* Crushed plant used to massage the muscles for cramps. (as *G. acerosa* 147:45)

Gilia subnuda, Coral Gilia
Navajo, Kayenta *Gynecological Aid* Ground flowers eaten to insure healthy pregnancy and ease labor. (179:38)

Glandularia bipinnatifida, Dakota Mock Vervain
Keres, Western *Snakebite Remedy* Leaves crushed with rocks and rubbed on snakebites. *Throat Aid* Infusion of leaves used as a gargle for sore throat. (as *Verbena lupinnatifida* 147:73)

Glandularia wrightii, Davis Mountain Mock
   Vervain
Navajo, Ramah *Panacea* Plant used as "life med-
icine." (as *Verbena wrightii* 165:41)

Glaux maritima, Sea Milkwort
Kwakiutl *Sedative* Boiled roots eaten to make
one very sleepy. (157:288)

Glechoma hederacea, Ground Ivy
Cherokee *Cold Remedy* Infusion used for colds.
Dermatological Aid Infusion used for babies'
hives. *Misc. Disease Remedy* Infusion used for
measles. *Pediatric Aid* Infusion used for babies'
hives. (66:37)

Gleditsia triacanthos, Honey Locust
Cherokee *Adjuvant* and *Anthelmintic* Pods used
to sweeten worm medicine. *Gastrointestinal Aid*
Compound taken for "dyspepsia from overeating."
(66:43) Infusion of bark taken and used as a bath
for dyspepsia. (152:32) *Misc. Disease Remedy* Infusion of pod taken for measles. *Pulmonary Aid*
Compound infusion of bark taken for whooping
cough. (66:43) **Creek** *Misc. Disease Remedy* Decoction of sprigs, thorns, and branches used as a
bath to prevent smallpox. (152:32) *Panacea* Pod
considered a good antidote for the complaints of
children. *Pediatric Aid* Pod considered a good antidote for the complaints of children. (148:669)
Delaware *Blood Medicine* Bark mixed with bark
of prickly ash, wild cherry, and sassafras and used
as a tonic to purify blood. *Cough Medicine* Bark
combined with bark of prickly ash, wild cherry,
and sassafras and used as a tonic for coughs.
(151:30) **Delaware, Oklahoma** *Blood Medicine*
Compound containing bark used as a blood purifier. *Cough Medicine* Compound containing bark
used for a severe cough. (150:25, 76) *Tonic* Compound containing bark used as a general tonic.
(150:25) **Meskwaki** *Cold Remedy* Infusion of
twig bark used for bad colds. *Febrifuge* Infusion
of bark used for fevers. *Misc. Disease Remedy*
Infusion of bark used for measles and especially
smallpox. *Tonic* Decoction of bark taken by patient to help regain flesh and strength. (129:228,
229) **Rappahannock** *Cold Remedy* Infusion of
roots and bark as a cold medicine. *Cough*

Medicine Infusion of roots and bark used as a
cough medicine. (138:31)

Glossopetalon spinescens var. aridum,
   Spiny Greasebush
Shoshoni *Tuberculosis Remedy* Decoction of
shrub taken regularly for tuberculosis. (as *Forsell-
esia nevadensis* 155:75)

Glyceria canadensis, Rattlesnake Mannagrass
Ojibwa *Gynecological Aid* Root used as a female
remedy. (130:371)

Glyceria fluitans, Water Mannagrass
Crow *Ceremonial Medicine* Burned as incense
during certain ceremonies. **Montana Indian**
Ceremonial Medicine Burned as incense during
certain ceremonies. (15:12)

Glyceria obtusa, Atlantic Mannagrass
Catawba *Analgesic* Infusion of beaten roots taken
for backaches. *Orthopedic Aid* Infusion of beaten
roots taken for backaches. (152:6)

Glycyrrhiza glabra, Cultivated Licorice
Cherokee *Cough Medicine* Used for coughs. *Expectorant* Used as an expectorant. *Respiratory Aid*
Used for asthma. *Throat Aid* Used for hoarseness.
(66:43) **Meskwaki** *Gynecological Aid* Compound
containing root, not a native plant, used for female
trouble. (129:229)

Glycyrrhiza lepidota, American Licorice
Bannock *Throat Aid* Root chewed for strong
throat for singing. Root boiled into a tonic and
taken for sore throat. (98:38) **Blackfoot** *Analgesic* Infusion of roots taken for chest pains. (72:72)
Antirheumatic (External) Infusion of roots applied to swellings. (72:76) *Cough Medicine* Infusion of roots taken for coughs. (72:72) *Oral Aid*
Burs kept in the mouth by buffalo runners to protect against thirst. (72:113) *Throat Aid* Infusion of
roots taken for sore throats. (72:72) *Veterinary
Aid* Roots used for horse windgalls. (72:88) **Cheyenne** *Antidiarrheal* Infusion of roots or leaves
used for diarrhea. (68:35) Infusion of roots or
leaves taken for diarrhea. (69:28) *Ceremonial
Medicine* Roots chewed to cool the body in the
Sweatlodge and Sundance Ceremonies. (68:35)

Roots chewed in the Sun Dance ceremony for the cooling effect. (69:28) *Gastrointestinal Aid* Infusion of roots or leaves used for stomachache. (68:35) Infusion of roots or leaves taken for upset stomach. (69:28) **Dakota** *Ear Medicine* Infusion of leaves applied to ears for earaches. (57:365) Poultice of steeped leaves applied to ears for earache. *Febrifuge* Decoction of root used for children with fevers. *Pediatric Aid* Decoction of root used as a febrifuge for children. (58:92) *Toothache Remedy* Root held in the mouth for toothaches. (57:365) Root chewed and held in mouth for toothache. (58:92) *Veterinary Aid* Poultice of chewed leaves applied to sores on horses. (57:365) Poultice of chewed leaves applied to sore backs of horses. (58:92) **Great Basin Indian** *Throat Aid* Roots chewed or decoction of roots taken for sore throats. (100:48) **Isleta** *Dermatological Aid* Leaves used in shoes to absorb moisture. (85:30) **Keres**, **Western** *Cough Medicine* Roots used as cough drops by singers or talkers. (147:45) **Keresan** *Febrifuge* Infusion of plant used as a wash for chills. (172:561) **Lakota** *Antihemorrhagic* Roots and Canadian milk vetch roots used for spitting of blood. *Misc. Disease Remedy* Roots chewed for the flu. (116:46) *Toothache Remedy* Roots chewed for toothache. *Unspecified* Roots used for "doctoring the sick." (88:40) **Montana Indian** *Throat Aid* Roots chewed and juice swallowed to strengthen the throat for singing. *Tonic* Infusion of roots taken as a tonic. (68:35) **Navajo, Ramah** *Cathartic* Decoction of root used as a cathartic. (165:32)

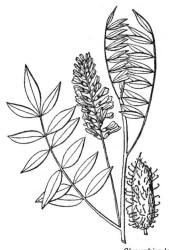

Glycyrrhiza lepidota

Paiute *Other* Infusion of plant used for some sicknesses. (144:317) **Pawnee** *Ear Medicine* Poultice of steeped leaves applied to ears for earache. *Febrifuge* Decoction of root used for children with fevers. *Pediatric Aid* Decoction of root used as a febrifuge for children. *Toothache Remedy* Root chewed and held in mouth for toothache. (58:92) **Sioux** *Ear Medicine* Infusion of leaves used for earache. *Febrifuge* and *Pediatric Aid* Infusion of roots used for children with fever. *Toothache Remedy* Roots chewed and used for toothache. *Veterinary Aid* Poultice of chewed root leaves applied to sore horse backs. (68:35) **Zuni** *Oral Aid* Root chewed to keep the mouth sweet and moist. (22:376)

Gnaphalium californicum, Ladies' Tobacco
Costanoan *Analgesic* Infusion of plant taken for stomach pain. *Cold Remedy* Infusion of plant taken for colds. *Gastrointestinal Aid* Infusion of plant taken for stomach pain. (17:26)

Gnaphalium canescens, Wright's Cudweed
Keres, **Western** *Cold Remedy* Ground, white flowers inhaled for head colds. *Dermatological Aid* Bruised leaves made into a paste and used as a liniment. (as *G. wrightii* 147:46)

Gnaphalium microcephalum, Smallhead
    Cudweed
Karok *Eye Medicine* Cold infusion of plant used as a wash for sore eyes. (125:390)

Gnaphalium obtusifolium, Rabbit Tobacco
Alabama *Sedative* Compound decoction of plant used many ways for nervousness or sleeplessness. (148:663, 664) Decoction of plant used as a face wash for nerves and insomnia. (152:61) **Cherokee** *Analgesic* Compound used for local pains, muscular cramps, and twitching. (66:51, 52) Infusion of plant rubbed into scratches made over muscle cramp pain. (152:61) *Antirheumatic (Internal)* Used with Carolina vetch for rheumatism. *Cold Remedy* Decoction taken for colds. *Cough Medicine* Used as a cough syrup. *Misc. Disease Remedy* Used in a sweat bath for various diseases. Warm liquid blown down throat for clogged throat (diphtheria). *Oral Aid* Chewed for sore mouth. *Orthopedic Aid* Compound used for muscular cramps and twitching. (66:51, 52) Infusion of

plant rubbed into scratches made over muscle cramp pain. (152:61) *Respiratory Aid* Smoked for asthma. *Throat Aid* Chewed for sore throat. (66:51, 52) **Choctaw** *Analgesic* Decoction of leaves and blossoms taken for lung pain. (as *G. polycephalum* 20:24) Decoction of leaves and blossoms taken for lung pain. (152:61) *Cold Remedy* Decoction of leaves and blossoms taken for colds. (as *G. polycephalum* 20:24) Decoction of leaves and blossoms taken for colds. (152:61) *Pulmonary Aid* Decoction of leaves and blossoms taken for lung pain. (as *G. polycephalum* 20:24) Decoction of leaves and blossoms taken for lung pain. (152:61) **Creek** *Adjuvant* Leaves added to medicines as a perfume. *Antiemetic* Decoction of leaves taken for vomiting. *Cold Remedy* Compound decoction of plant tops taken and used as inhalant for colds. *Misc. Disease Remedy* Poultice of decoction of leaves applied to throat for mumps. (148:661) Decoction of leaves used as a throat wash for mumps. (152:61) *Psychological Aid* Decoction of plant used as a wash for persons who "wanted to run away." (148:663, 664) *Sedative* Decoction of plant tops taken and used as a wash for old people unable to sleep. (148:661) *Witchcraft Medicine* Decoction of plant used as a wash for persons afflicted by ghosts. (148:663, 664) **Koasati** *Febrifuge* Decoction of leaves taken for fevers. *Pediatric Aid* Decoction of leaves used as a bath and given to children with fevers. (152:61) **Menominee** *Analgesic* Dried leaves steamed as an inhalant for headache. (44:129) *Disinfectant* Smudge of leaves used to fumigate premises to dispel ghost of a dead person. (as *G. polycephalum* 128:30) *Psychological Aid* Dried leaves steamed as an inhalant for "foolishness." (44:129) *Stimulant* Leaf smoke blown into nostrils to revive one who had fainted. *Witchcraft Medicine* Smudge of leaves used to fumigate premises to dispel ghost of a dead person. (as *G. polycephalum* 128:30) **Meskwaki** *Psychological Aid* Smudge of herb used to "bring back a loss of mind." *Stimulant* Smudged and used to revive an unconscious patient. (as *G. polycephalum* 129:214, 215) **Montagnais** *Cough Medicine* Decoction of plant taken for coughing. *Tuberculosis Remedy* Decoction of plant taken for consumption. (as *G. popycephalum* 133:314) **Rappahannock** *Febrifuge* Infusion of roots taken for chills. *Respiratory*

Aid Infusion of dried stems or dried leaves smoked in a pipe for asthma. (138:29)

Gnaphalium stramineum, Cotton Batting Plant
Kawaiisu *Analgesic* Hot poultice of leaves or stems applied to parts of body affected by pain. (as *G. chilense* 180:33) **Navajo, Ramah** *Ceremonial Medicine* and *Emetic* Plant used as a ceremonial emetic. *Panacea* Plant used as "life medicine." (as *G. chilense* 165:51) **Pomo** *Dermatological Aid* Poultice of boiled plant applied to a swollen face. (as *G. chilense* 54:15)

Gnaphalium uliginosum, Marsh Cudweed
Iroquois *Orthopedic Aid* Plants used for bruises. *Respiratory Aid* Compound infusion of plants used for asthma. (73:465)

Gnaphalium viscosum, Winged Cudweed
Miwok *Antirheumatic (External)* Poultice of leaves used for swelling. *Cold Remedy* Decoction of leaves taken for colds. *Gastrointestinal Aid* Decoction of leaves taken for stomach trouble. (as *G. decurrens* var. *californicum* 8:170)

Gonolobus sp., Milk Vine
Houma *Antiemetic* Infusion of root taken for "sick stomach." (135:63)

Goodyera oblongifolia, Western Rattlesnake Plantain
Cowlitz *Tonic* Infusion of plants taken as a tonic. (as *Peramium decipiens* 65:26) **Okanagan-Colville** *Dermatological Aid* Poultice of softened leaves applied to cuts and sores. *Reproductive Aid* Leaves split open and blown on several times by women wishing to become pregnant. (162:52) **Okanagon** *Gynecological Aid* Plant chewed by women before and at the time of childbirth. (as *Peramium decipiens* 104:41) **Saanich** *Antirheumatic (External)* Infusion of leaves used in the bath water of sprinters and canoers as a liniment for stiff muscles. (156:77) **Thompson** *Gynecological Aid* Plant chewed by women before and at the time of childbirth. (as *Peramium decipiens* 104:41) Plant chewed at childbirth to ease confinement. (as *Peramium decipiens* 141:462) Leaves chewed prenatally to determine the sex of a baby

and to insure an easy delivery. If the mother could swallow the chewed leaf, the baby was going to be a girl, but if she could not, then it was going to be a boy. (161:136)

Goodyera pubescens, Downy Rattlesnake Plantain
Cherokee *Blood Medicine* Compound decoction taken as a blood tonic. *Burn Dressing* Poultice of wilted leaves applied "to draw out burn." *Cold Remedy* Cold infusion of leaf taken for colds. *Dietary Aid* Cold infusion of leaf taken with whisky to improve the appetite. Compound decoction taken to build the appetite. *Emetic* Taken with whisky to improve the appetite and as an emetic. *Eye Medicine* Ooze dripped into sore eyes. *Kidney Aid* Cold infusion of leaf taken for kidneys. *Toothache Remedy* Infusion held in mouth for toothache. (66:50) **Delaware** *Antirheumatic (External)* Used as a medicine for rheumatism. *Gynecological Aid* Administered to women following childbirth. *Pulmonary Aid* Used for pleurisy. (as *Epipactis pubescens* 151:37) **Delaware, Oklahoma** *Antirheumatic (Internal)* Root used for rheumatism. *Gynecological Aid* Root given to women after childbirth. *Pulmonary Aid* Root used for pleurisy. (as *Epipactis pubescens* 150:31, 76) *Unspecified* Poultice of leaves used for unspecified purpose. (as *Epipactis pubescens* 150:76) **Mohegan** *Oral Aid* Poultice of mashed leaves used for babies with sore mouths. (as *Epipactis pubescens* 149:265) Mashed leaves used to wipe out infants' mouths to prevent soreness. (as *Epipactis pubescens* 151:72) *Pediatric Aid* Poultice of mashed leaves used for babies with sore mouths. (as *Epipactis pubescens* 149:265) Mashed leaves used to wipe out infants' mouths to prevent soreness. (as *Epipactis pubescens* 151:72)

Goodyera repens, Lesser Rattlesnake Plantain
Cherokee *Blood Medicine* Compound decoction taken as a blood tonic. *Burn Dressing* Poultice of wilted leaves applied "to draw out burn." *Cold Remedy* Cold infusion of leaf taken for colds. *Dietary Aid* Cold infusion of leaf taken with whisky to improve the appetite. Compound decoction taken to build the appetite. *Emetic* Taken with whisky to improve the appetite and as an emetic. *Eye Medicine* Ooze dripped into sore eyes. *Kidney Aid* Cold

infusion of leaf taken for kidneys. *Toothache Remedy* Infusion held in mouth for toothache. (66:50) **Potawatomi** *Gastrointestinal Aid* Root and leaves used for stomach diseases. *Gynecological Aid* Root and leaves used for female disorders. *Snakebite Remedy* Poultice of chewed leaves and swallowed juice used for snakebite, reference from 1796. *Urinary Aid* Root and leaves used for bladder diseases. (as *Epipactis repens* var. *ophioides* 131:67)

Gossypium herbaceum, Levant Cotton
Koasati *Gynecological Aid* Decoction of roots taken to ease childbirth. (152:42)

Grindelia camporum, Great Valley Gumweed
Costanoan *Dermatological Aid* Decoction of plant used for dermatitis, poison oak, boils, and wounds. (17:26) **Kawaiisu** *Analgesic* and *Orthopedic Aid* Decoction of leaves and flowers applied to sore parts of the body. (180:33) **Mewuk** *Blood Medicine* Fresh buds used extensively as a medicine for blood disorders. (97:338)

Grindelia decumbens, Reclined Gumweed
Keres, Western *Gastrointestinal Aid* Infusion of plant used for severe stomachache. (147:46)

Grindelia fastigiata, Pointed Gumweed
Keres, Western *Gastrointestinal Aid* Infusion of plant used for severe stomachache. (147:46)

Grindelia hallii, Hall's Gumweed
Diegueño *Blood Medicine* Decoction of leaves and stems taken as a blood tonic. (70:23)

Grindelia humilis, Hairy Gumweed
Mahuna *Dermatological Aid* Plant used for itching skin eruption caused by poison oak. (117:11)

Grindelia nana, Idaho Gumweed
Paiute *Cough Medicine* Decoction of plant said to be a good cough medicine. *Expectorant* Decoction of plant said to be a good expectorant. *Pulmonary Aid* Hot decoction of young shoots taken for pneumonia. *Urinary Aid* Infusion of plant taken for bladder trouble. (155:81, 82) **Sanpoil** *Tuberculosis Remedy* Decoction of roots used for tuberculosis. (109:218) **Shoshoni** *Analgesic* Decoction of plant taken for stomachaches. *Cough Medicine*

Decoction of plant said to be a good cough medicine. *Dermatological Aid* Poultice of boiled plant applied to swellings. *Disinfectant* Decoction of plant used as an antiseptic wash to help heal broken bones. *Emetic* Infusion of plant taken as an emetic. *Expectorant* Decoction of plant said to be a good expectorant. *Gastrointestinal Aid* Decoction of plant taken for stomachaches. *Misc. Disease Remedy* Decoction of plant taken for smallpox and measles. *Orthopedic Aid* Poultice of boiled plant applied to broken leg bones. *Urinary Aid* Infusion of plant taken for bladder trouble. *Venereal Aid* Decoction of plant taken for venereal disease. (155:81, 82)

Grindelia nuda var. *aphanactis*, Curlytop Gumweed

Navajo, Ramah *Dermatological Aid* Plant used to hold cuts together until they heal. *Emetic* Plant used as an emetic. *Gastrointestinal Aid* and *Pediatric Aid* Cold infusion of plant given to children to kill a swallowed ant. *Veterinary Aid* Cold infusion of plant given to lambs to kill a swallowed ant. (as *G. aphanactis* 165:51) **Zuni** *Poultice* Poultice of flower applied to ant bites. (as *G. aphanactis* 22:375) *Snakebite Remedy* Fresh or dried root chewed by medicine man before sucking snakebite and poultice applied to wound. (as *G. aphanactis* 22:374)

Grindelia robusta, Great Valley Gumweed

Miwok *Dermatological Aid* Decoction of leaves used to wash running sores. Infusion of pulverized leaves applied to sores. (8:170)

Grindelia squarrosa, Curlycup Gumweed

Blackfoot *Liver Aid* Infusion taken for the "liver." (68:32) Decoction of roots taken for liver troubles. (82:56) Decoction of root taken for liver trouble. (95:276) **Cheyenne** *Dermatological Aid* Decoction of flowering tops applied to skin diseases, scabs, and sores. *Eye Medicine* Gum rubbed on the outside of eyes for snow-blindness. (69:21) **Cheyenne, Northern** *Disinfectant* Decoction of flowering tops used to wash sores and other skin lesions. *Eye Medicine* Sticky, flower heads used for snow-blindness. (68:32) **Cree** *Abortifacient* Used to prevent childbearing. (12:485) *Gynecological Aid* Infusion of buds and flowers taken to ease and

lessen menses. *Kidney Aid* Plant and camomile used for kidney pains. (12:494) *Venereal Aid* Used for gonorrhea. (12:485) **Crow** *Cold Remedy* Taken for colds. *Cough Medicine* Taken for coughs. *Pulmonary Aid* Taken for whooping cough and pneumonia. *Respiratory Aid* Infusion sniffed up the nose for catarrh. Taken for bronchitis and asthma. (68:32) **Dakota** *Gastrointestinal Aid* and *Pediatric Aid* Infusion of plant tops given to children for stomachaches. (57:368) Decoction of plant given to children for colic. (58:133) **Flathead** *Cold Remedy* Taken for colds. *Cough Medicine* Taken for coughs. *Pulmonary Aid* Taken for whooping cough and pneumonia. *Respiratory Aid* Taken for bronchitis and asthma. *Tuberculosis Remedy* Infusion taken for tuberculosis. *Veterinary Aid* Flower heads rubbed on horses' hooves for protection against injury. (68:32) **Gosiute** *Cough Medicine* Roots used as a cough medicine. (31:371) **Lakota** *Antihemorrhagic* Decoction of blossoms and fetid marigold taken for the spitting of blood. (116:37) **Mahuna** *Dermatological Aid* Poultice of plants applied to cuts. *Disinfectant* Infusion used as a disinfectant wash. (117:15) **Montana Indian** *Venereal Aid* Decoction used as an antisyphilitic. (15:12) **Paiute** *Cough Medicine* Decoction of plant said to be a good cough medicine. *Expectorant* Decoction of plant said to be a good expectorant. *Pulmonary Aid* Hot decoction of young shoots taken for pneumonia. *Urinary Aid* Infusion of plant taken for bladder trouble. (155:81, 82) **Pawnee** *Veterinary Aid* Decoction of tops and

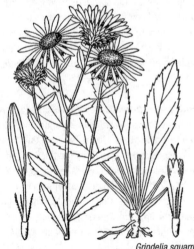

Grindelia squarrosa

leaves used as a wash for saddle galls and sores on horses. **Ponca** *Tuberculosis Remedy* Decoction of plant taken for consumption. (58:133) **Shoshoni** *Analgesic* Decoction of plant taken for stomachaches. (155:81, 82) *Cough Medicine* Dried buds used for coughs. (98:37) Decoction of plant said to be a good cough medicine. *Dermatological Aid* Poultice of boiled plant applied to swellings. *Disinfectant* Decoction of plant used as an antiseptic wash to help heal broken bones. *Emetic* Infusion of plant taken as an emetic. *Expectorant* Decoction of plant said to be a good expectorant. *Gastrointestinal Aid* Decoction of plant taken for stomachaches. *Misc. Disease Remedy* Decoction of plant taken for smallpox and measles. *Orthopedic Aid* Poultice of boiled plant applied to broken legs. *Urinary Aid* Infusion of plant taken for bladder trouble. *Venereal Aid* Decoction of plant taken for venereal disease. (155:81, 82) **Sioux** *Gastrointestinal Aid* Infusion taken for colic. (68:32) *Kidney Aid* Infusion taken for kidney trouble. (15:12) **Ute** *Cold Remedy* Used as a cough medicine. (30:34)

Grindelia squarrosa var. *serrulata*, Curlycup Gumweed

Blackfoot *Liver Aid* Infusion of root taken as a liver aid. (as *G. squarrosa serrulata* 98:45) **Shoshoni** *Kidney Aid* Dried upper third of plant and buds taken for dropsy. *Misc. Disease Remedy* Dried upper third of plant and buds taken for smallpox. (as *G. squarrosa serrulata* 98:43)

Guajacum coulteri

Seri *Unspecified* Berries used for medicine. (as *Guaiacum coulteri* 40:136)

Gutierrezia californica, San Joaquin Snakeweed

Kawaiisu *Orthopedic Aid* Poultice of heated plant applied to aching back or limbs. (180:33)

Gutierrezia microcephala, Threadleaf Snakeweed

Cahuilla *Toothache Remedy* Infusion of plant used as a gargle or plant placed inside the mouth for toothaches. (11:75) **Hopi** *Carminative* Used for "gastric disturbances." (34:323) **Navajo** *Veterinary Aid* Poultice of plant applied to the back and legs of horses. (as *G. lucida* 76:151) **Tewa** *Carminative* Used for "gastric disturbances." (34:323)

Gutierrezia sarothrae, Broom Snakeweed

Blackfoot *Herbal Steam* Roots used in herbal steam for unspecified ailments. (as *G. diversifolia* 95:276) *Respiratory Aid* Roots placed in boiling water and steam inhaled for respiratory ailments. (82:56) **Comanche** *Pulmonary Aid* Compound containing leaves used for whooping cough. (24:522) **Dakota** *Veterinary Aid* Decoction of flowers given to horses as a laxative. (57:368) **Diegueño** *Antidiarrheal* Decoction of fresh flowers or fresh roots taken for diarrhea. (74:220) **Isleta** *Dermatological Aid* Poultice of moistened leaves used for bruises. *Febrifuge* Infusion of leaves used as a bath for fevers. *Venereal Aid* Infusion of leaves used for venereal diseases. (as *G. furfuracea* 85:31) **Jemez** *Dermatological Aid* Decoction of plant used for sores. *Gynecological Aid* Decoction of plant taken by women after childbirth following the cedar decoction. (as *G. furfuracea* 36:23) **Keres, Western** *Antirheumatic (External)* Strong, black infusion of plant used as a rub for rheumatism. *Cathartic* Infusion of plant used as a cathartic. *Diaphoretic* Plant used as an ingredient in the sweat bath. *Emetic* Infusion of plant used as an emetic. *Eye Medicine* Infusion of plant used as an eyewash. *Snakebite Remedy* Chewed leaf juice taken for and rubbed on rattlesnake bites. *Veterinary Aid* Infusion of leaves used as a wash for horses after castration. (as *G. longifolia* 147:46)

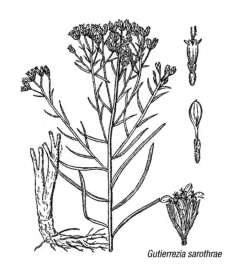

Gutierrezia sarothrae

Lakota *Cold Remedy* Decoction of plant taken for colds. *Cough Medicine* Decoction of plant taken for coughs. *Vertigo Medicine* Decoction of plant taken for dizziness. (116:37) **Navajo** *Analgesic* Plant ashes rubbed on the body for headaches. (45:86) Plant used for headaches. (76:151) *Ceremonial Medicine* Wood made into charcoal used in the medicines applied to the ailing gods. Two kinds of charcoal were used in the medicines which were applied to the ailing gods. The first was made from the bark of the pine and willow. The second was made from this plant and three-lobed sagebrush, to which were added the feathers dropped from a live crow and a live buzzard. (45:86) *Dermatological Aid* Plant used for wounds. (45:97) Poultice of chewed plant applied to ant, bee, and wasp sting swellings. (45:86) *Sedative* Plant used for "nervousness." (76:151) *Snakebite Remedy* Plant used for snakebites. *Veterinary Aid* Decoction of ground plant applied as poultice to sheep bitten by a snake. (45:86) **Navajo, Kayenta** *Antidiarrheal* Plant used for bloody diarrhea. *Ceremonial Medicine* and *Disinfectant* Plant used as a ceremonial fumigant ingredient. *Gastrointestinal Aid* Plant used for gastrointestinal disease. (179:48) **Navajo, Ramah** *Analgesic* Decoction of root taken for painful urination and stomachache. *Antidote* Compound decoction of plant used as an antidote for taking too much medicine. *Ceremonial Medicine* Decoction used ceremonially for snake infection or snakebite. *Dermatological Aid* Poultice or infusion of flowers and leaves applied to red ant bite and bee sting. *Disinfectant* Decoction used ceremonially for snake infection. *Febrifuge* Cold infusion of leaves applied to forehead for fever. *Gastrointestinal Aid* Decoction of root taken for stomachache. *Gynecological Aid* Decoction of root taken to hasten delivery of placenta. *Panacea* Root used as a "life medicine." *Snakebite Remedy* Decoction used ceremonially for snakebite. *Urinary Aid* Decoction of root taken for painful urination. *Veterinary Aid* Cold infusion of leaves used as a lotion on incisions and bites on lambs or colts. (165:51) **Paiute** *Antirheumatic* (*External*) Poultice of boiled leaves in cloth applied as a heat pack for rheumatism. *Hemostat* Poultice of boiled leaves applied to top of head for nosebleed. *Orthopedic Aid* Poultice of boiled leaves applied for sprains. **Shoshoni** *Cold Remedy*

Decoction of plant taken for colds. *Dermatological Aid* and *Disinfectant* Compound decoction of plant used as an antiseptic wash for measles and other rashes. *Misc. Disease Remedy* Compound decoction of plant used as an antiseptic wash for measles. (155:82, 83) **Tewa** *Analgesic* Plant used on hot coals to fumigate patient with painful menstruation. *Disinfectant* Plant used on hot coals to fumigate mother and newborn child. *Ear Medicine* Chopped, fresh plant rubbed around ear for earache. *Gastrointestinal Aid* Decoction of plant used for gastric disturbances, especially "gastric influenza." *Gynecological Aid* Compound containing plant used as snuff and as a fumigant for painful periods, and for women in labor. *Misc. Disease Remedy* Decoction of plant taken for gastric influenza. *Pediatric Aid* Plant used on hot coals to fumigate mother and newborn child. (as *G. longifolia* 115:56) **Zuni** *Antirheumatic* (*External*) Infusion of whole plant used for muscle aches. (as *G.* cf. *sarothrae* 22:375) *Diaphoretic* Infusion of blossoms taken as a diaphoretic. *Diuretic* Infusion of blossoms taken as a diuretic for "obstinate cases." *Strengthener* Infusion of blossoms taken to "make one strong in the limbs and muscles." (as *G. filifolia* 143:53) *Urinary Aid* Infusion of whole plant taken to increase strength for urinary retention. (as *G.* cf. *sarothrae* 22:375)

Gymnocarpium disjunctum, Pacific Oakfern
Abnaki *Other* Used as a demulcent. (as *Dryopteris disjuncta* 121:155)

Gymnocladus dioicus, Kentucky Coffee Tree
Dakota *Laxative* Infusion of root used as an enema and infallible remedy for constipation. *Stimulant* Pulverized root bark used as snuff to cause sneezing in comatose patient. (as *G. dioica* 58:89, 90) **Meskwaki** *Psychological Aid* Wax of pods "fed to a patient to cure him of lunacy." (as *G. dioica* 129:229) **Omaha** *Dietary Aid* Bark used as an appetizer. (as *G. dioica* 56:335) *Gynecological Aid* Powdered root mixed with water and given to women during protracted labor. *Hemostat* Root bark used for hemorrhages, especially from nose and during childbirth. *Kidney Aid* Root used "when kidneys failed to act." (as *G. canadensis* 48:584) *Laxative* Infusion of root used as an enema and infallible remedy for constipation. *Stimu-*

lant Pulverized root bark used as snuff to cause sneezing in comatose patient. (as *G. dioica* 58:89, 90) *Tonic* Bark used as a tonic. (as *G. dioica* 56:335) **Oto** *Laxative* Infusion of root used as an enema and infallible remedy for constipation. **Pawnee** *Analgesic* Pulverized pod sniffed to cause sneezing for headaches. *Stimulant* Pulverized root bark used as snuff to cause sneezing in comatose patient. **Ponca** *Laxative* Infusion of root used as an enema and infallible remedy for constipation. *Stimulant* Pulverized root bark used as snuff to cause sneezing in comatose patient. **Winnebago** *Laxative* Infusion of root used as an enema and infallible remedy for constipation. *Stimulant* Pulverized root bark used as snuff to cause sneezing in comatose patient. (as *G. dioica* 58:89, 90)

*H**abenaria odontopetala*, Toothpetal False Reinorchid **Seminole** *Strengthener* Plant used to make a medicine and given to students in medical training to make the body strong. (as *H. strictissima* var. *odontopetala* 145:102)

Hackelia floribunda, Manyflower Stickseed **Isleta** *Poison* Prickles from fruit caused skin irritation and swelling. (as *Lappula floribunda* 85:33) **Navajo, Ramah** *Orthopedic Aid* Root of this or any poisonous plant used for serious injury such as fracture. *Poison* Plant considered poisonous. (165:40, 41)

Hackelia hispida var. *hispida*, Showy Stickseed **Thompson** *Unspecified* Plant used medicinally for unspecified purpose. (as *Lappula hispida* 141:474)

Hackelia virginiana, Beggarslice **Cherokee** *Cancer Treatment* Bruised root with bear oil used as ointment for cancer. *Dermatological Aid* Compound decoction of root given for itch. (66:25) Decoction of roots used as a bath and taken for itching genitals. (as *Lappula virginiana* 152:52) *Kidney Aid* Decoction used for kidney trouble. *Love Medicine* Used for love charms. *Psychological Aid* Used for "good memory." (66:25)

Halosaccion glandiforme, Bladder Seaweed **Hesquiat** *Unspecified* Seaweed used as a medicine. (159:24) **Nitinaht** *Reproductive Aid* Sacs chewed by newly wed women wanting their first baby to be a boy. (160:51)

Hamamelis virginiana, American Witchhazel **Cherokee** *Analgesic* Infusion taken for periodic pains. *Cold Remedy* Infusion taken for colds. *Dermatological Aid* Infusion used as wash for sores and skinned places and leaves rubbed on scratches. *Febrifuge* Compound infusion taken for fevers. *Gynecological Aid* Infusion taken for periodic pains. *Throat Aid* Infusion taken for sore throat. *Tuberculosis Remedy* Infusion of bark taken for tuberculosis. (66:62) **Chippewa** *Dermatological Aid* Infusion of inner bark used as lotion for skin troubles. *Emetic* Inner bark used, especially in cases of poisoning, as an emetic. *Eye Medicine* Infusion of inner bark used as a wash for sore eyes. (59:131) **Iroquois** *Antidiarrheal* Infusion of twig bark taken for bloody dysentery. *Antiemetic* Poultice of branches applied to body part affected by colds and heaves. (73:346) *Antirheumatic (Internal)* Compound used for arthritis. (73:348) *Blood Medicine* Compound decoction of tips and sprouts taken as a blood purifier. (73:347) *Cold Remedy* Decoction of young branches taken or poultice applied for colds. *Cough Medicine* Decoction of young branches taken as medicine for coughs and colds. (73:348) *Dermatological Aid* Bark used as an astringent. (73:347) *Dietary Aid* Decoction of bark taken "when one can't eat," to stimulate the appetite. *Emetic* Decoction of bark taken as an emetic. (73:346) *Gynecological Aid* Compound decoction taken to prevent hemorrhage after childbirth. Decoction of shoots taken by a pregnant woman who has fallen or been hurt. (73:347) *Heart Medicine* Decoction of leaves and twigs taken for "cold around the heart." (73:346) *Kidney Aid* Decoction of twigs taken and poultice of bark used to regulate the kidneys. (73:348) *Misc. Disease Remedy* Infusion of twig bark taken for cholera. (73:346) *Orthopedic Aid* Decoction of shoots taken and poultice of bark used for bruises. *Panacea* Compound decoction of roots taken as a panacea. (73:347) *Pulmonary Aid* Decoction of bark taken for lung troubles or for spots and scars on lungs. *Respiratory Aid* Decoction of new growth

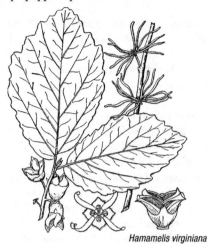

Hamamelis virginiana

twigs taken for chest colds and asthma. (73:348) *Toothache Remedy* Plant used as toothache medicine. *Tuberculosis Remedy* Compound decoction of roots or bark taken for consumption. (73:346) *Venereal Aid* Compound decoction of bark taken for venereal disease. (73:347) **Menominee** *Ceremonial Medicine* Seeds used as the sacred bead in the medicine ceremony. *Orthopedic Aid* Decoction rubbed on legs during sports, to keep legs limber. Infusion of twigs used to "cure a lame back." (128:37) *Other* Dried seeds used in a test to tell whether sick person would recover. (44:120) **Mohegan** *Dermatological Aid* Infusion of twigs and leaves used as a lotion for cuts, bruises, and insect bites. (151:72, 130) **Potawatomi** *Orthopedic Aid* Twigs used to create steam in the sweat bath for sore muscles. (131:59, 60)

Haplopappus sp.

Paiute *Antidiarrheal* Infusion of plant taken for diarrhea. *Gastrointestinal Aid* Infusion of plant taken for stomach troubles. (144:317)

Hazardia squarrosa var. *squarrosa*, Sawtooth Goldenbush

Diegueño *Antirheumatic* (*External*) Decoction of plant used for bathing the aches and pains of the body. (as *Aplopappus squarrosus* ssp. *grindelioides* 74:220)

Hedeoma drummondii, Drummond's Falsepennyroyal

Navajo *Analgesic* Plant used for pain. (45:72)

Navajo, Ramah *Misc. Disease Remedy* Infusion of plant taken in large quantities for influenza. (165:41)

Hedeoma hispida, Rough Falsepennyroyal

Dakota *Cold Remedy* Infusion of leaves used for colds. *Dietary Aid* Infusion of leaves used as a flavor and tonic appetizer in diet for the sick. (58:112)

Hedeoma nana, Falsepennyroyal

Navajo *Ceremonial Medicine* Used by assistant during the War Dance. At noon of the third day of the War Dance, the body of the patient was painted black. Medicine was then made of yarrow, red juniper, pine needles, and meadow rue, which were previously pulverized, then thrown into a bowl of water and stirred. This was then dabbed all over the patient who sipped the mixture before bathing his whole body in it. Foxtail grass and mock pennyroyal were then chewed by the assistant and sputtered on the patient. (45:72) **Shoshoni** *Cathartic* Decoction of plant taken as a physic. *Gastrointestinal Aid* Decoction of plant taken for indigestion. (155:83)

Hedeoma pulegioides, American Falsepennyroyal

Catawba *Cold Remedy* Decoction of roots used for colds. (134:188) Decoction of roots taken for colds. (152:53) **Cherokee** *Abortifacient* Infusion taken for "obstructed menses." *Analgesic* Poultice of leaves used for headaches. *Antidiarrheal* Infusion taken for "flux" and leaves rubbed on body as insect repellent. *Cold Remedy* Taken for colds. *Cough Medicine* Taken for coughs. *Diaphoretic* Decoction taken as a diaphoretic. *Expectorant* Decoction taken as an expectorant. *Febrifuge* Infusion taken for fever. *Pulmonary Aid* Taken for whooping cough. *Stimulant* Decoction taken as a stimulant. *Toothache Remedy* Beaten leaves held in mouth for toothache. (66:48) **Chickasaw** *Eye Medicine* Cold infusion of roots applied to forehead for itching eyes. (152:53) **Delaware** *Gastrointestinal Aid* Infusion of leaves used for stomach pains. (151:35) **Delaware, Oklahoma** *Analgesic* and *Gastrointestinal Aid* Infusion of leaves taken for stomach pains. (150:29, 76) **Iroquois** *Analgesic* Infusion of plants taken for headaches. (73:426)

Mahuna *Antidiarrheal* Plant used for dysentery. (117:7) **Mohegan** *Gastrointestinal Aid* Infusion of plant taken to warm the stomach. (149:265) Infusion of leaves said to be "warming and good for stomach." (151:72) **Nanticoke** *Diaphoretic* Whole plant used as a sudorific. (150:58, 84) *Kidney Aid* Plant considered an excellent remedy for kidney troubles. *Liver Aid* Plant considered an excellent remedy for liver troubles. (150:58) **Ojibwa** *Febrifuge* Infusion of plant taken for cold fevers. *Gastrointestinal Aid* Infusion of plant taken for upset stomachs. (4:2274) **Rappahannock** *Gynecological Aid* Infusion of fresh or dried plants taken for menstruation pains. (138:33) **Shinnecock** *Analgesic* Infusion of leaves taken for pains. (25:121)

Hedysarum boreale **ssp.** *mackenziei*,
Mackenzie's Sweetvetch
Alaska Native *Poison* Plant considered poisonous. (as *H. mackenzii* 71:155) **Eskimo, Inupiat** *Poison* Roots considered poisonous. (as *H. mackenzii* 83:142) **Tanana, Upper** *Poison* Plant considered poisonous. (as *H. mackenzii* 86:14) **Ute** *Unspecified* Roots used as medicine. (as *H. mackenzii* 30:35)

Helenium amarum **var.** *amarum*,
Yellowdicks
Koasati *Dermatological Aid* Decoction of entire plant used as a sweat bath for swellings. *Herbal Steam* Decoction of entire plant used as a sweat bath for dropsy and swellings. *Kidney Aid* Decoction of entire plant used as a sweat bath for dropsy. (as *H. tenuifolium* 152:62)

Helenium autumnale, Common Sneezeweed
Cherokee *Gynecological Aid* Compound infusion of roots given to prevent menstruation after childbirth. *Nose Medicine* Powdered, dry leaves used to induce sneezing. (66:56) **Comanche** *Febrifuge* Infusion of stems used as a wash for fever. (24:522) **Mahuna** *Respiratory Aid* Plant used for catarrh. (117:24) **Menominee** *Alterative* Compound infusion of flower heads taken "for its alterative effects." (128:30, 31) *Analgesic* Compound of dried flowers applied to small cuts made on temples for headache. Snuff of compounded flowers used to cause sneezing for headaches. (44:129) *Cold Remedy* Simple or compound snuff of flowers caused

sneezing to clear a stuffy head cold. (128:30, 31) **Meskwaki** *Cold Remedy* Disk florets used as snuff for colds or catarrh. *Gastrointestinal Aid* Infusion of florets taken for stomach catarrh. *Poison* Plant known to be poisonous to cattle. *Respiratory Aid* Snuff of dried disk florets inhaled for catarrh or colds. (129:215)

Helenium microcephalum, Littlehead
Tarweed
Comanche *Gynecological Aid* Pulverized flowers inhaled to cause sneezing and expulsion of afterbirth. (24:522) *Heart Medicine* Flowers dried, crushed, and inhaled for "heart flutter." *Hypotensive* Flowers dried, crushed, and inhaled for low blood pressure. (84:4) *Respiratory Aid* Pulverized flowers inhaled to cause sneezing and clear nasal passages. (24:522) Flowers dried, crushed, and inhaled for sinus congestion. (84:4)

Helenium puberulum, Rosilla
Costanoan *Cold Remedy* Dried, powdered plant rubbed on the forehead and nose for colds. *Dermatological Aid* Dried, powdered plant applied to wounds. (17:26) **Mendocino Indian** *Venereal Aid* Plant used for venereal diseases. (33:394)

Helianthella parryi, Parry's Dwarfsunflower
Navajo, Ramah *Dermatological Aid* Decoction of root taken and used as a lotion on arrow or bullet wound, a "life medicine." *Panacea* Decoction of root used as "life medicine," especially for arrow or bullet wounds. (165:51)

Helianthella uniflora, Oneflower Helianthella
Paiute *Dermatological Aid* Hot poultice of mashed root applied for swellings and sprains. *Orthopedic Aid* Poultice of mashed root applied for swellings and sprains. **Shoshoni** *Analgesic* Infusion of root used as a wash or compress for headaches. *Antirheumatic* (*External*) Poultice of mashed root applied for rheumatism of the shoulder or knee. (155:83, 84)

Helianthemum canadense, Longbranch
Frostweed
Cherokee *Kidney Aid* Infusion of leaf taken for kidneys. (66:35) **Delaware** *Throat Aid* Poultice of roots applied to sore throats. (151:32) **Delaware,**

Oklahoma *Analgesic* Infusion of plant taken and poultice of root applied for sore throat. (150:27, 76) *Tonic* Plant used as a "strengthening" medicine. (150:76)

Helianthus annuus, Common Sunflower
Apache, White Mountain *Snakebite Remedy* Poultice of crushed plants applied to snakebites. (113:158) **Dakota** *Analgesic* Infusion of flowers used for chest pains. (57:369) *Pulmonary Aid* Decoction of flower heads taken for pulmonary troubles. (58:130) **Gros Ventre** *Ceremonial Medicine* Oil from seeds used "to lubricate or paint the face or body." *Stimulant* Dried, powdered seeds mixed into cakes and taken on war party to combat fatigue. (15:12, 13) **Hopi** *Dermatological Aid* Plant used as a "spider bite medicine." (174:32, 96) **Jemez** *Dermatological Aid* Juice applied to cuts. (36:23) **Kiowa** *Oral Aid* Coagulated sap chewed, by the elders, to diminish thirst. (166:60) **Mandan** *Ceremonial Medicine* Oil from seeds used "to lubricate or paint the face or body." *Stimulant* Dried, powdered seeds mixed into cakes and taken on war party to combat fatigue. (15:12, 13) **Navajo** *Ceremonial Medicine* Plant, double bladderpod, sumac, and mistletoe used in the liniment for the War Dance. (45:87) *Dietary Aid* Seeds eaten to give appetite. (76:152) **Navajo, Kayenta** *Ceremonial Medicine* Plant used for sun sand-painting ceremony. *Disinfectant* Plant used for prenatal infection caused by solar eclipse. *Pediatric Aid* Plant used for prenatal infection caused by solar eclipse. (179:48) **Navajo, Ramah** *Dermatological Aid* Moxa of pith used on scratched wart for removal. *Other* Salve of pulverized seed and root used on injury from horse falling on person. (165:51) **Paiute** *Antirheumatic (External)* Decoction of root used as a warm wash for rheumatism. (155:84) **Pawnee** *Gynecological Aid* Dry seed compound eaten by pregnant nursing women to protect suckling child. (58:130) **Pima** *Anthelmintic* Poultice of warm ashes applied to stomach for worms. *Febrifuge* Decoction of leaves taken for high fevers. *Veterinary Aid* Decoction of leaves used as a wash for horses with sores caused by screwworms. (38:103) **Ree** *Ceremonial Medicine* Oil from seeds used "to lubricate or paint the face or body." *Stimulant* Dried, powdered seeds mixed into cakes and taken on war party to combat

fatigue. (15:12, 13) **Thompson** *Dermatological Aid* Powdered leaves alone or in ointment used on sores and swellings. (as *H. lenticularis* 141:469) **Zuni** *Snakebite Remedy* Fresh or dried root chewed by medicine man before sucking snakebite and poultice applied to wound. (22:375) Compound poultice of root applied with much ceremony to rattlesnake bite. (143:53, 54)

Helianthus anomalus, Western Sunflower
Hopi *Dermatological Aid* Plant used as a "spider medicine." (174:32, 96)

Helianthus cusickii, Cusick's Sunflower
Paiute *Heart Medicine* Infusion of roots taken for heart troubles. *Tuberculosis Remedy* Infusion of roots taken for tuberculosis. (93:116) **Shasta** *Analgesic* Pounded roots used in a steam bath for internal pain. *Carminative* Decoction of smashed roots taken for gas. *Dermatological Aid* Poultice of roots applied to swellings. *Disinfectant* Root burned in the house after a death. *Febrifuge* Poultice of roots applied for chills and fever. Root burned in the house for long, slow sickness with chills and fever. *Herbal Steam* Pounded roots used in a steam bath for internal pain. *Preventive Medicine* Roots burned to keep away disease. (79:340)

Helianthus decapetalus, Thinleaf Sunflower
Meskwaki *Dermatological Aid* Poultice of macerated root applied to sores of long standing. (129:215)

Helianthus giganteus, Giant Sunflower
Cherokee *Nose Medicine* Dry powder sprinkled to induce sneezing. (66:58)

Helianthus grosseserratus, Sawtooth Sunflower
Meskwaki *Burn Dressing* Poultice of blossoms used for burns. (129:215)

Helianthus niveus* ssp. *canescens, Showy Sunflower
Keres, Western *Hemostat* Stem juice applied to open bleeding wounds. (as *H. canus* 147:47)

Helianthus nuttallii, Nuttall's Sunflower
Navajo *Gastrointestinal Aid* Infusion of dried,

crushed leaves taken for stomach troubles. (45:87)

Helianthus occidentalis, Fewleaf Sunflower
Ojibwa, South *Dermatological Aid* Poultice of crushed root applied to "bruises and contusions." (77:199)

Helianthus petiolaris, Prairie Sunflower
Hopi *Dermatological Aid* Plant used as a "spider medicine." (174:32, 96) *Other* Used as a spider medicine. (34:324) **Navajo, Ramah** *Hunting Medicine* Cold infusion of flowers sprinkled on clothing for good luck in hunting. *Panacea* Cold infusion of whole plant used as "life medicine." (165:52) **Thompson** *Dermatological Aid* Powdered leaves alone or in ointment used on sores and swellings. (141:469)

Helianthus strumosus, Paleleaf Woodland Sunflower
Iroquois *Anthelmintic* Decoction of roots given to children and adults with worms. *Pediatric Aid* Decoction of roots given to children with worms. (73:469) **Meskwaki** *Pulmonary Aid* Infusion of root taken for lung troubles. (129:215)

Heliomeris longifolia var. ***annua***, Longleaf Falsegoldeneye
Navajo, Ramah *Panacea* Plant used as "life medicine." (as *Viguiera annua* 165:54)

Heliomeris longifolia var. ***longifolia***, Longleaf Falsegoldeneye
Navajo, Ramah *Panacea* Plant used as "life medicine." (as *Viguiera longifolia* 165:54)

Heliomeris multiflora var. ***multiflora***, Showy Goldeneye
Navajo, Ramah *Witchcraft Medicine* Plant designated as a witchcraft plant. (as *Viguiera multiflora* 165:54)

Heliopsis helianthoides var. ***scabra***, Smooth Oxeye
Chippewa *Stimulant* Decoction of dried root or chewed fresh root spit on limbs as stimulant. (as *H. scabra* 43:364) **Meskwaki** *Pulmonary Aid* Root used for lung troubles. (as *H. scabra* 129:215)

Heliotropium curassavicum, Salt Heliotrope
Paiute *Antidiarrheal* Plant used as a diarrhea medicine. (144:317) *Diuretic* Decoction of plant or roots taken in cases of "retention of urine." *Emetic* Decoction of root taken as an emetic. *Throat Aid* Decoction of root gargled for sore throat. (155:84, 85) **Pima** *Dermatological Aid* Poultice of dried, pulverized root applied to sores and wounds. (123:79) **Shoshoni** *Diuretic* Decoction of plant or roots taken in cases of "retention of urine." *Emetic* Decoction of root taken as an emetic. *Misc. Disease Remedy* Decoction of plant tops taken to aid in "bringing out" measles. *Throat Aid* Decoction of root gargled for sore throat. *Venereal Aid* Decoction of plant taken for venereal disease. (155:84, 85) **Tubatulabal** *Antidiarrheal* Decoction of entire plant taken for bloody flux. (167:59)

Hepatica nobilis var. ***acuta***, Sharplobe Hepatica
Cherokee *Analgesic* Infusion of plant taken as an emetic for abdominal pains. (as *H. acutiloba* 152:22) *Breast Treatment* Compound used for swollen breasts. (as *H. acutiloba* 66:38) *Emetic* Infusion of plant taken as an emetic for abdominal pains. (as *H. acutiloba* 152:22) *Gastrointestinal Aid* Compound decoction used for poor digestion. (as *H. acutiloba* 66:38) Infusion of plant taken as an emetic for abdominal pains. (as *H. acutiloba* 152:22) *Laxative* Infusion used as a laxative. *Liver Aid* Infusion used for the liver. (as *H. acutiloba* 66:38) **Iroquois** *Analgesic* Decoction of plants taken by pregnant women with side or labor pains. *Blood Medicine* Plant used as a blood purifier. *Contraceptive* Infusion of plants taken to prevent conception. *Gynecological Aid* Compound used for labor pains in parturition. Decoction of plants taken by middle-aged women to induce childbirth, and by pregnant women for sore abdomen or side pains. *Orthopedic Aid* Compound decoction of plants taken for stiff muscles. *Other* Compound decoction of roots given to children with "summer complaint." Roots used to tell fortune. *Pediatric Aid* Compound decoction of roots given to children with "summer complaint." (73:328) *Pulmonary Aid* Infusion of whole plant and another plant taken by forest runners with shortness of breath. (as *H. acutiloba* 118:42) *Witchcraft Medicine*

"Chewed by women to bewitch men and make them crazy by affecting their hearts." (73:328) **Menominee** *Gynecological Aid* Compound containing root used for female maladies, especially leukorrhea. (as *H. acutiloba* 128:48, 49) **Meskwaki** *Eye Medicine* and *Other* Infusion of root taken and used as a wash for twisted mouth or crossed eyes. (as *H. acutiloba* 129:239)

Hepatica nobilis var. *obtusa*, Roundlobed Hepatica

Chippewa *Abortifacient* Decoction of roots taken for amenorrhea. (as *H. triloba* 59:129) *Anticonvulsive* Decoction of root taken, especially by children, for convulsions. (as *H. americana* 43:336) *Dermatological Aid* Poultice of plants applied to inflammations and bruises. (as *H. triloba* 59:129) *Hunting Medicine* Roots used as charms on traps for fur-bearing animals. (as *H. triloba* 43:376) *Liver Aid* Plant used for liver ailments. (as *H. triloba* 59:129) *Pediatric Aid* Decoction of root taken for convulsions, "used chiefly for children." (as *H. americana* 43:336) **Menominee** *Antidiarrheal* Compound decoction of root used for dysentery. (as *H. triloba* 44:131) **Nanticoke** *Febrifuge* Petals chewed "to prevent fever in summer." (as *H. americana* 150:56, 84) **Potawatomi** *Other* Infusion of root and leaves taken for vertigo. (as *H. triloba* 131:74)

Heracleum maximum, Common Cow Parsnip

Aleut *Cold Remedy* Leaves used to make a tonic for colds. (as *H. lanatum* 6:427) *Dermatological Aid* Poultice of heated leaves applied to minor cuts. *Orthopedic Aid* Poultice of heated leaves applied to sore muscles. (as *H. lanatum* 6:425) *Throat Aid* Leaves used to make a soothing drink for sore throats. (as *H. lanatum* 6:427) **Bella Coola** *Analgesic* Poultice of compound containing roots used for lung or hip pains. *Antirheumatic* (*External*) Compound infusion of root used as poultice for pains like rheumatism. *Dermatological Aid* Poultice of crushed, boiled root, baked root, or raw root applied to boils. (as *H. lanatum* 127:61) Poultice of crushed and cooked roots applied to boils. (as *H. lanatum* 158:201) *Orthopedic Aid* Poultice of compound containing roots used for hip pains. *Pulmonary Aid* Poultice of compound containing roots used for lung pains.

(as *H. lanatum* 127:61) **Blackfoot** *Antidiarrheal* Infusion of fresh, young stems taken for diarrhea. (as *H. lanatum* 72:67) *Dermatological Aid* Infusion of young stems applied in the removal of warts. (as *H. lanatum* 72:76) Poultice of roots applied to bruises and chronic swellings. (as *H. lanatum* 82:48) **California Indian** *Antirheumatic* (*Internal*) Strong decoction of root used for rheumatism. (as *H. lanatum* 15:13) **Carrier** *Antirheumatic* (*External*) Poultice of ground roots applied for rheumatism. (as *H. lanatum* 26:82) **Carrier, Northern** *Dermatological Aid* Poultice of root applied to swellings and bruises. (as *H. lanatum* 127:61) **Chippewa** *Dermatological Aid* Poultice of boiled or dried root and flowers applied to boils. (as *H. lanatum* 43:350) *Throat Aid* Decoction of root gargled or dried root chewed for ulcerated sore throat. (as *H. lanatum* 43:342) **Cree** *Dermatological Aid* Powdered roots and lard used as an ointment or poultice of root paste applied to boils and swellings. (as *H. lanatum* 12:492) *Poison Plant* considered poisonous. *Toothache Remedy* Root held on the sore tooth for toothaches. (as *H. lanatum* 12:491) *Venereal Aid* Powdered roots and lard used as ointment or root paste poultice applied to venereal disease chancres. (as *H. lanatum* 12:494) **Cree, Woodlands** *Analgesic* Poultice of ground root, calamus, and yellow pond lily applied to the head for severe headaches. Decoction of root, calamus, and yellow pond lily used as a wash for severe headaches. *Antirheumatic* (*External*) Poultice of ground root, calamus, and

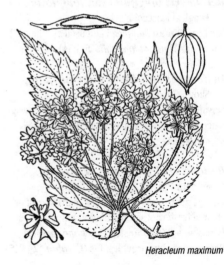

Heracleum maximum

yellow pond lily applied to painful limbs. Decoction of root, calamus, and yellow pond lily used as a wash for painful limbs. *Dermatological Aid* Poultice of root, calamus, root and yellow pond lily root applied to mancos, worms in the flesh. (as *H. lanatum* 91:40) **Gitksan** *Antirheumatic* (*External*) Poultice of fresh roots used for rheumatism. (as *H. lanatum* 62:25) Poultice of mashed root applied to rheumatic or other swellings. *Dermatological Aid* Poultice of mashed root applied to boils and other swellings. (as *H. lanatum* 127:61) *Witchcraft Medicine* Roots, red elder bark, and juniper boughs used as a smudge for evil witchcraft victims. (as *H. lanatum* 62:25) **Haisla** *Dermatological Aid* Poultice of roots, Indian hellebore, and Sitka spruce pitch applied to wounds. (as *H. lanatum* 35:214) **Iroquois** *Analgesic* Compound infusion of plant used as steam bath for headaches. *Antirheumatic* (*External*) Compound infusion of plant used as steam bath for rheumatism. *Dermatological Aid* Compound decoction used as wash or poultice applied to chancres or lumps on penis. *Diaphoretic* Infusion of plant used as steam bath to sweat out rheumatism and headaches. *Gastrointestinal Aid* Compound decoction of roots taken for bruises on the back of the stomach. *Hunting Medicine* Decoction of roots used as wash for rifles, a "hunting medicine." (as *H. lanatum* 73:400) *Misc. Disease Remedy* Plant used for influenza. (as *H. lanatum* 118:56) **Karok** *Poison* Roots poisonous to cattle. (as *H. lanatum* 125:387) **Klamath** *Unspecified* Roots used medicinally for unspecified purpose. (as *H. lanatum* 37:102) **Kwakiutl** *Dermatological Aid* Dried, pounded roots and oil used as a hair ointment. *Gynecological Aid* and *Pediatric Aid* Dried, pounded roots and oil rubbed on face and waist of girl at puberty. (as *H. lanatum* 157:276) **Makah** *Eye Medicine* Heated poultice of leaves applied for eye problems. *Tonic* Used as a spring tonic. *Unspecified* Central stalk considered strong medicine. (as *H. lanatum* 55:293) **Malecite** *Misc. Disease Remedy* Infusion of root shoots used for smallpox. Infusion used for cholera. (as *H. lanatum* 96:256) **Menominee** *Hunting Medicine* Herb used in the hunting bundle and smudged for 4 days to remove the charm. (as *H. lanatum* 128:81) *Witchcraft Medicine* An evil medicine used by sorcerers. (as *H. lanatum* 128:55) **Meskwaki** *Anal-*

gesic Seeds used for severe headache and root used for stomach cramps. *Dermatological Aid* Poultice of stems applied to wounds. *Gastrointestinal Aid* Root used for colic or any kind of stomach cramps. *Misc. Disease Remedy* Infusion of root used for erysipelas. (as *H. lanatum* 129:249) **Mewuk** *Antirheumatic* (*External*) Poultice of mashed roots applied to swellings. *Misc. Disease Remedy* Used for mumps. (as *H. lanatum* 97:366) **Micmac** *Misc. Disease Remedy* Root used for smallpox and cholera. (as *H. lanatum* 32:57) **Ojibwa** *Dermatological Aid* Poultice of pounded, fresh root applied to sores. (as *H. lanatum* 130:390) *Hunting Medicine* Root or seeds used to smudge a fire and drive away a bad spirit from the camp of the hunter. There is a bad spirit who is always present trying to steal away one's luck in hunting game. He must be driven away from the camp of the hunter by smudging a fire with the roots or seeds. This gets into the spirit's eyes and he cannot see the hunter leave the camp, so naturally does not follow and bother him. (as *H. lanatum* 130:432) **Okanagan-Colville** *Dermatological Aid* Decoction of roots, red willow, and chokecherry branches used as a cleansing medicine for the scalp. Decoction of branches used as a hair tonic to prevent gray hair and dandruff. *Orthopedic Aid* Heated poultice of sliced, pounded roots applied to sore backs. (as *H. lanatum* 162:62) **Okanagon** *Cathartic* Decoction of roots taken as a purgative. *Tonic* Decoction of roots taken as a tonic. (as *H. lanatum* 104:40) **Omaha** *Analgesic* Decoction of root taken for intestinal pains. *Cathartic* Decoction of root taken as a physic. *Gastrointestinal Aid* Decoction of root taken for intestinal pains. (as *H. lanatum* 58:107) **Paiute** *Antirheumatic* (*External*) Poultice of mashed root applied for rheumatism. (as *H. lanatum* 155:85, 86) *Cold Remedy* Decoction of roots taken for colds. (as *H. lanatum* 87:197) *Dermatological Aid* Roots used as a salve for sores. (as *H. lanatum* 87:196) Salve made from root applied to wounds. (as *H. lanatum* 155:85, 86) **Paiute, Northern** *Antirheumatic* (*External*) Poultice of roasted, split plants applied to aching joints for rheumatism. (as *H. lanatum* 49:130) **Pawnee** *Dermatological Aid* Poultice of scraped, boiled root applied to boils. (as *H. lanatum* 58:107) **Pomo** *Antirheumatic* (*External*) Decoction of plant used as a wash for rheumatism. Poultice of pounded, raw, or heated roots applied to rheumatism. *Dermatological Aid* Decoction of plant used as a wash for swellings. Poultice of pounded, raw, or heated roots applied to swellings. (as *H. lanatum* 54:14) **Pomo**, **Kashaya** *Antirheumatic (External)* Poultice of baked, pounded root used for rheumatism, arthritis, and other muscular pains. (as *H. lanatum* 60:87) **Quinault** *Analgesic* Poultice of warmed leaves applied to sore limbs. *Orthopedic Aid* Poultice of warmed leaves applied to sore limbs. (as *H. lanatum* 65:42) **Salish**, **Coast** *Dermatological Aid* Roots pounded, roasted, mixed with dogfish oil and used as a hair lotion to make hair grow long. (as *H. lanatum* 156:89) **Sanpoil** *Analgesic* Poultice of roots applied overnight to "painful parts, sore eyes, etc." *Dermatological Aid* Pounded root mixed with water and used as a hair wash for dandruff. *Eye Medicine* Poultice of roots applied overnight to "painful parts, sore eyes, etc." (as *H. lanatum* 109:220) **Shoshoni** *Cold Remedy* Decoction of root in whisky taken and smoke of root compound inhaled for colds. *Cough Medicine* Decoction of root in whisky taken for colds and coughs. *Throat Aid* Infusion of mashed root gargled and poultice applied for sore throat. *Toothache Remedy* Raw root placed in cavities for toothaches. *Tuberculosis Remedy* Decoction of root taken for tuberculosis. (as *H. lanatum* 155:85, 86) **Shuswap** *Dermatological Aid* Infusion of roots taken for sores. *Internal Medicine* Infusion of roots taken to kill all the internal germs. *Urinary Aid* Infusion of roots taken for the bladder. (as *Meracleum lanatum* 102:56) **Sikani** *Analgesic* Poultice of mashed roots applied to swellings of neuralgia or rheumatism. *Antirheumatic (External)* Poultice of mashed roots applied to swellings of rheumatism. *Dermatological Aid* Poultice of mashed roots applied to swellings of neuralgia. (as *H. lanatum* 127:61) **Tanaina** *Unspecified* Root used as a medicine. (as *H. lanatum* 126:329) **Thompson** *Cathartic* Decoction of roots taken as a purgative. (as *H. lanatum* 104:40) Decoction of root used as a purgative and tonic. (as *H. lanatum* 141:457) Decoction of roots taken by warriors and hunters as a purgative. (as *H. lanatum* 141:504) *Ceremonial Medicine* and *Disinfectant* Decoction of root used ceremonially as a wash for purification. (as *H. lanatum* 141:457) Decoction of roots taken by warriors and hunters as a purifier. (as *H.*

lanatum 141:504) *Tonic* Decoction of roots taken as a tonic. (as *H. lanatum* 104:40) Decoction of root used as a tonic and purgative. (as *H. lanatum* 141:457) *Unspecified* Plant used medicinally. (as *H. lanatum* 161:152) *Venereal Aid* Strong decoction of root used for syphilis. (as *H. lanatum* 141:457) **Washo** *Antidiarrheal* Decoction of root taken for diarrhea. *Toothache Remedy* Raw root placed in cavities for toothaches. (as *H. lanatum* 155:85, 86) **Winnebago** *Anticonvulsive* Plant tops used in smoke treatment for convulsions. *Stimulant* Plant tops used in smoke treatment for fainting. (as *H. lanatum* 58:107)

Heracleum sphondylium, Eltrot
Micmac *Gynecological Aid* Green and light-color plant used as medicine for women. (168:30) *Unspecified* Part of plant considered "good medicine." (32:57) *Urinary Aid* Dark and ripe plant used as medicine for men. (168:30)

Heteranthera reniformis, Kidneyleaf Mudplantain
Cherokee *Dermatological Aid* Hot poultice of root applied to inflamed wounds and sores. (66:45)

Heteromeles arbutifolia, Toyon
Costanoan (Olhonean) *Abortifacient* Infusion of leaves taken "for suppression of menses or irregular menses of girls." (97:373) **Diegueño** *Dermatological Aid* Infusion of bark and leaves used as wash for infected wounds. (74:217) **Mendocino Indian** *Analgesic* Decoction of leaves taken for various aches and pains. *Gastrointestinal Aid* Decoction of leaves taken for stomachaches. (33:355)

Heterotheca villosa var. *hispida*, Bristly Hairy Goldaster
Isleta *Poison* Plant, when touched, caused a skin irritation similar to ant bites. (as *Chrysopsis hirsutissima* 85:25) **Navajo**, **Ramah** *Dermatological Aid* Poultice of leaves applied to ant bites. *Nose Medicine* Poultice of leaves applied to sore nose. *Toothache Remedy* Poultice of root applied for toothache. (as *Chrysopsis hispida* 165:49)

Heterotheca villosa var. *villosa*, Hairy Goldenaster

Cheyenne *Disinfectant* Plant burned as incense to remove evil spirits from the house. (as *Chrysopsis villosa* 69:20) *Sedative* Infusion of plant tops and stems taken to sleep when feeling generally poor. (as *Chrysopsis foliosa* 63:187) Infusion of tops and stems taken for feeling poorly and made one sleepy. (as *Chrysopsis foliosa* 64:187) **Hopi** *Analgesic* Infusion of leaves and flowers used for chest pain. (as *Chrysopsis villosa* 174:95) **Navajo, Kayenta** *Ceremonial Medicine* Plant used in the corral dance. (as *Chrysopsis villosa* 179:46) **Navajo, Ramah** *Ceremonial Medicine* Plant used as a ceremonial emetic and chant lotion. *Emetic* Plant used alone as a sweat house emetic. Plant used as a ceremonial and sweat house emetic for various ailments. *Gastrointestinal Aid* Cold infusion of leaves used to kill a swallowed red ant. Plant used as a sweat house emetic for indigestion. *Heart Medicine* Plant used as an "aorta medicine." *Panacea* Root used as a "life medicine." *Toothache Remedy* Poultice of heated root applied for toothache. *Venereal Aid* Plant used as a sweat house emetic for sexual infection. (as *Chrysopsis villosa* 165:49)

Heuchera americana, American Alumroot

Cherokee *Antidiarrheal* Taken for dysentery. *Dermatological Aid* Powdered root used on malignant ulcers and infusion sprinkled on bad sores. Infusion of astringent root taken for bowel complaints. *Gastrointestinal Aid* Infusion of root taken for bowel complaints. *Gynecological Aid* Used for "immoderate flow of menses." *Hemorrhoid Remedy* Infusion of root taken for piles. *Oral Aid* Infusion used for "thrash" and sore mouth and root chewed to take coat off tongue. (66:23) **Chickasaw** *Dermatological Aid* Root used as a powerful astringent. *Tonic* Root used as a tonic. **Choctaw** *Dermatological Aid* Root used as a powerful astringent. *Tonic* Root used as a tonic. **Creek** *Dermatological Aid* Root used as a powerful astringent. *Tonic* Root used as a tonic. (23:286, 287) **Menominee** *Analgesic* Compound decoction of root used for stomach pain. *Gastrointestinal Aid* Raw root eaten for "disordered stomach." (44:130) **Meskwaki** *Dermatological Aid* Foliage used as an astringent for sores. *Panacea* Compound containing root used as a "healer." (129:246)

Heuchera americana var. *hispida*, Hairy Alumroot

Chippewa *Analgesic* Dried root chewed and juice swallowed for stomach pain. (as *H. hispida* 43:344) *Eye Medicine* Decoction of root used as a wash for sore eyes. (as *H. hispida* 43:360) *Gastrointestinal Aid* Dried root chewed and juice swallowed for stomach pain. (as *H. hispida* 43:344) **Menominee** *Antidiarrheal* Infusion of root used for diarrhea. (as *H. hispida* 128:53) **Sioux, Teton** *Antidiarrheal* Root, very powerful and small dose for children, used for chronic diarrhea. (as *H. hispida* 42:269)

Heuchera bracteata, Bracted Alumroot

Navajo *Gastrointestinal Aid* Plant chewed for indigestion. *Oral Aid* Plant chewed for sore gums. *Toothache Remedy* Compound poultice of crushed leaves applied to toothaches. (45:52)

Heuchera cylindrica, Roundleaf Alumroot

Blackfoot *Antidiarrheal* Decoction of roots used for diarrhea. *Dermatological Aid* Decoction of roots used as an astringent. (82:36) **Flathead** *Antidiarrheal* Roots infused or chewed for diarrhea. *Gastrointestinal Aid* Roots infused or chewed for stomach cramps. **Kutenai** *Antirheumatic* (*External*) Decoction of roots used for "aching bones." *Tuberculosis Remedy* Decoction of roots taken for tuberculosis. (68:31) **Okanagan-Colville** *Blood Medicine* Decoction of roots and Oregon grape roots used as a tonic for the "changing of the blood." *Dermatological Aid* Poultice of mashed, peeled roots applied to sores and cuts. Infusion of roots used to wash sores and cuts. Roots mixed with puffball spores and used as a salve for diaper rash. *Pediatric Aid* Decoction of roots used, especially for children and babies, to rinse out the mouth for sore throats. Roots mixed with puffball spores and used as a salve for diaper rash. *Throat Aid* Fresh root held in the mouth and sucked for sore throats. Decoction of roots used, especially for children and babies, to rinse out the mouth for sore throats. (162:138) **Shuswap** *Antidiarrheal* Decoction of leaves and roots taken for diarrhea. *Dermatological Aid* Decoction of leaves and roots used as a wash for sores. (102:68) **Thompson** *Dermatological Aid* Chewed leaves and roots spat on sores or wounds. Poultice of root with Douglas fir pitch used for wounds. *Liver Aid* Infusion of root taken for liver trouble. *Oral Aid* Small, peeled, cleaned root piece chewed for mouth sores and gum boils. *Throat Aid* Infusion of root taken for sore throats. *Unspecified* Root used for medicine. (161:282)

Heuchera cylindrica var. *alpina*, Alpine Alumroot

Cheyenne *Antirheumatic* (*External*) Powdered roots rubbed on the skin for rheumatism. (as *H. ovalifolia* 63:176) Powdered roots rubbed on the skin for rheumatism or sore muscles. (as *H. ovalifolia* 64:176) *Antirheumatic* (*Internal*) Infusion of roots taken for rheumatism. (as *H. ovalifolia* 63:176) Infusion of powdered plant tops taken for rheumatism or sore muscles. (as *H. ovalifolia* 64:176) *Dermatological Aid* Poultice of powdered roots applied for poison ivy and other skin rashes. (as *H. ovalifolia* 69:38) *Orthopedic Aid* Infusion of roots taken or powdered roots rubbed on skin for sore muscles. (as *H. ovalifolia* 63:176)

Heuchera cylindrica var. *glabella*, Beautiful Alumroot

Arapaho *Unspecified* Roots used medicinally for unspecified purpose. **Blackfoot** *Dermatological Aid* Pounded roots used for sores. (as *H. glabella* 100:47) *Eye Medicine* Infusion of root used as an eyewash. (as *H. glabella* 98:39) *Snakebite Remedy* Poultice of mashed, raw root applied to snakebites. *Veterinary Aid* Poultice of mashed, raw root applied to horses for snakebites. (*H. glabella* 98:49)

Heuchera flabellifolia, Bridger Mountain Alumroot

Blackfoot *Gastrointestinal Aid* Decoction of roots taken for stomach troubles and cramps. (82:36)

Heuchera glabra, Alpine Heuchera

Tlingit *Venereal Aid* Plant used for inflammation of testicles from syphilis. (as *H. devaricata* 89:284)

Heuchera micrantha, Crevice Alumroot

Skagit *Dermatological Aid* Pounded plants rubbed on hair to make it grow or applied to cuts. (65:31) **Thompson** *Dermatological Aid* Poultice of mashed root with Douglas fir pitch used for

wounds. The poultice was covered with a cloth and when it was taken off, all the poison was extracted from the open wound. Chewed leaves and roots spat on sores or wounds. *Liver Aid* Infusion of roots taken for liver trouble. *Oral Aid* Small, peeled, cleaned root piece chewed for mouth sores and gum boils. *Throat Aid* Infusion of root taken for sore throat. *Unspecified* Root used as medicine. (161:282)

Heuchera novomexicana, New Mexico Alumroot

Navajo, Ramah *Analgesic* Decoction of root taken as needed for internal pain. *Dermatological Aid* Poultice of split root applied to infected sores and swellings. *Disinfectant* Poultice of split root applied to infected sores. *Orthopedic Aid* Poultice of split root applied to infected sores, swellings, and fractures. *Panacea* Plant used as "life medicine." (165:29)

Heuchera parviflora, Littleflower Alumroot

Blackfoot *Dermatological Aid* Poultice of pounded root applied to sores and swellings. (95:274)

Heuchera parvifolia, Littleleaf Alumroot

Blackfoot *Antirheumatic* (*External*) Pounded, wetted root used for rheumatism. *Dermatological Aid* Pounded, wetted roots used for sores. (98:43) *Eye Medicine* Infusion of root used as an eyewash. (98:39) *Hemostat* Poultice of chewed roots applied to wounds and sores as a styptic. (72:76) Poultice of chewed roots applied to wounds as a styptic. (72:84) *Oral Aid* and *Pediatric Aid* Poultice of chewed roots applied to cold sores and children's mouth cankers. (72:76) *Veterinary Aid* Infusion of roots given to horses for respiratory troubles. (72:88) **Navajo, Kayenta** *Dermatological Aid* Plant used for rat bites. (179:25) **Navajo, Ramah** *Analgesic* Decoction of root taken for stomach-ache. *Gastrointestinal Aid* Decoction of root taken for stomachache. *Gynecological Aid* Decoction of split root taken to ease delivery of placenta. *Panacea* Root used as a "life medicine." *Venereal Aid* Infusion of root used as a lotion for venereal disease. (165:29, 30)

Heuchera richardsonii, Richardson's
   Alumroot
Blackfoot *Antidiarrheal* Rootstocks chewed for
diarrhea. (82:37) **Cree, Woodlands** *Antidiarrheal* Decoction of root or root chewed for diarrhea. *Eye Medicine* Infusion of root used to wash
sore eyes. (91:40) **Lakota** *Antidiarrheal* Infusion
of roots taken for diarrhea. *Dermatological Aid*
Poultice of powdered roots applied to sores.
(116:58)

Heuchera rubescens, Pink Alumroot
Gosiute *Dermatological Aid* Decoction of roots
used as an astringent. *Gastrointestinal Aid* and
Pediatric Aid Decoction of roots used for babies
and children with colic. (31:371) **Paiute** *Eye Medicine* Infusion of root used as an eyewash. *Venereal
Aid* Decoction of root taken for venereal disease.
Shoshoni *Antidiarrheal* Infusion of root taken
for diarrhea. *Febrifuge* Decoction of root taken for
high fever. *Heart Medicine* Decoction of root taken for heart trouble. *Liver Aid* Infusion of roots
taken for liver trouble or biliousness. *Tonic* Decoction of root taken as a tonic for general debility.
Venereal Aid Decoction of root taken for venereal
disease. *Veterinary Aid* Mashed, boiled leaves
used as a wash for horses' saddle sores. Soaked
roots given to horses and cows for cramps.
(155:87, 88)

Hexastylis arifolia, Littlebrownjug
Catawba *Analgesic* and *Gastrointestinal Aid* Infusion of leaves taken for stomach pains. *Heart Medicine* Infusion of leaves taken for heart troubles.
(as *Asarum apiifolia* 134:190)

Hexastylis arifolia* var. *arifolia, Littlebrownjug
Catawba *Analgesic* Leaves used for severe pain in
the heart from heart disease. (as *Asarum arifolia*
134:188) Infusion of leaves taken for stomach
pains or backaches. (as *Asarum arifolium* 152:20)
Gastrointestinal Aid Leaves used for stomach
trouble. (as *Asarum arifolia* 134:188) Infusion of
leaves taken for stomach pains. (as *Asarum arifolium* 152:20) *Heart Medicine* Leaves used for
severe pain in the heart from heart disease. (as
Asarum arifolia 134:188) Infusion of leaves taken
for heart troubles. *Orthopedic Aid* Plant used for

backache. (as *Asarum arifolium* 152:20) **Rappahannock** *Febrifuge* Infusion of leaves taken for
fever. *Pulmonary Aid* Infusion of leaves taken for
whooping cough. *Respiratory Aid* Decoction of
leaves with alcohol taken for asthma. (as *Asarum
arifolium* 138:25)

Hexastylis virginica, Virginia Heartleaf
Cherokee *Gastrointestinal Aid* Infusion taken "to
stop blood from passing." (66:37)

Hibiscus moscheutos* ssp. *moscheutos,
   Crimsoneyed Rosemallow
Shinnecock *Urinary Aid* Infusion of dried stalks
applied for inflammation of the bladder. (as *H.
palustris* 25:120)

Hibiscus tiliaceus, Sea Hibiscus
Hawaiian *Gynecological Aid* Slimy substance
from inner bark and water taken before or between the pain accompanying childbirth. *Laxative*
Slimy substance from bark or the flower bases
used as a laxative for adults and children. *Pediatric Aid* Slimy substance from bark or the flower
bases used as a laxative for adults and children.
Pulmonary Aid Bark and other plants crushed,
water added, strained, and resulting liquid taken
for congested chest. *Throat Aid* Shoots and buds
chewed and swallowed for dry throat. (2:39)

Hieracium canadense, Canadian Hawkweed
Ojibwa *Hunting Medicine* Flowers used to make a
hunting lure and mixed with other hunting charms.
Roots nibbled when hunting to attract a doe.
(130:429)

Hieracium cynoglossoides, Houndstongue
   Hawkweed
Okanagan-Colville *Tonic* Infusion of leaves and
roots taken as a general tonic. (162:84)

Hieracium fendleri, Yellow Hawkweed
Navajo, Ramah *Diuretic* Cold infusion of plant
taken by hunters for anuria. *Hunting Medicine*
Leaves chewed for good luck in hunting. (165:52)

Hieracium pilosella, Mouseear Hawkweed
Iroquois *Antidiarrheal* Infusion of plants taken
for diarrhea. (73:480)

Hieracium scabrum, Rough Hawkweed
Rappahannock *Antidiarrheal* Infusion of leaves taken or chewed for diarrhea. (138:27)

Hieracium scouleri, Woollyweed
Okanagan-Colville *Tonic* Infusion of leaves and roots taken as a general tonic. (162:84)

Hieracium venosum, Rattlesnakeweed
Cherokee *Gastrointestinal Aid* Compound infusion of root given for bowel complaints. (66:37)

Hierochloe occidentalis, California Sweet
   Grass
Karok *Gynecological Aid* Infusion of plant taken by women after miscarriage or to arrest fetus growth. *Veterinary Aid* Plant given to sick dogs. (as *Torresia macrophylla* 125:380)

Hierochloe odorata, Sweet Grass
Blackfoot *Cold Remedy* Smoke from burning leaves used for colds. (68:28) Burning leaf smoke inhaled for colds. (82:20) *Cough Medicine* Infusion of plant taken for coughs. (72:72) *Dermatological Aid* Leaves and boiled hoof sticky substance used as a hair tonic. (72:124) Stems soaked in water and used for chapping and windburn. (72:77) *Eye Medicine* Stems soaked in water and used as an eyewash. (72:81) *Strengthener* Grass chewed as a means of extended endurance in ceremonies involving prolonged fasting. (72:9) *Throat Aid* Infusion of plant taken for sore throats. (72:72) *Venereal Aid* Infusion of blades taken by

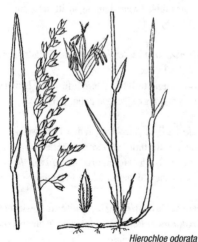
Hierochloe odorata

men for venereal infections. (72:69) *Veterinary Aid* Leaves used for saddle sores on horses. (82:20) **Cheyenne** *Ceremonial Medicine* Plant used as a ceremonial incense for purification. *Witchcraft Medicine* Plant burned in homes to prevent evil. (69:9) **Flathead** *Analgesic* Infusion used for "sharp pains inside." *Cold Remedy* Infusion used for colds. *Febrifuge* Infusion used for fevers. *Respiratory Aid* Infusion mixed with meadow rue seeds and used for congested nasal passages. (68:28) **Kiowa** *Dermatological Aid* Dried foliage employed as a perfume. (166:15) **Menominee** *Dermatological Aid* Grass used in basketry and as a perfume. (128:75) **Plains Indian** *Veterinary Aid* Leaves given to horses to make them long-winded on the chase. (82:20) **Thompson** *Dermatological Aid* Infusion or decoction of plant used as a wash for the hair and body. (141:476)

Hierochloe odorata ssp. odorata, Vanilla
   Grass
Blackfoot *Ceremonial Medicine* Plant burned as ceremonial incense. (as *Savastana odorata* 95:273, 274) *Dermatological Aid* Used to make a hair tonic. (as *Savastana odorata* 95:273) Leaves used as a hair wash and incense. (as *Sevastana odorata* 95:278) **Cheyenne** *Ceremonial Medicine* Dried plant burned in many ceremonies. (as *Torresia odorata* 63:170) **Dakota** *Ceremonial Medicine* Plant used in propitiatory rites. (as *Savastana odorata* 57:359) Plant used as incense in ceremony to invoke good powers and in peace ceremony. (as *Savastana odorata* 58:66) **Kiowa** *Dermatological Aid* Dried foliage employed as a perfume. (as *Torresia odorata* 166:15) **Omaha** *Ceremonial Medicine* Plant used in various rituals. (as *Savastana odorata* 56:322) Plant used as incense in ceremony to invoke good powers and in peace ceremony. **Pawnee** *Ceremonial Medicine* Plant used as incense in ceremony to invoke good powers and in peace ceremony. **Ponca** *Ceremonial Medicine* Plant used as incense in ceremony to invoke good powers and in peace ceremony. **Winnebago** *Ceremonial Medicine* Plant used as incense in ceremony to invoke good powers and in peace ceremony. (as *Savastana odorata* 58:66)

Hilaria jamesii, Galleta
Navajo, **Ramah** *Dietary Aid* and *Pediatric Aid*

Cold infusion given to babies to make them "want to eat a lot." (165:16)

Hoita macrostachya, Large Leatherroot
Luiseño *Dermatological Aid* Plant used for ulcers and sores. (as *Psoralea macrostachya* 132:231)

Hoita orbicularis, Roundleaf Leatherroot
Costanoan *Blood Medicine* Decoction of plant used for the blood. *Febrifuge* Decoction of plant used for fevers. (as *Psoralea orbicularis* 17:19)

Holocarpha virgata, Yellowflower Tarweed
Miwok *Febrifuge* Decoction of plant used as a bath for fevers. *Misc. Disease Remedy* Decoction of plant used as a bath for measles. (as *Hemizonia virgata* 8:170, 171)

Holodiscus discolor, Ocean Spray
Chehalis *Misc. Disease Remedy* Infusion of seeds taken for smallpox, black measles, and chickenpox. **Lummi** *Antidiarrheal* Blossoms used for diarrhea. *Eye Medicine* Infusion of inner bark used as an eyewash. *Oral Aid* Poultice of leaves applied to sore lips. *Orthopedic Aid* Poultice of leaves applied to sore feet. **Makah** *Tonic* Decoction of bark taken as a tonic by convalescents and athletes. (65:33) *Unspecified* Used to make medicine. (55:263) **Navajo, Ramah** *Misc. Disease Remedy* Decoction of leaves taken for influenza. (165:31) **Okanagan-Colville** *Burn Dressing* Bark dried, powdered, mixed with Vaseline, and used on burns. (162:126) **Sanpoil** *Dermatological Aid* Powder of dried leaves used for sores. (109:221) **Squaxin** *Blood Medicine* Seeds used as a blood purifier. (65:33)

Holodiscus dumosus, Rockspirea
Paiute *Antidiarrheal* Decoction of root taken for diarrhea. *Cold Remedy* Decoction of stems taken for colds. *Gastrointestinal Aid* Decoction of root taken for stomach disorders. **Shoshoni** *Disinfectant* Decoction of leaves, flowers, and stems used as an antiseptic wash. *Emetic* Decoction of leaves taken as an emetic. *Gastrointestinal Aid* Decoction of leaves and stems taken for stomachaches. *Unspecified* Decoction of leaf, flower, and stem taken for illnesses of "undefined cause." *Venereal Aid* Decoction of leaves or stems taken for venereal disease. (as *H. discolor* var. *dumosus* 155:88, 89)

Hordeum jubatum, Foxtail Barley
Chippewa *Eye Medicine* Dry root wrapped, moistened, and used as a compress for sties or inflammation of lid. (43:360) **Navajo, Ramah** *Poison* Plant considered poisonous and children taught to avoid it. (165:16) **Potawatomi** *Unspecified* Root used for unspecified ailments. (131:59)

Hordeum murinum ssp. *glaucum*, Smooth Barley
Costanoan *Urinary Aid* Decoction of plant used for bladder ailments. (as *H. glaucum* 17:30)

Horkelia californica, California Honeydew
Pomo, Kashaya *Blood Medicine* Decoction of root used as a blood purifier. (60:57)

Hosta lancifolia, Narrowleaf Plantainlily
Cherokee *Antihemorrhagic* Warm infusion of root taken for spitting blood. *Cough Medicine* Warm infusion of root taken for coughing. *Dermatological Aid* Leaf rubbed on swollen legs and feet after scratching insect bites. (as *H. japonica* 66:50)

Houstonia caerulea, Azure Bluet
Cherokee *Urinary Aid* Infusion given for bedwetting. (66:26)

Houstonia rubra, Red Bluet
Keres, Western *Eye Medicine* Infusion of plant used for sore eyes. *Gastrointestinal Aid* Infusion of plant used for the stomach. (147:48) **Navajo, Kayenta** *Gynecological Aid* Decoction of plant used for menstrual troubles. (179:43)

Houstonia wrightii, Pygmy Bluet
Navajo, Ramah *Ceremonial Medicine* Plant used as a ceremonial fumigant for "deer infection." *Dermatological Aid* Cold, compound infusion of plant taken and used as lotion for poison ivy rash. Dried, pulverized root used as dusting powder for sores on humans or livestock. *Disinfectant* Plant used as a ceremonial fumigant for "deer infection." *Panacea* Root used as a "life medicine." (165:45)

Hudsonia tomentosa, Woolly Beachheather
Montagnais *Blood Medicine* Decoction of plant taken by women to "purge the blood." (133:313)

Humulus lupulus, Common Hop
Cherokee *Analgesic* "Alleviates pain and produces sleep." *Antirheumatic* (*Internal*) Taken for
rheumatism. *Breast Treatment* Used for breast
and womb problems. *Gynecological Aid* Used for
"breast & female complaints where womb is debil-
itated." *Kidney Aid* Taken for inflamed kidneys.
Sedative "Alleviates pain and produces sleep."
Urinary Aid Taken for "gravel" and the bladder.
(66:39) **Dakota** *Analgesic* Decoction of fruits
taken for intestinal pains. *Febrifuge* Decoction of
fruits taken for fevers. *Gastrointestinal Aid* Decoction of fruits taken for intestinal pains. (57:362)
Delaware *Ear Medicine* Poultice of heated plants
in small bags applied for earache. *Sedative* Blossoms used for nervousness. *Stimulant* Infusion of
plants used as a tonic stimulant. *Toothache Remedy* Poultice of heated plants in small bags applied
for toothache. (151:31) **Delaware, Oklahoma**
Ear Medicine Poultice of heated herb in bag applied
for earache. *Sedative* Blossoms used in medicine
for "nervousness." *Stimulant* Infusion of plant
taken as a tonic and stimulant. (150:26, 76) *Tonic*
Infusion of plant taken as a "tonic-stimulant."
(150:26) *Toothache Remedy* Poultice of heated
herb in bag applied for toothache. (150:26, 76)
Meskwaki *Sedative* Root used for insomnia.
(129:250) **Mohegan** *Analgesic* Blossoms used
for pain. (151:130) *Ear Medicine* Dried blossoms
applied to earache. (149:266) *Sedative* Used in
making "nerve medicine." (25:120) Infusion of
blossoms used for nerves. (149:266) Infusion of
blossoms taken for nervous tension. (151:72, 130)
Toothache Remedy Dried blossoms applied to
toothache. (149:266) **Ojibwa** *Diuretic* Infusion
of herb taken as a diuretic and to reduce acidity
of urine. (130:391) **Omaha** *Dermatological Aid*
Root used for wounds. (48:584) **Round Valley
Indian** *Dermatological Aid* Poultice of soaked
hops applied to swellings and bruises. (33:344)
Shinnecock *Pulmonary Aid* Poultice of dried
hops heated in a cloth bag applied for pneumonia.
Sedative Used in making "nerve medicine" and
used as a poultice for pneumonia. (25:120)

Humulus lupulus var. **lupuloides**, Common
      Hop
Dakota *Analgesic* Infusion of fruit taken for intestinal pains. *Dermatological Aid* Simple or com-

pound poultice of chewed root applied to wounds.
Febrifuge Infusion of fruit taken for fevers. *Gastrointestinal Aid* Infusion of fruits taken "to allay
fevers and intestinal pains." (as *H. americana*
58:77) **Navajo, Ramah** *Cough Medicine* Plant
used for bad cough. *Hunting Medicine* Plant used
as a "big medicine" for "good luck" in hunting.
Misc. Disease Remedy Plant used for influenza.
Witchcraft Medicine Plant used for protection
against witches. (as *H. americanus* 165:22)

Huperzia lucidula, Shining Clubmoss
Iroquois *Blood Medicine* Compound used when
"blood is bad." *Cold Remedy* Decoction used
when woman catches cold due to suppressed menses. *Dermatological Aid* Compound used for neck
sores. (as *Lycopodium lucidulum* 73:263)

Huperzia selago var. **selago**, Fir Clubmoss
Nitinaht *Cathartic* Plant used as a purgative.
Emetic Plant used as a fast acting emetic. *Gastrointestinal Aid* Branches used to "clean . . . out"
the insides. (as *Lycopodium selago* 160:60)
Tanana, Upper *Analgesic* Poultice of the whole
plant applied to the head for headaches. (as *Lycopodium selago* 86:18)

Hybanthus concolor, Eastern Greenviolet
Iroquois *Veterinary Aid* Infusion of roots and
stems mixed with feed for mare with injured fetus.
(73:386)

Hydrangea arborescens, Wild Hydrangea
Cherokee *Abortifacient* Compound infusion taken
for menstrual period. *Antiemetic* Used as an antiemetic and cold infusion of bark used as antiemetic for children. *Burn Dressing* Poultice of scraped
bark used for burns. *Cancer Treatment* Used for
tumors. *Cathartic* Used as a purgative. *Dermatological Aid* Used for ulcers and poultice of scraped
bark used for "risings." *Disinfectant* Used as an
antiseptic. *Emetic* Infusion of bark given to induce
vomiting to "throw off disordered bile." *Gastrointestinal Aid* Bark chewed for stomach trouble.
Hypotensive Bark chewed for high blood pressure.
Liver Aid Infusion of bark given to induce vomiting
to "throw off disordered bile." *Orthopedic Aid*
Used for sprains and as poultice for sore or swollen muscles. *Pediatric Aid* Used as an antiemetic

and cold infusion of bark used as antiemetic for children. *Stimulant* Inner bark and leaves used as a stimulant. (66:54) **Delaware** *Kidney Aid* Roots and blue flag roots used for gallstones. (151:36) **Delaware, Oklahoma** *Liver Aid* Root combined with root of *Iris versicolor* and used for gallstones. (as *Hydranga aborescens* 150:30, 76)

Hydrangea cinerea, Ashy Hydrangea
Cherokee *Antiemetic* Infusion of bark scrapings taken for vomiting bile. *Cathartic* Infusion of roots taken as a cathartic by women during menses. *Emetic* Infusion of roots taken as an emetic by women during menses. *Gynecological Aid* Infusion of roots taken as an emetic and cathartic by women during menses. *Liver Aid* Infusion of bark scrapings taken for vomiting bile. (152:25)

Hydrastis canadensis, Golden Seal
Cherokee *Cancer Treatment* Used for cancer. *Dermatological Aid* Used as a tonic and wash for local inflammations. *Dietary Aid* Used to improve the appetite. *Gastrointestinal Aid* Used for "general debility" and "dyspepsy." *Stimulant* Used for cancer, general debility, dyspepsia, and to improve appetite. *Tonic* Used as a tonic and wash for local inflammations. (66:36) **Iroquois** *Antidiarrheal* Decoction of roots taken for whooping cough and diarrhea. *Carminative* Infusion of powdered root taken for gas. *Ear Medicine* Compound infusion with roots used as drops for earaches. *Emetic* Infusion of roots taken as an emetic for biliousness.

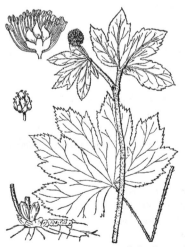

Hydrastis canadensis

Eye Medicine Compound decoction of plants taken for scrofula and used as drops for sore eyes. *Febrifuge* Infusion or decoction of roots taken for fevers. *Gastrointestinal Aid* Infusion of powdered root taken for sour stomach. *Heart Medicine* Infusion of roots with whisky taken for heart trouble. *Liver Aid* Infusion of powdered root taken for liver trouble, gall, sour stomach, and gas. *Pulmonary Aid* Infusion or decoction of roots taken for pneumonia. *Stimulant* Infusion of roots with whisky taken for run-down system. *Tuberculosis Remedy* Infusion or decoction of plants taken for tuberculosis, especially scrofula. (73:324) **Micmac** *Dermatological Aid* Root used for chapped or cut lips. (32:57)

Hydrocotyle poltata, Po-he-po-he
Hawaiian *Pulmonary Aid* Plant used for lung troubles. *Strengthener* Plant used for general body weakness. *Venereal Aid* Plant used for diseases of the sexual organs. (2:74)

Hydrocotyle umbellata, Manyflower Marsh-pennywort
Seminole *Cough Medicine, Respiratory Aid*, and *Sedative* Roots, or whole plant, used for turtle sickness: trembling, short breath and cough. (145:237)

Hydrophyllum canadense, Bluntleaf Waterleaf
Iroquois *Antidote* Compound infusion of roots taken as antidote for poisons. (73:420)

Hydrophyllum virginianum, Shawnee Salad
Iroquois *Oral Aid* Decoction or chewed roots used as wash for cracked lips and mouth sores. (73:420) **Menominee** *Analgesic* Compound decoction of root used for chest pain. (44:130) *Antidiarrheal* Astringent root used for flux. (128:37) **Ojibwa** *Antidiarrheal* and *Pediatric Aid* Root used by men, women, or children to "keep flux in check." (130:371)

Hymenopappus filifolius, Fineleaf Hymenopappus
Zuni *Dermatological Aid* Poultice of chewed root with lard applied to swellings. *Emetic* Warm decoction of root taken as an emetic. (143:54, 55)

Hymenopappus filifolius var. cinereus,
Fineleaf Hymenopappus
Navajo, **Ramah** *Cough Medicine* Decoction of
plant taken for cough. *Panacea* Cold infusion of
root used as "life medicine." (165:52)

Hymenopappus filifolius var. lugens,
Idaho Hymenopappus
Hopi *Ceremonial Medicine* and *Emetic* Compound containing plant used as a ceremonial
emetic. (as *H. lugens* 174:97) *Toothache Remedy*
Root chewed for decaying teeth. (as *H. lugens*
174:33, 97) **Navajo** *Blood Medicine* Decoction of
whole plant taken for blood poisoning. (as *H.
nudatus* 45:88) **Navajo**, **Kayenta** *Dermatological Aid* Poultice of plant applied to sores caused by
bird infections. *Other* Plant used for illness caused
by lunar eclipse. (as *H. lugens* 179:48) **Navajo**,
Ramah *Dermatological Aid* Infusion or decoction
of plant taken and used as a lotion for arrow or
bullet wound. (as *H. lugens* 165:52)

Hymenopappus newberryi, Newberry's
Hymenopappus
Isleta *Gastrointestinal Aid* Infusion of plant taken
for stomachache. Dried, ground plants made into
a powder and used on the stomach for stomachaches. *Pediatric Aid* Dried, ground plants made
into a powder and used on children's stomachs for
stomachaches. (as *Leucampyx newberri* 85:34)

Hymenopappus tenuifolius, Chalk Hill
Hymenopappus
Lakota *Veterinary Aid* Plant made into a tea and
salve used for horses' hooves. (116:38)

Hymenoxys bigelovii, Bigelow's Rubberweed
Hopi *Antirheumatic* (*External*) Used for severe
pains in hips and back. *Cathartic* Used as a purge.
Gynecological Aid Used for severe pains in hips
and back, especially in pregnant state. *Stimulant*
Used as a stimulant. *Unspecified* Infusion of plant
used for medicinal tea. (34:328)

Hymenoxys richardsonii, Pingue Hymenoxys
Zuni *Dermatological Aid* Poultice of chewed root
applied to sores and rashes. *Gastrointestinal Aid*
Infusion of root taken for stomachache. (as *H.
richarsonii* 22:375)

Hymenoxys richardsonii var. floribunda,
Colorado Rubberweed
Isleta *Psychological Aid* Leaves characterized as
making cattle crazy. (as *H. floribunda* 85:32)
Keres, **Western** *Poison* Plant considered poison-
ous to sheep. (as *H. floribunda* 147:48)

**Hymenoxys richardsonii var. richard-
sonii**, Pingue Hymenoxys
Navajo, **Ramah** *Ceremonial Medicine* Plant used
as a ceremonial emetic. *Dermatological Aid* Decoction of plant taken and used as lotion for red
ant bites. *Emetic* Plant used as a ceremonial
emetic. *Poison* Toxic to livestock, especially sheep.
(as *Actinea richardsoni* 165:47)

Hypericum ascyron, Great St. John's Wort
Menominee *Kidney Aid* Compounded with black-
cap raspberry root and used for kidney troubles.
Pulmonary Aid Compound containing root used
for weak lungs and as a specific for consumption.
Tuberculosis Remedy Root, thought to be a "specific," used in the first stages of consumption.
(128:37, 38) **Meskwaki** *Snakebite Remedy* Powder of boiled root applied to draw poison from
water moccasin bite. *Tuberculosis Remedy* Compound containing root used for consumption in
the first stages. (129:223)

Hypericum brachyphyllum, Coastalplain St.
John's Wort
Seminole *Cathartic* Plant used as a cathartic. (as
H. aspalathoides 145:275)

Hypericum concinnum, Gold Wire
Miwok *Dermatological Aid* Decoction of plant
used as a wash for running sores. (8:171)

Hypericum crux-andreae, St. Peter's Wort
Choctaw *Analgesic* Decoction of root used for
colic. *Eye Medicine* Decoction of leaves used as
wash for sore eyes. (as *Ascyrum crux–andreae*
20:23)

Hypericum ellipticum, Pale St. John's Wort
Iroquois *Abortifacient* Decoction of stems taken
after the remedy for the suppression of menses.
(73:386)

Hypericum fasciculatum, Peelbark St. John's Wort

Seminole *Cathartic* Infusion of roots taken for rat sickness: blocked urination and bowels. (145:231) Plant used as a cathartic. (145:275) *Urinary Aid* Infusion of roots taken for rat sickness: blocked urination and bowels. (145:231)

Hypericum gentianoides, Orangegrass

Cherokee *Abortifacient* Compound decoction taken "to promote menstruation." *Antidiarrheal* Infusion taken for bloody flux and bowel complaint. *Dermatological Aid* Milky substance rubbed on sores. *Febrifuge* Infusion taken for fever. *Gastrointestinal Aid* Infusion taken for bloody flux and bowel complaint. *Hemostat* Crushed plant sniffed for nosebleed. *Snakebite Remedy* Root chewed, a portion swallowed, and rest used as poultice for snakebite. *Strengthener* Infusion of root used as wash to give infants strength. *Venereal Aid* Milky substance used for venereal disease. (66:53)

Hypericum hypericoides, St. Andrew's Cross

Cherokee *Abortifacient* Compound decoction taken "to promote menstruation." *Antidiarrheal* Infusion taken for bloody flux and bowel complaint. *Dermatological Aid* Milky substance rubbed on sores. *Febrifuge* Infusion taken for fever. *Gastrointestinal Aid* Infusion taken for bloody flux and bowel complaint. *Hemostat* Crushed plant sniffed for nosebleed. *Snakebite Remedy* Root chewed, a portion swallowed, and rest used as poultice for snakebite. *Strengthener* Infusion of root used as wash to give infants strength. *Venereal Aid* Milky substance used for venereal disease. (66:53)

Hypericum hypericoides ssp. *hypericoides*, St. Andrew's Cross

Alabama *Antidiarrheal* Infusion of entire plant taken for dysentery. *Eye Medicine* Infusion of plant used as an eyewash. *Orthopedic Aid* Decoction of mashed plants used as a bath for children too weak to walk. *Pediatric Aid* Decoction of mashed plants used as a bath for children too weak to walk. **Choctaw** *Eye Medicine* Infusion of leaves used as a wash for sore eyes. *Gastrointestinal Aid* Decoction of roots taken for colic. (as *Ascyrum hypericoides* 152:42) **Houma** *Analgesic* Decoction of root taken, especially in childbirth, for severe

pain. *Febrifuge* Decoction of scraped roots and bark taken for fever. *Gynecological Aid* Decoction of root taken, especially in childbirth, for severe pain. *Toothache Remedy* Bark used to pack aching tooth. (as *Ascyrum hypericoides* 135:55) **Koasati** *Antirheumatic* (*Internal*) Decoction or infusion of leaves taken for rheumatism. (as *Ascyrum linifolium* 152:43) **Natchez** *Pediatric Aid* and *Urinary Aid* Infusion of plant given to children unable to urinate. (as *Ascyrum hypericoides* 152:42)

Hypericum multicaule, St. Peter's Wort

Alabama *Antidiarrheal* Decoction of whole plant taken for dysentery. *Eye Medicine* Infusion of plant used as an eyewash. (as *Ascyrum multicaule* 148:664)

Hypericum perforatum, Common St. John's Wort

Cherokee *Abortifacient* Compound decoction taken "to promote menstruation." *Antidiarrheal* Infusion taken for bloody flux and bowel complaint. *Dermatological Aid* Milky substance rubbed on sores. *Febrifuge* Infusion taken for fever. *Gastrointestinal Aid* Infusion taken for bloody flux and bowel complaint. *Hemostat* Crushed plant sniffed for nosebleed. *Snakebite Remedy* Root chewed, a portion swallowed, and rest used as poultice for snakebite. *Strengthener* Infusion of root used as wash to give infants strength. *Venereal Aid* Milky substance used for venereal disease. (66:53) **Iroquois** *Febrifuge* Plant used as a fever medicine. *Reproductive Aid* Roots used to prevent sterility. (73:385) **Montagnais** *Cough Medicine* Decoction of plant used as a cough medicine. (133:314)

Hypericum punctatum, Spotted St. John's Wort

Meskwaki *Unspecified* Compound containing root used as a medicine. (129:223)

Hypericum scouleri, Scouler's St. John's Wort

Paiute *Analgesic* Decoction of plant used as a bath for aching feet. (155:89) *Dermatological Aid* Flowers used for perfume. (93:90) *Orthopedic Aid* Decoction of plant used as a bath for aching feet. **Shoshoni** *Analgesic* Decoction of plant used as a bath for aching feet. *Dermatological Aid* Plant used several ways as a poultice for sores, swellings, wounds, and cuts. *Orthopedic Aid* Decoction of plant used as a bath for aching feet. *Toothache Remedy* Dried root used for toothache. *Venereal Aid* Infusion of tops taken over a long period of time for venereal disease. (155:89)

Hypoxis hirsuta, Common Goldstar
Cherokee *Heart Medicine* Infusion taken for the heart. (66:57)

Hyptis emoryi, Desert Lavender
Cahuilla *Antihemorrhagic* Infusion of blossoms and leaves taken for hemorrhages. (11:79)

Hyptis pectinata, Comb Bushmint
Seminole *Dermatological Aid* Infusion of roots applied to sores and ulcers on the legs and feet. (145:307) *Psychological Aid* Leaves and fruit used for insanity. (145:293)

Hyssopus officinalis, Hyssop
Cherokee *Abortifacient* Infusion taken to "bring on menses." *Cold Remedy* Syrup taken for colds. *Cough Medicine* Syrup taken for coughs. *Febrifuge* Infusion taken for fevers. *Pulmonary Aid* Syrup taken for "asthma and other lung and breast diseases." *Respiratory Aid* Syrup taken for "asthma and other lung and breast diseases." (66:40)

Ilex aquifolium, English Holly
Micmac *Cough Medicine* Root used for cough. *Febrifuge* Part of plant used for fevers and root used for consumption. *Tuberculosis Remedy* Root used for consumption. *Urinary Aid* Root used for gravel. (32:57)

Ilex cassine, Dahoon
Cherokee *Diaphoretic* Infusion, "black drink," caused sweating to purify physically and morally. *Emetic* Strong decoction called "black drink" induced vomiting for purification. *Kidney Aid* Used for "dropsy and gravel." *Urinary Aid* Plant prepared in unspecified manner and taken for "dropsy and gravel." (66:12, 62)

Ilex opaca, American Holly
Alabama *Eye Medicine* Decoction of bark used as a wash for sore eyes. (152:37) **Catawba** *Dermatological Aid* Infusion of leaves taken for sores. *Misc.*

Disease Remedy Infusion of leaves taken for measles. (134:188) Decoction of leaves taken for measles. (152:37) **Cherokee** *Gastrointestinal Aid* Berries chewed for "colics" and "dyspepsia." (66:38) Berries used for colics. (177:74) *Orthopedic Aid* Leaves used to scratch cramped muscles. (66:38) **Choctaw** *Eye Medicine* Decoction of leaves used as drops for sore eyes. **Koasati** *Dermatological Aid* Infusion of bark rubbed on areas affected by itching. (152:37)

Ilex verticillata, Common Winterberry
Iroquois *Cathartic* Decoction of bark taken as a physic. *Emetic* Decoction of bark taken as an emetic. *Gastrointestinal Aid* Plant taken for biliousness. *Other* Taken to retain vigor. *Psychological Aid* Decoction of bark taken as an emetic for craziness. (73:373) *Respiratory Aid* Compound decoction of roots taken for hay fever. (73:374) **Ojibwa** *Antidiarrheal* Bark used for diarrhea. (130:355)

Ilex vomitoria, Yaupon
Alabama *Ceremonial Medicine* Plant taken to "clear out the system and produce ceremonial purity." (148:666) *Emetic* Decoction of toasted leaves taken as an emetic. **Cherokee** *Emetic* Infusion of leaves taken as an emetic. (152:38) *Hallucinogen* Used to "evoke ecstasies." (66:12, 62) **Creek** *Cathartic* "Black drink" used to "clear out the system." (148:666) *Emetic* Decoction of leaves and shoots taken as an emetic. **Natchez** *Emetic* Plant used as an emetic. (152:38) **Seminole** *Psychological Aid* Bark used as medicine for old people's dance sickness: nightmarish dreams and waking up talking. (145:261)

Impatiens capensis, Jewelweed
Cherokee *Ceremonial Medicine* Used as an ingredient in green corn medicine. *Dermatological Aid* Juice rubbed on "ivy poisoning" and infusion of root used for babies with hives. *Gastrointestinal Aid* Crushed leaves rubbed on "child's sour stomach." *Gynecological Aid* Decoction taken and used to "bathe private parts" to aid in delivery. (66:41) Decoction of stems taken to ease childbirth. (as *I. biflora* 152:40) *Misc. Disease Remedy* Infusion of leaf taken for measles. *Pediatric Aid* Infusion of root used for babies with "bold hives"

and leaves used for "child's sour stomach." (66:41) **Chippewa** *Dermatological Aid* Poultice of bruised stems applied to rashes or other skin troubles. (as *I. biflora* 59:136) **Iroquois** *Dermatological Aid* Compound decoction of plants taken and used as a wash for liver spots. *Diuretic* Infusion of roots taken to increase urination. *Eye Medicine* Poultice of smashed stems applied to sore or raw eyelids. *Febrifuge* Cold infusion of plants taken for fevers. *Kidney Aid* Decoction of plants taken for kidney problems and dropsy. *Liver Aid* Compound decoction of plants taken and used as a wash for liver spots. *Urinary Aid* Decoction of plants taken for stricture or for difficult urination. (as *I. biflora* 73:380) **Malecite** *Liver Aid* Infusion of leaves used for jaundice. (as *I. biflora* 96:256) **Meskwaki** *Dermatological Aid* Poultice of fresh plant applied to sores and juice used for nettle stings. (as *I. biflora* 129:205) **Micmac** *Liver Aid* Herbs used for jaundice. (as *I. biflora* 32:57) **Mohegan** *Burn Dressing* Compound of balsam buds and rum used as ointment for burns. (as *I. biflora* 149:269) Poultice of crushed buds applied to burns. (as *I. biflora* 151:72) Poultice of crushed flower buds applied to burns. (as *I. biflora* 151:72, 130) *Dermatological Aid* Compound of balsam buds and rum used as ointment for cuts. (as *I. biflora* 149:269) Poultice of crushed flower buds applied to cuts and bruises. (as *I. biflora* 151:72, 130) *Orthopedic Aid* Compound of balsam buds and rum used as ointment for bruises. **Nanticoke** *Burn Dressing* Compound of balsam buds and rum used as ointment for burns. (as *I. biflora* 149:269) Infusion of plant taken and poultice of leaves applied to burns. (as

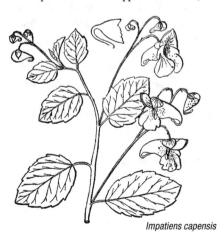

Impatiens capensis

I. biflora 150:57, 84) *Dermatological Aid* Compound of balsam buds and rum used as ointment for cuts. *Orthopedic Aid* Compound of balsam buds and rum used as ointment for bruises. (as *I. biflora* 149:269) **Ojibwa** *Analgesic* Juice of fresh plant rubbed on head for headache. *Unspecified* Infusion of leaves used medicinally for unspecified purpose. (as *I. biflora* 130:357, 358) **Omaha** *Dermatological Aid* Poultice of crushed stems and leaves applied to skin for rash and eczema. (as *I. biflora* 58:101) **Penobscot** *Burn Dressing* Compound of balsam buds and rum used as ointment for burns. *Dermatological Aid* Compound of balsam buds and rum used as ointment for cuts. *Orthopedic Aid* Compound of balsam buds and rum used as ointment for bruises. (as *I. biflora* 149:269) **Potawatomi** *Analgesic* Infusion of whole plant taken for stomach cramps and used as a liniment for soreness. *Dermatological Aid* Fresh juice of plant used as a wash on nettle stings or poison ivy rash. Infusion of whole plant used as a liniment for sprains and bruises. *Gastrointestinal Aid* Infusion of whole plant taken for stomach cramps. *Orthopedic Aid* Decoction of plant used as a liniment for sprains, bruises, and soreness. *Pulmonary Aid* Infusion of whole plant taken for chest cold. (as *I. biflora* 131:42) **Shinnecock** *Dermatological Aid* Salve made of balsam buds and Vaseline. (as *I. biflora* 25:122)

Impatiens pallida, Pale Touchmenot
Cherokee *Ceremonial Medicine* Used as an ingredient in green corn medicine. *Dermatological Aid* Juice rubbed on "ivy poisoning" and infusion of root used for babies with hives. *Gastrointestinal Aid* Crushed leaves rubbed on "child's sour stomach." *Gynecological Aid* Decoction taken and used to "bathe private parts" to aid in delivery. *Misc. Disease Remedy* Infusion of leaf taken for measles. *Pediatric Aid* Infusion of root used for babies with "bold hives" and leaves used for "child's sour stomach." (66:41) **Iroquois** *Dermatological Aid* Smashed stalks and juice rubbed on poison ivy blisters and mosquito bites. *Febrifuge* Cold infusion of plants taken for fevers. *Gynecological Aid* Infusion of plant taken to induce childbirth. Infusion of stalks taken to stop suffering while having a baby. Poultice of mashed plants applied to women's breast injury. (73:379) **Ojibwa** *Dermatologi-*

cal Aid Juice rubbed on sores. (4:2311) **Omaha** *Dermatological Aid* Poultice of crushed stems and leaves applied to skin for rash and eczema. (58:101)

Inula helenium, Elecampane Inula
Cherokee *Cough Medicine* Root used for coughs. *Gynecological Aid* "For female obstructions and pregnant women with weak bowels and wombs." *Pulmonary Aid* Root used for lung disorders. *Respiratory Aid* Root used for asthma. *Tuberculosis Remedy* Root used for "consumption." (66:33) **Delaware** *Gastrointestinal Aid* Roots made into a tonic and used to strengthen digestive organs. Roots made into a tonic and used to remove intestinal mucus. (151:37) *Tonic* Roots used with black snakeroot and stone root as a tonic. (151:33) **Delaware, Oklahoma** *Gastrointestinal Aid* Root used in a tonic to strengthen the digestive organs. *Laxative* Root used in a tonic to remove mucus from the intestines. (150:31) *Tonic* Root used in tonic taken for "strengthening digestive organs." (150:31, 76) **Delaware, Ontario** *Cold Remedy* Compound decoction of root or bark taken for colds. (150:67, 82) **Iroquois** *Analgesic* Compound roots used for chest pains. (73:465) *Antirheumatic* (*External*) Poultice of leaves or roots applied for rheumatism and arthritic sores. (73:467) *Carminative* Decoction or cold infusion of powdered roots taken for stomach gas. (73:465) *Cathartic* Compound roots used to clean out the intestines. (73:467) *Cold Remedy* Plant used for colds. *Cough Medicine* Compound decoction of roots taken for coughs or heaves. (73:466) *Dermatological Aid* Poultice of smashed plants applied to sores, cuts, or arthritic sores. (73:465) *Diuretic* Compound decoction of leaves and roots taken as a diuretic. *Febrifuge* Decoction of powdered plants or dried roots taken for fevers. *Gastrointestinal Aid* Compound decoction of roots and flowers taken for bruise on back of stomach. (73:466) Infusion of roots and other plant branches taken for large stomachs. (118:64) *Gynecological Aid* Compound decoction of dried roots taken by girls who "leak rotten." *Heart Medicine* Decoction of dried roots taken for fevers, tuberculosis, and heart troubles. (73:466) Decoction of roots taken for stroke. (73:467) *Misc. Disease Remedy* Compound decoction of powdered plants taken for fevers or typhoid. *Panacea* Plant

used as medicine for anything. (73:466) *Pediatric Aid* Dried leaves given to children for asthma. (73:467) *Pulmonary Aid* Compound roots used for chest pains. (73:465) *Respiratory Aid* Infusion of roots taken for asthma. (73:466) Dried leaves given to children for asthma. (73:467) *Tuberculosis Remedy* Decoction of leaf or root or infusion of one root taken for consumption. (73:466) *Veterinary Aid* Powdered roots mixed with horse's feed or decoction of root given for heaves. (73:465) **Malecite** *Analgesic* Dried roots finely powdered and snuffed for headaches. *Cold Remedy* Infusion of roots used for colds. *Heart Medicine* Infusion of roots used for heart trouble. (96:248) **Micmac** *Analgesic* Root used for headaches. *Cold Remedy* Root used for colds. *Heart Medicine* Root used for heart trouble. (32:57) **Mohegan** *Pulmonary Aid* Infusion of plant taken for lungs. (149:266) Leaves used for lung trouble. (151:130) *Tuberculosis Remedy* Infusion of leaves taken for tuberculosis. (151:72, 130) *Veterinary Aid* Infusion of plant given to horses for colic. (149:266) Infusion of leaves used for horses with colic. (151:72, 130)

Iodanthus pinnatifidus, Purple Rocket
Meskwaki *Love Medicine* Decoction of root used as a paint by women for a love medicine. (129:219, 220) *Poultice* Poultice used on head of old man who is cold, to bring warmth to whole body. (129:219)

Ipomoea indica, Oceanblue Morningglory
Hawaiian *Analgesic* Poultice of pounded flowers, leaves, and salt applied to the back for pain. *Dermatological Aid* Poultice of pounded roots, other plants, and the resulting liquid applied to flesh wounds. *Laxative* Whole plant and other plants baked and eaten as a laxative. *Orthopedic Aid* Poultice of pounded roots, other plants, and the resulting liquid applied to broken bones. *Pediatric Aid* and *Strengthener* Flowers chewed by mothers and given to infants for general weakness. (as *Impomea insularis* 2:52)

Ipomoea leptophylla, Bush Morningglory
Keres, Western *Gastrointestinal Aid* Infusion of staminate cones used as a stomach tonic. (147:48) **Keresan** *Veterinary Aid* Dried, ground root added to water and given to colts to cause them to be-

come large horses. Infusion of dried, pulverized root used for fertility of mares and growth of colts. (172:559) **Lakota** *Gastrointestinal Aid* Root scraped and eaten raw for stomach troubles. (116: 43) **Pawnee** *Analgesic* Pulverized root dusted on body for pain. *Sedative* Root used in smoke treatment for nervousness and bad dreams. *Stimulant* Pulverized root used to revive "one who had fainted." (58:110) **Sia** *Veterinary Aid* Infusion of ground roots used to promote the fertility of horses and the growth of the colts. (173:284)

Ipomoea pandurata, Man of the Earth
Cherokee *Antirheumatic* (*External*) Poultice of root applied to rheumatism. *Cough Medicine* Taken for coughs. *Diuretic* Taken as a diuretic. *Expectorant* Taken as an expectorant. *Kidney Aid* Taken for "dropsy." *Laxative* Taken as a laxative. *Misc. Disease Remedy* Infusion of root taken for cholera morbis. *Respiratory Aid* Taken for asthma. *Tuberculosis Remedy* Taken for consumption. *Urinary Aid* Taken for "gravel" and "suppression of urine." (66:51) **Creek** *Diuretic* Plant used as a diuretic. *Kidney Aid* Plant used "nephritic complaints." (148:670) **Iroquois** *Analgesic* Decoction of roots taken for abdominal pains. Infusion of powdered plants taken for headaches. *Blood Medicine* Compound infusion of bark, roots, and leaves taken as blood purifier. *Cough Medicine* Decoction of roots taken as a cough medicine. *Gastrointestinal Aid* Decoction of roots taken for abdominal pains. Infusion of powdered plants taken for upset stomachs. *Liver Aid* Plant used for the liver. *Misc. Disease Remedy* Infusion of dried roots taken for all kinds of diseases. *Other* Compound infusion taken or injured parts washed, a "Little Water Medicine." *Tuberculosis Remedy* Decoction of roots taken for initial stages of tuberculosis. *Witchcraft Medicine* Plant had magical potency. (73:419)

Ipomoea pes-caprae, Bayhops
Hawaiian *Reproductive Aid* Plant used by expectant mothers. (as *Impomea pes-caprae* 2:73)

Ipomoea sagittata, Saltmarsh Morningglory
Houma *Blood Medicine* Decoction of root taken to remove poison from the blood or heart. *Dermatological Aid* Poultice of boiled leaves applied to swellings. *Heart Medicine* Hot decoction of roots

taken to "take poison out of the blood or heart." *Snakebite Remedy* Leaf chewed and juice swallowed or poultice of chewed leaves used on snakebite. (135:62, 63)

Ipomoea tiliacea, Darkeye Morningglory
Hawaiian *Laxative* Plant used to make a laxative. (as *Argyreia tiliaefolia* 2:73)

Ipomopsis aggregata, Skyrocket Gilia
Great Basin Indian *Blood Medicine* Infusion of whole plant used for blood disease. (as *Gilia appregata* 100:49)

Ipomopsis aggregata ssp. **aggregata**,
Skyrocket Gilia
Hopi *Gynecological Aid* Plant used after birth when the mother lied in bed for 15 or 20 days. (as *Gilia aggregata* 34:321) **Navajo**, **Kayenta** *Cathartic* Plant used as a cathartic. *Dermatological Aid* Plant used for spider bites. *Emetic* Plant used as an emetic. *Gastrointestinal Aid* Plant used for stomach disease. (as *Gilia aggregata* 179:37) **Navajo**, **Ramah** *Hunting Medicine* Cold infusion taken and applied to body of hunter and weapons for good luck. (as *Gilia aggregata* 165:39) **Okanagan-Colville** *Febrifuge* Infusion of roots taken for high fevers. *Laxative* Infusion of leaves and stalks taken for constipation and to "clean out your system." Infusion of roots taken as a laxative. (as *Gilia aggregata* 162:111) **Paiute** *Cathartic* Simple or compound decoction of plant or root taken as a physic. *Cold Remedy* Decoction of root taken as a cold remedy. *Emetic* Simple or compound decoction of plant or root taken as an emetic. (as *Gilia aggregata* 155:76, 77) **Salish** *Dermatological Aid* Decoction of plants used as a face and hair wash by adolescent girls. *Eye Medicine* Decoction of plants used as an eyewash. *Pediatric Aid* Decoction of plants used as a face and hair wash by adolescent girls. (as *Gilia aggregata* 153:294) **Shoshoni** *Analgesic* Poultice of crushed, whole plant applied for rheumatic aches. *Antirheumatic* (*External*) Poultice of crushed plant applied for rheumatic aches. *Blood Medicine* Decoction of plant taken as a blood tonic. *Cathartic* Decoction of plant or root taken as a physic. *Dermatological Aid* Decoction of whole plant used as a disinfecting wash for the itch. *Disinfectant*

Decoction of whole plant used as a disinfectant wash for the itch. *Emetic* Compound decoction of roots used to induce vomiting. Decoction of plant or root taken as an emetic. *Tonic* Simple or compound decoction of whole plant taken as a blood tonic. *Venereal Aid* Simple or compound decoction of plant taken and used as a wash for gonorrhea and syphilis. (as *Gilia aggregata* 155:76, 77)

Ipomopsis aggregata ssp. *attenuata*, Scarlet Skyrocket

Navajo *Gastrointestinal Aid* Infusion of crushed, dried leaves taken for stomach troubles. (as *Gilia attenuata* 45:70)

Ipomopsis congesta ssp. *congesta*, Ballhead Gilia

Great Basin Indian *Analgesic* Poultice of dried, powdered blossoms applied for pain. (as *Gilia congesta* 100:49) **Paiute** *Antidiarrheal* Decoction of plant taken for diarrhea. *Cathartic* Decoction of plant taken as a physic. *Cold Remedy* Decoction of plant taken for colds. *Emetic* Decoction of plant taken as an emetic. *Gastrointestinal Aid* Decoction of plant taken for indigestion and stomach trouble. *Venereal Aid* Plant used in many ways for venereal diseases. **Shoshoni** *Antidiarrheal* Decoction of plant taken for diarrhea. *Cathartic* Decoction of plant taken as a physic. *Cold Remedy* Decoction of plant taken for colds. *Dermatological Aid* Decoction of plant used as an antiseptic wash for wounds, cuts, sores, and bruises. *Disinfectant* Decoction of plant used as an antiseptic wash for skin problems. *Emetic* Decoction of plant taken as an emetic. *Eye Medicine* Decoction or infusion of plant used as an eyewash. *Gastrointestinal Aid* Decoction of plant taken for indigestion and stomach trouble. *Kidney Aid* Decoction of plant taken for "kidney complaint." *Liver Aid* Decoction of plant taken for liver trouble. *Misc. Disease Remedy* Decoction of plant taken for influenza. Poultice of boiled, drained, and mashed plant applied for erysipelas. *Venereal Aid* Plant used in many ways for venereal diseases. *Veterinary Aid* Poultice of crushed, raw plants applied to back sores on horses. **Washo** *Antidiarrheal* Decoction of plant taken for diarrhea. *Cathartic* Decoction of plant taken as a physic. *Cold Remedy* Decoction of plant taken for colds. *Emetic* Decoc-

tion of plant taken as an emetic. *Gastrointestinal Aid* Decoction of plant taken for indigestion and stomach trouble. *Kidney Aid* Infusion of crushed plant taken and poultice applied for dropsy. (as *Gilia congesta* 155:77–80)

Ipomopsis gunnisonii, Sanddune Skyrocket

Navajo, **Kayenta** *Blood Medicine* Plant used as a blood purifier. *Dermatological Aid* Poultice of plant applied to sores. (as *Gilia gunnisoni* 179:37)

Ipomopsis laxiflora, Iron Skyrocket

Keres, **Western** *Emetic* Infusion of roots used as an emetic to eliminate the ozone in cases of lightning shock. (as *Gilia laxiflora* 147:45)

Ipomopsis longiflora ssp. *longiflora*, Flaxflowered Gilia

Hopi *Analgesic* Decoction of leaves used for stomachache. (as *Gilia longiflora* 174:87) *Gastrointestinal Aid* Decoction of leaves taken for stomachache. (as *Gilia longiflora* 174:33, 87) **Keres**, **Western** *Emetic* Infusion of roots used as an emetic to eliminate the ozone in cases of lightning shock. (as *Gilia longiflora* 147:45) **Navajo** *Ceremonial Medicine* Plant used as medicine in the Wind and Female Shooting Chants. *Emetic* Decoction of pounded plant taken to vomit. *Gastrointestinal Aid* Decoction of pounded plant taken for the bowels. *Veterinary Aid* Infusion of flowers mixed with feed and given to sheep for stomach troubles. (as *Gilia longiflora* 45:70) **Navajo**, **Kayenta** *Blood Medicine* and *Gynecological Aid* Plant used for postpartum septicemia. (as *Gilia longiflora* 179:38) **Navajo**, **Ramah** *Analgesic* Plant used for stomachache and arthritis. *Antirheumatic* (*Internal*) Plant used for arthritis. *Ceremonial Medicine* Plant used as ceremonial eyewash and chant lotion. *Dermatological Aid* Infusion of plant used as hair tonic to lengthen hair and prevent baldness. *Disinfectant* Plant used for "deer infection" and "snake infection." *Eye Medicine* Plant used as ceremonial eyewash and chant lotion. *Gastrointestinal Aid* Plant chewed with salt for heartburn. Plant used for stomachache. *Gynecological Aid* Plant used to facilitate delivery of placenta. *Panacea* Plant used as "life medicine." *Veterinary Aid* Cold infusion of plant applied daily to heal incision in castrated colt. (as *Gilia longiflora* 165:40) **Tewa** *Analgesic* Infusion of pulverized flowers and leaves used for headache. *Dermatological Aid* Infusion of pulverized flowers and leaves used on sores. (as *Gilia longiflora* 115:55) **Zuni** *Dermatological Aid* and *Pediatric Aid* Poultice of dried, powdered flowers and water applied to remove hair on newborns and children. (as *Gilia longiflora* 22:378)

Ipomopsis multiflora, Manyflowered Gilia
Navajo, Ramah *Ceremonial Medicine* Decoction of plant used as a ceremonial medicine. (as *Gilia multiflora* 165:40) **Zuni** *Analgesic* Powdered, whole plant applied to face for headache. *Dermatological Aid* Powdered plant applied to wounds. *Pulmonary Aid* Crushed blossoms smoked in corn husks to "relieve strangulation." (as *Gilia multiflora* 143:52)

Ipomopsis polycladon, Manybranched Gilia
Navajo, Kayenta *Sedative* Plant used as a soporific. *Tonic* Plant used as a tonic. (as *Gilia polycladon* 179:38)

Iresine diffusa, Juba's Bush
Houma *Pulmonary Aid* Syrup of leaves and stems taken for whooping cough. (as *I. paniculata* 135:66)

Iris cristata, Dwarf Crested Iris
Cherokee *Dermatological Aid* Compound decoction of pulverized root used as salve for ulcers. *Liver Aid* Infusion taken for liver. *Urinary Aid* Compound decoction of root used for "yellowish urine." (66:41)

Iris douglasiana, Douglas Iris
Yokia *Oral Aid* and *Pediatric Aid* Leaves used to wrap babies during berry gathering trips to retard perspiration and prevent thirst. (33:330)

Iris macrosiphon, Bowltube Iris
Pomo *Gynecological Aid* Roots used to hasten the birth of a baby. (97:284)

Iris missouriensis, Rocky Mountain Iris
Great Basin Indian *Toothache Remedy* Root put in a hollow tooth for toothaches. (100:47) **Klamath** *Emetic* Dried rootstocks used by medicine

men as smoking material to cause nausea. Dried rootstocks sometimes used by medicine men as a smoking material, mixed with poison camas and a little tobacco, to give a person a severe nausea, in order to secure a heavy fee for making him well again. (37:93) **Montana Indian** *Emetic* Decoction of rootstocks used by medicine men to induce vomiting. (15:13) **Navajo, Ramah** *Ceremonial Medicine* and *Emetic* Decoction of plant used as a ceremonial emetic. (165:21) **Nevada Indian** *Kidney Aid* Infusion of roots taken for kidney troubles. *Urinary Aid* Infusion of roots taken for bladder troubles. (100:47) **Paiute** *Analgesic* Decoction of root taken for stomachaches. *Dermatological Aid* Paste of ripe seeds applied to sores. *Ear Medicine* Warm decoction of root dropped into ear for earache. *Gastrointestinal Aid* Decoction of root taken for stomachaches. *Toothache Remedy* Raw root placed in cavity or against gum for toothache. *Urinary Aid* Decoction of root taken for bladder troubles. *Venereal Aid* Decoction of root used for gonorrhea. **Shoshoni** *Analgesic* Decoction of root taken for stomachaches. Poultice of mashed roots applied for rheumatic pains. *Antirheumatic (External)* Poultice of mashed roots applied to rheumatic pains. *Burn Dressing* Paste of ripe seeds applied to burns. *Dermatological Aid* Pulped root applied as a salve for venereal sores. *Ear Medicine* Warm decoction of root dropped into ear for earache. *Gastrointestinal Aid* Decoction of root taken for stomachaches. *Toothache Remedy* Raw root placed in cavity or against gum for toothache. *Venereal Aid* Decoction of root taken for gonorrhea and root salve used for venereal sores. (155:89, 90) **Yavapai** *Cathartic* Decoction of root taken as a purgative. (53:261) **Zuni** *Pediatric Aid* Poultice of chewed root applied to increase strength of newborns and infants. *Strengthener* Poultice of chewed root used for newborns and infants to increase strength. (22:373)

Iris setosa, Beachhead Iris
Aleut *Laxative* Decoction of root taken as a laxative. (6:428) **Eskimo, Inupiat** *Poison* Whole plant considered poisonous. (83:140)

Iris tenuissima, Longtube Iris
Pomo *Gynecological Aid* Roots used to hasten the birth of a baby. (97:284)

Iris verna, Dwarf Violet Iris
Cherokee *Dermatological Aid* Compound decoction of pulverized root used as salve for ulcers. *Liver Aid* Infusion taken for liver. *Urinary Aid* Compound decoction of root used for "yellowish urine." (66:41) **Creek** *Cathartic* Plant used as a powerful cathartic. (148:669, 670)

Iris versicolor, Harlequin Blueflag
Abnaki *Poison* Plant considered poisonous. (121:155) Plant considered poisonous. (121:175) **Algonquin**, **Tête-de-Boule** *Burn Dressing* Poultice of smashed roots applied to burns. *Dermatological Aid* Poultice of smashed roots applied to wounds. (110:129) **Chippewa** *Dermatological Aid* Poultice of root, very strong, applied to swellings. (43:366) Poultice of roots applied to scrofulous sores. *Tuberculosis Remedy* Poultice of roots applied to scrofulous sores. (59:126) **Cree**, **Hudson Bay** *Cathartic* Plant used as a purgative. *Liver Aid* Plant used to increase the flow of bile. (78:303) **Creek** *Cathartic* Plant used as a powerful cathartic. (148:669, 670) Plant used as a cathartic. (152:10) **Delaware** *Antirheumatic* (*External*) Roots used for rheumatism. *Kidney Aid* Roots used for kidney disorders. *Liver Aid* Roots used for liver disorders. *Venereal Aid* Roots used for scrofula. (151:36) **Delaware**, **Oklahoma** *Antirheumatic* (*Internal*) Root taken for rheumatism. (150:30, 76) *Kidney Aid* Root used for disorders of the kidneys. *Liver Aid* Root used for disorders of the liver. (150:30) Root combined with root of *Hydrangea arborescens* and used for gallstones. *Tuberculosis*

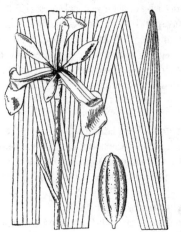

Iris versicolor

Remedy Root taken for "scrofula." (150:30, 76) **Iroquois** *Blood Medicine* Poultice of crushed rhizomes applied for blood poisoning caused by contusions. (118:67) *Cathartic* Infusion of plant taken as a physic. *Gynecological Aid* Infusion of smashed roots taken at menses to induce pregnancy. *Orthopedic Aid* Infusion of smashed roots taken to induce paralysis. *Respiratory Aid* Compound decoction with roots taken for hay fever. (73:287) **Malecite** *Throat Aid* Infusion of plants and bulrush used as a gargle for sore throats. (96:248) **Meskwaki** *Burn Dressing* Poultice of freshly macerated root applied to burns. *Cold Remedy* Root used for colds. *Dermatological Aid* Poultice of freshly macerated root applied to sores. *Pulmonary Aid* Root used for lung trouble. (129:224) **Micmac** *Dermatological Aid* Root used for wounds and herb used for sore throat. *Misc. Disease Remedy* Root used for cholera and the prevention of disease. *Panacea* Root used as a "basic medical cure" and for cholera. *Throat Aid* Herbs used for sore throat and root used for wounds. (32:57) **Mohegan** *Analgesic* Poultice of pulverized root mixed with flour applied to pain. (151:72, 130) **Montagnais** *Analgesic* Poultice of crushed plant mixed with flour applied to any pain. (133:315) Compound poultice of plant and flour applied to pain. (149:268) **Ojibwa** *Cathartic* Decoction of root taken as a "quick physic." *Emetic* Decoction of root taken as an emetic. (130:371) **Omaha** *Dermatological Aid* Paste of pulverized rootstock applied to sores and bruises. *Ear Medicine* Pulverized rootstock mixed with water or saliva and dropped in ear for earache. *Eye Medicine* Rootstock used to medicate "eye-water." (58:72) **Penobscot** *Herbal Steam* Plant steamed throughout the house to keep away "disease in general." (133:311) *Misc. Disease Remedy* Infusion of root taken for cholera. (133:308, 309) *Preventive Medicine* Root chewed to keep disease away; the plant is thought to "kill" sickness. (133:311) **Ponca** *Dermatological Aid* Paste of pulverized rootstock applied to sores and bruises. *Ear Medicine* Pulverized rootstock mixed with water or saliva and dropped in ear for earache. *Eye Medicine* Rootstock used to medicate "eye-water." (58:72) **Potawatomi** *Dermatological Aid* Poultice of root used to allay inflammation. (131:60) **Rappahannock** *Panacea* Infusion of dried roots taken for "every complaint." (138:28)

Iris virginica, Virginia Iris
Cherokee *Dermatological Aid* Compound decoction of pulverized root used as salve for ulcers. *Liver Aid* Infusion taken for liver. *Urinary Aid* Compound decoction of root used for "yellowish urine." (66:41)

Isocoma acradenia var. *acradenia*, Alkali Goldenbush
Cahuilla *Dermatological Aid* Poultice of boiled leaves applied to sores. *Throat Aid* Leaves soaked in a pan of boiling water and steam inhaled for sore throats. (as *Haplopappus acradenius* 11:75)

Isocoma pluriflora, Southern Jimmyweed
Navajo, Kayenta *Dermatological Aid* and *Pediatric Aid* Plant used as a lotion to heal infant's navel. (as *Aplopappus heterophyllus* 179:44) **Pima** *Analgesic* Poultice of plant applied for muscular pain. *Cough Medicine* Leaves chewed for coughs. *Orthopedic Aid* Poultice of plant applied for muscular pain. (as *Aplopappus heterophyllus* 38:101)

Iva axillaris, Poverty Weed
Mahuna *Abortifacient* Plant used to cause abortions. *Contraceptive* Plant used to prevent conception. (117:67) **Paiute** *Dermatological Aid* Leaves used as a plaster or infusion used as a wash for sores or skin irritations. **Shoshoni** *Analgesic* Infusion or decoction of plant taken, especially by children, for stomachaches or cramps. *Antidiarrheal* Decoction of plant taken for diarrhea. *Cold Remedy* Infusion or decoction of plant used by children for colds. (155:90, 91) *Gastrointestinal Aid* Root soaked in cold water for tea and taken for bowel disorders. (98:42) Infusion or decoction of plant taken, especially by children, for stomachaches or cramps. Raw, roasted, or boiled root eaten for indigestion. *Pediatric Aid* Infusion or decoction of plant taken, especially by children, for stomachaches or cramps. Infusion or decoction of plant used by children for colds. (155:90, 91) **Ute** *Unspecified* Used as medicine. (30:35)

Iva xanthifolia, Giant Sumpweed
Navajo, Kayenta *Dermatological Aid* Poultice of plant applied to boils. *Veterinary Aid* Plant used to heal castration incision in sheep. (179:48) **Navajo, Ramah** *Cough Medicine* Infusion or decoction

taken and used as lotion for cough. *Misc. Disease Remedy* Infusion or decoction taken and used as lotion for influenza. *Witchcraft Medicine* Infusion or decoction taken and used as lotion for protection from witches. (165:52)

Ivesia gordonii, Gordon's Ivesia
Arapaho *Tonic* Infusion of root used as a tonic. (as *Horkelia gordonii* 98:40) Infusion of resinous roots used as a general tonic. (100:48)

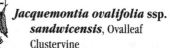 *Jacquemontia ovalifolia* ssp. *sandwicensis*, Ovalleaf Clustervine
Hawaiian *Dermatological Aid* Plant mixed with taro leaves and salt and used for cuts. *Pediatric Aid* and *Strengthener* Plant used for babies with general body weakness. (as *J. sandwicensis* 2:73)

Jeffersonia diphylla, Twinleaf
Cherokee *Dermatological Aid* Poultice used for sores, ulcers, and inflamed parts. *Kidney Aid* Infusion taken for dropsy. *Urinary Aid* Infusion taken for gravel and urinary problems. (66:59) **Iroquois** *Antidiarrheal* Decoction of whole plant taken by adults and children with diarrhea. *Liver Aid* Decoction of whole plant taken for gall. *Pediatric Aid* Decoction of whole plant taken by adults and children with diarrhea. (73:332)

Juglans californica, California Walnut
Costanoan *Blood Medicine* Infusion of leaves taken for thin blood. (17:20)

Juglans cinerea, Butternut
Cherokee *Antidiarrheal* Infusion of bark taken to check bowels. *Cathartic* Pills from inner bark used as a cathartic and compound infusion used for toothache. (66:61) Pills prepared from inner bark and used as a cathartic. (177:75) *Toothache Remedy* Pills from inner bark taken as a cathartic (66:61) **Chippewa** *Cathartic* Decoction of plant sap taken as a cathartic. (59:127) **Iroquois** *Analgesic* Compound decoction of plants taken for urinating pain. *Anthelmintic* Compound decoction with bark taken to kill worms in adults. *Blood Medicine* Compound decoction taken as a blood puri-

fier and for venereal disease. (73:295) *Cathartic* Decoction of bark taken as a physic and cathartic. (73:296) *Dermatological Aid* Compound decoction taken when skin becomes thin. Infusion or chewed bark applied to bleeding wounds. (73:295) Nutmeat oil formerly used for the hair, either alone or mixed with bear grease. (170:123) *Emetic* Infusion of plant and other plant wood and bark used as an emetic to remove yellow from the stomach. (118:39) *Gynecological Aid* Compound decoction with bark taken to induce pregnancy. (73:294) *Hemostat* Infusion or chewed bark applied to bleeding wounds. *Laxative* Compound decoction of bark or shoots taken as a laxative. *Liver Aid* Compound decoction taken for yellow skin and too much gall. *Oral Aid* Compound infusion of buds used as mouthwash for mouth ulcers. *Psychological Aid* Compound decoction with plant taken for "loss of senses during menses." *Toothache Remedy* Juice used for toothache. *Tuberculosis Remedy* Compound decoction used as poultice for infected and swollen tubercular glands. *Urinary Aid* Compound decoction of plants taken for urinating pain. *Venereal Aid* Decoction of shoots taken as a laxative and for venereal disease. (73:295) **Malecite** *Cathartic* Infusion of bark used as a purgative. (96:254) **Menominee** *Cathartic* Syrup from sap used as a standard "physic." (128:38, 39) **Meskwaki** *Cathartic* Decoction of twig bark or decoction of wood and bark taken as a cathartic. (129:224) **Micmac** *Cathartic* Bark used as a purgative. (32:57) **Potawatomi** *Cathartic* Bark used as a physic and infusion of inner bark taken as a tonic. *Tonic* Infusion of inner bark taken as a tonic and bark used as a physic. (131:60, 61)

Juglans nigra, Black Walnut
Cherokee *Dermatological Aid* Infusion used as a wash for sores. *Misc. Disease Remedy* Infusion of inner bark taken for smallpox and infusion of leaves used for goiter. *Poison* "Bark used cautiously in medicine because it is poisonous." *Toothache Remedy* Bark chewed for toothache. (66:61) **Comanche** *Dermatological Aid* Pulverized leaves rubbed on affected part for ringworm. (24:522) **Delaware** *Anthelmintic* Juice from green hulls of fruits rubbed over areas infected by ringworm. *Dermatological Aid* Sap used in applications for inflammations. *Gastrointestinal Aid* Three bun-

dles of bark boiled to make a strong tea and used for 2 days to remove intestinal bile. (151:29) **Delaware, Oklahoma** *Cathartic* Strong decoction of bark taken as a cathartic. *Dermatological Aid* Juice from green hull of fruit rubbed on skin for ringworm. Sap applied to any inflammation. *Emetic* Strong decoction of bark taken as an emetic. (150:24, 76) *Gastrointestinal Aid* and *Liver Aid* Decoction of bark taken "to remove bile from the intestines." (150:24) **Houma** *Dermatological Aid* Infusion of nutshells used as a wash for "the itch." *Hypotensive* Decoction of mashed leaves taken for relief from "blood pressure." (135:66) **Iroquois** *Analgesic* Poultice of bark applied for headache. *Blood Medicine* Compound decoction with brandy taken as a blood purifier. (73:296) *Dermatological Aid* Nutmeat oil formerly used for the hair, either alone or mixed with bear grease. (170:123) *Laxative* Compound decoction of bark taken as a laxative. *Psychological Aid* Poultice of bark applied for "craziness." *Witchcraft Medicine* Infusion of bark used as a medicine for rain. (73:296) **Kiowa** *Anthelmintic* Decoction of root bark taken to kill "worms." (166:21) **Meskwaki** *Cathartic* Inner bark used as a very strong physic. *Snakebite Remedy* Coiled and charred twig bark and old bark applied in water for snakebite. (129:224, 225) **Rappahannock** *Antidiarrheal* Infusion of root bark taken to prevent dysentery. (138:32) *Febrifuge* Compound with north side bark used as a poultice for chills. (138:31) *Gastrointestinal Aid* Infusion of root bark taken to "roughen the intestines." (138:32)

Juncus bufonius, Toad Rush
Iroquois *Emetic* Infusion of plant taken as an emetic by runners. The runner drank about 2 quarts the first time, vomited, drank the same quantity, and vomited again. The face and body were also washed with the liquid. This was done about three times during the week before the race. (170:89)

Juncus bufonius var. *bufonius*, Toad Rush
Iroquois *Dermatological Aid* Compound decoction used as wash for the entire body. *Emetic* Compound decoction taken as an emetic. *Strengthener* Compound decoction taken to "give strength to runners and other athletes." (73:279)

Juncus effusus, Common Rush
Cherokee *Emetic* Decoction of plant taken as an emetic. (152:7) *Oral Aid* Decoction used "to dislodge spoiled saliva." *Orthopedic Aid* Infusion given to babies to prevent lameness. *Pediatric Aid* Infusion used as a wash to strengthen babies and given to babies to prevent lameness. *Strengthener* Infusion used as a wash to strengthen babies. (66:53) **Karok** *Unspecified* Stems and leaves placed in the fire and the medicine man prayed over it. (5:33)

Juncus ensifolius, Swordleaf Rush
Hoh *Unspecified* Used as a medicine. **Quileute** *Unspecified* Used as a medicine. (114:59)

Juncus mertensianus, Mertens's Rush
Okanagan-Colville *Witchcraft Medicine* Plant used for "witchcraft" or "plhax." (162:38)

Juncus tenuis, Poverty Rush
Cherokee *Oral Aid* Decoction used "to dislodge spoiled saliva." *Orthopedic Aid* Infusion given to babies to prevent lameness. *Pediatric Aid* Infusion used as a wash to strengthen babies and given to babies to prevent lameness. *Strengthener* Infusion used as a wash to strengthen babies. (66:53) **Iroquois** *Emetic* Decoction or infusion of plant taken by lacrosse players and runners to vomit. *Sports Medicine* Infusion of plant taken to vomit and used as a wash by lacrosse players. *Veterinary Aid* Infusion of plant given to "colt that has had too much feed." (73:279)

Juniperus californica, California Juniper
Apache, White Mountain *Anticonvulsive* Scorched twigs rubbed on body for fits. *Cold Remedy* Infusion of leaves taken for colds. *Cough Medicine* Infusion of leaves taken for coughs. *Gynecological Aid* Infusion of leaves taken by women previous to childbirth to relax muscles. (113:158) **Costanoan** *Analgesic* Decoction of leaves taken for pain. *Diaphoretic* Decoction of leaves taken to cause sweating. (17:6) **Diegueño** *Analgesic* Infusion of leaves and bark taken for hangovers. *Hypotensive* Infusion of leaves and bark taken for high blood pressures. (74:216) **Gosiute** *Cold Remedy* Infusion of leaves used for colds. *Cough Medicine* Infusion of leaves used for coughs. (31:372)

Mahuna *Febrifuge* and *Misc. Disease Remedy* Infusion of berries taken or berries chewed for grippe fevers. (117:9)

Juniperus communis, Common Juniper
Algonquin *Other* Used for "cold" conditions, since plant was regarded as "hot." (18:142) **Bella Coola** *Analgesic* Decoction of roots, leaves, branches, and bark taken for stomach pain. *Cough Medicine* Decoction of root, leaves, branches, and bark taken for "cough from the lungs." *Gastrointestinal Aid* Decoction of roots, leaves, branches, and bark taken for stomach pain. (127:49) Infusion of roots, leaves, branches, and bark taken for stomach pains, for ulcers, and for heartburn. *Pulmonary Aid* Infusion of roots, leaves, branches, and bark taken for lung cough. (158:197) **Blackfoot** *Pulmonary Aid* Used for lung diseases. (68:37) Decoction of berries used for lung diseases. (82:17) *Venereal Aid* Used for venereal diseases. (68:37) Decoction of berries used for venereal diseases. (82:17) **Carrier** *Tuberculosis Remedy* Decoction of berries and kinnikinnick leaves or balsam strained and taken for tuberculosis. (26:71) **Carrier, Northern** *Cathartic* Decoction of tips taken as a purgative and for coughs. *Cough Medicine* Decoction of tips taken for coughs and as a purgative. **Carrier, Southern** *Analgesic* Steam from boiling branches inhaled for headache and chest pain. (127:49) **Cheyenne** *Ceremonial Medicine* Leaves burned as incense in ceremonies, especially to remove fear of thunder. *Cold Remedy* Cones chewed, infusion of boughs or cones taken

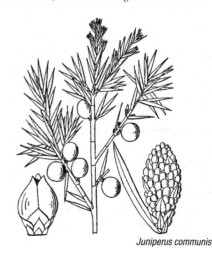

Juniperus communis

or used as steam bath for colds. *Cough Medicine* Infusion of boughs or fleshy cones taken for coughing. *Febrifuge* Infusion of boughs or fleshy cones taken for high fevers. *Gynecological Aid* Leaves burned at childbirth to promote delivery. *Herbal Steam* Cones chewed, infusion of boughs or cones taken or used as steam bath for colds. *Love Medicine* Wood flutes used to "charm a girl whom a man loved to make her love him." *Sedative* Infusion of boughs or fleshy cones taken as a sedative. *Throat Aid* Infusion of boughs or cones taken for tickles in the throat or tonsillitis. (69:4) **Chippewa** *Respiratory Aid* Decoction of twigs and leaves taken for asthma. (59:124) **Cree, Hudson Bay** *Dermatological Aid* Poultice of bark applied to wounds. *Disinfectant* Plant used for the antiseptic qualities on wounds. (78:302) **Cree, Woodlands** *Antidiarrheal* Decoction of barked procumbent stem or branch used for diarrhea. *Cough Medicine* Decoction of branch or wood and other herbs used for coughs. *Febrifuge* Decoction of branch or wood and other herbs used for fevers. *Gynecological Aid* Decoction of branch or wood and other herbs used for "woman's troubles," and for sickness after giving birth. *Kidney Aid* Decoction of green berries taken for sore backs from kidney troubles. *Pediatric Aid* Decoction of branch or wood and other herbs used for teething sickness. *Pulmonary Aid* Decoction of barked procumbent stem or branch used for sore chest from lung infections. *Respiratory Aid* Blue berries smoked in a pipe for asthma. *Toothache Remedy* Decoction of branch or wood and other herbs used for teething sickness. (91:41) **Delaware, Ontario** *Gynecological Aid* Compound infusion of bark taken for women's diseases. (151:110) *Tonic* Compound infusion of bark taken as a tonic. (150:68, 82) **Eskimo, Inupiat** *Cold Remedy* Infusion of berries taken or one berry a day eaten to prevent colds, and for colds. *Cough Medicine* Decoction of berries, needles, and twigs taken one cup a day for coughing. *Misc. Disease Remedy* Infusion of berries taken or one berry a day eaten to prevent flu, and for the flu. *Respiratory Aid* Decoction of berries, needles, and twigs taken one cup a day for respiratory ailments. (83:110) **Gitksan** *Unspecified* Plant used for many medicinal applications. (35:314) **Hanaksiala** *Dermatological Aid* Heated poultice of branch and "berry" paste applied to

wounds and cuts. (35:160) **Iroquois** *Cold Remedy* Decoction taken for colds caused by overheating and chills. *Cough Medicine* Decoction taken for coughs caused by overheating and chills. (73:271) *Kidney Aid* Infusion of boughs used for kidney pain. *Tonic* Infusion of boughs used as a tonic. (119:83) **Kwakiutl** *Antidiarrheal* Compound decoction of berries taken for diarrhea. *Blood Medicine* Decoction of wood and bark taken to purify the blood. *Respiratory Aid* Decoction of wood and bark taken for short breath. (157:266) **Malecite** *Dermatological Aid* Infusion of boughs used as a hair wash. (96:250) *Tonic* Infusion of boughs used as a tonic. *Tuberculosis Remedy* Infusion of roots and prince's pine used for consumption. (96:252) **Micmac** *Antirheumatic (Internal)* Part of plant used for rheumatism and bark used for tuberculosis. *Dermatological Aid* Stems used in hair wash, gum used for wounds, and cones used for ulcers. *Orthopedic Aid* Gum used for sprains and bark used for tuberculosis. *Tonic* Stems used in a tonic and bark used for tuberculosis. *Tuberculosis Remedy* Root or bark used for consumption and stems used as a tonic. (32:57) **Navajo, Ramah** *Emetic* Used as an emetic for all ceremonials. (165:11) **Okanagan-Colville** *Cold Remedy* Infusion of bark and needles taken for colds. *Tonic* Infusion of bark and needles taken as a tonic before entering the sweat house. *Tuberculosis Remedy* Infusion of bark and needles taken for consumption. (162:18) **Okanagon** *Eye Medicine* Infusion of twigs used as a wash for sore eyes. *Kidney Aid* Berries eaten for kidney disorders. *Tonic* Decoction of small branches used as a tonic. (104:42) **Potawatomi** *Urinary Aid* Compound containing berries used for urinary tract diseases. (131:69) **Shuswap** *Diaphoretic* Used in the sweat house. *Panacea* Decoction of stems and needles taken for any sickness. (102:50) **Tanana, Upper** *Antirheumatic (External)* Decoction of branches and fruit used as a wash for body aches and pains. *Cold Remedy* Decoction of branches and fruit taken for colds. Raw fruit eaten for colds. Decoction of branches taken for colds. Decoction of berries taken for colds. *Cough Medicine* Decoction of branches and fruit taken for coughs. Raw fruit eaten for coughs. *Kidney Aid* Decoction of branches and fruit taken for kidney problems. Raw fruit eaten for kidney problems. *Panacea* Branches

Juniperus monosperma ·

burned on top of the wood stove to keep sickness away. *Throat Aid* Decoction of branches taken for sore throats. *Tuberculosis Remedy* Decoction of branches taken for tuberculosis. (86:4) **Thompson** *Antirheumatic* (*Internal*) Infusion of branches taken for aching muscles. *Cathartic* Decoction of branches taken as a physic. *Cold Remedy* Decoction of branches used for colds. (161:92) *Eye Medicine* Infusion of twigs used as a wash for sore eyes. (104:42) Infusion or decoction of twigs used as a wash for sore eyes. *Gastrointestinal Aid* Decoction of twigs taken as a tonic for the stomach. (141:474) Infusion of three 10-cm-long branches taken to "make your insides nice." *Heart Medicine* Infusion of boughs taken for "leakage of the heart." *Hypotensive* Infusion of branches taken for high blood pressure. The branches were steeped in boiling water until the water cooled. The cool infusion was taken for 2 weeks after which the blood pressure returned to normal. (161:92) *Kidney Aid* Berries eaten for kidney disorders. (104:42) Decoction of branches used for kidney ailments. (161:92) *Tonic* Decoction of small branches used as a tonic. (104:42) Decoction of twigs taken as a tonic for the stomach. (141:474) Decoction of branches taken as a tonic. *Tuberculosis Remedy* Branches used for tuberculosis. It was said that for the medicine to be really effective, the boughs should be taken from a plant growing all by itself. (161:92)

Juniperus communis var. *montana*, Common Juniper

Arapaho *Disinfectant* Needles burned as a disinfectant. *Gastrointestinal Aid* Infusion of needles taken for bowel troubles. (as *J. sibirica* 100:46) *Misc. Disease Remedy* Ground needles scent used to drive smallpox away. (as *J. sibirica* 98:50) **Cheyenne** *Cough Medicine* Infusion of leaves used for coughs. (as *J. sibirica* 63:169) Infusion of leaves used for coughs. One or two berries chewed and the juice swallowed for bad coughs. (as *J. sibirica* 64:169) *Throat Aid* Infusion of leaves used for a tickling in the throat. (as *J. sibirica* 63:169) Infusion of leaves used for a tickling in the throat. (as *J. sibirica* 64:169) **Gitksan** *Witchcraft Medicine* Boughs, red elder bark, and cow parsnip roots used for evil witchcraft victims. (62:25) **Navajo, Ramah** *Ceremonial Medicine* Decoction of plant used as a ceremonial emetic. *Cough Medicine* Decoction taken and used as lotion for fever or "big cough." *Emetic* Decoction of plant used as a ceremonial emetic. *Febrifuge* Decoction of plant used internally and externally for fever. (as *J. sibirica* 165:12) **Paiute** *Blood Medicine* Seeds from dried fruit eaten as a blood tonic. *Orthopedic Aid* Seeds from dried fruit eaten for lumbago. *Tonic* Seeds from dried fruit eaten as a blood tonic. *Venereal Aid* Cold decoction of twigs taken for venereal disease. **Shoshoni** *Blood Medicine* and *Tonic* Decoction of branches taken as a blood tonic. (155:91, 92)

Juniperus horizontalis, Creeping Juniper

Blackfoot *Kidney Aid* Used for kidney problems. (68:37) *Veterinary Aid* Roots soaked in water and used as a bath on horses for shiny hair. (72:89) **Cheyenne** *Ceremonial Medicine* Leaves burned as incense in ceremonies, especially to remove fear of thunder. *Cold Remedy* Cones chewed, infusion of boughs or cones taken or used as steam bath for colds. *Cough Medicine* Infusion of boughs or fleshy cones taken for coughing. *Febrifuge* Infusion of boughs or fleshy cones taken for high fevers. *Gynecological Aid* Leaves burned at childbirth to promote delivery. *Herbal Steam* Cones chewed, infusion of boughs or cones taken or used as steam bath for colds. *Love Medicine* Wood flutes used to "charm a girl whom a man loved to make her love him." *Sedative* Infusion of boughs or fleshy cones taken as a sedative. *Throat Aid* Infusion of boughs or cones taken for tickles in the throat or tonsillitis. (69:4) **Crow** *Ceremonial Medicine* Young twigs and leaves burned as incense during incantations. **Montana Indian** *Kidney Aid* Infusion of seeds taken for kidney trouble. (as *J. sabina procumbens* 15:13)

Juniperus monosperma, Oneseed Juniper

Apache, White Mountain *Anticonvulsive* Scorched twigs rubbed on body for fits. *Cold Remedy* Infusion of leaves taken for colds. *Cough Medicine* Infusion of leaves taken for coughs. *Gynecological Aid* Infusion of leaves taken by women previous to childbirth to relax muscles. (113:158) **Hopi** *Antirheumatic* (*External*) Poultice of heated twigs bound over a bruise or sprain for swelling. *Gastrointestinal Aid* Decoction of plant and sagebrush taken for indigestion. *Gynecological Aid* Infusion of leaves taken and used for many purposes. *Laxative* Decoction of leaves taken as a laxative. *Pediatric Aid* Plant ashes rubbed on newborn baby. *Reproductive Aid* Decoction of leaves taken by women who desire a female child. (34:330) **Isleta** *Antirheumatic* (*External*) Infusion of cedar bark used for bathing and washing sore feet. *Emetic* Strong infusion of leaves given in large quantities as an emetic. *Gynecological Aid* Infusion of leaves given to mothers after childbirth. (85:32) **Jemez** *Gastrointestinal Aid* Decoction of leaves taken for stomach or bowel disorders. *Gynecological Aid* Decoction of leaves taken by women after the birth of an infant. (36:24) **Keres, Western** *Antidiarrheal* Infusion of staminate cones used for diarrhea. *Dermatological Aid* Chewed bark taken for or applied to spider bites. *Diaphoretic* Plant used as an ingredient in the sweat bath. *Ear Medicine* Ground leaves mixed with salt and used in ears to eliminate bugs. *Emetic* Infusion of twigs or chewed twigs used as an emetic before breakfast. *Gastrointestinal Aid* Infusion of staminate cones used as a stomach tonic. *Laxative* Infusion of staminate cones used as a laxative. Bark chewed as a laxative. (147:48) **Navajo, Ramah** *Analgesic* Decoction used for postpartum or menstrual pain and cold infusion used for stomachache. *Ceremonial Medicine* Decoction used in "bath for purification of burial party." *Cough Medicine* Compound decoction, sometimes salted, taken for cough. (165:11, 12) *Dermatological Aid* Bark highly prized as a medicine for burns. (165:11) *Diaphoretic* Compound used as sweat bath medicine. *Emetic* Infusion of inner bark given to newborns "to clean out impurities." *Febrifuge* Cold infusion of plant used for fever. *Gastrointestinal Aid* Cold infusion of plant used for stomachache. *Gynecological Aid* Decoction or smoke of various plant parts used for childbirth difficulties. *Pediatric Aid* Infusion of inner bark used as an emetic for newborn "to clean out all impurities." Plant used as bed and coverlet for baby, "to make him strong and healthy." *Stimulant* Wet twigs or pulverized needles used as stimulant in postpartum fainting. *Veterinary Aid* Decoction given to sheep for bloating from eating "chamiso." (165:11, 12) **Paiute** *Cold Remedy* Decoction of twigs taken and fumes from burning branches

inhaled for colds. *Dermatological Aid* and *Misc. Disease Remedy* Heated twigs rubbed on measles eruptions to relieve the discomfort. **Shoshoni** *Cold Remedy* Decoction of twigs taken and fumes from burning branches inhaled for colds. *Dermatological Aid* and *Misc. Disease Remedy* Heated twigs rubbed on measles eruptions to relieve the discomfort. (155:92) **Tewa** *Analgesic* Poultice of toasted leafy twigs applied to bruise or sprain pains. (115:39, 40) *Antirheumatic* (*External*) Poultice of heated twigs bound over a bruise or sprain for swelling. (34:330) *Dermatological Aid* Poultice of leafy twigs used for the pain and swellings of bruises or sprains. *Disinfectant* Leaves placed on hot coals as an herbal steam to "fumigate" new mother. *Diuretic* Berries used as an "active diuretic." (115:39, 40) *Gastrointestinal Aid* Decoction of plant and sagebrush taken for indigestion. *Gynecological Aid* Infusion of leaves taken and used for many purposes. (34:330) Decoction of leaves taken and used as a postpartum wash. *Herbal Steam* Leaves placed on hot coals as an herbal steam to "fumigate" new mother. *Internal Medicine* Berries eaten or decoction of berries used "for every kind of internal chill." (115:39, 40) *Laxative* Decoction of leaves taken as a laxative. (34:330) *Orthopedic Aid* Poultice of toasted leafy twigs applied to bruise or sprain pains. (115:39, 40) *Pediatric Aid* Plant ashes rubbed on newborn baby. *Reproductive Aid* Decoction of leaves taken by women who desire a female child. (34:330) *Toothache Remedy* Gum used as a filling for decayed teeth. (115:39, 40) **Zuni** *Antirheumatic* (*External*) Infusion of leaves used for muscle aches. *Contraceptive* Infusion of leaves taken to prevent conception. *Gynecological Aid* Infusion of leaves taken postpartum to prevent uterine cramps and stop vaginal bleeding. (22:373) Simple or compound infusion of twigs used to promote muscular relaxation at birth, and after childbirth to stop blood flow. *Hemostat* Simple or compound infusion of twigs taken after childbirth to stop blood flow. (143:55)

Juniperus occidentalis, Western Juniper
Apache, White Mountain *Anticonvulsive* Scorched twigs rubbed on body for fits. *Cold Remedy* Infusion of leaves taken for colds. *Cough Medicine* Infusion of leaves taken for coughs. *Gyne-*

cological Aid Infusion of leaves taken by women previous to childbirth to relax muscles. (113:158) **Paiute** *Analgesic* Decoction of berries taken for menstrual cramps. Decoction of young twigs taken for stomachaches. Fumes from burning twigs or leaves inhaled for headaches. *Antihemorrhagic* Decoction of young twigs taken for hemorrhages. *Antirheumatic* (*External*) Branches used in the sweat bath for rheumatism. Decoction of berries taken or poultice of decoction applied for rheumatism. Poultice of boiled twigs applied and cooled decoction used as a wash for rheumatism. *Blood Medicine* Decoction of berries or young twigs taken as a blood tonic. (155:92–96) *Cold Remedy* Infusion of leaves taken as a cold medicine. (93:47) Branches used in the sweat bath for "heavy colds." Fumes from burning twigs or leaves inhaled for colds. Simple or compound decoction of twigs or berries taken for colds. *Cough Medicine* Decoction of twigs or berries taken for coughs. *Dermatological Aid* Compound poultice of twigs used as a drawing agent for boils or slivers. Poultice of mashed twigs applied for swellings or rheumatism. Strong decoction used as an antiseptic wash for sores. *Disinfectant* Branches burned as a fumigant after illness. Decoction of twigs used as an antiseptic wash for sores. *Diuretic* Decoction of berries taken to induce urination. *Febrifuge* Simple or compound decoction of young twigs taken for fevers. *Gastrointestinal Aid* Decoction of young twigs taken for stomachaches. *Gynecological Aid* Decoction of berries taken for menstrual cramps. *Kidney Aid* Decoction of berries taken for kidney ailments. Simple or compound decoction of young twigs taken for kidney trouble. (155:92–96) *Misc. Disease Remedy* Bed of hot coals and branches used for malaria and other diseases. (93:47) Compound decoction of young twigs taken for smallpox. Decoction of young twigs taken for influenza. (155:92–96) *Pulmonary Aid* Bed of hot coals and branches used for pneumonia. (93:47) Compound decoction of twigs taken for fever, pneumonia, and influenza. *Tonic* Decoction of berries taken as a blood tonic. Decoction of young twigs taken as a blood tonic. *Venereal Aid* Decoction of shaved root taken for venereal disease. Decoction of twig or compound decoction of berry taken for venereal disease. (155:92–96) *Veterinary Aid* Boughs placed in a pan of coals and fumes inhaled by

horses that have eaten poison camas. (93:47) **Shoshoni** *Anthelmintic* Strained cold water infusion of pulverized terminal twigs taken for worms. *Burn Dressing* Poultice of mashed twigs applied to burns. *Cold Remedy* Simple or compound decoction of twigs or berries taken for colds. *Cough Medicine* Decoction of twigs taken for coughs. *Dermatological Aid* Poultice of mashed twigs applied to swellings. Strong decoction used as an antiseptic wash for measles and smallpox. *Disinfectant* Branches burned as a fumigant after illness. Decoction of twigs used as an antiseptic wash for measles and smallpox. *Diuretic* Decoction of berries taken to induce urination. *Heart Medicine* Decoction of berries taken for heart trouble. *Kidney Aid* Simple or compound decoction of twigs or decoction of berry used for kidney trouble. *Misc. Disease Remedy* Compound decoction of young twigs taken for influenza or smallpox. Decoction of twigs used as an antiseptic wash for measles and smallpox. *Oral Aid* Poultice of pounded, moistened leaves applied to jaw for swollen and sore gums. *Throat Aid* Poultice of twigs applied to neck for sore throat. *Tonic* Decoction of young twigs taken as a general tonic. *Toothache Remedy* Poultice of leaves applied to jaw for toothache. *Venereal Aid* Decoction of twigs taken for venereal disease. **Washo** *Analgesic* Fumes from burning twigs inhaled for headaches. *Cold Remedy* Fumes from burning twigs inhaled for colds. *Disinfectant* Branches burned as a fumigant after illness. (155:92–96)

Juniperus osteosperma, Utah Juniper

Havasupai *Cold Remedy* Green branches used singly or together with other plants for colds. (171:206) **Hopi** *Gynecological Aid* Decoction of branches used especially by women during confinement. (as *J. utahensis* 164:157) *Other* Misbehaving youngsters held in a blanket over a smoldering fire of plant. (as *J. utahensis* 174:37) **Navajo** *Analgesic* Seeds eaten for headaches. *Dermatological Aid* Used to wash the hair. (76:152) **Paiute** *Analgesic* Decoction of berries taken for menstrual cramps. Decoction of young twigs taken for stomachaches. Fumes from burning twigs inhaled for headaches and colds. *Antihemorrhagic* Decoction of young twigs taken for hemorrhages. *Antirheumatic* (*External*) Branches used in the sweat bath for rheumatism. Decoction of berries taken or poultice of decoction applied for rheumatism. Poultice of boiled twigs applied and cooled decoction used as a wash for rheumatism. *Blood Medicine* Decoction of berries or young twigs taken as a blood tonic. *Cold Remedy* Branches used in the sweat bath for heavy colds. Fumes from burning twigs or leaves inhaled for headaches and colds. Simple or compound decoction of twigs or berries taken for colds. *Cough Medicine* Decoction of twigs or berries taken for coughs. *Dermatological Aid* Compound poultice of twigs used as a drawing agent for boils or slivers. Poultice of mashed twigs applied for swellings or rheumatism. Strong decoction used as an antiseptic wash for sores. *Disinfectant* Branches burned as a fumigant after illness. Strong decoction of twigs used as an antiseptic wash for sores. *Diuretic* Decoction of berries taken to induce urination. *Febrifuge* Simple or compound decoction of young twigs taken for fevers. *Gastrointestinal Aid* Decoction of young twigs taken for stomachaches. *Gynecological Aid* Decoction of berries taken for menstrual cramps. *Kidney Aid* Decoction of berries taken for kidney ailments. Simple or compound decoction of young twigs taken for kidney trouble. *Misc. Disease Remedy* Compound decoction of twigs taken for smallpox. Decoction of young twigs taken for influenza. *Pulmonary Aid* Compound decoction of twigs taken for fevers, pneumonia, and influenza. *Tonic* Decoction of young twigs or berries taken as a blood tonic. *Venereal Aid* Decoction of shaved root taken for venereal disease. Decoction of twig or compound decoction of berry taken for venereal disease. (as *J. utahensis* 155:93–96) **Paiute, Northern** *Analgesic* Roasted berry steam used for pains. *Antirheumatic* (*External*) Roasted berry steam used for rheumatism. *Cold Remedy* Infusion of leaves taken and burning leaf scent inhaled for colds. (49:130) **Shoshoni** *Anthelmintic* Strained cold water infusion of pulverized terminal twigs taken for worms. *Burn Dressing* Poultice of mashed twigs applied to burns. *Cold Remedy* Simple or compound decoction of twigs or berries taken for colds. *Cough Medicine* Decoction of twigs taken for coughs. *Dermatological Aid* Poultice of mashed twigs applied to swellings. Strong decoction used as an antiseptic wash for measles and smallpox. *Disin-*

fectant Branches burned as a fumigant after illness. Strong decoction of twigs used as an antiseptic wash for measles and smallpox. *Diuretic* Decoction of berries taken to induce urination. *Heart Medicine* Decoction of berries taken for heart trouble. *Kidney Aid* Compound decoction of twigs or decoction of berry taken for kidney ailments. Simple or compound decoction of young twigs taken for kidney trouble. *Misc. Disease Remedy* Compound decoction of twigs taken for influenza and smallpox. Strong decoction of twigs used as an antiseptic wash for measles and smallpox. *Oral Aid* Poultice of pounded leaves held to the jaw for swollen and sore gums. *Throat Aid* Poultice of twigs applied to neck for sore throat. *Tonic* Decoction of young twigs taken as a general tonic. *Toothache Remedy* Poultice of leaves applied to jaw for toothache. *Venereal Aid* Decoction of twigs taken for venereal disease. **Washo** *Analgesic* Fumes from burning twigs inhaled for headaches. *Cold Remedy* Fumes from burning twigs inhaled for colds. *Disinfectant* Branches burned as a fumigant after illness. (as *J. utahensis* 155:93–96)

Juniperus pinchotii, Pinchot's Juniper
Comanche *Analgesic* Dried leaves sprinkled on live coals and smoke inhaled for headache. *Ceremonial Medicine* Dried leaves sprinkled on live coals and smoke inhaled for ghost sickness. *Gynecological Aid* Decoction of dried and pulverized roots taken for menstrual complaints. *Other* Dried leaves sprinkled on live coals and smoke inhaled for vertigo. (84:3)

Juniperus scopulorum, Rocky Mountain Juniper
Blackfoot *Antiemetic* Infusion of berries taken for vomiting. (82:17) Infusion of berries taken for vomiting. (95:276) *Antirheumatic* (*External*) Leaves boiled, turpentine added, mixture cooled and used for arthritis and rheumatism. (68:36) Decoction of leaves and turpentine rubbed on parts affected by arthritis and rheumatism. (82:17) **Cheyenne** *Ceremonial Medicine* Leaves burned as incense in ceremonies, especially to remove fear of thunder. (69:4) *Cold Remedy* Infusion of boughs, branches, and cones used for colds. Fleshy cones chewed for colds. (68:36) Cones chewed, infusion of boughs or cones taken or used

as steam bath for colds. (69:4) *Cough Medicine* Infusion of leaves used for coughs. (63:170) Infusion of leaves taken for constant coughing. (64:170) Infusion taken for coughs. (68:36) Infusion of boughs or fleshy cones taken for coughing. (69:4) *Febrifuge* Infusion of boughs, branches, and cones used for fevers. (68:36) Infusion of boughs or fleshy cones taken for high fevers. *Gynecological Aid* Leaves burned at childbirth to promote delivery. *Herbal Steam* Cones chewed, infusion of boughs or cones taken or used as steam bath for colds. *Love Medicine* Wood flutes used to "charm a girl whom a man loved to make her love him." (69:4) *Pulmonary Aid* Infusion of boughs, branches, and cones used for pneumonia. *Sedative* Infusion used for sedating hyperactive persons. (68:36) Infusion of boughs or fleshy cones taken as a sedative. (69:4) *Throat Aid* Infusion of leaves used for a tickling in the throat. (63:170) Infusion of leaves taken for a tickling in the throat. (64:170) Infusion taken for "tickling of the throat." (68:36) Infusion of boughs or cones taken for tickles in the throat or tonsillitis. (69:4) **Crow** *Antidiarrheal* Infusion taken for diarrhea. *Antihemorrhagic* Infusion taken for lung or nose hemorrhages. *Dietary Aid* Fleshy cones chewed to increase the appetite. *Gastrointestinal Aid* Fleshy cones chewed for upset stomach. *Gynecological Aid* Infusion taken after birth for cleansing and healing. **Flathead** *Ceremonial Medicine* Plant burned and smoke used to purify the air and ward off illness. *Cold Remedy* Infusion of boughs, branches, and cones used for colds. *Febrifuge* Infusion of boughs, branches, and cones used for fevers. *Pulmonary Aid* Infusion of boughs, branches, and cones used for pneumonia. *Veterinary Aid* Leaves placed on hot coals and smoke used for sick horses. **Kutenai** *Cold Remedy* Infusion of boughs, branches, and cones used for colds. Plant burned and smoke used for colds. *Febrifuge* Infusion of boughs, branches, and cones used for fevers. *Misc. Disease Remedy* Infusion taken for sugar diabetes. *Pulmonary Aid* Infusion of boughs, branches, and cones used for pneumonia. **Montana Indian** *Antirheumatic (External)* Concoction used for arthritis and rheumatic pain. (68:36) *Ceremonial Medicine* Aromatic twigs burned as incense. (15:14) **Navajo** *Ceremonial Medicine* Plant taken as a "War Dance medicine." *Dermatological Aid* Plant

rubbed on the hair for dandruff. *Unspecified* Pounded mixture of herbs given to patient during the blackening ceremony of the War Dance. (45:20) **Navajo, Kayenta** *Analgesic* Plant used for pain. (179:15) **Navajo, Ramah** *Analgesic* Decoction of needles taken and used as lotion for headache and stomachache. *Ceremonial Medicine* Cold infusion used as a ceremonial medicine to protect from enemies and witches. *Cold Remedy* Decoction of needles taken and used as lotion for colds. *Febrifuge* Decoction of needles taken and used as lotion for fever. *Gastrointestinal Aid* Decoction of needles taken and used as lotion for stomachache. *Kidney Aid* Decoction of needles taken and used as lotion for kidney trouble. *Witchcraft Medicine* Cold infusion taken and used as lotion in ceremony for protection from witches. (165:12) **Nez Perce** *Cold Remedy* Infusion of boughs, branches, and cones used for colds. *Febrifuge* Infusion of boughs, branches, and cones used for fevers. *Pulmonary Aid* Infusion of boughs, branches, and cones used for pneumonia. (68:36) **Okanagan-Colville** *Antihemorrhagic* Decoction of branch tips and needles taken for internal hemorrhaging. *Antirheumatic (External)* Poultice of mashed and dampened branches applied to arthritic joints. *Dermatological Aid* Poultice of mashed and dampened branches applied to skin sores. *Misc. Disease Remedy* Decoction of sap used for the flu and colds. Five strips of bark each about 5 cm by 10 cm were boiled in about 2 liters of water in order to obtain the sap. Only bark from the bottom part of the tree could be used. *Other* Decoction of branch tips and needles considered a good emergency medicine. *Poison* Berries believed to be poisonous. (162:19) **Okanagon** *Urinary Aid* Fruit eaten for bladder troubles. (104:41) **Saanich** *Misc. Disease Remedy* Scented branches hung around the house during disease epidemics to "drive the germs away." (156:70) **Sanpoil** *Dermatological Aid* Decoction of leaves, stems, and berries used as a wash for sores. *Tuberculosis Remedy* Berries eaten or decoction taken for tuberculosis. *Unspecified* Berries eaten or decoction taken for general illnesses. (109:221) **Shoshoni** *Venereal Aid* Decoction of twigs taken over a long period of time for venereal disease. (155:92) **Shuswap** *Diaphoretic* Used in the sweat house. *Misc. Disease Remedy* Decoction of plant used as a steam bath for the flu. *Panacea*

Decoction of stems and needles taken for any sickness. (102:50) **Sioux** *Cold Remedy* Infusion of boughs, branches, and cones used for colds. Plant burned and smoke used for colds. *Febrifuge* Infusion of boughs, branches, and cones used for fevers. *Misc. Disease Remedy* Infusion of leaves formerly used for cholera. *Pulmonary Aid* Infusion of boughs, branches, and cones used for pneumonia. **Stony Indian** *Antihemorrhagic* Infusion taken for hemorrhages. (68:36) **Swinomish** *Antirheumatic (External)* Infusion of roots used as a foot soak for rheumatism. *Disinfectant* Decoction of leaves used to disinfect the house. *Panacea* Infusion of leaves used as a wash for all ailments. *Tonic* Infusion of leaves taken as a general tonic. (65:21) **Thompson** *Antirheumatic (External)* Decoction of berries used externally for rheumatism. *Cold Remedy* Decoction of branches and berries taken for colds. *Dermatological Aid* Decoction of berries used as a wash for all types of bites and stings. Decoction of boughs taken or used as a wash for hives or sores. The informant said that she used a decoction of mashed boughs and Douglas fir to bathe her children when they had the "seven year itch" and that it worked, but not as well as modern medicine. *Disinfectant* Decoction or infusion of plant used to disinfect the house after an illness or death. The decoction was used to scrub the floors, walls, and furniture after an illness or death in the house. It was also used to wash the deceased person's bedding and clothing as well as serving as a protective wash for other members of the household. The steam from the infusion was also said to have a disinfecting effect. If they knew that an illness was going to arrive, they broke the branches and burned them in the house for the strong smoke which they said would keep the air fresh so that the sickness would not affect them. They also burned the branches after a death in the house to freshen the air. (161:92) *Diuretic* Fresh berries eaten as a diuretic. (141:465) Fresh or dried berries eaten as a diuretic. *Gastrointestinal Aid* Decoction of berries used externally for stomach ailments. *Gynecological Aid* Decoction of branches and berries taken every morning just before childbirth. The decoction was taken every morning just before childbirth to promote muscular relaxation. *Heart Medicine* Decoction of branches and berries taken for heart trouble.

Kidney Aid Infusion of plant taken for kidney trouble. *Misc. Disease Remedy* Decoction of boughs used for "black measles" or chickenpox. *Other* Plant considered effective in combating evil "spirits" associated with illness and death. *Tuberculosis Remedy* Decoction of branches and berries taken for tuberculosis. (161:92) *Urinary Aid* Fruit eaten for bladder troubles. (104:41) Fresh berries eaten as a medicine for the bladder. (141:465) Fresh or dried berries eaten for bladder trouble. (161:92) *Veterinary Aid* Strong decoction of berries used to kill ticks on horses. (141:512)

Juniperus virginiana, Eastern Red Cedar
Cherokee *Abortifacient* Used for "female obstructions." *Anthelmintic* Decoction of berries given for worms. *Antirheumatic (Internal)* Used for rheumatism and "female obstructions." *Cold Remedy* Infusion taken for colds. *Dermatological Aid* Used as an ointment for itch, skin diseases, and "white swelling." *Diaphoretic* Used as a diaphoretic. *Misc. Disease Remedy* Used as a diaphoretic and for measles. (66:28) **Chippewa** *Antirheumatic (External)* Compound decoction of twigs used as herbal steam for rheumatism. *Antirheumatic (Internal)* Compound decoction of twigs taken for rheumatism. *Herbal Steam* Compound decoction of twigs taken or used as herbal steam for rheumatism. (43:362) **Comanche** *Disinfectant* Smoke from leaves inhaled for purifying effect. (24:522) **Cree**, **Hudson Bay** *Diuretic* Leaves used as a diuretic. (78:303) **Dakota** *Cold Remedy* Smoke from burned twigs inhaled as a cold remedy. *Cough*

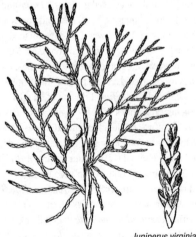

Juniperus virginiana

Medicine Decoction of fruits and leaves taken for coughs. *Misc. Disease Remedy* Decoction of leaves taken and used as a wash for cholera. *Veterinary Aid* Decoction of fruits and leaves given to horses for coughs. (58:63, 64) **Delaware**, **Oklahoma** *Antirheumatic* (*External*) Infusion of twigs used as herbal steam for rheumatism. (150:30, 76) *Herbal Steam* Infusion of roots or twigs used as herbal steam for rheumatism. (150:30) **Iroquois** *Antirheumatic* (*Internal*) Compound decoction taken for rheumatism. *Cold Remedy* Compound decoction taken for colds. *Cough Medicine* Compound decoction taken for coughs. *Diuretic* Compound decoction taken as a diuretic. (73:271) **Kiowa** *Oral Aid* Berries chewed for canker sores in the mouth. (166:13) **Lakota** *Cold Remedy* Leaves burned and smoke inhaled for head colds. (88:30) **Meskwaki** *Adjuvant* Wood prepared in warm water and used as a seasoner for other medicines. *Other* Decoction of leaves taken by convalescent patients. *Stimulant* Decoction of leaves taken for weakness and as a convalescent medicine. (129:234) **Ojibwa**, **South** *Analgesic* Bruised leaves and berries used internally for headache. (77:198) **Omaha** *Ceremonial Medicine* Plant used in the sun dance ceremony and various rituals. Plant used in the vapor bath of the purificatory rites. (56:320) *Cold Remedy* Smoke from burned twigs inhaled as a cold remedy. *Cough Medicine* Decoction of fruits and leaves taken for coughs. (58:63, 64) *Diaphoretic* Plant used in the vapor bath of the purificatory rites. (56:320) *Herbal Steam* Twigs used on hot stones in vapor bath, especially in purification rites. *Veterinary Aid* Decoction of fruits and leaves given to horses for coughs. **Pawnee** *Cold Remedy* Smoke from burned twigs inhaled as a cold remedy. *Cough Medicine* Decoction of fruits and leaves taken for coughs. *Sedative* Smoke from burning twigs used for nervousness and bad dreams. *Veterinary Aid* Decoction of fruits and leaves given to horses for coughs. **Ponca** *Cold Remedy* Smoke from burned twigs inhaled as a cold remedy. *Cough Medicine* Decoction of fruits and leaves taken for coughs. *Herbal Steam* Twigs used on hot stones in vapor bath, especially in purification rites. *Veterinary Aid* Decoction of fruits and leaves given to horses for coughs. (58:63, 64) **Rappahannock** *Other* Infusion of bark taken for summer complaint (sum-

mer cholera). *Pulmonary Aid* Compound infusion with berries taken for shortness of breath. (138:30) *Respiratory Aid* Compound infusion with berries taken for asthma. (138:33) **Salish** *Disinfectant* Plant used for fumigation. (153:294)

Juniperus virginiana var. *silicicola*, Southern Red Cedar

Seminole *Analgesic* Infusion of leaves taken as an emetic for rainbow sickness: fever, stiff neck, and backache. (as *J. silicicola* 145:210) Infusion of leaves taken as an emetic for thunder sickness: fever, dizziness, headache, and diarrhea. (as *J. silicicola* 145:213) Leaves used for scalping sickness: severe headache, backache, and low fever. (as *J. silicicola* 145:262) *Antidiarrheal* Infusion of leaves taken as an emetic for thunder sickness: fever, dizziness, headache, and diarrhea. (as *J.silicicola* 145:213) *Antirheumatic* (*External*) Decoction of leaves used as a body rub and steam for joint swellings. (as *J. silicicola* 145:193) *Cold Remedy* Infusion of leaves and bark taken and steam inhaled for runny nose, stuffy head, and sore throat. *Cough Medicine* Infusion of leaves and bark taken and steam inhaled for coughs. (as *J. silicicola* 145:279) *Emetic* Infusion of leaves taken as an emetic for rainbow sickness: fever, stiff neck, and backache. (as *J. silicicola* 145:210) Infusion of leaves taken as an emetic for thunder sickness: fever, dizziness, headache, and diarrhea. (as *J. silicicola* 145:213) Plant used as an emetic during religious ceremonies. (as *J. silicicola* 145:409) *Eye Medicine* Infusion of leaves taken and used as a bath for mist sickness: eye disease, fever, and chills. *Febrifuge* Infusion of leaves taken and used as a bath for mist sickness: eye disease, fever, and chills. (as *J. silicicola* 145:209) Infusion of leaves taken as an emetic for rainbow sickness: fever, stiff neck, and backache. (as *J. silicicola* 145:210) Infusion of leaves taken as an emetic for thunder sickness: fever, dizziness, headache, and diarrhea. (as *J. silicicola* 145:213) Leaves used for scalping sickness: severe headache, backache, and low fever. *Orthopedic Aid* Leaves used for scalping sickness: severe headache, backache, and low fever. (as *J. silicicola* 145:262) Leaves used to smoke the body for eagle sickness: stiff neck or back. Leaves used to smoke the body for fawn sickness: swollen legs and face. (as *J. silicicola* 145:305) *Other*

Leaves burned for ghost sickness: dizziness and staggering. (as *J. silicicola* 145:260) *Pediatric Aid* Plant and other plants used as a baby's charm for fear from dreams about raccoons or opossums. (as *J. silicicola* 145:221) *Psychological Aid* Plant burned to smoke the body for insanity. (as *J. silicicola* 145:293) *Sedative* Plant and other plants used as a baby's charm for fear from dreams about raccoons or opossums. (as *J. silicicola* 145:221) *Stimulant* Decoction of leaves used as a bath for hog sickness: unconsciousness. (as *J. silicicola* 145:229) *Unspecified* Plant used for medicinal purposes. (as *J. cilicicola* 145:161) Leaves used as medicine. (as *J. silicicola* 145:156) Plant used as medicine. (as *J. silicicola* 145:158) Plant used medicinally. (as *J. silicicola* 145:164) *Vertigo Medicine* Infusion of leaves taken as an emetic for thunder sickness: fever, dizziness, headache, and diarrhea. (as *J. silicicola* 145:213) *Witchcraft Medicine* Leaves used to make a witchcraft medicine. (as *J. bilicicola* 145:394)

Justicia crassifolia, Thickleaf Waterwillow
Seminole *Reproductive Aid* Plant used to restore virility. (145:319)

Kallstroemia californica, California Caltrop
Tewa *Antidiarrheal* Root used for diarrhea. *Dermatological Aid* Poultice of chewed leaves applied to sores or swellings. (as *K. brachystylis* 115:56, 57)

Kalmia angustifolia, Sheep Laurel
Abnaki *Cold Remedy* Used for head colds. (121:154) *Nose Medicine* Powdered leaves mixed with bark from another plant and used as snuff for nasal inflammation. (121:170) **Algonquin, Quebec** *Cold Remedy* Singed, crushed leaves used like snuff for colds. *Poison* Plant considered poisonous. (14:215) **Algonquin, Tête-de-Boule** *Analgesic* Leaves boiled and used for headaches. *Poison* Infusion of leaves taken in great quantities caused death. (110:129) **Cree, Hudson Bay** *Gastrointestinal Aid* Decoction of twigs with leaves and flowers taken for bowel complaints. *Tonic* Decoction of twigs with leaves and flowers taken as a tonic. (78:303) **Malecite** *Dermatological Aid* Salve of

pounded, fresh plant used for swellings. *Orthopedic Aid* Salve of pounded, fresh plant used for sprains. (96:244) **Micmac** *Analgesic* Herb used for pain, swellings, and sprains. (32:57) Poultice of crushed leaves bound to head for headache. (133:316) *Dermatological Aid* and *Orthopedic Aid* Herb used for swellings, pain, and sprains. (32:57) *Panacea* Infusion of leaves considered valuable as a "non-specific remedy." *Poison* Plant considered very poisonous. (133:316) **Montagnais** *Analgesic* Infusion of leaves taken sparingly for backache. *Cold Remedy* Infusion of leaves taken sparingly for colds. (133:314) *Gastrointestinal Aid* Infusion of leaves taken, poisonous if too strong, for stomach complaints. (133:317) *Poison* Leaves considered poisonous. (133:314) **Penobscot** *Analgesic* Compound poultice of plant used on cuts made in painful area to treat pain. *Panacea* Compound poultice of plant applied "for all kinds of trouble." (133:311)

Kalmia latifolia, Mountain Laurel
Cherokee *Analgesic* Infusion of leaves put on scratches made over location of the pain. (152:48) *Antirheumatic* (*External*) "Bristly edges of ten to twelve leaves" rubbed over skin for rheumatism. *Dermatological Aid* Crushed leaves used to "rub brier scratches." *Disinfectant* Infusion used as a wash "to get rid of pests" and as a liniment. *Orthopedic Aid* "Leaf ooze rubbed into scratched skin of ball players to prevent cramps." Compound used as liniment. *Panacea* Leaf salve used "for healing." (66:42) **Cree, Hudson Bay** *Antidiarrheal* Decoction of leaves taken for diarrhea. *Poison* Plant considered poisonous. (78:303) **Mahuna** *Dermatological Aid* Plant used as a body deodorizer. *Poison* Plant considered poisonous. (117:52)

Kalmia microphylla, Alpine Laurel
Kwakwaka'wakw *Antiemetic* and *Antihemorrhagic* Decoction of leaves used for vomiting and spitting blood. (35:241)

Kalmia polifolia, Bog Laurel
Gosiute *Unspecified* Leaves used as medicine. (as *K. glauca* 31:373) **Hesquiat** *Poison* Leaves could be poisonous and should never be used to make tea. (159:65) **Kwakiutl** *Antihemorrhagic* Decoction of leaves taken for "spitting of blood." (as *K. glauca* 16:380) Decoction of leaves taken for

blood-spitting. (157:283) *Dermatological Aid* Decoction of leaves used as a wash for open sores and wounds that do not heal. (as *K. glauca* 16:380, 382) Decoction of leaves used as a wash for open sores and wounds. (157:283) **Thompson** *Unspecified* Decoction of plant used medicinally. (141: 465) **Tlingit** *Dermatological Aid* Infusion of whole plant used for skin ailments. (as *K. glauca* 89:284)

Keckiella breviflora ssp. *breviflora*, Bush Beardtongue
Miwok *Cold Remedy* Infusion taken for colds. (as *Pentstemon breviflorus* 8:171) **Paiute** *Dermatological Aid* Ground, dry leaves used for running sores. (as *Pentstemon berviflorus* 98:44)

Keckiella cordifolia, Heartleaf Penstemon
Mahuna *Dermatological Aid* Infusion used as a wash or poultice of plant applied for fistulas and ulcers. (as *Pentstemon cordifolius* 117:12)

Kochia americana, Greenmolly
Navajo, Kayenta *Venereal Aid* Plant used for venereal disease. (179:21)

Kochia scoparia, Common Kochia
Navajo *Ceremonial Medicine* Used by the medicine man for painting a patient during a healing ceremony. *Dermatological Aid* Plant used for sores. (as *K. trichophylla* 76:152)

Koeleria macrantha, Prairie Junegrass
Cheyenne *Ceremonial Medicine* Plant used in the Sun Dance ceremony. *Dermatological Aid* Plant used for cuts. *Stimulant* Plant tied to Sun Dancers head to prevent him from getting tired. (as *K. cristata* 69:10)

Krameria erecta, Littleleaf Ratany
Pima *Dermatological Aid* Poultice of powdered root applied to sores. (as *K. parvifolia* 123:80)

Krameria grayi, White Ratany
Paiute *Dermatological Aid* Infusion of root used as a wash for gonorrheal sores. Root powder or decoction of root applied to sores. *Disinfectant* and *Eye Medicine* Infusion of root used as a wash for gonorrheal eye infections. *Venereal Aid* Decoc-

tion of root taken and used as a wash for gonorrheal eye infections and sores. (155:96) **Pima** *Analgesic* Infusion of roots taken for pain. *Cough Medicine* Infusion of roots taken for coughs. *Dermatological Aid* Poultice of powdered roots applied to prevent infection on newborn's navel. Decoction of roots applied as poultice to sores caused by "bad disease." *Disinfectant* Poultice of powdered roots applied to prevent infection on newborn's navel. *Eye Medicine* Infusion of twigs used for sore eyes. *Febrifuge* Infusion of roots taken for fevers. *Pediatric Aid* Poultice of powdered roots applied to prevent infection on newborn's navel. *Throat Aid* Root chewed for sore throats. (38:91) **Shoshoni** *Dermatological Aid* Infusion of pulverized root used as a wash for swellings. (155:96)

Krascheninnikovia lanata, Winter Fat
Gosiute *Febrifuge* Plant used for intermittent fevers. (as *Eurotia lanata* 31:369) **Hopi** *Burn Dressing* Powdered root used for burns. *Febrifuge* Decoction of leaves used for fever. (as *Eurotia lanata* 34:317) Compound containing plant used for fever. (as *Eurotia lanata* 174:32, 74) *Orthopedic Aid* Plant used for sore muscles. (as *Eurotia lanata* 174:32) **Navajo** *Antihemorrhagic* Decoction of leaves taken for blood-spitting. (as *Eurotia lanata* 45:44) *Dermatological Aid* Plant used for sores and boils. *Misc. Disease Remedy* Plant used for smallpox. (as *Eurotia lanata* 76:151) **Navajo, Ramah** *Antidote* Cold infusion of plant taken as needed for *Datura* poisoning. *Dermatological Aid* Poultice of chewed leaves applied to poison ivy rash. *Panacea* Cold infusion of plant used as "life medicine." (as *Eurotia lanata* 165:25) **Paiute** *Dermatological Aid* Decoction of plant used as a head and scalp tonic and prevents graying. (as *Eurotia lanata* 155:74, 75) *Eye Medicine* Decoction of leaves alone or with stems used as a wash or compress for sore eyes. (as *Eurotia lanata* 155:74, 75) **Shoshoni** *Dermatological Aid* Decoction of plant used as a head and scalp tonic. *Eye Medicine* Decoction of leaves alone or with stems used as a wash or compress for sore eyes. (as *Eurotia lanata* 155:74, 75) **Tewa** *Burn Dressing* Powdered root used for burns. *Febrifuge* Decoction of leaves used for fever. (as *Eurotia lanata* 34:317) **Zuni** *Burn Dressing* Poultice of ground root applied to burns

and bound with cotton cloth. (as *Eurotia lanata* 143:51)

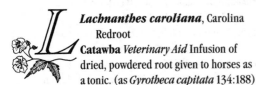 **_Lachnanthes caroliana_**, Carolina Redroot
Catawba *Veterinary Aid* Infusion of dried, powdered root given to horses as a tonic. (as *Gyrotheca capitata* 134:188) **Cherokee** *Antihemorrhagic* Taken for "spitting blood." *Cancer Treatment* Strong decoction used as a wash for cancer. *Dermatological Aid* Strong decoction of astringent root used as a wash for cancer. *Gastrointestinal Aid* Taken for bowel complaints. *Gynecological Aid* Taken for "flooding." *Hemorrhoid Remedy* Used for bloody piles. *Oral Aid* Used for sore mouth. *Throat Aid* Used for sore throat. *Venereal Aid* Compound decoction taken for venereal disease. (66:52)

Lactuca biennis, Tall Blue Lettuce
Bella Coola *Analgesic* Decoction of root taken for body pain, but not pain in the limbs. *Antidiarrheal* Decoction of root taken for diarrhea. *Antiemetic* Decoction of root taken for vomiting. *Antihemorrhagic* Decoction of root taken for hemorrhage, body pain, and heart trouble. *Heart Medicine* Decoction of root taken for heart trouble, hemorrhage, and pain. (as *L. spicata* 127:65) **Ojibwa** *Gynecological Aid* Infusion of plant used for caked breast and to ease lactation. (as *L. spicata* 130:364, 365) **Potawatomi** *Unspecified* Plant used as a medicine for unspecified illnesses. (as *L. spicata* 131:52)

Lactuca canadensis, Canada Lettuce
Cherokee *Analgesic* Used for pain and infusion given "for calming nerves." *Ceremonial Medicine* Used as an ingredient in a green corn medicine. *Sedative* Infusion given "for calming nerves" and "produces sleep." *Stimulant* Infusion used as a stimulant. *Veterinary Aid* Infusion given for "milk-sick." (66:42) **Chippewa** *Dermatological Aid* Milky sap from fresh plant rubbed on warts. (43:350) **Iroquois** *Analgesic* Compound infusion of roots and bark taken for back pain. *Eye Medicine* Compound infusion of roots and bark taken for dark circles and puffy eyes. *Hemostat* Poultice of smashed roots applied to severe bleeding from

a cut. *Kidney Aid* Compound infusion of roots and bark taken for kidney trouble. *Orthopedic Aid* Compound infusion of roots and bark taken for back pain. (73:478) **Menominee** *Dermatological Aid* Milky juice of plant rubbed on poison ivy eruptions. (128:31)

Lactuca sativa, Garden Lettuce
Isleta *Gastrointestinal Aid* Fresh leaves eaten for stomachaches. (as *L. integrata* 85:33) **Meskwaki** *Gynecological Aid* Infusion of leaves taken after childbirth to hasten the flow of milk. (as *L. scariola* var. *integrata* 129:215)

Lactuca serriola, Prickly Lettuce
Navajo, **Ramah** *Ceremonial Medicine* and *Emetic* Compound decoction of plant used as a ceremonial emetic. (165:52)

Lactuca tatarica var. **_pulchella_**, Blue Lettuce
Iroquois *Hemorrhoid Remedy* Poultice of plants applied to piles. (as *L. pulchella* 73:478) **Okanagan-Colville** *Antidiarrheal* and *Pediatric Aid* Infusion of roots and stems given to children for diarrhea. (as *L. pulchella* 162:84)

Lactuca virosa, Bitter Lettuce
Navajo *Antidiarrheal*, *Antiemetic*, and *Gastrointestinal Aid* Plant used for gastroenteritis (nausea, vomiting, and diarrhea). (76:152)

Lagenaria siceraria, Bottle Gourd
Cherokee *Dermatological Aid* Poultice of soaked seeds used for boils. (as *L. vulgaris* 66:37) **Houma** *Analgesic* Poultice of crushed leaves applied to the forehead for headaches. (135:62) **Seminole** *Analgesic* Seeds used for adult's sickness caused by adultery: headache, body pains, and crossed fingers. (145:256) *Psychological Aid* Seeds burned to smoke the body for insanity. (145:293)

Lamarckia aurea, Goldentop
Diegueño *Analgesic* Decoction of grass with "small tassels" taken for headaches. (70:23)

Laportea canadensis, Canadian Woodnettle
Houma *Febrifuge* Decoction of plant taken for fever. (135:60) **Iroquois** *Antidote* Decoction taken to counteract poison made from menstrual blood

and fruit. *Emetic* Decoction of roots taken to vomit to neutralize a love medicine. (73:307) *Gynecological Aid* Infusion of smashed roots taken to facilitate childbirth. (73:306) *Psychological Aid* Decoction taken to counteract loneliness because your woman has left. *Tuberculosis Remedy* Compound infusion of smashed roots taken for tuberculosis. *Witchcraft Medicine* Decoction taken "when your woman goes off and won't come back." (73:307) **Meskwaki** *Diuretic* and *Urinary Aid* Root used as a "diurient" and for urine incontinence. (129:250, 251) **Ojibwa** *Diuretic* Infusion of root taken as a diuretic. *Urinary Aid* Infusion of root used for various urinary ailments. (130:391, 392)

Lappula occidentalis var. *cupulata*,
Flatspine Stickseed

Navajo *Gynecological Aid* Parts of the plant used at confinement. *Hemostat* Parts of the plant used for nosebleeds. (as *L. texana* 76:153) **Navajo, Kayenta** *Dermatological Aid* Plant used as a lotion for itching. (as *L. texana* 179:40)

Lappula occidentalis var. *occidentalis*,
Desert Stickseed

Navajo, Kayenta *Dermatological Aid* Poultice of plant applied to sores caused by insects. (as *L. redowskii* 179:40) **Navajo, Ramah** *Dermatological Aid* Cold infusion used as lotion for sores or swellings. (as *L. redowskii* 165:41)

Lappula squarrosa, European Stickseed
Ojibwa, South *Analgesic* Roots on hot stones use as an inhalant or snuff of raw root used for headache. (as *Echinospermum lappula* 77:201)

Larix americana
Micmac *Dermatological Aid* Poultice of boiled inner bark applied to sores and swellings. *Diuretic* Decoction of boughs taken as a diuretic. (as *Pinus microcarpa* 133:317)

Larix laricina, Tamarack
Abnaki *Cough Medicine* Used for coughs. (121:154) Decoction of plant and bark from another plant used for coughs. Infusion of bark and roots from other plants taken for persistent coughs. (121:163) **Algonquin, Quebec** *Cough Medicine* Needles and inner bark used for cough

medicine. *Disinfectant* Poultice of needles and inner bark applied to infections. *Unspecified* Used with ground pine as a medicinal tea. (14:127) **Algonquin, Tête-de-Boule** *Laxative* Infusion of young branches used as a laxative. (110:129) **Anticosti** *Kidney Aid* Decoction of bark and bark from another plant taken for kidney troubles. (120:63) **Chippewa** *Blood Medicine* Infusion of bark taken for anemic conditions. (59:123) *Burn Dressing* Poultice of chopped inner bark applied to burns. (43:352) **Cree, Woodlands** *Antiemetic* Used with eight different trees for vomiting. *Dermatological Aid* Decoction used as a wash and poultice of boiled inner bark and wood applied to frostbite or deep cuts. Poultice of warm, boiled inner bark applied to wounds to draw out infection. (91:41) **Iroquois** *Analgesic* Fermented compound decoction taken for soreness. *Antirheumatic (Internal)* Compound decoction taken for rheumatism. *Blood Medicine* Fermented compound decoction taken when "blood gets bad and cold." *Cold Remedy* Compound decoction taken for colds. *Cough Medicine* Compound decoction taken for coughs. *Febrifuge* Fermented compound decoction taken for fever. *Stimulant* Fermented compound decoction taken when one is tired from complaint. *Venereal Aid* Compound decoction taken for gonorrhea. Compound powder poultice "put in bag, place penis in bag and tie around waist." (73:268) **Malecite** *Cold Remedy* Infusion of bark used for colds. *Strengthener* Infusion of bark used for general debility. *Tuberculosis Remedy* Infusion of

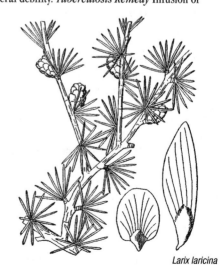

Larix laricina

bark used for consumption. (96:249) *Unspecified* Bark used as medicine. (137:6) *Venereal Aid* Infusion of bark, spruce bark, and balsam bark used for gonorrhea. (96:257) **Menominee** *Dermatological Aid* Poultice of bark used for unspecified ailments. *Other* Infusion of bark "drives out inflammation and generates heat." *Veterinary Aid* Infusion of bark given to horses "to better their condition from distemper." (128:45) **Micmac** *Cold Remedy* Bark used for colds. *Dermatological Aid* Bark used for "suppurating wounds" and colds. *Stimulant* Bark used for physical weakness. *Tuberculosis Remedy* Bark used for consumption. *Venereal Aid* Bark used for gonorrhea. (32:58) **Montagnais** *Expectorant* Infusion of buds and bark taken as an expectorant. (19:14) **Ojibwa** *Disinfectant* Dried leaves used as an inhalant and fumigator. (130:378, 379) *Unspecified* Infusion of roots and bark used as a general medicine. (as *L. americana* 112:244) **Ojibwa, South** *Analgesic* Boiled, crushed leaves, and bark used as herbal steam for headache and backache. Poultice of crushed leaves and bark applied for headache. *Herbal Steam* Boiled, crushed leaves and bark used as herbal steam for headache and backache. (as *L. americana* 77:198) **Potawatomi** *Dermatological Aid* Poultice of fresh inner bark applied to wounds and inflammations. *Other* Infusion of bark taken to drive out inflammation and to warm body. *Veterinary Aid* Shredded inner bark mixed with feed to make horse's hide loose. (131:69, 70)

Larix occidentalis, Western Larch
Kutenai *Dermatological Aid* Gum used for cuts and bruises. *Tuberculosis Remedy* Infusion of bark used for tuberculosis. **Nez Perce** *Cold Remedy* Infusion of bark used for colds. *Cough Medicine* Infusion of bark used for coughs. *Throat Aid* Sap chewed for sore throat. (68:22) **Okanagan-Colville** *Antirheumatic (External)* Decoction of plant tops used to soak arthritic limbs. *Antirheumatic (Internal)* Decoction of plant taken for severe arthritis. *Blood Medicine* Decoction of plant tops taken to help "changing of the blood." Decoction of plant tops and Oregon grapes used as a blood purifier. *Cancer Treatment* Decoction of plant taken for cancer. *Dermatological Aid* Decoction of plant tops used as an antiseptic wash for cuts and sores, and to soak severe skin sores.

(162:25) **Thompson** *Burn Dressing* Poultice of pitch mixed with fat or Vaseline and used for sores, cuts, and burns. *Cancer Treatment* Decoction of small pieces of branches and tops used for cancer. A decoction of plant tops was used to wash the areas affected by cancer. A second decoction of branch pieces was taken internally. It made the emaciated patient get better and gain weight. This treatment was used after a "western" doctor diagnosed the breast cancer patient as being terminal. *Cough Medicine* Branches used for dry coughs. *Dermatological Aid* Decoction of bark used as a wash for wounds, such as bullet wounds. Poultice of pitch used for sores, cuts, and burns. The pitch was mixed with tallow and used as a poultice for sores or it was mixed with fat or Vaseline and used for cuts and burns. *Dietary Aid* Decoction of small pieces of branches and bark used to stimulate the appetite. *Gastrointestinal Aid* Decoction of small pieces of branches and bark used for ulcers. *Gynecological Aid* Decoction of small pieces of branches and bark taken as a form of birth control after childbirth. *Orthopedic Aid* Pitch considered a valuable bone setter for broken bones that would not heal. Branches used for broken bones. *Panacea* Branches used as a medicine for any type of illness. (161:99) *Pediatric Aid* Decoction of leaves used as a healthful, strengthening wash for infants. Decoction of plant used as a wash to make babies strong and healthy. (141:475) Decoction of bark used as a wash or bath for babies, to make them strong and healthy. *Respiratory Aid* Poultice of pitch used or infusion of pitch taken for respiratory diseases. *Strengthener* Decoction of bark used as a wash or bath for babies, to make them strong and healthy. *Tuberculosis Remedy* Poultice of pitch used or infusion of pitch taken for tuberculosis. (161:99)

Larrea tridentata, Creosote Bush
Coahuilla *Gastrointestinal Aid* Infusion of leaves taken for bowel complaints and consumption. *Tuberculosis Remedy* Infusion of leaves taken for consumption and bowel complaints. (as *L. mexicana* 9:78) *Veterinary Aid* Plant given to horses for colds, distemper, or runny nose. (as *L. mexicana* 9:79) **Diegueño** *Antirheumatic (External)* Decoction of leaves used as a bath for rheumatism and painful arthritis. *Orthopedic Aid* Decoction of

leaves used as a bath for aching bones and sprains. (70:23) **Hualapai** *Cold Remedy* Infusion of leaves taken or leaves steamed for colds. *Disinfectant* Infusion of leaves used as a disinfecting skin cleanser. *Respiratory Aid* Infusion of leaves taken or leaves steamed for congestion and asthma. (169:28) **Kawaiisu** *Analgesic* Decoction of leaves used as a wash for sore and aching parts of the body. *Disinfectant* Plant used for the antiseptic properties. *Orthopedic Aid* Decoction of leaves used as a wash for sore and aching parts of the body. Poultice of heated leaves applied to aching limbs. *Unspecified* Plant used for medicinal purposes. *Veterinary Aid* Decoction of leaves used for collar sores on draft animals. (180:36) **Mahuna** *Dermatological Aid* Infusion of plant used for dandruff. *Disinfectant* Infusion of plant used as a disinfectant and deodorizer. (as *L. mexicana* 117:37) *Gastrointestinal Aid* Plant used for stomach cramps from delayed menstruation. (as *L. mexicana* 117:14) **Paiute** *Cold Remedy* Infusion of leaves taken as a cold medicine. (98:37) **Pima** *Analgesic* Decoction of twigs taken for gas pains or headaches caused by upset stomachs. Infusion of leaves taken for pain or used as bath and rub for rheumatic pains. Poultice of heated branches and leaves applied for pain. *Antidiarrheal* Plant gum chewed and swallowed as an antidysenteric and intestinal antispasmodic. *Antirheumatic (External)* Infusion of leaves used as bath and rub or poultice applied to rheumatic pains. *Antirheumatic (Internal)* Infusion of plant taken for rheumatism. *Carminative* Decoction of branches taken for gas caused by upset stomach or gas pains. *Cold Remedy* Decoction of gum taken for colds. *Dermatological Aid* Infusion of plant used as wash for impetigo sores or dandruff. Poultice of leaves applied to prevent feet from perspiring or as a deodorant. Poultice of leaves applied to scratches, wounds, sores, and bruises. *Emetic* Decoction of leaves taken as an emetic for high fevers. (38:61) Decoction of leaves taken as an emetic. (as *L. mexicana* 123:79) *Febrifuge* Decoction of leaves taken as an emetic for high fevers. *Gastrointestinal Aid* Decoction of plant taken for stomachaches and cramps. Plant gum chewed and swallowed as an intestinal antispasmodic. *Oral Aid* Decoction of gum used as a gargle. *Panacea* Plant used to cure everything. *Strengthener* Smoke from plant used for weakness

and laziness. *Toothache Remedy* Infusion of plant held in the mouth for toothaches. *Tuberculosis Remedy* Decoction of gum taken for tuberculosis. (38:61) *Unspecified* Poultice of boiled leaves used for unspecified purpose. (as *L. mexicana* 123:79) *Urinary Aid* Infusion of leaves taken for dysuria (difficulty in passing urine). (38:61) **Yavapai** *Antirheumatic (External)* Decoction of leaves and stems used as wash for rheumatism. *Dermatological Aid* Decoction of leaves and stems used as a wash for cuts and sores. Dried, pulverized leaves used for sores. *Throat Aid* Decoction of leaves and stems taken for sore throat. *Venereal Aid* Decoction of leaves and stems used as a wash for gonorrhea. Whole leaves used on penis for gonorrhea. (as *L. mexicana* 53:261)

Larrea tridentata var. *tridentata*, Creosote Bush

Cahuilla *Antirheumatic (External)* Plant made into liniment used by elderly people for swollen limbs caused by poor blood circulation. *Cancer Treatment* Infusion of stems and leaves used for cancer. *Cold Remedy* Infusion of stems and leaves used for colds. *Dermatological Aid* Decoction or poultice of leaves used on open wounds. Crushed leaf powder applied to sores and wounds. *Disinfectant* Decoction or poultice of leaves used to draw out poisons and for infections. *Emetic* Infusion of stems and leaves used, in heavy doses, to induce vomiting. *Gastrointestinal Aid* Infusion of stems and leaves used for bowel complaints. *Gynecological Aid* Infusion of stems and leaves used for stomach cramps from delayed menstruation. *Pulmonary Aid* Infusion of stems and leaves used for chest infections, and as a decongestant for clearing lungs. *Respiratory Aid* Leaves boiled or heated and the steam inhaled for congestion. *Tonic* Infusion of stems and leaves mixed with honey and used as a general health tonic before breakfast. (as *L. divaricata* 11:83) **Isleta** *Antirheumatic (External)* Decoction of leaves used as a body bath for rheumatism. *Dermatological Aid* Leaves used in shoes to absorb moisture. *Disinfectant* Decoction of leaves used as a disinfectant. (as *Covillea glutinosa* 85:26) **Paiute** *Analgesic* Decoction of leaves taken for bowel cramps. *Antirheumatic (External)* Infusion of leaves used as a wash for rheumatism. *Burn Dressing* Compound decoction of leaves with badger oil used as a salve for burns. *Cold Remedy* Decoction of leaves taken for colds. *Dermatological Aid* Dried, powdered leaves sprinkled on sores. *Gastrointestinal Aid* Decoction of leaves taken for bowel cramps. *Misc. Disease Remedy* Infusion of leaves used as a wash for chickenpox. *Panacea* Plant used for many different illnesses and considered a "cure-all." *Venereal Aid* Compound decoction of leaves taken for gonorrhea. (as *L. divaricata* 155:96, 97) **Papago** *Analgesic* Branches used as bed for women with menstrual cramps or after childbirth. *Antirheumatic (External)* Poultice of heated branches applied for rheumatism. Poultice of heated branches applied to joints. *Dermatological Aid* Plant used for poisonous bites and sores. Dried, powdered leaf rubbed on infant's navel to promote healing. Poultice of chewed leaves placed on insect bites, snakebites, and sores. Poultice of chewed plant applied to spider or scorpion bites. Poultice of dried, powdered leaves applied to infant's navel. *Emetic* Decoction of leaves taken as an emetic. *Gynecological Aid* Branches used as bed for women with menstrual cramps or after childbirth. Infusion of leaves rubbed on breasts to start milk flow. Infusion of leaves used as wash on breasts to start milk flow. Poultice of heated branches applied to facilitate childbirth. *Orthopedic Aid* Plant used for stiff limbs. Green branches laid on ashes, aching feet, and stiff limbs held in smoke. Smoke from smoldering green branches used for sore feet. *Pediatric Aid* Dried, powdered leaf rubbed on infant's navel to promote healing. Poultice of dried, powdered leaves applied to infant's navel. *Snakebite Remedy* Poultice of chewed leaves placed on snakebites, insect bites, and sores. Poultice of chewed plant applied to snakebites. (as *Covillea glutinosa* 29:64, 65) **Shoshoni** *Cold Remedy* Decoction of leaves taken for colds. *Diuretic* Decoction of leaves taken to "stimulate urination." *Venereal Aid* Decoction of leaves taken for venereal disease. (as *L. divaricata* 155:96, 97)

Lathyrus eucosmus, Bush Vetchling
Navajo, Kayenta *Gynecological Aid* Plant used to remove placenta. (179:28) **Navajo, Ramah** *Disinfectant* Cold infusion taken and used as a lotion for "deer infection." *Veterinary Aid* Cold infusion

used as lotion on horses for swellings or injuries. (165:32)

Lathyrus japonicus var. **maritimu**s, Sea Peavine
Eskimo, Inupiat *Poison* Peas considered poisonous. (as *L. maritimus* 83:141) **Iroquois** *Antirheumatic (External)* Stalks cooked as greens and used for rheumatism. (as *L. maritimus* 103:93)

Lathyrus jepsonii ssp. **californicus**, California Peavine
Mendocino Indian *Orthopedic Aid* Poultice of boiled plants applied to swollen joints. (as *L. watsoni* 33:357)

Lathyrus ochroleucus, Cream Peavine
Ojibwa *Gastrointestinal Aid* Plant used for stomach trouble. *Veterinary Aid* Foliage fed to a pony to make him lively for a race. (130:372, 373)

Lathyrus palustris, Slenderstem Peavine
Ojibwa *Veterinary Aid* Plant fed to a sick pony to make him fat. (130:373)

Lathyrus venosus, Veiny Peavine
Chippewa *Anticonvulsive* Simple or compound decoction of root taken or applied to chest for convulsions. (43:336) *Emetic* Decoction of root taken as an emetic for internal blood accumulation. *Hemostat* Poultice of boiled root applied to bleeding wounds. (43:356) *Stimulant* Decoction of root taken as a stimulant. *Tonic* Decoction of root taken as a tonic. (43:364)

Lathyrus vestitus, Pacific Peavine
Costanoan *Emetic* Decoction of roots used as an emetic for internal injuries. *Panacea* Decoction of roots used as a general remedy. (17:19)

Leathesia difformis, Bubble Seaweed
Hesquiat *Unspecified* Used for some kind of medicine. (159:24)

Lechea minor, Thymeleaf Pinweed
Seminole *Analgesic* Decoction of leaves taken for headaches. (145:282) *Antidiarrheal* Plant used as an astringent for diarrhea. (145:168) Decoction of plant taken by babies and adults for bird sickness:

diarrhea, vomiting, and appetite loss. (145:234) Plant used as a diarrhea medicine. (145:275) *Antiemetic* and *Dietary Aid* Decoction of plant taken by babies and adults for bird sickness: diarrhea, vomiting, and appetite loss. (145:234) *Febrifuge* Decoction of leaves taken for fevers. *Gastrointestinal Aid* Decoction of leaves taken for stomachaches. (145:282) *Pediatric Aid* Decoction of plant taken by babies and adults for bird sickness: diarrhea, vomiting, and appetite loss. (145:234)

Ledum groenlandicum, Bog Labradortea
Abnaki *Cold Remedy* Used for head colds. (121:154) *Nose Medicine* Powdered leaves mixed with bark from another plant and used as snuff for nasal inflammation. (121:170) **Algonquin, Quebec** *Analgesic* Infusion of plant used for headaches. *Ceremonial Medicine* Infusion of plant taken for colds. *Tonic* Infusion of plant used as a tonic. (14:214) *Unspecified* Leaves used to make tea and medicinal tea. (14:116) **Anticosti** *Unspecified* Infusion of plant used medicinally. (120:68) **Bella Coola** *Analgesic* and *Gastrointestinal Aid* Decoction of leaves taken for stomach pain. (127:63) **Chippewa** *Burn Dressing* Powder containing powdered root applied to burns. *Dermatological Aid* Powder containing powdered root applied to ulcers. (43:354) **Cree** *Burn Dressing* Poultice of powdered leaf ointment applied to burns and scalds. (12:492) *Diuretic* Infusion of leaves used as a diuretic. (12:493) *Emetic* Used as an emetic. (12:484) **Cree, Hudson Bay** *Analgesic* Infusion of flowering tops used for insect sting pain. *Antirheumatic (External)* Infusion of flowering tops used for rheumatism. *Dermatological Aid* Boiled, powdered wood applied to chafed skin. Poultice of fresh, chewed leaves applied to wounds. *Orthopedic Aid* Infusion of flowering tops used for tender feet. (as *L. latifolium* 78:303) **Cree, Woodlands** *Breast Treatment* Poultice of leaves applied to cracked nipples. *Burn Dressing* Poultice of leaves and grease applied to burns. Decoction of plant used to wash burns before application of burn ointment. *Dermatological Aid* Decoction of plant used as a wash for itchy skin, hand sores, and chapped skin. Poultice of leaves and fish oil applied to the umbilical scab. Powdered leaves applied directly to a baby's skin for rashes in the skin folds. *Diuretic* Plant used as a diuretic. *Pediatric Aid*

Poultice of leaves and fish oil applied to the umbilical scab. Powdered leaves applied directly to a baby's skin for rashes in the skin folds. *Pulmonary Aid* Decoction of plant used for pneumonia. Decoction of plant and calamus used for whooping cough. (91:42) **Gitksan** *Diuretic* Decoction of leaves used as a diuretic and beverage. (127:63) **Haisla & Hanaksiala** *Cold Remedy* Infusion of leaves taken for colds. *Dietary Aid* Decoction of leaves and small branches taken to increase the appetite. *Tuberculosis Remedy* Infusion of leaves taken for tuberculosis. (35:241) **Kitasoo** *Cold Remedy* and *Respiratory Aid* Decoction of dried leaves used for colds and other respiratory ailments. (35:333) **Kwakiutl** *Narcotic* Leaves considered narcotic. (157:283) **Makah** *Blood Medicine* Infusion of leaves taken as a blood purifier. (65:43) *Gynecological Aid* Infusion of leaves and sugar given to mothers after childbirth to gain their strength. *Kidney Aid* Infusion of leaves used as a kidney medicine. (55:301) *Unspecified* Infusion of fresh or dried plant used as a medicine. (160:106) **Malecite** *Kidney Aid* Infusion of plant used for kidney trouble. (96:257) **Micmac** *Cold Remedy* Leaves used for the common cold. (as *L. latifolium* 32:58) *Diuretic* Decoction of leaves taken as a diuretic. (as *L. latifolium* 133:317) *Kidney Aid* Leaves used for kidney trouble and to make a beverage. *Misc. Disease Remedy* Leaves used for scurvy and as a beverage. *Respiratory Aid* Leaves used for asthma. (as *L. latifolium* 32:58) *Tonic*

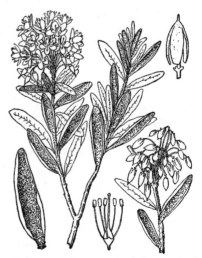

Ledum groenlandicum

Infusion of leaves taken for a "beneficial effect on the system." (133:316) **Montagnais** *Blood Medicine* Infusion of leaves and twigs taken to purify the blood. (133:313) *Febrifuge* Poultice of plant applied or infusion taken for fever. (19:14) Infusion of leaves and twigs "taken in case of chill." (133:313) *Liver Aid* and *Pediatric Aid* Poultice of plant applied or infusion given to children for jaundice. (19:14) **Nitinaht** *Dietary Aid* Infusion of leaves used as an appetite stimulant. (55:301) Infusion of fresh or dried plant taken as a tonic for increased appetite. *Strengthener* Infusion of fresh or dried plant taken as a tonic when "run down." **Nootka** *Unspecified* Infusion of fresh or dried plant used as a medicine. (160:106) **Okanagan-Colville** *Kidney Aid* Infusion of leaves and twigs taken for the kidneys. (162:102) **Oweekeno** *Cold Remedy* Infusion of leaves taken as a cold medicine. *Throat Aid* Infusion of leaves taken for sore throat. (35:96) **Potawatomi** *Unspecified* Compound containing leaves used to correct unspecified ailment. (131:57) **Quinault** *Antirheumatic* (*Internal*) Infusion of leaves taken for rheumatism. (65:43) **Salish** *Tonic* Decoction of plants taken as a tonic. (153:294) **Shuswap** *Dermatological Aid* Infusion or decoction of leaves taken for poison ivy. (102:56) *Eye Medicine* Decoction of plants used for blindness, sore eyes, and poison ivy. (102:62)

Ledum palustre, Marsh Labradortea
Eskimo, **Inupiat** *Poison* Plant contains ledol, a poisonous substance known to cause cramps, diarrhea, and paralysis. *Unspecified* Infusion of young, dried, stored leaves used as a medicinal tea. (83:60) **Tanana, Upper** *Antirheumatic* (*External*) Decoction of leaves and stems used for arthritis. *Antirheumatic* (*Internal*) Fresh or dried leaves chewed for body aches. *Blood Medicine* Decoction of leaves and stems used for weak blood. *Cold Remedy* Decoction of stems and leaves taken for colds. *Cough Medicine* Decoction of stems and leaves taken for coughs. *Dermatological Aid* Decoction of stems and leaves used as a wash for rashes and dandruff. Dried leaves ground into a powder or leaf ash used on sores. *Disinfectant* Decoction of stems and leaves used as a wash for infections. Fresh or dried leaves chewed for infections. *Gastrointestinal Aid* Decoction of leaves and stems used for heartburn. *Misc. Disease Rem-*

edy Decoction of leaves and stems used for flu. *Panacea* Decoction of stems and leaves, blackberry leaves, and spruce inner bark taken for sickness in general. *Respiratory Aid* Fresh or dried leaves chewed for congestion. *Throat Aid* Decoction of stems and leaves taken for sore throats. *Vertigo Medicine* Decoction of leaves and stems used for dizziness. (86:16) **Tlingit** *Venereal Aid* Compound infusion of sprouts and bark taken for syphilis. (89:283)

Ledum palustre ssp. **decumbens**, Marsh Labradortea
Eskimo, Alaska *Antihemorrhagic* Infusion of plant used for spitting up blood. *Gastrointestinal Aid* Infusion of plant used for upset stomach. (1:37) *Unspecified* Infusion of leaves used for medicinal purposes. (as *L. decumbens* 3:715) **Eskimo, Inupiat** *Poison* Plant contains ledol, a poisonous substance known to cause cramps, diarrhea, and paralysis. *Unspecified* Infusion of young, dried, stored leaves used as a medicinal tea. (as *L. decumbens* 83:60) **Eskimo, Kuskokwagmiut** *Pediatric Aid* Burning dried stalk shaken around head and shoulders of sick child. (as *L. decumbens* 101:32) **Eskimo, Nunivak** *Unspecified* Infusion of stems and leaves used for the medicinal value. (as *L. decumbens* 126:325) **Eskimo, Western** *Analgesic* and *Gastrointestinal Aid* Compound decoction of stem and leaf used for stomachache and intestinal discomfort. (as *L. decumbens* 90:5)

Leiophyllum buxifolium, Sand Myrtle
Nanticoke *Tonic* Berries used to make spring tonic. (150:58, 84)

Lemna trisulca, Star Duckweed
Iroquois *Antirheumatic* (*External*) Poultice of wetted plant and another plant applied to swellings. (118:71)

Leonurus cardiaca, Common Motherwort
Cherokee *Gastrointestinal Aid* Taken for "disease of the stomach." *Sedative* Given for "nervous and hysterical affections" and taken as a stimulant. *Stimulant* Taken as a stimulant for fainting. (66:45) **Delaware** *Gynecological Aid* Infusion of leaves used for female diseases. (151:38) **Delaware, Oklahoma** *Gynecological Aid* Infusion of

leaves taken for "female diseases." (150:32, 76) **Iroquois** *Gastrointestinal Aid* Infusion of dried plant taken to facilitate digestion. *Sedative* Infusion of dried plant taken as a tonic for nerves. *Tonic* Infusion of dried plant taken as a tonic. (119:98) **Micmac** *Gynecological Aid* Part of plant used for obstetric cases. (32:58) **Mohegan** *Gynecological Aid* Infusion taken for "female ills." (25:121) Infusion of plant taken for peculiar ills of women. (149:265) Infusion of leaf, highly regarded herb, taken for diseases peculiar to women. (151:72, 130) *Tonic* Complex compound infusion including motherwort taken as spring tonic. (149:266) **Shinnecock** *Gynecological Aid* Infusion taken for "female ills." (25:121)

Lepechinia calycina, Woodbalm
Miwok *Analgesic* Decoction of leaves taken for headaches. *Febrifuge* Decoction of leaves taken for fever. *Misc. Disease Remedy* Decoction of leaves taken for ague. (as *Sphacele calycina* 8:173)

Lepidium densiflorum, Common Pepperweed
Isleta *Analgesic* Leaves chewed for headaches. (as *L. apetalum* 85:34) **Lakota** *Kidney Aid* Infusion of plant used for the kidneys. (116:41) **Mahuna** *Dietary Aid* Infusion of plant taken as a reducing aid. (as *L. apetalum* 117:66) **Navajo, Kayenta** *Gastrointestinal Aid* Plant used for effects of swallowing an ant. *Pediatric Aid* and *Sedative* Plant rubbed on baby's face to put infant to sleep. (179:24)

Lepidium lasiocarpum, Shaggyfruit Pepperweed
Navajo *Disinfectant* Plant used as a "disinfectant." (76:153)

Lepidium montanum, Mountain Pepperweed
Navajo, Kayenta *Gastrointestinal Aid* Plant used for biliousness and gastrointestinal disorders. *Other* Plant used for palpitations and dizziness. (179:24)

Lepidium nitidum, Shining Pepperweed
Cahuilla *Dermatological Aid* Decoction of leaves used to wash hair, kept the scalp clean and prevented baldness. (11:85) **Diegueño** *Gastrointestinal Aid* Tablespoon of seeds in water used, fol-

lowed the next day by a physic, for indigestion. (70:23)

Lepidium virginicum, Virginia Pepperweed
Cherokee *Dermatological Aid* Poultice of bruised root applied to "draw blister quickly." *Pulmonary Aid* Used as a poultice for croup. *Veterinary Aid* Infusion given to sick chickens and mixed with feed to make chickens lay. (66:48) **Houma** *Tuberculosis Remedy* Compound decoction of plant with whisky taken for tuberculosis. (135:64) **Menominee** *Dermatological Aid* Infusion of plant used as a wash or bruised plant used for poison ivy. (128:33)

Leptarrhena pyrolifolia, Fireleaf Leptarrhena
Aleut *Misc. Disease Remedy* Infusion of leaves taken for "sicknesses such as influenza." (6:427) **Thompson** *Dermatological Aid* Poultice of chewed, fresh leaves applied to wounds and sores. (as *Leptarrhenia amplexifolia* 141:465)

Leptodactylon pungens, Granite Pricklygilia
Navajo, Kayenta *Dermatological Aid* Plant used for scorpion stings. *Kidney Aid* Plant used for kidney disease. (as *Gilia pungens* 179:38) **Navajo, Ramah** *Disinfectant* Decoction of plant used for "snake infection." *Gynecological Aid* Decoction of plant taken during pregnancy keeps baby small, for easy labor. (as *Gilia pungens* 165:40) **Shoshoni** *Eye Medicine* Decoction or infusion of plant used as a wash for sore or swollen eyes. (as *Gilia pungens* 155:81)

Lespedeza capitata, Roundhead Lespedeza
Meskwaki *Antidote* Root used as antidote for poison. (129:229) **Omaha** *Analgesic* Moxa of stems used in cases of neuralgia. *Antirheumatic (External)* Moxa of stems used in cases of rheumatism. **Ponca** *Analgesic* Moxa of stems used in cases of neuralgia. *Antirheumatic (External)* Moxa of stems used in cases of rheumatism. (58:97, 98)

Lesquerella douglasii, Douglas's Bladderpod
Okanagan-Colville *Antidiarrheal* Roots chewed, juice swallowed, and pulp spat out for diarrhea. *Gastrointestinal Aid* Roots chewed, juice swallowed, and pulp spat out for "heartburn." (162:92) **Shuswap** *Dermatological Aid* Poultice of mashed

plants applied to sores. *Diaphoretic* Plant used to produce sweating. (102:61)

Lesquerella fendleri, Fendler's Bladderpod
Keres, Western *Antirheumatic* (*External*)
Bruised plant mixed with salt and used as a rub for swellings. *Emetic* Infusion of plant used as an emetic. (147:52) **Navajo** *Dermatological Aid* Infusion of plants taken to counteract the effects of spider bites. (45:49)

Lesquerella intermedia, Mid Bladderpod
Hopi *Ceremonial Medicine* and *Emetic* Infusion of root taken as a ceremonial emetic. (174:77) *Gynecological Aid* Root rubbed on abdomen when uterus failed to contract after childbirth. (174:36, 77) *Snakebite Remedy* Root eaten and poultice of chewed root used for snakebite. (174:32, 77) **Navajo, Kayenta** *Ceremonial Medicine* Plant used as a Nightway medicine. *Eye Medicine* Poultice of roots applied to sore eyes. (179:24)

Lesquerella rectipes, Straight Bladderpod
Navajo, Ramah *Ceremonial Medicine* Cold infusion used as a ceremonial eyewash and pulverized plant used as a ceremonial snuff. *Eye Medicine* Cold infusion of plant used as a ceremonial eyewash. *Respiratory Aid* Finely ground leaves used ceremonially as snuff to clear nasal passages. *Toothache Remedy* Poultice of crushed or chewed leaves applied for toothache. (165:29)

Lessingia glandulifera var. glandulifera,
   Valley Vinegarweed
Kawaiisu *Analgesic* Moxa of dried stem bark used for pain. (as *L. germanorum* var. *vallicola* 180:36)

Lessoniopsis littoralis, Short Kelp
Nitinaht *Strengthener* Burned stipes made into a salve and used to strengthen young boys. (160:51)

Leucanthemum vulgare, Ox Eye Daisy
Iroquois *Eye Medicine* Infusion of flowers and roots with other plants used as an eyewash. (as *Chrysanthemum leucanthemum* var. *pinnatifidum* 118:64) **Menominee** *Febrifuge* Plant used as a fever medicine. (as *Chrysanthemum leucanthemum* 128:29) **Mohegan** *Tonic* Dandelion and

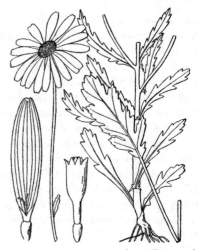

Leucanthemum vulgare

white daisy used to make wines and taken as tonics. (as *Chrysanthemum leucanthemum* 25:121) Compound decoction or infusion of plants taken as a spring tonic. (as *Chrysanthemum leucanthemum* 149:266) Flowers used to make a tonic. (as *Chrysanthemum leucanthemum* 151:72, 128) **Quileute** *Dermatological Aid* Decoction of dried flowers and stems used as a wash for chapped hands. (as *Chrysanthemum leucanthemum* 65:49) **Shinnecock** *Tonic* Dandelion and white daisy used to make wines and taken as tonics. (as *Chrysanthemum leucanthemum* 25:121)

Leucocrinum montanum, Common Starlily
Paiute *Dermatological Aid* Poultice of pulverized roots applied to sores or swellings. **Shoshoni** *Dermatological Aid* Poultice of pulverized roots applied to sores or swellings. (155:100)

Leucothoe axillaris, Coastal Doghobble
Cherokee *Analgesic* Infusion used for "shifting pains." *Antirheumatic* (*External*) Infusion rubbed on for rheumatism. *Antirheumatic* (*Internal*) Compound decoction of leaf used for rheumatism. *Dermatological Aid* Infusion of leaf and stem used to bathe itch. (66:32) *Other* Decoction of leaves rubbed into scratches made on legs as preliminary treatment. (as *L. catesbaei* 152:49) *Stimulant* Infusion rubbed on for "languor." *Veterinary Aid* Root ooze applied to mangy dog. (66:32)

Lewisia pygmaea, Pigmy Bitterroot
Thompson *Psychological Aid* Some believed that eating the roots caused insanity. (141:479)

Lewisia rediviva, Oregon Bitterroot
Blackfoot *Throat Aid* Pounded, dry root chewed for sore throat. (98:38) **Flathead** *Breast Treatment* Roots eaten for increased milk flow after childbirth. *Gynecological Aid* Infusion of roots taken for increased milk flow after childbirth. *Heart Medicine* Infusion of roots taken for heart pain. *Pulmonary Aid* Infusion of roots taken for pleurisy pain. **Nez Perce** *Blood Medicine* Plant used for impure blood. *Gynecological Aid* Roots eaten for increased milk flow after childbirth. Infusion of roots taken for increased milk flow after childbirth. (68:46) **Okanagan-Colville** *Dermatological Aid* Poultice of raw roots applied to sores. Raw roots eaten for poison ivy rashes. *Misc. Disease Remedy* Dried or fresh roots eaten for diabetes. *Witchcraft Medicine* "Hearts" used in some type of witchcraft. (162:114)

Leymus cinereus, Basin Wildrye
Okanagan-Colville *Antihemorrhagic* Decoction of roots taken for internal hemorrhaging. *Dermatological Aid* Decoction of roots used as a wash to stimulate hair growth. *Venereal Aid* Infusion of mashed roots taken for gonorrhea. (as *Elymus cinereus* 162:55) **Thompson** *Veterinary Aid* Hollow straw used to clear the blocked nipple of a cow. The udder was splashed with warm water, massaged, and the straw poked into it to clear the blockage. (as *Elymus cinereus* 161:140)

Leymus condensatus, Giant Wildrye
Paiute *Eye Medicine* Dried leaves used to scrape pimples from the underside of the eyelid. (as *Elymus condensatus* 93:51) Decoction or infusion of leaves used as a wash for sore eyes. Sharp edges of leaf blades used to scrape granulated eyelids. **Shoshoni** *Eye Medicine* Decoction or infusion of leaves used as a wash for sore eyes. Sharp edges of leaf blades used to scrape granulated eyelids. (as *Elymus condensatus* 155:67)

Leymus mollis ssp. *mollis*, American Dunegrass
Makah *Unspecified* Bundles of roots used to rub the body after bathing. (as *Elymus mollis* 65:21) **Nitinaht** *Strengthener* Rootstocks twisted together and rubbed on bodies of young men while bathing for strength. (as *Elymus mollis* var. *mollis* 160:88) **Quileute** *Unspecified* Roots braided, tied into bundles, and used to rub the body after bathing. (as *Elymus mollis* 65:21)

Liatris acidota, Sharp Gayfeather
Koasati *Antirheumatic* (*Internal*) Decoction of roots taken for rheumatism. (152:62)

Liatris laxa, Rattlesnake Master
Seminole *Analgesic* Decoction of roots used for cow sickness: lower chest pain, digestive disturbances, and diarrhea. *Antidiarrheal* Decoction of roots used for cow sickness: lower chest pain, digestive disturbances, and diarrhea. (145:191) Decoction of roots taken by babies and adults for bird sickness: diarrhea, vomiting, and appetite loss. *Antiemetic* Decoction of roots taken by babies and adults for bird sickness: diarrhea, vomiting, and appetite loss. (145:234) *Antirheumatic* (*External*) Decoction of plant used as a body rub and steam for joint swellings. (145:193) *Dietary Aid* Decoction of roots taken by babies and adults for bird sickness: diarrhea, vomiting, and appetite loss. (145:234) *Gastrointestinal Aid* Decoction of roots used for cow sickness: lower chest pain, digestive disturbances, and diarrhea. (145:191) *Pediatric Aid* Decoction of roots taken by babies and adults for bird sickness: diarrhea, vomiting, and appetite loss. (145:234)

Liatris punctata, Dotted Gayfeather
Blackfoot *Dermatological Aid* Poultice of boiled roots applied to swellings. *Gastrointestinal Aid* Infusion of roots taken for stomachaches. (82:59) **Comanche** *Urinary Aid* Root chewed and juice swallowed for swollen testes. (24:522) **Meskwaki** *Dermatological Aid* Infusion of root applied locally for itch. *Urinary Aid* Infusion of root used for bloody urine and by women for bladder trouble. *Venereal Aid* Infusion of root used for gonorrhea. *Veterinary Aid* Infusion of root used for ponies to make them spirited for hunting in hot weather. (129:216)

Liatris punctata var. punctata, Dotted
  Gayfeather
Blackfoot *Analgesic* Infusion of root taken for
stomachache. *Dermatological Aid* Boiled root applied to swellings. *Gastrointestinal Aid* Infusion of
root taken for stomachache. (as *Lacinaria punctata* 95:274)

Liatris scariosa, Devil's Bite
Meskwaki *Kidney Aid* Used for kidney troubles.
Urinary Aid Used for bladder troubles. (129:216)

Liatris scariosa var. scariosa, Devil's Bite
Chippewa *Veterinary Aid* Decoction of root used
as a horse stimulant before a race. (as *Laciniaria
scariosa* 43:366) **Omaha** *Dermatological Aid*
Poultice of powdered plants applied to external
inflammation. *Dietary Aid* Roots used as an appetizer. *Gastrointestinal Aid* Plant taken for abdominal troubles. *Tonic* Roots used as a tonic. (as *Lacinaria scariosa* 56:335) *Veterinary Aid* Chewed
corm blown into nostrils of horses to strengthen
them and help them. **Pawnee** *Antidiarrheal* and
Pediatric Aid Decoction of leaves and corms given
to children for diarrhea. (as *Laciniaria scariosa*
58:133, 134)

Liatris spicata, Dense Gayfeather
Cherokee *Analgesic* Used as an anodyne and
decoction or tincture used for backache and limb
pains. *Carminative* Used as a carminative. *Diaphoretic* Root used as a sudorific. *Diuretic* Root
used as a diuretic. *Expectorant* Root used as an
expectorant. *Gastrointestinal Aid* Decoction or
tincture taken for colic. *Kidney Aid* Root used
for dropsy. *Stimulant* Root used as a stimulant.
(66:27) **Menominee** *Heart Medicine* Compound
decoction of root used for a "weak heart." (as
Lacinaria spicata 44:129)

Licania michauxii, Gopher Apple
Seminole *Analgesic* Plant used for wolf sickness:
vomiting, stomach pain, diarrhea, and frequent
urination. Infusion of plant taken for wolf sickness: vomiting, stomach pain, diarrhea, and frequent urination. Roots and leaves used for labor
pains and hasten the birth. (as *Chrysobalanus oblongifolius* 145:165, 227, 323) *Antidiarrheal* Plant
used for wolf sickness: vomiting, stomach pain,

diarrhea, and frequent urination. Infusion of plant
taken for wolf sickness: vomiting, stomach pain,
diarrhea, and frequent urination. (as *Chrysobalanus oblongifolius* 145:165, 227) *Antiemetic* Plant
used for wolf sickness: vomiting, stomach pain,
diarrhea, and frequent urination. Infusion of plant
taken for wolf sickness: vomiting, stomach pain,
diarrhea, and frequent urination. (as *Chrysobalanus oblongifolius* 145:166, 227) *Gastrointestinal
Aid* Plant used for wolf sickness: vomiting, stomach pain, diarrhea, and frequent urination. Infusion of plant taken for wolf sickness: vomiting,
stomach pain, diarrhea, and frequent urination.
(as *Chrysobalanus oblongifolius* 145:165, 227)
Other Complex infusion of leaves and roots taken
for chronic conditions. (as *Chrysobalanus oblongifolia* 145:272) *Psychological Aid* Infusion of
plant used to steam and bathe the body for insanity. (as *Chrysobalanus oblongifolia* 145:292)
Reproductive Aid Roots and leaves used for labor
pains and hasten the birth. (as *Chrysobalanus
oblongifolius* 145:323) *Unspecified* Plant used for
medicinal purposes. (as *Chrysobalanus oblongifolius* 145:162) *Urinary Aid* Plant used for wolf
sickness: vomiting, stomach pain, diarrhea, and
frequent urination. Infusion of plant taken for wolf
sickness: vomiting, stomach pain, diarrhea, and
frequent urination. (as *Chrysobalanus oblongifolius* 145:165, 227)

Ligusticum apiifolium, Celeryleaf Licoriceroot
Karok *Dietary Aid* Infusion of roots taken by
person who lacks an appetite. (as *L. apiodorum*
125:387) **Pomo** *Antihemorrhagic* and *Pulmonary
Aid* Decoction of roots taken for lung hemorrhages.
(as *L. apiodorum* 54:14) **Pomo, Kashaya** *Blood
Medicine* Decoction of root taken for anemia. *Pulmonary Aid* Decoction of root taken for lung hemorrhage. *Tuberculosis Remedy* Decoction of root
taken for the beginning of tuberculosis. (60:64)

Ligusticum canadense, Canadian Licoriceroot
Cherokee *Gastrointestinal Aid* Roots chewed or
smoked for all stomach disorders. **Creek** *Gastrointestinal Aid* Roots chewed or smoked for all
stomach disorders. (as *Lingusticum canadense*
145:276)

Ligusticum canbyi, Canby's Licoriceroot
Cree *Heart Medicine* Used for heart troubles.
Crow *Cold Remedy* Roots chewed for colds. *Cough Medicine* Roots chewed for coughs. *Ear Medicine* Infusion of roots used for earache. *Respiratory Aid* Root shavings added to boiling water and steam inhaled for sinus infection and congestion.
Flathead *Anticonvulsive* Roots chewed, rubbed on the body, or smoked for seizures. *Unspecified* Plants used as herbal medicine. **Kutenai** *Unspecified* Plants used as herbal medicine. (68:24)
Okanagan-Colville *Ceremonial Medicine* Roots burned and smoke used to revive singers from a trance, considered ceremonially dead. Roots burned and smoke used to revive a subdued person possessed by the "bluejay spirit." *Cold Remedy* Root tied in a cheesecloth and kept near a baby's face to prevent a cold. *Internal Medicine* Roots used as a good general internal medicine. *Other* Roots burned and smoke used for unconsciousness, trances, or "possession" by spirits. *Pediatric Aid* Root tied in a cheesecloth and kept near a baby's face to prevent a cold. (162:64) **Thompson** *Unspecified* Roots used medicinally whenever obtainable. (161:153)

Ligusticum filicinum, Fernleaf Licoriceroot
Menominee *Panacea* Root used for many ailments. (128:55) **Paiute** *Cough Medicine* Root used in a cough remedy. (155:100, 101)

Ligusticum grayi, Gray's Licoriceroot
Atsugewi *Analgesic* Roots used to avoid pains. *Cold Remedy* Infusion of root taken or roots chewed for colds. *Cough Medicine* Infusion of root taken or roots chewed for coughs. *Gastrointestinal Aid* Infusion of root taken or roots chewed for children's stomachaches. *Panacea* Infusion of root taken or roots chewed for ailments. *Pediatric Aid* Infusion of root taken or roots chewed for children's stomachaches. (50:140)

Ligusticum porteri, Porter's Licoriceroot
Zuni *Antirheumatic* (*External*) Infusion of root used for body aches. *Ceremonial Medicine* Root chewed by medicine man and patient during curing ceremonies for various illnesses. *Throat Aid* Crushed root and water used as wash and taken for sore throat. (22:379)

Ligusticum scothicum, Scottish Licoriceroot
Bella Coola *Unspecified* Leaves spread over hot stones and used as medicinal bed for the sick. (127:61)

Ligusticum scothicum ssp. hultenii,
    Hultén's Licoriceroot
Eskimo, Western *Poison* Mature plant in late summer considered mildly poisonous. (as *L. hultenii* 90:60)

Lilium canadense, Canadian Lily
Algonquin, Quebec *Gastrointestinal Aid* Root used for stomach disorders. (14:138) **Cherokee** *Antidiarrheal* Infusion of root given for "flux." *Antirheumatic* (*Internal*) Infusion of root used in various ways for rheumatism. *Dietary Aid* and *Pediatric Aid* Decoction of boiled tubers given "to make child fleshy and fat." (66:43) **Chippewa** *Snakebite Remedy* Decoction of root applied to snakebites. (43:352) **Malecite** *Abortifacient* Infusion of plant and sweet viburnum roots used for irregular menstruation. (96:258) **Micmac** *Abortifacient* Parts of plant used for irregular menstruation. (32:58)

Lilium columbianum, Columbian Lily
Okanagan-Colville *Witchcraft Medicine* Bulbs dried, mashed with "stink bugs," powdered, and used against "plhax," that is, witchcraft. (162:46)

Lilium philadelphicum, Wood Lily
Algonquin, Quebec *Gastrointestinal Aid* Root used for stomach disorders. (14:138) **Chippewa** *Dermatological Aid* Poultice of boiled bulbs applied to wounds, contusions, and dog bites. *Witchcraft Medicine* Poultice of bulbs applied to dog bites and caused dog's fangs to drop out. (59:125)
Iroquois *Gynecological Aid* Decoction of whole plant taken "to bring away placenta after childbirth." *Love Medicine* "Dry plants in sun, if twists together, wife is unfaithful; determines love." Decoction of roots taken by wife as emetic and used as a wash "if husband is unfaithful." (73:282)
Malecite *Adjuvant* Roots used to strengthen other medicines. (96:245) *Cough Medicine* Roots used with roots of blackberry and mountain raspberry, staghorn sumac for coughs. (96:251) *Dermatological Aid* Poultice of ground roots used for swell-

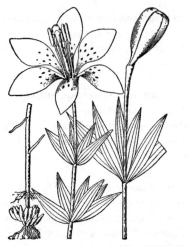

Lilium philadelphicum

ings and bruises. (96:245) *Febrifuge* Roots used with roots of blackberry and mountain raspberry, staghorn sumac for fevers. *Tuberculosis Remedy* Roots used with roots of blackberry and mountain raspberry, staghorn sumac for consumption. (96: 251) **Menominee** *Dermatological Aid* Poultice of boiled, mashed root applied to sores. (44:132) **Micmac** *Cough Medicine* Roots used for coughs. *Dermatological Aid* Roots used for swellings and bruises. *Febrifuge* Roots used for fever. *Tuberculosis Remedy* Roots used for consumption and fever. (32:58)

Lilium philadelphicum var. andinum,
　Wood Lily
Dakota *Dermatological Aid* Pulverized or chewed flowers applied as antidote for spider bites. (as *L. umbellatum* 58:71)

Limonium californicum, California Sea-
　lavender
Costanoan *Blood Medicine* Decoction of plant used to clean the blood. *Respiratory Aid* Powdered plant placed in nostrils to cause sneezing for congestion. *Urinary Aid* Decoction of plant used for internal injuries or urinary problems. *Venereal Aid* Decoction of plant used for venereal disease. (17:11)

Limonium carolinianum, Carolina Sea-
　lavender
Micmac *Tuberculosis Remedy* Roots pounded,

ground, added to boiling water, and used for consumption with hemorrhage. (96:259)

Limonium vulgare, Mediterranean Sea-
　lavender
Micmac Roots used for consumption with hemorrhage. (as *Statice limonium* 32:62)

Limosella aquatica, Water Mudwort
Navajo, Ramah *Ceremonial Medicine* Leaves ceremonially rubbed on body for protection in hunting and from witches. *Dermatological Aid* Roll of washed leaves used to plug a bullet or arrow wound. *Hunting Medicine* Leaves ceremonially rubbed on body for protection while hunting. *Witchcraft Medicine* Leaves rubbed on body ceremonially for protection against witches. (165:44)

Linanthus ciliatus, Whiskerbrush
Pomo, Calpella *Blood Medicine* Cold decoction of plant taken to purify the blood. *Cold Remedy* Infusion of plant given to children for colds. *Cough Medicine* Infusion of plant given to children for coughs. *Pediatric Aid* Infusion of plant given to children for coughs and colds. (33:381)

Linanthus nuttallii ssp. nuttallii, Nuttall's
　Desert Trumpets
Navajo, Ramah *Panacea* Plant used as "life medicine." (165:40)

Linaria vulgaris, Butter and Eggs
Iroquois *Antidiarrheal* Cold infusion of leaves taken for diarrhea. *Emetic* Infusion of plants taken to vomit as an anti-love medicine and remove bewitching. *Love Medicine* Compound infusion of smashed plants taken to vomit as an anti-love medicine. *Pediatric Aid* and *Sedative* Compound infusion of plants and flowers given to babies that cry too much. *Witchcraft Medicine* Compound infusion of smashed plants taken to vomit and remove bewitching. (73:433) **Ojibwa** *Herbal Steam* Compound containing plant used as a bronchial inhalant in the sweat lodge. *Respiratory Aid* Compound containing dried plant used as a bronchial inhalant in the sweat lodge. (130:389)

Lindera benzoin, Northern Spicebush
Cherokee *Abortifacient* Taken for female obstruc-

tions. *Blood Medicine* Taken for the blood and female obstructions. *Cold Remedy* Taken for colds. *Cough Medicine* Taken for coughs. *Dermatological Aid* Infusion of bark taken for "bold hives." *Diaphoretic* Compound decoction of bark taken as a diaphoretic, any part is a diaphoretic. *Misc. Disease Remedy* Infusion of bark taken to break out measles. *Pulmonary Aid* Taken for croup. *Respiratory Aid* Taken for phthisic. *Tonic* Used for "white swellings" and infusion taken as a spring tonic. (66:56) **Creek** *Analgesic* and *Diaphoretic* Infusion of branches taken and steam bath used to cause perspiring for aches. *Emetic* Plant used as an emetic. (152:24) **Iroquois** *Cold Remedy* Decoction or infusion of stripped leaves and twigs taken for colds. *Febrifuge* Compound decoction of plants used as a steam bath for cold sweats. *Misc. Disease Remedy* Decoction of stripped leaves and twigs taken for colds and measles. *Panacea* Compound decoction of roots taken as a panacea. (73:335) *Venereal Aid* Compound decoction of roots taken for gonorrhea and syphilis. Compound poultice of bark applied to lumps that remain after having syphilis. (73:334)

Lindera benzoin var. *benzoin*, Northern Spicebush

Chippewa *Unspecified* Leaves used medicinally. (as *Benzoin aestivale* 59:131) **Creek** *Antirheumatic* (*Internal*) Infusion of branches taken or used as herbal steam to cause sweating for pains. *Blood Medicine* Compound containing plant taken to cause vomiting which purifies the blood. *Diaphoretic* Infusion of branches taken or used as herbal steam to cause sweating for pains. *Emetic* Compound containing plant taken to cause vomiting which purifies the blood. *Herbal Steam* Infusion of branches used as herbal steam for aches and pains. (as *Benzoin aestivale* 148:657) **Rappahannock** *Abortifacient* Infusion taken to correct delayed menses. *Gynecological Aid* Infusion taken for menstruation pains. (as *Benzoin aestivale* 138:33)

Linnaea borealis, Twinflower

Montagnais *Orthopedic Aid* Mashed plant used for "inflammation of the limbs." (133:314) **Tanana, Upper** *Analgesic* Poultice of the whole plant applied to the head for headaches. *Pediatric*

Aid and *Psychological Aid* Poultice of the whole plant applied to the child's head to insure him a long life. (86:18) **Thompson** *Unspecified* Decoction of plant used as a medicine for unspecified purpose. (141:458)

Linnaea borealis ssp. *longiflora*, Longtube Twinflower

Algonquin, Quebec *Gynecological Aid* Infusion of entire plant used for menstrual difficulties. Infusion of entire plant used by pregnant women to insure the good health of the child. (14:235) **Iroquois** *Febrifuge* Decoction of twigs given to children with fever. *Gastrointestinal Aid* Decoction of twigs given to children with cramps. *Pediatric Aid* Decoction of twigs given to children with cramps, fever, or for crying. *Sedative* Decoction of twigs given to children for crying. (73:444) **Potawatomi** *Gynecological Aid* Entire plant used for unspecified female troubles. (131:45, 46) **Snohomish** *Cold Remedy* Decoction of leaves taken for colds. (65:47)

Linum australe, Southern Flax

Hopi *Gastrointestinal Aid* Infusion of plant taken for stomach disorders. (174:83) *Gynecological Aid* Decoction of plant taken and used as a wash to ease protracted labor. (174:36, 83)

Linum australe var. *australe*, Southern Flax

Navajo, Kayenta *Kidney Aid* Infusion of plant used for kidney disease. (as *L. aristatum* var. *australe* 179:30)

Linum lewisii, Prairie Flax

Gosiute *Dermatological Aid* Infusion of flax used for bruise swellings. (31:349) Poultice of plant applied to bruises for the swelling. (31:373) **Great Basin Indian** *Eye Medicine* Seeds used to make an eye medicine. (100:48) **Navajo, Kayenta** *Analgesic* Plant used for headaches. *Disinfectant* Plant used as a fumigant. (179:30) **Navajo, Ramah** *Gastrointestinal Aid* Decoction of leaves taken for heartburn. (165:33, 34) **Okanagon** *Dermatological Aid* and *Pediatric Aid* Infusion of flowers, leaves, and stem used as skin and hair wash by young females. (104:42) **Paiute** *Carminative* Infusion of whole stem used for gas. (98:44) *Dermatological Aid* Poultice of leaves alone or stems and leaves applied to swellings. *Eye Medicine* Infusion or decoction of plant parts used as an eyewash. (155:101, 102) *Gastrointestinal Aid* Infusion of whole stem used for a disordered stomach. (98:44) *Poultice* Poultice of leaves applied for goiter. (155:101, 102) *Unspecified* Infusion of roots used as an medicinal tea. (100:48) **Shoshoni** *Dermatological Aid* Poultice of leaves applied to swellings. (155:101, 102) *Eye Medicine* Infusion of root used as an eye medicine. (98:39) Infusion or decoction of plant parts used as an eyewash. *Liver Aid* Poultice of crushed leaves applied for "gall trouble." (155:101, 102) **Thompson** *Dermatological Aid* Infusion of flowers, leaves, and stem used as skin and hair wash by young females. (104:42) Infusion of flowers, leaves, and stems used as wash for adolescents' skin and hair. (141:467) Decoction of stems and flowers used as wash by girls for beautiful hair and face. (141:507) Decoction of whole plant with the roots used to wash the hair and scalp if hair loss occurred. (161:234) *Pediatric Aid* Infusion of flowers, leaves, and stem used as skin and hair wash by young females. (104:42)

Linum puberulum, Plains Flax
Apache, **White Mountain** *Eye Medicine* Berry juice used as an eye medicine. (113:158) **Navajo**, **Ramah** *Gastrointestinal Aid* Decoction of leaves taken for heartburn. Infusion of plant taken to kill a swallowed red ant. *Panacea* Plant used as "life medicine." (165:35) **Zuni** *Eye Medicine* Berry juice squeezed into eye for inflammation. (143:56)

Linum rigidum, Stiffstem Flax
Keres, **Western** *Psychological Aid* Infusion of plant used by racers to make them speedy. (147:52)

Linum usitatissimum, Common Flax
Cherokee *Cold Remedy* and *Cough Medicine* Taken for "violent colds, coughs and diseases of lungs." *Febrifuge* Decoction poured over body for "fever attacks." (66:34) Decoction of plant poured over patient for fevers. (152:34) *Pulmonary Aid* Taken for "violent colds, coughs and diseases of lungs." *Urinary Aid* Seeds used for "gravel" or burning during urination. (66:34)

Liparis loeselii, Yellow Widelip Orchid
Cherokee Compound infusion of root taken for urinary problems. (66:59)

Liquidambar styraciflua, Sweet Gum
Cherokee *Antidiarrheal* Rosin or inner bark used for diarrhea, flux, and dysentery. *Dermatological Aid* Salve used for wounds, sores, and ulcers and mixed with sheep or cow tallow for itch. *Gynecological Aid* Infusion of bark taken to stop flooding. *Other* Gum used as drawing plaster and compound infusion of bark taken for bad disease. *Sedative* Infusion of bark given to nervous patients. (66:58) Gum used as a "drawing plaster" and infusion of inner bark used for nervous patients. (177:74) **Choctaw** *Dermatological Aid* Compound decoction of root used as a dressing for cuts and wounds. (20:23) Decoction of plant used as a poultice for cuts and bruises. (152:26) **Houma** *Dermatological Aid* Decoction of root applied to skin sores thought to be caused by worms. *Diaphoretic* and *Febrifuge* Decoction of Spanish moss from this tree taken as a diaphoretic for fever. (135:61, 62) **Koasati** *Other* Decoction of bark taken for "night sickness." (152:26) **Rappahannock** *Antidiarrheal* Compound infusion with dried bark taken for dysentery. (138:34) *Veterinary Aid* Rolled, hardened sap placed in dog's nose for distemper. (138:27)

Liriodendron tulipifera, Tuliptree
Cherokee *Anthelmintic* Infusion of bark taken for pinworms. Used for cholera infantum and infusion of bark given for pinworms. *Antidiarrheal* Bark used for cholera infantum, "dyspepsy, dysentery and rheumatism." *Antirheumatic* (*Internal*) Bark used for "dyspepsy, dysentery and rheumatism." *Cough Medicine* Bark used in cough syrup. *Dermatological Aid* Decoction blown onto wounds and boils. *Febrifuge* Infusion of root bark taken for fever. (66:50) Infusion of root bark taken for fevers. (177:74) *Gastrointestinal Aid* Bark used for "dyspepsy, dysentery and rheumatism." Compound used as steam bath for indigestion or biliousness. *Misc. Disease Remedy* Given for cholera infantum and infusion of bark given for pinworms. *Orthopedic Aid* Decoction blown onto fractured limbs. *Pediatric Aid* Given for cholera infantum and infusion of bark given for pinworms. *Poultice*

Used as a poultice and infusion of bark given for pinworms. (66:50) Infusion of root bark used in poultices. (177:74) *Sedative* Used for "women with hysterics and weakness." *Snakebite Remedy* Decoction used as a wash for snakebite. *Stimulant* Used for "women with hysterics and weakness." (66:50) **Rappahannock** *Analgesic* Poultice of bruised leaves bound to head for neuralgic pain. *Love Medicine* Raw, green bark chewed as a sex invigorant. *Stimulant* Raw, green bark chewed as a stimulant. (138:25)

Lithocarpus densiflorus, Tan Oak
Costanoan *Dermatological Aid* Infusion of bark used as a wash for face sores. *Toothache Remedy* Infusion of bark held in the mouth to tighten loose teeth. (17:20) **Pomo**, **Kashaya** *Cough Medicine* Acorns, the tannin soothed the cough, used as cough drops. (60:83) **Yurok** *Strengthener* Acorn mush taken by old people on their death bed to survive the day. (5:35)

Lithophragma affine, Common Woodlandstar
Mendocino Indian *Cold Remedy* Root chewed for colds. *Gastrointestinal Aid* Root chewed for stomachaches. (as *Tellima affinis* 33:353)

Lithospermum canescens, Hoary Puccoon
Menominee *Sedative* Compound infusion taken and rubbed on body to quiet person near convulsions. (44:128)

Lithospermum caroliniense, Hairy Puccoon
Lakota *Pulmonary Aid* Root powder taken for chest wounds. (116:40)

Lithospermum incisum, Narrowleaf
    Gromwell
Blackfoot *Ceremonial Medicine* Dried tops burned as incense in ceremonials. (as *L. linearifolium* 95:277) **Cheyenne** *Orthopedic Aid* Powdered leaves, roots, and stems rubbed on paralyzed part. (as *L. linearifolium* 63:185) Finely ground leaves rubbed on paralyzed part. (as *L. linearifolium* 63:40, 41) Leaf, root, and stem powder rubbed on body for paralysis. *Psychological Aid* Infusion of roots, leaves, and stems rubbed on head and face for irrational behavior from any illness. (as *L. linearifolium* 64:185) Infusion of

stems, leaves, and roots used as a wash for "irrationalness." (as *L. linearifolium* 69:15) *Sedative* Infusion of plant parts rubbed on face when irrational from illness. (as *L. linearifolium* 63:185) Decoction of root rubbed on one who was "irrational by reason of illness." *Stimulant* Plant chewed, then spit and blown in face or rubbed on chest as a stimulant. (as *L. linearifolium* 63:40, 41) Chewed plant spit and blown into face and rubbed over the heart by the doctor for sleepiness. (as *L. linearifolium* 64:185) Chewed plant spit and blown onto face to keep a very sleepy person awake. (as *L. linearifolium* 69:15) **Great Basin Indian** *Unspecified* Roots used medicinally for unspecified purpose. (as *L. angustifolium* 100:50) **Hopi** *Antihemorrhagic* Plant used for hemorrhages. *Blood Medicine* Plant used for building up the blood. (34:331) *Unspecified* Used as a medicinal plant. Used as a medicinal plant. (as *L. linearifolium* 164:165) **Navajo** *Cold Remedy* Plant chewed for colds. (as *L. angustifolium* 45:71) Plant used for colds. *Contraceptive* Plant used as an oral contraceptive. (76:161) *Cough Medicine* Plant chewed for coughs. (as *L. angustifolium* 45:71) Plant used for coughs. (as *L. angustifolium* 76:161) *Dermatological Aid* Roots used for soreness at the attachment of the umbilical cord. *Pediatric Aid* Roots used for soreness at the attachment of the umbilical cord. (as *L. angustifolium* 45:71) **Navajo**, **Ramah** *Eye Medicine* Cold infusion of pulverized root and seeds used as an eyewash. *Panacea* Root used as a "life medicine" and considered a "big medicine." (165:41) **Sioux**, **Teton** *Pulmonary Aid*

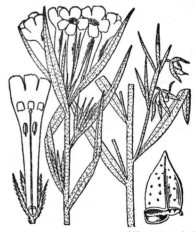

Lithospermum incisum

Fragrant herb used for lung hemorrhages. (as *L. linearifolium* 42:269, 270) **Zuni** *Ceremonial Medicine* Salve of powdered root applied ceremonially to swelling of any body part. (as *L. linearifolium* 143:56) *Dermatological Aid* Powdered root mixed with bum branch resin and used for abrasions and skin infections. (22:374) Poultice of root used and decoction of plant taken for swelling. (as *L. linearifolium* 143:56) *Gastrointestinal Aid* Infusion of root taken for stomachache. *Kidney Aid* Infusion of root taken for kidney problems. (22:374) *Throat Aid* Poultice of root used and decoction of plant taken for sore throat. (as *L. linearifolium* 143:56)

Lithospermum multiflorum, Manyflowered Gromwell

Navajo, Ramah *Panacea* Root used as a "life medicine" and considered a "big medicine." (165:41)

Lithospermum officinale, European Gromwell

Iroquois *Diuretic* and *Pediatric Aid* Infusion of dried, powdered seeds given to children as a diuretic. (118:56)

Lithospermum ruderale, Western Gromwell

Cheyenne *Analgesic* Poultice of dried, powdered leaves and stems applied for rheumatic pains. *Antirheumatic (External)* Poultice of dried, powdered leaves and stems applied for rheumatic pains. (63:185) Poultice of dried, pulverized leaves and stems applied for rheumatic pains. (64:185) **Gosiute** *Diuretic* Infusion or decoction of roots used as a diuretic. (as *L. pilosum* 31:351) Roots used as a diuretic for kidney troubles. (as *L. pilosum* 31:373) *Kidney Aid* Infusion or decoction of roots used for kidney troubles. (as *L. pilosum* 31:351) Roots used as a diuretic for kidney troubles. (as *L. pilosum* 31:373) **Navajo** *Contraceptive* Plant used as an oral birth control. (82:51) **Okanagan-Colville** *Antihemorrhagic* Infusion of roots taken for internal hemorrhaging. (162:91) **Shoshoni** *Antidiarrheal* Infusion or decoction of root taken for diarrhea. (155:102) *Contraceptive* Plant used as an oral birth control. (82:51) Infusion of root taken for 6 months as a permanent birth control. (98:46) Cold water infusion of root taken daily for 6 months as a contraceptive. (155:102) **Shuswap** *Dermatological Aid* Plant used for sores. *Disinfectant*

Decoction of plant used as a bath to "clean the germs off the body." (102:60) **Thompson** *Witchcraft Medicine* Root used to "inflict sickness or bad luck on persons." (as *L. pilosum* 141:508) **Ute** *Diuretic* Decoction of roots used as a diuretic. (as *L. pilosum* 30:35)

Lobelia cardinalis, Cardinal Flower

Cherokee *Analgesic* Compound given for pain and poultice of crushed leaves used for headache. *Anthelmintic* Infusion of root taken for worms. *Antirheumatic (Internal)* Infusion given for rheumatism. *Cold Remedy* Infusion of leaf taken for colds. *Dermatological Aid* Poultice of root used for "risings" and infusion used for "sores hard to heal." *Febrifuge* Infusion of leaf taken for fever. *Gastrointestinal Aid* Infusion of root taken for stomach trouble. *Hemostat* Cold infusion "snuffed" for nosebleed. *Pulmonary Aid* Used for croup. *Venereal Aid* Used for syphilis. (66:28) **Delaware** *Misc. Disease Remedy* Infusion of roots used for typhoid. (151:34) **Delaware, Oklahoma** *Misc. Disease Remedy* Infusion of root, considered to be very strong medicine, taken for typhoid. (150:28, 76) **Iroquois** *Adjuvant* Plant strengthened all medicines. (73:453) *Analgesic* Infusion of roots taken or poultice applied for pain. *Anticonvulsive* Compound decoction of plants taken by women for epilepsy. (73:452) *Basket Medicine* Infusion of stalks and flowers used as wash for baskets, a "basket medicine." (73:453) *Dermatological Aid* Decoction of roots used as a wash and poultice applied to chancres and fever sores. (73:452) *Febrifuge* Plant used as a fever medicine. *Gastrointestinal Aid* Compound decoction of plants taken for bad stomach caused by consumption. (73:453) *Gynecological Aid* Decoction or infusion taken and poultice or wash used for breast troubles. (73:452) *Love Medicine* Decoction of plants or infusion of roots used as a wash for love medicine. (73:453) *Other* Compound infusion of plants taken for stricture caused by menstruating women. Decoction of roots, plants, and blossoms taken for cramps. (73:452) Infusion of roots taken or washed on injured parts, "Little Water Medicine." *Panacea* Plant used for every ailment. (73:453) *Psychological Aid* Compound decoction of whole plant taken for sickness caused by grieving. (73:452) *Tuberculosis Remedy* Compound decoction of plants taken for bad stomach caused by consumption. (73:453) *Witchcraft Medicine* Infusion of roots taken or poultice applied for trouble caused by witchcraft. (73:452) **Meskwaki** *Love Medicine* Roots used as a love medicine. (129:231) Ground roots used in food to end quarrels, a love medicine and anti-divorce remedy. (129:273) **Pawnee** *Love Medicine* Compound containing roots and flowers used as a love charm. (58:129)

Lobelia cardinalis ssp. *graminea* var. *propinqua*, Cardinal Flower

Zuni *Antirheumatic* (*External*) Ingredient of "schumaakwe cakes" and used externally for rheumatism. *Dermatological Aid* Ingredient of "schumaakwe cakes" and used externally for swelling. (as *L. splendens* 143:56)

Lobelia inflata, Indian Tobacco

Cherokee *Analgesic* Poultice of root used for body aches and leaves rubbed on aches and stiff neck. *Dermatological Aid* Used for bites and stings and roots and leaves used on boils and sores. *Emetic* Plant used as a strong emetic. *Gastrointestinal Aid* Tincture in small doses prevented colics. *Orthopedic Aid* Poultice of root used for body aches and leaves rubbed on aches and stiff neck. *Other* Smoked "to break tobacco habit." *Pulmonary Aid* Given for croup and tincture in small doses prevented croup. *Respiratory Aid* Plant taken for "asthma and phthisic." *Throat Aid* Chewed for sore throat. (66:40) **Crow** *Ceremonial Medicine* Used in religious ceremonies. (15:14, 15) **Iroquois** *Cathartic* Cold infusion of whole plant taken as a physic. (73:455) *Dermatological Aid* Infusion of roots or leaves used as a wash or poultice on abscesses or sores. *Emetic* Infusion of plant taken to vomit and cure tobacco or whisky habit. (73:454) Cold infusion of whole plant taken as an emetic. (73:455) *Love Medicine* Infusion of plant taken as a love or anti-love medicine. (73:454) *Other* Cold infusion of whole plant used as a divining agent. (73:455) *Psychological Aid* Infusion of plant taken to vomit and cure tobacco or whisky habit. *Venereal Aid* Infusion of smashed roots used as wash and poultice for venereal disease sores. *Witchcraft Medicine* Decoction of plant taken to counteract sickness produced by witchcraft. (73:454)

Lobelia kalmii, Ontario Lobelia

Cree, Hudson Bay *Emetic* Plant used as an emetic. (78:303) **Iroquois** *Dermatological Aid* Infusion of smashed plants used as drops for abscesses. *Ear Medicine* Infusion of smashed plants used as drops for earaches. *Emetic* Infusion of plants taken to vomit to remove the effect of a love medicine. *Love Medicine* Infusion of plants taken to vomit to remove the effect of a love medicine. (73:455)

Lobelia siphilitica, Great Blue Lobelia

Cherokee *Analgesic* Compound given for pain and poultice of crushed leaves used for headache. *Anthelmintic* Infusion of root taken for worms. *Antirheumatic* (*Internal*) Infusion given for rheumatism. *Cold Remedy* Infusion of leaf taken for colds. *Dermatological Aid* Poultice of root used for "risings" and infusion used for "sores hard to heal." *Febrifuge* Infusion of leaf taken for fever. *Gastrointestinal Aid* Infusion of root taken for stomach trouble. *Hemostat* Cold infusion "snuffed" for nosebleed. *Pulmonary Aid* Used for croup. *Venereal Aid* Used for syphilis. (66:28) **Iroquois** *Cough Medicine* Plant used as a gargle for coughs. (73:454) *Witchcraft Medicine* Infusion of smashed plants taken for anti-bewitchment. (73:453) **Meskwaki** *Love Medicine* Finely chopped roots eaten by couple to avert divorce and renew love. (129:231, 232) Ground roots used in food to end quarrels, a love medicine and anti-divorce remedy. (129:273)

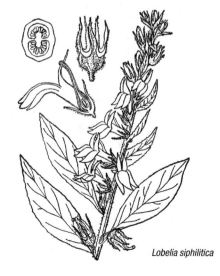

Lobelia siphilitica

Lobelia spicata, Palespike Lobelia
Cherokee *Orthopedic Aid* Compound taken for "arm shakes and trembles." (66:43) Cold infusion of roots put into scratches made for shaking arms. (152:60) **Iroquois** *Blood Medicine* Decoction of stalks used as wash for bad blood. *Dermatological Aid* Decoction of stalks used as wash for neck and jaw sores. *Emetic* and *Love Medicine* Infusion of plants taken as an emetic for the lovelorn. (73:454)

Loeseliastrum matthewsii, Desert Calico
Tubatulabal *Cold Remedy* Decoction of plant taken for colds. (as *Langloisia matthewsii* 167:59)

Lomatium ambiguum, Wyeth Biscuitroot
Okanagan-Colville *Cold Remedy* Infusion of flowers and upper leaves taken for colds and sore throats. *Throat Aid* Infusion of flowers and upper leaves taken for sore throats. (162:70)

Lomatium californicum, California Lomatium
Karok *Dietary Aid* Decoction of roots taken by person who does not feel like eating. (as *Leptotaenia californica* 125:387) **Kawaiisu** *Cold Remedy* and *Emetic* Decoction of dried roots taken for colds, but caused vomiting. *Gastrointestinal Aid* Pounded root rubbed on the stomach for stomachaches. *Throat Aid* Root chewed for sore throat. (180:37) **Yuki** *Analgesic* and *Antirheumatic* (*External*) Root moxa used for arthritic pains. *Cold Remedy* Dried root smoked or decoction of roots taken for colds. *Other* Root dried, ground, and smoked in a pipe for severe colds; this occasionally caused dizziness. (39:44)

Lomatium dissectum, Fernleaf Biscuitroot
Nez Perce *Dermatological Aid* Root oil used for sores. *Dietary Aid* Infusion of cut roots taken to increase the appetite. *Eye Medicine* Root oil used for sore eyes. *Respiratory Aid* Roots mixed with tobacco and smoked for sinus trouble. *Tuberculosis Remedy* Infusion of cut roots taken for tuberculosis. (68:26) **Okanagan-Colville** *Antirheumatic* (*Internal*) Infusion or decoction of roots taken for arthritis. *Blood Medicine* Shoots used to "change the blood" to adapt to the summer's heat. *Dermatological Aid* Poultice of peeled, pounded

roots applied to open cuts, sores, boils, or bruises. Roots soaked in cold water and used for dandruff. *Dietary Aid* Infusion of roots taken to increase the appetite. *Orthopedic Aid* Poultice of peeled, pounded roots applied to sore backs. *Other* Infusion or decoction of roots taken for some general illness. *Poison* Purple shoots considered poisonous. Mature tops and roots considered poisonous. Strong infusion or decoction of roots considered poisonous. *Tuberculosis Remedy* Infusion or decoction of roots taken for tuberculosis. *Veterinary Aid* Plant tops rubbed on cattle to kill lice. (162:66) **Paiute, Northern** *Analgesic* Roots smoked and decoction of roots taken or used as a head wash for head pains. Roots mixed with tobacco and smoked for headaches. *Antirheumatic* (*External*) Decoction of plant rubbed on the joints for rheumatism and aches. *Cold Remedy* Decoction of roots taken and roots smoked for colds. Root chips thrown on the fire and fumes inhaled or roots sliced, boiled, and eaten for colds. Roots mixed with tobacco and smoked for colds. *Dermatological Aid* Poultice of roasted roots applied to sores. Decoction of plant rubbed on pimples and sores. *Diuretic* Decoction of plant taken to pass water stopped by venereal disease. *Panacea* Plant used for all the common ailments and injuries. *Throat Aid* Roots chewed and juice swallowed for sore throats. *Vertigo Medicine* Roots smoked and decoction of roots taken or used as a head wash for dizziness. (49:129) **Shuswap** *Dermatological Aid* Poultice of mashed roots or decoction of mashed roots applied to sores. (102:56) **Thompson** *Cold Remedy* Infusion of dried root used for colds. *Orthopedic Aid* Poultice of washed, pounded root used for sprains and as a bone setter for broken bones. (161:154)

Lomatium dissectum var. dissectum, Fernleaf Biscuitroot
Thompson *Burn Dressing* Root powder mixed with grease and used as a salve for burns. *Dermatological Aid* Dried root powder sprinkled on wounds and sores to aid healing. (as *Leptotaenia dissecta* 141:472) *Veterinary Aid* Dried, crushed root sprinkled on horses' sores or wounds. (as *Leptotaenia dissecta* 141:513)

Lomatium dissectum var. *multifidum*,
Carrotleaf Biscuitroot

Blackfoot *Ceremonial Medicine* Pulverized root burned as incense. *Dietary Aid* Root used to make a drink taken as a tonic to help weakened people gain weight. *Stimulant* and *Tonic* Root used to make a drink taken as a tonic for "people in a weakened condition." *Veterinary Aid* Root smoke inhaled by horses for distemper. (as *Leptotaenia multifida* 95:274) **Cheyenne** *Analgesic* Infusion of dried roots taken for stomach pains or internal disorders. (as *Leptotoenia multifida* 63:182) Infusion of dried, powdered roots taken for stomach pains or any internal disorder. Infusion of pulverized stems and leaves taken for stomach pains or any internal disorder. (as *Leptotaenia multifida* 64:182) *Gastrointestinal Aid* Infusion of dried roots taken for stomach pains or internal disorders. (as *Leptotoenia multifida* 63:182) Infusion of dried, powdered roots taken for stomach pains or any internal disorder. Infusion of pulverized stems and leaves taken for stomach pains or any internal disorder. (as *Leptotaenia multifida* 64:182) *Tonic* Infusion of dried roots taken as a tonic. (as *Leptotoenia multifida* 63:182) Infusion of dried, powdered roots taken as a tonic. Infusion of pulverized stems and leaves used as a tonic. (as *Leptotaenia multifida* 64:182) **Gosiute** *Dermatological Aid* Poultice of roots applied to wounds, cuts, or bruises. (as *Ferula multifida* 31:348) Poultice of roots applied to wounds and bruises. (as *Ferula multifida* 31:369) *Disinfectant* and *Orthopedic Aid* Poultice of roots applied to infected, compound fractures. (as *Ferula multifida* 31:348) Poultice of roots applied to foot crushed under the wheel of a wagon. *Veterinary Aid* Burning root smoke inhaled by horse for distemper. (as *Ferula multifida* 31:369) **Great Basin Indian** *Cold Remedy* Decoction of roots taken or steam inhaled for colds. *Cough Medicine* Infusion of roots taken for coughs. *Dermatological Aid* Poultice of powdered roots used on sores. *Misc. Disease Remedy* Decoction of roots taken or steam inhaled for flu. Decoction of roots taken for colds and flu. *Other* Plant used to make a scent for a sick person. *Respiratory Aid* Dried roots burned on coals and smoke inhaled for asthma or bronchial troubles. *Tonic* Infusion of roots taken as a tonic. *Unspecified* Decoction of root water used to sponge a sick person. Dried, pounded roots and grease massaged on affected parts. (as *Leptotaenia multifida* 100:49) **Kawaiisu** *Analgesic* Pounded roots applied as a salve to sore limbs. *Dermatological Aid* Infusion of roots used as a wash or poultice applied to cuts and open wounds. Pounded roots applied as a salve to cuts and wounds. *Orthopedic Aid* Pounded roots applied as a salve to sore limbs. (180:37) **Montana Indian** *Poison* Young sprouts eaten, but poisonous to stock in early spring. (as *Leptotaenia multifida* 15:14) **Navajo** *Ceremonial Medicine* Infusion of dried, ground plant mixed with other plants and taken by patients for Mountain Top Chant. (as *Leptotaenia dissecta* var. *multifida* 45:67) **Nevada Indian** *Veterinary Aid* Poultice of ground chips given to horses for head trouble and sores. **Oregon Indian** *Veterinary Aid* Roots used in a wash for horse ticks and dandruff. (as *Leptotaenia multifida* 98:49) **Paiute** *Antirheumatic* (*External*) Poultice of root applied and decoction of root used as a wash for rheumatism. *Cold Remedy* Compound decoction of root taken for colds. Compound of pulverized roots smoked for colds. *Cough Medicine* Decoction of root taken as a cough remedy. (as *Leptotaenia multifida* 155:97–100) *Dermatological Aid* Smashed roots used for sores and swellings. (as *Leptotaenia multifida* 87:196) Poultice of root applied and decoction used as a wash for swellings. Poultice of root applied or decoction used as a wash for rashes, cuts, or sores. Sap from cut roots or oil from decoction used as a salve on cuts and sores. *Disinfectant* Root used as "the basis of a number of antiseptics." *Herbal Steam* Compound of roots used as herbal steam for lung or nasal congestion and asthma. *Misc. Disease Remedy* Decoction of dried root taken for influenza. Decoction of root and sometimes leaves used as an antiseptic wash for smallpox. *Orthopedic Aid* Poultice of root applied and decoction used as a wash for sprains. *Panacea* Root used for a wide variety of ailments, usually as a decoction. *Pulmonary Aid* Compound of roots used as herbal steam for lung congestion. Pulverized roots smoked to clear lungs and nasal passages. Root used in various ways for pneumonia. *Respiratory Aid* Compound of roots used as herbal steam for nasal congestion and asthma. Decoction of dried root taken for hay fever, bronchitis, and pneumonia. Pulverized roots smoked alone or in compound for asthma. *Throat Aid* Raw root chewed and decoction of root taken for sore throat. (as *Leptotaenia multifida* 155:97–100) *Tuberculosis Remedy* Decoction of roots taken for tuberculosis. (as *Leptotaenia multifida* 87:198) Compound of pulverized roots smoked for tuberculosis. Decoction of dried root taken for tuberculosis. *Venereal Aid* Simple or compound decoction of root taken for venereal diseases. *Veterinary Aid* Root smoke inhaled by horses for distemper. **Shoshoni** *Antirheumatic* (*External*) Poultice of root applied and decoction of root used as a wash for rheumatism. *Cold Remedy* Compound decoction of root taken for colds. *Cough Medicine* Decoction of root taken as a cough remedy. *Dermatological Aid* Poultice of root applied and decoction used as a wash for swellings. Sap from cut roots or oil from decoction used as a salve on cuts and sores. *Disinfectant* Root used as "the basis of a number of antiseptics." (as *Leptotaenia multifida* 155:97–100) *Eye Medicine* Root oil used as eye drops for "trachoma." (82:48) Oil of root used for trachoma. (as *Leptotaenia multifida* 98:39) Sap from cut roots used as eye drops for trachoma or gonorrheal eye infections. *Herbal Steam* Compound of roots used as herbal steam for lung or nasal congestion and asthma. *Misc. Disease Remedy* Decoction of dried root taken for influenza. Decoction of root and sometimes leaves used as an antiseptic wash for smallpox. *Orthopedic Aid* Poultice of root applied and decoction used as a wash for sprains. *Panacea* Root used for a wide variety of ailments, usually as a decoction. *Pulmonary Aid* Compound of roots used as herbal steam for lung congestion. Decoction of dried root taken for pneumonia. Pulverized roots smoked to clear lungs and nasal passages. *Respiratory Aid* Compound of roots used as herbal steam for nasal congestion and asthma. Decoction of dried root taken for hay fever and bronchitis. Pulverized roots smoked for asthma. *Throat Aid* Raw root chewed for sore throat. *Tuberculosis Remedy* Compound of pulverized roots smoked for tuberculosis. Decoction of dried root taken for tuberculosis. *Venereal Aid* Simple or compound decoction of root taken for venereal diseases. *Veterinary Aid* Smoke from root alone or in compound inhaled by horses for distemper. (as *Leptotaenia multifida* 155:97–100) **Ute** *Dermato-*

logical Aid Poultice of root pulp applied to wounds and bruises. *Veterinary Aid* Roots burned in a pan and held beneath the horse's nose for distemper. (as *Ferula multifida* 30:34) **Washo** *Cold Remedy* Decoction of root taken as a cold remedy. *Cough Medicine* Decoction of root taken as a cough remedy. *Dermatological Aid* Pulverized root applied as powder to infant's severed umbilical cord. Sap from cut roots or oil from decoction used as a salve on cuts and sores. *Herbal Steam* Compound of roots used as herbal steam for lung or nasal congestion and asthma. *Misc. Disease Remedy* Decoction of dried root taken for influenza. *Panacea* Root used for a wide variety of ailments, usually as a decoction. *Pediatric Aid* Poultice of fresh root pulp applied to severed umbilical cord. *Pulmonary Aid* Compound of roots used as herbal steam for lung congestion. Decoction of dried root taken for pneumonia. Pulverized roots smoked to clear lungs and nasal passages. *Respiratory Aid* Compound of roots used as herbal steam for nasal congestion and asthma. Decoction of dried root taken for hay fever and bronchitis. Pulverized roots smoked for asthma. *Throat Aid* Raw root chewed for sore throat. *Tuberculosis Remedy* Decoction of dried root taken for tuberculosis. (as *Leptotaenia multifida* 155:97–100)

Lomatium foeniculaceum ssp. *daucifolium*, Desert Biscuitroot

Dakota *Love Medicine* Compound containing seeds used by men as a love charm. **Omaha** *Love Medicine* Compound containing seeds used by men as a love charm. **Pawnee** *Love Medicine* Compound containing seeds used by men as a love charm. **Ponca** *Love Medicine* Compound containing seeds used by men as a love charm. **Winnebago** *Love Medicine* Compound containing seeds used by men as a love charm. (as *Cogswellia daucifolia* 58:107)

Lomatium graveolens var. *graveolens*, King Desertparsley

Gosiute *Cold Remedy* Compound decoction of roots taken for biliousness with severe colds. (as *Peucedanum graveolens* 31:351) Decoction of plant used for severe colds. (as *Peucedanum graveolens* 31:376) *Gastrointestinal Aid* Compound decoction of roots taken for biliousness with severe colds. (as *Peucedanum graveolens* 31:351) Decoction of plant used for biliousness. (as *Peucedanum graveolens* 31:376) *Throat Aid* Decoction of roots used or poultice of root pulp applied for sore throats. (as *Peucedanum graveolens* 31:351) Poultice of mashed plant applied to throat for a sore throat. *Unspecified* Root used as medicine. (as *Peucedanum graveolens* 31:376)

Lomatium macrocarpum, Bigseed Biscuitroot
Blackfoot *Strengthener* Infusion of roots taken for weakness. *Veterinary Aid* Smoke from burning roots or decoction of roots inhaled by horses for distemper. **Crow** *Antirheumatic* (*External*) Poultice of boiled root shavings used for swellings. *Cold Remedy* Infusion of root shavings mixed with animal fat and used for colds. *Throat Aid* Roots chewed and juice used for sore throats. (68:26) **Okanagan-Colville** *Cold Remedy* Dried roots soaked overnight and chewed for colds. *Misc. Disease Remedy* Dried roots soaked overnight and chewed for flu. *Oral Aid* and *Pediatric Aid* Poultice of pounded roots applied to the inside of babies mouths for mouth sores or "thrush." *Respiratory Aid* Dried roots soaked overnight and chewed for bronchitis. (162:69) **Thompson** *Pediatric Aid* Leaves used in babies' bath water to make them sleep a lot. (161:155) *Reproductive Aid* Root eaten by childless women for infertility. (as *Peucedanum macrocarpum* 141:508) Roots eaten by elderly couples to help them conceive. *Sedative* Leaves used in babies' bath water to make them sleep a lot. Leaves used as padding, especially in children's cradles, to cause them to sleep a lot. (161:155)

Lomatium nudicaule, Barestem Biscuitroot
Cowichan *Cold Remedy* Seeds chewed for colds. *Throat Aid* Seeds chewed for sore throats. (156:89) **Kwakiutl** *Analgesic* Poultice of chewed seeds applied or chewed seeds blown on head for headaches. (157:276) *Antirheumatic* (*External*) Poultice of chewed seeds applied to back for sore places, pains, or itching. (as *Peucedanum lecocarpum* 16:382) *Cold Remedy* Poultice of chewed seeds applied for colds. (157:276) *Cough Medicine* Seeds kept in the mouth and the saliva swallowed to loosen the phlegm for hoarseness and coughs. (as *Penoedanum leiocarpum* 16:381)

Seeds sucked for coughs. *Dermatological Aid* Poultice of chewed seeds applied to carbuncles. *Gastrointestinal Aid* Poultice of chewed seeds applied for stomachaches. *Gynecological Aid* Infusion of seeds taken by pregnant women to insure an easy delivery. Poultice of chewed seeds applied for swelling of a woman's breasts. *Herbal Steam* Compound with seeds used in a steam bath for general sickness. *Hunting Medicine* Seeds used by hunters for protection. *Laxative* Seeds eaten for constipation. *Orthopedic Aid* Poultice of chewed seeds applied for backaches and swollen knees and feet. *Panacea* Compound with seeds used in a steam bath for general sickness. (157:276) *Throat Aid* Seeds kept in the mouth and the saliva swallowed to loosen the phlegm for hoarseness and coughs. (as *Penoedanum leiocarpum* 16:381) Seeds sucked for sore throats. (157:276) **Nitinaht** *Ceremonial Medicine* Seeds burned as a protective fumigant against bad spirits and illness. *Cold Remedy* Poultice of warm, soaked seeds applied to the chest for colds. (160:92) **Saanich** *Cold Remedy* Seeds chewed for colds. *Throat Aid* Seeds chewed for sore throats. **Salish, Coast** *Internal Medicine* Seeds swallowed for internal complaints. **Songish** *Cold Remedy* Seeds chewed for colds. *Throat Aid* Seeds chewed for sore throats. (156:89) **Thompson** *Cold Remedy* Strong decoction of whole plant or stems and leaves taken for colds. (as *Peucedanum nudicaulis* 141:473) Decoction of leaves, strawberry leaves, and ginger root used as a vitamin supplement for colds. *Diaphoretic* Infusion of 2 teaspoons of dried seeds used to "sweat the cold out." (161:156) *Febrifuge* Strong decoction of whole plant or stems and leaves taken for fevers. (as *Peucedanum nudicaulis* 141:473)

Lomatium nuttallii, Nuttall's Biscuitroot
Creek *Poison* Plant considered poisonous if eaten in winter. *Unspecified* Used as a medicine in summer. (148:667)

Lomatium orientale, Northern Idaho Biscuitroot
Cheyenne *Analgesic* Infusion of roots and leaves used by children and adults for bowel pain and diarrhea. (as *Cogswellia orientalis* 63:182) Infusion of pounded roots and leaves taken for bowel pain. (as *Cogswellia orientalis* 64:182) Infusion

of roots and leaves used or dried roots and leaves eaten for bowel pain. (68:26) *Antidiarrheal* Infusion of roots and leaves used by children and adults for bowel pain and diarrhea. (as *Cogswellia orientalis* 63:182) Infusion of pounded roots and leaves taken for diarrhea. (as *Cogswellia orientalis* 64:182) Roots and leaves infused or eaten dry for diarrhea. (68:26) *Gastrointestinal Aid* Infusion of roots and leaves used by children and adults for bowel pain and diarrhea. (as *Cogswellia orientalis* 63:182) Infusion of pounded roots and leaves taken for bowel pain. (as *Cogswellia orientalis* 64:182) *Pediatric Aid* Infusion of roots and leaves used by children and adults for bowel pain and diarrhea. (as *Cogswellia orientalis* 63:182) Infusion of pounded roots and leaves given to children for bowel pain or diarrhea. (as *Cogswellia orientalis* 64:182)

Lomatium triternatum, Nineleaf Biscuitroot
Blackfoot *Panacea* Chewed roots blown onto affected part by the diviner. The healing qualities of the spray were believed to penetrate the body at that place. (72:83) *Pulmonary Aid* Infusion of roots and leaves taken for chest troubles. (72:72) *Strengthener* Fruit chewed by long distance runners to avoid side aches. (72:67) **Okanagan-Colville** *Cold Remedy* Infusion of flowers and upper leaves taken for colds. *Throat Aid* Infusion of flowers and upper leaves taken for sore throats. (162:70)

Lomatium utriculatum, Common Lomatium
Kawaiisu *Dermatological Aid* Decoction of plant used as a wash for swollen limbs. *Orthopedic Aid* Decoction of plant used as a wash for broken limbs. (180:38) **Salish, Coast** *Analgesic* Roots chewed or soaked in water and taken for headaches. *Gastrointestinal Aid* Roots chewed or soaked in water and taken for stomach disorders. (156:89)

Lonicera arizonica, Arizona Honeysuckle
Navajo, Ramah *Ceremonial Medicine* and *Emetic* Leaves used as a ceremonial emetic. (165:45)

Lonicera canadensis, American Fly Honeysuckle
Iroquois *Blood Medicine* Complex compound

taken as blood purifier. *Dermatological Aid* Decoction of shoots taken for chancres caused by syphilis. *Pediatric Aid* Infusion of bark given to children who cry all night. *Psychological Aid* Infusion of bark taken for homesickness. *Sedative* Infusion of bark given to children who cry all night. *Venereal Aid* Decoction of shoots taken for chancres caused by syphilis. (73:443) **Menominee** *Urinary Aid* Bark used for urinary diseases. *Venereal Aid* Compound containing bark used for gonorrhea. (128:27) **Montagnais** *Diuretic* Infusion of vines taken as a diuretic. (133:315) **Potawatomi** *Diuretic* Compound infusion of bark used as a diuretic. (131:46)

Lonicera ciliosa, Orange Honeysuckle
Chehalis *Contraceptive* Infusion of leaves taken as a contraceptive. *Dermatological Aid* Infusion of crushed leaves used as a hair wash to make it grow. (65:48) **Cowichan** *Unspecified* Leaves used for medicine. (156:79) **Klallam** *Dermatological Aid* Poultice of chewed leaves applied to bruises. **Lummi** *Tuberculosis Remedy* Decoction of leaves taken for tuberculosis. **Skagit** *Tonic* Decoction of leaves applied to the body as a strengthening tonic. **Squaxin** *Gynecological Aid* Infusion of leaves taken for womb trouble. **Swinomish** *Cold Remedy* Infusion of bark or chewed leaf juice taken for colds. *Gynecological Aid* Infusion of leaves used as a steam bath to stimulate lacteal flow. *Throat Aid* Infusion of bark taken for colds and sore throats. (65:48) **Thompson** *Anticonvulsive* Infusion of woody part of vine taken in small amounts or used as a bath for epilepsy. Infusion of woody part of vine taken in small amounts or used as a bath for children with epilepsy. Flowers sucked for epilepsy. *Reproductive Aid* Decoction of chopped, cooked vine stems taken by women who could not become pregnant. *Sedative* Vine pieces used under the pillow to induce sound sleep. (161:196) *Tonic* Decoction of peeled stems taken as a tonic. (141:471)

Lonicera dioica, Limber Honeysuckle
Algonquin, Quebec *Cathartic* Infusion of bark used as a cathartic. *Gynecological Aid* Infusion of bark used for menstrual difficulties. *Kidney Aid* Infusion of bark used for kidney stones. (14:234) **Chippewa** *Diuretic* Infusion of stems taken as a

diuretic. *Urinary Aid* Infusion of stems taken for dysuria. (as *L. divica* 59:141) **Iroquois** *Emetic* Decoction of vines taken as an emetic to throw off effects of love medicine. *Love Medicine* Decoction of vines taken as an emetic, love or anti-love medicine. *Venereal Aid* Compound decoction of roots taken for gonorrhea. (73:443) **Meskwaki** *Anthelmintic* Infusion of berry and root bark taken by pregnant women for worms. (129:207)

Lonicera dioica var. *glaucescens*, Limber Honeysuckle

Cree, Woodlands *Diuretic* Infusion of inner bark, either scraped from or attached to the stem, used as a diuretic. Infusion of peeled, internodal stem lengths used for urine retention. *Gynecological Aid* Decoction of stems used for blood clotting after childbirth. *Misc. Disease Remedy* Infusion of peeled, internodal stem lengths used for flu. *Venereal Aid* Decoction of stems used for venereal disease. (91:43) **Iroquois** *Febrifuge* Decoction of plants given to children for fevers and sickness. *Gynecological Aid* Decoction taken by pregnant women for internal and leg soreness. *Pediatric Aid* Decoction of plants given to children for fevers and sickness. *Tuberculosis Remedy* Compound decoction of roots taken for consumption. (73:444)

Lonicera interrupta, Chaparral Honeysuckle

Mendocino Indian *Eye Medicine* Infusion of leaves taken and used as a wash for sore eyes. (33:388) **Shoshoni** *Antirheumatic (External)* Poultice of raw root applied to swellings. **Yuki** *Dermatological Aid* Leaves used in a wash for sores. (98:44)

Lonicera involucrata, Twinberry Honeysuckle

Bella Coola *Cough Medicine* Decoction of bark taken for cough. *Dermatological Aid* Poultice of chewed leaves used on itch, boils, and gonorrheal sores and bark used for sores. (127:63) Leaves chewed and used for itchy skin and boils. (158:203) *Venereal Aid* Poultice of chewed leaves or toasted bark applied to gonorrheal sores. (127:63) **Blackfoot** *Cathartic* and *Emetic* Infusion of berries used as a cathartic and emetic to cleanse the body. *Gastrointestinal Aid* Infusion of berries used for stomach troubles. *Pulmonary Aid* Infusion of berries used for chest troubles. (72:67)

Carrier *Dermatological Aid* Poultice of crushed leaves applied to open sores. *Eye Medicine* Decoction of leaves used to bathe sore eyes. (26:77) **Carrier, Northern** *Dermatological Aid* Compound decoction of stems taken for body sores. *Orthopedic Aid* Compound decoction of stems taken for constitutional weakness or paralysis. *Stimulant* Compound decoction of stems taken for constitutional weakness. **Carrier, Southern** *Eye Medicine* Decoction of bark used daily as an eyewash. (127:63) **Gitksan** *Eye Medicine* Fruit juice used for sore eyes. Infusion of inner bark used for sore eyes. (35:229) Fresh juice of berries or infusion of inner bark used in sore eyes. (127:63) **Kwakiutl** *Analgesic* Compound infusion of bark used as foot bath for painful legs and feet. (16:380) Chewed leaves with yellow cedar rubbed on painful places. (16:382) *Antirheumatic (External)* Plant used in sweat baths for arthritis and rheumatism. (157:266) *Dermatological Aid* Leaves chewed with yellow cedar and rubbed on painful places. (16:380) Chewed leaves rubbed on sores. Poultice of bark, berries, or leaves and grease applied to swellings or sores. *Gynecological Aid* Decoction of bark applied to women's breasts to make milk flow. (157:279) *Herbal Steam* Plant used in sweat baths for arthritis and rheumatism. (157:266) *Orthopedic Aid* Compound decoction of bark used as foot bath for leg and foot pains. (16:380) Compound infusion of bark used as a soak for sore feet and legs. Infusion of leaves or roots applied as poultice to swollen shoulders and feet. (157:279) **Kwakiutl, Southern** *Analgesic* Poultice of bark and berries or leaves, fresh sea

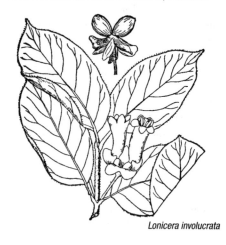

Lonicera involucrata

wrack, and alder bark applied for aches and pains. (157:260) **Makah** *Dermatological Aid* Mashed fruit applied to the scalp for dandruff. *Emetic* Fruit used as an emetic. (55:317) *Gynecological Aid* Leaves chewed by women during confinement. (65:48) *Poison* Fruit considered poisonous. (55:317) **Navajo, Ramah** *Ceremonial Medicine* and *Emetic* Leaves used as a ceremonial emetic. (165:45) **Nitinaht** *Psychological Aid* Buds eaten in spring or bark rubbed on body as a tonic for nervous breakdowns. **Nootka, Manhousat** *Love Medicine* Decoction of bark or fresh bark eaten by whalers to relieve effects of sexual abstinence. (160:99) **Nuxalkmc** *Cough Medicine* Leaves or bark used for coughs. *Dermatological Aid* Leaves or bark used for boils and itchy areas. *Venereal Aid* Leaves or bark used for gonorrhea. (35:229) **Okanagan-Colville** *Gynecological Aid* Branches used to make a medicine for mothers after childbirth. *Poison* Berries considered poisonous. (162:94) **Poliklah** *Poison* Berries considered poisonous. (97:173) **Quileute** *Antidote* and *Emetic* Leaves chewed as an emetic when poisoned. (65:48) **Quinault** *Dermatological Aid* Leaves chewed or rubbed on sores. (175:276) *Gynecological Aid* Leaves chewed by women during confinement. (65:48) *Oral Aid* Leaves chewed for sore mouth. (175:276) **Thompson** *Dermatological Aid* Poultice of boiled leaves applied to swellings. (141:457) Decoction of sticks, leaves and all, used for scabs and sores. *Dietary Aid* Decoction of stems and leaves taken as a tonic "for vitamins." (161:197) *Orthopedic Aid* Decoction of leaves and twigs used as a liniment. (141:457) Decoction of sticks, leaves and all, used for broken bones. (161:197) *Poison* Berries considered poisonous if more than two or three eaten. (141:489) *Throat Aid* Decoction of sticks, leaves and all, taken for sore throat. *Urinary Aid* Decoction of sticks, leaves and all, taken for bladder trouble. (161:197) **Tolowa** *Poison* "Not good to eat, poison." (5:37) **Wet'suwet'en** *Burn Dressing* Bark used for burns. *Dermatological Aid* Bark used for wounds. *Disinfectant* Bark used for infections. (61:152)

Lonicera oblongifolia, Swamp Fly Honeysuckle
Iroquois *Analgesic* Poultice of hot bark applied to abdomen for urinating pain. *Gynecological Aid*

Compound decoction of branches taken for falling of the womb. *Psychological Aid* Infusion of bark taken for loneliness. *Sedative* Infusion of bark taken for restlessness. *Urinary Aid* Poultice of hot bark applied to abdomen for urinating pain. (73:443)

Lonicera subspicata var. *johnstonii*,
Johnston's Honeysuckle
Diegueño *Veterinary Aid* Decoction of plant used to wash sores on horses. (70:24)

Lonicera utahensis, Utah Honeysuckle
Navajo, Ramah *Hunting Medicine* Chewed leaves blown on weapons for good luck in hunting. (165:45) **Okanagan-Colville** *Blood Medicine* Infusion of branches taken as a tonic to "change the blood" in the spring and fall. *Dermatological Aid* Infusion of branches and leaves used to wash sores and infections. *Laxative* Infusion of branches taken as a mild laxative. (162:94)

Lophophora williamsii, Peyote
Comanche *Ceremonial Medicine* and *Narcotic* Plant used in ceremonies as a narcotic. (24:522) **Delaware** *Panacea* Carried in small beaded bags and worn around the neck to protect against illness. *Tuberculosis Remedy* Used for tuberculosis. (151:39) **Kiowa** *Analgesic* and *Antirheumatic* (*External*) Poultice of plants applied for rheumatic pains. *Cold Remedy* Decoction of plants taken for colds. *Dermatological Aid* Poultice of plants applied for cuts. *Febrifuge* Decoction of plants taken for fevers. *Gastrointestinal Aid* Decoction of plants taken for intestinal ills. *Misc. Disease Remedy* Decoction of plants taken for grippe and scarlet fever. *Narcotic* Plant used as a narcotic. *Orthopedic Aid* Poultice of plants applied for bruises. *Panacea* Decoction of plants taken as a panacea. *Pulmonary Aid* Decoction of plants taken for pneumonia and scarlet fever. *Tuberculosis Remedy* Decoction of plants taken for tuberculosis. *Venereal Aid* Decoction of plants taken for venereal disease. (166:43) **Omaha** *Ceremonial Medicine* Plant revered and used in important ritual and ceremonial sacraments. (58:104, 110) **Paiute** *Unspecified* Plant used by one shaman for curing. (93:91) **Ponca** *Hallucinogen* Dried flesh "buttons" eaten to cause auditory and visual hallucinations. *Un-*

specified Decoction of dried flesh "buttons" taken for illness. (80:48) **Winnebago** *Ceremonial Medicine* Plant revered and used in important ritual and ceremonial sacraments. (58:104, 110)

Lotus humistratus, Foothill Deervetch
Karok *Gynecological Aid* Infusion of plant taken and used as a wash by women in labor. (125:385)

Lotus scoparius, Common Deerweed
Costanoan *Cough Medicine* Decoction of foliage used for coughs. (17:19)

Lotus scoparius var. *scoparius*, Common Deerweed
Mahuna *Blood Medicine* Infusion of plant taken to build the blood. (as *Hosackia glabra* 117:34)

Lotus wrightii, Wright's Deervetch
Navajo, Ramah *Analgesic* Decoction of leaves used for stomachache. *Cathartic* Decoction of leaves used as a cathartic. *Disinfectant* Decoction of leaves used for "deer infection." *Gastrointestinal Aid* Decoction of leaves used for stomachache. *Panacea* Plant used as "life medicine." (165:32)
Zuni *Witchcraft Medicine* Poultice of chewed root applied to swellings caused by being witched by a bullsnake. (22:376)

Ludwigia bonariensis, Carolina Primrose-willow
Hawaiian *Blood Medicine* Infusion of pounded whole plants and other plants strained and taken to purify the blood. *Dermatological Aid* and *Pediatric Aid* Seeds or root pulp used by children on small cuts or scratches. (as *Jussiaea villosa* 2:48)

Ludwigia virgata, Savannah Primrosewillow
Seminole *Dermatological Aid* Decoction of root taken and used as a body steam for snake sickness: itchy skin. (145:239)

Luetkea pectinata, Partridgefoot
Okanagon *Analgesic* Decoction of plant taken for abdominal pains. *Dermatological Aid* Poultice of crushed plant applied to sores. *Gastrointestinal Aid* Decoction of plant taken for abdominal pains. *Gynecological Aid* Decoction of plant taken by women for profuse or prolonged menstruation.

(104:42) **Thompson** *Analgesic* Decoction of plant taken for abdominal pains. (141:472) *Dermatological Aid* Poultice of crushed plant applied to sores. (104:42) Poultice of crushed, fresh plant applied to sores. (141:472) *Gastrointestinal Aid* Decoction of plant taken for abdominal pains. (104:42) Decoction of plant taken for abdominal pain. (141:472) *Gynecological Aid* Decoction of plant taken by women for profuse or prolonged menstruation. (104:42) Decoction of plant taken for profuse or prolonged menstruation. (141:472)

Lupinus albifrons, Silver Lupine
Karok *Gastrointestinal Aid* Decoction of plant taken and used as a steam bath for stomach troubles. (125:385)

Lupinus arcticus, Arctic Lupine
Eskimo, Inupiat *Poison* Seeds considered poisonous. (83:143)

Lupinus argenteus ssp. *ingratus*, Silvery Lupine
Navajo, Ramah *Dermatological Aid* Poultice of crushed leaves applied to poison ivy blisters. (as *L. ingratus* 165:32)

Lupinus brevicaulis, Shortstem Lupine
Navajo *Dermatological Aid* Plant rubbed on as a liniment for boils. *Reproductive Aid* Plant used for sterility. (45:56)

Lupinus caudatus ssp. *argophyllus*, Kellogg's Spurred Lupine
Navajo, Ramah *Ceremonial Medicine* Leaves used as a ceremonial emetic. *Dermatological Aid* Cold infusion of leaves used as a lotion on poison ivy blisters. *Emetic* Leaves used as a ceremonial emetic. (as *L. aduncus* 165:32)

Lupinus kingii, King's Lupine
Hopi *Eye Medicine* Plant used as an eye medicine. (174:33, 80) **Navajo, Ramah** *Dermatological Aid* Poultice of crushed leaves used for poison ivy blisters and other skin irritations. *Panacea* Leaves used as "life medicine." (165:32)

Lupinus littoralis, Seashore Lupine
Kwakiutl *Pediatric Aid* and *Sedative* Root ash

rubbed into a newborn baby's cradle to make infant sleep well. (157:284)

Lupinus lyallii, Dwarf Mountain Lupine
Navajo *Dermatological Aid* Plant used for boils. (45:97)

Lupinus nootkatensis, Nootka Lupine
Alaska Native *Poison* Roots considered poisonous. (71:157)

Lupinus perennis, Sundial Lupine
Cherokee *Antiemetic* Cold infusion taken and used as wash "to check hemorrhage and vomiting." *Antihemorrhagic* Cold infusion taken and used as wash "to check hemorrhage and vomiting." (66:43, 44) **Menominee** *Veterinary Aid* Plant used to fatten a horse and make him spirited and full of fire. *Witchcraft Medicine* Plant rubbed on hands or body to give person power to control horses. (128:40)

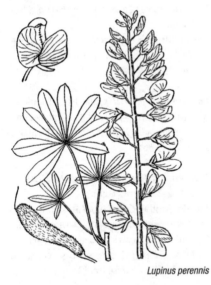

Lupinus perennis

Lupinus polyphyllus, Bigleaf Lupine
Salish *Tonic* Decoction of plants used as a tonic. (153:293) **Thompson** *Poison* Plant considered poisonous. (161:224) *Unspecified* Plant used medicinally for unspecified purpose. (141:461) *Veterinary Aid* Plant eaten by horses as medicine. (161:224)

Lupinus pusillus, Rusty Lupine
Hopi *Ear Medicine* Plant used as an ear medicine. *Eye Medicine* Plant used as an eye medicine. (34:333)

Lupinus pusillus* ssp. *intermontanus, Intermountain Lupine
Navajo, Kayenta *Disinfectant* Plant used as a fumigant ingredient. *Ear Medicine* Plant used for earaches. *Hemostat* Plant used for nosebleeds. (179:28)

Lupinus rivularis, Riverbank Lupine
Thompson *Unspecified* Plant used medicinally for unspecified purpose. (141:461)

Lupinus sericeus, Silky Lupine
Okanagan-Colville *Eye Medicine* Seeds pounded, mixed with water, strained, and resulting liquid used as an eye medicine. (162:105)

Lupinus sericeus* var. *sericeus, Silky Lupine
Thompson *Poison* Plant considered poisonous. *Veterinary Aid* Plant eaten by horses as medicine. (161:224)

Lupinus sulphureus, Sulphur Lupine
Okanagan-Colville *Eye Medicine* Seeds pounded, mixed with water, strained, and resulting liquid used as an eye medicine. (162:105)

Lupinus wyethii, Wyeth's Lupine
Okanagan-Colville *Eye Medicine* Seeds pounded, mixed with water, strained, and resulting liquid used as an eye medicine. (162:105)

Luzula multiflora, Common Woodrush
Navajo, Ramah *Ceremonial Medicine* Plant used as a ceremonial emetic and for other ceremonial purposes. *Emetic* Plant used as a ceremonial emetic. (165:20)

Lycium pallidum, Pale Wolfberry
Hopi *Ceremonial Medicine* Plant used at the annual "Niman-katcina" ceremony. (46:19) **Navajo, Kayenta** *Toothache Remedy* Ground root placed in cavity for toothaches. (179:41) **Navajo, Ramah** *Ceremonial Medicine* and *Emetic* Leaves or root used as ceremonial emetic. *Misc. Disease Remedy*

Plant used for chickenpox and poultice of plant used for toothaches. *Panacea* Bark and dried berries used as "life medicine." *Toothache Remedy* Poultice of heated root applied for toothache. (165:42)

Lycium torreyi, Squawthorn
Navajo, Ramah *Ceremonial Medicine* and *Emetic* Leaves or root used as ceremonial emetic. *Misc. Disease Remedy* Plant used for chickenpox and poultice of plant used for toothaches. *Panacea* Bark and dried berries used as "life medicine." *Toothache Remedy* Poultice of heated root applied for toothache. (165:42)

Lycoperdon sp., Puffball
Blackfoot *Antihemorrhagic* Spores mixed with water and taken for internal hemorrhage. *Hemostat* Poultice of spores applied to wounds as a styptic. Plant pieces held to the nose for nosebleeds. (72:84) *Veterinary Aid* Plant pieces applied as a styptic on castration wounds and other cuts. (72:89) **Haisla & Hanaksiala** *Poison* Spores dangerous, especially harmful to the eyes. (35:134) **Pomo, Kashaya** *Poison* Plant considered poisonous. (60:132)

Lycopodium clavatum, Running Clubmoss
Aleut *Analgesic* and *Gynecological Aid* Infusion of plant taken for postpartum pain. (6:427) **Carrier, Southern** *Analgesic* Moss inserted into the nose to cause bleeding for headaches. (127:48) **Montagnais** *Febrifuge* "Brew" from plant used for weakness and fever. *Stimulant* Compound containing plant used for weakness and fever. (133:315) **Potawatomi** *Hemostat* Spores of fruiting spikes used as a styptic and coagulant. (131:64)

Lycopodium complanatum, Groundcedar
Blackfoot *Dermatological Aid* Spores applied as an antiseptic dust on wounds. *Hemostat* Spores snuffed for nosebleed. *Pulmonary Aid* Decoction of plant used for lung diseases. *Venereal Aid* Decoction of plant used for venereal diseases. (82:16) **Iroquois** *Reproductive Aid* Compound decoction taken to induce pregnancy. (73:263) **Ojibwa** *Stimulant* Dried leaves used as a reviver. (130:375)

Lycopodium dendroideum, Tree Groundpine
Montagnais *Cathartic* and *Gastrointestinal Aid* Decoction of plant taken as a purgative "in case of biliousness." (133:316) **Penobscot** *Unspecified* Plant thought to have "some medicinal value." (133:309)

Lycopodium obscurum, Rare Clubmoss
Chippewa *Antirheumatic* (*External*) Compound decoction of moss used as herbal steam for rheumatism. (43:362) **Iroquois** *Blood Medicine* Cold, compound decoction taken for weak blood. *Gynecological Aid* Decoction of root taken for change of life and resulting blindness and deafness. (73:263) **Ojibwa** *Diuretic* Plant combined with *Diervilla lonicera* and taken as a diuretic. (130:375) **Potawatomi** *Hemostat* Spores of fruiting spikes used as a styptic and coagulant. (131:64)

Lycopodium sabinifolium, Savinleaf Groundpine
Iroquois *Venereal Aid* Compound decoction with plant taken for gonorrhea. (73:263)

Lycopus americanus, American Waterhorehound
Meskwaki *Analgesic* and *Gastrointestinal Aid* Compound containing entire plant used for stomach cramps. (129:225)

Lycopus asper, Rough Bugleweed
Iroquois *Laxative* and *Pediatric Aid* Decoction of plants given to children as a laxative. *Poison* Plant considered poisonous. (as *L. lucidus* ssp. *americanus* 73:427)

Lycopus virginicus, Virginia Waterhorehound
Cherokee *Ceremonial Medicine* Infusion taken at green corn ceremony. *Other* and *Pediatric Aid* Chewed root given to infants to give them "eloquence of speech." *Snakebite Remedy* Root chewed, a portion swallowed, the rest applied to snakebite wound. *Veterinary Aid* Decoction fed to snakebitten dog. (66:39) **Iroquois** *Poison* Roots and leaves considered poisonous. (73:426)

Lygodesmia grandiflora, Largeflower Skeletonplant
Gosiute *Veterinary Aid* Plant used as a horse

medicine. (31:374) **Hopi** *Gynecological Aid* Leaves chewed to increase mother's milk supply. (174:36, 97) **Navajo, Kayenta** *Dermatological Aid* Plant milk applied to sores caused by sunburn. (179:48)

Lygodesmia juncea, Rush Skeletonplant
Blackfoot *Cough Medicine* Infusion of stems taken for burning coughs. (72:72) *Dermatological Aid* Infusion of stems mixed with grease and applied as a hair tonic. (72:124) *Diuretic* Infusion of powdered galls taken as a diuretic. (72:70) *Gastrointestinal Aid* Decoction of plant taken for heartburn. (82:61) *Gynecological Aid* Decoction of plant taken for symptoms resembling heartburn caused by pregnancy. (72:61) *Kidney Aid* Infusion of plant taken for kidney trouble. (72:70) *Orthopedic Aid* Crushed stems used as foot pads in moccasins. (72:115) *Pediatric Aid* and *Tonic* Infusion of plant used as a general tonic for children. (72:67) *Veterinary Aid* Infusion of plant rubbed on saddle sores and leg wounds. Infusion of plant given to horses with coughs. (72:89) **Cheyenne** *Breast Treatment* Infusion of dried stems taken to increase milk flow. (68:27) *Gynecological Aid* Infusion of plants taken by women to increase the supply of milk. (63:191) Simple or compound decoction of plant taken to increase maternal milk flow. (63:41) Infusion of plant taken by women after childbirth to increase milk flow. (64:191) Infusion of stems taken by pregnant and nursing mothers to increase milk flow. (69:22) *Misc. Disease Remedy* Infusion of leaves taken for smallpox and measles. (63:191)

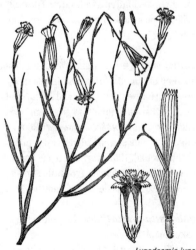

Lygodesmia juncea

Pediatric Aid Infusion of stems taken by pregnant and nursing mothers for a healthy baby. (69:22) *Psychological Aid* Infusion of dried stems taken to bring feelings of contentment to mothers. (68:27) **Keres, Western** *Antirheumatic (External)* Poultice of crushed plant, warmed with rocks, applied to swellings. (147:53) **Lakota** *Antidiarrheal* and *Pediatric Aid* Infusion of whole plant used for children with diarrhea. (116:38) **Omaha** *Eye Medicine* Infusion of stems used as a wash for sore eyes. *Gynecological Aid* Infusion of stems taken by nursing mothers to increase milk flow. (58:136) **Ponca** *Antidiarrheal* Infusion of plant taken for diarrhea. (80:152) *Eye Medicine* Infusion of stems used as a wash for sore eyes. (58:136) Infusion of plant applied to sore eyes. (80:152) *Gynecological Aid* Infusion of stems taken by nursing mothers to increase milk flow. (58:136) Infusion of plant used to increase milk flow of mothers. (80:152) **Sioux** *Eye Medicine* Infusion of dried stems used for sore eyes. *Gynecological Aid* Infusion of dried stems taken to increase milk flow. (68:27)

Lyonia mariana, Piedmont Staggerbush
Cherokee *Dermatological Aid* Infusion used for toe itch, "ground-itch," and ulcers. (66:57)

Lysichiton americanus, American Skunk-
    cabbage
Bella Coola *Gastrointestinal Aid* Decoction of root taken for stomach trouble. (as *L. kamtschatcense* 127:52, 53) **Clallam** *Dermatological Aid* Poultice of roots used for sores. (47:196) **Cowlitz** *Antirheumatic (External)* Poultice of heated blossoms applied to the body for rheumatism. (65:22) **Gitksan** *Antihemorrhagic* Compound containing root used as plaster on the chest for lung hemorrhages. *Antirheumatic (External)* Compound containing root used for rheumatism. Poultice applied or leaves sat on or lain on in sweat bath for rheumatism. *Antirheumatic (Internal)* Smoke of root inhaled for influenza, rheumatism, and bad dreams. *Dermatological Aid* Simple or compound poultice of mashed root applied for blood poisoning and boils. *Misc. Disease Remedy* Smoke from burning roots inhaled for influenza and bad dreams. *Poison* Roots considered poisonous. *Pulmonary Aid* Compound containing root used as plaster on the chest for lung hemorrhages. *Seda-*

tive Smoke of root inhaled for bad dreams, influenza, and rheumatism. (as *L. kamtschatcense* 127:52, 53) **Haisla & Hanaksiala** *Burn Dressing* Poultice of pounded root paste applied to burns. *Urinary Aid* Roots used experimentally for bloody urine. (35:189) **Hesquiat** *Burn Dressing* Poultice of cold and fresh leaves applied for burns. (160:78) *Dermatological Aid* Poultice of cool leaves used for bad burns. *Unspecified* Roots used as a medicine. (159:48) **Klallam** *Dermatological Aid* Poultice of baked roots applied to carbuncles. *Tuberculosis Remedy* Poultice of leaves applied to parts of the body sore with scrofula. (65:22) **Kwakiutl** *Dermatological Aid* Poultice of leaf, oil, down, and Douglas fir bark applied to carbuncles. (157:270) Heated leaves used to draw out thorns and splinters. Poultice of steamed, mashed roots applied to swellings. Poultice of washed, heated leaves applied to boils, carbuncles, and sores. Pulverized root rubbed into a child's head to make his hair grow. *Herbal Steam* Leaves used in a sweat bath for general weakness or undefined sickness. *Other* Leaves used in a sweat bath for undefined sickness. *Pediatric Aid* Pulverized root rubbed into a child's head to make his hair grow. *Stimulant* Leaves used in a sweat bath for general weakness. (157:271) **Makah** *Abortifacient* Raw root chewed by women to effect an abortion. (65:22) Roots chewed to induce an abortion. (160:78) *Analgesic* Poultice of warmed leaves applied for chest pain. (65:22) Warmed leaves applied to chest for pain. (160:78) *Antirheumatic (External)* Roots used for arthritis. (55:336) *Blood Medicine* Decoction of roots taken as a blood purifier. *Gastrointestinal Aid* Root chewed to soothe the stomach after taking an emetic. *Pulmonary Aid* Poultice of warmed leaves applied for chest pain. (65:22) *Unspecified* Roots used medicinally for unspecified purpose. (55:336) **Nitinaht** *Burn Dressing* Poultice of one leaf applied for severe burns. (160:78) **Quileute** *Analgesic* Leaves used for headaches. *Dermatological Aid* Poultice of leaves applied to cuts and swellings. *Febrifuge* Leaves used for fevers. *Gynecological Aid* Decoction of pounded root taken to bring about easy delivery. **Quinault** *Panacea* Poultice of leaves applied for many ailments. *Urinary Aid* Decoction of roots taken to clean out the bladder. **Samish** *Other* Infusion of roots used as a wash for invalids. (65:22) **Shuswap** *Analgesic* Poultice of

leaves applied for pain, particularly pains in the knees. *Dermatological Aid* Poultice of leaves applied to sores. *Orthopedic Aid* Poultice of leaves applied for pain, particularly pains in the knees. *Panacea* Cold infusion of roots taken for any sickness. (102:53) **Skokomish** *Analgesic* Leaves used for headaches. *Cathartic* Infusion of roots taken as a physic. *Dermatological Aid* Poultice of leaves applied to cuts and swellings. *Febrifuge* Leaves used for fevers. **Swinomish** *Other* Infusion of roots used as a wash for invalids. (65:22) **Thompson** *Dermatological Aid* Powdered, charred rhizome mixed with bear grease, used as an ointment for animal bites and infections. Charcoal used for wounds. The charcoal was applied four times, the fourth time being mixed with bear grease. *Psychological Aid* Leaves placed under pillows during sleep or the head washed with charcoal to induce "power dreams." (161:113) **Tolowa** *Antirheumatic (External)* Roots used in a steam for arthritis and lumbago. *Other* Roots used in a steam for stroke. **Yurok** *Antirheumatic (External)* Roots used in a steam for arthritis and lumbago. *Misc. Disease Remedy* Roots used in a steam for stroke. (5:38)

Lysimachia quadrifolia, Whorled Yellow
    Loosestrife
Cherokee *Gastrointestinal Aid* Decoction of root taken for "bowel trouble" and "kidney problems." *Gynecological Aid* Infusion taken for "female trouble." *Kidney Aid* Taken "for kidney problems." (66:43) *Urinary Aid* Infusion of roots taken for urinary troubles. (152:50) **Iroquois** *Emetic* Infusion of roots taken as an emetic. (73:411)

Lysimachia thyrsiflora, Tufted Loosestrife
Iroquois *Gynecological Aid* Compound decoction used as wash and applied as poultice to stop milk flow. (73:411)

Lythrum alatum var. *lanceolatum*, Winged
    Lythrum
Cherokee *Kidney Aid* Infusion taken "for kidneys." (as *L. lanceolatum* 66:43)

Lythrum californicum, California Loosestrife
Kawaiisu *Dermatological Aid* Plant used for washing hair. *Unspecified* Plant used medicinally. (180:40)

Lythrum salicaria, Purple Loosestrife
Iroquois *Febrifuge* and *Witchcraft Medicine*
Compound decoction of plants taken for fever and
sickness caused by the dead. (73:389)

 Machaeranthera alta, Purple
Aster
Navajo *Dermatological Aid* Plant
used as a rub on pimples. (45:88)

Machaeranthera canescens ssp. cane-
scens var. canescens, Cutleaf Goldenweed
Navajo *Nose Medicine* Dried and pulverized plant
used as a snuff for nose troubles. *Throat Aid* Dried
and pulverized plant used as a snuff for throat
troubles. (as *Aster canescens* 45:82) **Okanagan-**
Colville *Witchcraft Medicine* Used for witchcraft.
(as *Aster canescens* 162:79) **Zuni** *Emetic* Infusion of whole plant taken and rubbed on abdomen
as an emetic. (as *M. glabella* 143:56)

Machaeranthera canescens ssp. cane-
scens var. leucanthemifolia, Whiteflower
Machaeranthera
Paiute *Throat Aid* Poultice of mashed leaves
applied to swollen jaw or neck glands. **Shoshoni**
Analgesic Decoction of fresh or dried leaves taken
for headaches. *Blood Medicine* Decoction of whole
plant taken as a blood tonic. *Cathartic* Warm infusion of plant tops taken as a physic. *Eye Medicine*
Infusion of scraped roots taken as an eyewash.
Tonic Decoction of whole plant taken as a blood
tonic. (as *Aster leucanthemifolius* 155:49)

Machaeranthera canescens ssp. glabra
var. aristata, Hoary Tansyaster
Hopi *Gynecological Aid* Decoction of plant taken
by parturient women for any disorder. (as *Aster
cichoriaceus* 174:36, 94) *Stimulant* Decoction of
plant taken as a strong stimulant. (as *Aster cichoriaceus* 174:31, 94)

Machaeranthera gracilis, Slender Goldenweed
Navajo, **Ramah** *Dermatological Aid* Cold infusion used as lotion for pimples, boils, and sores.
Eye Medicine Cold, compound infusion of plant
used as an eyewash. *Internal Medicine* Decoction

of plant taken for internal injury. *Respiratory Aid*
Plant used as snuff to cause sneezing, clearing
congested nose. (as *Aplopappus gracilis* 165:47)

Machaeranthera grindelioides var.
grindelioides, Rayless Aster
Hopi *Cough Medicine* Decoction of root taken for
cough. (as *Aplopappus nuttallii* 174:35, 94)

Machaeranthera parviflora, Smallflower
Tansyaster
Navajo *Cathartic* Plant used as a purgative. (as
Aster parviflorus 76:148)

Machaeranthera pinnatifida ssp. pinnati-
fida, Lacy Tansyaster
Navajo *Analgesic* Plant or some part of it used for
headaches. (as *Haplopappus spinulosus* **ssp.** *typ-
icus* 76:151)

Machaeranthera tanacetifolia, Tanseyleaf
Aster
Hopi *Gynecological Aid* Decoction of plant taken
by parturient women for any disorder. (as *Aster
tanacetifolius* 174:36, 94) *Stimulant* Decoction
of plant taken as a strong stimulant. (as *Aster tanacetifolius* 174:31, 94) **Navajo**, **Ramah** *Gastrointestinal Aid* Decoction of whole plant taken for
stomachache. *Respiratory Aid* Dried root used as
snuff to cause sneezing to relieve congested nose.
(as *Aster tanacetifolius* 165:49) **Zuni** *Unspecified*
Infusion of flowers taken with other flowers for
unspecified illnesses. (22:375)

Maclura pomifera, Osage Orange
Comanche *Eye Medicine* Decoction of root used
as a wash for sore eyes. (24:522)

Macranthera sp.
Jemez *Veterinary Aid* Decoction of plant given to
horses with blood poisoning. (36:25)

Macromeria viridiflora, Gianttrumpets
Hopi *Anticonvulsive* Dried plant and mullein
smoked for "fits," craziness, and witchcraft. (as
Onosmodium thurberi 174:33, 88) *Psychological
Aid* Compound of plant smoked by persons not in
their "right mind." *Witchcraft Medicine* Compound of plant smoked as a cure for persons with

"power to charm." (as *Onosmodium thurberi* 174:88)

Madia glomerata, Mountain Tarweed
Cheyenne *Ceremonial Medicine* Dried plant used in special ceremony for perverted, oversexed people. *Herbal Steam* Infusion of stems and leaves taken and used as a steam bath for venereal disease. *Love Medicine* Dried plant aroma used as a love medicine to attract a woman. *Psychological Aid* Dried plant used for perverted, oversexed people. *Venereal Aid* Infusion of stems and leaves taken and used as a steam bath for venereal disease. (69:22) **Crow** *Ceremonial Medicine* Dried herbs burned as incense in some ceremonies. (15:15)

Magnolia acuminata, Cucumber Tree
Cherokee *Analgesic* Infusion of bark taken for stomachache or cramps. *Antidiarrheal* Compound medicine containing bark taken for "bloody flux." *Gastrointestinal Aid* Infusion of bark used for toothache. Used in steam bath for "indigestion or biliousness with swelling abdomen." *Respiratory Aid* Hot infusion of bark snuffed for sinus and used for toothache. *Toothache Remedy* Warm compound decoction of bark held in mouth for toothache. (66:44) **Iroquois** *Anthelmintic* Compound decoction taken by men for worms caused by venereal disease. *Toothache Remedy* Infusion of inner bark "chewed" for toothaches. *Venereal Aid* Compound decoction taken by men for worms caused by venereal disease. (73:330)

Magnolia grandiflora, Southern Magnolia
Choctaw *Dermatological Aid* Decoction of bark used as wash for prickly heat itching. (20:23) Decoction of plant used as a bath for prickly heat. *Kidney Aid* Infusion of mashed bark used as a steam bath for dropsy. **Koasati** *Dermatological Aid* Decoction of bark used as a wash for sores. (152:23)

Magnolia macrophylla, Bigleaf Magnolia
Cherokee *Analgesic* Infusion of bark taken for stomachache or cramps. *Antidiarrheal* Compound medicine containing bark taken for "bloody flux." *Gastrointestinal Aid* Infusion of bark taken for stomachache or cramps. Used in steam bath for

"indigestion or biliousness with swelling abdomen." *Respiratory Aid* Hot infusion of bark snuffed for sinus and used for toothache. *Toothache Remedy* Warm compound decoction of bark held in mouth for toothache. (66:44)

Magnolia virginiana, Sweet Bay
Houma *Blood Medicine* Decoction of leaves and twigs taken to warm the blood. *Cold Remedy* Decoction of leaves and twigs taken for colds. *Febrifuge* Decoction of leaves and twigs taken for chills. (135:56) **Rappahannock** *Hallucinogen* Leaves or bark placed in cupped hands over nose and inhaled as "mild dope." (as *M. glauca*, laurel *138*:28)

Mahonia aquifolium, Hollyleaved Barberry
Blackfoot *Antihemorrhagic* Decoction of root used for hemorrhages. *Gastrointestinal Aid* Decoction of root used for stomach trouble. (as *Berberis aquifolium* 95:275) **Karok** *Misc. Disease Remedy* Leaves and roots used as a steam bath for "yellow fever." (as *Berberis aquifolium* 125:383) *Other* Fruits, if eaten, caused diarrhea. (5:38) *Panacea* Decoction of roots taken as a good medicine for all kinds of sickness. *Poison* Plant considered poisonous. (as *Berberis aquifolium* 125:383) **Keres, Western** *Other* Plant chewed for sickness that occurred during hunting when approached by a dying deer. *Preventive Medicine* Infusion of leaves used to prevent sickness that occurred while hunting and approached by dying deer (as *Berberis aquifolium* 147:32) **Nitinaht** *Laxative* Used as a laxative. (160:98) *Tuberculosis Remedy* Used with

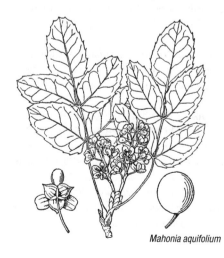

Mahonia aquifolium

hemlock and alder as drink for tuberculosis. *Unspecified* Bark used medicinally. (as *Berbaris aquifolium* 55:254) **Okanagan-Colville** *Blood Medicine* Decoction of branches and chokecherry branches taken for the "changing of the blood." Infusion of branches taken as a blood tonic. *Eye Medicine* Infusion of plant used to wash out blurry or bloodshot eyes. *Kidney Aid* Roots used to make a tonic for the kidneys. Decoction of roots and chokecherry or kinnikinnick branches taken for bad kidneys. (as *Berberis aquifolium* 162:85) **Samish** *Tonic* Infusion of roots taken as a general tonic. (as *Berberis aquifolium* 65:30) **Sanpoil** *Antiemetic* Decoction of stem tips taken for vomiting. *Eye Medicine* Infusion of root parts used as a wash for the eyes. *Gastrointestinal Aid* Decoction of stem tips taken "to relieve a disturbed stomach." *Tuberculosis Remedy* Decoction of roots used for tuberculosis. (as *Berberis aquifolium* 109:219) **Squaxin** *Blood Medicine* Infusion of roots taken to purify the blood. *Throat Aid* Infusion of roots used as a gargle for sore throats. **Swinomish** *Tonic* Infusion of roots taken as a general tonic. (as *Berberis aquifolium* 65:30) **Thompson** *Antirheumatic* (*External*) Decoction of peeled, chopped root bark used as a wash for arthritis. *Antirheumatic* (*Internal*) Decoction of peeled, chopped root bark taken for arthritis. *Blood Medicine* Decoction of peeled, chopped root bark taken as a blood tonic. *Eye Medicine* Infusion of stems and bark used to make an eyewash for red, itchy eyes. *Laxative* Fruit considered an "excellent laxative." *Tonic* Fruit eaten as a "tonic." *Venereal Aid* Decoction of peeled, chopped roots taken for syphilis. (161:187)

Mahonia dictyota, Shining Netvein Barberry **Kawaiisu** *Venereal Aid* Decoction of roots taken for gonorrhea. (as *Berberis dictyota* 180:15)

Mahonia fremontii, Frémont's Mahonia **Apache**, **White Mountain** *Ceremonial Medicine* Plant used for ceremonial purposes. (as *Berberis fremontii* 113:155) **Hopi** *Oral Aid* Plant used for gums. (as *Odostemon fremontii* 174:33, 76) **Hualapai** *Gastrointestinal Aid* Roots used as a bitter tonic to promote digestion. *Laxative* Roots made into a bitter tonic and used as a laxative.

Liver Aid Roots used as a bitter tonic for the liver. (as *Berberis fermontii* 169:5)

Mahonia haematocarpa, Red Barberry **Apache**, **Mescalero** *Eye Medicine* Inner wood shavings soaked in water and used as an eyewash. (as *Berberis haematocarpa* 10:49)

Mahonia nervosa, Cascade Oregongrape **Nitinaht** *Laxative* Used as a laxative. (160:98) **Thompson** *Antirheumatic* (*External*) Decoction of peeled, chopped root bark used as wash for arthritis. *Antirheumatic* (*Internal*) Decoction of peeled, chopped root bark taken for arthritis. *Blood Medicine* Decoction of peeled, chopped root bark taken as a blood tonic. *Eye Medicine* Infusion of woody stems and bark used as an eyewash for red, itchy eyes. *Laxative* Fruit considered an "excellent laxative." *Psychological Aid* Plant induced dreams of someone sleeping when brought into the house. *Venereal Aid* Decoction of peeled, chopped roots taken for syphilis. (161:187)

Mahonia nervosa* var. *nervosa, Cascade Oregongrape **Hoh** *Blood Medicine* Infusion of roots used as a blood remedy. (as *Berberis nervosa* 114:61) **Nitinaht** *Tuberculosis Remedy* Used with hemlock and alder as drink for tuberculosis. *Unspecified* Bark used medicinally. (as *Berbaris nervosa* 55:254) **Paiute** *Blood Medicine* Infusion of roots and leaves taken as a general tonic "to make the blood good." *Hemostat* Infusion of roots and leaves taken as a general tonic for nosebleeds. (as *Berberis nervosa* 93:72) **Quileute** *Blood Medicine* Infusion of roots used as a blood remedy. (as *Berberis nervosa* 114:61) **Skagit** *Venereal Aid* Decoction of roots taken for venereal disease. (as *Berberis nervosa* 65:30)

Mahonia pinnata* ssp. *pinnata, California Barberry **Miwok** *Antirheumatic* (*Internal*) Decoction of root taken for rheumatism. *Dermatological Aid* Chewed root liquid placed on cuts, wounds, and abrasions to prevent swelling. Decoction of root used as a wash for cuts and bruises. (as *Berberis pinnata* 8:168) *Gastrointestinal Aid* Decoction of root taken for heartburn. *Misc. Disease Remedy*

Decoction of root taken for ague. (as *Berberis pinnata* 8:167) Leaves chewed as a preventative of ague. *Tuberculosis Remedy* Decoction of roots taken for consumption. (as *Berberis pinnata* 8:168)

Mahonia pumila, Dwarf Barberry
Karok *Tonic* Root used in a tonic. **Tolowa** *Blood Medicine* Roots used in a concoction for blood purification. *Cough Medicine* Roots used in a concoction for coughs. (5:38)

Mahonia repens, Oregongrape
Blackfoot *Antihemorrhagic* Decoction of roots used for hemorrhages. (as *Berberis repens* 98:45) *Dermatological Aid* Poultice of fresh berries applied to boils. Infusion of roots applied to boils. (as *Berberis repens* 72:75) *Disinfectant* Infusion of roots applied as an antiseptic to wounds. (as *Berberis repens* 72:83) *Gastrointestinal Aid* Decoction of roots used for stomach trouble. (as *Berberis repens* 98:45) *Kidney Aid* Infusion of berries used for kidney troubles. (as *Berberis repens* 72:66) *Veterinary Aid* Berries mixed with water and given to horses with coughs. Infusion or roots used for body sores on horses. (as *Berberis repens* 72:88) **Cheyenne** *Unspecified* Fruit used in medicinal preparations. (as *Berberis repens* 69:15) **Flathead** *Antirheumatic* (*External*) Infusion of roots used for rheumatism. *Contraceptive* Infusion of roots used as a contraceptive. *Cough Medicine* Infusion of roots used for coughs. *Dermatological Aid* Roots crushed and used for wounds and cuts. *Gynecological Aid* Infusion of roots used for delivery of the placenta. *Venereal Aid* Infusion of roots taken for gonorrhea and syphilis. (as *Berberis repens* 68:18) **Great Basin Indian** *Antidiarrheal* Infusion of roots taken for dysentery. *Blood Medicine* Infusion of roots taken to thicken the blood for bleeders. (as *Berberis repens* 100:47) **Havasupai** *Analgesic* Cooled decoction of roots taken three times a day for headaches. *Antirheumatic* (*External*) Cooled decoction of roots used as a wash for aches. *Cold Remedy* Cooled decoction of roots used as a wash for colds. *Gastrointestinal Aid* Cooled decoction of roots taken three times a day for stomach upsets. *Laxative* Cooled decoction of roots taken as a laxative for colds and stomach ailments. *Pediatric Aid* and

Unspecified Cooled decoction of roots given to sick babies. (as *Berberis repens* 171:219) **Kutenai** *Blood Medicine* Taken to "enrich" the blood. *Kidney Aid* Infusion of roots taken for kidney trouble. (as *Berberis repens* 68:18) **Mendocino Indian** *Blood Medicine* Decoction of root bark taken as a blood purifier. *Gastrointestinal Aid* Decoction of root bark taken for stomach troubles. (as *Berberis repens* 33:348) **Montana Indian** *Febrifuge* Decoction of root bark used for mountain fever. *Gastrointestinal Aid* Decoction of root bark used for stomach trouble. *Kidney Aid* Decoction of root bark used for kidney trouble. *Tonic* Decoction of root bark used as a tonic. (as *Berberis repens* 15:8) **Navajo** *Antirheumatic* (*Internal*) Decoction of leaves and twigs taken for rheumatic stiffness. (as *Berberis repens* 45:48) **Navajo, Kayenta** *Panacea* Infusion of plant taken and poultice of plant applied as a cure-all. (as *Berberis repens* 179:23) **Navajo, Ramah** *Ceremonial Medicine* Whole plant used as a ceremonial emetic. *Dermatological Aid* Cold infusion of plant used as a lotion on scorpion bites. *Emetic* Whole plant used as a ceremonial emetic. *Laxative* Decoction of root used for constipation. (as *Berberis repens* 165:28) **Paiute** *Antidiarrheal* Decoction of root taken to prevent or stop bloody dysentery. *Blood Medicine* Decoction of root taken as a blood tonic or purifier. Decoction of root taken to "thicken the blood of haemophilic persons." *Cough Medicine* Decoction of root, sometimes with whisky, taken for coughs. *Gastrointestinal Aid* Decoction of stems taken as a tonic for stomach troubles. *Urinary Aid* Decoction of root taken for bladder difficulties. (as *Berberis repens* 155: 51, 52) *Venereal Aid* Decoction of roots taken for venereal disease. (as *Berberis repens* 87:198) Decoction of roots taken for venereal diseases. **Shoshoni** *Analgesic* Decoction of leaves taken or root used for general aches or rheumatic pains. *Antidiarrheal* Decoction of root taken to prevent or stop bloody dysentery. *Antirheumatic* (*Internal*) Decoction of roots or leaves taken for general aches or rheumatic pains. *Blood Medicine* Infusion or decoction of root taken as a blood tonic or purifier. *Cough Medicine* Decoction of root, sometimes with whisky, taken for coughs. *Kidney Aid* Decoction of root taken as a kidney medicine. *Venereal Aid* Decoction of roots taken for venereal diseases.

(as *Berberis repens* 155:51, 52) **Shuswap** *Blood Medicine* Decoction of leaves and stems taken as a blood tonic. (as *Berberis repens* 102:59)

Maianthemum canadense, Canada Beadruby
Iroquois *Kidney Aid* Compound decoction of roots taken for the kidneys. (73:284) **Montagnais** *Analgesic* Infusion of plant taken for headache. (133:314) **Ojibwa** *Analgesic* Plant used for headache and sore throat. *Gynecological Aid* and *Kidney Aid* Plant used "to keep the kidneys open during pregnancy." *Throat Aid* Plant used for sore throat and headache. *Unspecified* Smoke inhaled for unspecified purpose. (130:373, 374) **Potawatomi** *Throat Aid* Root used for sore throat. (131:62, 63)

Maianthemum dilatatum, Twoleaf False
　　Solomon's Seal
Hesquiat *Dermatological Aid* Poultice of whole or mashed leaves used for boils and cuts. *Tuberculosis Remedy* Fruit used as a good medicine for tuberculosis. (159:55) **Makah** *Reproductive Aid* Chewed roots taken to correct sterility. (65:25) **Nitinaht** *Burn Dressing* Poultice of leaves used for minor burns. *Dermatological Aid* Poultice of leaves used for sores, boils, cuts, and wounds. (160:86) **Oweekeno** *Dermatological Aid* Poultice of water-soaked, bruised leaves applied to wounds. (35:78) **Quinault** *Eye Medicine* Infusion of pounded roots used as a wash for sore eyes. (65:25) Poultice of chewed roots applied to sore eyes. (as *M. bifolium* 175:276)

Maianthemum racemosum ssp. *amplexicaule*, Western Solomon's Seal
Karok *Dermatological Aid* and *Pediatric Aid* Poultice of root applied to the severed umbilical cord of child. (as *Smilacina amplexicaulis* 125:381)

Maianthemum racemosum ssp. *racemosum*, Feather Solomon's Seal
Abnaki *Antihemorrhagic* Used by men for spitting up blood. Used for spitting up blood. (as *Smilacina racemosa* 121:154) Decoction of plant taken for spitting up blood. (as *Smilacina racemosa* 121:174) **Algonquin, Quebec** *Antirheumatic* (*Internal*) Infusion of plant used as a tea for sore backs.

(as *Smilacina racemosa* 14:139) **Cherokee** *Eye Medicine* Cold infusion of root used as a wash for sore eyes. (as *Smilacina racemosa* 66:56) **Chippewa** *Analgesic* Compound decoction of root taken for back pain. (as *Vagnera racemosa* 43:356) Burning root fumes inhaled for headaches and pain. (as *Smilacina racemosa* 59:125) *Gynecological Aid* Compound decoction of root taken for "female weakness." (as *Vagnera racemosa* 43:356) **Costanoan** *Contraceptive* Decoction of leaves used as a contraceptive. (as *Smilacina racemosa* 17:28) **Delaware, Oklahoma** *Tonic* Compound containing root used as a tonic. (as *Smilacina racemosa* 150:80) **Gitksan** *Antirheumatic* (*Internal*) Decoction of root, a very strong medicine, taken for rheumatism. *Cathartic* Decoction of root, a very strong medicine, taken as a purgative. *Dermatological Aid* Poultice of mashed roots bound on cuts. *Kidney Aid* Decoction of root taken for sore back and kidney trouble. *Orthopedic Aid* Decoction of roots taken as a very strong medicine for sore back. (as *Smilacina racemosa* 127:53) **Iroquois** *Anthelmintic* Compound infusion with whisky taken for tapeworms. (as *Smilacina racemosa* 73:284) *Antidote* Compound infusion taken as remedy for poison. *Antirheumatic* (*External*) Compound infusion used as foot soak. *Antirheumatic* (*Internal*) Compound decoction taken for rheumatism. (as *Smilacina racemosa* 73:283) *Blood Medicine* Compound infusion with whisky taken as a blood remedy. (as *Smilacina racemosa* 73:284) *Dermatological Aid* Poultice used for

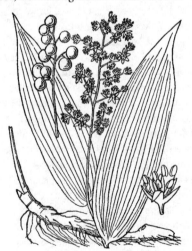

Maianthemum racemosum ssp. *racemosum*

swellings. (as *Smilacina racemosa* 73:283) *Gynecological Aid* Compound decoction of roots used "when woman has miscarriage." (as *Smilacina racemosa* 73:284) *Hunting Medicine* Cold, compound infusion used to "get a fish on each hook, every cast." *Other* Compound decoction of roots used as a "rooster fighting medicine." *Snakebite Remedy* Roots bound to spoiled snakebites. (as *Smilacina racemosa* 73:283) *Witchcraft Medicine* Compound used for witching. (as *Smilacina racemosa* 73:284) **Kitasoo** *Unspecified* Plant used for medicinal purposes. (as *Smilacina racemosa* 35:321) **Malecite** *Dermatological Aid* Leaves and stalks boiled and used for rashes or itching. (as *Smilacina racemosa* 96:250) **Menominee** *Herbal Steam* and *Respiratory Aid* Root used in herbal steam inhaled for catarrh. (as *Smilacina racemosa* 128:41) **Meskwaki** *Anticonvulsive* Smudge of root used in cases of a fit, to bring back to normal. *Ceremonial Medicine* Root used in meeting when medicine man wants to perform trick or cast spells. *Laxative* Compound containing root used to loosen the bowels. *Misc. Disease Remedy* Root cooked in kettle to prevent sickness during time of plague. *Pediatric Aid* Smudge used "to hush a crying child." *Psychological Aid* Smudge of root used in cases of insanity, to bring back to normal. *Sedative* Smudge used "to hush a crying child." *Stimulant* Smudge used to "smoke patient for five minutes" and revive him. *Veterinary Aid* Root mixed with food fed to hogs to prevent hog cholera. (as *Smilacina racemosa* 129:230, 231) **Micmac** *Dermatological Aid* Leaves and stems used for rashes and itch. (as *Smilacina racemosa* 32:62) **Mohegan** *Cough Medicine* Infusion of leaves used for cough. (as *Smilacina racemosa* 149:265) Infusion of leaves used as a cough remedy. (as *Smilacina racemosa* 151:75, 132) *Gastrointestinal Aid* Infusion of root used for "a stronger stomach." (as *Smilacina racemosa* 149:265) Infusion of root taken for stomach disorders. (as *Smilacina racemosa* 151:75, 132) *Tonic* Complex compound infusion including spikenard root taken as spring tonic. (as *Smilacina racemosa* 149:266) **Ojibwa** *Analgesic* Compound containing root used for headache. *Gynecological Aid* and *Kidney Aid* Compound containing root taken "to keep kidneys open during pregnancy." *Stimulant* Root used as a reviver. *Throat Aid* Compound containing root

used for sore throat. (as *Smilacina racemosa* 130:374) **Ojibwa, South** *Analgesic* Roots used as an inhalant for headache. *Gynecological Aid* Decoction of leaves used by "lying-in women." *Hemostat* Poultice of crushed, fresh leaves applied to bleeding cuts. (as *Smilacina racemosa* 77:199) **Okanagan-Colville** *Cold Remedy* Decoction of rhizomes taken for colds. *Dietary Aid* Decoction of rhizomes taken to increase the appetite. (as *Smilacina racemosa* 162:48) **Potawatomi** *Stimulant* Root smudged on coals and used to revive comatose patient. (as *Smilacina racemosa* 131:63) **Shuswap** *Blood Medicine* Decoction of roots taken as a blood purifier. (as *Smilacina racemosa* 102:55) **Thompson** *Analgesic* Compound decoction of root taken for internal pains. (as *Vagnera racemosa* 141:459) *Antirheumatic* (*Internal*) Decoction of leaves taken two or three times a day for rheumatism. *Cancer Treatment* Decoction of rhizomes taken in several doses over a period of several days for cancer. (as *Smilacina racemosa* 161:127) *Gastrointestinal Aid* Decoction of rhizomes taken as a stomach medicine. *Gynecological Aid* Decoction of rhizomes taken during the menstrual period. (as *Vagnera racemosa* 141:458) Decoction of leaves and roots taken during pregnancy for internal soreness. *Heart Medicine* Decoction of rhizomes taken in several doses over a period of several days for heart trouble. *Throat Aid* Decoction of rhizomes taken for a sore or ulcerated throat. The decoction was taken in several doses over a period of several days. (as *Smilacina racemosa* 161:127)

Maianthemum stellatum, Starry False
    Solomon's Seal
Delaware *Cathartic* Roots combined with others and used to cleanse the system. *Gastrointestinal Aid* Roots combined with others and used to stimulate the stomach. *Gynecological Aid* Roots combined with others and used for leukorrhea. (as *Smilacina stellata* 151:38) **Delaware, Oklahoma** *Cathartic* Compound containing root taken to "cleanse the system." (as *Smilacina stellata* 150:32, 80) *Gastrointestinal Aid* Compound containing root taken to stimulate the stomach and cleanse the system. (as *Smilacina stellata* 150:32) *Gynecological Aid* Compound containing root taken for leukorrhea. *Stimulant* Compound contain-

ing root taken to "stimulate the stomach." (as *Smilacina stellata* 150:32, 80) *Tuberculosis Remedy* Root used alone or in compound for scrofula. *Venereal Aid* Root used alone or in compound for venereal disease. (as *Smilacina stellata* 150:80) **Gosiute** *Antirheumatic* (*External*) Pounded roots rubbed on limbs affected by rheumatism. (as *Smilacina stellata* 31:382) **Iroquois** *Gynecological Aid* Compound infusion taken for stricture caused when a woman has her changes. (as *Smilacina stellata* 73:283) **Navajo, Kayenta** *Ceremonial Medicine* Plant used in the Fire Dance. (as *Smilacina stellata* 179:17) **Navajo, Ramah** *Ceremonial Medicine* and *Emetic* Decoction of plant used as a ceremonial emetic. (as *Smilacina stellata* 165:20) **Paiute** *Cough Medicine* Exudate from plant used as a cough syrup. *Dermatological Aid* Poultice of fresh or dried roots applied to boils or swellings. *Ear Medicine* Pulped root squeezed into ear for earache. *Eye Medicine* Infusion of root used as a wash for eye inflammations. *Gastrointestinal Aid* Decoction of root taken for stomach trouble. *Gynecological Aid* Decoction of root taken to regulate menstrual disorders. *Orthopedic Aid* Poultice of fresh or dried roots applied to sprains. **Shoshoni** *Eye Medicine* Infusion of root used as a wash for eye inflammations. *Gastrointestinal Aid* Decoction of root taken for stomach trouble. *Gynecological Aid* Decoction of leaf taken daily for a week by women as a contraceptive. Decoction of root taken to regulate menstrual disorders. *Venereal Aid* Decoction of root taken for venereal disease. (as *Smilacina stellata* 155:139, 140) **Thompson** *Analgesic* Compound decoction of roots taken for internal pains. (as *Vagnera stellata* 141:459) *Antirheumatic* (*Internal*) Decoction of leaves taken two or three times a day for rheumatism. *Cold Remedy* Decoction of crushed, dried leaves and fruits taken for colds. (as *Smilacina stellata* 161:129) **Washo** *Blood Medicine* and *Dermatological Aid* Infusion of root used as an antiseptic wash in cases of blood poisoning. *Hemostat* Powdered root applied to bleeding wounds. *Tonic* Decoction of root taken as a tonic. (as *Smilacina stellata* 155:139, 140)

Malacothrix fendleri, Fendler's Desert-
　dandelion
Navajo, Ramah *Dermatological Aid* Poultice of

leaves applied to sores. *Eye Medicine* Cold infusion used as wash for sore eyes. (165:52)

Malacothrix glabrata, Smooth Desert-
　dandelion
Apache, White Mountain *Blood Medicine* Roots used as a blood medicine. (113:158)

Malacothrix sonchoides, Sowthistle Desert-
　dandelion
Navajo, Kayenta *Antiemetic* Plant used for vomiting. (179:49)

Malaxis unifolia, Green Addersmouth Orchid
Ojibwa *Diuretic* Compound containing root used as a diuretic. (as *Microstylis unifolia* 130:377)

Malus coronaria, Sweet Crabapple
Cherokee *Gastrointestinal Aid* Infusion of bark taken for gallstones and piles and infusion used for sore mouth. *Hemorrhoid Remedy* Infusion of bark taken for gallstones and "piles" and infusion used for sore mouth. *Oral Aid* Infusion of bark taken for gallstones and infusion used as a wash for sore mouth. (66:31)

Malus coronaria* var. *coronaria, Sweet
　Crabapple
Iroquois *Abortifacient* Decoction of roots taken for suppressed menses. (as *Pyrus coronaria* 73:351) *Dermatological Aid* Cold infusion of bark used as wash for black eyes. *Eye Medicine* Cold infusion of bark used as wash for snow-blindness and black or sore eyes. *Gynecological Aid* Cold, compound infusion of twig bark taken for difficult birth. *Tuberculosis Remedy* Compound decoction of roots taken for consumption. (as *Pyrus coronaria* 73:350)

Malus fusca, Oregon Crabapple
Bella Coola *Eye Medicine* Compound decoction of bark or root used as an eyewash for soreness. (as *Pyrus diversifolia* 127:60) **Cowichan** *Panacea* Infusion of bark and wild cherry bark taken as a cure-all tonic. (as *Pyrus fusca* 156:87) **Gitksan** *Antirheumatic* (*Internal*) Decoction of trunk and branch or inner bark taken for rheumatism. *Dietary Aid* Decoction of trunk, branches, or inner bark taken as a "fattening medicine." *Diuretic* De-

coction of trunk and branches or inner bark taken as a laxative and diuretic. *Eye Medicine* Juice, scraped from peeled trunk, used as an eye medicine. *Laxative* Decoction of trunk and branch or inner bark taken as a laxative and diuretic. *Tuberculosis Remedy* Decoction of trunk and branch or inner bark taken for consumption. (as *Pyrus diversifolia* 127:60) **Haisla & Hanaksiala** *Antirheumatic* (*Internal*) Fruit eaten after a long day of hunting, "kills poison in muscles." *Ceremonial Medicine* Afterbirth of a child tied to a young tree to ensure the child would grow up strong. (35:265) **Hoh** *Venereal Aid* Infusion used for gonorrhea. (as *Pyrus diversifolia* 114:64) **Klallam** *Eye Medicine* Infusion of bark used as an eyewash. (as *Pyrus diversifolia* 65:38) **Kwakiutl** *Antihemorrhagic* Shredded bark used for blood-spitting. *Dermatological Aid* Tree used for eczema or skin troubles. (as *Pyrus fusca* 157:290) **Makah** *Antidiarrheal* Infusion of bark taken for dysentery and diarrhea. (as *Pyrus diversifolia* 65:38) *Blood Medicine* Bark used as a "blood purifier" and it "puts something in your blood that cuts down the clots." (as *Pyrus fusca* 55:268) *Dermatological Aid* Poultice of chewed bark applied to wounds. (as *Pyrus diversifolia* 65:38) *Gastrointestinal Aid* Bark used for ulcers. (as *Pyrus fusca* 55:268) Infusion of bark taken for intestinal disorders. (as *Pyrus diversifolia* 65:38) *Heart Medicine* Bark used for the heart. *Internal Medicine* Bark used for any internal ailment. Bark used for internal organs. *Laxative* Bark of larger trees used as a laxative. *Orthopedic Aid* Used for fractures. *Panacea* Bark used for any illness and considered a complete medicine, all in itself. (as *Pyrus fusca* 55:268) *Pulmonary Aid* Soaked leaves chewed for lung trouble. (as *Pyrus diversifolia* 65:38) Leaves chewed for lung trouble. (as *Pyrus fusca* 160:121) *Tonic* Used as a tonic. (as *Pyrus fusca* 55:268) Infusion of bark used as a tonic. (as *Pyrus fusca* 160:121) *Tuberculosis Remedy* Used for tuberculosis. *Unspecified* Bark used to make the most popular and healing medicine. (as *Pyrus fusca* 55:268) **Nitinaht** *Cough Medicine* Infusion of bark taken for coughs. *Dietary Aid* Infusion of bark taken for losing weight. *Panacea* Infusion of bark taken for "any kind of sickness." (as *Pyrus fusca* 160:121) *Tonic* Bark and roots used as a tonic for young men in training. Used as a tonic to "repair the

damage done by the elder" during puberty rites. *Unspecified* Used as a medicine. (as *Pyrus fusca* 55:268) **Oweekeno** *Oral Aid* Bark chewed by hunters to suppress thirst. (35:109) **Quileute** *Pulmonary Aid* Infusion of bark taken for lung trouble. (as *Pyrus diversifolia* 65:38) *Venereal Aid* Infusion used for gonorrhea. (as *Pyrus diversifolia* 114:64) **Quinault** *Analgesic* and *Blood Medicine* Infusion of bark taken for "soreness inside, for it is throughout the blood." *Eye Medicine* Infusion of bark used as an eyewash. (as *Pyrus diversifolia* 65:38) **Saanich** *Panacea* Infusion of bark and wild cherry bark taken as a cure-all tonic. (as *Pyrus fusca* 156:87) **Samish** *Dermatological Aid* Decoction of bark used as a wash for cuts. *Gastrointestinal Aid* Decoction of bark taken for stomach disorders. **Swinomish** *Dermatological Aid* Decoction of bark used as a wash for cuts. *Gastrointestinal Aid* Decoction of bark taken for stomach disorders. (as *Pyrus diversifolia* 65:38) **Thompson** *Analgesic* Decoction of bark and cascara bark taken for sciatica. (161:262)

Malus ioensis* var. *ioensis, Prairie Crabapple
Meskwaki *Misc. Disease Remedy* Used 50 years ago for smallpox. (as *Pyrus ioensis* 129:242)

Malus pumila, Cultivated Apple
Cherokee *Gastrointestinal Aid* and *Hemorrhoid Remedy* Infusion of bark taken for gallstones and "piles." *Pulmonary Aid* Used with other ingredients to give ballplayers wind during the game. *Throat Aid* Infusion of inner bark used for lost voice and used as an ingredient in drink for dry throat. (66:23)

Malus sylvestris, Apple
Cherokee *Throat Aid* Decoction of inner bark taken to loosen phlegm for hoarseness. (as *Pyrus malus* 152:29) **Iroquois** *Ear Medicine* Decoction of bark used as drops for earaches. *Eye Medicine* Compound poultice of bark and fruit peelings used for black eyes. Compound infusion of bark and leaves used as drops for blindness. *Orthopedic Aid* Compound poultice of bark and fruit peelings used for bruises. (as *Pyrus malus* 73:350)

Malva moschata, Musk Mallow
Iroquois *Febrifuge* Infusion of plant taken for

chills. *Stimulant* Infusion of plant taken for lassitude. (73:385)

Malva neglecta, Common Mallow
Cherokee *Dermatological Aid* Flowers put in oil and mixed with tallow for use on sores. (66:44) **Iroquois** *Dermatological Aid* Compound infusion of plants applied as poultice to swellings of all kinds. (73:384) *Emetic* Infusion of smashed plant taken to vomit for a love medicine. *Gastrointestinal Aid* Compound decoction of plants applied as poultice to baby's swollen stomach. *Love Medicine* Infusion of smashed plant taken to vomit for a love medicine. *Orthopedic Aid* Cold, compound infusion of leaves applied as poultice to broken bones. Compound decoction of plants applied as poultice to baby's sore back. *Pediatric Aid* Compound decoction of plants applied to baby's swollen stomach or sore back. (73:385) **Mahuna** *Analgesic* Plant used for painful congestion of the stomach. *Gastrointestinal Aid* Plant used for painful congestion of the stomach. (as *M. rotundifolia* 117:8) **Navajo, Ramah** *Other* Cold infusion of plant taken and used as a lotion for injury or swelling. (165:36)

Malva nicaeensis, Bull Mallow
Costanoan *Analgesic* Decoction of plant taken for migraine headaches. Poultice of heated leaves applied to the stomach or head for pain. *Dermatological Aid* Decoction of roots used as a hair rinse. *Emetic* Decoction of plant taken as an emetic. *Febrifuge* Decoction of roots used, especially for children, for fevers. *Gastrointestinal Aid* Poultice of heated leaves applied to stomach or head for pain. *Other* Decoction of plant taken for migraine headaches. *Pediatric Aid* Decoction of roots used, especially for children, for fevers. (17:8)

Malva parviflora, Cheeseweed Mallow
Diegueño *Dermatological Aid* Decoction of leaves or roots used as a rinse for dandruff and to soften the hair after the hair wash. *Febrifuge* Decoction of leaves or roots used as an enema and bath for babies with fevers. (70:24) **Miwok** *Antirheumatic (External)* Infusion of leaves, soft stems, and flowers used as poultice on swellings. *Dermatological Aid* Infusion of leaves, soft stems, and flowers used as poultice on running sores and

boils. (8:171) **Pima** *Dermatological Aid* Decoction of plant used as a shampoo. (38:79)

Malvella leprosa, Alkali Mallow
Choctaw *Antidiarrheal, Burn Dressing,* and *Gastrointestinal Aid* Root used for "dysentery, diarrhea, inflammation of the bowels, burns, etc." (as *Sida hederacea* 23:287)

Mammillaria grahamii var. **grahamii**, Graham's Nipple Cactus
Pima *Ear Medicine* Plant boiled and placed warm in the ear for earaches and suppurating ears. (as *M. microcarpa* 38:57)

Manfreda virginica, False Aloe
Catawba *Kidney Aid* Infusion of pounded roots taken and used externally for dropsy. (as *Agave virginica* 134:191) Infusion of pounded roots taken and used as a wash for dropsy. (as *Agave virginica* 152:10) *Snakebite Remedy* Infusion of roots taken and used externally for snakebite. (as *Agave virginica* 134:191) Infusion of roots taken and used as a wash for snakebites. (as *Agave virginica* 152:10) **Cherokee** *Anthelmintic* Root chewed for worms. *Antidiarrheal* Root chewed for diarrhea. (as *Agave virginica* 66:23) Root, a very strong medicine, chewed for persistent diarrhea. (as *Agave virginica* 177:74) *Liver Aid* Root chewed for the liver. (as *Agave virginica* 66:23) **Creek** *Snakebite Remedy* Decoction of root in sweet milk taken or used as wash for rattlesnake bite. Root chewed and swallowed or used externally for rattlesnake bite. (23:289) **Seminole** *Snakebite Remedy* Plant used for snakebites. (as *Agave virginica* 145:297)

Marah fabaceus, California Manroot
Pomo *Dermatological Aid* Pounded nuts and grease rubbed on the head for falling hair. (as *Echinocystis fabacea* 54:14) **Pomo, Kashaya** *Dermatological Aid* Raw, pounded root mixed with pounded pepper nuts and skunk grease applied to head to prevent baldness. (60:41)

Marah horridus, Sierran Manroot
Kawaiisu *Dermatological Aid* Mashed, roasted seeds used as a salve for skin irritations and sores, and as a salve to eliminate baldness. *Ear Medicine* Roasted seeds placed in the ear for earaches.

(180:40) Tubatulabal *Dermatological Aid*
Burned, ripe seeds rubbed on pimples and newborn baby's navel. *Pediatric Aid* Burned, ripe
seeds rubbed on newborn baby's navel. (as *Echinocystis horrida* 167:59)

Marah macrocarpus, Cucamonga Manroot
Costanoan *Dermatological Aid* Seeds used as a
paste for pimples and skin sores. (17:24) **Luiseño**
Cathartic Roots used as a purgative. (as *Echinocystis macrocarpa* 132:229)

Marah macrocarpus var. *major*, Cucamonga
Manroot
Mahuna *Dermatological Aid* Plant juices rubbed
on parts afflicted by ringworm. Seed oil rubbed on
the head for diseased scalps and hair roots. (as
Micrapelis micracarpa 117:38)

Marah oreganus, Coastal Manroot
Chehalis *Dermatological Aid* and *Tuberculosis
Remedy* Salve of root ash and grease applied to
scrofula sores. (as *Echinocystis oregana* 65:48)
Karok *Dermatological Aid* Poultice of roots applied to bruises and boils. (5:39) *Poison* Plant
considered poisonous. (as *Echinocystis oregana*
125:386) **Mendocino Indian** *Antirheumatic*
(*External*) Seeds and roots used for rheumatism
or root rubbed on rheumatic joints. *Dermatological Aid* Root rubbed on rheumatic joints, boils,
and swellings. *Poison* Roots and seeds considered
poisonous. *Urinary Aid* Seeds eaten for urinary
troubles. *Venereal Aid* Seeds and roots used for
rheumatism and venereal disease. (as *Micrampe-
lis marah* 33:390) **Paiute** *Eye Medicine* Decoction of peeled, sliced, and dried root used for
"sore eyes." (as *Echinocystis oreganas* 93:113)
Squaxin *Analgesic* and *Orthopedic Aid* Infusion
of smashed stalks used as a soak for aching hands.
Poison Plant considered poisonous. (as *Echinocystis oregana* 65:48)

Marrubium vulgare, Horehound
Cahuilla *Kidney Aid* Infusion of whole plant used
for flushing the kidneys. (11:88) **Cherokee** *Breast
Treatment* Infusion used for "breast complaints."
Cold Remedy Taken for colds. *Cough Medicine*
Mixed with sugar to make cough syrup. *Pediatric
Aid* Infusion given to babies. *Throat Aid* Taken for

hoarseness. (66:39) **Costanoan** *Cough Medicine*
Decoction of leaves used for coughs. *Dermatological Aid* Heated leaf salve used on boils. *Pulmonary Aid* Decoction of leaves used for whooping
cough. (17:16) **Diegueño** *Cold Remedy* Infusion
of leaves taken for colds. *Pediatric Aid* Infusion of
leaves mixed with honey and given to children for
colds and whooping cough. *Pulmonary Aid* Infusion of leaves taken for whooping cough. (70:25)
Hopi *Unspecified* Used as a medicinal plant.
(164:165) **Isleta** *Antirheumatic* (*External*) Poultice of crushed leaves used for swellings. (85:34)
Kawaiisu *Cold Remedy* Hot or cold infusion of
leaves and flowering tops taken for colds. *Cough
Medicine* Hot or cold infusion of leaves and flowering tops taken for coughs. *Respiratory Aid* Plant
used as a syrup for respiratory ailments. (180:40)
Mahuna *Cough Medicine* Infusion of leaves and
flowers taken for coughs. *Throat Aid* Infusion of
leaves and flowers taken for sore throats. (117:18)
Navajo *Throat Aid* Infusion of plant taken for sore
throats. (45:73) **Navajo, Ramah** *Analgesic* Decoction of plant used for stomachache and influenza.
Disinfectant Strong infusion used for "lightning
infection." *Gastrointestinal Aid* Decoction of plant
taken for stomachache. *Gynecological Aid* Root
used before and after childbirth. *Misc. Disease
Remedy* Decoction of plant taken for influenza.
(165:41) **Paiute** *Analgesic* Branches used to whip
aching body parts to stimulate circulation. (155:
103) **Rappahannock** *Cold Remedy* Infusion of
roots taken for colds. *Cough Medicine* Compound
decoction taken for coughs. (138:27) **Round
Valley Indian** *Antidiarrheal* Decoction of leaves
taken for diarrhea. *Cold Remedy* Decoction of
leaves taken for colds. (33:383) **Yuki** *Cough Medicine* Infusion of plant taken for coughs. (39:47)

Marshallia obovata, Spoonshape Barbara's
Buttons
Catawba *Misc. Disease Remedy* Plant used in cer-
tain diseases. (134:191)

Matelea biflora, Star Milkvine
Comanche *Ceremonial Medicine* Decoction of
thick, white roots used for ghost sickness. *Dermatological Aid* Decoction of thick, white roots used
for bruises. *Gastrointestinal Aid* Root paste used
for severe stomach pains. *Gynecological Aid*

Decoction of thick, white roots used for menstrual cramps. *Misc. Disease Remedy* Root paste used for diphtheria and other throat closing ailments in children. *Orthopedic Aid* Decoction of thick, white roots used for broken bones. *Pediatric Aid* Root paste used for diphtheria and other throat closing ailments in children. (84:9)

Matelea cynanchoides, Prairie Milkvine
Comanche *Ceremonial Medicine* Decoction of thick, white roots used for ghost sickness. *Dermatological Aid* Decoction of thick, white roots used for bruises. *Gastrointestinal Aid* Root paste used for severe stomach pains. *Gynecological Aid* Decoction of thick, white roots used for menstrual cramps. *Misc. Disease Remedy* Root paste used for diphtheria and other throat closing ailments in children. *Orthopedic Aid* Decoction of thick, white roots used for broken bones. *Pediatric Aid* Root paste used for diphtheria and other throat closing ailments in children. (84:9)

Matricaria discoidea, Disc Mayweed
Aleut *Analgesic* and *Carminative* Infusion of leaves taken for stomach pains, especially from gas. *Gastrointestinal Aid* Infusion of leaves taken for stomach pain, especially for gas on the stomach. *Laxative* Infusion of leaves taken as a laxative. *Panacea* Plant used as a cure-all. *Tonic* Plant used to make a tonic. (as *M. matricarioides* 6:426) **Blackfoot** *Antidiarrheal* Decoction of plant and flowers used for diarrhea. (as *M. matri-*

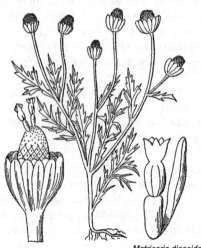
Matricaria discoidea

carioides 82:61) **Cahuilla** *Antidiarrheal* Infusion of plant used for diarrhea. *Gastrointestinal Aid* Infusion of plant used for colic and to settle upset stomachs. (as *M. matricarioides* 11:88) **Cherokee** *Gastrointestinal Aid* Infusion taken "to keep regular." (as *M. matricarioides* 66:49) **Cheyenne** *Ceremonial Medicine* Plant used in the Sun Dance ceremony. (as *M. matricarioides* 69:22) *Dermatological Aid* Dried, pulverized flowers, leaves, sweet grass, horse mint, and sweet pine used as a perfume. (as *M. matricarioides* 64:189) *Unspecified* Plant tops used as an ingredient in many medicines. (as *M. matricarioides* 69:22) **Costanoan** *Analgesic* Decoction of plant taken for stomach pain. *Anticonvulsive* Decoction of plant used for infant convulsions. *Dermatological Aid* and *Disinfectant* Seeds used as salve for infected sores. *Febrifuge* Decoction of plant taken for fever. *Gastrointestinal Aid* Decoction of plant taken for stomach pain and indigestion. *Pediatric Aid* Decoction of plant used for infant convulsions. (as *M. matricarioides* 17:27) **Diegueño** *Febrifuge* Decoction of plant mixed with mallow and elderberry blossoms and used as an enema for babies with fever. *Gynecological Aid* Decoction of whole plant taken by women following childbirth. *Pediatric Aid* Decoction of plant mixed with mallow and elderberry blossoms and used as an enema for babies with fever. (as *M. matricarioides* 70:25) **Eskimo, Alaska** *Antihemorrhagic* Plant tops chewed for spitting up blood. (as *M. matricarioides* 1:38) **Eskimo, Inuktitut** *Unspecified* Used for medicinal purposes. (as *M. matricarioides* 176:183) **Eskimo, Kuskokwagmiut** *Adjuvant* Plant used in the steam bath for the pleasant odor. *Cold Remedy* Decoction of dried seed heads taken for colds. *Gastrointestinal Aid* Decoction of dried seed heads taken for indigestion. (as *M. suaveolens* 101:22, 23) **Eskimo, Western** *Adjuvant* Plants added to sweat bath water container to impart fragrance. (as *M. suaveolens* 90:39) *Cold Remedy* and *Gastrointestinal Aid* Decoction of dried seed heads used "for either indigestion or a cold." (as *M. suaveolens* 90:13) **Flathead** *Antidiarrheal* Infusion of herb used for diarrhea. *Cold Remedy* Infusion of herb used for children with colds. *Gastrointestinal Aid* Infusion of herb used for upset stomach. *Pediatric Aid* Infusion of herb used for children with colds. (as *M. matricarioi-*

des 68:23) **Montana Indian** *Antidiarrheal* Decoction of herbs and flowers used for diarrhea. (15:15) *Gynecological Aid* Infusion of herb used for building up blood at childbirth and delivering the placenta. Infusion of herb used by young girls for menstrual cramps. (as *M. matricarioides* 68:23) **Okanagan-Colville** *Love Medicine* Tops and human hair buried on range to prevent loved ones or relations from going away. *Veterinary Aid* Tops, horse and human hair, and musk gland material buried on range to prevent horses from running away. *Witchcraft Medicine* Plant used for witchcraft. (as *M. matricarioides* 162:84) **Shuswap** *Cold Remedy* Dried plants used for colds. *Heart Medicine* Dried plants used for the heart. (as *M. matricarioides* 102:59) **Ute** *Unspecified* Used as a medicine. (30:35) **Yokia** *Antidiarrheal* Decoction of leaves and flowers taken for diarrhea. (33:395)

Matteuccia struthiopteris, Ostrich Fern
Cree, Woodlands *Gynecological Aid* Decoction of leaf stalk base from the sterile frond taken to speed expulsion of the afterbirth. *Orthopedic Aid* Decoction of leaf stalk base from the sterile frond taken for back pain. (91:44)

Medeola virginiana, Indian Cucumberroot
Iroquois *Anticonvulsive* Infusion of crushed dried berries and leaves given to babies with convulsions. *Panacea* Compound infusion taken or placed on injured part, a "Little Water Medicine." *Pediatric Aid* Infusion of crushed dried berries and leaves given to babies with convulsions. *Witchcraft Medicine* Raw root chewed and spit on hook to "make fish bite." (73:285)

Medicago sativa, Alfalfa
Costanoan *Ear Medicine* Poultice of heated leaves applied to the ear for earaches. (17:19)

Melampyrum lineare, Narrowleaf Cowwheat
Ojibwa *Eye Medicine* Infusion of plant used as a "little medicine for the eyes." (130:389)

Melia azedarach, Chinaberrytree
Cherokee *Anthelmintic* Infusion of root and bark given for worms. *Dermatological Aid* Used for "scald head," ringworm, and "tetterworm." (66:29)

Melica imperfecta, Smallflower Melicgrass
Kawaiisu *Toothache Remedy* Plant clump used to discard children's milk teeth, "then another one will grow in." (180:40)

Melicope cinerea, Manena
Hawaiian *Venereal Aid* Plant used for venereal diseases. (as *Pelea cinerea* 2:72)

Melilotus indicus, Annual Yellow Sweetclover
Pomo, Kashaya *Laxative* Decoction of whole plant taken as a purgative, a very strong laxative. (60:37)

Melilotus officinalis, Yellow Sweetclover
Iroquois *Dermatological Aid* Infusion of flowers and rhizomes from another plant applied to the face for pimples and sunburn. (as *M. alba* 118:49) *Febrifuge* Infusion taken for typhoid-like fever caused by odor from killed snake. (as *M. alba* 73:364) **Navajo, Ramah** *Cold Remedy* Cold infusion taken and used as lotion for colds caused by becoming chilled. (as *M. alba* 165:33)

Melissa officinalis, Common Balm
Cherokee *Cold Remedy* Used for old colds. *Febrifuge* Used for typhus fevers, chills, and fevers. *Misc. Disease Remedy* Plant used for typhus fevers, chills, and fevers. *Stimulant* Used as a stimulant. *Tonic* Used as a tonic. (66:24) **Costanoan** *Gastrointestinal Aid* Decoction of plant used for infants' colic and stomachaches. *Pediatric Aid* Decoction of plant used for infants with colic. (17:16)

Melothria pendula, Guadeloupe Cucumber
Houma *Snakebite Remedy* Poultice of pulverized leaves and gunpowder applied to moccasin bite. (135:64)

Menispermum canadense, Common Moonseed
Cherokee *Antidiarrheal* Taken for weak stomachs and bowels. *Dermatological Aid* Root used for skin diseases. *Gastrointestinal Aid* Taken for weak stomachs and bowels. *Gynecological Aid* Taken by "weakly females." *Laxative* Root used as a laxative. *Stimulant* Taken by "weakly females." *Venereal Aid* Taken for venereal diseases and as a laxative. (66:54) **Delaware, Oklahoma** *Dermatological*

Aid Salve containing plant used on chronic sores. (150:27)

Menodora scabra, Rough Menodora
Navajo, Ramah *Analgesic* Decoction of root used for backbone pain. *Gastrointestinal Aid* Cold infusion taken for heartburn. *Gynecological Aid* Decoction of plant taken to facilitate labor. *Orthopedic Aid* Decoction of root used for "pain in backbone." *Panacea* Plant used as "life medicine." (165:39)

Mentha arvensis, Wild Mint
California Indian *Kidney Aid* Infusion of leaves taken for kidney complaint. (98:41) **Cherokee** *Febrifuge* Infusion given for fever. (66:45) **Cheyenne** *Antiemetic* Infusion of ground leaves and stems taken for vomiting. (68:64) *Ceremonial Medicine* Plant used in the Sun Dance ceremony. *Dermatological Aid* Decoction of plant used as a hair oil. *Heart Medicine* Infusion of ground leaves and stems taken to strengthen heart muscles. (69:27) *Love Medicine* Leaves chewed and placed on body for improved love life. (68:64) Infusion of ground leaves and stems used to improve one's love life. *Stimulant* Infusion of ground leaves and stems taken to stimulate vital organs. (69:27) **Flathead** *Cold Remedy* Infusion taken for colds. *Cough Medicine* Infusion taken for coughs. *Febrifuge* Infusion taken for fevers. *Tonic* Infusion taken as a tonic. *Toothache Remedy* Leaves used for carious teeth. **Gros Ventre** *Analgesic* Infusion

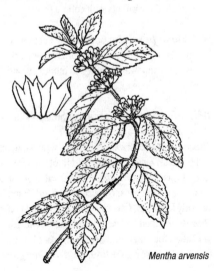

Mentha arvensis

taken for headaches. (68:64) **Iroquois** *Antidote* Compound decoction of plants taken to vomit as cure for poison. (73:428) **Kawaiisu** *Analgesic* Poultice of leaves and stems applied to areas of pain. *Dermatological Aid* Poultice of leaves and stems applied to areas of swelling. (180:40) **Kutenai** *Antirheumatic* (*External*) Poultice of leaves used for rheumatism and arthritis. *Cold Remedy* Infusion taken for colds. *Cough Medicine* Infusion taken for coughs. *Febrifuge* Infusion taken for fevers. *Kidney Aid* Infusion taken for kidney problems. *Tonic* Infusion taken as a tonic. (68:64) **Menominee** *Pulmonary Aid* Compound infusion taken and poultice applied to chest for pneumonia. (128:39) **Navajo, Kayenta** *Dermatological Aid* Plant used as a lotion for swellings. *Disinfectant* and *Pediatric Aid* Roots used for prenatal snake infection. (179:40) **Navajo, Ramah** *Febrifuge* Cold infusion taken and used as lotion for fever. *Misc. Disease Remedy* Cold infusion taken and used as lotion for influenza. *Stimulant* Cold infusion given to counteract effects of being struck by a whirlwind. (165:41) **Okanagan-Colville** *Analgesic* Infusion of stems taken for pains. *Antirheumatic* (*Internal*) Infusion of stems taken for swellings. *Cold Remedy* Infusion of stems taken for colds. *Febrifuge* Infusion of stems taken for fevers. *Gastrointestinal Aid* and *Pediatric Aid* Infusion of stems taken for colic in children. (162:109) **Paiute** *Other* Plant chewed or infusion of entire plant, except root, taken to keep cool. (144:317) **Thompson** *Cold Remedy* Infusion of plant taken for colds. *Misc. Disease Remedy* Infusion of plant taken to prevent influenza. One informant said that during the flu epidemic after the First World War, her grandmother made a big potful of mint tea. She and her family drank this and did not get sick. (161:233)

Mentha canadensis, Canadian Mint
Abnaki *Panacea* Used by children for maladies. *Pediatric Aid* Used by children for maladies. (121:155) Used for crying babies. *Sedative* Used for crying babies. (121:171) **Algonquin, Tête-de-Boule** *Febrifuge* Plant used as a fever medicine. (110:129) **Bella Coola** *Analgesic* Decoction of entire plant taken for stomach pain. *Gastrointestinal Aid* Decoction of entire plant taken for stomach pain. (127:63) **Blackfoot** *Analgesic* Dried leaves

chewed and swallowed for chest pains. *Heart Medicine* Dried leaves chewed and swallowed for heart ailments. (as *M. arvensis* var. *villosa* 82:51) **Carrier, Southern** *Cold Remedy* Decoction of entire plant taken for colds and the stomach. *Gastrointestinal Aid* Decoction of entire plant taken for the stomach and various ailments. *Pulmonary Aid* Decoction of entire plant taken for "lung affections" and colds. (127:63) **Cheyenne** *Antiemetic* Decoction of leaves and stems taken to prevent vomiting. (63:186) Decoction of finely ground leaves and stems taken to prevent vomiting. (63:39) Decoction of ground stems and leaves taken to prevent vomiting. (64:186) **Chippewa** *Carminative* Plant used as a carminative. (59:140) **Cree, Hudson Bay** *Gastrointestinal Aid* Infusion of plant used as a stomachic. (78:303) **Cree, Woodlands** *Analgesic* Infusion of leaves taken for headaches. *Antihemorrhagic* Infusion of plant taken for coughing up blood. *Cold Remedy* Infusion of plant taken to prevent the onset of a cold and for prolonged colds. Infusion of leaves taken for colds. *Febrifuge* Infusion of leaves taken for fevers. *Hemostat* Leafy stems and flowers inserted into the nostril for serious nosebleeds. *Oral Aid* Ground flowers and yarrow placed in a cloth, moistened, and rubbed on infected gums to remove pus. *Toothache Remedy* Poultice of ground leaves or leafy stems applied to the gums for toothaches. (as *M. arvensis* var. *villosa* 91:45) **Dakota** *Carminative* Sweetened infusion taken as a carminative or beverage. (58:112, 113) **Gosiute** *Analgesic*, *Cold Remedy*, and *Cough Medicine* Decoction of plant taken for coughs and colds with headaches. (31:351) **Great Basin Indian** *Gastrointestinal Aid* Infusion of whole plant taken for indigestion. (100:50) **Hoh** *Unspecified* Used as smelling and rubbing medicine. (114:68) **Iroquois** *Emetic* Compound decoction of plants taken to vomit as cure for poison. (as *M. arvensis* var. *canadensis* 73:428) *Febrifuge* Infusion of plant given to children for fevers. (118:58) *Hemorrhoid Remedy* Compound decoction of roots taken and used as a wash for piles. (as *M. arvensis* var. *canadensis* 73:428) *Pediatric Aid* Infusion of plant given to children for fevers. (118:58) **Isleta** *Eye Medicine* Poultice of moistened, crushed leaves used for eye trouble. (as *M. penardi* 85:34) **Keres, Western** *Analgesic* Infusion of dried plants used for headaches. *Febrifuge* Infusion of

dried plants used for fevers. (147:53) **Keresan** *Febrifuge* Infusion of plant used for fever. (172:562) **Mahuna** *Sedative* Plant used as a sedative. (117:23) **Malecite** *Gastrointestinal Aid* Infusion of plants used by children with stomach trouble. *Pediatric Aid* Infusion of plants used to quiet children suffering from croup, and used by children with stomach trouble. *Pulmonary Aid* Infusion of plants used by children with croup. *Sedative* Infusion of plants used to quiet children suffering from croup. (96:250) **Menominee** *Febrifuge* Infusion of whole plant used for fever. (44:132) **Micmac** *Antiemetic* and *Pediatric Aid* Herb used for children with an upset stomach. *Pulmonary Aid* Herb used for croup. (32:58) **Mohegan** *Gastrointestinal Aid* Infusion of leaves considered beneficial to the stomach. (151:73, 130) **Montana Indian** *Unspecified* Infusion of leaves used for various complaints. (15:15) **Ojibwa** *Blood Medicine* Infusion of entire plant taken as a blood remedy. *Diaphoretic* Plant used in the sweat bath. *Febrifuge* Infusion of leaves taken for fevers. (as *M. arvensis* var. *canadensis* 130:371, 372) *Gastrointestinal Aid* Infusion of plants taken for stomach troubles. (112:231) **Okanagon** *Analgesic* Infusion of leaves and plant tips given to children with colicky pains. Infusion of leaves and plant tips taken for pains. *Cold Remedy* Infusion of leaves and plant tips taken for colds. *Dermatological Aid* Infusion of leaves and plant tips taken for swellings. *Gastrointestinal Aid* and *Pediatric Aid* Infusion of leaves and plant tips given to children with colicky pains. (104:42) **Omaha** *Carminative* Plant used as a carminative. (56:334) Sweetened infusion taken as a carminative or beverage. (58:112, 113) **Paiute** *Analgesic* Decoction of various plant parts taken for headaches. Leaves used in several ways for headaches. (155:104, 105) *Carminative* Infusion of leaves and stems taken for gas pains. (as *M. penardi* 98:45) *Cold Remedy* Infusion of fresh or dried leaves taken for colds. (as *M. arvensis* var. *glabrata* 93:107) Decoction of various plant parts taken for colds. *Dermatological Aid* Poultice of crushed leaves applied to swellings. *Febrifuge* Decoction of various plant parts taken and used as a wash for fevers. *Gastrointestinal Aid* and *Pediatric Aid* Infusion and/or decoction of plant parts used for stomachache, indigestion, and babies' colic. *Throat Aid* Leaves chewed for sore throats.

(155:104, 105) **Paiute, Northern** *Cold Remedy* Fresh leaves put in the nostrils for colds. Plant spread out on the ground and lied on for a cold. *Febrifuge* Plant spread out on the ground and lied on for a fever. (49:129) **Pawnee** *Carminative* Sweetened infusion taken as a carminative or beverage. **Ponca** *Carminative* Sweetened infusion taken as a carminative or beverage. (58:112, 113) **Potawatomi** *Febrifuge* Leaves or plant top used for fevers. *Pulmonary Aid* Decoction of leaves used for pleurisy. (as *M. arvensis* var. *canadensis* 131:61) **Quileute** *Unspecified* Used as smelling and rubbing medicine. (114:68) **Salish** *Unspecified* Decoction of plants used as a medicine. (as *M. borealis* 153:294) **Sanpoil** *Cold Remedy* Decoction of leaves taken by adults for colds and infusion given to children. Decoction of plant given to infants for colds. *Panacea* Decoction of leaves taken by adults and given to children for "illnesses of a general nature." *Pediatric Aid* Decoction of leaves taken by adults for colds and infusion given to children. Decoction of plant given to infants for colds. Infusion of leaves given to children for "illnesses of a general nature." (109:218) **Shoshoni** *Carminative* Infusion of leaves and stems taken for gas pains. (as *M. penardi* 98:45) *Cold Remedy* Decoction of various plant parts taken for colds. *Febrifuge* Decoction of various plant parts taken and used as a wash for fevers. *Gastrointestinal Aid* Decoction of plant parts used for stomachache, indigestion, or babies' colic. (155:104, 105) *Pediatric Aid* Decoction of plant parts used for stomachache, indigestion, or babies' colic. (155:104, 105) **Sia** *Febrifuge* Infusion of leaves taken for fevers. (173:284) **Thompson** *Analgesic* Infusion of leaves and plant tips given to children with colicky pains. Infusion of leaves and plant tips taken for pains. (104:42) Decoction of leaves and tops taken for pains. *Antirheumatic* (*External*) Leaves used in the sweat bath for rheumatism. Plant steamed in the sweat bath for rheumatism and severe colds. (141:475) *Cold Remedy* Infusion of leaves and plant tips taken for colds. (104:42) Decoction of leaves and tops taken and used as herbal steam for colds. Plant steamed in the sweat bath for severe colds. (141:475) *Dermatological Aid* Infusion of leaves and plant tips taken for swellings. (104:42) Decoction of leaves and tops taken for swellings. (141:475) *Gastrointestinal Aid* Infusion of leaves

and plant tips given to children with colicky pains. (104:42) *Herbal Steam* Plant steamed in the sweat bath for rheumatism and severe colds. (141:475) *Pediatric Aid* Infusion of leaves and plant tips given to children with colicky pains. (104:42) *Unspecified* Plant used as a charm for unspecified purpose. (141:507) **Washo** *Antidiarrheal* Decoction of various plant parts taken for diarrhea. *Cold Remedy* Decoction of various plant parts taken for colds. *Febrifuge* Decoction of various plant parts taken for fevers. *Gastrointestinal Aid* and *Pediatric Aid* Decoction of plant parts used for stomachache, indigestion, and babies' colic. (155:104, 105) **Winnebago** *Carminative* Sweetened infusion taken as a carminative or beverage. (58:112, 113)

Mentha ×piperita, Peppermint

Cherokee *Adjuvant* Plant used to flavor medicine and foods. *Analgesic* Taken for colic pains, cramps, and used for nervous headache. *Antiemetic* Taken for vomiting. *Carminative* Taken to "dispel flatulence and remove colic pains." *Cold Remedy* Infusion taken for colds. *Febrifuge* Infusion taken for fevers. *Gastrointestinal Aid* Taken for "affections of stomach and bowels" and infusion used for upset stomach. Taken for bowel problems. *Hemorrhoid Remedy* Tincture applied externally to piles. *Misc. Disease Remedy* Given for cholera infantum. *Pediatric Aid* Given for cholera infantum. *Sedative* Taken for hysterics. *Stimulant* Used as a stimulant. *Urinary Aid* Taken for "suppression of urine and gravelly affection." (water mint 66:48, 49) **Delaware, Oklahoma** *Tonic* Compound containing leaves used as a tonic. (water mint 150:76) **Hoh** *Unspecified* Used as smelling and rubbing medicine. **Quileute** *Unspecified* Used as smelling and rubbing medicine. (peppermint 114:68) **Iroquois** *Cold Remedy* Infusion of whole plant taken for colds. *Febrifuge* Infusion of whole plant taken for fevers. *Other* Compound infusion used as wash on injured parts, a "Little Water Medicine." *Witchcraft Medicine* Infusion of plant will throw off witchcraft. (water mint 73:428) **Menominee** *Pulmonary Aid* Compound infusion taken and poultice applied to chest for pneumonia. (water mint 128:39) **Mohegan** *Anthelmintic* Infusion of plant given to babies for worms. (water mint 149:265) Infusion of leaves taken by children and adults as a vermifuge. (water mint 151:73, 130) *Pediatric*

Aid Infusion given to babies for worms. (water mint 149:265) Infusion of leaves used as a vermifuge for children and adults. (water mint 151:73)

Mentha spicata, Spearmint

Cherokee *Adjuvant* Plant used to flavor medicine and foods. *Analgesic* Taken for colic pains, cramps, and used for nervous headache. *Antiemetic* Taken for vomiting. *Carminative* Taken to "dispel flatulence and remove colic pains." *Cold Remedy* Infusion taken for colds. *Febrifuge* Infusion taken for fevers. *Gastrointestinal Aid* Taken for "affections of stomach and bowels" and infusion used for upset stomach. Taken for bowel problems. *Hemorrhoid Remedy* Tincture applied externally to piles. *Misc. Disease Remedy* and *Pediatric Aid* Given for cholera infantum. *Sedative* Taken for hysterics. *Stimulant* Used as a stimulant. *Urinary Aid* Taken for "suppression of urine and gravelly affection." (66:48, 49) **Iroquois** *Analgesic* Cold infusion applied to forehead or powdered plant snuffed for headaches. (73:427) *Cold Remedy* Infusion of whole plant taken as a cold remedy. (73:428) *Emetic* Infusion of plants given to children as an emetic. *Febrifuge* Compound infusion of powdered plants taken for fevers. *Gastrointestinal Aid* Infusion of plants given to children for a bad stomach. *Misc. Disease Remedy* Compound infusion of powdered plants taken for typhoid. *Other* Compound infusion used as wash on injured parts, a "Little Water Medicine." *Pediatric Aid* Infusion of plants given to children as an emetic or for a bad stomach. *Respiratory Aid* Compound decoction of roots and berries taken for hay fever. (73:427) **Mahuna** *Sedative* Plant used as a sedative. (117:23) **Miwok** *Antidiarrheal* Infusion of leaves taken for diarrhea. *Gastrointestinal Aid* Infusion of leaves taken for stomach trouble. (8:171) **Mohegan** *Anthelmintic* Infusion of plant taken as a worm medicine. (149:265) Infusion of leaves taken as a vermifuge. (151:73, 130)

Mentzelia albicaulis, Whitestem Blazingstar

Gosiute *Burn Dressing* Seeds used for burns. (31:375) **Hopi** *Toothache Remedy* Plant used as toothache medicine. (34:335) **Navajo, Ramah** *Snakebite Remedy* Compound containing leaves used for snakebite. *Toothache Remedy* Poultice of crushed, soaked seeds applied for toothache. (165:36)

Mentzelia albicaulis var. veatchiana, Whitestem Blazingstar

Kawaiisu *Burn Dressing* Pounded seeds made into a salve and rubbed on burned skin. (as *M. veatchiana* 180:41)

Mentzelia laciniata, Cutleaf Blazingstar

Navajo, Ramah *Eye Medicine* Infusion of flowers used as an eyewash. (165:36)

Mentzelia laevicaulis, Smoothstem Blazingstar

Cheyenne *Antirheumatic* (*Internal*) Roots used for rheumatism and arthritis. *Dietary Aid* Roots chewed for thirst prevention. *Ear Medicine* Roots used for earaches. *Febrifuge* Roots used for fevers. *Misc. Disease Remedy* Infusion of roots taken for mumps, measles, and smallpox. *Unspecified* Plant used as an ingredient in medicinal preparations. Roots used for complicated illnesses. (69:30) **Gosiute** *Dermatological Aid* Infusion of roots used for bruise swellings. (31:349) **Mendocino Indian** *Dermatological Aid* Decoction of leaves used as a wash for skin diseases. *Gastrointestinal Aid* Decoction of leaves taken for stomachaches. (33:369) **Montana Indian** *Dermatological Aid* Decoction of leaves applied as a lotion for certain skin diseases. *Gastrointestinal Aid* Decoction of leaves taken for stomach trouble. (15:16) **Thompson** *Unspecified* Plant used medicinally for unspecified purpose. (141:474)

Mentzelia multiflora, Manyflowered Mentzelia

Keres, Western *Diuretic* Infusion of plant used as a diuretic. *Psychological Aid* Plants used to make infants good horseback riders. Plants used to whip 3- or 4-month-old infants, or ground leaves rubbed on their thighs so that they will become good horseback riders when they grow up. *Tuberculosis Remedy* Leaves and roots used as the strongest tuberculosis medicine by the strongest patients. (147:54) **Navajo** *Emetic* Plant used as an emetic. (76:161)

Mentzelia multiflora var. multiflora, Adonis Blazingstar

Navajo, Kayenta *Ceremonial Medicine* Plant used as fumigant for collared lizard ceremony.

Dermatological Aid Plant used to keep smallpox sores from pitting. *Disinfectant* Plant used as fumigant for collared lizard ceremony. *Gastrointestinal Aid* Plant used for abdominal swellings. (as *M. pumila* var. *multiflora* 179:32) **Navajo, Ramah** *Eye Medicine* Infusion of flowers used as an eyewash. (as *M. pumila* var. *multiflora* 165:37)

Mentzelia nuda var. nuda, Bractless Blazing-star

Dakota *Febrifuge* Boiled, strained sap applied externally for fever. (as *Nuttallia nuda* 58:103)

Mentzelia pumila, Dwarf Mentzelia
Apache, White Mountain *Laxative* Powdered roots used for constipation. (113:158) **Hopi** *Toothache Remedy* Plant used as "a toothache medicine." (174:85) **Zuni** *Laxative* Powdered root inserted into rectum as a suppository for constipation. (143:57) *Pediatric Aid* and *Strengthener* Plant used to whip children to make them strong so they could hold on to a horse without falling. (143:84)

Menyanthes trifoliata, Common Buckbean
Aleut *Analgesic* Infusion of roots taken for gas pains, constipation, and rheumatism. *Antirheumatic* (*Internal*) Compound containing roots taken as a tonic for gas pains and rheumatism. *Carminative* Compound containing roots taken as a tonic for gas pains. *Laxative* Compound containing roots taken as a tonic for constipation. *Tonic*

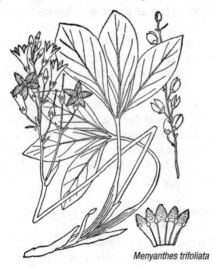

Menyanthes trifoliata

Roots used as a powerful ingredient in a tonic. (6:427) **Kwakiutl** *Antiemetic* Decoction of roots or leaves taken when sick to the stomach. (157:287) *Antihemorrhagic* Decoction of root and stem used for "spitting of blood and other internal diseases." (16:380) Decoction of ground stem and roots taken for blood-spitting. *Dietary Aid* Decoction of roots or leaves taken to put on weight. *Gastrointestinal Aid* Decoction of roots or leaves taken when sick to the stomach. *Misc. Disease Remedy* Decoction of roots or leaves taken to put on weight during the flu. (157:287) **Menominee** *Unspecified* Plant used in medicines. (128:36) **Micmac** *Unspecified* Strong decoction of root taken for unspecified purpose. (as *Mergantnes trifolia* 133:317) **Tlingit** *Unspecified* Plant used for the medicinal value. (126:330)

Menziesia ferruginea, Rusty Menziesia
Hesquiat *Oral Aid* Nectar sucked from flowers to sweeten the mouth. (159:65) **Kwakiutl** *Analgesic* Leaves chewed for heart pain. *Dermatological Aid* Poultice of heated leaves applied to sores and swellings. *Gastrointestinal Aid* Leaves chewed for stomach troubles. *Heart Medicine* Leaves chewed for heart pain. (157:283) **Nitinaht** *Witchcraft Medicine* Bark used to counteract evil spells and doctor remedies. (160:107) **Quinault** *Love Medicine* Forked twig waved in the air by a woman to make a man fall in love with her. (65:43)

Merremia dissecta, Noyau Vine
Hawaiian *Analgesic* Poultice of pounded flowers, leaves, and salt applied to the back for pain. *Dermatological Aid* Poultice of pounded roots, other plants, and the resulting liquid applied to flesh wounds. *Laxative* Roots and other plants pounded, mixed with water and an egg, and taken as a laxative. *Orthopedic Aid* Poultice of pounded roots, other plants, and the resulting liquid applied to broken bones. *Pediatric Aid* and *Strengthener* Flowers chewed by mothers and given to infants for general weakness. (as *Impomea dissecta* 2:52)

Mertensia ciliata, Mountain Bluebells
Cheyenne *Breast Treatment* Infusion of plant used to increase milk flow of mothers. (as *Mestensia ciliata* 69:16) *Dermatological Aid* Infusion of powdered roots taken for itching from smallpox.

(64:184) *Gynecological Aid* Infusion of plant taken by women to increase supply of milk. (63:184) Infusion of plant taken by women after childbirth to increase milk flow. (64:184) *Misc. Disease Remedy* Infusion of leaves taken for smallpox and measles. (63:184) Infusion of leaves taken for smallpox and measles. (64:184) Infusion of leaves used for measles and smallpox. (as *Mestensia ciliata* 69:16)

Mertensia virginica, Virginia Bluebells
Cherokee *Pulmonary Aid* Taken for whooping cough. *Tuberculosis Remedy* Taken for consumption. (66:26) **Iroquois** *Antidote* Compound infusion of roots taken as an antidote for poisons. *Venereal Aid* Decoction of roots taken for venereal disease. (73:421)

Metrosideros polymorpha var. **polymorpha**, 'Ohi'a
Hawaiian *Analgesic* Flowers and other plants rubbed, squeezed, and the resulting liquid taken for severe childbirth pain. (as *Metrosideros collins polym* 2:31)

Microlepia setosa, Pa-la-pa-la-i
Hawaiian *Psychological Aid* Plant used for insanity. (as *M. strigosa* 2:73)

Mikania batatifolia, Southern Hempvine
Seminole *Dermatological Aid* Plant used for snake sickness: itchy skin. (145:166) Decoction of plant taken and used as a body steam for snake sickness: itchy skin. (145:239)

Mimulus cardinalis, Crimson Monkeyflower
Karok *Pediatric Aid* Infusion of plant used as a wash for newborn baby. (125:389)

Mimulus eastwoodiae, Eastwood's Monkeyflower
Navajo, **Kayenta** *Anticonvulsive* Plant used for hiccups. (179:42)

Mimulus glabratus var. **jamesii**, James's Monkeyflower
Potawatomi *Unspecified* Leaves used as treatment for unspecified ailments. (131:83)

Mimulus guttatus, Seep Monkeyflower
Kawaiisu *Analgesic, Herbal Steam*, and *Orthopedic Aid* Decoction of stems and leaves used as steam bath for chest and back soreness. (180:41) **Shoshoni** *Dermatological Aid* Poultice of crushed leaves applied to wounds or rope burns. (155:105) **Yavapai** *Gastrointestinal Aid* Decoction taken as tea for stomachache. (as *M. nasutus* 53:261)

Mimulus ringens, Ringen Monkeyflower
Iroquois *Anticonvulsive* Compound decoction of roots taken by women for epilepsy. *Antidote* Compound decoction of plants used as wash to counteract poison. (73:435)

Mirabilis alipes, Winged Four O'Clock
Paiute *Analgesic* Decoction of root taken and used as a wash for headaches. Decoction of root used as a wash for neuralgia. Poultice of crushed, fresh leaves applied for headaches. *Antiemetic* Decoction of root taken or used as a wash for fainting spells and nausea. *Burn Dressing* Dried root powder moistened and used as a salve for burns. *Cathartic* Decoction of root taken as a physic. *Dermatological Aid* Dried root powder sprinkled on sores or made into a wash for impetigo. Poultice of mashed leaves applied to swellings. *Psychological Aid* Decoction of root used as a wash for "delirium," neuralgia, and dizziness. *Stimulant* Decoction of root taken or used as a wash for fainting spells and dizziness. (as *Hermidium alipes* 155:86, 87) **Paiute, Northern** *Dermatological Aid* Poultice of dried, powdered roots applied and decoction of powdered roots used as a wash for sores. (as *Hermidium alipes* 49:125)

Mirabilis bigelovii var. **retrorsa**, Bigelow's Four O'Clock
Paiute *Dermatological Aid* Powdered root used as shampoo and infusion of root taken simultaneously. (as *Hesperonia retrorsa* 98:46) Powdered root used as shampoo and infusion taken simultaneously. (as *Hesperonia retrorsa* 98:57)

Mirabilis californica, California Four O'Clock
Luiseño *Cathartic* Decoction of leaves taken as a purgative. (132:232) **Mahuna** *Febrifuge* Plant used for eruptive fevers. (117:10)

Mirabilis coccineus, Scarlet Four O'Clock
Hopi *Dermatological Aid* Decoction of plant used as a wash for wounds. (as *Oxybaphus coccinea* 174:32, 75) **Yavapai** *Venereal Aid* Pounded, boiled root taken for gonorrhea. (as *Allionia coccinea* 53:260)

Mirabilis greenei, Greene's Four O'Clock
Karok *Pediatric Aid* Plant used to make a newborn baby healthy. (125:383)

Mirabilis linearis, Narrowleaf Four O'Clock
Lakota *Diuretic* Infusion of roots taken for urinating difficulties. (116:52) **Navajo**, **Kayenta** *Gastrointestinal Aid* Root used for stomach disorders. *Gynecological Aid* Infusion of roots used for postpartum treatment. *Panacea* Plant used as a life medicine. (as *Oxybaphus linearis* 179:21) **Navajo**, **Ramah** *Burn Dressing* Poultice of soaked, split root applied to burns. *Cough Medicine* Decoction of plant used for coughs. *Hunting Medicine* Cold infusion of plant used as a lotion for good luck in trading or hunting. *Veterinary Aid* Decoction of plant used for sheep and horses with coughs. (as *Oxybaphus linearis* 165:26) **Zuni** *Diuretic* Root eaten to induce urination. *Emetic* Root eaten to induce vomiting. *Gastrointestinal Aid* Infusion of root taken for stomachache. (as *Oxybaphus linearis* 22:377)

Mirabilis multiflora, Colorado Four O'Clock
Hopi *Gynecological Aid* Used to push up the blood in the woman during the pregnant stage. *Hallucinogen* Root chewed by medicine man to induce visions while making a diagnosis. *Veterinary Aid* Used as antiseptic to wash out wounds in horses. (as *Nirabilis multiflora* 34:334) **Navajo** *Antirheumatic (Internal)* Plant used for rheumatism. *Dermatological Aid* Plant used for "swellings." *Oral Aid* Plant used for various mouth disorders. (76:161) **Navajo**, **Ramah** *Dermatological Aid* Poultice of root applied to swellings. (165:26) **Zuni** *Dietary Aid* Powdered root mixed with flour, made into a bread and used to decrease appetite. (22:377)

Mirabilis multiflora var. multiflora,
Colorado Four O'Clock
Hopi *Hallucinogen* Roots chewed by doctor to induce visions while making diagnosis. (as *Quamoclidion multiflorum* 174:31, 75) **Tewa** *Kidney Aid* Infusion of pulverized root taken for swellings "of dropsical origin." (as *Quamoclidion multiflorum* 115:60) **Zuni** *Dietary Aid* Infusion of root taken and rubbed on abdomen of hungry adults and children. (as *Quamoclidion multiflorum* 143:58, 59) *Gastrointestinal Aid* and *Pediatric Aid* Infusion of powdered root taken by adults or children after overeating. (as *Quamoclidion multiflorum* 143:58)

Mirabilis nyctaginea, Heartleaf Four O'Clock
Cherokee *Dermatological Aid* Poultice of beaten root used for boils and milk poured over leaves used as fly poison. (66:34, 35) **Chippewa** *Orthopedic Aid* Decoction of root or poultice of root applied to sprain or strained muscles. (as *Allionia nyctaginea* 43:362) **Dakota** *Anthelmintic* Decoction of roots taken as a vermifuge. (as *Allionia nyctaginea* 57:361) Compound decoction of root taken as a vermifuge. *Dermatological Aid* Compound decoction of root used as wash for swollen arms or legs. (as *Allionia nyctaginea* 58:78) *Febrifuge* Decoction of roots taken as a febrifuge. (as *Allionia nyctaginea* 57:361) Decoction of root taken for fever. (as *Allionia nyctaginea* 58:78) **Meskwaki** *Burn Dressing* Poultice of macerated root applied to burns. *Urinary Aid* Root or whole herb used for bladder troubles. (as *Oxybaphus nyctaginea* 129:232) **Ojibwa** *Orthopedic Aid* Root used for sprains and swellings. (as *Oxybaphus nyctagineus* 130:375) **Pawnee** *Gynecological Aid* Decoction of root taken after childbirth for abdominal swelling. *Oral Aid* Dried, ground root applied to baby's sore mouth. *Pediatric Aid* Pulverized dried root applied to babies for sore mouth. **Ponca** *Dermatological Aid* Chewed root blown into wounds. (as *Allionia nyctaginea* 58:78) **Sioux**, **Teton** *Dermatological Aid* Moistened, grated root rubbed on skin for swelling. *Orthopedic Aid* Herb used externally for broken bones. (as *Allionia nyctaginea* 42:270)

Mirabilis oblongifolia, Mountain Four O'Clock
Navajo, **Ramah** *Burn Dressing* Poultice of soaked, split root applied to burns. (as *Oxybaphus comatus* 165:26)

Mirabilis oxybaphoides, Smooth Spreading Four O'Clock

Navajo, Kayenta *Dermatological Aid* Plant used for spider bites or as a hair lotion for dandruff. (179:21) **Navajo, Ramah** *Orthopedic Aid* Poultice of whole plant applied to fractures. (165:26)

Mirabilis pumila, Dwarf Four O'Clock

Navajo, Kayenta *Dermatological Aid* Plant used as a lotion for sores and skin eruptions. (as *Oxybaphus pumilus* 179:21)

Mitchella repens, Partridge Berry

Abnaki *Antirheumatic (External)* Used for swellings. (121:155) Poultice of plant applied to swellings. (121:173) **Cherokee** *Analgesic* Taken for "monthly period pains." *Antidiarrheal* Decoction made with milk taken for dysentery. *Dermatological Aid* Infusion taken for hives and used for sore nipples. *Diaphoretic* Taken as a diaphoretic. *Dietary Aid* Given to baby before it "takes the breast." *Diuretic* Taken as a diuretic. *Gastrointestinal Aid* Infusion of root taken with rattlesnake weed for bowel complaint. *Gynecological Aid* Used to facilitate childbirth, for sore nipples, and taken for menstrual cramps. *Hemorrhoid Remedy* Decoction made with milk taken for piles. *Pediatric Aid* Given to baby before it "takes the breast." *Veterinary Aid* Given to pregnant cat and her kittens. (66:47) **Chippewa** *Unspecified* Infusion of whole plant used for medicinal purposes. (59:141) **Delaware** *Abortifacient* Infusion used for suppressed menstruations to strengthen the female generative organs. *Antirheumatic (External)* Hot infusion of roots or twigs used as a steam treatment for muscular swellings and stiff joints. (151:36) **Delaware, Oklahoma** *Abortifacient* Infusion of plant taken for "suppressed menses." *Antirheumatic (External)* Strong infusion of roots or twigs used as herbal steam for rheumatism. (150:30, 76) *Gynecological Aid* Infusion of plant taken to strengthen the "female generative organs." *Herbal Steam* Infusion of roots or twigs used as herbal steam for rheumatism. (150:30) **Iroquois** *Analgesic* Compound decoction of roots taken for urinating pain. Decoction of plants taken by pregnant women with side or labor pains. (73:441) Compound infusion of roots and bark taken for back pain. (73:442) Berries used to prevent severe labor pains.

(103:96) *Anticonvulsive* Compound infusion given to children with convulsions. (73:440) *Antiemetic* Compound infusion of roots and bark taken for vomiting. (73:442) *Blood Medicine* Compound decoction of plants taken as blood purifier. Decoction of plants taken to "remove chill from the blood." (73:441) *Carminative* Decoction of plant taken for stomach gas. (73:442) *Cathartic* Decoction of roots given to newborn babies as a physic for stomachaches. *Dermatological Aid* Decoction of plants given to babies with rashes. Poultice of smashed plant applied to bleeding cuts. (73:441) *Febrifuge* Compound infusion given to children with inward fever. Compound infusion of plants taken for typhoid-like fever or inward fever. (73:440) Poultice of hot plant applied to chest for fevers. (73:442) *Gastrointestinal Aid* Compound infusion taken for inward fever from stomach trouble. (73:440) Decoction of roots given to newborn babies as a physic for stomachaches. Poultice applied or decoction of vines given to babies with swollen abdomens. *Gynecological Aid* Compound decoction of leaves and roots taken for leukorrhea (sick womb). Compound decoction of plants taken by pregnant women with side pains. (73:441) Compound of plants taken for labor pain in parturition. (73:442) Berries used to prevent severe labor pains and to facilitate delivery. (103:96) *Hemostat* Poultice of smashed plant applied to bleeding cuts. (73:441) *Kidney Aid* Infusion or decoction of roots and bark taken for kidney troubles. (73:442) *Love Medicine* Compound of plant used as love medicine. (73:441) *Misc. Disease Remedy* Decoction of plant taken by pregnant mother to prevent rickets in baby. *Orthopedic Aid* Compound infu-

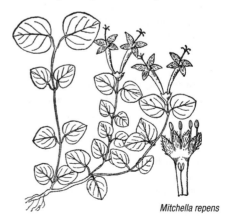

Mitchella repens

sion of roots and bark taken for back pain.
(73:442) *Pediatric Aid* Compound infusion given
to children with inward fever and convulsions. Decoction of vines given to babies when they will not
suckle. (73:440) Decoction of plants given to babies with rashes. Decoction of roots given to newborn babies as a physic for stomachaches. Poultice
applied or decoction of vines given to babies with
swollen abdomens. (73:441) Decoction of plant
taken by pregnant mother to prevent rickets in
baby. (73:442) *Psychological Aid* Compound infusion of plants taken for typhoid-like fever or craziness. (73:440) *Urinary Aid* Compound decoction
of plants taken for swollen testicles or ruptures.
Compound decoction of roots taken for urinating
pain. Decoction of plants taken for bladder stricture. *Venereal Aid* Compound decoction of plants
taken for venereal disease. (73:441) **Menominee**
Gynecological Aid Decoction of leaves used for
"diseases of women." (44:133) *Sedative* Infusion
of leaves taken "to cure insomnia." (128:51)
Montagnais *Febrifuge* Berries cooked into a jelly
and used for fevers. (133:313) **Ojibwa** *Ceremonial Medicine* Leaves smoked during ceremonies.
(112:239) **Penobscot** *Unspecified* Infusion of
leaves used as a medicine for unspecified purpose.
(133:309) **Seminole** *Kidney Aid* Plant used for
kidney disorders. (145:274)

Mitella diphylla, Twoleaf Miterwort
Iroquois *Emetic* Decoction of whole plants taken
to vomit and counteract bad luck. *Eye Medicine*
Infusion of plant used as drops for sore eyes.
(73:345)

Mitella nuda, Naked Miterwort
Cree, Woodlands *Ear Medicine* Crushed leaf
wrapped in a cloth and inserted in the ear for earaches. (91:45)

Mitella trifida, Threeparted Miterwort
Gosiute *Gastrointestinal Aid* and *Pediatric Aid*
Infusion of roots used for babies with colic.
(31:375)

Mnium affine
Carrier, Southern *Antirheumatic* (*External*)
Decoction of plant used to bathe a swollen face.
(35:53)

Mnium punctatum
Makah *Antirheumatic* (*External*) Leaves used for
swellings. (35:53)

Modiola caroliniana, Carolina Bristlemallow
Houma *Misc. Disease Remedy* Compound infusion gargled and decoction taken for sore throat
or diphtheria. *Throat Aid* Compound infusion gargled and decoction taken for tonsillitis or sore
throat. (135:64)

Monarda didyma, Scarlet Beebalm
Cherokee *Abortifacient* Used for female obstructions. *Analgesic* Poultice of leaves used for headache. *Carminative* Used carminative for colic and
flatulence. *Cold Remedy* Poultice of leaves used for
colds. *Diaphoretic* Used as a diaphoretic. *Diuretic*
Used as a diuretic. *Febrifuge* Hot infusion of leaf
used to "bring out measles" and infusion used as
febrifuge. *Gastrointestinal Aid* Infusion of leaf
and plant top taken for weak bowels and stomach.
Heart Medicine Infusion used for heart trouble.
Hemostat Infusion of leaf or root taken orally and
wiped on head for nosebleed. *Misc. Disease Remedy* Infusion of leaf used to "bring out measles"
and infusion used to "sweat off flu." *Sedative* Used
for hysterics and restful sleep. (66:39)

Monarda fistulosa, Wildbergamot Beebalm
Blackfoot *Cough Medicine* Infusion of plant taken
for coughs. (72:72) *Dermatological Aid* Poultice
of a flower head applied to a burst boil and removed after the wound healed. (72:77) Poultice of
plant pieces applied to cuts. (72:84) *Emetic* Infusion of plant and another plant taken and used as
a steam to serve as an emetic. (72:65) *Eye Medicine* Used to make a solution for sore eyes. (68:70)
Kidney Aid Infusion of plant taken for aching kidneys. (72:67) *Throat Aid* Root chewed for swollen
neck glands. (72:77) **Cherokee** *Abortifacient*
Used for female obstructions. *Analgesic* Poultice of
leaves used for headache. *Carminative* Used as a
carminative for colic and flatulence. *Cold Remedy*
Poultice of leaves used for colds. *Diaphoretic*
Used as a diuretic, diaphoretic, and especially for
"sweating off flu." *Diuretic* Used as a carminative
for colic, diuretic, and diaphoretic. *Febrifuge* Hot
infusion of leaf used to "bring out measles" and
infusion used as febrifuge. *Gastrointestinal Aid*

Infusion of leaf and plant top taken for weak bowels and stomach. *Heart Medicine* Infusion used for heart trouble. *Hemostat* Infusion of leaf or root taken orally and wiped on head for nosebleed. *Misc. Disease Remedy* Infusion of leaf used to "bring out measles" and infusion used to "sweat off flu." *Sedative* Used for hysterics and restful sleep. (66:39) **Chippewa** *Analgesic* Chewed leaves placed in nostrils for headaches. *Cold Remedy* Plant tops used for colds. (59:140) **Choctaw** *Analgesic* Plant rubbed on child's chest for pain. *Cathartic* Infusion of leaves taken as a cathartic. *Pediatric Aid* Plant rubbed on child's chest for pain. (152:54) **Crow** *Respiratory Aid* Infusion taken for respiratory problems. (68:70) **Dakota** *Analgesic* Infusion of flowers and leaves taken for abdominal pains. (57:363) Decoction of flowers and leaves taken for abdominal pains. (58:111) *Gastrointestinal Aid* Infusion of flowers and leaves taken for abdominal pains. (57:363) Decoction of leaves and flowers taken for abdominal pains. (58:111) **Flathead** *Cold Remedy* Infusion taken for colds. Plants hung on walls for colds. *Cough Medicine* Used for coughs. *Eye Medicine* Used to make a solution for sore eyes. *Febrifuge* Infusion taken for fevers. *Misc. Disease Remedy* Infusion taken for flu and chills. *Pulmonary Aid* Infusion taken for pneumonia. *Toothache Remedy* Used for toothache. (68:70) **Koasati** *Febrifuge* Decoction of leaves used as a bath for chills. (152:54) **Kutenai** *Kidney Aid* Infusion used for kidney problems. (68:70) **Lakota** *Cough Medicine* Infusion of leaves used as a cough remedy. *Eye Medicine* Infusion of leaves used on a cloth placed on sore eyes overnight. *Hemostat* Poultice of chewed leaves applied to stop the flow of blood. *Pulmonary Aid* Infusion of leaves used for whooping cough. *Stimulant* Infusion of leaves used for fainting. (116:50) **Menominee** *Pediatric Aid* Decoction of stem and leaves used as strengthening bath for infants. (44:133) *Respiratory Aid* Simple or compound infusion of leaves and flowers used as a universal remedy for catarrh. (128:39) **Meskwaki** *Cold Remedy* Compound used for colds. (129:225) **Montana Indian** *Gynecological Aid* Infusion taken for expulsion of the afterbirth. (68:70) **Navajo** *Analgesic* Cold infusion of plant used as a wash for headaches. (45:73) **Ojibwa** *Anticonvulsive* Infusion of plant taken or used as a bath for

infant convulsions. *Febrifuge* Infusion of flowers taken for fevers. *Pediatric Aid* Infusion of plant taken or used as a bath for infant convulsions. (4:2274) *Respiratory Aid* Plant boiled and steam inhaled "to cure catarrh and bronchial affections." (130:372) **Ojibwa, South** *Analgesic* and *Gastrointestinal Aid* Decoction of root taken for "pain in the stomach and intestines." (77:201) **Sioux** *Gastrointestinal Aid* Infusion taken for stomach pains. (68:70) **Sioux, Teton** *Cold Remedy* Infusion of blossoms used for "hard cold." *Febrifuge* Infusion of blossoms used for fever. (42:270) **Winnebago** *Dermatological Aid* Decoction of leaves used on pimples and other skin eruptions on the face. (58:111)

Monarda fistulosa ssp. *fistulosa* var. *menthifolia*, Mintleaf Beebalm

Cheyenne *Ceremonial Medicine* Plant used in ceremonies. (as *M. menthoefolia* 63:186) *Dermatological Aid* and *Veterinary Aid* Chewed or dried leaves used as a perfume for horses, bodies, and clothing. (as *M. menthoefolia* 64:186) **Navajo, Ramah** *Dermatological Aid* Cold infusion taken and used as lotion for gunshot or arrow wounds. (as *M. menthaefolia* 165:41) **Tewa** *Analgesic* Pulverized plant rubbed on the head for headache. *Eye Medicine* Plant used for sore eyes. *Febrifuge* Dried plant or leaves rubbed over body and infusion taken for fever. *Throat Aid* Dried leaves worn around neck and decoction taken for sore throat. (as *M. menthaefolia* 115:57, 58)

Monarda fistulosa ssp. *fistulosa* var. *mollis*, Oswego Tea

Blackfoot *Eye Medicine* Infusion of blossoms used as an eyewash to allay inflammation. (as *M. scabra* 95:275) **Chippewa** *Anthelmintic* Decoction of root and blossoms taken for worms. (as *M. mollis* 43:346) *Burn Dressing* Poultice of moistened, dry flowers and leaves applied to scalds and burns. (as *M. mollis* 43:354) *Dermatological Aid* Infusion of flower and leaf used as a wash, especially for children, for "eruptions." (as *M. mollis* 43:350) **Flathead** *Gynecological Aid* Infusion of leaves used by women after confinement. **Sioux** *Gynecological Aid* Infusion of leaves used by women after confinement. (as *M. scabra* 15:16)

Monarda pectinata, Pony Beebalm

Kiowa *Dermatological Aid* Flowers gathered, placed in water, and the liquid sprinkled on the hair as a perfume. Infusion of flowers used as a wash for insect bites and stings. Flowers gathered, placed in water, and the liquid sprinkled on the hair as a perfume. (166:49) **Navajo** *Analgesic* Plant used for headaches. (76:153) **Navajo, Kayenta** *Gastrointestinal Aid* Plant used for stomach disease. (179:41) **Navajo, Ramah** *Analgesic* Cold infusion taken and used as poultice for headache. *Ceremonial Medicine* Plant used in a ceremonial lotion. *Cough Medicine* Cold infusion taken and used as poultice for cough. *Febrifuge* Cold infusion taken and used as poultice for fever. *Misc. Disease Remedy* Cold infusion taken and used as poultice for influenza. (165:41)

Monarda punctata, Spotted Beebalm

Delaware *Dermatological Aid* Infusion of plant used to bathe patients' faces. *Febrifuge* Infusion of plant used for fever. (151:35) **Delaware, Oklahoma** *Febrifuge* Infusion of whole plant taken and used as a face wash for fever. (150:29, 76) **Meskwaki** *Analgesic* Compound containing leaves snuffed up nostrils for sick headache. Compound containing leaves used for stomach cramps. *Cold Remedy* Compound used as a snuff for head colds and catarrh. *Gastrointestinal Aid* Compound containing leaves used for stomach cramps. *Respiratory Aid* Compound used as a snuff for catarrh and used for head cold. *Stimulant* Compound applied at nostrils of patient to rally him when at

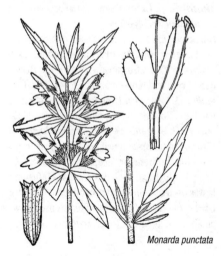

Monarda punctata

point of death. (129:225, 226) **Mohegan** *Febrifuge* Infusion of leaves used for fevers. (151:73, 130) **Nanticoke** *Cold Remedy* Infusion of whole plant taken as a cold remedy. (150:55, 84) **Navajo, Ramah** *Analgesic* Cold infusion taken and used as poultice for headache. *Cough Medicine* Cold infusion taken and used as poultice for cough. *Febrifuge* Cold infusion taken and used as poultice for fever. (165:42) **Ojibwa** *Gastrointestinal Aid* Decoction of plants taken for stomach or bowel troubles. *Laxative* Decoction of plants taken for sick stomach, bowels, or for constipation. (112:231) *Unspecified* Plant used as a rubbing medicine. (112:240)

Monardella lanceolata, Mustang Mountainbalm

Diegueño *Unspecified* Infusion of plant used as a medicinal tea and beverage. (70:25) **Luiseño** *Unspecified* Infusion of plant used for medicinal purposes. (132:229) **Miwok** *Analgesic* Decoction of leaves, upper stems, and flowers taken for headaches. *Cold Remedy* Decoction of leaves, upper stems, and flowers taken for colds. (8:171)

Monardella odoratissima, Pacific Monardella

Karok *Diaphoretic* Plant used as a sweat medicine. *Love Medicine* Plant used as a love medicine by women. (125:389) **Miwok** *Cold Remedy* Decoction of stems and flower heads taken for colds. *Febrifuge* Decoction of stems and flower heads taken for fevers. (8:171) **Okanagan-Colville** *Cold Remedy* and *Pediatric Aid* Infusion of leaves and stems given to children and adults for the common cold. (162:109) **Paiute** *Analgesic* Decoction of plant taken for gas pains. *Cold Remedy* Decoction of plant taken for colds. *Eye Medicine* Decoction of branches used as an eyewash for soreness or inflammation. *Gastrointestinal Aid* Decoction of plant taken for indigestion, gas pain, or minor digestive upset. (155:105, 106) **Sanpoil** *Cold Remedy* and *Pediatric Aid* Decoction of stems and leaves taken by adults and children for severe colds. (as *M. adoratissima* 109:218) **Shoshoni** *Analgesic* Decoction of plant taken for gas pains. *Blood Medicine* Decoction of branches taken as a blood tonic. *Cathartic* Decoction of branches taken as a physic. *Cold Remedy* Decoction of plant taken for colds. *Gastrointestinal Aid* Decoction of plant taken for indigestion, gas pain, or minor digestive upset. *Tonic* Decoction of branches taken as a general tonic. **Washo** *Analgesic* Decoction of plant taken for gas pains. *Cold Remedy* Decoction of plant taken for colds. *Gastrointestinal Aid* Decoction of plant taken for indigestion, gas pain, or minor digestive upset. (155:105, 106)

Monardella villosa, Coyote Mint
Cahuilla *Gastrointestinal Aid* Infusion of leaves taken for stomachaches. (11:89) **Costanoan** *Blood Medicine* and *Pulmonary Aid* Poultice of plant applied to back cuts to draw out "bad blood" for pneumonia. *Respiratory Aid* Decoction of plant and plant salve used for respiratory conditions. (17:16) **Mahuna** *Gastrointestinal Aid* Plant used for stomachaches. (117:8)

Monardella villosa* ssp. *sheltonii, Shelton's Mountainbalm
Mendocino Indian *Blood Medicine* Infusion of dried leaves taken to purify the blood. *Gastrointestinal Aid* Infusion of dried leaves taken for colic. (as *M. sheltonii* 33:384)

Moneses uniflora, Single Delight
Cowichan *Dermatological Aid* Poultice of leaves applied to draw out the pus from boils or abscesses. (156:83) **Eskimo, Alaska** *Cold Remedy* Infusion of dried plants used for colds. *Cough Medicine* Infusion of dried plants used for coughs. (126:331) **Haisla & Hanaksiala** *Throat Aid* Plant chewed for sore throats. (35:261) **Kwakiutl** *Analgesic* Poultice of chewed or pounded plant applied to pains. (157:283) *Dermatological Aid* Poultice of chewed plant applied to swellings to draw blisters. (16:382) Plant used to draw blisters. Poultice of chewed or pounded plant applied to swellings. (157:283) **Kwakwaka'wakw** *Dermatological Aid* Poultice of chewed plant applied to swellings and blisters. (35:261) **Montagnais** *Orthopedic Aid* Infusion of plant used as a medicine for paralysis. (as *Monensis uniflora* 133:314) **Salish, Coast** *Dermatological Aid* Poultice of leaves applied to draw out the pus from boils or abscesses. (156:83)

Moneses uniflora* ssp. *reticulata, Single Delight
Haisla & Hanaksiala *Throat Aid* Plant chewed

for sore throats. **Kwakwaka'wakw** *Dermatological Aid* Poultice of chewed plant applied to swellings and blisters. (35:261)

Monolepis nuttalliana, Nuttall's Povertyweed
Navajo, Ramah *Ceremonial Medicine* Plant used as ceremonial emetic. *Dermatological Aid* Poultice of moist leaves applied to skin abrasions. *Emetic* Plant used as ceremonial emetic. *Hunting Medicine* Pinch of dried plant eaten by hunters to prevent "buck fever." (165:25)

Monotropa hypopithys, Pinesap
Kwakiutl *Love Medicine* Plant used in a love potion. (as *Hypopites monotropa* 157:283)

Monotropa uniflora, Indian Pipe
Cherokee *Anticonvulsive* Pulverized root given to children for fits, epilepsy, and convulsions. *Dermatological Aid* Crushed plant rubbed on bunions or warts. *Eye Medicine* Juice and water used to wash sore eyes. *Pediatric Aid* Pulverized root given to children for fits, epilepsy, and convulsions. (66:40) **Cree, Woodlands** *Toothache Remedy* Flower chewed for toothaches. (91:46) **Mohegan** *Analgesic* and *Cold Remedy* Infusion of root or leaves taken for pain due to colds. (151:73, 130) *Febrifuge* Leaves used for colds and fever. (151:130) **Potawatomi** *Gynecological Aid* Infusion of root taken for female troubles. (131:57) **Thompson** *Dermatological Aid* Poultice of plant used for sores that would not heal. Dried powdered stems applied to sores or burned stalk rubbed on sores. (161:215)

Moricandia arvensis, Purple Mistress
Hoh *Unspecified* Plants used for medicine.
Quileute *Unspecified* Plants used for medicine. (as *Brassica arvensis* 114:61)

Morinda citrifolia, Indian Mulberry
Hawaiian *Dermatological Aid* Young fruit thoroughly pounded with salt or fruit juice and used for broken bones and deep cuts. *Orthopedic Aid* Young fruit thoroughly pounded with salt or fruit juice used for broken bones and deep cuts. *Unspecified* Leaves used to make medicine. (2:73)

Morus alba, White Mulberry
Cherokee *Anthelmintic* Infusion of bark taken for worms. *Antidiarrheal* Infusion of bark taken to "check dysentery." *Cathartic* Infusion of bark used as a purgative. *Laxative* Infusion of bark taken as a laxative. (66:45)

Morus nigra, Black Mulberry
Delaware, **Oklahoma** *Cathartic* Decoction of bark taken as a cathartic. *Emetic* Decoction of bark taken as an emetic. *Gastrointestinal Aid* and *Liver Aid* Decoction of bark taken "to remove bile from the intestines." (150:25, 76)

Morus rubra, Red Mulberry
Alabama *Urinary Aid* Decoction of roots taken for passing yellow urine. (152:19) **Cherokee** *Anthelmintic* Infusion of bark taken for worms. *Antidiarrheal* Infusion of bark taken to "check dysentery." *Cathartic* Infusion of bark used as a purgative. *Laxative* Infusion of bark taken as a laxative. (66:45) **Creek** *Emetic* Roots used as an emetic. *Stimulant* Infusion of root taken for weakness. *Urinary Aid* Infusion of root taken for urinary problems. (148:659) **Meskwaki** *Panacea* Root bark used as a medicine for any sickness. (129:251) **Rappahannock** *Dermatological Aid* Tree sap rubbed on skin for ringworm. (138:30)

Mucuna gigantea, Seabean
Hawaiian *Laxative* Fruit meat and other plants chewed, mixed with salt water, and injected with an enema as a laxative. (2:45)

Muhlenbergia dubia, Pine Muhly
Navajo *Veterinary Aid* Compound poultice with roots applied to make sheep's blood cake. (76:153)

Muhlenbergia richardsonis, Mat Muhly
Blackfoot *Veterinary Aid* Roots used as a horse medicine. (82:22)

Murdannia nudiflora, Nakedstem Dewflower
Hawaiian *Blood Medicine* Infusion of pounded leaves and other plants strained and taken to purify the blood. (as *Commelina nudiflora* 2:70)

Musa ×paradisiaca, Paradise Banana
Hawaiian *Strengthener* Bud or young flower juice rubbed on tongue and mouth interior for body weakness from stomach disorder. (as *M. sapientum* 2:65)

Myosotis laxa, Bay Forget Me Not
Makah *Dermatological Aid* Plant rubbed on the hair to act like a hair spray. (55:312)

Myosurus aristatus, Bristle Mousetail
Navajo, **Ramah** *Panacea* Plant used as "life medicine." *Witchcraft Medicine* Cold infusion of plant taken to protect from witches. (165:27)

Myosurus cupulatus, Arizona Mousetail
Navajo, **Ramah** *Dermatological Aid* Cold infusion used internally or externally for ant bites. *Gastrointestinal Aid* Cold infusion of plant taken and used as a lotion for effects of swallowing an ant. (165:27)

Myosurus minimus, Tiny Mousetail
Navajo, **Ramah** *Dermatological Aid* Cold infusion taken or poultice of chewed plant applied to ant bite. (165:27)

Myrica cerifera, Southern Bayberry
Choctaw *Febrifuge* Decoction of leaves and stems taken "during attacks of fever." (20:23) Decoction of leaves and stems taken for fevers. *Throat Aid* Decoction of roots used as a gargle for inflamed tonsils. (152:13) **Houma** *Anthelmintic* Decoction of leaves taken as a vermifuge. (135:56) **Koasati** *Gastrointestinal Aid* and *Pediatric Aid* Decoction of roots given to children with stomachaches. (152:13) **Micmac** *Analgesic* Roots used for headaches. (32:58) *Antirheumatic (External)* Hot poultice of pounded, water-soaked roots applied to inflammations. (168:30) *Dermatological Aid* Roots used for inflammations. *Stimulant* Berries, bark, and leaves used as an exhilarant and beverage. (32:58) **Seminole** *Analgesic* Decoction of leaves taken for headaches. *Febrifuge* Decoction of leaves taken for fevers. *Gastrointestinal Aid* Decoction of leaves taken for stomachaches. (145:282) *Love Medicine* Decoction of wood ashes placed on the tongue to cleanse the body and strengthen the marriage. (145:250)

Myrica gale, Sweet Gale
Bella Coola *Diuretic* Decoction of pounded branches taken as a diuretic and for gonorrhea. *Venereal Aid* Decoction of pounded branches taken for gonorrhea and as a diuretic. (127:55) Infusion of pounded branches and fruits taken as a diuretic for gonorrhea. (158:206)

Myriophyllum sibiricum, Shortspike Watermilfoil
Iroquois *Blood Medicine* Infusion of whole plant and two other plants taken by adolescents for poor blood circulation. (as *M. exalbescens* 118:51) *Emetic* Infusion of plant taken as a strong emetic. (as *M. exalbescens* 118:51). *Pediatric Aid* Infusion of whole plant and two other plants taken by adolescents for poor blood circulation. (as *M. exalbescens* 118:51)

Myriophyllum spicatum, Spike Watermilfoil
Menominee *Unspecified* Some plants of this class used in medicines. (128:37)

Myriophyllum verticillatum, Whorlleaf
   Watermilfoil
Iroquois *Other* Compound infusion of plants used as a "snowsnake medicine." *Pediatric Aid* and *Stimulant* Decoction of plant given to children when they lie very quiet and never move. (73:391)

Ｎ *Nama hispidum*, Bristly Nama
Navajo, Kayenta *Dermatological Aid* Plant used as a lotion for spider or tarantula bites. (179:39)

Napaea dioica, Glade Mallow
Meskwaki *Dermatological Aid* Poultice of root applied to keep old sores soft and boiled root used for swellings. *Gynecological Aid* Root used to ease childbirth and for female troubles. *Hemorrhoid Remedy* Roots used as a special remedy for piles. *Hunting Medicine* Root used as a hunting charm and for female troubles. (129:232)

Navarretia atractyloides, Hollyleaf
   Pincushionplant
Costanoan *Burn Dressing* Toasted, powdered plant or plant ash applied to burns. (17:13)

Navarretia cotulifolia, Cotulaleaf Pincushionplant
Miwok *Antirheumatic* (*External*) Decoction applied to swelling. (8:171)

Nemopanthus mucronatus, Catberry
Malecite *Cough Medicine* Used with blackberry roots, staghorn sumac, lily roots, and mountain raspberry roots for coughs. *Febrifuge* Used with blackberry roots, staghorn sumac, lily roots, and mountain raspberry roots for fevers. (96:251) *Kidney Aid* Infusion of root scrapings used for gravel. (96:257) *Tuberculosis Remedy* Used with blackberry roots, staghorn sumac, lily roots, and mountain raspberry roots for consumption. (96:251) **Ojibwa** *Unspecified* Berries used medicinally for unspecified purpose. (130:355) **Potawatomi** *Panacea* Compound decoction boiled down to syrup and used for many kinds of diseases. *Tonic* Decoction of small branches reduced to syrup and taken as a tonic. (131:39)

Nepeta cataria, Catnip
Cherokee *Abortifacient* Infusion used for female obstructions. *Anthelmintic* Infusion used for worms. *Anticonvulsive* Infusion used for spasms. *Cold Remedy* "Syrup" and honey used for colds and infusion used for babies' colds. *Cough Medicine* "Syrup" and honey used for coughs. *Dermatological Aid* Infusion taken for hives and poultice of leaf used for boils and swellings. *Febrifuge* Infusion taken for fevers and poultice of leaf used for boils. *Gastrointestinal Aid* Infusion used for colic and infusion of leaves used for stomach. *Pediatric Aid* Infusion used for babies' colds. *Sedative* Infusion used for hysterics. *Stimulant* Infusion of leaf used as a stimulant. *Tonic* Infusion of leaf used as a tonic. (66:28) **Chippewa** *Febrifuge* Simple or compound decoction of leaves taken for fever. (43:354) **Delaware** *Pediatric Aid* Leaves used with peach seeds to make a beneficial syrup for children. (151:37) **Delaware, Oklahoma** *Pediatric Aid* Leaves used with peach pits to make a tonic for children. (150:31, 82) *Tonic* Leaves prepared with peach pit and given as a pediatric tonic. (150:31, 76) **Delaware, Ontario** *Pediatric Aid* and *Sedative* Infusion of leaves given to soothe infants. (150:67) **Hoh** *Pediatric Aid* Infusion used as medicine for infants. (114:68) **Iroquois** *Anal-*

gesic Cold infusion of plants taken for headaches. Decoction of plant tips given to children with headaches. (73:423) *Antidiarrheal* Compound decoction of stems given to children with diarrhea. (73:422) Plant used as a laxative and astringent for diarrhea. *Antiemetic* Infusion of plants taken for vomiting from fever or unknown cause. *Cold Remedy* Infusion of stems taken for colds. *Cough Medicine* Infusion of stems taken for coughs. *Febrifuge* Cold infusion of plants taken or applied to forehead for fevers and chills. *Gastrointestinal Aid* Infusion of plant given to children for stomachaches due to colds. Infusion of plants taken for trouble caused by eating rich foods. *Laxative* Plant used as a laxative and astringent for diarrhea. (73:423) *Oral Aid* Flowers and roots used for excess saliva. (118:58) *Other* Cold infusion of plants taken for fever and "summer complaint." (73:423) *Pediatric Aid* Compound decoction of stems given to children with diarrhea. (73:422) Decoction of plant tips given to children when peevish or with headaches. Infusion of plant given to children for stomachaches due to colds. Infusion of plant tips given to babies who are restless and cannot sleep. Plant used for babies with fevers. *Sedative* Decoction of plant tips given to children when peevish. *Throat Aid* Infusion of stems taken for sore throats and chills. (73:423) **Keres, Western** *Stimulant* Infusion of plant used as a bath for tiredness. (147:55) **Menominee** *Diaphoretic* Decoction of whole plant, except root, taken to produce perspiration. (44:132) *Pulmonary Aid* Compound infusion taken and poultice applied to chest for pneumonia.

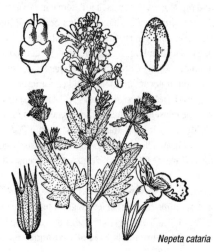

Nepeta cataria

(128:39) *Sedative* Decoction of whole plant, except root, taken to produce restful sleep. (44:132) **Mohegan** *Gastrointestinal Aid* Infusion of plant given to babies for colic. (149:266) Infusion of leaves taken for the stomach and given to infants for colic. (151:74, 130) *Pediatric Aid* Infusion given to babies for colic. (149:266) Infusion of leaves given to infants for colic. (151:74, 13) **Ojibwa** *Blood Medicine* Infusion of leaves taken as a blood purifier. *Other* Infusion of leaves used to bathe a patient to raise the body temperature. (130:372) **Okanagan-Colville** *Cold Remedy* Infusion of plant tops taken for colds. (162:110) **Quileute** *Pediatric Aid* Infusion used as medicine for infants. (114:68) **Rappahannock** *Analgesic* Infusion of leaves given to babies for pains. *Antirheumatic (Internal)* Infusion of leaves given to babies for rheumatism. *Pediatric Aid* Infusion of leaves given to babies for pains, rheumatism, and measles. Weak infusion of plant given to children as a tonic. *Tonic* Weak infusion of plant given to children as a tonic. (138:25) **Shinnecock** *Antirheumatic (Internal)* Dried leaves smoked in a pipe for rheumatism. (25:119)

Nephroma arcticum, Arctic Kidney Lichen
Eskimo, Inuktitut *Strengthener* Infusion of plant used for "weakness." (176:187)

Nereocystis luetkeana
Kwakiutl, Southern *Burn Dressing* Leaves used for burns. *Dermatological Aid* Leaves used for scabs and nonpigmented spots. Leaves dried, pulverized, and rubbed into children's heads to make hair grow long. *Orthopedic Aid* Leaves used for swollen feet. *Pediatric Aid* Leaves dried, pulverized, and rubbed into children's heads to make hair grow long. (common kelp 157:261) **Nitinaht** *Dermatological Aid* Bulbs dried, melted, hardened, and used as skin cream for protection from sun, wind, and cold. (common kelp 160:52) **Pomo, Kashaya** *Expectorant* Dried, salty stalk strips sucked for colds with sore throats and to clear mucus. *Throat Aid* Dried, salty stalk strips sucked for colds with sore throats. (as *N. luetkeama*, bull kelp 60:124)

Nicotiana attenuata, Coyote Tobacco
Apache, White Mountain *Ceremonial Medicine*

Plant smoked in the medicine ceremonies. (113: 158) **Hopi** *Ceremonial Medicine* Plant smoked for all ceremonial occasions. (46:19) **Navajo, Kayenta** *Hemostat* Plant used for nosebleed. *Narcotic* Plant used as a narcotic. (179:41) **Navajo, Ramah** *Analgesic* Leaves smoked in corn husks for headache. *Ceremonial Medicine* Plant smoked in corn husks for ceremonial purposes. *Cough Medicine* Leaves smoked in corn husks for cough. *Veterinary Aid* Plant used to heal castration cuts on a young racehorse. (165:43) **Paiute** *Anthelmintic* Decoction of leaves taken sparingly to expel worms. (155:106, 107) *Antirheumatic (External)* Infusion of stems and leaves used as a wash for aches and pains. (93:108) Crushed seeds used as a liniment for rheumatic swellings. Poultice of crushed leaves applied to swellings, especially from rheumatism. *Cathartic* Weak decoction of leaves taken as a physic. (155:106, 107) *Cold Remedy* Leaves smoked during sweat house bathing and prayer, connected with spiritual power. (93:108) Dried leaves smoked alone or in a compound for colds and asthma. *Dermatological Aid* Decoction of leaves used as a healing wash for hives or other skin irritations. Poultice of chewed leaves applied to cuts. Poultice of crushed leaf applied or crushed seed used as a liniment for swellings. Poultice of crushed leaves applied to eczema or other skin infections. Pulverized dust of plant sprinkled on sores. (155:106, 107) *Emetic* Infusion of stems and leaves taken as an emetic. (93: 108) Weak decoction of leaves taken as an emetic. *Kidney Aid* Decoction of leaves used as a wash for "dropsical conditions." (155:106, 107) *Misc. Disease Remedy* Infusion of plant taken for measles. *Respiratory Aid* Infusion of stems and leaves taken for respiratory diseases. (93:108) Compound containing dried leaves smoked for asthma. *Snakebite Remedy* Poultice of chewed leaves bound on snakebite after removing poison. (155:106, 107) *Tuberculosis Remedy* Infusion of stems and leaves taken for tuberculosis. (93:108) Compound containing dried leaves smoked for tuberculosis. (155:106, 107) **Salish** *Dermatological Aid* Plant used as a head wash for dandruff. (153:294) **Shoshoni** *Anthelmintic* Decoction of leaves taken sparingly to expel worms. *Antirheumatic (External)* Poultice of crushed leaves applied to swellings, especially from rheumatism. *Cathartic* Weak decoction of

leaves taken as a physic. *Dermatological Aid* Decoction of leaves used as a healing wash for hives or other skin irritations. Poultice of chewed leaves applied to cuts. Poultice of crushed leaf applied to reduce swellings. *Emetic* Weak decoction of leaves taken as an emetic. *Toothache Remedy* Poultice of crushed leaves applied to gum for toothache. *Tuberculosis Remedy* Compound of dried leaves smoked for tuberculosis. (155:106, 107) **Shuswap** *Urinary Aid* Plant used for the bladder. (102:69) **Tewa** *Ceremonial Medicine* Dried leaves and other plant parts smoked ceremonially. (115:103, 104) *Cough Medicine* Poultice of leaves mixed with oil and soot applied to neck and chest for cough. *Gynecological Aid* Snuff containing leaves used by women in labor. (115:106) *Nose Medicine* Snuff of leaves used for "a discharge from the nose." (115:103, 104) *Toothache Remedy* Leaves placed on or in a tooth for toothache. (115:106) **Thompson** *Dermatological Aid* Decoction of plant used as a wash to remove dandruff and prevent falling hair. (141:467, 468) **Zuni** *Snakebite Remedy* Smoke blown over body for throbbing from rattlesnake bite. (143:54)

Nicotiana clevelandii, Cleveland's Tobacco
Cahuilla *Dermatological Aid* Poultice of leaves applied to cuts, bruises, swellings, and other wounds. *Ear Medicine* Leaf smoke blown into the ear and covered with a warm pad for earaches. *Emetic* Infusion of leaves used as an emetic. *Hunting Medicine* Leaves smoked as part of a hunting ritual. (11:90)

Nicotiana glauca, Tree Tobacco
Cahuilla *Dermatological Aid* Poultice of leaves applied to cuts, bruises, swellings, and other wounds. *Ear Medicine* Leaf smoke blown into the ear and covered with a warm pad for earaches. *Emetic* Infusion of leaves used as an emetic. *Hunting Medicine* Leaves smoked as part of a hunting ritual. (11:90) **Hawaiian** *Dermatological Aid* Plant used for removing the pus from scrofulous sores or boils. Plant used for sores and the smoke used for cuts. *Tuberculosis Remedy* Plant used for removing the pus from scrofulous sores. (2:73) **Mahuna** *Antirheumatic (External)* Infusion of leaves used as a steam bath for rheumatism. *Throat Aid* Poultice of leaves applied to inflamed

throat glands. *Tuberculosis Remedy* Poultice of leaves applied for scrofula. (117:60)

Nicotiana quadrivalvis var. bigelovii,
Bigelow's Tobacco

Costanoan *Cathartic* Leaves smoked as a general purgative in social and ritual contexts. *Ceremonial Medicine* Leaves smoked as a general purgative in social and ritual contexts. *Ear Medicine* Plant smoke blown into the ear for earaches. *Emetic* Fresh leaves chewed as an emetic. (as *N. bigelovii* 17:14) **Karok** *Unspecified* Used for medicine. (as *N. bigelovi* 97:209) **Kawaiisu** *Analgesic* Chewed plant put in the nostril for headaches. Poultice of plant applied to the chest for internal pains. *Dermatological Aid* Poultice of plant applied to itchy bites. Poultice of plant applied to bleeding cuts. *Ear Medicine* Chewed plant put in the ear for earaches. *Emetic* Plant eaten to cause vomiting. Plant induced vomiting. *Gastrointestinal Aid* Plant eaten to clean out the stomach. *Gynecological Aid* Poultice of plant applied to woman's stomach during parturition. *Hallucinogen* Plant eaten to cause dreams. *Hemostat* Poultice of plant applied to bleeding cuts. *Other* Plant used for infanticide and suicide. *Poison* Plant considered poisonous. *Psychological Aid* Plant blown in the air to prevent bad dreams. *Respiratory Aid* Plant used as snuff for stuffy noses. *Sedative* Plant used as a soporific. *Stimulant* Plant used for fatigue. *Toothache Remedy* Plant held between the teeth for toothaches. (as *N. bigelovii* 180:43)

Nicotiana rustica, Aztec Tobacco

Cherokee *Analgesic* Used for cramps and sharp pains. (66:59) Chewed plant used for headaches. (152:56) *Anthelmintic* Used as an anthelmintic. *Anticonvulsive* Used as an antispasmodic. *Cathartic* Used as a cathartic. *Ceremonial Medicine* Used extensively in rituals. *Dermatological Aid* Poultice of beaten plant used for boils and applied to insect bites. *Diaphoretic* Used as a sudorific. *Diuretic* Used as a diuretic. *Emetic* Used as an emetic. *Expectorant* Used as an expectorant. *Gastrointestinal Aid* Taken for colic. *Kidney Aid* Taken for dropsy. *Misc. Disease Remedy* Decoction of leaf used for ague, "locked-jaw," and "black-yellow disease." *Other* Compound used for apoplexy, dizziness, and fainting. (66:59) Decoction of leaves

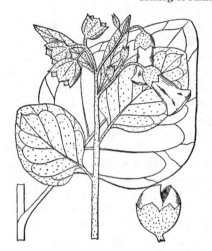

Nicotiana rustica

rubbed in scratches made on the patient for apoplexy. (152:56) *Snakebite Remedy* Juice applied to snakebite. *Toothache Remedy* Smoke blown on toothache. *Vertigo Medicine* Used for dizziness and fainting. (66:59) **Iroquois** *Antidote* Compound decoction of plants used as wash to counteract poison. *Dermatological Aid* Poultice of chewed plant applied to all insect bites. *Psychological Aid* Decoction of plants taken for insanity caused by masturbation. *Tuberculosis Remedy* Plant used for consumption. (73:430)

Nicotiana tabacum, Cultivated Tobacco

Cherokee *Analgesic* Used for cramps and sharp pains. *Anthelmintic* Used as an anthelmintic. *Anticonvulsive* Used as an antispasmodic. *Cathartic* Used as a cathartic. *Ceremonial Medicine* Used extensively in rituals. *Dermatological Aid* Poultice of beaten plant used for boils and applied to insect bites. *Diaphoretic* Used as a sudorific. *Diuretic* Used as a diuretic. *Emetic* Used as an emetic. *Expectorant* Used as an expectorant. *Gastrointestinal Aid* Taken for colic. *Kidney Aid* Taken for dropsy. *Misc. Disease Remedy* Decoction of leaf used for ague, "locked-jaw," and "black-yellow disease." *Other* Compound used for apoplexy, dizziness, and fainting. *Snakebite Remedy* Juice applied to snakebite. *Toothache Remedy* Smoke blown on toothache. *Vertigo Medicine* Used for dizziness and fainting. (66:59) **Haisla & Hanaksiala** *Antirheumatic* (*External*) Juice rubbed on the hands and feet for rheumatism. (35:291)

Hawaiian *Dermatological Aid* Plant used for removing the pus from scrofulous sores or boils. Plant used for sores and the smoke used for cuts. *Tuberculosis Remedy* Plant used for removing the pus from scrofulous sores. (2:73) **Hesquiat** *Dermatological Aid* Chewed leaves used as a poultice or rubbed on bruises and cuts. (159:76) **Micmac** *Ear Medicine* Leaves used for earache. *Hemostat* Leaves used for bleeding. (32:58) **Mohegan** *Ear Medicine* Smoke blown into the ear for an earache. **Montauk** *Toothache Remedy* Tobacco placed in tooth for toothache. **Rappahannock** *Ear Medicine* Smoke blown into the ear for an earache. *Toothache Remedy* Tobacco placed in tooth for toothache. **Shinnecock** *Ear Medicine* Smoke blown into the ear for an earache. *Toothache Remedy* Tobacco placed in tooth for toothache. (25:120) **Thompson** *Dermatological Aid* Poultice of plant used on cuts and sores. (161:288)

Nicotiana trigonophylla, Desert Tobacco
Cahuilla *Dermatological Aid* Poultice of leaves applied to cuts, bruises, swellings, and other wounds. *Ear Medicine* Leaf smoke blown into the ear and covered with a warm pad for earaches. *Emetic* Infusion of leaves used as an emetic. *Hunting Medicine* Leaves smoked as part of a hunting ritual. (11:90)

Nolina microcarpa, Sacahuista
Isleta *Antirheumatic* (*Internal*) Decoction of root taken for rheumatism. *Pulmonary Aid* Decoction of root taken for pneumonia and lung hemorrhages. (85:35)

Nothochelone nemorosa, Woodland Beardtongue
Paiute *Dermatological Aid* Green, mashed plant juice applied to sores "like iodine." (as *Penstemon nemorosus* 93:109)

Nuphar lutea ssp. *advena*, Yellow Pondlily
Iroquois *Analgesic* Compound decoction taken for pain between shoulder blades. *Anticonvulsive* Compound decoction with plant taken by men with epilepsy. *Blood Medicine* Compound infusion of dried roots taken for blood disease. *Febrifuge* Compound decoction with roots taken for recurring chills followed by fever. (as *N. luteum* ssp.

macrophyllum 73:319) *Gastrointestinal Aid* Poultice of roots or decoction taken and used as wash for swollen abdomen. (as *N. luteum* ssp. *macrophyllum* 73:318) *Heart Medicine* Infusion of dried, grated plant taken for heart trouble. (as *N. luteum* ssp. *macrophyllum* 73:319) *Misc. Disease Remedy* Infusion of roots taken to dry up smallpox. (as *N. luteum* ssp. *macrophyllum* 73:318) *Other* Cold infusion of roots used as a "ghost medicine." *Pulmonary Aid* Compound decoction taken for swollen lungs. *Witchcraft Medicine* "Hung up inside to keep witches away" as an anti-witch remedy. Compound used to "detect bewitchment." Poultice of roots applied to sore areas caused by witchcraft diseases. (as *N. luteum* ssp. *macrophyllum* 73:319) **Menominee** *Dermatological Aid* Poultice of dried, powdered root applied to cuts and swellings. (as *Nymphaea advena* 128:42, 43) **Micmac** *Dermatological Aid* Poultice of bruised root with flour or meal applied to swellings and bruises. (as *Nuphar advena* 133:317) *Orthopedic Aid* Leaves used for limb swellings. (as *Nymphaea advena* 32:58) **Ojibwa** *Dermatological Aid* Poultice of grated root applied to sores and powdered root used for cuts and swellings. (as *Nymphaea advena* 130:376) **Penobscot** *Dermatological Aid* Poultice of mashed leaves applied to swollen limbs. (as *Nymphaea advena* 133:310) **Potawatomi** *Dermatological Aid* Poultice of pounded root applied for "many inflammatory diseases." (as *Nymphaea advena* 131:65) **Rappahannock** *Dermatological Aid* Poultice of parched and bruised leaf used to remove fever and inflammation from sores. Warmed leaves applied to boils. *Febrifuge* Poultice of parched and bruised leaf used to remove fever and inflammation from sores. (as *Nymphaea advena* 138:32) **Sioux** *Hemostat* Dry, porous rhizomes ground fine and applied to wounds as a styptic. (as *Nuphar advena* 15:17) **Thompson** *Analgesic* Cold decoction of stems or roots taken for internal pains. *Dermatological Aid* Poultice of fresh or dried leaves applied to wounds, cuts, or sores. (as *Nymphaea advena* 141:460)

Nuphar lutea ssp. *polysepala*, Rocky
 Mountain Pondlily
Bella Coola *Analgesic* Decoction of root taken for pain in any part of the body. *Antirheumatic*

(*Internal*) Decoction of root taken for rheumatic pain. *Blood Medicine* Decoction of root considered "good for the blood." *Heart Medicine* Decoction of root taken for heart disease pain. *Tuberculosis Remedy* Decoction of root taken for consumption pain. (as *Nymphaea polysepala* 127:56) Rhizomes used for tuberculosis. (as *Nuphar polysepalum* 158:206) *Venereal Aid* Decoction of root taken for gonorrheal pain. **Gitksan** *Antihemorrhagic* Infusion of toasted root scrapings taken for lung hemorrhages. *Gynecological Aid* Infusion of toasted root or decoction of root heart used as a contraceptive. *Pulmonary Aid* Decoction of root taken for lung hemorrhage. (as *Nymphaea polysepala* 127:56) **Haisla & Hanaksiala** *Tuberculosis Remedy* Decoction of rhizomes taken for tuberculosis. *Unspecified* Decoction of rhizomes taken as medicine. (35:256) **Hesquiat** *Unspecified* Pond lily was a good medicine. (as *Nuphar polysepalum* 159:70) **Kitasoo** *Gynecological Aid* Decoction of plant and devil's club used for unspecified woman's illness. (35:339) **Kwakiutl** *Analgesic* Poultice of heated leaves applied or rhizome extract taken for chest pains. *Orthopedic Aid* Rhizomes used as a medicine for internal swellings or sickness in the bones. *Respiratory Aid* Rhizome extract taken for asthma and chest pains. (as *N. polysepalum* 157:287) **Nitinaht** *Other* Large rhizomes placed in hot water and liquid taken to prevent sickness during epidemics. (as *N. polysepalum* 160:114) *Unspecified* Decoction of rhizomes used as a medicinal drink. (as *N. polysepalum* 55:251) Rhizomes used as a medicine. (as *N. polysepalum* 159:70) **Okanagan-Colville** *Poison* Roots considered poisonous. *Toothache Remedy* Stems placed directly on the tooth for toothaches. (as *N. polysepalum* 162:110) **Quinault** *Analgesic* Poultice of heated roots applied for pain. *Antirheumatic* (*External*) Poultice of heated roots applied for rheumatism. (as *Nymphozanthus polysepalus* 65:29) **Shuswap** *Analgesic* Infusion of mashed roots applied for sore back pain. *Antirheumatic* (*External*) Infusion of mashed roots applied for rheumatism. *Dermatological Aid* Infusion of mashed roots taken for sores. *Orthopedic Aid* Infusion of mashed roots applied for sore back pain. (as *Nuphar polysepalum* 102:64) **Tanana**, **Upper** *Analgesic* Poultice of sliced, warmed rhizomes applied for pain. (as *N. polysepalum* 86:17)

Thompson *Antirheumatic* (*External*) Powdered, dried leaves mixed with bear grease and used as an ointment for swellings. *Dermatological Aid* Powdered, dried leaves mixed with bear grease and used as an ointment for bites and infections. *Gastrointestinal Aid* Large rhizomes chewed for ulcers. (161:235)

Nuphar lutea* ssp. *variegata, Variegated Yellow Pondlily
Algonquin, **Quebec** *Dermatological Aid* Poultice of mashed rhizomes applied to swellings. *Disinfectant* Poultice of mashed rhizomes applied to infections. (as *N. variegatum* 14:163) **Cree**, **Woodlands** *Analgesic* Poultice of grated rhizome, calamus, water or grease, and sometimes cow parsnip applied for headaches. *Antirheumatic* (*External*) Poultice of grated rhizomes and other ingredients applied to sore joints, swellings, and painful limbs. Poultice consisted of grated rhizomes, grated calamus rootstocks, and occasionally cow parsnip with the addition of water or grease. *Dermatological Aid* Poultice of roots with calamus and cow parsnip roots applied to mancos, worms in the flesh. Poultice of fresh or rehydrated, dried rhizome slice applied to infected skin lesions. Poultice of sliced, dried roots soaked in water and applied to infected wounds. *Panacea* Powdered rhizomes added to a many-herb remedy for various ailments. (as *N. variegatum* 91:46) **Flathead** *Antirheumatic* (*External*) Decoction of rootstocks added to bath water for rheumatism. *Dermatological Aid* Poultice of baked rootstocks used for sores. *Venereal Aid* Infusion of rootstocks taken for venereal disease. *Veterinary Aid* Poultice of rootstocks used for horses with cuts and bruises. (as *N. variegatum* 68:33) **Iroquois** *Blood Medicine* and *Pediatric Aid* Infusion of rhizomes and two other plants taken by adolescents for poor blood circulation. *Veterinary Aid* Infusion of plant, other plant fragments, and milk given to pigs that drool and have sudden movements. (as *N. variegatum* 118:43) **Kutenai** *Dermatological Aid* Poultice of baked rootstocks used for sores. **Sioux** *Hemostat* Rootstocks powdered and used as a styptic for wounds. (as *N. variegatum* 68:33)

Nymphaea odorata, American White Waterlily
Chippewa *Oral Aid* Dried, pulverized root put in

the mouth for sores. (as *Castalia odorata* 43:342) **Micmac** *Cold Remedy* Leaves used for colds. (32:58) *Cough Medicine* Juice of root taken for coughs. *Dermatological Aid* Poultice of boiled root applied to swellings. (133:317) *Gland Medicine* Roots used for suppurating glands and leaves used for colds. *Misc. Disease Remedy* Leaves used for grippe. *Orthopedic Aid* Leaves used for limb swellings and colds. (32:58) **Ojibwa** *Cough Medicine* Root used as a cough medicine for tuberculosis. *Tuberculosis Remedy* Root used as a cough medicine for tuberculosis. (as *Castalia odorata* 130:376) **Okanagan-Colville** *Poison* Roots considered poisonous. *Toothache Remedy* Stems placed directly on the tooth for toothaches. (162:110) **Penobscot** *Dermatological Aid* Compound poultice of mashed leaves applied to limb swellings. (as *Castalia odorata* 133:310) **Potawatomi** *Unspecified* Poultice of pounded root used for unspecified ailments. (as *Castalia odorata* 131:65)

Nymphoides cordata, Little Floatingheart
Seminole *Cough Medicine* Plant used for turtle sickness: trembling, short breath, and cough. (as *N. lacunosum* 145:237) *Other* Complex infusion of roots taken for chronic conditions. (as *N. lacunosum* 145:272) *Respiratory Aid* and *Sedative* Plant used for turtle sickness: trembling, short breath, and cough. (as *N. lacunosum* 145:237)

Nyssa sylvatica, Black Gum
Cherokee *Anthelmintic* Compound given for worms. (66:26) Infusion of bark used as a bath and given to children with worms. (152:47) *Antidiarrheal* Compound decoction given for diarrhea. *Emetic* Inner bark used as part of "drink to vomit bile." (66:26) Decoction of inner bark taken to cause vomiting when unable to retain food. (152:47) *Eye Medicine* Strong ooze from root dripped into eyes. (66:26) *Gastrointestinal Aid* Decoction of inner bark taken to cause vomiting when unable to retain food. (152:47) *Gynecological Aid* Infusion given for childbirth and infusion of bark given for "flooding." *Other* Compound infusion of bark used for "bad disease." (66:26) *Pediatric Aid* Infusion of bark used as a bath and given to children with worms. (152:47) *Urinary Aid* Used as ingredient in drink for "milky urine." (66:26) **Creek** *Tuberculosis Remedy* Decoction of bark used as

a bath and taken for pulmonary tuberculosis. (152:47) **Houma** *Anthelmintic* Decoction of root or bark taken for worms. (135:55) **Koasati** *Dermatological Aid* Decoction of bark taken and applied to gun wounds. (152:47)

Obolaria virginica, Virginia Pennywort
Cherokee *Cold Remedy* Taken for colds. *Cough Medicine* Taken for coughs. *Diaphoretic* Taken as a diaphoretic. *Gastrointestinal Aid* Taken for colic. (66:48) **Choctaw** *Dermatological Aid* Simple or compound decoction of root used as a wash or dressing for cuts and bruises. (20:23) Decoction of root used as bath or poultice of root applied to cuts and bruises. (152:51)

Ochrosia compta, Ho-le-i
Hawaiian *Herbal Steam* Infusion of bark and leaves used for steam in the sweat bath. *Pediatric Aid* and *Strengthener* Nuts and other plants chewed and fed to infants for general debility. (as *Ochorosia sandwicensis* 2:44)

Octoblephorum albidum, Moss
Seminole *Antirheumatic* (*External*) and *Febrifuge* Plant used for fire sickness: fever and body aches. (145:203)

Odontoglossum chinensis, Pa-la-a
Hawaiian *Laxative* Infusion of plant used for softening the bowels and constipation. (as *Odontoglossum chineusis* 2:73)

Oemleria cerasiformis, Indian Plum
Kwakiutl *Analgesic* and *Dermatological Aid* Poultice of chewed, burned plant and oil applied to sore places. (as *Osmaronia cerasiformis* 157:289) **Makah** *Laxative* Bark used as a mild laxative. *Tuberculosis Remedy* Decoction of bark taken for tuberculosis. *Unspecified* Bark used as a healing agent. (55:264)

Oenanthe sarmentosa, Water Parsley
Haisla & Hanaksiala *Poison* Plant considered highly toxic. (35:216) **Kitasoo** *Cathartic* Roots used as a purgative. *Emetic* Roots used as an

emetic. (35:326) **Kwakiutl** *Emetic* Seeds and roots used as an emetic. (157:277) **Kwakwaka' wakw** *Emetic* Plant used as an emetic. (35:216) Roots used as an emetic. (35:326) **Makah** *Laxative* Pounded roots used as a laxative. (65:42) **Nitinaht** *Gynecological Aid* Roots squashed and swallowed to facilitate and speed up delivery. (160:93) **Nuxalkmc** *Emetic* Plant used as an emetic. (35:216) **Tsimshian** *Ceremonial Medicine* Roots eaten as an emetic to seek supernatural powers and purify. (35:326)

Oenothera albicaulis, Whitest Eveningprimrose
Hopi *Ceremonial Medicine* Used to ward out the cold through prayer. (34:336) **Keres, Western** *Antirheumatic* (*External*) Poultice of plant used for swellings. (as *Anogra albicaulis* 147:27) **Navajo, Ramah** *Ceremonial Medicine* Dried flowers used as ceremonial medicine. (as *O. ctenophylla* 165:37, 38) *Orthopedic Aid* Decoction of root taken and used as a lotion for strain from carrying heavy load. *Panacea* Decoction of root taken and used as a lotion for muscle strain, a "life medicine." (165:37) Root used as a "life medicine." (as *O. ctenophylla* 165:37, 38) *Throat Aid* Compound poultice of plant applied for "throat trouble." (165:37)

Oenothera biennis, Common Eveningprimrose
Cherokee *Dietary Aid* Infusion taken for "overfatness." *Hemorrhoid Remedy* Hot root poultice used for piles. (66:33) **Iroquois** *Dermatological Aid* Compound used for boils. *Hemorrhoid Remedy* Compound decoction of roots taken and used as a wash for piles. *Stimulant* Compound used for laziness. *Strengthener* Chewed roots rubbed on arms and muscles to provide athletes great strength. (73:390) **Ojibwa** *Dermatological Aid* Poultice of soaked, whole plant applied to bruises. (130:376) **Potawatomi** *Unspecified* Tiny seeds used as a valuable medicine for unspecified ailment. (131:66, 67)

Oenothera brachycarpa, Shortfruit Eveningprimrose
Navajo, Kayenta *Dermatological Aid* Plant used as a lotion for sores. (179:33)

Oenothera cespitosa, Tufted Eveningprimrose
Blackfoot *Dermatological Aid* Wet poultice of crushed roots applied to sores and swellings. (82:48) **Gosiute** *Unspecified* Root used as medicine. (31:375) **Isleta** *Dermatological Aid* Poultice of dried, ground leaves used on sores for rapid healing. (as *Pachylophus hirsutus* 85:36) **Navajo, Kayenta** *Ceremonial Medicine* Plant used in various ceremonies. *Dermatological Aid* Plant used as dusting powder for chafing. *Gynecological Aid* Poultice of ground plant applied for prolapse of the uterus. (179:33)

Oenothera cespitosa* ssp. *cespitosa, Tufted
Eveningprimrose
Blackfoot *Dermatological Aid* Poultice of pounded root applied to inflamed sores and swellings. (as *Pachylobus caespitosus* 95:274) Poultice of pounded, wetted root applied to inflamed sores. (as *Pachylophus caespitosus* 98:44)

Oenothera cespitosa* ssp. *marginata,
Tufted Eveningprimrose
Hopi *Eye Medicine* Plant used with Kachina ears for sore eyes. *Toothache Remedy* Plant used as toothache medicine. (34:337) **Navajo, Ramah** *Panacea* Poultice of plant or root used only for large swellings, a "life medicine." (165:37)

Oenothera coronopifolia, Crownleaf Eveningprimrose
Navajo, Ramah *Adjuvant* Dried leaves added to improve the flavor of wild tobacco. *Analgesic* and *Gastrointestinal Aid* Cold infusion of leaves taken for stomachache. *Panacea* Poultice of plant or root used only for large swellings, a "life medicine." (165:37) **Zuni** *Antirheumatic* (*External*) Poultice of powdered flower and saliva applied at night to swellings. (22:377)

Oenothera elata* ssp. *hookeri, Hooker's
Eveningprimrose
Navajo, Kayenta *Ceremonial Medicine* Plant used as a Plumeway emetic. *Cold Remedy* Plant used for colds. *Dermatological Aid* Poultice of plant applied to sores. *Emetic* Plant used as a Plumeway emetic. *Misc. Disease Remedy* Hot poultice of plant applied for mumps. (as *O. hookeri* 179:33) **Navajo, Ramah** *Panacea* Poultice of root

used only for large swellings, a "life medicine." (as *O. bookeri* var. *hirsutissima* 165:37) **Zuni** *Antirheumatic* (*External*) Poultice of powdered flower and saliva applied at night to swellings. (as *O. bookeri* 22:377)

Oenothera flava, Yellow Eveningprimrose
Navajo, Ramah *Burn Dressing* Seedpod ashes applied to burns. *Panacea* Poultice of plant or root used only for large swellings, a "life medicine." Poultice of root used for swellings and internal injuries, a "life medicine." *Throat Aid* Poultice of compound containing whole plant used for "throat trouble." (165:38)

Oenothera pallida, Pale Eveningprimrose
Navajo, Kayenta *Ceremonial Medicine* Plant used as a Beadway emetic. *Dermatological Aid* Plant used as dusting powder for venereal disease sores. Poultice of plant applied to spider bites. *Emetic* Plant used as a Beadway emetic. *Kidney Aid* Infusion of plant used for kidney disease. *Venereal Aid* Plant used as dusting powder for venereal disease sores. *Veterinary Aid* Plant used for livestock with colic. (179:34)

Oenothera pallida* ssp. *runcinata, Pale Eveningprimrose
Navajo, Ramah *Ceremonial Medicine* and *Emetic* Plant used as a ceremonial emetic. *Snakebite Remedy* Decoction of root and leaves used as a lotion for snakebites. *Throat Aid* Soaked plant rubbed on throat and infusion taken for sore throat. (as *O. runcinata* 165:38)

Oenothera perennis, Small Eveningprimrose
Iroquois *Orthopedic Aid* Decoction of plants taken for paralysis. (73:390)

Oenothera primiveris, Desert Eveningprimrose
Navajo, Ramah *Ceremonial Medicine* Fresh or dried flowers used as ceremonial lotion and medicine. *Dermatological Aid* Poultice of plant applied to swellings. (165:38)

Oenothera triloba, Stemless Eveningprimrose
Zuni *Antirheumatic* (*External*) Ingredient of "schumaakwe cakes" and used externally for rheumatism. *Dermatological Aid* Ingredient of "schumaakwe cakes" and used externally for swelling. (as *Lavauxia triloba* 143:55)

Oenothera villosa* ssp. *strigosa, Hairy Eveningprimrose
Navajo, Ramah *Disinfectant* Cold infusion of dried root taken for "deer infection." *Hunting Medicine* Dried leaves and tobacco smoked for good luck in hunting. (as *O. procera* 165:38)

Onoclea sensibilis, Sensitive Fern
Iroquois *Antirheumatic* (*Internal*) Used for arthritis and infection. (73:256) *Blood Medicine* Fermented compound decoction taken before meals and bed to "make blood." (73:254) Compound decoction of roots taken for "cold in blood." Decoction used as a hair wash and taken for the blood which caused the hair to fall out. (73:255) Infusion of rhizomes given to children when "the blood doesn't have a determined path." (118:34) *Dermatological Aid* Poultice of plant top used for deep cuts. (73:256) *Gastrointestinal Aid* Used "for trouble with the intestines, when you catch cold and get inflated and sore." (73:255) *Gynecological Aid* Infusion of root taken for pain after childbirth. Infusion of whole plant or roots applied to full, nonflowing breasts. (73:254) Decoction of roots taken for fertility in women and the blood, to give strength after childbirth, and to start menses and for swellings, cramps, and sore abdomen. (73:255) *Pediatric Aid* Infusion of rhizomes given to children when "the blood doesn't have a determined path." (118:34) *Tuberculosis Remedy* Compound decoction of roots taken during the early stages of consumption. (73:256) *Venereal Aid* Compound decoction used for venereal disease. (73:254) Cold, compound infusion of plant washed on sores and taken for gonorrhea. (73:255) Infusion of plant and female fern rhizomes used by men for venereal diseases. (118:34) **Ojibwa** *Gynecological Aid* Decoction of powdered, dried root used by patients with caked breast for milk flow. (130:382)

Onopordum acanthium, Scotch Cottonthistle
Iroquois *Emetic* Decoction used as an emetic to counter witchcraft. *Poison* Decoction used for witchcraft poison. *Witchcraft Medicine* Decoction

used for witchcraft poison and as an emetic to counter witchcraft. (73:476)

Onosmodium molle, Smooth Onosmodium
Lakota *Antirheumatic* (*External*) Infusion of roots and seeds used by men for swellings. *Veterinary Aid* Infusion of roots and seeds given to horses or used as a rubbing solution. (116:41)

Onosmodium molle* ssp. *occidentale,
    Western Onosmodium
Cheyenne *Antirheumatic* (*External*) Pulverized leaves and stems mixed with grease and used as a rub for lumbago. (as *O. occidentale* 64:185) *Dermatological Aid* Smashed leaves and stems rubbed on numb skin. (as *O. occidentale* 63:185) Pulverized leaves and stems mixed with grease and rubbed on numb skin. (as *O. occidentale* 64:185) *Orthopedic Aid* Smashed leaves and stems rubbed on back for lumbago. (as *O. occidentale* 63:185)

Oplopanax horridus, Devil's Club
Bella Coola *Antirheumatic* (*Internal*) Decoction of root bark and stems taken for rheumatism. *Cathartic* Root bark chewed as purgative and decoction of root bark and stems taken. (as *Fatsia horrida* 127:62) *Emetic* Inner bark chewed as an emetic. (as *O. horridum* 158:201) **Carrier** *Analgesic* Poultice of bark scrapings applied or bark pills taken for pain. (as *O. horridum* 26:82) **Carrier, Northern** *Analgesic* Inner bark taken for stomach and bowel cramps. *Cathartic* Inner bark

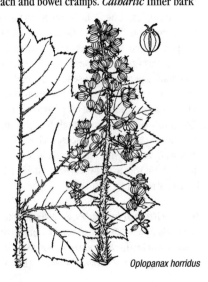
Oplopanax horridus

acts as a purgative, especially if taken with hot water. *Gastrointestinal Aid* Inside layer of inner bark taken for stomach and bowel cramps. **Carrier, Southern** *Cathartic* and *Gynecological Aid* Decoction of bark taken as a purgative before and after childbirth. (as *Fatsia horrida* 127:62) **Cheyenne** *Analgesic* Root mixed with tobacco and smoked for headache. (as *Fatsia horrida* 15:12) **Cowlitz** *Antirheumatic* (*External*) Infusion of bark used as wash for rheumatism. *Cold Remedy* Infusion of bark taken for colds. *Poison* Plant considered poisonous. (as *O. horridum* 65:41) **Crow** *Analgesic* Root mixed with tobacco and smoked for headache. (as *Fatsia horrida* 15:12) **Gitksan** *Analgesic* Fresh or dried inner bark used for stomach ulcers and pain. Infusion of dried bark used for stomach pain and ulcers. (as *O. horridum* 62:16) *Antihemorrhagic* Poultice of compound containing bark used as a chest plaster for lung hemorrhage. (as *Fatsia horrida* 127:62) *Antirheumatic* (*External*) Bark and other plants used for arthritis. (61:152) Poultice of compound containing bark used for rheumatism. (as *Fatsia horrida* 127:62) *Cancer Treatment* Bark and other plants used for cancer. (61:152) *Cathartic* Compound decoction taken as a diuretic and purgative for "strangury." (as *Fatsia horrida* 127:62) *Cold Remedy* Decoction of inner bark used for colds. *Cough Medicine* Decoction of inner bark used for coughs. *Dermatological Aid* Poultice of inner bark applied to wounds. Bark and other plants used as a skin wash. (61:152) Poultice of compound containing bark applied to boils and ulcers. *Diuretic* Compound decoction taken as a diuretic and purgative for "strangury." (as *Fatsia horrida* 127:62) *Gastrointestinal Aid* Bark used as a "cleanser." *Misc. Disease Remedy* Bark and other plants used for diabetes. Decoction of inner bark used for flu. (61:152) *Orthopedic Aid* Decoction taken to aid the knitting of broken bones. *Other* Compound decoction taken continuously for rupture. *Pulmonary Aid* Poultice of compound containing bark used as a chest plaster for lung hemorrhage. (as *Fatsia horrida* 127:62) *Respiratory Aid* Bark and other plants used for bronchitis. *Tonic* Decoction of inner bark used as a tonic. *Tuberculosis Remedy* Bark and other plants used for tuberculosis. (61:152) *Venereal Aid* Decoction taken as a purgative for gonorrhea. (as *Fatsia horrida* 127:62) **Green River**

Group *Cold Remedy* Infusion of roots taken for colds. *Dermatological Aid* Dried bark used as a deodorant. (as *O. horridum* 65:41) **Haisla** *Antirheumatic (External)* Bark and other plants used for arthritis. *Cancer Treatment* Bark and other plants used for cancer. *Cold Remedy* Decoction of inner bark used for colds. *Cough Medicine* Decoction of inner bark used for coughs. *Dermatological Aid* Poultice of inner bark applied to wounds. Bark and other plants used as a skin wash. *Gastrointestinal Aid* Bark used as a "cleanser." *Misc. Disease Remedy* Bark and other plants used for diabetes. Decoction of inner bark used for flu. *Respiratory Aid* Bark and other plants used for bronchitis. *Tonic* Decoction of inner bark used as a tonic. *Tuberculosis Remedy* Bark and other plants used for tuberculosis. (61:152) **Haisla & Hanaksiala** *Antirheumatic (External)* Infusion of pounded leaves applied to arthritic joints. *Dermatological Aid* Inner bark placed in wounds followed by an application of Sitka spruce pitch. Juice used for sores. *Emetic* Decoction or infusion of plant and sea water taken as an emetic. *Eye Medicine* Decoction of stem bark, stems, or winter roots used as an eyewash for cataracts. Decoction of plant used as an eyewash for cataracts. *Gastrointestinal Aid* Juice taken for stomach sickness. *Laxative* Decoction or infusion taken as a laxative. **Hanaksiala** *Cold Remedy* Infusion or decoction of plant taken for winter colds. (35:217) **Hoh** *Unspecified* Used as medicine. (as *Echinopanax horridum* 114:65) **Kwakiutl** *Analgesic* Bark used in a steam bath for body pains. Root held in the mouth and juice swallowed for stomach pains. *Dermatological Aid* Rotten stem ash and oil rubbed on swellings. *Gastrointestinal Aid* Root held in the mouth and juice swallowed for stomach pains. *Herbal Steam* Bark used in a steam bath for body pains. *Laxative* Root held in the mouth and juice swallowed for constipation. *Poison* Spines considered poisonous. *Tuberculosis Remedy* Bark extract taken for tuberculosis. *Witchcraft Medicine* Plant used for the magical powers. (as *O. horridum* 157:278) **Lummi** *Gynecological Aid* Poultice of bark applied to woman's breast to stop an excessive flow of milk. (as *O. horridum* 65:41) **Makah** *Antirheumatic (External)* Poultice of cooked or boiled plant applied to sore spots. Plant used for arthritis. *Unspecified* Bark and roots used medici-

nally. (as *O. horridum* 55:289) **Montana Indian** *Ceremonial Medicine* Used by medicine men in their incantations. (as *Fatsia horrida* 15:12) **Nitinaht** *Antirheumatic (Internal)* Infusion of bark taken for arthritis and rheumatism. (as *O. horridum* 55:289) Infusion of stem pieces taken for arthritis. (160:95) *Orthopedic Aid* Infusion of bark taken for bone ailments. *Unspecified* Used for medicine. (as *O. horridum* 55:289) **Okanagan-Colville** *Cough Medicine* Infusion of roots and stems taken for dry coughs. *Tuberculosis Remedy* Infusion of roots and stems taken for consumption. (as *O. horridum* 162:73) **Okanagon** *Blood Medicine* Infusion of crushed stems taken as a blood purifier. *Dermatological Aid* Burned stems and grease salve rubbed on swollen parts. *Gastrointestinal Aid* Infusion of crushed stems taken for stomach troubles and indigestion. *Tonic* Infusion of crushed stems taken as a tonic. (as *Fatsia horrida* 104:40) **Oweekeno** *Analgesic* Decoction of inner bark from young spring growth taken for general aches and pains. *Antirheumatic (External)* Roots used in a bath for rheumatism. *Cold Remedy* Decoction of inner bark from young spring growth taken for colds. Plant boiled and vapor inhaled for colds. *Dermatological Aid* Berries mashed into a foam and rubbed into the scalp for head lice. *Panacea* Decoction of inner bark from young spring growth taken for any kind of sickness. *Poison* Berries considered poisonous. *Tonic* Decoction of inner bark from young spring growth used as a tonic. (35:85) **Quileute** *Unspecified* Used as medicine. (as *Echinopanax horridum* 114:65) **Salish, Coast** *Analgesic* Poultice of pounded, boiled roots used for rheumatism and other aches and pains. *Antirheumatic (External)* Poultice of pounded, boiled roots used for rheumatism. Prickly stems beaten against the skin as a counterirritant for sore limbs. (as *O. horridum* 156:78) **Sanpoil** *Cold Remedy* Infusion of inner pith of stalk taken for colds. (as *Echinopanax horridum* 109:220) **Skagit** *Gynecological Aid* Decoction of bark taken by women to start menstrual flow after childbirth. *Tuberculosis Remedy* Decoction of bark taken for tuberculosis. (as *O. horridum* 65:41) **Thompson** *Blood Medicine* Infusion of crushed stems taken as a blood purifier. (as *Fatsia horrida* 104:40) Decoction of stems taken as a blood purifier. (as *Echinopanax horridum*

141:459) *Dermatological Aid* Burned stems and grease salve rubbed on swollen parts. (as *Fatsia horrida* 104:40) Stem ash with grease used as an ointment for swellings. (as *Echinopanax horridum* 141:459) *Dietary Aid* Infusion of sticks, with the spines and outer bark removed, taken to cease weight loss. The infusion was taken in doses of about ½ cup before meals, to replace milk and other beverages. It was noted that if the infusion was taken for too great a period of time, one could gain too much weight. Infusion of whole plant taken to give one a good appetite. (161:164) *Gastrointestinal Aid* Infusion of crushed stems taken for stomach troubles and indigestion. (as *Fatsia horrida* 104:40) Infusion of crushed stems taken for indigestion and stomach troubles. (as *Echinopanax horridum* 141:459) Infusion of whole plant taken for ulcers. (161:164) *Laxative* Decoction of stems taken as a laxative. (as *Echinopanax horridum* 141:459) *Misc. Disease Remedy* Infusion of sticks, with the spines and outer bark removed, taken for influenza and other illnesses. Infusion of roots taken for diabetes. *Panacea* Infusion of sticks, with the spines and outer bark removed, taken for everything. (161:164) *Tonic* Infusion of crushed stems taken as a tonic. (as *Fatsia horrida* 104:40) Decoction of stems taken as a tonic. (as *Echinopanax horridum* 141:459) **Tlingit** *Dermatological Aid* Compound containing plant ash used for sores. (as *Panax horridum* 89:284) **Wet'suwet'en** *Antirheumatic* (*External*) Bark and other plants used for arthritis. *Cancer Treatment* Bark and other plants used for cancer. *Cold Remedy* Decoction of inner bark used for colds. *Cough Medicine* Decoction of inner bark used for coughs. *Dermatological Aid* Poultice of inner bark applied to wounds. Bark and other plants used as a skin wash. *Gastrointestinal Aid* Bark used as a "cleanser." *Misc. Disease Remedy* Bark and other plants used for diabetes. Decoction of inner bark used for flu. *Respiratory Aid* Bark and other plants used for bronchitis. *Tonic* Decoction of inner bark used as a tonic. *Tuberculosis Remedy* Bark and other plants used for tuberculosis. (61:152)

Opuntia acanthocarpa, Buckhorn Cholla
Cahuilla *Burn Dressing* Stem ash applied to burns. *Dermatological Aid* Stem ash applied to cuts. (11:95) **Pima** *Gastrointestinal Aid* Plant used for stomach troubles. (38:58)

Opuntia basilaris var. aurea, Golden Pricklypear
Shoshoni *Analgesic* Poultice of inner pulp applied to cuts and wounds and for the pain. *Dermatological Aid* Fuzz-like spines rubbed into warts or moles to remove them. Poultice of inner pulp applied to cuts and wounds and for the pain. (155:107, 108)

Opuntia clavata, Club Cholla
Keres, **Western** *Dermatological Aid* Dried joints ground or burned into a powder and used on open sores or bad wounds. *Veterinary Aid* Dried joints ground or burned into a powder and used on open sores or bad wounds on horses. (147:56)

Opuntia engelmannii, Cactus Apple
Pima *Gynecological Aid* Poultice of heated plant applied to breasts to encourage the flow of milk. (38:60)

Opuntia ficus-indica, Tuna Cactus
Cahuilla *Cathartic* Boiled fruit used as a purgative. *Dermatological Aid* Plugs made from the plant and inserted into wounds as healing agents. *Laxative* Boiled fruit used for constipation. (as *O. megacantha* 11:96)

Opuntia fragilis, Brittle Pricklypear
Okanagan-Colville *Dermatological Aid* Poultice of flesh applied to skin sores and infections. *Diuretic* Flesh eaten to cause urination. (162:92) **Shuswap** *Dermatological Aid* Poultice of heated quills applied to cuts, sores, and boils. *Throat Aid* Poultice of heated quills applied to swollen throats. (102:60)

Opuntia humifusa, Pricklypear
Dakota *Dermatological Aid* Poultice of peeled stems bound on wounds. (58:104) **Lakota** *Snakebite Remedy* Cut stems used for rattlesnake bites. (88:32) **Nanticoke** *Dermatological Aid* Juice of fruit rubbed on warts. (150:56, 84) **Pawnee** *Dermatological Aid* Poultice of peeled stems bound on wounds. (58:104)

Opuntia imbricata var. *imbricata*, Tree
Cholla
Keres, Western *Dermatological Aid* Ground needle coverings made into a paste and used for boils.
Ear Medicine Dried stem pith used for earache
and running ear. *Strengthener* Thorn coverings
eaten by men in times of war to make them tough.
(as *O. arborescens* 147:55)

Opuntia leptocaulis, Christmas Cactus
Apache, Chiricahua & Mescalero *Narcotic*
Fruits crushed and mixed with a beverage to pro-
duce narcotic effects. (28:55)

Opuntia macrorhiza var. *macrorhiza*,
Twistspine Pricklypear
Navajo, Ramah *Dermatological Aid* Cactus spines
formerly used to pierce ears and lance small skin
abscesses. *Gynecological Aid* Stem roasted and
material used to lubricate midwife's hand for placenta removal. (as *O. plumbea* 165:37)

Opuntia phaeacantha, Tulip Pricklypear
Pima *Gynecological Aid* Poultice of heated plant
applied to breasts to encourage the flow of milk.
(38:60)

Opuntia polyacantha, Plains Pricklypear
Flathead *Analgesic* Stems smashed and used for
backache. *Antidiarrheal* Infusion of stems taken
for diarrhea. (68:39) **Navajo** *Poison* Plant used as
a poison for hunting. (45:65) **Okanagan-Colville**
Dermatological Aid Poultice of flesh applied to
skin sores and infections. *Diuretic* Flesh eaten to
cause urination. (162:92) **Sioux** *Dermatological
Aid* Stems peeled and used for wounds. (68:39)

Opuntia tunicata, Thistle Cholla
Hawaiian *Laxative* Leaf juice and roots used for
constipation. *Reproductive Aid* Leaf juice and
roots used by expectant mothers. (as *O. tuna* 2:73)

Opuntia versicolor, Staghorn Cholla

Opuntia whipplei, Whipple Cholla
Hopi *Antidiarrheal* Root chewed or compound
decoction taken for diarrhea. (174:34, 86)

Orbexilum pedunculatum var. *pedunculatum*, Sampson's Snakeroot
Catawba *Dermatological Aid* Root used as salve
for boils, sores, and wounds. (as *Psorglea pedunculata* 134:188) Poultice of boiled roots applied to
sores. (as *Psoralea pedunculata* 152:32) *Orthopedic Aid* Root used as salve for broken bones.
(as *Psorglea pedunculata* 134:188)

Orbexilum pedunculatum var. *psoralioides*, Sampson's Snakeroot
Cherokee *Abortifacient* Infusion taken for obstructed menstruation. *Diaphoretic* Taken as a
diaphoretic. *Gastrointestinal Aid* Taken for colic
and indigestion. *Gynecological Aid* Infusion taken
to "check discharge." *Tonic* Taken as a tonic. (as
Psoralea psoralioides 66:55)

Oreoxis alpina ssp. *alpina*, Alpine Oreoxis
Navajo *Ceremonial Medicine* Plant, greasewood,
and wild privet used as a medicine for the Coyote
Chant. (as *Cymopterus alpinus* 45:67)

Orobanche californica, California Broomrape
Paiute *Cold Remedy* Decoction of plant taken for
colds. *Pulmonary Aid* Decoction of plant taken
for pneumonia or pulmonary trouble. (155:108)

Orobanche fasciculata, Clustered Broomrape
Blackfoot *Dermatological Aid* Chewed root blown
onto wounds by medicine men. (as *Thalesia fasciculata* 95:276) **Keres, Western** *Pulmonary Aid*
Roots eaten as a lung medicine. (as *Thalesia fasciculata* 147:72) **Montana Indian** *Cancer Treatment* Parasite (cancer root) on sweet sage roots
used for cancer. *Poison* Plant poisonous to stock.
(as *Aphyllon fasciculatum* 15:6) **Navajo** *Dermatological Aid* Infusion of leaves used as wash for
sores. (45:77) Poultice of plant applied to wounds
and open sores. (76:153) **Navajo, Ramah** *Panacea* Plant used as "life medicine." *Pediatric Aid*
Plant used for birth injuries. (165:45) **Zuni** *Hemorrhoid Remedy* Powdered plant inserted into rectum as a specific for hemorrhoids. (as *Thalesia
fasciculata* 143:61)

Orobanche ludoviciana, Louisiana Broomrape
Blackfoot *Dermatological Aid* Plant chewed by medicine men and blown upon wounds. (82:53) **Pima** *Dermatological Aid* Poultice of stems applied to ulcerated sores. (38:49)

Orobanche ludoviciana ssp. **ludoviciana**, Sand Broomrape
Navajo, Kayenta *Dermatological Aid* Powdered plant applied to gunshot wounds. (as *O. multiflora* var. *arenosa* 179:43)

Orthilia secunda, Sidebells Wintergreen
Carrier, Southern *Eye Medicine* Strong decoction of root used as an eyewash. (as *Pyrola secunda* 127:62)

Orthocarpus purpureoalbus, Purplewhite Owlclover
Navajo, Ramah *Cathartic* Decoction of whole plant taken as a cathartic. *Ceremonial Medicine* Compound decoction used as ceremonial medicine. *Gastrointestinal Aid* Cold infusion of plant taken for heartburn. (165:44)

Osmorhiza berteroi, Sweetcicely
Bella Coola *Cathartic* Infusion of ground root pieces taken as a purgative. *Emetic* Infusion of ground root pieces taken as an emetic. (as *O. chilensis* 158:201) **Blackfoot** *Cold Remedy* Hot drink containing root taken for colds. *Throat Aid* Hot drink containing root taken for tickling in throat. (as *Washingtonia divaricata* 95:276) *Veterinary*

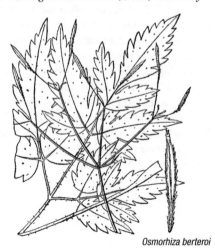

Osmorhiza berteroi

Aid Whole plant fed to mares in the winter to put them into condition for foaling. (as *O. chilensis* 82:49) Plant given to mares to put them in good foaling condition. (as *Washingtonia divaricata* 95:276) Roots placed in mares' mouths and chewed to put them in good condition for foaling. (as *Washingtonia divaricata* 98:49) **Cheyenne** *Adjuvant* Plant used as an ingredient in all medicines. *Cold Remedy* Root chewed or infusion of leaves taken for colds. *Stimulant* Root chewed to "bring one around." (as *O. chilensis* 69:40) **Karok** *Analgesic* Root chewed for headaches. *Panacea* Roots used for any illness. *Preventive Medicine* Roots placed under pillow to prevent sickness. *Psychological Aid* Infusion of roots used as a bath for grieving person. (as *Osmorrhiza nuda* var. *brevipes* 125:386) **Kwakiutl** *Emetic* Seeds and roots used as an emetic. *Poison* Plant "sure to kill" if eaten. (as *Osmorhiza chilensis* 157:277) **Swinomish** *Love Medicine* Roots chewed and used as powerful love charms. (as *O. chilensis* 65:41)

Osmorhiza brachypoda, California Sweetcicely
Kawaiisu *Cold Remedy* Decoction of roots taken for colds. *Cough Medicine* Decoction of roots taken for coughs. *Dermatological Aid* Infusion of mashed plant used as a hair wash to kill fleas. (180:47)

Osmorhiza claytonii, Clayton's Sweetroot
Chippewa *Dermatological Aid* Poultice of moistened, pulverized root used for ulcers, especially running sores. (43:354) *Throat Aid* Decoction of root gargled or root chewed for sore throat. (43:342) **Menominee** *Dietary Aid* Root eaten "to enable one to put on flesh." (128:55) Branch or piece of root eaten cautiously for losing flesh, a fattener. (128:72) *Eye Medicine* Decoction of root used as an eyewash for sore eyes. (44:133) **Ojibwa** *Gynecological Aid* Infusion of root used to ease parturition. *Throat Aid* Infusion of root taken for sore throat. (130:391) **Tlingit** *Cough Medicine* Warm infusion of whole plant taken for coughs. (as *Osmorhyza brevistyla* 89:283)

Osmorhiza longistylis, Longstyle Sweetroot
Cheyenne *Gastrointestinal Aid* Infusion of leaves, stems, and roots taken for bloated or disordered

stomach. (63:181) Infusion of pulverized leaves, stems, and roots taken for bloated stomachs or disordered stomachs. (64:181) *Kidney Aid* Infusion of leaves, stems, and roots taken by men for dysfunctioning kidneys. (63:181) Infusion of pulverized leaves, stems, and roots taken for kidney troubles. (64:181) **Chippewa** *Gynecological Aid* Infusion of roots taken for amenorrhea. *Veterinary Aid* Decoction of roots used as nostril wash to increase dog's sense of scent. (59:137) **Meskwaki** *Dietary Aid* Compound infusion of leaves taken "to regain flesh and strength." *Eye Medicine* Used chiefly as an eye remedy. *Panacea* Used as a "good medicine for everything." *Veterinary Aid* Grated root mixed with salt for distemper in horses. (129: 249) **Ojibwa** *Gynecological Aid* Infusion of root used to ease parturition. *Throat Aid* Infusion of root taken for sore throat. (130:391) **Omaha** *Dermatological Aid* Poultice of pounded root applied to boils. **Pawnee** *Stimulant* Decoction of root taken for weakness and general debility. (as *Washingtonia longistylis* 58:107) **Potawatomi** *Eye Medicine* Root used to make an eye lotion. *Gastrointestinal Aid* Infusion of root used as a stomachic. (131:86) **Winnebago** *Dermatological Aid* Poultice of pounded root applied to wounds. (as *Washingtonia longistylis* 58:107)

Osmorhiza occidentalis, Western Sweetroot
Blackfoot *Breast Treatment* Infusion of roots applied to swollen breasts. (72:77) *Cough Medicine* Infusion of plant taken for coughs. (72:72) *Dermatological Aid* Infusion of roots applied to sores. (72:77) *Eye Medicine* Infusion of roots used for eye troubles. (72:81) *Gynecological Aid* Roots used by women as a feminine deodorant. (72:124) Infusion of roots taken by women to induce labor. (72:61) *Nose Medicine* Infusion of roots used for nose troubles. (72:81) **Okanagan-Colville** *Febrifuge* Infusion of roots taken for fevers. *Toothache Remedy* Roots applied to the tooth for toothaches. (162:70) **Paiute** *Analgesic* Decoction of root taken for stomachaches and gas pains. *Cathartic* Decoction of root taken as a physic. *Cold Remedy* Decoction of root taken for colds. *Dermatological Aid* Decoction of root used as a wash for venereal sores and skin rashes. Hot decoction of root applied to kill head lice. Poultice of pulped roots applied to cuts, sores, swellings, and bruises. *Dis-*

infectant Decoction of root used as an antiseptic wash for venereal sores. *Eye Medicine* Decoction of root used as an eyewash. *Febrifuge* Decoction of root taken for fever, and for chills. *Gastrointestinal Aid* Decoction of root taken for stomachaches, indigestion, or gas pains. *Misc. Disease Remedy* Decoction of root taken for colds and influenza. (155:109, 110) *Pulmonary Aid* Infusion of roots taken "when sick in the chest, not feeling well." (93:93) Decoction of root taken for pulmonary disorders and pneumonia. *Snakebite Remedy* Poultice of pulped roots applied to snakebites. *Throat Aid* Root chewed for sore throat. *Venereal Aid* Decoction of root used as an antiseptic wash for venereal sores. Simple or compound decoction of root taken for venereal disease. (155:109, 110) **Paiute, Northern** *Analgesic* Roots chewed for chest pains. *Antirheumatic* (*External*) Roots used to make a liniment. *Cold Remedy* Roots chewed for colds. *Dermatological Aid* Decoction of roots taken for sores. *Eye Medicine* Decoction of roots taken for sore eyes. (49:128) **Shoshoni** *Analgesic* Decoction of root taken for stomachaches and gas pains. Fresh root inserted into nostrils for headaches. *Antidiarrheal* Decoction of root taken for diarrhea. (155:109, 110) *Cathartic* Infusion of roots taken as a general physic. (98:41) Decoction of root taken as a physic. (155:109, 110) *Cold Remedy* Infusion of aromatic roots with Indian balsam taken for heavy colds. (98:38) Simple or compound decoction of root taken or pulverized root smoked for colds. *Cough Medicine* Compound decoction of roots taken for coughs, "heavy colds," and fevers. *Dermatological Aid* Hot decoction of root applied to kill head lice. Poultice of pulped roots applied to cuts, sores, swellings, and bruises. *Disinfectant* Decoction of root used as an antiseptic wash for measles. *Eye Medicine* Decoction of root used as an eyewash. *Febrifuge* Simple or compound decoction of root taken for fevers. *Gastrointestinal Aid* Decoction of root taken for stomachaches, indigestion, or gas pains. *Gynecological Aid* Decoction of root taken to regulate menstrual disorders. *Misc. Disease Remedy* Decoction of root taken for colds and influenza. Decoction of root used as an antiseptic wash for measles. (155: 109, 110) *Pulmonary Aid* Infusion of aromatic roots with Indian balsam taken for pneumonia. (98:38) Decoction of root used for pulmonary disorders, pneumonia, and whooping cough. *Snakebite Remedy* Poultice of pulped roots applied to snakebites. *Throat Aid* Root chewed for sore throat. *Tonic* Decoction of root taken as a tonic to protect against illness. *Toothache Remedy* Poultice of raw root applied for toothaches. *Venereal Aid* Infusion or decoction of root taken for venereal disease. (155:109, 110) **Thompson** *Cold Remedy* Root chewed for colds. (161:158) **Washo** *Analgesic* Decoction of root taken for stomachaches and gas pains. *Cathartic* Decoction of root taken as a physic. *Cold Remedy* Decoction of root taken for colds. *Gastrointestinal Aid* Decoction of root taken for stomachaches, indigestion, or gas pains. *Misc. Disease Remedy* Decoction of root taken for colds and influenza. *Pulmonary Aid* Decoction of root taken for pulmonary disorders and pneumonia. (155:109, 110)

Osmorhiza purpurea, Purple Sweetroot
Songish *Love Medicine* Roots used by girls as love charms. (156:89)

Osmunda cinnamomea, Cinnamon Fern
Cherokee *Antirheumatic* (*External*) Compound decoction of root applied with warm hands for rheumatism. (66:8) Decoction of roots rubbed on area affected by rheumatism. (152:4) *Febrifuge* Compound decoction used for chills. *Snakebite Remedy* Root chewed, a portion swallowed, and remainder applied to the wound. *Tonic* Cooked fronds eaten as "spring tonic." (66:33) **Iroquois** *Analgesic* Decoction taken for headache and joint pain. *Antirheumatic* (*External*) Decoction taken for rheumatism. *Cold Remedy* Decoction taken for colds. *Gynecological Aid* Roots used for "woman's troubles." *Orthopedic Aid* Decoction taken for joint pain. *Panacea* Decoction taken for malaise. *Venereal Aid* Cold, compound infusion used as a wash and decoction taken for affected parts. *Veterinary Aid* Compound chopped and added to cows food for difficult birth of a calf. (73:261) **Menominee** *Gynecological Aid* Used to promote the flow of milk and for caked breasts. (128:70)

Osmunda claytoniana, Interrupted Fern
Iroquois *Blood Medicine* Cold, compound decoction taken for weak blood. *Venereal Aid* Compound decoction taken for gonorrhea. (73:260)

Osmunda regalis, Royal Fern
Iroquois *Anticonvulsive* Infusion of fronds and wild ginger rhizomes used by children with convulsions from intestinal worms. (118:33) *Blood Medicine* Decoction taken by women for watery blood. *Gynecological Aid* Decoction taken by women for strong menses. Decoction used when "girls leak rotten; affected women can't raise children." *Kidney Aid* Decoction taken by women for cold in kidneys. (73:260) *Pediatric Aid* Infusion of fronds and wild ginger rhizomes used by children with convulsions from intestinal worms. (118:33) **Menominee** *Unspecified* Roots used medicinally for unspecified purpose. (128:44) **Seminole** *Other* Complex infusion of roots taken for chronic conditions. (145:272) *Pediatric Aid* Plant used for chronically ill babies. (145:329) *Psychological Aid* Infusion of plant used to steam and bathe the body for insanity. (145:292) *Unspecified* Plant used for medicinal purposes. (145:162)

Osteomeles anthyllidifolia, Hawaii Hawthorn
Hawaiian *Dermatological Aid* Leaves, root bark and salt pounded and the resulting liquid used on deep cuts. *Laxative* Seeds and buds chewed and given to children as a laxative for general debility of the body. (2:38)

Ostrya virginiana, Eastern Hop Hornbeam
Cherokee *Blood Medicine* Infusion of bark taken to build up blood. *Orthopedic Aid* Decoction of bark used to bathe sore muscles. *Toothache Remedy* Infusion of bark held in mouth for toothache. (66:39) **Chippewa** *Antihemorrhagic* Compound infusion of heartwood taken for lung hemorrhages. (43:340) *Antirheumatic* (*External*) Compound decoction of heartwood used as herbal steam for rheumatism. (43:362) *Cough Medicine* Compound liquid made from wood taken as a cough syrup. (43:340) *Kidney Aid* Decoction of wood taken for kidney trouble. (43:346) *Pulmonary Aid* Compound infusion of inner wood taken for lung hemorrhage. (43:340) **Delaware**, **Ontario** *Gynecological Aid* Compound containing root used for "female weakness." *Tonic* Compound containing root used as a tonic. (150:82) **Iroquois** *Cancer Treatment* Decoction of bark used for rectum cancer. (73:299) *Cough Medicine* Decoction of heart

chips taken for catarrh coughs. (73:298) *Dermatological Aid* Infusion used for swellings. (73:299) *Tuberculosis Remedy* Compound decoction of bark taken for consumption. (73:298) **Potawatomi** *Antidiarrheal* Infusion of bark used for flux. *Antihemorrhagic* Compound decoction of heartwood chips taken for hemorrhages. (131:44)

Oxalis corniculata, Creeping Woodsorrel
Cherokee *Anthelmintic* Infusion taken and used as a wash for children with hookworms. *Antiemetic* Cold infusion of leaf taken to stop vomiting. *Blood Medicine* Infusion taken for blood. *Cancer Treatment* Used for cancer "when it is first started." *Dermatological Aid* Salve of infusion of leaf mixed with sheep grease used for sores. *Oral Aid* Leaves chewed for "disordered saliva" and sore mouth. *Pediatric Aid* Infusion taken and used as a wash for children with hookworms. *Throat Aid* Chewed for sore throat. (66:56)

Oxalis drummondii, Drummond's Woodsorrel
Navajo, Ramah *Analgesic* Decoction of bulb used for pain. *Dermatological Aid* Poultice of bulbs, alone or in compound, applied to sores. (as *O. amplifolia* 165:34)

Oxalis oregana, Oregon Oxalis
Cowlitz *Eye Medicine* Fresh juice from plant applied to sore eyes. (65:39) **Karok** *Dietary Aid* Plant used by anyone who does not feel like eating. (125:385) **Makah** *Other* Decoction of plants taken for "summer complaint." (65:39) **Pomo** *Antirheumatic (External)* Decoction of whole plant used as a wash for rheumatism. (54:13) **Pomo, Kashaya** *Antirheumatic (External)* Decoction of whole plant used to wash parts of the body afflicted with rheumatism. (60:108) **Quileute** *Dermatological Aid* Poultice of wilted leaves applied to boils. **Quinault** *Eye Medicine* Chewed root juice applied to sore eyes. (65:39) **Tolowa** *Antirheumatic (External)* Poultice of plant applied to swollen areas on the skin. *Dermatological Aid* Poultice of plant applied to sores. *Disinfectant* Poultice of plant applied to draw out infections. (5:42)

Oxalis stricta, Common Yellow Oxalis
Iroquois *Blood Medicine* Compound decoction of roots taken as a blood medicine. (as *O. europaea*

73:366) *Febrifuge* Infusion of plant taken for fever. *Gastrointestinal Aid* Infusion of plant taken for cramps and nausea. (as *O. europaea* 73:365) *Oral Aid* Infusion of plant used as wash to refresh the mouth. (as *O. europaea* 73:366) *Other* Infusion of plant taken for "summer complaint." *Witchcraft Medicine* Compound used as an anti-witch medicine. (as *O. europaea* 73:365) **Kiowa** *Oral Aid* Leaves chewed on long walks to relieve thirst. The Kiowa name means "salt weed." This name may indicate that there was an early realization that the loss of salt through perspiration may be counteracted by chewing the leaves of this plant. (166:35) **Omaha** *Dermatological Aid* Poultice of plants applied for swellings. (56:335)

Oxalis violacea, Violet Woodsorrel
Cherokee *Anthelmintic* Infusion taken and used as a wash for children with hookworms. *Antiemetic* Cold infusion of leaf taken to stop vomiting. *Blood Medicine* Infusion taken for blood. *Cancer Treatment* Used for cancer "when it is first started." *Dermatological Aid* Salve of infusion of leaf mixed with sheep grease used for sores. *Oral Aid* Leaves chewed for "disordered saliva" and sore mouth. *Pediatric Aid* Infusion taken and used as a wash for children with hookworms. *Throat Aid* Chewed for sore throat. (66:56) **Pawnee** *Veterinary Aid* Pounded bulbs fed to horses to make them run faster. (as *Ionoxalis violacea* 58:98)

Oxydendrum arboreum, Sourwood
Catawba *Gynecological Aid* Cold infusion of plant taken by women to check excessive flow of blood. Cold infusion of plant taken by women when very sick from the change of life. (134:188) Cold infusion of plant taken to regulate flow of blood during menopause. (152:49) **Cherokee** *Antidiarrheal* Compound infusion taken for diarrhea. *Dermatological Aid* Bark ooze used for itch. *Gastrointestinal Aid* Taken as a tonic for "dyspepsy." *Oral Aid* Bark chewed for mouth ulcers. *Pulmonary Aid* Taken as a tonic for lung diseases. *Respiratory Aid* Taken as a tonic for phthisic and asthma. *Sedative* Infusion taken for nerves. (66:56)

Oxytropis campestris, Cold Mountain Crazyweed
Thompson *Disinfectant* Decoction of roots taken

and poured on head in sweat house for purification. (141:504)

Oxytropis lagopus, Haresfoot Pointloco
Blackfoot *Dermatological Aid* Plant chewed to allay swelling. *Throat Aid* Plant chewed for sore throat. (as *Aragallus lagopus* 95:274) Plant chewed for sore throat and swelling. (as *Aragallus lagopus* 98:38)

Oxytropis lambertii, Lambert's Crazyweed
Hopi *Poison* Plant poisonous to cattle. (174:80)
Lakota *Poison* Plant, in quantities, poisonous to livestock and horses. (116:47) **Navajo, Kayenta** *Laxative* Plant used for constipation. (179:28)

Oxytropis monticola, Yellowflower Locoweed
Thompson *Dermatological Aid* Decoction of whole plant used as a wash for the head, hair, and whole body. (141:473, 474)

Oxytropis sericea, Silvery Oxytrope
Blackfoot *Dermatological Aid* Infusion of leaves applied to sores. (72:77) *Ear Medicine* Infusion of leaves used for ear troubles. (72:81)

Paeonia brownii, Brown's Peony
Costanoan *Gastrointestinal Aid* Decoction of roots or plants used for stomachaches and indigestion. *Laxative* Decoction of plants taken for constipation. *Pulmonary Aid* Decoction of roots used for pneumonia. (17:7) **Mahuna** *Febrifuge* and *Pulmonary Aid* Infusion of roots taken for complicated lung fevers. (117:9) **Paiute** *Cough Medicine* Seeds used to make cough medicine. (11:98) Cold infusion of seeds used as a cough medicine. (87:197) Decoction of root taken as a cough remedy. *Dermatological Aid* Decoction of root used as a liniment for swellings. (155:110, 111) *Dietary Aid* Decoction of sun dried roots used to make people grow fat. (93:71) *Eye Medicine* Infusion of root used as a wash for sore eyes. (155:110, 111) *Heart Medicine* Fresh roots chewed and the juice swallowed for heart trouble. (93:71) *Kidney Aid* Decoction of root taken for kidney trouble. *Tuberculosis Remedy* Decoction of root taken for tuberculosis. (155:110, 111) *Veterinary Aid* Decoction of sun

dried roots given to make horses grow fat. (93:71)
Shoshoni *Antidiarrheal* Decoction of root taken for diarrhea. *Burn Dressing* Powder of pulverized, dried roots applied to burns. *Cough Medicine* Decoction of root taken as a cough remedy. *Dermatological Aid* Powdered, dried roots used on cuts, wounds, sores, and burns. Poultice of mashed root applied to boils and deep cuts or wounds. *Eye Medicine* Infusion or decoction of root used as a wash for sore eyes. *Kidney Aid* Decoction of root taken for kidney trouble. *Throat Aid* Decoction of root gargled for sore throat. *Tuberculosis Remedy* Decoction of root taken for tuberculosis. *Venereal Aid* Decoction of root taken for venereal disease.
Washo *Analgesic* Decoction of root used as a lotion for headaches. *Tuberculosis Remedy* Decoction of root taken for tuberculosis. (155:110, 111)

Paeonia californica, California Peony
Diegueño *Gastrointestinal Aid* Infusion of sliced, oven baked roots taken for indigestion. (70:28)

Panax quinquefolius, American Ginseng
Cherokee *Analgesic* Used for headache. *Anticonvulsive* Root used for convulsions and palsy. *Expectorant* Root used as an expectorant. *Gastrointestinal Aid* Root chewed for colic. *Gynecological Aid* Used for "weakness of the womb and nervous affections." *Oral Aid* Infusion used for "thrush." *Other* Root used as a tonic and expectorant and for palsy and vertigo. *Tonic* Root used as a tonic. (66:36) **Creek** *Dermatological Aid* Poultice of plant applied to bleeding cuts. *Diaphoretic* and *Febrifuge* Decoction of plant taken to produce sweating for fevers. *Hemostat* Poultice of plant applied to bleeding cuts. *Pulmonary Aid* Decoction of roots taken for short-windedness. (152:44)
Delaware *Tonic* Roots and other plant parts used as a general tonic. *Unspecified* Plants used to effect cures where all others have failed. (151:32)
Delaware, Oklahoma *Panacea* Infusion of root used in any severe illness as a cure when others have failed. *Tonic* Infusion of root and other plant parts taken as a general tonic. (150:27, 76) **Houma** *Antiemetic* Decoction of root taken for vomiting. *Antirheumatic (Internal)* Decoction of root with whisky taken for rheumatism. (135:61) **Iroquois** *Anthelmintic* Compound infusion of roots taken for tapeworms. *Antiemetic* Decoction of roots

taken for vomiting from cholera morbus. Infusion of roots taken for vomiting gall. *Blood Medicine* Compound infusion of roots taken as a blood remedy. *Dermatological Aid* Infusion of roots taken for sores on body and boils. *Dietary Aid* Infusion of roots taken for a bad appetite. *Ear Medicine* Compound infusion of roots used as drops for earaches. *Eye Medicine* Infusion of roots used as a wash for 2-year-old children with sore eyes. (73:395) *Febrifuge* Infusion of roots used for night fevers. (118:55) *Gastrointestinal Aid* Decoction of roots taken for upset stomach and vomiting gall. *Gynecological Aid* Compound infusion of seedpods taken by women having difficulty with labor. *Liver Aid* Decoction or infusion of roots taken to stop vomiting gall. *Misc. Disease Remedy* Decoction of roots taken for vomiting from cholera morbus. *Panacea* Compound decoction of roots taken or dried roots smoked as a panacea. (73:395) Dried roots smoked for every ailment or fainting spells. (73:396) *Pediatric Aid* Infusion of roots used as a wash for 2-year-old children with sore eyes. *Respiratory Aid* Smashed root smoked for asthma. (73:395) *Stimulant* Plant used for laziness and as a stimulant. *Tonic* Plant used as a tonic. (73:396) *Tuberculosis Remedy* Compound infusion of roots taken for tuberculosis. (73:395) *Venereal Aid* Plant used for gonorrhea. (73:396) **Menominee** *Hunting Medicine* Root used in some war bundles and hunting bundles. (128:80) *Psychological Aid* and *Tonic* Plant acted as a tonic and "strengthener of mental powers." (128:24) **Meskwaki** *Adjuvant* Used chiefly as a seasoner to render other remedies powerful. *Love Medicine*

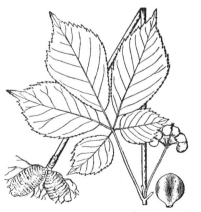

Panax quinquefolius

Compound called a "bagger" and used by a woman to get a husband. *Panacea* and *Pediatric Aid* Used as a "universal remedy for children and adults." (129:204) **Micmac** *Blood Medicine* Roots used as a "detergent for the blood." (32:58) **Mohegan** *Panacea* Herb highly valued as a cure-all. (151:74, 130) *Tonic* Complex compound infusion including ginseng root taken as spring tonic. (149:266) Root used alone or in combination to make a tonic. (151:74, 130) **Pawnee** *Love Medicine* Compound containing root used by men as a love charm. (58:106) **Penobscot** *Reproductive Aid* Infusion of root taken by women to increase fertility. (133:310) **Potawatomi** *Adjuvant* Root used as a seasoner in many powdered medicines. *Ear Medicine* Poultice of pounded root applied to earache. *Eye Medicine* Infusion of pounded root used as wash for sore eyes. (131:41) **Seminole** *Antirheumatic (External)* Decoction of roots used as a body rub and steam for joint swellings. (145:193) *Dermatological Aid* Poultice of roots applied to burst and drain boils and carbuncles. (145:243) Plant used for gunshot wounds. (145:302) Plant used in medicine bundles for bullet wounds. (145:422) *Love Medicine* Plant rubbed on the body and clothes to get back a divorced wife. (145:401) *Pediatric Aid* Plant and other plants used as a baby's charm for fear from dreams about raccoons or opossums. (145:221) *Respiratory Aid* Infusion of roots taken for shortness of breath. Four bits of root were floated on water in a container. If none sank, the water was drunk and the patient would recover immediately. If one or two sank, the recovery would be slower, and if all four sank the patient was certain to die. (145:278) *Sedative* Plant and other plants used as a baby's charm for fear from dreams about raccoons or opossums. (145:221) *Tonic* Plant used as a general tonic. (145:318) *Unspecified* Plant used for medicinal purposes. (145:161) Plant used as medicine. (145:158) Plant used medicinally. (145:164) *Witchcraft Medicine* Plant used to make a witchcraft medicine. (145:394)

Panax trifolius, Dwarf Ginseng

Cherokee *Analgesic* An "ingredient to relieve sharp pains in the breast." (66:36) Chewed plant used for headaches. Infusion of plant taken for breast pains and chewed plant used for headaches. (152:44) *Antirheumatic (Internal)* Used for rheumatism. (66:36) *Breast Treatment* Infusion of plant taken for breast pains. (152:44) *Dermatological Aid* Compound infusion given to children for "bold hives." *Gastrointestinal Aid* Root chewed for short breath and colic and infusion taken for colic. Used for "nervous debility," "dyspepsia," and apoplexy. *Kidney Aid* Root used for "dropsy" and gout. *Liver Aid* Used for the liver. *Misc. Disease Remedy* Used for "diseases induced by mercury" and pox. *Other* Taken for "nervous debility, dyspepsia and apoplexy." (66:36) Decoction of roots rubbed into scratches made for apoplexy. (152:44) *Pediatric Aid* Compound infusion given to children for "bold hives." *Pulmonary Aid* Root chewed for short breath and colic and infusion used for colic. *Stimulant* Cold, compound infusion of beaten roots given for fainting. *Tuberculosis Remedy* Infusion used for tuberculosis and "scrofulous sores." *Venereal Aid* Root used for stubborn venereal disease. (66:36) **Iroquois** *Analgesic* Compound used for chest pains. *Hunting Medicine* Infusion of roots used as a wash for fishing equipment, a "fishing medicine." *Pulmonary Aid* Compound used for chest pains. *Sports Medicine* Decoction of plant rubbed on the arms and legs of lacrosse players. (73:396) **Ojibwa, South** *Hemostat* Poultice of chewed root applied to cuts as a coagulant. (as *Aralia trifolia* 77:201)

Pandanus tectorius, Tahitian Screwpine
Hawaiian *Analgesic* Roots and other plants pounded, squeezed, resulting liquid heated and taken for chest pains. *Laxative* and *Pediatric Aid* Flowers chewed by the mothers and given to infants with constipation. *Strengthener* Roots and other plants pounded, resulting liquid heated and taken for weakness from too many births. (as *P. odoratissimus* 2:41)

Panicum capillare, Witch Grass
Keres, Western *Emetic* Infusion of leaves used as an emetic before breakfast. (147:57) **Mahuna** *Dietary Aid* Infusion of plant taken as a reducing aid. (117:66)

Panicum obtusum, Obtuse Panicgrass
Isleta *Dermatological Aid* Grass characterized as making the hair grow rapidly. (85:36)

Papaver somniferum, Opium Poppy
Cherokee *Analgesic* Large dose used to produce sleep, for pain and cramps. *Anticonvulsive* Large dose given as antispasmodic, to produce sleep and for pain. *Sedative* Large dose used for pain, to produce sleep and soothe and tranquilize the system. *Stimulant* Small doses given as a stimulant and larger dose produced sleep and used for pain. (66:50, 51)

Parnassia fimbriata, Rocky Mountain Parnassia
Cheyenne *Gastrointestinal Aid* Infusion of powdered leaves given to babies for stomach trouble. (63:176) Infusion of powdered leaves given to small babies for dullness or sick to the stomach. (64:176) *Pediatric Aid* Infusion of powdered leaves given to babies when dull or for stomach trouble. (63:176) Infusion of powdered leaves given to small babies for dullness or sick to the stomach. (64:176) *Stimulant* Infusion of powdered leaves given to babies when dull. (63:176) **Gosiute** *Venereal Aid* Poultice of plant applied or plant used as wash for venereal diseases. (31:351)

Parryella filifolia, Common Dunebroom
Hopi *Toothache Remedy* Beans used for toothaches. (34:339) Beans used for toothaches. (174:33, 80) **Navajo, Ramah** *Ceremonial Medicine* and *Emetic* Leaves used as a ceremonial emetic. (165:33) **Tewa** *Toothache Remedy* Beans used for toothaches. (34:339)

Parthenium hysterophorus, Santa Maria Feverfew
Koasati *Antidiarrheal* Decoction of roots taken for dysentery. (152:63)

Parthenium integrifolium, Wild Quinine
Catawba *Burn Dressing* Poultice of fresh leaves applied to burns. *Veterinary Aid* Leaf ash rubbed on horse's sore back. (134:191)

Parthenocissus quinquefolia, Virginia Creeper
Cherokee *Liver Aid* Infusion taken for yellow jaundice. (66:60) **Iroquois** *Antidote* Compound decoction of twigs taken and used as wash to counteract poison sumac. *Orthopedic Aid* Poultice of

vines applied to bunches (swellings) on wrists. *Other* Compound decoction of bark taken for stricture caused by menstruating woman. *Poison* Plant considered poisonous. *Urinary Aid* Compound decoction of plants taken for difficult urination. (73:382)

Parthenocissus quinquefolia var. *quinquefolia*, Virginia Creeper

Houma *Dermatological Aid* Hot decoction of stems and leaves applied to reduce swellings. Poultice of crushed leaves and vinegar applied to wounds. *Misc. Disease Remedy* Poultice of crushed leaves and vinegar applied for lockjaw. (as *Psedera quinquefolia* 135:63) **Meskwaki** *Antidiarrheal* Decoction of root taken for diarrhea. (as *Psedera quinquefolia* 129:252)

Parthenocissus vitacea, Woodbine

Iroquois *Urinary Aid* Compound decoction of plants taken for difficult urination caused by gall. (73:382) **Navajo** *Ceremonial Medicine* Used as part of the medicine the patient takes in the Mountain Chant Ceremony. (45:62) **Navajo, Ramah** *Dermatological Aid* Infusion of leaves and berries used as a lotion for swollen arm or leg. (165:36)

Paspalidium geminatum var. *paludivagum*, Egyptian Panicum

Seminole *Dermatological Aid* Plant used for snake sickness: itchy skin. (as *Panicum paludivagum* 145:166) Decoction of whole plant taken and used as a body steam for snake sickness: itchy skin. (as *Panicum paludivagum* 145:239)

Passiflora incarnata, Purple Passionflower

Cherokee *Dermatological Aid* Compound infusion of root used for boils. Pounded root applied to "draw out inflammation" of brier or locust wounds. *Dietary Aid* Infusion of root given to babies to aid in weaning. *Ear Medicine* Warm infusion of beaten root dropped into ear for earache. *Liver Aid* Infusion taken for liver and compound infusion of root used for boils. *Pediatric Aid* Infusion of root given to babies to aid in weaning. (66:47) **Houma** *Blood Medicine* Infusion of roots taken as a blood tonic. (135:63)

Pastinaca sativa, Wild Parsnip

Cherokee *Analgesic* Taken for "sharp pains." (66:47) **Iroquois** *Dermatological Aid* Compound decoction used as wash or poultice applied to chancres or lumps on penis. (73:399) **Ojibwa** *Gynecological Aid* Compound infusion of minute quantity of root taken for female troubles. *Poison* Root powerful in small amounts and poisonous in large amounts. (130:391) **Paiute** *Tuberculosis Remedy* Root medicine taken "for their all over inside—when they have this awful, maybe TB." (93:93) **Potawatomi** *Dermatological Aid* Poultice of root applied to inflammation and sores. *Poison* Root considered poisonous when taken internally. (131:86)

Paxistima myrsinites, Boxleaf Myrtle

Bella Coola *Unspecified* Formerly used for medicine. (158:203) **Navajo, Ramah** *Ceremonial Medicine* and *Emetic* Plant used as an emetic in various ceremonies. (165:36) **Okanagan-Colville** *Cold Remedy* Decoction of branches taken for colds. *Kidney Aid* Decoction of branches taken for kidney troubles. *Tuberculosis Remedy* Decoction of branches taken for tuberculosis. (162:95) **Thompson** *Analgesic* Poultice of leaves used for pain in any part of the body. *Dermatological Aid* Poultice of boiled leaves applied to swellings and body pains. (141:468) *Internal Medicine* Decoction or infusion of plant used for internal ailments. *Orthopedic Aid* Decoction or infusion of plant used for broken bones. *Tuberculosis Remedy* Decoction or infusion of branches taken for tuberculosis. (161:202)

Pectis angustifolia, Narrowleaf Pectis

Keres, Western *Gastrointestinal Aid* Blossoms and salt eaten for stomach trouble. *Psychological Aid* Infusion of plant used as an emetic before breakfast to relieve sadness and worry. (147:58) **Navajo** *Carminative* Plant used as a carminative. *Ceremonial Medicine* Plant used in the liniment for the Chiricahua Apache Wind Chant. *Gastrointestinal Aid* Crushed leaves used for stomachaches. (45:88)

Pectis papposa, Cinchweed Fetidmarigold

Pima *Laxative* Decoction of plant or dried plant taken as a laxative. (38:104) **Zuni** *Carminative*

Infusion of whole plant taken as a carminative. *Eye Medicine* Infusion of blossoms used as eye drops for snow-blindness. (143:57)

Pedicularis attollens, Attol Lousewort
Washo *Dermatological Aid* Poultice of plant applied to cuts, sores, and swellings. *Tonic* Decoction of leaves taken as a tonic. (155:112)

Pedicularis bracteosa, Bracted Lousewort
Thompson *Unspecified* Plant used medicinally for unspecified purpose. (141:467)

Pedicularis canadensis, Canadian Lousewort
Catawba *Analgesic* Infusion of roots used for stomach pains. *Gastrointestinal Aid* Infusion of roots used for stomach pains and disorders. (134:190) **Cherokee** *Antidiarrheal* Taken "for bloody discharge from bowels" and used to rid sheep of lice. *Cough Medicine* Used as an ingredient in cough medicine. *Dermatological Aid* Infusion of root rubbed on sores. *Gastrointestinal Aid* Decoction of root taken for stomachache and infusion taken for "flux." *Veterinary Aid* Put in dog bed to delouse pups and used to rid sheep of lice. (66:43) **Chippewa** *Blood Medicine* Infusion of dried roots used for anemic conditions. (59:140) **Iroquois** *Emetic* and *Gastrointestinal Aid* Decoction taken to vomit for stomachaches caused by menstruating women. *Heart Medicine* Infusion of smashed roots taken for heart troubles. *Orthopedic Aid* Compound decoction of plants used as steam bath for sore legs or knees. *Tuberculosis Remedy* Compound infusion of whole plants taken for consumption with bad hemorrhage. (73:436) **Menominee** *Love Medicine* Root carried on the person who is contemplating making love advances. (128:81) *Veterinary Aid* Chopped root added to feed to make pony fat and vicious to all but its owner. (128:53) **Meskwaki** *Cancer Treatment* Poultice of root applied to tumors. *Dermatological Aid* Poultice of root applied to external swellings. *Internal Medicine* Decoction of plant taken for internal swelling and poultice applied for external swelling. (129:247) *Love Medicine* Root used in food to make estranged married people congenial and a love medicine used to return love (129:273) **Mohegan** *Abortifacient* Infusion of leaves taken to induce abortion. (151:74, 130) **Ojibwa** *Gastrointestinal Aid* Infusion of roots taken for stomach ulcers. (4:2304) *Love Medicine* Finely cut root secretly added to another's food as an aphrodisiac. (130:389, 390) Chopped root added to food as a love charm. The root was added to some dish of food that was cooking, without the knowledge of the people who were going to eat it, and if they had been quarrelsome, then they became lovers again. However, the informant said that it was too often put to bad uses. (130:432) *Throat Aid* Infusion of fresh or dried leaves taken for sore throats. (4:2304) **Potawatomi** *Cathartic* Root used as a physic. *Internal Medicine* Root used by Prairie Potawatomi for both internal and external swellings. (131:83)

Pedicularis centranthera, Dwarf Lousewort
Shoshoni *Gastrointestinal Aid* and *Pediatric Aid* Decoction of root given to children for stomachaches. (155:112)

Pedicularis groenlandica, Elephanthead Lousewort
Cheyenne *Cough Medicine* Infusion of powdered leaves and stems taken to stop or loosen a cough. (63:187) Infusion of powdered leaves and stems taken to stop or loosen a long-lasting cough. (64:187) Infusion of smashed leaves and stems taken for coughs. (69:39)

Pedicularis racemosa, Sickletop Lousewort
Thompson *Unspecified* Plant used medicinally for unspecified purpose. (141:467)

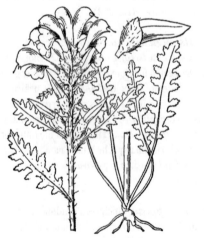

Pedicularis canadensis

Pediomelum argophyllum, Silverleaf
  Scurfpea
Cheyenne *Febrifuge* Decoction of plant taken for fever and salve of plant used for high fever. (as *Psoralea argophylla* 63:40) Infusion of ground leaves and stems taken for fevers. (as *Psoralea argophylla* 63:178) Ground leaf and stem powder mixed with grease and rubbed over the body for high fevers. (as *Psoralea argophylla* 64:178) **Chippewa** *Veterinary Aid* Compound infusion of root applied to chest and legs of horse as a stimulant. (as *Psoralea argophylla* 43:366) **Lakota** *Unspecified* Plant used as a medicine. *Veterinary Aid* Roots fed to tired horses. (as *Psoralea argophylla* 116:47) **Meskwaki** *Laxative* Infusion of root used for chronic constipation. (as *Psoralea argophylla* 129:230) **Montana Indian** *Dermatological Aid* Decoction of plant used as a wash for wounds. (as *Psoralea argophylla* 15:20)

Pediomelum canescens, Buckroot
Seminole *Analgesic* Poultice of warmed roots applied externally as an analgesic. (as *Psoralea canescens* 145:167) Poultice of wet, warm tuberous roots applied for pains. *Antirheumatic* (*External*) Poultice of wet, warm tuberous roots applied for rheumatism. (as *Psoralea canescens* 145:285) *Cold Remedy* Infusion of tuberous roots taken and steam inhaled for runny nose, stuffy head, and sore throat. *Cough Medicine* Infusion of tuberous roots taken and steam inhaled for coughs. (as *Psoralea canescens* 145:279) *Unspecified* Plant used as medicine. (as *Psoralea canescens* 145:158)

Pediomelum cuspidatum, Largebract Indian
  Breadroot
Lakota *Unspecified* Used as a medicine. (as *Psoralea cuspidata* 116:47)

Pediomelum esculentum, Breadroot
  Scurfpea
Blackfoot *Antirheumatic* (*External*) Poultice of chewed roots applied to sprains. (as *Psoralea esculenta* 72:80) *Ear Medicine* Chewed root spittle used for earaches. *Eye Medicine* Chewed root spittle applied to the eye to remove matter. (as *Psoralea esculenta* 72:82) *Gastrointestinal Aid* Infusion of dried roots taken for gastroenteritis. Chewed roots blown into a baby's rectum for colic. (as

Psoralea esculenta 72:68) Roots chewed by children for bowel complaints. (as *Psoralea esculenta* 82:41) *Orthopedic Aid* Poultice of chewed roots applied to fractures. (as *Psoralea esculenta* 72:80) *Pediatric Aid* Chewed roots blown into a baby's rectum for colic. (as *Psoralea esculenta* 72:68) *Pulmonary Aid* Infusion of roots taken for chest troubles. (as *Psoralea esculenta* 72:73) *Throat Aid* Infusion of dried roots taken for sore throats. (as *Psoralea esculenta* 72:68) Roots chewed for sore throat. (as *Psoralea esculenta* 72:73) *Toothache Remedy* Roots chewed by teething children. (as *Psoralea esculenta* 82:41) *Unspecified* Root pieces dried and attached to clothing and robes as ornamentation and medicine. (as *Psoralea esculenta* 72:119) **Cheyenne** *Antidiarrheal* Plant used as a diarrhea medicine. *Burn Dressing* Plant used as a burn medicine. *Unspecified* Plant used as an ingredient for medicinal mixtures. (as *Psoralea esculenta* 69:29)

Pelea sp., Alani-kuahiwi
Hawaiian *Blood Medicine* Infusion of pounded bark and other ingredients taken to purify the blood. *Ceremonial Medicine* Leaves placed on the bed as a beauty remedy for king, queens, and their sons and daughters. The alani was the Hawaiian beauty remedy and was dedicated to the exclusive use of the kings and queens and their sons and daughters. The leaves, in sufficient quantity, were taken and laid on the bed, covering the space, from the neck to the feet. A sheeting of tapa, tightly drawn, was laid over the leaves. In the meantime, 20 leaves were allowed to remain in the water overnight and placed in the sun during the day. This was for bathing. Towards evening, the royal child, or the one chosen for beauty, was given a bath of this water. In it were put the alani flowers. After the bath the child was fed a fattening ration. After feeding, and when the child became sleepy, it was placed in the bed covered with the alani leaves. This was repeated for five consecutive days. The bedding was then changed, the old alani leaves were removed and new ones took their place, and the process continued from that point on for 5 days more. Not only did this treatment improve the appearance, but it made the skin immune to certain diseases, especially skin diseases. *Dermatological Aid* Leaves placed in beds of kings, queens,

their sons, and daughters to make the skin immune to diseases. *Pediatric Aid* and *Strengthener* Young shoots or buds used for children with general debility. (2:15)

Pellaea atropurpurea, Purple Cliffbrake
Mahuna *Blood Medicine* Infusion of plants taken to tone and thin the blood. *Kidney Aid* Infusion of plants taken to flush the kidneys. *Preventive Medicine* Infusion of plants taken as a preventative against sunstroke. (117:22)

Pellaea mucronata, Birdfoot Cliffbrake
Costanoan *Antihemorrhagic* and *Blood Medicine* Decoction of plant used for internal injuries to cough up "bad blood." *Dermatological Aid* Infusion of leaves used as a wash for facial sores. *Emetic* Decoction of plant used for internal injuries to cough up "bad blood." *Febrifuge* Infusion of sprouts taken for fevers. (17:5) **Yavapai** *Dermatological Aid* Dried, pulverized leaves dusted on sores. *Gynecological Aid* Decoction taken as tea by women after childbirth. (53:261)

Pellaea mucronata ssp. mucronata, Birdfoot Cliffbrake
Diegueño *Antihemorrhagic* Decoction of rhizomes taken for hemorrhage. (as *P. mucronata* var. *mucronata* 70:28) **Luiseño** *Unspecified* Decoction of fronds used for medicinal purposes. (as *P. ornithopus* 132:234) **Miwok** *Antihemorrhagic* Infusion taken for nosebleed. *Blood Medicine* Infusion taken as a blood purifier. *Other* Infusion taken as a spring medicine. (as *P. ornithopus* 8:171)

Peltandra virginica, Green Arrow Arum
Nanticoke *Pediatric Aid* and *Unspecified* Grated root in milk given to babies for unspecified purpose. (150:58)

Peltigera aphthosa
Nitinaht *Tuberculosis Remedy* Plants chewed and eaten for tuberculosis. *Urinary Aid* Formerly used to facilitate urination. (160:55)

Peltigera canina, Dogtooth Lichen
Nitinaht *Urinary Aid* Formerly used to facilitate urination. (160:55)

Peniocereus greggii var. greggii, Night-blooming Cereus
Nevada Indian *Heart Medicine* Infusion of root taken as a cardiac stimulant. (as *Cereus greggii* 98:40) **Papago** *Dermatological Aid* Seedpod and deer grease salve rubbed on sores. Seedpod mixed with deer grease as salve for sores. (as *Cereus greggii* 29:65) **Pima** *Misc. Disease Remedy* Decoction of roots taken for diabetes. (as *Cereus greggii* 38:55)

Pennellia micrantha, Mountain Mock Thelypody
Navajo, Ramah *Gynecological Aid* Decoction of root taken to expedite delivery. *Toothache Remedy* Poultice of crushed, heated roots applied for toothache. (165:29)

Pennisetum glaucum, Pearl Millet
Navajo, Ramah *Dermatological Aid* Fruits rubbed on open facial pimples. (as *Setaria lutescens* 165:17)

Penstemon acuminatus, Sharpleaf Penstemon
Blackfoot *Analgesic* Decoction of plant taken for stomach pain. (as *Pentstemon acuminatus* 95:276) *Antiemetic* Infusion of leaves taken for vomiting. (82:53) Decoction of plant taken for vomiting. *Gastrointestinal Aid* Decoction of plant taken for cramps and stomach pain. (as *Pentstemon acuminatus* 95:276)

Penstemon ambiguus, Gilia Beardtongue
Keres, Western *Emetic* Infusion of plant used as an emetic. (as *Pentstemon ambiguus* 147:58) **Navajo, Kayenta** *Dermatological Aid* Plant used for solpugid (wind scorpion) bites or poultice of plant applied to eagle bites. *Disinfectant* and *Veterinary Aid* Plant used as a fumigant for livestock with snakebites. (179:42)

Penstemon barbatus, Beardlip Penstemon
Navajo, Ramah *Analgesic* Decoction of root taken for menstrual pain and stomachache. *Burn Dressing* Cold infusion or powdered plant applied to burns. *Cough Medicine* Decoction of plant taken for cough. *Dermatological Aid* Poultice of root applied to swellings, gun wounds, and arrow

wounds, a "life medicine." *Gastrointestinal Aid* Simple or compound decoction of root taken for stomachache. *Gynecological Aid* Honey sucked from flower by pregnant woman to keep baby small for easy labor. Simple or compound decoction of root taken for menstrual pain. *Panacea* Decoction of plant taken for internal injuries, a "life medicine." Poultice of root applied to gun wounds, arrow wounds, and swellings, a "life medicine." *Veterinary Aid* Poultice of plant applied to sheep for fractured legs. (165:44)

Penstemon barbatus* ssp. *torreyi, Torrey's Penstemon
Apache, White Mountain *Witchcraft Medicine* Plant used as a magic medicine. (as *Pentstemon torreyi* 113:159) **Navajo** *Diuretic* Infusion of plants taken as a diuretic. (as *Penstemon torreyi* 45:77) **Tewa** *Dermatological Aid* Plant used as a dressing for sores. (as *Pentstemon torreyi* 115:58) **Zuni** *Hunting Medicine* Chewed root rubbed over the rabbit stick to insure success in the hunt. (as *Pentstemon torreyi* 143:95)

Penstemon centranthifolius, Scarlet Bugler
Costanoan *Dermatological Aid* and *Disinfectant* Poultice of plant applied to deep, infected sores. (as *Pentstemon centranthifolius* 17:15)

Penstemon confertus, Yellow Penstemon
Thompson *Cathartic* Decoction of root taken as a purgative. (as *Pentstemon confertus* 141:467) Decoction used as a beverage, but if too strong acted as a purgative. (as *Pentstemon confertus* 141:493) *Dermatological Aid* Toasted, powdered stems and leaves sprinkled on sores, cuts, and wounds. (as *Pentstemon confertus* 141:473) *Gastrointestinal Aid* Decoction of outer bark taken for stomach troubles. (as *Pentstemon confertus* 141:467)

Penstemon deustus, Scabland Penstemon
Paiute *Dermatological Aid* Poultice of smashed leaves applied to sores. (87:196) Poultice of mashed, fresh leaves applied to boils, mosquito bites, tick bites, and open sores. (93:109) Poultice of green leaves or leaf powder applied to various skin problems. Poultice of green or dried plant applied for swellings. *Eye Medicine* Decoction of plant used as an eyewash. *Gastrointestinal Aid*

and *Pediatric Aid* Decoction of plant taken for stomachaches, especially children's. (155:112, 113) **Paiute, Northern** *Dermatological Aid* Poultice of dried, ground leaves and stalks applied to chapped and cracked skin. (49:129) **Shoshoni** *Analgesic* Decoction of plants used as a hot bath for sore feet and swollen legs and veins. Decoction of plants taken for colds and rheumatic aches. *Antirheumatic (Internal)* Decoction of whole plant taken for rheumatic aches. *Cold Remedy* Decoction of whole plant taken for colds. (155:112, 113) *Dermatological Aid* Powdered root used for sores. (as *Penstemon deustus* 98:44) Poultice of green leaves or leaf powder applied to various skin problems. *Disinfectant* Decoction of stems and leaves dropped into the ear for ear infections. *Ear Medicine* Strong decoction of stems and leaves dropped into ear for ear infection. *Eye Medicine* Decoction of plant used as an eyewash. *Gastrointestinal Aid* Decoction of plant taken for stomachaches, especially children's. *Orthopedic Aid* Decoction of plants used as a hot bath for sore feet and swollen legs and veins. *Pediatric Aid* Decoction of plant taken for stomachaches, especially children's. (155:112, 113) *Venereal Aid* Juice of mashed, raw leaves used as wash for venereal disease. (as *Penstemon deustus* 98:47) Compound infusion of plant used as a wash for gonorrheal sores. Plant used in various ways both internally and externally for venereal disease. (155:112, 113)

Penstemon eatonii, Eaton's Penstemon
Navajo, Kayenta *Dermatological Aid* Plant used for spider bites. *Disinfectant* Plant used as a fumigant and Lightning infection emetic. *Emetic* Plant used as a Lightning infection emetic. *Gastrointestinal Aid* Plant used for stomach troubles. *Hemostat* Plant used as a hemostatic. *Orthopedic Aid* Plant used for backache. *Snakebite Remedy* Poultice of plant applied to snakebites. *Veterinary Aid* Plant used for livestock with colic. (179:42) **Shoshoni** *Analgesic* Decoction of whole plant used as a wash for pain and healing of burns. *Burn Dressing* Decoction of whole plant used as a wash for pain and healing of burns. (155:114)

Penstemon fendleri, Fendler's Penstemon
Navajo, Ramah *Dermatological Aid* Plant used for arrow or gunshot wounds. (165:44)

Penstemon fruticosus, Bush Penstemon
Iroquois *Emetic* Compound decoction of plants
taken as an emetic to cure a love medicine. *Gynecological Aid* Compound decoction used as wash
by women who are bothered by milk flow. *Love
Medicine* Compound decoction of plants taken as
an emetic to cure a love medicine. (as *P. pubescens* 73:434) **Okanagan-Colville** *Analgesic*
Infusion of plant tops taken for headaches. *Cold
Remedy* Infusion of plant tops taken for colds.
Dermatological Aid Infusion of plant tops used for
sore and itchy scalp and to bathe the skin for acne
and pimples. *Gastrointestinal Aid* Infusion of
plant tops taken for internal disorders. *Misc. Disease Remedy* Infusion of plant tops taken for flu.
Toothache Remedy Raw roots placed on the tooth
for severe toothaches. *Veterinary Aid* Infusion of
plant tops used on animals for skin problems.
(162:139) **Salish** *Unspecified* Decoction of plants
used as a medicine. (as *Pentstemon douglassii*
153:294) **Shuswap** *Urinary Aid* Plant used for
the bladder. (102:69) **Thompson** *Antirheumatic*
(*External*) Whole plant used to make bathing
water for rheumatism. Decoction of plant used as
a wash for arthritis or as a bath for any kind of
aches and sores. (161:286) *Eye Medicine* Infusion
of fresh plant used as a wash for sore eyes. (as
Pentstemon douglasii 141:468) Infusion of plant
used as an eyewash. The informant used the infusion as an eyewash after she had gotten glass
splinters in her eye. Decoction of leaves used as
an eyewash for sore, red eyes. *Gastrointestinal
Aid* Decoction of plant taken for ulcers and "to
clean you out." (161:286) *Kidney Aid* Decoction
of stems, flowers, and leaves taken for kidney trouble. *Orthopedic Aid* Decoction of stems, flowers,
and leaves taken for sore back. (as *Pentstemon
douglasii* 141:468) Decoction of plant with other
"weeds" used as a poultice for broken bones. *Veterinary Aid* Decoction of plant used on horses'
legs. The decoction was used to wash a horse's leg,
and after just a couple of days the horse was able
to walk again. (161:286)

Penstemon fruticosus var. **scouleri**, Little-
    leaf Bush Penstemon
Okanagon *Eye Medicine* Decoction of stems, flow-
ers, and leaves used as a wash for inflamed eyes.
Kidney Aid Decoction of stems, flowers, and leaves

taken for kidney troubles. *Orthopedic Aid* Decoction of stems, flowers, and leaves taken for sore
back. **Thompson** *Eye Medicine* Decoction of
stems, flowers, and leaves used as a wash for inflamed eyes. *Kidney Aid* Decoction of stems, flowers, and leaves taken for kidney troubles. *Orthopedic Aid* Decoction of stems, flowers, and leaves
taken for sore back. (as *Pentstemon scouleri*
104:41)

Penstemon grandiflorus, Large Beardtongue
Dakota *Analgesic* Decoction of roots used for
chest pains. (as *Pentstemon grandiflorus* 57:363)
Kiowa *Gastrointestinal Aid* Decoction of roots
taken for stomachaches. (166:51) **Pawnee** *Febrifuge* Decoction of leaves taken for chills and fever.
(as *Pentstemon grandiflorus* 58:114)

Penstemon jamesii, James's Beardtongue
Navajo, Kayenta *Emetic* and *Pediatric Aid* Plant
used as an emetic and lotion to purify a newborn
infant before nursing. (179:43) **Navajo, Ramah**
Analgesic Cold, compound infusion of plant taken
for headache caused by hunting. *Ceremonial Medicine* Plant used ceremonially for headache and
sore throat. *Throat Aid* Cold infusion taken and
used as lotion for sore throat. (165:44)

Penstemon laetus, Mountain Blue Penstemon
Karok *Psychological Aid* Infusion of plant taken
and used as a steam bath by grieving person. (as
Pentstemon laetus 125:389)

Penstemon laevigatus, Eastern Smooth
Beardtongue
Cherokee *Gastrointestinal Aid* Infusion taken for
cramps. (66:25)

Penstemon linarioides ssp. **colorado-
    ensis**, Colorado Penstemon
Navajo, Ramah *Gynecological Aid* Decoction of
plant taken early in pregnancy to insure birth of
female child. Decoction of plant taken to facilitate
labor and delivery of placenta. (165:44)

Penstemon palmeri, Palmer's Penstemon
Navajo, Kayenta *Snakebite Remedy* Poultice of
plant applied to snakebite sores. (179:43)

Penstemon richardsonii, Cutleaf Beardtongue
Okanagan-Colville *Misc. Disease Remedy* Infusion of stalks with leaves and flowers taken for
typhoid fever. (162:139) **Paiute** *Dermatological
Aid* Poultice of crushed leaves applied to sores.
(93:109)

Penstemon rostriflorus, Bridge Penstemon
Kawaiisu *Orthopedic Aid* Poultice of mashed
roots applied to swollen limbs. (as *P. bridgesii*
180:47)

Penstemon virgatus, Upright Blue Beardtongue
Navajo, Ramah *Panacea* Whole plant or root
used as "life medicine." (165:45)

**Pentagrama triangularis ssp. triangu-
laris**, Western Goldfern
Karok *Analgesic* and *Gynecological Aid* Plant
used to mitigate the afterpains of childbirth. (as
Gymnogramme triangularis 125:377) **Miwok**
Toothache Remedy Chewed for toothache. (as
Gymnogramma triangularis 8:170)

Pentaphylloides floribunda, Shrubby
Cinquefoil
Cheyenne *Ceremonial Medicine* Dried, powdered
leaves rubbed over hands, arms, and body for Con-
trary dance. (as *Dasiphora fruticosa* 63:176)
Other Plant used as a medicine against an enemy.
Poison Plant considered poisonous. (as *Potentilla
fruticosa* 69:35) **Tanana, Upper** *Gynecological
Aid* Branches placed under the mattress to lessen
first menstruation and number of years of menstruation. (as *Potentilla fruticosa* 86:8)

Penthorum sedoides, Ditch Stonecrop
Meskwaki *Cough Medicine* Seeds used to make a
cough syrup. (129:219)

Peperomia sp., Ala-ala-waionui-pehu
Hawaiian *Gynecological Aid* Whole plant with
other ingredients and coconut milk taken by
women with sexual organ afflictions. *Laxative*
Buds chewed by the mother and given to the newborn infant as a laxative. *Other* Stems and other
ingredients pounded and the resulting liquid taken

for wasting away of the body. *Pediatric Aid* Buds
chewed by the mother and given to the newborn
infant as a laxative. *Pulmonary Aid* Leaves with
other ingredients and water taken for pulmonary
diseases. (2:13) *Respiratory Aid* Buds and other
plants pounded, the resulting liquid heated and
taken for asthma. (2:57) *Strengthener* Stems and
other ingredients taken for general debility. Stems
and other ingredients pounded and the resulting
liquid taken for general weakness. (2:13)

Perezia sp.
Yavapai *Dermatological Aid* and *Pediatric Aid*
Cotton-like material at root base placed on baby's
umbilicus. (53:261)

Pericome caudata, Mountain Leaftail
Navajo, Ramah *Analgesic* Decoction of root
taken for general body pain. Fresh leaves "smelled"
for headache. *Ceremonial Medicine* Cold infusion
of leaves used as a ceremonial chant lotion and
emetic. *Cough Medicine* Decoction of root taken
for cough. *Dermatological Aid* Compound containing stems used as shampoo to prevent falling
hair. *Diaphoretic* Decoction of root used as a
sweat bath medicine. *Emetic* Cold infusion of
leaves used as a ceremonial chant lotion and
emetic. *Febrifuge* Cold infusion of leaves taken for
fever. *Gynecological Aid* Decoction of root taken
to facilitate delivery of placenta. *Misc. Disease
Remedy* Cold infusion of leaves taken for influenza.
Toothache Remedy Poultice of heated root applied
for toothache. *Witchcraft Medicine* Decoction of
root used for protection from witches. (165:52)

Perideridia gairdneri, Gairdner's Yampah
Blackfoot *Antidiarrheal* and *Antiemetic* Infusion
of roots taken to counteract cathartic and emetic
effects of another infusion. (72:67) *Breast Treatment* Infusion of roots used to massage sore
breasts with warm stones. (72:77) *Cough Medicine* Infusion of roots or roots chewed for coughs.
Root smudge smoke inhaled for nagging coughs.
(72:72) *Dermatological Aid* Infusion of roots applied to sores and wounds. (72:77) *Diuretic* Roots
eaten in quantity as a diuretic. (72:67) Infusion of
roots taken as a diuretic. (72:70) *Laxative* Roots
eaten in quantity as a mild laxative. (72:67) *Panacea* Chewed roots sprayed onto affected part by the

diviner. A diviner, like Dog Child, would find the root mysteriously during the rituals. While he sang, often with a drum, he would dig the ground with a special bear claw, coming up with the root every time and anywhere. (72:83) *Respiratory Aid* Infusion of roots used as a nostril wash for catarrh. (72:72) *Strengthener* Roots chewed by buffalo runners to extend their endurance. (72:116) *Throat Aid* Infusion of roots or roots chewed for sore throats. (72:72) *Veterinary Aid* Infusion of roots given to horses as a diuretic. Roots chewed by lazy horses to enliven them. Infusion of roots used for horses with nasal gleet. (72:89) **Cheyenne** *Unspecified* Roots used as an ingredient in medicines. (69:41)

Perideridia gairdneri ssp. *gairdneri*,
Gairdner's Yampah

Blackfoot *Dermatological Aid* Root used to draw inflammation from swellings. *Throat Aid* Root used for sore throat. (as *Carum gairdneri* 95:274) **Cheyenne** *Unspecified* Plant used for medicinal purposes. (as *Carum gairdneri* 63:182) Decoction of roots, stems, and leaves used as a medicine. (as *Carum gairdneri* 64:182)

Perideridia kelloggii, Kellogg's Yampah
Pomo *Antiemetic* Decoction of flowers taken for vomiting. (as *Carum kelloggii* 54:14) **Pomo, Kashaya** *Antiemetic* Decoction of flowers used for vomiting. (60:89)

Perilla frutescens, Beefsteakplant
Rappahannock *Blood Medicine* An ingredient of a blood medicine. (as *P. fructescens* 138:31)

Persea borbonia, Red Bay
Seminole *Abortifacient* Infusion of leaves taken to abort a fetus up to about 4 months old. (145:320) *Analgesic* Infusion of leaf taken for bear sickness: fever, headache, thirst, constipation, and blocked urination. (145:198) Infusion of leaves taken for sun sickness: eye disease, headache, high fever, and diarrhea. (145:206) Infusion of leaves taken as an emetic for rainbow sickness: fever, stiff neck, and backache. (145:210) Infusion of leaves taken as an emetic for thunder sickness: fever, dizziness, headache, and diarrhea. (145:213) Infusion of plant taken for wolf sickness:

vomiting, stomach pain, diarrhea, and frequent urination. (145:227) Leaves used for baby sickness caused by adultery: appetite loss, fever, headache, and diarrhea. (145:253) Leaves used for adult's sickness caused by adultery: headache, body pains, and crossed fingers. (145:256) Decoction of leaves taken for dead people's sickness. (145:257) Leaves used for scalping sickness: severe headache, backache, and low fever. (145:262) Decoction of leaves taken for headaches. (145:282) *Antidiarrheal* Leaves used for bird sickness: diarrhea, vomiting, and appetite loss. (145:156) Infusion of leaves taken for sun sickness: eye disease, headache, high fever, and diarrhea. (145:206) Infusion of leaves taken as an emetic for thunder sickness: fever, dizziness, headache, and diarrhea. (145:213) Leaves burned and smoke "smelled" by the baby for raccoon sickness: diarrhea. (145:218) Infusion of leaves taken by babies and adults for otter sickness: diarrhea and vomiting. (145:222) Infusion of plant taken for wolf sickness: vomiting, stomach pain, diarrhea, and frequent urination. (145:227) Decoction of leaves taken by babies and adults for bird sickness: diarrhea, vomiting, and appetite loss. (145:234) Leaves used for baby sickness caused by adultery: appetite loss, fever, headache, and diarrhea. (145:253) *Antiemetic* Leaves used for bird sickness: diarrhea, vomiting, and appetite loss. (145:156) Infusion of leaves taken by babies and adults for otter sickness: diarrhea and vomiting. (145:222) Infusion of leaves taken as an emetic and rubbed on the body for cat sickness: nausea.

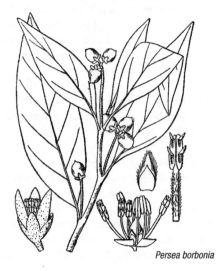

Persea borbonia

(145:224) Infusion of plant taken for wolf sickness: vomiting, stomach pain, diarrhea, and frequent urination. (145:227) Decoction of leaves taken by babies and adults for bird sickness: diarrhea, vomiting, and appetite loss. (145:234) Infusion of leaves taken by children for buzzard sickness: vomiting. (145:305) *Antirheumatic (External)* Decoction of leaves rubbed on body and body steamed for deer sickness: numb, painful limbs and joints. (145:192) Plant used for fire sickness: fever and body aches. (145:203) *Ceremonial Medicine* Leaf used as an emetic in purification after funerals, at doctor's school, and after death of patient. (145:167) Infusion of leaves added to food after a recent death. (145:342) *Dietary Aid* Leaves used for bird sickness: diarrhea, vomiting, and appetite loss. (145:156) Infusion of leaves taken by babies for opossum sickness: appetite loss, and drooling. (145:220) Decoction of leaves taken by babies and adults for bird sickness: diarrhea, vomiting, and appetite loss. (145:234) Leaves used for baby sickness caused by adultery: appetite loss, fever, headache, and diarrhea. (145:253) Decoction of leaves taken for dead people's sickness. (145:257) Infusion of leaves taken as emetic for ghost sickness: grief, lung cough, appetite loss, and vomiting. (145:260) *Emetic* Decoction of plant and other plants taken as an emetic by doctors to strengthen his internal medicine. (145:145) Leaves used as an emetic to "clean the insides." (145:167) Leaves used as an emetic by the doctor to prevent the next patient from getting worse. (145:184) Infusion of leaves taken as an emetic for rainbow sickness: fever, stiff neck, and backache. (145:210) Infusion of leaves taken as an emetic for thunder sickness: fever, dizziness, headache, and diarrhea. (145:213) Infusion of leaves taken as an emetic and rubbed on the body for cat sickness: nausea. (145:224) Plant used as an emetic during religious ceremonies. (145:409) *Eye Medicine* Infusion of leaves taken for sun sickness: eye disease, headache, high fever, and diarrhea. (145:206) Infusion of leaves taken and used as a bath for mist sickness: eye disease, fever, and chills. (145:208) *Febrifuge* Infusion of leaf taken for bear sickness: fever, headache, thirst, constipation, and blocked urination. (145:198) Plant used for fire sickness: fever and body aches. (145:203) Infusion of leaves taken for sun sickness: eye disease, head-

ache, high fever, and diarrhea. (145:206) Infusion of leaves taken and used as a bath for mist sickness: eye disease, fever, and chills. (145:208) Infusion of leaves taken as an emetic for rainbow sickness: fever, stiff neck, and backache. (145:210) Infusion of leaves taken as an emetic for thunder sickness: fever, dizziness, headache, and diarrhea. (145:213) Leaves used for baby sickness caused by adultery: appetite loss, fever, headache, and diarrhea. (145:253) Decoction of leaves taken for dead people's sickness. (145:257) Leaves used for scalping sickness: severe headache, backache, and low fever. (145:262) Decoction of leaves taken for fevers. (145:282) *Gastrointestinal Aid* Infusion of plant taken for wolf sickness: vomiting, stomach pain, diarrhea, and frequent urination. (145:227) Infusion of leaves taken as emetic for ghost sickness: grief, lung cough, appetite loss, and vomiting. (145:260) Decoction of leaves taken for stomachaches. (145:282) *Laxative* Infusion of leaf taken for bear sickness: fever, headache, thirst, constipation, and blocked urination. (145:198) *Love Medicine* Leaves sung over to get the love of a particular girl. (145:400) *Oral Aid* Infusion of leaf taken for bear sickness: fever, headache, thirst, constipation, and blocked urination. (145:198) Infusion of leaves taken by babies for opossum sickness: appetite loss and drooling. (145:220) *Orthopedic Aid* Decoction of leaves taken for dead people's sickness. (145:257) Leaves used for scalping sickness: severe headache, backache and low fever. (145:262) *Other* Leaves burned for ghost sickness: dizziness and staggering. (145:260) Infusion of leaves taken and rubbed on the body for "mythical wolf" sickness. (145:306) *Panacea* Leaves used medicinally for everything and could be added to any medicine. (145:161) *Pediatric Aid* Leaves burned and smoke "smelled" by the baby for raccoon sickness: diarrhea. (145:218) Infusion of leaves taken by babies for opossum sickness: appetite loss and drooling. (145:220) Leaves with other plants used as a baby's charm for fear from dreams about raccoons or opossums. (145:221) Infusion of leaves taken by babies and adults for otter sickness: diarrhea and vomiting. (145:222) Decoction of leaves taken by babies and adults for bird sickness: diarrhea, vomiting, and appetite loss. (145:234) Leaves used for baby sickness caused by adultery: appetite loss, fever, headache, and diarrhea. (145:253) Infusion of leaves taken by children for buzzard sickness: vomiting. (145:305) Whole plant used for chronically ill babies. (145:329) *Psychological Aid* Infusion of leaves taken as emetic for ghost sickness: grief, lung cough, appetite loss, and vomiting. (145:260) Infusion of leaves used to steam and bathe the body for insanity. (145:292) Plant burned to smoke the body for insanity. (145:293) *Pulmonary Aid* Infusion of leaves taken as emetic for ghost sickness: grief, lung cough, appetite loss, and vomiting. (145:260) *Reproductive Aid* Infusion of leaves taken and rubbed on the body for protracted labor. (145:323) *Respiratory Aid* Decoction of leaves taken for dead people's sickness. (145:257) *Sedative* Leaves with other plants used as a baby's charm for fear from dreams about raccoons or opossums. (145:221) Infusion of leaves taken and used as a steam for turkey sickness: dizziness or "craziness." (145:236) *Stimulant* Decoction of leaves used as a bath for hog sickness: unconsciousness. (145:229) Decoction of leaves taken for dead people's sickness. (145:257) *Unspecified* Leaves used for medicinal purposes. (145:161) Plant used medicinally. (145:164) *Urinary Aid* Infusion of leaf taken for bear sickness: fever, headache, thirst, constipation, and blocked urination. (145:198) Infusion of plant taken for wolf sickness: vomiting, stomach pain, diarrhea, and frequent urination. (145:227) *Vertigo Medicine* Infusion of leaves taken as an emetic for thunder sickness: fever, dizziness, headache, and diarrhea. (145:213)

Persea palustris, Swamp Bay
Creek *Alterative* Root used as a "hydragogue" and alterant. *Diaphoretic* and *Febrifuge* Decoction of root used as a diaphoretic in "fevers of all descriptions." *Kidney Aid* Decoction of root used for dropsy. (as *P. pubescens* 23:289)

Persea planifolia, American Avocado
Mahuna *Oral Aid* Powdered seeds used for pyorrhea. *Toothache Remedy* Infusion used for toothaches. (117:25)

Petasites frigidus, Arctic Sweet Coltsfoot
Eskimo, Inupiat *Cold Remedy* Infusion of dried, stored leaves used for colds and head congestion.

Respiratory Aid Infusion of dried, stored leaves used for chest congestion. (83:62)

Petasites frigidus var. nivalis, Arctic Sweet Coltsfoot
Eskimo, Inupiat *Cold Remedy* Infusion of dried, stored leaves used for colds and head congestion. *Respiratory Aid* Infusion of dried, stored leaves used for chest congestion. (as *P. hyperboreus* 83:62)

Petasites frigidus var. palmatus, Arctic Sweet Coltsfoot
Concow *Dermatological Aid* Dried, grated roots applied to boils and running sores. *Misc. Disease Remedy* Root used for the first stages of grippe. *Tuberculosis Remedy* Root used for the first stages of consumption. (as *P. palmata* 33:395) **Delaware** *Cough Medicine* Combined with great mullein, plum root, and glycerin and used as a syrup for coughs. *Pulmonary Aid* Combined with great mullein, plum root, and glycerin and used as a syrup for lung trouble. *Respiratory Aid* Combined with great mullein, plum root, and glycerin and used as a syrup for catarrh. (as *P. palmatus* 151:36) **Delaware, Oklahoma** *Cough Medicine* Compound decoction of leaves taken for coughs. *Pulmonary Aid* Compound decoction of leaves taken for catarrh and lung trouble. *Respiratory Aid* Compound containing plant taken for catarrh, coughs, and lung trouble. (as *P. palmata* 150:30, 31) **Karok** *Panacea* Plant used for sickly babies. *Pediatric Aid* Plant used for sickly babies. (as *P. palmata* 125:390) **Lummi** *Emetic* Decoction of roots taken as an emetic. (as *P. speciosus* 65:49) **Menominee** *Dermatological Aid* Decoction of root used for itch. (as *P. palmatus* 128:31) **Quileute** *Cough Medicine* Decoction of roots or raw roots eaten as a cough medicine. **Quinault** *Dermatological Aid* Infusion of smashed roots used as a wash for swellings. *Eye Medicine* Infusion of smashed roots used as a wash for sore eyes. **Skagit** *Antirheumatic* (*External*) Poultice of warmed leaves applied to parts afflicted with rheumatism. *Tuberculosis Remedy* Decoction of roots taken for tuberculosis. (as *P. speciosus* 65:49) **Tanaina** *Antirheumatic* (*Internal*) and *Misc. Disease Remedy* Plant used for diseases from rheumatism to tuberculosis. *Tuberculosis*

Remedy Plant used for diseases from rheumatism to tuberculosis. (as *P. palmatus* 126:329) **Tlingit** *Dermatological Aid* Compound containing plant used for sores. (as *Nardosmia palmata* 89:284) **Tolowa** *Antirheumatic* (*External*) Leaves placed in hot water and used for arthritic joints. (as *P. palmatum* 5:42)

Petasites sagittatus, Arrowleaf Sweet Coltsfoot
Cree, **Woodlands** *Dermatological Aid* Poultice of leaves applied to worms eating the flesh and itchy skin. (91:48)

Peteria scoparia, Rush Peteria
Navajo, **Ramah** *Ceremonial Medicine* Cold infusion of root used by family to protect hogan and livestock. *Dermatological Aid* Plant used as a lotion for injury inflicted by porcupine. *Misc. Disease Remedy* Compound infusion of tops taken for influenza. *Veterinary Aid* Smoke from dried tops inhaled by sheep for cough. *Witchcraft Medicine* Compound infusion of tops taken for protection from witches. (165:33)

Petradoria pumila ssp. *pumila*, Grassy Rockgoldenrod
Hopi *Analgesic* Plant considered a good remedy for breast pain. (as *Solidago petradoria* 174:98) *Breast Treatment* Plant used for breast pain and to dry up flow of milk. (as *Solidago petradoria* 34:361) *Gynecological Aid* Plant used to decrease milk flow and ease breast pain. (as *Solidago petradoria* 174:36, 98) **Navajo**, **Kayenta** *Dermatological Aid* Plant used for ant bites. (as *Solidago petradoria* 179:50) **Navajo**, **Ramah** *Cathartic* Strong decoction taken as a cathartic. *Ceremonial Medicine* Plant used as a ceremonial emetic. *Dermatological Aid* Cold infusion used as a lotion for injuries. *Emetic* Plant used as a ceremonial emetic. (as *Solidago petradoria* 165:53)

Petrophyton caespitosum var. *caespitosum*, Rocky Mountain Rockspirea
Gosiute *Burn Dressing* Poultice of boiled roots applied to burns. (as *Spiraea caespitosa* 31:349) Boiled roots used as a salve for burns. *Gastrointestinal Aid* Leaves used as a bowel medicine. (as *Spiraea caespitosa* 31:382) **Navajo**, **Kayenta** *Ceremonial Medicine* Plant used as a charm or

prayer in the "Pleiades rite." *Narcotic* Plant used as a narcotic. (as *Spiraea caespitosa* 179:27)

Petroselinum crispum, Parsley
Cherokee *Abortifacient* Infusion of top and root taken as an abortive for "female obstructions." *Gynecological Aid* Infusion taken by "lying-in women whose discharges are too scant." *Kidney Aid* Infusion of top and root taken for kidneys and "dropsy." *Urinary Aid* Infusion of top and root taken for the bladder. (66:47) **Micmac** *Urinary Aid* Herb used for "cold in the bladder." (as *P. sativum* 32:58)

Peucedanum sandwicense, Makou
Hawaiian *Laxative* and *Pediatric Aid* Bark eaten by children and adults as a mild laxative. *Reproductive Aid* Bark taken by expectant mother for the healthy effect on the growing life. (2:71)

Phacelia californica, California Scorpionweed
Costanoan *Febrifuge* Decoction of root used for fevers. (17:13) **Kawaiisu** *Cold Remedy* Infusion of roots taken for colds. *Cough Medicine* Infusion of roots taken for coughs. *Gastrointestinal Aid* Infusion of roots taken for stomach problems. *Stimulant* Infusion of roots taken when weak and not feeling good. (180:48) **Pomo**, **Kashaya** *Dermatological Aid* Fresh, crushed leaf juice rubbed on cold sores and impetigo. (60:48)

Phacelia crenulata, Cleftleaf Wildheliotrope
Hopi *Veterinary Aid* Plant used for injury in animals, especially horses. (34:344)

Phacelia crenulata var. *corrugata*, Cleftleaf Wildheliotrope
Hopi Plant used for injury in animals, especially horses. (as *P. corrugata* 34:343) **Keres**, **Western** *Antirheumatic* (*External*) Infusion of root used as a rub for swellings. *Throat Aid* Infusion of plant used for sore throat. (as *P. corrugata* 147:59)

Phacelia hastata var. *hastata*, Silverleaf Phacelia
Thompson *Gynecological Aid* Decoction of plant taken for difficult menstruation. (as *P. leucophylla* 141:470)

Phacelia heterophylla, Varileaf Phacelia
Miwok *Dermatological Aid* Poultice of pulverized, dried plant put in fresh wounds. (8:171, 172)

Phacelia linearis, Threadleaf Phacelia
Shuswap *Cold Remedy* Infusion of plant taken for a bad cold. (102:64) **Thompson** *Unspecified* Decoction of plant used medicinally. (as *P. menziesii* 141:468)

Phacelia neomexicana, New Mexico Scorpionweed
Zuni *Dermatological Aid* Powdered root mixed with water and used for rashes. (22:376)

Phacelia purshii, Miami Mist
Cherokee *Antirheumatic (External)* Poultice of plant used for swollen joints. (66:49)

Phacelia ramosissima, Branching Phacelia
Kawaiisu *Emetic* Decoction of roots taken to cause vomiting. *Gastrointestinal Aid* Decoction of roots taken to clear the "bad stomach." *Venereal Aid* Decoction of roots taken for gonorrhea. (180:48)

Phaseolus acutifolius, Tepary Bean
Papago *Toothache Remedy* Plant bitten and held between teeth for toothache. (29:65)

Phaseolus angustissimus, Slimleaf Bean
Zuni *Pediatric Aid* and *Strengthener* Crushed leaves, blossoms, and powdered root rubbed on a child's body as a strengthener. (143:85)

Phegopteris sp., Ako-lea
Hawaiian *Dietary Aid* Young shoots or buds and bark mixed with cooked leaves and eaten to restore the loss of appetite. *Gynecological Aid* Inner bark scraped or buds mixed with cooked taro leaves and water and eaten during childbirth. (2:12)

Philadelphus lewisii, Lewis's Mockorange
Okanagan-Colville *Cathartic* Decoction of plant taken as a physic in the morning and evening. (162:108) **Thompson** *Antirheumatic (External)* Powdered, burned wood mixed with pitch or bear grease and rubbed on the skin for swellings. Dried, powdered leaves mixed with pitch or bear

grease and rubbed on the skin for swellings. *Breast Treatment* Poultice of bruised leaves used by women for infected breasts. *Dermatological Aid* Powdered, burned wood mixed with pitch or bear grease and rubbed on the skin for sores. Dried, powdered leaves mixed with pitch or bear grease and rubbed on the skin for sores. Strained decoction of branches, sometimes with the blossoms, used as a soaking solution for eczema. *Hemorrhoid Remedy* Strained decoction of branches, sometimes with the blossoms, used to soak bleeding hemorrhoids. *Pulmonary Aid* Strained decoction of branches taken for sore chest. (161:230)

Philadelphus lewisii var. gordonianus, Gordon's Mockorange
Snohomish *Dermatological Aid* Soapy lather from bruised leaves rubbed on sores. (as *P. gordonianus* 65:31)

Phlebodium aureum, Golden Polypody
Seminole *Other* Complex infusion of tuberous roots taken for chronic conditions. (145:272) *Pediatric Aid* Plant used for chronically ill babies. (145:329) *Psychological Aid* Infusion of plant used to steam and bathe the body for insanity. (145:292) *Unspecified* Plant used for medicinal purposes. (145:162)

Phlox austromontana, Desert Phlox
Havasupai *Antirheumatic (External)* Decoction of pounded roots rubbed all over the body for aches. *Cold Remedy* Decoction of pounded roots rubbed all over the body for colds. *Gastrointestinal Aid* and *Pediatric Aid* Decoction of pounded roots given to babies with stomachaches. (171:238) **Navajo, Kayenta** *Toothache Remedy* Crushed plant placed in cavity for toothaches. (179:38)

Phlox caespitosa, Tufted Phlox
Navajo *Burn Dressing* Plant used for burns. *Cathartic* Plant used as a cathartic. (as *P. douglasii* var. *diffusa* 76:162) *Ceremonial Medicine* Crushed plant and other plants used to make the Night Chant liniment. (45:70) Plant used in medicine ceremonies. *Diuretic* Plant used as a diuretic. *Gynecological Aid* Plant used for childbirth. *Toothache Remedy* Plant used as toothache medicine. (as *P. douglasii* var. *diffusa* 76:162)

Phlox gracilis* ssp. *gracilis, Slender Phlox
Gosiute *Dermatological Aid* Poultice of mashed plant applied to wounds and bruises. (as *Gilia gracilis* 31:370) **Navajo, Ramah** *Dermatological Aid* Poultice of plant applied to sores on body. *Oral Aid* Cold infusion used as mouthwash for mouth sores. (as *Gilia gracilis* 165:40) **Ute** *Dermatological Aid* Poultice of plant applied to bruised or sore legs. (as *Gilia gracilis* 30:34)

Phlox hoodii, Spiny Phlox
Blackfoot *Laxative* and *Pediatric Aid* Infusion of plant given to children as a mild laxative. (72:67) *Pulmonary Aid* Infusion of plant taken for chest pains. (72:73)

Phlox longifolia, Longleaf Phlox
Havasupai *Antirheumatic* (*External*) Decoction of pounded roots rubbed all over the body for aches. *Cold Remedy* Decoction of pounded roots rubbed all over the body for colds. *Gastrointestinal Aid* and *Pediatric Aid* Decoction of pounded roots given to babies with stomachaches. (171:238) **Okanagan-Colville** *Blood Medicine* and *Pediatric Aid* Infusion of whole plant given to "anemic" children. (162:112) **Paiute** *Cathartic* Decoction of root taken as a physic. *Eye Medicine* Infusion or decoction of root used as an eyewash. *Gastrointestinal Aid* and *Pediatric Aid* Decoction of root given to children for stomachaches. *Venereal Aid* Decoction of root taken for venereal disease. **Shoshoni** *Antidiarrheal* Infusion of mashed root taken for diarrhea. (155:115) *Dermatological Aid* Decoction of leaves used for boils. (98:44) *Eye Medicine* Infusion or decoction of root used as an eyewash. *Gastrointestinal Aid* Decoction of entire plant taken for stomach disorders. Infusion of root given to children for stomachaches. *Pediatric Aid* Infusion of root given to children for stomachaches. **Washo** *Eye Medicine* Infusion or decoction of root used as an eyewash. (155:115)

Phlox maculata, Wild Sweetwilliam
Cherokee *Dietary Aid* and *Pediatric Aid* Infusion of root used as a wash to make children grow and fatten. (66:58)

Phlox multiflora, Flowery Phlox
Cheyenne *Stimulant* Infusion of smashed leaves and flowers taken as a stimulant. (63:184) Infusion of pulverized leaves and flowers used as a wash and taken as a stimulant for body numbness. (64:184)

Phlox pilosa, Downy Phlox
Meskwaki *Blood Medicine* Infusion of leaves taken to cure and purify blood. *Dermatological Aid* Infusion of leaves used as wash for eczema. *Love Medicine* Compound containing root used as a love medicine. (129:235)

Phlox stansburyi, Colddesert Phlox
Navajo, Ramah *Contraceptive* Decoction of leaves taken during menstruation as a contraceptive. *Dermatological Aid* Decoction of leaves used as a lotion for sores. *Disinfectant* Plant used as a fumigant for "deer infection." *Gynecological Aid* Decoction of leaves taken during pregnancy to insure birth of female baby. Decoction of leaves taken to facilitate delivery of placenta. (165:40)

Phlox subulata, Moss Phlox
Mahuna *Antirheumatic* (*Internal*) Plant used for rheumatism. (117:59)

Phoenicaulis cheiranthoides, Wallflower Phoenicaulis
Paiute *Gynecological Aid* and *Tonic* Decoction of root taken as a tonic after childbirth. (as *Parrya menziesii* 155:112)

Phoradendron californicum, Mesquite Mistletoe
Pima *Cathartic* Decoction of berries taken as a purge. *Dermatological Aid* Infusion of plant used as a wash for sores. *Gastrointestinal Aid* Decoction of berries taken for stomachaches. (38:82)

Phoradendron juniperinum, Juniper Mistletoe
Hopi *Gastrointestinal Aid* Plant used as "medicine for the stomach." (174:34, 72) *Unspecified* Plant used medicinally. (34:345) *Witchcraft Medicine* Plant used as "medicine for the stomach and bad medicine of wizards." (174:72) **Keres, Western** *Antidiarrheal* Crushed plant given to children for diarrhea. *Antirheumatic* (*External*) Crushed plant used as a rub for rheumatism. *Pediatric Aid*

Crushed plant given to children for diarrhea. (147:59) **Navajo** *Dermatological Aid* Plant used for warts. (76:162) **Navajo, Ramah** *Gastrointestinal Aid* Cold infusion taken to relieve distress caused by eating too much meat. (165:23) **Tewa** *Gastrointestinal Aid* Infusion of pulverized plant taken for "chill in the stomach." (115:47) **Zuni** *Emetic* Infusion of whole plant taken as an emetic for stomachaches. (22:377) *Gynecological Aid* Compound infusion of plant taken to promote muscular relaxation at birth. Simple or compound infusion of twigs taken after childbirth to stop blood flow. *Hemostat* Simple or compound infusion of twigs taken after childbirth to stop blood flow. (143:55)

Phoradendron juniperinum ssp. juniperinum, Juniper Mistletoe
Navajo *Dermatological Aid* Plant used for warts. (as *P. ligatum* 76:162)

Phoradendron leucarpum, Oak Mistletoe
Cherokee *Analgesic* "Tea ooze" used to bathe head for headache. *Anticonvulsive* Dried and pulverized plant "good for epilepsy or fits, best if from oak." *Gynecological Aid* Hot infusion used as "medicine for pregnant women." *Hypotensive* Infusion used for high blood pressure. *Love Medicine* Infusion taken after vomiting for 4 days, to cure "love sickness." (as *P. serotinum* 66:45) **Creek** *Pulmonary Aid* Compounds containing leaves and branches used for lung trouble. (as *P. flavescens* 148:659) Leaves and branches used for lung trou-

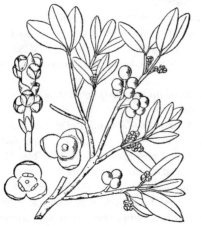

Phoradendron leucarpum

bles. (as *P. flavescens* 152:20) *Tuberculosis Remedy* Compounds containing leaves and branches used for consumption. (as *P. flavescens* 148:659) **Houma** *Orthopedic Aid* Decoction of plant taken for debility and paralytic weakness. *Panacea* Decoction of plant said to be good for sickness in general, a panacea. (as *P. flavescens* 135:58) **Mendocino Indian** *Abortifacient* Infusion of roots taken for abortions. *Poison* Plant considered poisonous. *Toothache Remedy* Root chewed for toothaches. (as *P. flavescens* 33:344) **Seminole** *Antirheumatic (External)* Decoction of leaves rubbed on body and body steamed for deer sickness: numb, painful limbs and joints. (as *P. flavescens* 145:192) *Emetic* Plant used as an emetic during religious ceremonies. (as *P. flavescens* 145:409) *Pediatric Aid* Plant used for chronically ill babies. (as *P. flavescens* 145:329)

Phoradendron macrophyllum ssp. macrophyllum, Colorado Desert Mistletoe
Diegueño *Dermatological Aid* Decoction of entire, fresh plant used for dandruff. (as *P. tomentosum* ssp. *macrophyllum* 70:28)

Phoradendron villosum, Pacific Mistletoe
Kawaiisu *Abortifacient* Infusion of plant taken first 2 months of pregnancy to cause an abortion. *Antirheumatic (External)* Infusion of plant used as a wash on limbs affected by rheumatism. (as *P. flavescens* var. *villosum* 180:49) **Pomo** *Abortifacient* Decoction of leaves taken to bring on delayed menstruation. (54:13)

Phoradendron villosum ssp. villosum, Pacific Mistletoe
Pomo, Kashaya *Abortifacient* Decoction of leaves used for delayed menstruation. (as *P. flavescens* var. *villosum* 60:72)

Phragmites australis, Common Reed
Apache, White Mountain *Antidiarrheal* Root used for diarrhea and kindred diseases. *Gastrointestinal Aid* Root used for stomach troubles and kindred diseases. (as *P. communis* 113:159) **Blackfoot** *Emetic* Decoction of whole plant taken as an emetic. (as *P. communis* 82:22) **Cahuilla** *Orthopedic Aid* Used as a splint for broken limbs. (as *P. communis* var. *berlandieri* 11:101) **Iro-**

quois *Ceremonial Medicine* Decoction of root-stocks and bottle brush grass used as medicine to soak corn seeds before planting. (as *P. communis* 170:18) *Other* Compound used as a "corn medicine." (73:273) **Keres, Western** *Pediatric Aid* Crushed plant given to children for diarrhea. (as *P. communis* 147:59) **Paiute** *Analgesic* Sugary sap taken by pneumonia patients to loosen phlegm and soothe lung pain. *Expectorant* Sugary sap taken by pneumonia patients to loosen phlegm. *Pulmonary Aid* Sugary sap taken by pneumonia patients to loosen phlegm and soothe lung pain. (as *P. communis* 155:116) **Seminole** *Dermatological Aid* Poultice of plant applied to dry up boils and carbuncles. (as *P. communis* 145:243)

Phryma leptostachya, American Lopseed
Chippewa *Throat Aid* Decoction of root gargled or root chewed for sore throat. (43:342) **Ojibwa, South** *Antirheumatic (Internal)* Decoction of root taken for rheumatic leg pains. (77:201)

Phyla cuneifolia, Fogfruit
Navajo, Kayenta *Dermatological Aid* Poultice of plants applied to spider bites. (as *Lippia cuneifolia* 179:40)

Phyla lanceolata, Lanceleaf Fogfruit
Mahuna *Antirheumatic (Internal)* Plant used for rheumatism. (as *Lippia lanceolata* 117:60)

Phyla nodiflora, Turkey Tangle Fogfruit
Houma *Orthopedic Aid* and *Pediatric Aid* Decoction of plant used as a wash to make weak, lazy babies walk. (as *Lippia nodiflora* 135:65)

Phyllodoce empetriformis, Pink Mountain-heath
Thompson *Tuberculosis Remedy* Decoction of plant taken over a period of time for tuberculosis and spitting up blood. (161:215)

Phyllospadix torreyi, Torrey's Surfgrass
Kwakiutl *Pediatric Aid* and *Strengthener* Leaves placed in the bottom of child's cradle to make him grow strong. (157:274)

Physalis heterophylla, Clammy Groundcherry
Iroquois *Burn Dressing* Compound infusion of dried leaves and roots used as wash for scalds and burns. *Emetic* and *Gastrointestinal Aid* Compound infusion of leaves and roots taken to vomit for bad stomachaches. *Venereal Aid* Compound infusion of dried leaves and roots used as wash for venereal disease. (73:430) **Lakota** *Dietary Aid* Three or five berries used for lack of appetite. (116:60) **Meskwaki** *Unspecified* Root used as a medicine. (129:247)

Physalis lanceolata, Lanceleaf Groundcherry
Omaha *Analgesic* Decoction of root used for headache and stomach trouble. *Dermatological Aid* Root used as a dressing for wounds. *Gastrointestinal Aid* Decoction of root used for stomach trouble and headache. *Unspecified* Root used in smoke treatment for unspecified ailments. **Ponca** *Analgesic* Decoction of root used for headache and stomach trouble. *Dermatological Aid* Root used as a dressing for wounds. *Gastrointestinal Aid* Decoction of root used for stomach trouble and headache. *Unspecified* Root used in smoke treatment for unspecified ailments. **Winnebago** *Analgesic* Decoction of root used for headache and stomach trouble. *Dermatological Aid* Root used as a dressing for wounds. *Gastrointestinal Aid* Decoction of root used for stomach trouble and headache. *Unspecified* Root used in smoke treatment for unspecified ailments. (58:113)

Physalis philadelphica, Mexican Groundcherry
Diegueño *Eye Medicine* Berries squeezed and the juice used as an eyewash. (70:28)

Physalis pubescens, Husk Tomato
Navajo, Ramah *Panacea* Dried leaves and root used as "life medicine." (165:43)

Physalis virginiana., Virginia Groundcherry
Meskwaki *Stimulant* Infusion of whole plant taken for dizziness. (129:247, 248)

Physalis viscosa, Starhair Groundcherry
Omaha *Dermatological Aid* Root used to dress wounds. (as *P. viscora* 48:584)

Physaria chambersii, Chambers's Twinpod
Paiute *Eye Medicine* Infusion or decoction of var-

ious plant parts used as a wash for sore eyes or sties. **Shoshoni** *Eye Medicine* Infusion or decoction of various plant parts used as a wash for sore eyes and sties. (155:116)

Physaria didymocarpa, Common Twinpod
Blackfoot *Abortifacient* Infusion of plant taken in small amounts to abort. (72:61) *Analgesic* Plant chewed for cramps and stomach trouble. (95:274) *Antirheumatic (External)* Infusion of roots applied to aching parts of the body. (72:78) Strong infusion of plant used as a liniment on sprains. (72:79) Decoction of plant used for swellings. (82:35) *Dermatological Aid* Weak decoction of plant used for diaper rash. Weak decoction of leaf used on newborn's umbilical. (72:77) Infusion of plant applied to wounds to heal with less irritation. (72:84) Infusion of plant used to allay swelling. (95:274) *Dietary Aid* Decoction of plant taken slowly to gradually expand the stomach until food was eaten without pain. This decoction was used by a person who had not eaten for a long time. (72:104) *Ear Medicine* Infusion of leaves used as drops for ear infections. *Eye Medicine* Infusion of leaves used as drops for bloodshot eyes. (72:81) *Gastrointestinal Aid* Plant chewed for cramps and stomach troubles. (82:35) Plant chewed for cramps, stomach trouble, and sore throat. (95:274) Infusion of leaves taken for stomach trouble. (98:38) *Orthopedic Aid* Strong infusion of plant used as a liniment on dislocations. (72:79) *Pediatric Aid* Weak decoction of leaf used on newborn's umbilical. (72:77) *Throat Aid* Plant chewed for sore throats. (82:35) Plant chewed for sore throat. (95:274) Infusion of leaves taken for sore throat. (98:38) *Toothache Remedy* Leaf clenched between the teeth for toothache. (72:77) Plant used as toothache medicine. (72:78) *Veterinary Aid* Infusion of plant applied as a liniment to the shoulders of work and wagon horses. (72:89)

Physaria didymocarpa* var. *lanata,
    Common Twinpod
Blackfoot *Gastrointestinal Aid* Plant chewed for stomach troubles. *Throat Aid* Plant chewed for sore throats. (100:47)

Physaria newberryi, Newberry's Twinpod
Hopi *Antidote* and *Ceremonial Medicine* Plant

taken as an antidote after the snake dance. (46:16) **Navajo** *Respiratory Aid* Plant used as a snuff for catarrh. (45:49)

Physocarpus capitatus, Pacific Ninebark
Bella Coola *Emetic* Decoction of 3-foot stick taken alternatively with large amounts of water as an emetic. (158:208) **Green River Group** *Emetic* Young shoots, peeled of bark, used as an emetic. (65:33) **Hesquiat** *Antidote* Decoction of bark taken as an antidote for poisoning, caused vomiting. *Antirheumatic (External)* Decoction of bark used as a wash or soaking solution for rheumatic pain. *Antirheumatic (Internal)* Decoction of bark taken for rheumatic fever. *Emetic* Decoction of bark taken as an antidote for poisoning, caused vomiting. Bark chewed and juice swallowed to induce vomiting. *Laxative* Decoction of bark taken in small doses as a laxative. (159:73) **Kwakiutl** *Cathartic* Root extract used as a purgative. *Emetic* Decoction of bark taken to induce vomiting. *Laxative* Decoction of bark taken for constipation. *Venereal Aid* Root extract used for locomotor ataxia. (157:289) **Saanich** *Laxative* Infusion of macerated roots taken as a quick laxative. (156:86)

Physocarpus malvaceus, Mallow Ninebark
Okanagan-Colville *Hunting Medicine* Infusion of bark used to wash arrows and other hunting equipment to protect them from spells. (162:126)

Physocarpus opulifolius, Common Ninebark
Bella Coola *Analgesic* and *Emetic* Decoction of inner bark taken as an emetic by persons "dizzy with pain." *Laxative* Decoction of inner bark taken as a laxative for gonorrhea. *Tuberculosis Remedy* Decoction of inner bark taken and used as a wash for scrofulous glands in neck. *Venereal Aid* Decoction of inner bark taken and used as wash for gonorrhea. **Carrier, Southern** *Cathartic* and *Emetic* Decoction of bark taken as an emetic, a large dose fatal. (127:59) **Chippewa** *Emetic* Infusion of roots taken as an emetic. (59:132) **Iroquois** *Gynecological Aid* Poultice used when women swell after copulation; caused by bad medicine. (73:349) **Menominee** *Gynecological Aid* Bark used to make a drink for female maladies, to cleanse system and enhance fertility. (128:49)

Physostegia parviflora, Western False Dragonhead
Meskwaki _Cold Remedy_ Infusion of leaves taken for bad cold. (129:226)

Phytolacca americana, American Pokeweed
Cherokee _Antirheumatic (Internal)_ Infusion of berry taken for arthritis. Roots and berries or berry wine used for rheumatism. _Blood Medicine_ Cooked greens eaten or infusion of root taken to build the blood. _Dermatological Aid_ Poultice used for ulcers and swellings and infusion of root used for eczema. Salve used on "ulcerous sores" and dried, crushed roots sprinkled on old sores. _Febrifuge_ Poultice used for "nervous fevers, ulcers and swellings." _Kidney Aid_ Cold infusion of powdered root taken for kidneys. (66:50) _Laxative_ Plant used in a side dish with laxative properties. (178:251) _Other_ Compound used for "white swelling." (66:50) _Poison_ Roots and berries considered poisonous. _Unspecified_ Berries used for medicine. (105:51) **Delaware** _Antirheumatic (External)_ Roasted, crushed roots used with sarsaparilla and mountain grape barks for rheumatism. _Blood Medicine_ Roasted, crushed roots used with sarsaparilla and mountain grape barks as a blood purifier. _Dermatological Aid_ Roots roasted and the salve used for chronic sores. _Gland Medicine_ Roots roasted and the salve used for glandular swellings. _Stimulant_ Roasted, crushed roots used with sarsaparilla and mountain grape barks as a stimulant. (as _P. decandra_ 151:32) **Delaware, Oklahoma**

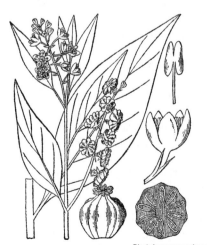

Phytolacca americana

Antirheumatic (External) Strong infusion of roots or twigs used as herbal steam for rheumatism. (as _P. decandra_ 150:30, 78) _Antirheumatic (Internal)_ Compound containing root used for rheumatism. _Blood Medicine_ Compound containing root used as a blood purifier. (as _P. decandra_ 150:27, 78) _Herbal Steam_ Infusion of roots or twigs used as herbal steam for rheumatism. (as _P. decandra_ 150:30) _Stimulant_ Compound containing root used as a stimulant. (as _P. decandra_ 150:27, 78) **Iroquois** _Antirheumatic (External)_ Stalks cooked as greens and used for rheumatism. (as _P. decandra_ 103:93) _Cathartic_ Plant used as a cathartic. (73:316) _Cold Remedy_ Decoction of stems taken for chest colds. (73:317) _Dermatological Aid_ Compound with undried roots applied as a salve on bunions. Poultice of crushed roots applied to bruises. Raw berries rubbed on skin lumps. _Emetic_ Plant used as an emetic. _Expectorant_ Plant used as an expectorant. (73:316) _Liver Aid_ Compound infusion of whole roots used for liver sickness. (73:317) _Love Medicine_ "Tie in a poplar tree, then place among roots," as a love medicine. _Orthopedic Aid_ Decoction of roots applied as poultice to sprains, bruises, and swollen joints. _Witchcraft Medicine_ Plant used for bewitchment. (73:316) **Mahuna** _Analgesic_ Roots used for severe, neuralgic pains. _Dermatological Aid_ Leaves used for skin diseases or to remove pimples and blackheads. _Poison_ Plant considered poisonous. (as _P. decandra_ 117:65) **Micmac** _Hemostat_ Leaves used for bleeding wounds. (as _P. decandra_ 32:59) **Mohegan** _Gynecological Aid_ Poultice of mashed berries applied to sore breasts. (as _P. decandra_ 151:74, 130) _Poison_ Root considered poisonous. (as _P. decandra_ 151:74) **Rappahannock** _Antidiarrheal_ Infusion of berries taken for dysentery. _Antirheumatic (Internal)_ Fermented infusion of leaves taken for rheumatism. _Dermatological Aid_ Compound infusion with roots applied to ivy poison. Poultice of mashed root applied to wart until it bleeds. _Hemorrhoid Remedy_ Steam from decoction of roots used for piles. (138:29) **Seminole** _Analgesic_ Berries eaten as an analgesic. (145:167) Berries eaten for pains. _Antirheumatic (Internal)_ Berries eaten for rheumatism. (145:285)

Picea abies, Norway Spruce
Mohegan _Analgesic_ Poultice of sap or gum applied

for boil and abscess pains. (151:74) *Dermatological Aid* Sap or gum applied to boil or abscess pains. (151:74, 130)

Picea engelmannii, Engelmann's Spruce

Navajo, Ramah *Ceremonial Medicine* and *Emetic* Plant used as a ceremonial emetic. (165:12) **Okanagan-Colville** *Respiratory Aid* Infusion of bark used for respiratory ailments. *Tuberculosis Remedy* Infusion of bark used for tuberculosis. (162:27) **Thompson** *Cancer Treatment* Decoction of needles and gum taken for cancer. It was said that if this treatment did not work, nothing would work. The decoction was taken with a spoon directly from the bark blisters and in concentrated form. *Cough Medicine* Decoction of needles and gum taken for coughs. (161:100) *Dermatological Aid* Twig ashes mixed with grease and used as an ointment or salve. (141:475) Pitch used for eczema. *Psychological Aid* Tree and red cedar tree caused vivid dreams for anyone who slept under it. (161:100)

Picea glauca, White Spruce

Abnaki *Urinary Aid* Infusion of cones taken for urinary troubles. (121:164) **Algonquin, Quebec** *Cough Medicine* Inner bark chewed and infusion of inner bark taken for coughs. *Dermatological Aid* Gum used as a salve. *Gynecological Aid* Used in the sudatory, this is taken by women after childbirth and for other complaints. *Internal Medicine* Infusion of branch tips taken to "heal the insides."

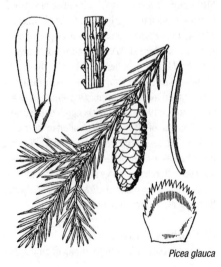

Picea glauca

Laxative Gum chewed as a laxative. (14:126) Resin chewed as a laxative. (14:73) *Unspecified* Used in the sudatory, this is taken by women after childbirth and for other complaints. (14:126) **Chippewa** *Antirheumatic (External)* Compound decoction of twigs used as herbal steam for rheumatism. (as *P. canadensis* 43:362) **Cree, Woodlands** *Antirheumatic (Internal)* Decoction of inner bark used for arthritis. *Blood Medicine* Poultice of gum and lard applied for blood poisoning. *Dermatological Aid* Pitch and grease used as an ointment for skin rashes, scabies, persistent scabs, and growing boils. Rotten, dried, finely powdered wood used as baby powder and for skin rashes. Poultice of gum and lard applied to infections. Rotten wood used in baby dusting powder. *Pediatric Aid* Rotten, dried, finely powdered wood used as baby powder and for skin rashes. Rotten wood used in baby dusting powder. (91:48) **Eskimo, Alaska** *Dermatological Aid* Poultice of resin applied to wounds. *Unspecified* Infusion of needles used as medicine for all purposes. (as *P. canadensis* 3:716) **Eskimo, Inuktitut** *Dermatological Aid* Poultice of gum and grease applied to pustulant wounds. *Respiratory Aid* Decoction of gum or needles taken for respiratory infections. (176:188) **Eskimo, Kuskokwagmiut** *Cough Medicine* Decoction of green needles taken or raw needles chewed as cough medicine. (101:28, 29) **Eskimo, Nunivak** *Dermatological Aid* Resin applied to wounds. *Panacea* Infusion of needles used as a medicine for all purposes. (as *P. canadensis* 126:325) **Eskimo, Western** *Cough Medicine* Decoction of needles taken or raw needles chewed as a cough medicine. (90:24) **Gitksan** *Cold Remedy* Decoction of bark or inner bark used for colds. *Cough Medicine* Decoction of bark or inner bark used for coughs. *Misc. Disease Remedy* Decoction of bark or inner bark used for flu. *Tonic* Decoction of bark or inner bark used as a tonic. (as *P. glauca × engelmannii* 61:152) **Iroquois** *Gastrointestinal Aid* Gum chewed to facilitate digestion. (119:83) **Koyukon** *Ceremonial Medicine* Pitch, swan feathers, and slender grass tops burned by shamans when making medicine for a sick person. (99:50) *Dermatological Aid* Infusion of needles used as a rub or bath for dry skin or sores. (99:49) Pitch applied to sores and cuts. (99:50) *Hunting Medicine* Tops put in animal track by girls before stepping over it, to avoid alienating animals from hunters. *Kidney Aid* Infusion of needles taken for kidney problems. *Panacea* Infusion of needles taken to promote general good health. *Unspecified* Tree tops used by the shamans to brush people and remove their sickness. (99:49) **Malecite** *Unspecified* Pitch used in medicines. (137:6) **Menominee** *Dermatological Aid* Poultice of cooked, beaten inner bark applied to wounds, cuts, or swellings. *Internal Medicine* Infusion of inner bark taken for "inward troubles for either man or woman." (as *P. canadensis* 128:45) **Micmac** *Cough Medicine* Bark used as a cough remedy. *Dermatological Aid* Bark used to prepare a salve for cuts and wounds. Gum used for scabs and sores. *Gastrointestinal Aid* Parts of plant used for stomach trouble. *Misc. Disease Remedy* Bark, leaves, and stems used for scurvy. (as *P. canadensis* 32:59) **Montagnais** *Tonic* Infusion of twigs taken "for generally beneficial effects." (as *P. canadensis* 133:314) **Ojibwa** *Disinfectant* Dried leaves used as an inhalant and fumigator. (as *P. canadensis* 130:379) **Ojibwa, South** *Antidiarrheal* Compound containing outer bark taken for diarrhea. (as *Abies canadensis* 77:198) **Okanagan-Colville** *Respiratory Aid* Infusion of bark used for respiratory ailments. *Tuberculosis Remedy* Infusion of bark used for tuberculosis. (162:27) **Shuswap** *Dermatological Aid* Poultice of soft pitch applied to sores. *Panacea* Decoction of bark taken for tuberculosis and other sickness. *Toothache Remedy* Hard pitch chewed to clean the teeth. *Tuberculosis Remedy* Decoction of bark taken for tuberculosis. (102:51) **Tanana, Upper** *Antirheumatic* (*Internal*) Decoction of tree top, young birch tip, and Hudson Bay tea taken for body aches. *Cold Remedy* Decoction of young tips, Hudson Bay tea, and blackberry stems taken for colds. Raw cambium chewed for colds. Decoction of tree top, young birch tip, and Hudson Bay tea taken for colds. Decoction of tree tip, Hudson Bay tea, and blackberry stems used for colds. *Cough Medicine* Raw cambium chewed for coughs. *Dermatological Aid* Poultice of raw or boiled cambium applied to sores and infected areas or used to bandage cuts. Decoction of tree tip used as a wash for rashes and sores. Pitch and moose fat warmed into an ointment and used for sores. Pitch boiled in water and applied to sores. Soft pitch, sometimes mixed with grease, used as an ointment

for sores. *Disinfectant* Decoction of tree top and cottonwood taken for infections. Soft pitch, sometimes mixed with grease, used as an ointment for external infections. *Hemorrhoid Remedy* Chewed pitch applied to bleeding cuts. *Oral Aid* Decoction of young tips, Hudson Bay tea, and blackberry stems taken for mouth sores. Decoction of tree tip, Hudson Bay tea, and blackberry stems used for mouth sores. *Pulmonary Aid* Decoction of wood ash taken for chest problems. *Respiratory Aid* Decoction of tree top, young birch tip, and Hudson Bay tea taken for congestion. *Throat Aid* Pitch chewed for sore throats. *Tuberculosis Remedy* Raw cambium chewed for tuberculosis. Decoction of wood ash taken for tuberculosis. (86:2) **Tlingit** *Antidiarrheal* Sap mixed with mountain goat tallow and used for diarrhea. (as *Pinus canadensis* 89:283) **Wet'suwet'en** *Cold Remedy* Decoction of bark or inner bark used for colds. *Cough Medicine* Decoction of bark or inner bark used for coughs. *Misc. Disease Remedy* Decoction of bark or inner bark used for flu. *Tonic* Decoction of bark or inner bark used as a tonic. (as *Picea glauca* × *engelmannii* 61:152)

Picea mariana, Black Spruce
Algonquin, Quebec *Dermatological Aid* Gum used as a salve. *Internal Medicine* Infusion of branch tips used for "healing the insides." *Unspecified* Used in the medicinal sudatory. (14:127) **Cree, Woodlands** *Antidiarrheal* Decoction of cones taken for diarrhea. *Burn Dressing* Pitch mixed with grease and used as ointment for bad burns. *Dermatological Aid* Pitch mixed with grease and used as ointment for skin rashes, scabies, and persistent scabs. *Oral Aid* Cone chewed for a sore mouth. *Throat Aid* Decoction of cones used as a gargle for sore throats. *Toothache Remedy* Cone chewed for toothaches. *Venereal Aid* Decoction of cones and other herbs taken for venereal disease. (91:49) **Eskimo, Inuktitut** *Dermatological Aid* Poultice of gum and grease applied to pustulant wounds. *Respiratory Aid* Decoction of gum or needles taken for respiratory infections. (176:188) **Iroquois** *Gastrointestinal Aid* Gum chewed to facilitate digestion. (119:83) **Koyukon** *Dermatological Aid* Infusion of needles used as a rub or bath for dry skin or sores. *Hunting Medicine* Tops put in animal track by girls before stepping over it,

to avoid alienating animals from hunters. *Kidney Aid* Infusion of needles taken for kidney problems. *Panacea* Infusion of needles taken to promote general good health. *Unspecified* Tree tops used by the shamans to brush people and remove their sickness. (99:49) **Malecite** *Unspecified* Pitch used in medicines. (137:6) **Montagnais** *Cough Medicine* Decoction of twigs taken for coughs. (133:314) **Ojibwa** *Analgesic* Infusion of roots and bark used for stomach pain. *Anticonvulsive* Infusion of roots and bark used for trembling and fits. *Gastrointestinal Aid* Infusion of roots and bark used for stomach pain. (as *P. nigra* 112:244) *Stimulant* Leaves used as a reviver and bark used as a medicinal salt. *Unspecified* Bark used as a medicinal salt. (130:379) **Ojibwa, South** *Unspecified* Decoction of leaves and crushed bark taken for unspecified ailments. (as *Abies nigra* 77:198) **Potawatomi** *Dermatological Aid* Poultice of inner bark applied to infected inflammations. *Disinfectant* Poultice of inner bark applied to infected inflammations. (131:70)

Picea parryana, Spruce
Keres, Western *Antirheumatic* (*External*) Infusion of leaves used as a bath for rheumatism. *Cold Remedy* Infusion of leaves used for colds. *Gastrointestinal Aid* Infusion of plant used to clean the stomach. (147:60)

Picea rubens, Red Spruce
Cherokee *Cold Remedy* Infusion of bough taken for colds. *Misc. Disease Remedy* Infusion of bough taken to break out measles. (66:57) **Montagnais** *Pulmonary Aid* Compound decoction of bark taken for lung trouble. *Throat Aid* Compound decoction of bark taken for throat trouble. (133:315)

Picea sitchensis, Sitka Spruce
Bella Coola *Analgesic* Decoction of cones taken for pain and bark used as steam bed for backache. *Antirheumatic* (*External*) Poultice of compound containing gum applied to the arms for rheumatism. Steam bed of ripe cones or bark on hot stones used by rheumatics. (127:51, 52) Sapling bark and ripe cones used to make steam baths for rheumatism. (158:198) *Burn Dressing* "Branches used to whip a burned arm or leg until the blood came." (127:51, 52) *Ceremonial Medicine* Boughs

used ritually for protection from death and illness. (158:198) *Dermatological Aid* Gum applied to "small cuts, broken skin and suppurating sores." (127:51, 52) Poultice of gum applied to cuts. *Disinfectant* Poultice of gum applied to infections. (158:198) *Diuretic* Decoction of gum taken as a diuretic for gonorrhea. (127:51, 52) *Gastrointestinal Aid* Sapling bark and ripe cones used to make steam baths for stomach troubles. (158:198) *Heart Medicine* Poultice of compound containing gum applied to the chest for heart trouble. *Laxative* Sap from peeled trunk taken in large doses as a laxative. (127:51, 52) Cambium eaten as a laxative. (158:198) *Venereal Aid* Compound decoction of tips of small spruces taken for gonorrhea. Decoction of gum taken as a diuretic for gonorrhea. (127:51, 52) Decoction of branch tips and other herbs taken for gonorrhea. Gum taken for gonorrhea. (158:198) **Carrier, Southern** *Analgesic* Decoction of new shoots and bark taken for stomach pain. *Eye Medicine* Gum from new shoots and small branches placed in the eyes for snow-blindness. *Gastrointestinal Aid* Decoction of new shoots and bark taken for stomach pain. **Gitksan** *Antirheumatic* (*Internal*) Compound decoction of twigs with leaves and bark taken for rheumatism. *Tuberculosis Remedy* Compound containing gum taken before meals for consumption. (127:51, 52) **Haisla & Hanaksiala** *Antirheumatic* (*External*) Poultice of pitch, Indian hellebore roots and rhizomes applied to sore areas. *Cold Remedy* Inner bark chewed for colds. *Cough Medicine* Inner bark chewed for coughs. *Dermatological Aid* Poultice of boiled pitch applied to cuts, sores, boils, and wounds. *Oral Aid* Pitch chewed as a breath freshener. *Tuberculosis Remedy* Pitch chewed everyday for tuberculosis. **Hanaksiala** *Laxative* Infusion of dried bough tips taken for constipation. (35:175) **Hesquiat** *Analgesic* Boughs used to scrub skin, until it bled, for aches and pains. *Dermatological Aid* Rendered pitch and deer oil used as salve for sores and sunburn. (159:41) **Kwakiutl** *Analgesic* Head struck with branches until it bled for headaches. (157:269) *Antidiarrheal* Compound decoction of roots taken for diarrhea. (157:264) Decoction of roots used for diarrhea. *Cold Remedy* Bud extract taken for coughs and colds. *Cough Medicine* Bud extract or pitch and grease taken for coughs. *Dermatologi-*

cal Aid Poultice of pitch applied to boils, swellings, cuts, and abrasions. *Disinfectant* Branches in house of sick person to prevent anything unclean from entering. *Kidney Aid* Compound poultice of boiled root bark applied to woman's kidney swellings. *Other* Branch tips rubbed to cleanse person contaminated with menstrual blood. (157:269) **Makah** *Blood Medicine* Decoction of plants used to "take out bad blood." *Dermatological Aid* Compound poultice of ashes applied to infant's navel. (65:17) *Gastrointestinal Aid* Pitch used as a stomach medicine. (55:234) *Pediatric Aid* Compound poultice of ashes applied to infant's navel. *Strengthener* Decoction of plants used as a strengthening bath. (65:17) **Oweekeno** *Antirheumatic (External)* Decoction of bark used as a soak for soreness. Pitch mixed with badge moss and used for arthritic joints. *Dermatological Aid* Pitch boiled and used for dermatitis. Pitch mixed with pounded dogtooth lichens and used for wounds. *Gastrointestinal Aid* Decoction of bark used for gastrointestinal difficulties. *Unspecified* Pitch eaten as medicine. (35:68) **Quinault** *Dermatological Aid* Poultice of gum applied to cuts and wounds. *Throat Aid* Infusion of inner bark taken for throat problems. (65:17) **Sikani** *Cough Medicine* Inner bark chewed for a cough. (127:51, 52) **Thompson** *Antidiarrheal* Decoction of burned cone ashes taken for dysentery. *Eye Medicine* Needles used to restore eyesight. A blind person, or one with poor eyesight, rubbed his hands with the needles and then rubbed his eyes with his hands to restore his eyesight. *Panacea* Decoction of boughs used for any kind of illness. *Unspecified* Infusion of bark taken as a medicine. Decoction of inner bark taken as a medicine. Evergreen tops considered good medicine. (161:100) **Tlingit** *Toothache Remedy* Compound containing warmed seeds used for toothache. *Venereal Aid* Compound poultice of sap applied for syphilis. (89:284) **Tsimshian** *Hunting Medicine* Boughs used by shamans, hunters, and fishers during preparatory and purification rituals. (35:317)

Picradeniopsis oppositifolia, Oppositeleaf Bahia
Navajo, **Ramah** *Dermatological Aid* Poultice of chewed leaves applied to red ant bites. *Gastrointestinal Aid* Cold infusion of leaves taken after swallowing a red ant. *Herbal Steam* Steam from compound containing plant used medicinally. *Panacea* Plant used as "life medicine." (as *Bahia oppositifolia* 165:49)

Picradeniopsis woodhousei, Woodhouse's Bahia
Zuni *Dermatological Aid* Poultice of chewed root applied to sores and rashes. (as *Bahia woodhousei* 22:374) *Emetic* Infusion of whole plant taken, vomiting ensued, for "sick stomach." (as *Bahia woodhousei* 143:44) *Gastrointestinal Aid* Infusion of root taken for stomachache. (as *Bahia woodhousei* 22:374)

Pilea pumila, Canadian Clearweed
Cherokee *Dermatological Aid* Stems rubbed between the toes for itching. *Dietary Aid* and *Pediatric Aid* Infusion given to children to reduce excessive hunger. (66:52, 53) **Iroquois** *Respiratory Aid* "Squeeze water out of stem and inhale for sinus problems." (73:308)

Piloblephis rigida, Wild Pennyroyal
Seminole *Ceremonial Medicine* Infusion of leaves added to food after a recent death. (as *Pycnothymus rigidus* 145:342) *Cold Remedy* Infusion of plant taken for colds. (as *Pycnothymus rigidus* 145:283) *Dermatological Aid* Infusion of roots applied to sores and ulcers on the legs and feet. (as *Pycnothymus rigidus* 145:307) *Emetic* Plant used as an emetic during religious ceremonies. (as *Pycnothymus rigidus* 145:409) *Febrifuge* Infusion of plant taken for fevers. (as *Pycnothymus rigidus* 145:283) *Pediatric Aid* Plant used for chronically ill babies. (as *Pycnothymus rigidus* 145:329) *Stimulant* Decoction of whole plant minus the roots used as a bath for hog sickness: unconsciousness. (as *Pycnothymus rigidus* 145:229)

Pimpinella anisum, Anise Burnet Saxifrage
Cherokee *Respiratory Aid* Infusion of half a teaspoonful in a cup of hot water taken for catarrh. (66:23) **Delaware** *Cathartic* Roots used as a cathartic. *Gastrointestinal Aid* Roots used as a stomach tonic. (151:33) **Delaware, Oklahoma** *Cathartic* Root used as a cathartic. (150:28, 78) *Gastrointestinal Aid* and *Tonic* Root used as a stomach tonic. (150:28)

Pinguicula lutea, Yellow Butterwort
Seminole *Analgesic* and *Gastrointestinal Aid* Infusion of whole plant taken for raw meat sickness: severe abdominal pains. (145:276, 277)

Pinguicula pumila, Small Butterwort
Seminole *Analgesic* and *Gastrointestinal Aid* Infusion of whole plant taken for raw meat sickness: severe abdominal pains. (145:276, 277)

Pinus aristata, Bristlecone Pine
Shoshoni *Dermatological Aid* Poultice of heated pitch applied to sores and boils. (155:117)

Pinus banksiana, Jack Pine
Cree, Woodlands *Dermatological Aid* Poultice of inner bark applied to deep cuts. (91:50) **Menominee** *Unspecified* Every part of tree used as a medicine. (128:45) **Ojibwa** *Anticonvulsive* Plant used for fits. *Stimulant* Plant used for fainting. (as *P. baksiana* 112:244) Leaves used as a reviver. (130:379) **Potawatomi** *Dermatological Aid* Pitch from boiled cones used as an ointment for unspecified ailment. *Pulmonary Aid* Leaves used as a fumigant to clear congested lungs. *Stimulant* Leaves used as a fumigant to revive a comatose patient. (131:70)

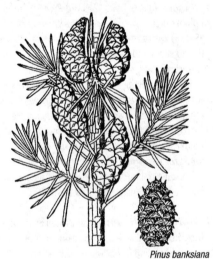

Pinus banksiana

Pinus contorta, Lodgepole Pine
Bella Coola *Antirheumatic* (*External*) Compound containing gum used as poultice on arms for rheumatism. *Dermatological Aid* Gum applied to cuts and chewed gum applied to broken skin.

Heart Medicine Compound containing gum used as poultice on chest for heart trouble. *Tuberculosis Remedy* Decoction of gum taken for consumption. (127:49, 50) **Blackfoot** *Tuberculosis Remedy* Infusion of pitch taken for tubercular coughs. Here is a fine example of the origin and use of a "personal medicine" which was later expanded to include general therapeutic practice. There was once a woman named Last Calf who was riddled with tuberculosis. While she and her husband were camped near a beaver lodge, she noticed the animal's tracks in the mud and left some food for it. The beaver took the gift and returned the favor by appearing to her in a vision. He gave her a cure for tuberculosis. She was to collect the pitch of the lodgepole pine, boil it in water, and drink the infusion while uttering a special song. (The song had no words.) Last Calf's husband was alarmed at this treatment and cautioned her against poisoning but she went ahead and drank the brew. She said she felt as though she were going to die and began vomiting profusely. She drank again with the same result, but the next morning her chest was cleared as never before. (72:73) **Carrier, Northern** *Dermatological Aid* Compound decoction of needle tips taken for paralysis and body sores. *Eye Medicine* Gum painted on eye "to remove white scum" and for snow-blindness. *Orthopedic Aid* Compound decoction of needle tips taken for paralysis, weakness, or sores. *Stimulant* Compound decoction of needle tips taken for constitutional weakness. **Carrier, Southern** *Analgesic* Decoction of new shoots taken for stomach pain. *Gastrointestinal Aid* Decoction of new shoots taken for stomach pain. (127:49, 50) **Eskimo, Alaska** *Cold Remedy* Juice taken for colds. *Cough Medicine* Juice taken for coughs. *Unspecified* Sap used as a medicine. (126:331) **Flathead** *Burn Dressing* Poultice of heated sap and bone marrow used for burns. *Dermatological Aid* Poultice of sap, red axle grease, and Climax chewing tobacco used for boils. (68:52) **Gitksan** *Blood Medicine* Inner bark eaten as a blood purifier and used as a cathartic. *Cathartic* Needles or inner bark eaten or decoction of inner bark taken as a purgative. *Diuretic* Needles eaten or decoction of inner bark taken as a purgative and diuretic. (127:49, 50) *Tonic* Decoction of bark used as a tonic. (61:152) *Tuberculosis Remedy* Decoction of inner bark taken for consumption and gonorrhea. (127:49, 50) *Unspecified* Bark used for medicines. (61:152) *Venereal Aid* Decoction of inner bark taken for gonorrhea and other "serious ailments." (127:49, 50) **Kutenai** *Tuberculosis Remedy* Inner bark eaten for tuberculosis. (68:52) **Kwakiutl** *Cough Medicine* Decoction of buds and pitch taken for coughs. *Gastrointestinal Aid* Decoction of buds and pitch taken for stomachaches. (157:269) **Okanagan-Colville** *Gastrointestinal Aid* Cambium layer eaten for stomach troubles such as ulcers. Decoction of sap taken for ulcers. *Throat Aid* Pitch sucked and juice swallowed for sore throats. (162:28) **Okanagon** *Cold Remedy* Gum used for colds. *Cough Medicine* Gum used for coughs. *Orthopedic Aid* Decoction of bark gum and fat rubbed on the body for muscle and joint aches. *Throat Aid* Gum used for sore throats. (104:40) **Quinault** *Dermatological Aid* Poultice of pitch applied to open sores. *Throat Aid* Buds chewed for sore throats. (65:17) **Salish, Coast** *Dermatological Aid* Sap mixed with deer tallow and used for psoriasis and other diseases. *Misc. Disease Remedy* Sap mixed with deer tallow and used for psoriasis and other diseases. (156:69, 70) **Shuswap** *Cough Medicine* Infusion of inner bark taken for coughs. *Tuberculosis Remedy* Infusion of inner bark taken for tuberculosis. (102:51) **Sikani** *Cough Medicine* Pitch chewed and saliva swallowed for a cough. (127:49, 50) **Thompson** *Analgesic* Salve of boiled sap and grease applied for pains. *Antirheumatic* (*External*) Salve of boiled sap and grease applied for rheumatism. (141:461) *Cold Remedy* Gum used for colds. (104:40) Salve of boiled sap and grease used for colds. (141:461) *Cough Medicine* Gum used for coughs. (104:40) Salve of boiled sap and grease used for coughs. (141:461) *Dermatological Aid* Pitch mixed with bear tallow, rose petals, and red ocher and used as face cream or for blemishes. (161:102) *Disinfectant* Salve of resin with animal fat applied to body as a purifier after sweat bath. (141:504) Pitch used as a sort of "cold cream" with disinfectant properties. *Misc. Disease Remedy* Infusion of twigs with needles attached used for influenza. (161:102) *Orthopedic Aid* Decoction of bark gum and fat rubbed on the body for muscle and joint aches. (104:40) Salve of boiled sap and grease applied for muscle and joint soreness. (141:461) *Pediatric Aid* Pitch mixed with bear tallow, rose

petals, and red ocher and rubbed on the skin of newborn babies. (161:102) *Pulmonary Aid* Salve of boiled sap and grease applied to back and chest for congestion. (141:461) *Throat Aid* Gum used for sore throats. (104:40) Salve of boiled sap and grease used for sore throats. (141:461) **Tlingit** *Venereal Aid* Compound infusion of sprouts and bark taken for syphilis. (as *P. inops* 89:283)

Pinus contorta var. *contorta*, Lodgepole Pine
Haisla & Hanaksiala *Antirheumatic* (*External*) Smoldering twigs applied to arthritic or injured joints for the pain and swelling. (35:178) **Kwakwaka'wakw** *Unspecified* Buds and pitch used medicinally. (35:70) **Nitinaht** *Dermatological Aid* Pitch mixed with melted deer tallow and used as a skin cosmetic. (160:73)

Pinus contorta var. *murrayana*, Murray Lodgepole Pine
Klamath *Eye Medicine* Pitch placed inside the lid for sore eyes. (as *P. murrayana* 37:89)

Pinus echinata, Shortleaf Pine
Choctaw *Anthelmintic* Cold infusion of buds taken for worms. (152:5) **Nanticoke** *Analgesic* "Pellets of tar" considered "beneficial for soreness of the back." (150:55) *Cathartic* "Pellets of tar" used as a cathartic. (150:55, 84) *Orthopedic Aid* "Pellets of tar" considered "beneficial for soreness of the back." (150:55) **Rappahannock** *Dermatological Aid* Compound infusion or decoction of top branches used as wash for swellings. *Emetic* Compound with grated dried bark taken to induce vomiting. *Veterinary Aid* Compound with dried bark fed to dogs with distemper to induce vomiting. (138:27)

Pinus edulis, Twoneedle Pinyon
Apache, Mescalero *Cold Remedy* Needles burned and smoke inhaled for colds. (10:35) **Apache, Western** *Dermatological Aid* Heated pitch applied to the face to remove facial hair. (21:185) **Apache, White Mountain** *Venereal Aid* Leaves chewed for venereal diseases. (113:159) **Havasupai** *Dermatological Aid* Poultice of melted gum applied to cuts. *Veterinary Aid* Poultice of melted gum applied to horses for cuts. (171:205)

Hopi *Dermatological Aid* Poultice of gum used to exclude air from cuts and sores. (174:32) *Disinfectant* Gum smoke used as disinfectant for family of dead person. (174:63) *Tuberculosis Remedy* Plant used for "consumption." (174:35, 63) *Witchcraft Medicine* Gum applied to forehead as a protection from sorcery. (174:63) **Hualapai** *Expectorant* Decoction of inner bark taken as an expectorant tea. *Other* Fresh, white pitch burned to purify the air. (169:35) **Isleta** *Dermatological Aid* Gum mixed with tallow and used as a salve for cuts and open sores. (85:37) **Keres, Western** *Dermatological Aid* Pitch used on open sores. *Gastrointestinal Aid* Infusion of foliage used as an emetic to clean the stomach. (147:60) **Navajo** *Ceremonial Medicine* Needles used in the medicine for the "War Dance." Pitch painted all over the patient in the War Dance. (45:21) *Dermatological Aid* Plant used for cuts and sores. (45:97) Gum with tallow and red clay and used as a salve on open cuts and sores. (45:21) *Emetic* Resin used as an emetic. (76:162) **Navajo, Ramah** *Analgesic* Compound decoction used for headache. *Burn Dressing* Poultice of chewed buds applied to burns. *Ceremonial Medicine* Decoction of wood or needles used as ceremonial emetic. *Cold Remedy* Compound decoction used for colds. Fumes from burning resin inhaled for head colds. *Cough Medicine* Compound decoction used for cough. *Ear Medicine* Pulverized, dried buds used as fumigant for earache. *Emetic* Decoction of wood or needles used as ceremonial emetic. *Febrifuge* Compound decoction used for fever. *Misc. Disease Remedy* Compound decoction used for influenza. *Other* Compound containing inner bark used for injuries. (165:12, 13) **Tewa** *Dermatological Aid* Poultice of gum used to exclude air from cuts and sores. (34:347) Resin applied to cuts and sores to keep out the air. (115:41) **Zuni** *Dermatological Aid* Powdered resin sprinkled in opened abscess or mixed with lard or Vaseline and placed in abscess. Powdered resin used for skin infections. (22:373) *Diaphoretic* Needles chewed and swallowed as a diaphoretic. *Disinfectant* Powdered gum sprinkled on lanced groin swellings as an antiseptic. *Diuretic* Needles eaten and infusion of twigs used as a diuretic and diaphoretic for syphilis. *Venereal Aid* Needles eaten and infusion of twigs used as a diuretic and diaphoretic for syphilis. Powdered

gum sprinkled on scraped syphilitic ulcers. (143:57, 58)

***Pinus elliottii*, Slash Pine**
Seminole *Analgesic* Decoction of wood bits or bark applied externally as an analgesic. (as *P. caribaea* 145:167) *Antirheumatic (External)* Decoction of wood or bark used as a bath for aches and pains. (as *P. caribaea* 145:286) *Dermatological Aid* Decoction of roots and buds used for ball-game sickness: sores, back or limb pains, and hemorrhoids. (as *P. caribaea* 145:269) Decoction of wood or bark used as a bath for sores and cuts. (as *P. caribaea* 145:286) *Hemorrhoid Remedy* and *Orthopedic Aid* Decoction of roots and buds used for ballgame sickness: sores, back or limb pains, and hemorrhoids. (as *P. caribaea* 145:269)

***Pinus flexilis*, Limber Pine**
Navajo, Ramah *Ceremonial Medicine* Plant used as a ceremonial emetic. *Cough Medicine* Plant used as a cough medicine. *Emetic* Plant used as a ceremonial emetic. *Febrifuge* Plant used as medicine for fever. *Hunting Medicine* Plant smoked by hunters for "good luck." (165:13)

***Pinus glabra*, Spruce Pine**
Cherokee *Anthelmintic* Given for worms. *Antidiarrheal* Bark chewed "to check bowels." *Antirheumatic (External)* Oil used to bathe painful joints. *Antirheumatic (Internal)* Syrup taken for chronic rheumatism. *Cold Remedy* Infusion, steam, and oil used in various ways as cold remedy. *Cough Medicine* Syrup taken by pregnant women with cough. *Dermatological Aid* Poultice of tar used on scald head, tetterworm, stone bruises, and ulcers. *Febrifuge* Compound infusion of needles to "break out fever." *Gastrointestinal Aid* Taken for colics and gout. *Gynecological Aid* Compound infusion of needles for "child-bed-fevers." Syrup taken by pregnant women with cough and poultice used for swollen breasts. *Hemorrhoid Remedy* Compound infusion of root taken for piles. *Kidney Aid* Taken for "weak back or kidneys." *Laxative* Taken as a gentle laxative. *Misc. Disease Remedy* Taken for gout, to break out measles, and for complications from mumps. *Orthopedic Aid* Taken for "weak back or kidneys." *Other* Skim turpentine off root decoction and use on deer's skin for drawing plas-

ter. *Respiratory Aid* Compound infusion of needles in apple juice taken by ballplayers "for wind." Syrup taken for "catarrh (ulcer of the lungs)." *Sedative* Given for hysterics. *Stimulant* Compound infusion of root taken as a stimulant. *Tuberculosis Remedy* Tar used for consumption. *Urinary Aid* Syrup used as poultice for swollen testicles caused by mumps. *Venereal Aid* Syrup taken for chronic rheumatism and venereal disease. (66:49)

Pinus lambertiana, Sugar Pine
Kawaiisu *Carminative* Dried sap powder eaten for stomach gas. *Eye Medicine* Powdered sap and milk used as drops for sore eyes and gives infants good eyes. *Laxative* Dried sap powder eaten to loosen the bowels. *Pediatric Aid* Powdered sap and milk used as drops for sore eyes and gives infants good eyes. (180:50) **Mendocino Indian** *Cathartic* Plant used as a cathartic. (33:306) **Miwok** *Eye Medicine* Sugar pine sugar used as a wash for sore or blind eyes. (8:151) **Pomo** *Unspecified* Sugar found in bark wounds ground up, molded into cakes, and used as a medicine. (7:79)

Pinus monophylla, Singleleaf Pinyon
Apache, Western *Dermatological Aid* Heated pitch applied to the face to remove facial hair. (21:185) **Cahuilla** *Dermatological Aid* Pitch used as a face cream by girls to prevent sunburn. (11:102) **Gosiute** *Anthelmintic* Decoction of gum taken for worms or other intestinal parasites. (31:350) **Havasupai** *Dermatological Aid* Poultice of melted gum applied to cuts. *Veterinary Aid* Poultice of melted gum applied to horses for cuts. (171:205) **Hopi** *Dermatological Aid* Poultice of gum used to exclude air from cuts and sores. *Disinfectant* Gum smoke used as disinfectant for family of dead person. *Witchcraft Medicine* Gum applied to forehead as a protection from sorcery. (174:63) **Kawaiisu** *Contraceptive* Cooked pitch taken by women who wanted no more children. *Dermatological Aid* Pitch used as salve on cuts. *Gynecological Aid* Cooked pitch taken by women to stop menstruation. *Pediatric Aid* Cooked pitch given to adolescent girls to keep youthful and increase life span. (180:50) **Paiute** *Analgesic* Poultice of heated resin applied for general muscular soreness. *Antidiarrheal* Decoction of resin or simple or compound pills of resin taken for diarrhea.

Antiemetic Decoction of resin taken for nausea. *Antirheumatic* (*Internal*) Decoction of resin taken for rheumatism. *Cold Remedy* Compound poultice of heated resin applied for chest congestion from colds. Simple or compound decoction of several plant parts taken for colds. *Dermatological Aid* Compound poultice of pitch applied to sores, cuts, swellings, and insect bites. Simple or compound poultice of heated resin applied to draw boils or slivers. *Febrifuge* Decoction of resin taken for fevers. *Gastrointestinal Aid* Decoction of resin taken for indigestion, nausea, or bowel troubles. *Gynecological Aid* Decoction of resin taken as a tonic after childbirth and for general debility. *Misc. Disease Remedy* Decoction of resin taken for influenza. *Orthopedic Aid* Poultice of heated resin applied to treat any general muscular soreness. *Pulmonary Aid* Compound poultice of heated resin applied for chest congestion from colds. Poultice of heated resin applied for pneumonia. *Throat Aid* Resin chewed or pulverized resin applied with swab for sore throat. *Tonic* Decoction of resin taken as a tonic after childbirth and for general debility. *Tuberculosis Remedy* Decoction of resin taken for tuberculosis and influenza. *Venereal Aid* Compound decoction of resin taken for venereal disease. Decoction of resin taken, resin chewed or used as pills for venereal disease. Pulverized resin dusted on syphilitic sores. (155:117, 118) **Shoshoni** *Analgesic* Poultice of heated resin applied for sciatic pains or muscular soreness. Poultice of heated resin used for sciatic pains and general muscular soreness. *Antiemetic* Decoction of resin taken for nausea. *Cold Remedy* Compound decoction of several plant parts taken for colds. Smoke of pitch compound inhaled for colds. *Cough Medicine* Compound decoction of pitch taken for coughs. *Dermatological Aid* Compound decoction of needles used as antiseptic wash for rashes. Compound poultice of pitch applied to sores, cuts, swellings, and insect bites. Poultice of heated resin applied to draw boils or imbedded slivers. *Disinfectant* Compound decoction of needles used as antiseptic wash for measles and other rashes. *Febrifuge* Decoction of resin taken for fevers. *Gastrointestinal Aid* Decoction of resin taken for indigestion, nausea, or bowel troubles. *Kidney Aid* Compound decoction of resin taken for the kidneys. *Misc. Disease Remedy* Compound decoction of needles used as antiseptic wash for measles. Compound decoction of pitch taken for smallpox. *Orthopedic Aid* Poultice of heated resin applied for sciatic pains or muscular soreness. *Poultice* Poultice of heated resin applied for ruptures. *Pulmonary Aid* Poultice of heated resin applied for pneumonia. *Venereal Aid* Decoction of resin taken for venereal disease. *Veterinary Aid* Smoke from root compound inhaled by horses for distemper. (155:117, 118) **Washo** *Cold Remedy* Compound decoction of resin taken for colds. *Venereal Aid* Decoction of needles or wood taken or fresh resin used as pills for gonorrhea. (155:117, 118)

Pinus monticola, Western White Pine
Hoh *Cough Medicine* Gum used for coughs. (114:58) **Kwakiutl** *Cough Medicine* Pitch used for coughs. *Dermatological Aid* Pitch used for sores. *Gastrointestinal Aid* Pitch used for stomachaches. *Reproductive Aid* Gum chewed by women for fertility and by girls to become pregnant without sex. (157:270) **Lummi** *Tuberculosis Remedy* Infusion of bark taken for tuberculosis. (65:16) **Mahuna** *Antirheumatic* (*Internal*) Plant used for rheumatism. (117:60) **Nitinaht** *Dermatological Aid* Pitch mixed with melted deer tallow and used as a skin cosmetic. (160:73) **Quileute** *Cough Medicine* Gum used for coughs. (114:58) **Quinault** *Blood Medicine* Infusion of bark taken to purify the blood. *Gastrointestinal Aid* Infusion of bark taken for stomach disorders. (65:16) **Shuswap** *Tuberculosis Remedy* Bark used for tuberculosis. (102:51) **Skagit** *Antirheumatic* (*External*) Decoction of young shoots used as a soak for rheumatism. *Dermatological Aid* Decoction of bark used for cuts and sores. *Tuberculosis Remedy* Infusion of bark taken for tuberculosis. (65:16) **Thompson** *Panacea* Infusion of boughs used for any kind of illness by old people. *Unspecified* Pitch used medicinally. (161:103)

Pinus ponderosa, Ponderosa Pine
Cheyenne *Dermatological Aid* Pitch used to hold the hair in place. (68:50) Gum used as a salve or ointment for sores and scabby skin. (69:6) **Flathead** *Analgesic* Poultice of pitch and melted animal tallow or lard used for backache. *Antirheumatic* (*External*) Poultice of pitch and melted animal tallow or lard used for rheumatism.

Boughs used in sweat lodges for muscular pain. *Dermatological Aid* Pitch warmed and used for boils and carbuncles. Needles jabbed into the scalp for dandruff. *Gynecological Aid* Needles heated and used for faster delivery of the placenta. (68:50) **Navajo** *Ceremonial Medicine* Pollen used in the "Night Chant" medicine. (45:23) **Navajo, Ramah** *Ceremonial Medicine* Cones with seeds removed used as a ceremonial medicine. Needles used as a ceremonial emetic. *Cough Medicine* Compound decoction of needles taken for bad coughs and fever. *Emetic* Needles used as a ceremonial emetic. *Febrifuge* Compound decoction of needles taken for fever and bad cough. (165:13, 14) **Okanagan-Colville** *Abortifacient* Green buds never chewed by pregnant women because it would cause a miscarriage. *Antihemorrhagic* Decoction of plant tops taken for internal hemorrhaging. *Dermatological Aid* Poultice of pitch applied to boils. *Eye Medicine* Infusion of dried buds used as an eyewash. *Febrifuge* Decoction of plant tops taken for high fevers. *Gastrointestinal Aid* Good medicine for the stomach. *Witchcraft Medicine* Needles spread on the floor of the sweat house to fight off "plhax," witchcraft. (162:29) **Okanagon** *Eye Medicine* Decoction of gum used as an ointment for sore eyes. (104:41) **Paiute** *Dermatological Aid* Poultice of dry, chewed pitch used on boils. (93:40) **Shuswap** *Dermatological Aid* Plant used to remove underarm odors. *Panacea* and *Pediatric Aid* Infusion of plant used as a wash for sick babies. *Stimulant* Used in the sweat house to hit oneself at the hottest point. (102:52) **Thompson** *Antirheu-*

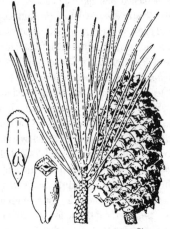

Pinus ponderosa

matic (*External*) Pitch used for aching backs, joints, and limbs. (161:104) *Dermatological Aid* Boiled gum mixed with grease and used as an ointment for sores. (141:466) Decoction of tops used in washing the face and head by girls who want fair and smooth skin. (141:508) Poultice of gum applied to boils, sores, and chapped skin. White gum was used as a poultice with buckskin on boils and chronic sores while reddish gum was used on hard, red sores. The reddish gum was mixed with any kind of lard, such as deer fat, strained, and used on sores. Pitch made into a salve and used for boils or cuts. The pitch ointment was left on the skin for 3 or 4 days. It was said to get quite itchy, but after a while, the pitch was removed with the bandage and then took effect. If the pitch stuck to the skin, it was not ready to remove. *Ear Medicine* Poultice of warmed gum applied to the ear for earache. (161:104) *Eye Medicine* Decoction of gum used as an ointment for sore eyes. (104:41) Boiled gum mixed with grease and used as an ointment for inflamed eyes. (141:466) *Pediatric Aid* Gum used on babies' skin like baby oil. The ointment caused the baby to sleep all the time, just like aspirin. *Sedative* Gum used on babies' skin like baby oil causing them to sleep all the time. (161:104) *Veterinary Aid* Hot gum and animal fat poured on horses' sores or wounds. (141:514)

Pinus quadrifolia, Parry Pinyon
Cahuilla *Dermatological Aid* Pitch used as a face cream by girls to prevent sunburn. (11:102)

Pinus resinosa, Red Pine
Algonquin, Tête-de-Boule *Cold Remedy* Poultice of wetted, inner bark applied to the chest for strong colds. (110:129) **Ojibwa** *Stimulant* Powdered, dried leaves used as a reviver or inhalant. *Unspecified* Bark and cones used medicinally. (130:379) **Ojibwa, South** *Analgesic* Decoction of leaves and bark used as herbal steam for headache and backache. Poultice of crushed leaves and bark applied for headache. (77:198) **Potawatomi** *Stimulant* Leaves used as a fumigant to revive a comatose patient. (131:70)

Pinus rigida, Pitch Pine
Iroquois *Antirheumatic* (*Internal*) Pitch taken for rheumatism. *Burn Dressing* Pitch used for burns. *Dermatological Aid* Compound infusion applied as a poultice to break open boils. Pitch applied to cuts in joints and boils. *Laxative* Pitch taken as a laxative. (73:267) **Shinnecock** *Dermatological Aid* Poultice applied to boils and abscesses. (25:121)

Pinus sabiniana, California Foothill Pine
Costanoan *Antirheumatic* (*Internal*) Pitch chewed for rheumatism. (17:6) **Mendocino Indian** *Burn Dressing* Pitch applied to burns. *Dermatological Aid* Pitch applied to sores. (33:307) **Miwok** *Burn Dressing* Crushed nuts' charcoal applied to burns. *Dermatological Aid* Crushed nuts' charcoal applied to sores and abrasions. (8:149) **Wailaki** *Antirheumatic* (*Internal*) Gum chewed for rheumatism. **Yokia** *Analgesic* Burning twigs and leaves used as sweat bath for rheumatism pain. *Antirheumatic* (*External*) Burning twigs and leaves used as sweat bath for rheumatism pain. *Dermatological Aid* Burning twigs and leaves used as sweat bath for bruises. *Diaphoretic* Burning twigs and leaves used as sweat bath for rheumatism pain and bruises. *Tuberculosis Remedy* Infusion of bark taken for consumption. (33:307)

Pinus strobus, Eastern White Pine
Abnaki *Cough Medicine* Decoction of bark and another plant used for coughs. (121:163) **Algonquin, Tête-de-Boule** *Cold Remedy* Poultice of wetted, inner bark applied to the chest for strong colds. (110:129) **Chippewa** *Dermatological Aid* Compound poultice of trunk of young tree applied to cuts and wounds. (43:352) Poultice of pitch applied to felons and similar inflammations. (59:123) **Delaware, Ontario** *Analgesic* Poultice of pitch applied to draw out the poison and pain from boils. (150:68) *Dermatological Aid* Pitch applied to boils to "draw out the poison and reduce the pain." *Kidney Aid* Infusion of twigs taken for kidney disorders. (150:68, 82) *Pediatric Aid* Powder from decayed plant used on babies "because of its healing properties." (150:68) *Pulmonary Aid* Infusion of twigs taken for pulmonary diseases. (150:68, 82) *Unspecified* Powder from decayed plant used on babies "because of its healing properties." (150:68) **Iroquois** *Antirheumatic* (*Internal*) Decoction of raw bark taken for rheumatism. (73:264) *Blood Medicine* Infusion of young trees

taken as a blood tonic, "don't vomit." (73:266) *Cold Remedy* Compound decoction taken for colds, coughs, and rheumatism. (73:264) Steam from decoction of bark inhaled for head cold. (73:267) *Cough Medicine* Compound decoction or infusion taken for colds, coughs, or rheumatism. (73:264) *Dermatological Aid* Powdered wood used on chafed babies, sores, and improperly healed navels. (73:265) Compound decoction used as wash and compound poultice applied to deep cuts. Decoction of bark used for skin eruptions and scabs. Poultice used for drawing thorns and slivers. Strained, compound poultice used for cuts, bruises, sores, and scabs on face. (73:266) Compound decoction used as salve for cuts and wounds. Decoction of shaved knots, "better than penicillin," used for poison ivy. (73:267) *Dietary Aid* Decoction of knots taken to increase the appetite. *Emetic* Decoction of one knot taken to vomit for regular consumption. (73:265) Decoction of branches taken as a spring emetic. Decoction used as an emetic "when someone dies and you can't forget it." (73:266) *Gastrointestinal Aid* Raw bark taken for the stomach and cramps. (73:265) Compound decoction taken to clean the stomach. *Liver Aid* Compound decoction taken for gall. (73:266) *Misc. Disease Remedy* Raw bark taken to prevent typhoid. (73:265) *Orthopedic Aid* Decoction of leaves used as a wash for nonwalking 2- or 3-year-old infants. (73:264) Compound poultice of leaves bound to broken bones. Poultice of gum applied to broken coccyx. Raw bark taken for rheumatism and stiff limbs. (73:265) *Other* Compound used as

a sugar medicine. (73:267) *Panacea* Leaves burned in spring and fall, smoke used to fill the house and prevent all sickness. (73:265) *Pediatric Aid* Decoction of leaves used as a wash for non-walking 2- or 3-year-old infants. (73:264) Powdered wood used on chafed babies, sores, and improperly healed navels. (73:265) *Psychological Aid* Decoction used as an emetic "when someone dies and your can't forget it." (73:266) *Pulmonary Aid* Compound decoction of bark taken by fat people for breathing difficulties. (73:264) Compound decoction taken for shortness of wind. (73:266) Salve applied to chest for chest cold. *Throat Aid* Taken for infections and sore throats. (73:267) *Tuberculosis Remedy* Decoction of knots taken for consumption. Decoction of one knot taken to vomit for regular consumption. (73:265) Decoction of twigs taken for scrofula. (73:267) *Venereal Aid* Compound decoction used as a salve on dry, cracked, venereal diseased penis. (73:265) *Veterinary Aid* Decoction of twigs used for boils on horses' necks. (73:267) *Witchcraft Medicine* Burning branch smoke drove away ghosts from the house of returning people. Smoke from plant used as a wash for a person who has seen a dead person. (73:266) **Menominee** *Analgesic* Infusion of bark, an important medicine, taken for chest pain. (128:46) *Dermatological Aid* Poultice of pounded inner bark applied to sores. (44:132) Poultice of pounded bark applied to wounds, sores, or ulcers. (128:46) **Micmac** *Cold Remedy* Bark, leaves, and stems used for colds. *Cough Medicine* Bark, leaves, and stems used for coughs. *Dermatological Aid* Bark used for wounds and sap used for hemorrhaging. (32:59) Boiled inner bark used for sores and swellings. (133:317) *Hemostat* Sap used for hemorrhaging. *Kidney Aid* Plant parts used for kidney trouble. *Misc. Disease Remedy* Bark, leaves, and stems used for grippe. Inner bark, bark, and leaves used for scurvy. (32:59) **Mohegan** *Analgesic* Poultice of sap or gum applied for boil and abscess pains. (151:74) *Cold Remedy* Cold infusion of bark taken for colds. (149:264) Bark, sap, or gum used for coughs, colds, and boils. (151:130) *Cough Medicine* Infusion of bark used for stubborn cough and pitch chewed for cough. (25:121) Infusion of bark taken for coughs and colds. (149:269) Infusion of dried inner bark used as a cough remedy. *Dermatological Aid* Sap or gum

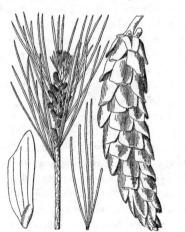

Pinus strobus

applied to boil or abscess pains. (151:74, 130) **Montagnais** *Cold Remedy* Boiled gum taken for colds. *Throat Aid* Boiled gum taken for sore throats. *Tuberculosis Remedy* Boiled gum taken for consumption. (133:315) **Ojibwa** *Stimulant* Dried leaves used as a reviver or inhalant. (130: 379) *Unspecified* Plant used for medicinal purposes. (112:244) Bark and cones used medicinally. (130:379) **Ojibwa, South** *Analgesic* Boiled, crushed leaves used as herbal steam for headache and backache. Poultice of crushed leaves applied for headaches. *Herbal Steam* Boiled, crushed leaves used as herbal steam for headache and backache. (77:198) **Potawatomi** *Dermatological Aid* Pitch or resin of wood and bark used as the base for a salve. (131:70) **Shinnecock** *Cough Medicine* Infusion of bark used for stubborn cough and pitch chewed for cough. (25:121)

Pinus virginiana, Virginia Pine
Cherokee *Anthelmintic* Given for worms. *Antidiarrheal* Bark chewed "to check bowels." *Antirheumatic* (*External*) Oil used to bathe painful joints. *Antirheumatic* (*Internal*) Syrup taken for chronic rheumatism. *Ceremonial Medicine* Branches burned and ashes thrown on hearth fire after a death in the home. *Cold Remedy* Infusion, steam, and oil used in various ways as cold remedy. *Cough Medicine* Syrup taken by pregnant women with cough. *Dermatological Aid* Poultice of tar used on scald head, tetterworm, stone bruises, and ulcers. *Febrifuge* Compound infusion of needles used to "break out fever." *Gastrointestinal Aid* Taken for colics and gout. *Gynecological Aid* Compound infusion of needles used for "childbed-fevers." Syrup taken by pregnant women with cough and poultice used for swollen breasts. *Hemorrhoid Remedy* Compound infusion of root taken for piles. *Kidney Aid* Taken for "weak back or kidneys." *Laxative* Taken as a gentle laxative. *Misc. Disease Remedy* Taken for gout, to break out measles, and for complications from mumps. *Orthopedic Aid* Taken for "weak back or kidneys." *Other* Skim turpentine off root decoction and use on deer's skin for drawing plaster. *Respiratory Aid* Compound infusion of needles in apple juice taken by ballplayers "for wind." Syrup taken for "catarrh (ulcer of the lungs)." *Sedative* Given for hysterics. *Stimulant* Compound infusion of root taken as a

stimulant. *Tuberculosis Remedy* Tar used for consumption. *Urinary Aid* Syrup used as poultice for swollen testicles caused by mumps. *Venereal Aid* Syrup taken for chronic rheumatism and venereal disease. (66:49) **Choctaw** *Anthelmintic* Infusion of buds taken for worms. (as *P. mitis* 20:24) **Rappahannock** *Kidney Aid* Rolled, hardened sap used as pills and taken for kidney trouble. (138:27)

Piper methysticum, Kava
Hawaiian *Analgesic* Roots chewed for sharp, blinding headaches. *Cold Remedy* Plant and other plants pounded, squeezed, the resulting juice heated and taken for chills and hard colds. *Dermatological Aid* and *Eye Medicine* Roots chewed to prevent contagious diseases of all sorts, especially skin diseases and eye troubles. *Gastrointestinal Aid* Plant ashes and other ashes rubbed on children for a disorderly stomach. *Gynecological Aid* Plant pieces and other plants mixed with water and taken for weaknesses arising from virginity. Plant pieces and other plants mixed with coconut milk and taken for displacement of the womb. *Misc. Disease Remedy* Roots chewed to prevent contagious diseases of all sorts, especially skin diseases and eye troubles. *Oral Aid* Plant ashes and other ashes rubbed on children for thick white coatings on the tongue. *Pediatric Aid* Buds chewed by children for general debility. Plant ashes and other ashes rubbed on children with general weakness of the body, rubbed on children for a disorderly stomach, and for thick white coatings on the tongue. *Pulmonary Aid* Decoction of whole plant and other plants taken for lung and kindred troubles. *Sedative* Decoction of plant and other plants taken for sleeplessness. *Stimulant* Buds chewed by children for general debility. *Strengthener* Plant ashes and other ashes rubbed on children with general weakness of the body. *Urinary Aid* Infusion of plant, other plants, and coconut milk taken for difficulty in passing urine. (2:17)

Piper nigrum, Black Pepper
Cherokee *Dermatological Aid* Used as an astringent. *Stimulant* Used as a stimulus. (66:48)

Piperia sp.
Mahuna *Dermatological Aid* Plant used for black widow and scorpion bites. *Eye Medicine* Plant

used for trachoma. *Snakebite Remedy* Plant used for rattlesnake bites. (117:34)

Pipturus sp., Mamaki
Hawaiian *Pediatric Aid* Seeds eaten by infants for general debility of the body. *Strengthener* Seeds eaten by expectant mothers for general debility of the body. Seeds eaten by infants for general debility of the body. (2:71)

Pittosporum sp., Ho-a-wa
Hawaiian *Tuberculosis Remedy* Fruit and other plants pounded and resulting liquid used as a wash for scrofulous neck swellings. (2:44)

Pityopsis graminifolia var. graminifolia, Narrowleaf Silkgrass
Choctaw *Oral Aid* Burned plant ashes used for mouth sores. (as *Chrysopsis graminea* 20:24) Plant ashes used as powder for mouth sores. (as *Chrysopsis graminifolia* 152:60) **Seminole** *Cold Remedy* Infusion of plant taken for colds. *Febrifuge* Infusion of plant taken for fevers. (as *Chrysopsis graminifolia* 145:283)

Plagiomnium insigne, Badge Mnium
Bella Coola *Antirheumatic* (*External*) Poultice of crushed "leaves" applied to infections and swellings. *Blood Medicine* Poultice of "leaves" used for blood blisters. *Breast Treatment* Poultice of "leaves" used for breast abscesses in women. *Dermatological Aid* Poultice of "leaves" used for boils. (158:196) **Oweekeno** *Antirheumatic* (*External*) Heated or cooled poultice of boiled plant and Sitka spruce pitch applied to sore and swollen joints. *Dermatological Aid* Poultice of boiled plant and Sitka spruce pitch applied to cuts for the swelling. *Internal Medicine* Plant dried, chewed for the juice, and swallowed for internal ailments. (35:52)

Plagiomnium juniperinum, Hair Cap Moss
Heiltzuk *Antirheumatic* (*External*) Plant used as an anti-swelling medicine. (35:53)

Plantago aristata, Largebracted Plantain
Cherokee *Analgesic* Poultice of leaf applied for headache. *Antidiarrheal* Infusion of root taken for dysentery and infusion given to check babies' bowels. *Antidote* Infusion used for poisonous bites and

stings. *Burn Dressing* Poultice of wilted or scalded leaf applied to burns. *Dermatological Aid* Poultice used for blisters, ulcers, insect stings, and infusion used orally and as wash. *Eye Medicine* Juice used for sore eyes. *Gastrointestinal Aid* Taken for bowel complaints. *Gynecological Aid* Infusion taken to "check discharge" and used as a douche. *Orthopedic Aid* Compound infusion of leaf given to strengthen a child learning to walk. *Pediatric Aid* Compound infusion of leaf given to strengthen a child learning to walk. Infusion given to check babies' bowels. *Snakebite Remedy* Infusion used for snakebites. *Urinary Aid* Taken for "bloody urine." (66:50)

Plantago australis ssp. hirtella, Mexican Plantain
Tolowa *Dermatological Aid* Poultice of leaves applied to cuts and boils. **Yurok** *Dermatological Aid* Poultice of steamed leaves applied to boils. (as *P. hirtella* 5:45)

Plantago cordata, Heartleaf Plantain
Houma *Burn Dressing* and *Dermatological Aid* Poultice of raw leaves and oil or grease used on cuts, sores, burns, and boils. (135:62)

Plantago lanceolata, Narrowleaf Plantain
Cherokee *Analgesic* Poultice of leaf applied for headache. *Antidiarrheal* Infusion of root taken for dysentery and infusion given to check babies' bowels. *Antidote* Infusion used for poisonous bites, stings, and snakebites. *Burn Dressing* Poultice of wilted or scalded leaf applied to burns. *Dermatological Aid* Poultice used for blisters, ulcers, insect stings, and infusion used orally and as wash. *Eye Medicine* Juice used for sore eyes. *Gastrointestinal Aid* Taken for bowel complaints. *Gynecological Aid* Infusion taken to "check discharge" and used as a douche. *Orthopedic Aid* Compound infusion of leaf given to strengthen a child learning to walk. *Pediatric Aid* Compound infusion of leaf given to strengthen a child learning to walk. Infusion given to check babies' bowels. *Snakebite Remedy* Infusion used for snakebites. *Urinary Aid* Taken for "bloody urine." (66:50) **Kawaiisu** *Ear Medicine* Infusion of leaves put in the ear for earaches. (180:52)

Plantago macrocarpa, Seashore Plantain
Aleut *Tonic* Decoction of root taken as a tonic.
(6:428)

Plantago major, Common Plantain
Abnaki *Analgesic* Poultice of leaves applied for
pain. *Antirheumatic* (*External*) Poultice of leaves
applied to the foot for rheumatism or swellings.
(121:172) **Algonquin**, **Quebec** *Poultice* Leaves
used as poultices. (14:231) **Algonquin**, **Tête-de-
Boule** *Burn Dressing* Poultice of leaves applied to
burns. *Dermatological Aid* Poultice of leaves applied to wounds and contusions. (110:130) **Carrier** *Cough Medicine* Decoction of plant taken for
coughs. *Gastrointestinal Aid* Decoction of plant
taken for stomach problems. *Laxative* Decoction
of plant taken as a laxative. (26:86) **Cherokee**
Analgesic Poultice of leaf applied for headache.
Antidiarrheal Infusion of root taken for dysentery
and infusion given to check babies' bowels. *Antidote* Infusion used for poisonous bites, stings, and
snakebites. *Burn Dressing* Poultice of wilted or
scalded leaf applied to burns. *Dermatological Aid*
Poultice used for blisters, ulcers, insect stings, and
infusion used orally and as wash. *Eye Medicine*
Juice used for sore eyes. *Gastrointestinal Aid*
Taken for bowel complaints. *Gynecological Aid*
Infusion taken to "check discharge" and used as
a douche. *Orthopedic Aid* Compound infusion of
leaf given to strengthen a child learning to walk.
Pediatric Aid Compound infusion of leaf given to
strengthen a child learning to walk. Infusion given
to check babies' bowels. *Snakebite Remedy* Infusion used for snakebites. *Urinary Aid* Taken for
"bloody urine." (66:50) **Chippewa** *Antirheumatic* (*External*) Poultice of chopped, fresh leaves applied for rheumatism. (43:362) *Dermatological
Aid* Simple or compound poultice of chopped root
or fresh leaf used for inflammations. (43:348)
Snakebite Remedy Poultice of chopped, fresh
leaves, and root applied to snakebites. (43:353)
Costanoan *Febrifuge* Decoction of roots taken for
fever. *Laxative* Decoction of roots taken for constipation. (17:11) **Delaware** *Gynecological Aid* Plant
combined with other plant parts and used for female diseases. *Unspecified* Poultice of crushed
leaves used medicinally. (151:37) **Delaware**,
Oklahoma *Gynecological Aid* Compound containing plant used for "female diseases." *Unspecified*

Poultice of crushed leaves used for unspecified ailments. (150:31, 82) **Delaware**, **Ontario** *Dermatological Aid* Poultice of crushed leaves applied to
bruises. (150:66, 82) **Hesquiat** *Dermatological
Aid* Poultice of leaves used for drawing out the pus
from sores, cuts, and infections. (159:70) **Iroquois** *Blood Medicine* Infusion of roots with other
roots used to purify the blood. (118:59) *Dermatological Aid* Poultice of leaves applied to sores. Poultice of boiled flower stems applied to abscesses.
Gastrointestinal Aid Infusion of seeds taken to
facilitate digestion and reduce intestinal inflammation. *Gynecological Aid* Infusion of seeds taken
to regulate and shorten menses. (119:98) *Respiratory Aid* Infusion of roots with other roots used for
difficult breathing caused by lower chest pains.
(118:59) **Isleta** *Gastrointestinal Aid* Infusion of
leaves used as a stomach tonic. (85:38) **Kawaiisu**
Ear Medicine Infusion of leaves put in the ear for
earaches. (180:52) **Keres**, **Western** *Blood Medicine* Roots used for blood medicine. (147:61)
Kwakiutl *Dermatological Aid* Poultice of leaves
applied to draw blisters on sores and swellings.
(157:287) **Mahuna** *Dermatological Aid* Plant
used to dislodge and draw out poisonous thorns
and splinters. (117:16) **Meskwaki** *Burn Dressing*
Infusion of leaves used for burns. *Dermatological
Aid* Fresh leaf used for swellings. *Diuretic* Infusion
of leaves taken for bowel troubles and as a urinary.
Gastrointestinal Aid Infusion of leaves used for
bowel troubles and as a urinary. (129:234, 235)
Mohegan *Burn Dressing* Leaves bound over burns.
Dermatological Aid Leaves bound over bruises.

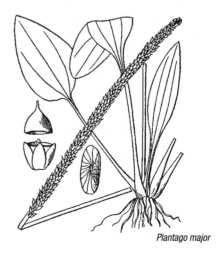

Plantago major

(149:266) Poultice of fresh leaves applied to insect bites, cuts, or swellings. (151:74, 130) *Snakebite Remedy* Leaves bound over snakebites to draw out poison. (149:266) Poultice of fresh leaves applied to snake and insect bites to remove poison. (151:74) **Navajo, Ramah** *Disinfectant* Cold infusion of plant taken for "lightning infection." *Panacea* Root used as a "life medicine." (165:45) **Nitinaht** *Dermatological Aid* Poultice of moist leaves placed on cuts, boils, and open sores. *Disinfectant* Poultice of moist leaves placed on infections and boils. *Gastrointestinal Aid* Leaves chewed and swallowed for stomach ulcers. (160:115) **Ojibwa** *Burn Dressing* Poultice of soaked leaves bound on burns, scalds, and snakebites. *Dermatological Aid* Poultice of soaked leaves bound on bruises, sprains, sores, and bee stings. *Orthopedic Aid* Poultice of soaked leaves bound on bruises, sprains, or sores. *Snakebite Remedy* Poultice of soaked leaves bound on snakebites. (130:380, 381) *Unspecified* Poultice of pounded leaves applied for medicinal purposes. (4:2317) **Okanagan-Colville** *Dermatological Aid* Poultice of mashed leaves applied to kill the germs of sores. (162:111) **Paiute** *Cold Remedy* Decoction of root taken for colds. *Dermatological Aid* Poultice of leaves bound onto cuts and wounds to promote healing without scars. *Pulmonary Aid* Decoction of root taken for pneumonia. (155:119, 120) **Ponca** *Dermatological Aid* Hot leaves applied to foot to draw out thorns or splinters. (58:115) **Potawatomi** *Dermatological Aid* Poultice of heated leaf bound on swellings and inflammations. *Throat Aid* Decoction of root taken to lubricate throat for removal of lodged bone. (131:71, 72) **Rappahannock** *Febrifuge* Poultice of ground leaves used for fever. (138:25) **Shinnecock** *Dermatological Aid* Poultice of pounded leaves applied to draw out inflammation from sore spots. *Eye Medicine* Infusion of leaves used as a wash for sore eyes. (25:119) **Shoshoni** *Antirheumatic (External)* Compound poultice of leaves applied to wounds, swellings, and rheumatism. (155:119, 120) *Dermatological Aid* Poultice and infusion of whole plant used for battle bruises. Poultice of raw leaves with wild clematis applied to wounds. (98:43) Compound poultice of leaves applied for wounds, bruises, swellings, and boils. Poultice of mashed leaves applied to dropsical swellings and infections. *Disinfectant* Poultice of mashed leaves

applied to dropsical swellings and infections. *Gastrointestinal Aid* Decoction of root taken for stomach trouble. *Kidney Aid* Poultice of mashed leaves applied to dropsical swellings and infections. (155:119, 120) **Shuswap** *Dermatological Aid* Poultice of mashed plants applied to sores. *Diaphoretic* Leaf rubbed on the body to produce sweating. (102:64) **Thompson** *Dermatological Aid* Poultice of chewed leaves used for sores and carbuncles. *Hemorrhoid Remedy* Poultice of chewed leaves used for hemorrhoids. (161:236) **Yurok** *Dermatological Aid* Poultice of steamed leaves applied to boils. (5:46)

***Plantago ovata*, Desert Indianwheat**
Pima *Antidiarrheal* Cold infusion of seeds taken for diarrhea. (as *P. fastigiata* 38:96)

***Plantago patagonica*, Woolly Plantain**
Hopi *Psychological Aid* Plant given to a person to make him more agreeable. (as *P. purshii* 34:349) Used to make a person more agreeable. (as *P. purshii* 174:37) Plant given to a person "to make him more agreeable." (as *P. purshii* 174:92) **Keres, Western** *Analgesic* Infusion of plant used for headaches. *Antidiarrheal* Infusion of plant used for diarrhea. (as *P. purshii* 147:61) **Navajo** *Gastrointestinal Aid*, *Laxative*, and *Pediatric Aid* Infusion of seeds given to babies when they "spoil" (colic or constipation). (as *P. purshii* 76:154) **Navajo, Ramah** *Dietary Aid* Cold infusion of plant parts taken to reduce appetite and prevent obesity. (as *P. purshii* 165:45) **Okanagan-Colville** *Dermatological Aid* Poultice of mashed leaves applied to sores. (162:111) **Zuni** *Antidiarrheal* Infusion of whole plant taken three times a day for bloody diarrhea. (22:377)

***Plantago rugelii* var. *asperula*, Blackseed Plantain**
Menominee *Burn Dressing* Poultice of fresh leaves applied to burn or any inflammation. (44:132) *Dermatological Aid* Poultice of fresh leaves applied to any inflammation. (44:131) Poultice of specific sides of leaf applied to swellings and other ailments. (128:46, 47)

***Platanthera ciliaris*, Yellow Fringed Orchid**
Cherokee *Analgesic* Cold infusion used for head-

ache. *Antidiarrheal* Infusion of root taken every hour for "flux." (as *Habenaria ciliaris* 66:47) **Seminole** *Snakebite Remedy* Roots used for snakebites. (as *Habenaria ciliaris* 145:297)

Platanthera dilatata var. *dilatata*, Scent-bottle
Micmac *Urinary Aid* Root juice taken with water for gravel. (as *Havernaria dilatata* 133:317) **Shuswap** *Poison* Leaves considered poisonous. (as *Habenaria dilatata* 102:55)

Platanthera leucostachys, Bog Orchid
Thompson *Analgesic* Plant used in the sweat bath for rheumatism and various joint and muscle aches. *Antirheumatic* (*External*) Heated decoction of plant used as a wash for rheumatism. Plant used in the sweat bath for rheumatism and various joint and muscle aches. (as *Habenaria leucostachys* 141:467) *Disinfectant* Decoction of whole plant used as a wash after the purifying sweat bath. (as *Habenaria leucostachys* 141:504) *Herbal Steam* Plant used in the sweat bath for rheumatism and various joint and muscle aches. Plant steamed in the sweat bath for rheumatism and other joint and muscle aches. (as *Habenaria leucostachys* 141:467) *Hunting Medicine* Plant used to wash guns "to insure good luck when hunting." *Love Medicine* Plant used in wash by women "hoping to gain a mate and have success in love." (as *Habenaria leucostachys* 141:506) *Orthopedic Aid* Plant used in the sweat bath for sprains, stiff and aching muscles and joints. (as *Habenaria leucostachys* 141:467)

Platanthera ×*media*, Bog Orchid
Potawatomi *Love Medicine* Women rubbed this plant on their cheek as a love charm to enable them to secure a good husband. (as *Habenaria dilatata* var. *media* 131:121)

Platanthera orbiculata var. *orbiculata*, Large Roundleaved Orchid
Iroquois *Dermatological Aid* Poultice of leaves applied to sores caused by scrofula and cuts. *Tuberculosis Remedy* Poultice of leaves bound to sore caused by scrofula. (as *Habenaria orbiculata* 73:289) **Montagnais** *Dermatological Aid* Poultice of leaves applied to blisters on hands or feet. (as *Habenaria orbiculata* 133:313)

Platanthera psycodes, Lesser Purple Fringed Orchid
Iroquois *Analgesic* Infusion of single root and flowers given to young children for cramps. (as *Habenaria psycodes* 73:289) *Gynecological Aid* Infusion of root taken as a parturition medicine. *Panacea* Compound infusion taken or placed on injured part, a "Little Water Medicine." (as *Habenaria psycodes* 73:290) *Pediatric Aid* Infusion of single root and flowers given to young children for cramps. (as *Habenaria psycodes* 73:289)

Platanthera stricta, Modoc Bog Orchid
Kwakiutl *Love Medicine* Compound with plant used as a love charm. (as *Habenaria saccata* 157:275)

Platanus occidentalis, American Sycamore
Cherokee *Abortifacient* Compound decoction taken "for menstrual period." *Antidiarrheal* Taken for dysentery. (66:58) Infusion of inner bark taken for dysentery. (152:26) *Cathartic* Taken as a purgative. (66:58) Decoction of roots taken by women during menses as a cathartic. (152:26) *Cough Medicine* Infusion of inner bark taken for cough. *Dermatological Aid* Bark ooze used as wash for infected sores and infusion given for infant rash. *Emetic* Taken as an emetic. (66:58) Decoction of roots taken by women during menses as an emetic. (152:26) *Gastrointestinal Aid* Compound used in steam bath for indigestion or biliousness. *Gynecological Aid* Compound decoction used to aid in expelling afterbirth. (66:58) Decoction of roots taken by women during menses as an emetic and cathartic. (152:26) *Misc. Disease Remedy* Infusion of inner bark taken for measles. *Other* Compound infusion of bark taken for "bad disease." *Pediatric Aid* Infusion given for infant rash. *Urinary Aid* Taken for milky urine. (66:58) Infusion of inner barks taken for difficult urination with yellow discharge. (152:26) **Creek** *Tuberculosis Remedy* Bark used in medicine taken for pulmonary tuberculosis. (148:659) Decoction of bark taken for pulmonary tuberculosis. (152:26) **Delaware** *Cold Remedy* Infusion of three chips from east side of honey locust and sycamore trees used as drinks for colds.

Throat Aid Infusion of bark mixed with honey locust bark and used as a gargle for hoarseness and sore throat. (151:30) **Delaware, Oklahoma** *Cold Remedy* Compound infusion of bark taken for colds. (as *P. occidentalis* 150:25) *Throat Aid* Compound infusion of bark gargled for hoarseness and sore throat. (as *P. occidentalis* 150:25, 78) **Iroquois** *Antirheumatic* (*External*) Compound infusion of bark and roots used as foot soak for rheumatism. *Dermatological Aid* Compound decoction used for skin eruptions, scabs, and eczema. (73:348) **Mahuna** *Gastrointestinal Aid* Plant used for internal ulcers. *Respiratory Aid* Plant used for catarrh. (117:24) **Meskwaki** *Analgesic* Bark eaten for internal pains. *Blood Medicine* Infusion of bark taken as a blood purifier and used for colds. *Cold Remedy* Infusion of bark used for colds and to purify the blood. *Dermatological Aid* Compound containing bark used on knife or ax wounds. *Dietary Aid* Bark eaten to become fat. *Hemostat* Bark used for hemorrhages and lung troubles. *Misc. Disease Remedy* Infusion of bark used as wash to dry smallpox pustules and prevent scars. *Pulmonary Aid* Bark used for lung troubles and hemorrhages. (129:235)

Platanus racemosa, California Sycamore **Costanoan** *Panacea* Infusion of plant used as a general remedy. (17:20) **Diegueño** *Blood Medicine* Decoction of bark used as a tonic for the blood. (74:217) *Respiratory Aid* Decoction of bark taken for a week for asthma. (70:30) **Kawaiisu** *Unspecified* Infusion of bark taken for the relief of some indisposition. Decoction of small bark pieces taken for an unrecorded indisposition. (180:53)

Pleomele aurea, Golden Hala Pepe **Hawaiian** *Febrifuge* Buds, bark, root bark, and other plants pounded and resulting liquid taken for chills and high fever. *Pulmonary Aid* Leaves, bark, root bark, and other plants pounded and resulting liquid taken for lung troubles. *Respiratory Aid* Leaves, bark, root bark, and other plants pounded and resulting liquid taken for asthma. (as *Dracaena aurea* 2:42)

Pleopeltis polypodioides* ssp. *polypodioides, Resurrection Fern **Houma** *Analgesic* Decoction of fronds taken for

headaches. *Oral Aid* Cold decoction of fronds used as a wash for babies' sore mouth or thrush. Decoction of fronds used for bleeding gums. *Pediatric Aid* Cold decoction of fronds used as a wash for babies' sore mouth or thrush. *Vertigo Medicine* Decoction of fronds taken for dizziness. (as *Marginaria polypodioides* 135:55)

Pluchea foetida, Stinking Camphorweed **Choctaw** *Febrifuge* Decoction of leaves taken "during attacks of fever." (20:23) Decoction of leaves taken for fevers. (152:63)

Pluchea sericea, Arrow Weed **Havasupai** *Throat Aid* Leaves chewed or boiled for throat irritations. (139:285) **Paiute** *Antidiarrheal* Decoction of root taken for diarrhea, especially bloody diarrhea. *Gastrointestinal Aid* Raw root chewed or decoction of root taken for indigestion. (155:120) **Pima** *Antidiarrheal* Decoction of roots taken for diarrhea. (38:105) *Dermatological Aid* Infusion of root bark used as a wash for the face and sore eyes. (as *P. borealis* 123:79) *Eye Medicine* Decoction of roots used for sore eyes. (38:105) Infusion of bark used as a wash for the face and sore eyes. (as *P. borealis* 123:79) *Gastrointestinal Aid* Decoction of roots taken for stomachaches. *Pediatric Aid* and *Sedative* Poultice of roots applied to soothe nervous child that cried while sleeping. *Veterinary Aid* Poultice of chewed roots applied to snakebites on horses. (38:105)

Plumbago zeylanica, Wild Leadwort **Hawaiian** *Antirheumatic* (*External*) Poultice of pounded bark, leaves, and roots applied to swollen parts of the body. *Dermatological Aid* Leaves, stems, other plant parts, and fruit juice made into a paste and applied to sores. (as *Chunbago zelanica* 2:25)

Poa fendleriana, Mutton Grass **Hopi** *Ceremonial Medicine* Pollen used in prayer medicine. (34:350)

Podophyllum peltatum, May Apple **Cherokee** *Anthelmintic* Root used as anthelmintic. *Antirheumatic* (*Internal*) Root soaked in whisky and taken for rheumatism and as a purgative. *Cathartic* Boiled root eaten as a purgative.

(66:44) Decoction of root boiled into a syrup, made into pills, and given as a purgative. (177:74) *Dermatological Aid* Powdered root used on ulcers and sores. *Ear Medicine* "Drop of juice of fresh root" put in ear for deafness. (66:44) Juice of fresh root dropped into the ear for deafness. (177:74) *Laxative* Powdered root eaten "to correct constipation." *Poison* Root joints considered poisonous. (66:44) **Delaware** *Laxative* Roots used to make a laxative. *Tonic* Roots used to make a spring tonic. (151:38) **Delaware, Oklahoma** *Laxative* Root used to make a laxative. *Love Medicine* Plant used as a love charm. *Tonic* Root used to make a spring tonic. (150:32, 78) **Iroquois** *Cathartic* Cold infusion of smashed root taken or raw root chewed for a strong physic. (73:331) *Ceremonial Medicine* Decoction of leaves with other plants used as medicine to soak corn seeds before planting. (170:19) *Dermatological Aid* Compound decoction of roots taken for boils. *Laxative* Decoction or infusion of roots taken or raw root chewed as a laxative. *Poison* Root considered poisonous. *Strengthener* Compound decoction of plants taken to increase strength. (73:331) *Veterinary Aid* Seeds and pulp of fruit placed in cut of atrophied shoulder muscle of horse. (73:330) Decoction of plant used as a laxative for horses bound up on green grass. (73:331) **Meskwaki** *Antirheumatic (Internal)* Root used for rheumatism and as a physic. *Cathartic* Compound containing root used as a physic and for rheumatism. *Emetic* Decoction of root taken as an emetic. (129:206)

Pogogyne douglasii ssp. *parviflora*, Douglas's Mesamint
Concow *Analgesic* and *Gastrointestinal Aid* Leaves used as a counterirritant for stomach and bowel pains. (as *P. parviflora* 33:384)

Polemonium elegans, Elegant Jacobsladder
Thompson *Dermatological Aid* Compound decoction containing several species used as a wash for the head and hair. (141:467)

Polemonium pulcherrimum ssp. *lindleyi*, Lindley's Polemonium
Thompson *Dermatological Aid* Decoction of plant used as a wash for the head and hair. (as *P. humile* 141:467)

Polemonium reptans, Greek Valerian
Meskwaki *Cathartic* Compound containing root used as powerful physic. *Diuretic* Compound containing root used as powerful urinary. (129:235, 236)

Poliomintha incana, Hoary Rosemarymint
Comanche *Adjuvant* Leaves chewed by medicine woman retaining other drugs in her mouth to sweeten the taste. Used to increase the efficacy of other medicine plants. (as *Poliomentha ineana* 84:7) **Hopi** *Antirheumatic (External)* Plant used for rheumatism. *Ear Medicine* Plant used for ear trouble. (34:351) **Navajo, Kayenta** *Dermatological Aid* Plant used for sores. (179:41) **Tewa** *Antirheumatic (External)* Plant used for rheumatism. *Ear Medicine* Plant used for ear trouble. (34:351)

Polygala alba, White Milkwort
Sioux *Ear Medicine* Decoction of root used for earache. (15:18)

Polygala cornuta, Sierran Milkwort
Miwok *Analgesic* Decoction used for pains. *Cold Remedy* Decoction used for colds. *Cough Medicine* Decoction used for coughs. *Emetic* Decoction used as an emetic. (8:172)

Polygala lutea, Orange Milkwort
Choctaw *Dermatological Aid* Poultice of dried blossoms mixed with water applied to swellings. (20:24) Poultice of dried blossoms applied to swellings. (152:35) **Seminole** *Antirheumatic (External)*, *Blood Medicine*, and *Heart Medicine* Plant used for sapiyi sickness: heart palpitations, yellow skin, body swelling, and short breath. (145:264) *Other* Complex infusion of whole plant taken for chronic conditions. (145:272) *Respiratory Aid* Plant used for sapiyi sickness: heart palpitations, yellow skin, body swelling, and short breath. (145:264)

Polygala paucifolia, Gaywings
Iroquois *Dermatological Aid* Infusion of plant taken and poultice of leaves applied to abscesses on limbs. (73:368) Decoction of plant used as a wash for boils and syphilitic sores. (73:369) *Orthopedic Aid* Compound poultice of plants applied to sore legs. (73:368) *Pediatric Aid* and *Venereal*

Aid Decoction of plant used as a wash for babies with syphilitic sores. (73:369)

Polygala polygama, Racemed Milkwort
Montagnais *Cough Medicine* Decoction of plant used as a cough medicine. (133:314)

Polygala rugelii, Yellow Milkwort
Seminole *Antirheumatic (External)*, *Blood Medicine*, *Heart Medicine*, and *Respiratory Aid* Plant used for sapiyi sickness: heart palpitations, yellow skin, body swelling, and short breath. (145:264) *Snakebite Remedy* Infusion of plant taken for snakebites. (145:297)

Polygala senega, Seneca Snakeroot
Blackfoot *Respiratory Aid* Decoction of roots used for respiratory diseases. (82:42) **Cherokee** *Abortifacient* Used as an emmenagogue. *Antirheumatic (Internal)* Used for rheumatism. *Cathartic* Infusion of root or root powder taken as a cathartic. *Cold Remedy* Used for colds. *Diaphoretic* Used as a sudorific. *Diuretic* Used as a diuretic and cathartic. *Expectorant* Infusion of root or root powder taken as an expectorant. *Kidney Aid* Used for "dropsy" and infusion of root or root powder used as an expectorant. *Other* Used for "inflammatory complaints" and swellings. *Pulmonary Aid* Used for pleurisy and croup. *Snakebite Remedy* Root chewed, "sufficient quantity" swallowed, and wound poulticed with the rest. (66:55) **Chippewa** *Anticonvulsive* Compound infusion or decoction of root taken for "fits." (41:63, 64) Compound decoction of root taken for convulsions. (43:336) *Heart Medicine* Compound decoction of root prepared ceremonially and taken for heart trouble. (43:338) *Hemostat* Compound infusion or decoction of root used on bleeding wounds. (41:63, 64) Compound decoction of root used on bleeding wounds. (43:336) *Stimulant* Compound infusion or decoction of root taken or used externally as stimulant. (41:63, 64) Compound decoction of root taken as a stimulant. (43:364) *Tonic* Compound decoction of root or dried root alone taken as a tonic. (43:336) *Unspecified* Roots carried for general health and safe journeys. (43:376) **Cree, Woodlands** *Blood Medicine* Infusion of blooms taken as a blood medicine. *Oral Aid* Root used for sore mouths. *Panacea* Powdered roots added to a many-herb remedy and used for various ailments. *Throat Aid* Chewed root juice swallowed for sore throats. *Toothache Remedy* Root applied directly to a tooth for toothache. (91:51) **Malecite** *Cold Remedy* Dried roots chewed for colds. (96:244) **Meskwaki** *Heart Medicine* Decoction of root taken for heart trouble. (129:236) **Micmac** *Cold Remedy* Root used for colds. (32:59) **Ojibwa** *Unspecified* Plant used for medicinal purposes. (112:235) **Ojibwa, South** *Cold Remedy* Decoction of root used for colds. *Cough Medicine* Decoction of root used for cough. *Gastrointestinal Aid* Infusion of leaves taken to "destroy water bugs that have been swallowed." *Throat Aid* Infusion of leaves taken for sore throat. (77:199)

Polygala verticillata, Whorled Milkwort
Cherokee *Other* Infusion taken for "summer complaint." (66:45) **Iroquois** *Other* and *Pediatric Aid* Infusion of plant given to babies with "summer complaint." (73:369)

Polygonatum biflorum, King Solomon's Seal
Cherokee *Antidiarrheal* Taken for dysentery. *Breast Treatment* Used for breast diseases. *Dermatological Aid* Hot poultice of bruised root used to draw risings or carbuncles. *Gastrointestinal Aid* Infusion of roasted roots taken for stomach trouble. *Gynecological Aid* Taken by females afflicted with "whites or profuse menstruation." *Pulmonary Aid* Used for lung diseases. *Tonic* Root used as a mild tonic for "general debility." (66:56) **Chippewa** *Sedative* Plant used to insure sound

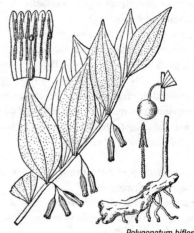

Polygonatum biflorum

sleep. (59:126) **Menominee** *Analgesic* Compound poultice of boiled, mashed root applied for sharp pains. (44:134) *Stimulant* Smudge of compound containing dried root used to revive unconscious patient. (128:41) **Meskwaki** *Stimulant* Root heated on coals and fumes inhaled by unconscious patient to revive him. (129:230) **Ojibwa** *Cathartic* Root used as a physic and decoction used as cough remedy. *Cough Medicine* Decoction of root used as a cough remedy and root used as a physic. (130:374) **Rappahannock** *Dermatological Aid* Decoction of roots applied as a salve to cuts, bruises, and sores. *Orthopedic Aid* Decoction of roots applied as a salve to cuts and bruises. (138:30)

Polygonatum biflorum var. *commutatum*, King Solomon's Seal
Chippewa *Analgesic* Decoction of root steamed and inhaled for headache. *Herbal Steam* Decoction of root sprinkled on hot stones and used as an herbal steam for headache. (as *P. commutatum* 43:336) *Misc. Disease Remedy* Roots used to prevent measles and other diseases. (as *P. commutatum* 59:125)

Polygonatum pubescens, Hairy Solomon's Seal
Abnaki *Antihemorrhagic* Used by women for spitting up blood. Used for spitting up blood. (121:154) Decoction of plant taken for spitting up blood. (121:174) **Iroquois** *Carminative* Compound decoction of plant taken for "gas on the stomach." (73:284) *Eye Medicine* Infusion of roots used to wash the eyes for snow-blindness. *Hunting Medicine* Compound infusion of roots used to "get a fish on each hook, every cast." (73:285)

Polygonum alpinum, Alaska Wild Rhubarb
Tanana, Upper *Cold Remedy* Raw roots and stem bases chewed for colds. *Cough Medicine* Raw roots and stem bases chewed for coughs. (as *P. alaskanum* 86:15)

Polygonum amphibium, Water Knotweed
Cree, Woodlands *Oral Aid* Poultice of fresh roots applied directly to blisters in the mouth. *Panacea* Powdered roots added to a many-herb remedy and used for various ailments. (91:51) **Okanagan-Colville** *Cold Remedy* Infusion of dried, pounded

roots taken or raw root eaten for chest colds. (162:113)

Polygonum amphibium var. *emersum*, Longroot Smartweed
Meskwaki *Antidiarrheal* Infusion of leaves and stems used for children with flux. *Gynecological Aid* Compound decoction of root taken for injured womb. *Oral Aid* Root used for mouth sores. *Pediatric Aid* Infusion of leaves and stems used for children with flux. (as *P. muhlenbergii* 129:236) **Ojibwa** *Analgesic* Infusion of plant taken for stomach pain. *Gastrointestinal Aid* Infusion of plant used for stomach pain. *Hunting Medicine* Plant used as hunting medicine. (as *P. muhlenbergii* 130:381) Dried flowers included in the hunting medicine and smoked to attract deer to the hunter. (as *P. muhlenbergii* 130:431)

Polygonum amphibium var. *stipulaceum*, Water Smartweed
Potawatomi *Unspecified* Root used for unspecified ailments. (131:72)

Polygonum arenastrum, Ovalleaf Knotweed
Iroquois *Gynecological Aid* Decoction of whole plant used for miscarriage injuries. *Love Medicine* Powdered, dry root placed in other person's tea as a love medicine. *Orthopedic Aid* Decoction of whole plant used for lame back. *Veterinary Aid* Decoction of plant mixed with feed and given to heifers to restore their milk. (73:314)

Polygonum aviculare, Prostrate Knotweed
Cherokee *Analgesic* Taken for painful urination. Infusion mixed with meal used as poultice for pain. *Antidiarrheal* Infusion of root given to children for diarrhea. *Dermatological Aid* Used for "scaldhead." *Pediatric Aid* Infusion of root given to children for diarrhea. Leaves rubbed on children's thumb to prevent thumb sucking. *Poison* Used to poison fish and infusion mixed with meal used as poultice for pain. *Poultice* Used as a poultice for "swelled and inflamed parts." *Urinary Aid* Taken for "gravel," painful urination, and bloody urine. (66:55) **Choctaw** *Gynecological Aid* Strong infusion of whole plant taken freely to prevent abortion. (23:286) **Iroquois** *Antidiarrheal* Infusion of plant and another plant given to children

for diarrhea. (118:40) *Dermatological Aid* Compound poultice of raw plants applied to cuts and wounds. *Orthopedic Aid* Compound decoction taken and poultice used for baby's broken coccyx. *Pediatric Aid* Compound decoction taken and poultice used for baby's broken coccyx. (73:313) Infusion of plant and another plant given to children for diarrhea. (118:40) **Mendocino Indian** *Dermatological Aid* Decoction of whole plant used as an astringent. (33:345) **Navajo, Ramah** *Analgesic* and *Gastrointestinal Aid* Warm infusion of plant taken for stomachache. (165:23) **Thompson** *Antidiarrheal* and *Pediatric Aid* Decoction of whole plant taken, especially by children, for diarrhea. (161:238)

Polygonum bistorta, Meadow Bistort
Aleut *Tonic* Root used as a tonic. (163:263)

Polygonum bistortoides, American Bistort
Miwok *Dermatological Aid* Poultice of root used on sores and boils. (8:172)

Polygonum careyi, Carey's Smartweed
Potawatomi *Cold Remedy* and *Febrifuge* Infusion of entire plant taken for cold accompanied by fever. (131:72)

Polygonum densiflorum, Denseflower Knotweed
Hawaiian *Blood Medicine* Infusion of pounded whole plants and other plants strained and taken to purify the blood. (as *P. glabrum* 2:48)

Polygonum douglasii ssp. *johnstonii*, Johnston's Knotweed
Navajo, Ramah *Nose Medicine* Plant used as snuff for nose troubles. (as *P. sawatchense* 165:24)

Polygonum hydropiper, Marshpepper Knotweed
Cherokee *Analgesic* Taken for painful urination. Infusion mixed with meal used as poultice for pain. *Antidiarrheal* Infusion of root given to children for diarrhea. *Dermatological Aid* Used for "scaldhead." *Pediatric Aid* Infusion of root given to children for diarrhea. Leaves rubbed on children's thumb to prevent thumb sucking. *Poison* Used to poison fish and infusion mixed with meal

used as poultice for pain. *Poultice* Used as a poultice for "swelled and inflamed parts." *Urinary Aid* Taken for "gravel," painful urination, and bloody urine. (66:55) **Iroquois** *Analgesic* Poultice of wetted plant applied to the forehead for headaches. (118:40) *Febrifuge* Decoction of plant taken for fever, chills, and "when cold." *Gastrointestinal Aid* Decoction of small piece of plant taken for indigestion. Whole plant used for children with swollen stomachs. *Pediatric Aid* Whole plant used for children with swollen stomachs. (73:314) **Malecite** *Kidney Aid* Infusion of dried leaves used for dropsy. (96:244)

Polygonum lapathifolium, Curlytop Knotweed
Apache, White Mountain *Unspecified* Plant used for medicinal purposes. (113:159) **Keres, Western** *Gastrointestinal Aid* Infusion of plant taken for stomach trouble. (147:62) **Navajo, Ramah** *Ceremonial Medicine* Cold infusion of plant used as ceremonial chant lotion. (165:23, 24) **Potawatomi** *Febrifuge* Infusion of whole plant used for fever. (131:72) **Zuni** *Cathartic* Decoction of plant taken as an emetic and purgative. *Emetic* Decoction of root taken as an emetic and purgative. (143:58)

Polygonum pensylvanicum, Pennsylvania Smartweed
Chippewa *Anticonvulsive* Infusion of plant tops taken for epilepsy. (59:129) **Iroquois** *Veterinary Aid* Decoction of plant given to horses for colic and "when urine is bound up." (73:314) **Menominee** *Antihemorrhagic* Infusion of leaf taken for "hemorrhage of blood from the mouth." *Gynecological Aid* Compound infusion of leaf taken to aid postpartum healing. (128:47) **Meskwaki** *Antidiarrheal* Used to wipe anus for bloody flux. *Hemorrhoid Remedy* Used for piles. (129:236, 237)

Polygonum persicaria, Spotted Ladysthumb
Cherokee *Analgesic* Decoction mixed with meal and used as poultice for pain. *Dermatological Aid* Crushed leaves rubbed on poison ivy. *Urinary Aid* Infusion taken for "gravel." (66:26) **Chippewa** *Analgesic* Decoction of leaves and flowers taken for stomach pain. *Gastrointestinal Aid* Simple or compound decoction of flowers and leaves taken for stomach pain. (43:344) **Iroquois** *Antirheu-*

matic (*External*) Decoction of plant used as a foot and leg soak for rheumatism. *Heart Medicine* Plant used for heart trouble. *Veterinary Aid* Plant rubbed over horses to keep flies away. (73:315)

Polygonum punctatum, Dotted Smartweed **Chippewa** *Analgesic* and *Gastrointestinal Aid* Compound decoction of leaves and flowers taken for stomach pain. (43:344) **Houma** *Analgesic* and *Orthopedic Aid* Decoction of root taken for pains and swellings in the legs and joints. (135:58) **Iroquois** *Psychological Aid* Compound decoction taken for "loss of senses during menses." (73:315)

Polygonum ramosissimum, Bushy Knotweed **Navajo, Ramah** *Analgesic* and *Gastrointestinal Aid* Warm infusion of plant taken for stomachache. *Panacea* Plant used as a "life medicine." (165:24)

Polygonum virginianum, Jumpseed **Cherokee** *Pulmonary Aid* Hot infusion of leaves with bark of honey locust given for whooping cough. (as *Tovara virginiana* 66:42)

Polymnia canadensis, Whiteflower Leafcup **Houma** *Dermatological Aid* Poultice of crushed leaves applied to swellings. (135:63) **Iroquois** *Toothache Remedy* Plant used as toothache medicine. (73:468)

Polypodium californicum, California Polypody **Mendocino Indian** *Eye Medicine* Infusion of roots used as a wash for sore eyes. **Wailaki** *Antirheumatic* (*External*) Root juice rubbed on areas affected by rheumatism. *Dermatological Aid* Root juice rubbed on sores. (33:303) **Yurok** *Disinfectant* Rhizomes used as an "antibiotic" for infections. (5:46)

Polypodium glycyrrhiza, Licorice Fern **Bella Coola** *Oral Aid* Rhizomes chewed to flavor the mouth. *Throat Aid* Rhizomes chewed and juice swallowed for sore throat. (158:196) **Haisla** *Analgesic* Rhizomes used for chest pains. *Respiratory Aid* Rhizomes used for shortness of breath. **Haisla & Hanaksiala** *Cold Remedy* Rhizomes used for colds. *Cough Medicine* Rhizomes used for coughs. *Throat Aid* Rhizomes chewed or sucked for sore

throats. (35:158) **Hesquiat** *Carminative* Rhizomes growing on the wild crabapple used for gas. *Cough Medicine* Long, slender rhizomes eaten as a medicine for coughs. *Oral Aid* Long, slender rhizomes eaten raw to sweeten the mouth. *Throat Aid* Long, slender rhizomes eaten as a medicine for sore throats. (159:30) **Kitasoo** *Cough Medicine* Rhizomes used for coughs. *Throat Aid* Rhizomes used for sore throats. (35:312) **Kwakiutl** *Antidiarrheal* Compound decoction of plants or roots taken for diarrhea. (157:266) **Antiemetic** and *Antihemorrhagic* Roots sucked and juice swallowed for vomiting blood. (157:264) **Makah** *Unspecified* Rhizomes used for internal ailments. (55:220) **Nitinaht** *Cough Medicine* Licorice flavored rhizomes chewed and juice swallowed for coughs. *Respiratory Aid* Licorice flavored rhizomes chewed and juice swallowed for sore chest. (160:64) **Nootka** *Alterative* and *Venereal Aid* Plant used as an excellent alterative for venereal complaints. (as *P. falcatum* 146:80, 81) **Oweekeno** *Cough Medicine* Rhizomes chewed for coughs. *Throat Aid* Rhizomes chewed for sore throats. (35:59) **Thompson** *Cold Remedy* Rhizomes chewed or infusion of rhizomes taken for colds. *Oral Aid* Rhizomes used as medicine for sore gums. *Throat Aid* Rhizomes chewed or infusion of rhizomes taken for sore throats. (161:91)

Polypodium hesperium, Western Polypody **Thompson** *Cold Remedy* Rhizomes chewed or infusion of rhizomes taken for colds. *Oral Aid* Rhizomes used as medicine for sore gums. *Throat Aid* Rhizomes chewed or infusion of rhizomes taken for sore throats. (161:91)

Polypodium incanum, Resurrection Fern **Seminole** *Other* Complex infusion of leaves taken for chronic conditions. (145:272) *Psychological Aid* Infusion of plant used to steam and bathe the body for insanity. (145:291)

Polypodium virginianum, Rock Polypody **Abnaki** *Gastrointestinal Aid* Used for stomachaches. (121:154) Decoction of whole plant used for stomachaches. (121:162) **Algonquin, Quebec** *Heart Medicine* Used to make a medicinal tea for heart disease. (14:123) **Bella Coola** *Analgesic* Simple or compound decoction taken for stomach pains. *Gastrointestinal Aid* Compound decoction of root taken for stomach pain, not vomiting or diarrhea. *Throat Aid* Roots chewed for swollen, sore throat and compound decoction used for stomach pain. (as *P. vulgare* 127:48) **Cherokee** *Dermatological Aid* Poultice used for inflamed swellings and wounds and infusion taken for hives. (66:60, 61) **Cowichan** *Cold Remedy* Rhizomes used for colds. *Gastrointestinal Aid* Rhizomes used for stomach ailments. *Throat Aid* Rhizomes used for sore throat. (as *P. vulgare* 156:69) **Cowlitz** *Misc. Disease Remedy* Infusion of crushed stems taken for the measles. (as *P. vulgare* 65:13) **Cree, Woodlands** *Tuberculosis Remedy* Decoction of leaf taken for tuberculosis. (91:51) **Green River Group** *Cough Medicine* Baked or raw roots used as a cough medicine. (as *P. vulgare* 65:13) **Iroquois** *Misc. Disease Remedy* Compound decoction taken for cholera. (73:260) **Klallam** *Cough Medicine* Baked or raw roots used as a cough medicine. **Makah** *Cough Medicine* Peeled stems chewed for coughs. (as *P. vulgare* 65:13) **Malecite** *Pulmonary Aid* Infusion of pounded roots used for pleurisy. (as *P. vulgare* 96:252) **Micmac** *Diuretic* Infusion of plant used for urine retention. (122:55) *Pulmonary Aid* Roots used for pleurisy. (32:59) **Quinault** *Cough Medicine* Baked or raw roots used as a cough medicine. (as *P. vulgare* 65:13) **Saanich** *Cold Remedy* Rhizomes used for colds. *Gastrointestinal Aid* Rhizomes used for stomach ailments. *Throat Aid* Rhizomes used for sore throat. (as *P. vulgare* 156:69) **Skagit, Upper** *Dermatological Aid* Plant used to make a demulcent. *Expectorant* Plant used to make an expectorant. *Laxative* Plant used to make a laxative. (as *P. vulgare* 154:42)

Polypogon monspeliensis, Annual Rabbitsfoot Grass
Navajo, Kayenta *Heart Medicine* Infusion of ashes taken for palpitations. (179:16)

Polyporus sp.
Blackfoot *Antidiarrheal* Infusion of plant taken for diarrhea and dysentery. (72:67)

Polystichum acrostichoides, Christmas Fern
Cherokee *Antirheumatic* (*External*) Compound decoction of root applied with warm hands for rheumatism. (as *Aspidium acrostichoides* 66:8) Roots used in "medicine rubbed on skin for rheumatism after scratching." (66:33) Decoction of roots rubbed on area affected by rheumatism. (152:3) *Antirheumatic* (*Internal*) Infusion taken for rheumatism. *Emetic* Roots used as an ingredient in an emetic and infusion taken for rheumatism. *Febrifuge* Compound decoction taken for chills and infusion taken for fever. *Gastrointestinal Aid* Cold infusion of root used for "stomachache or bowel complaint." *Pulmonary Aid* Infusion taken for pneumonia. *Toothache Remedy* Compound decoction used for toothache and chills. (66:33) **Iroquois** *Analgesic* Decoction of plant used by children for cramps. (73:256) *Anticonvulsive* Poultice of wet, smashed roots used on children's back and head for convulsions. *Antidiarrheal* Compound decoction taken for diarrhea. (73:257) *Antirheumatic* (*External*) Infusion of smashed roots used as a foot soak for "rheumatism" in back and legs. (73:256) *Blood Medicine* Cold, compound decoction taken for weak blood and as a blood purifier. *Dermatological Aid* Poultice of wet, smashed roots used on children's back and head for red spots. (73:257) *Emetic* Infusion of roots taken as an emetic for dyspepsia and consumption. *Febrifuge* Decoction of vine with small leaves used for children with fevers. (73:256) *Gynecological Aid* Plant taken before and after baby to clean womb. Roots used as a "Lady's medicine" for the insides. (73:257) *Orthopedic Aid* Poultice applied to back and feet for spinal trouble and sore back of babies. *Pediatric Aid* Decoction of plant used by children for cramps. Decoction of vine with small leaves used for children with fevers. (73:256) Poultice applied to back and feet for spinal trouble and sore back of babies. (73:256) Poultice of wet, smashed roots used on children's back and head for convulsions, and for red spots. *Stimulant* Decoction of plant given to children (sometimes mother too) for listlessness. *Throat Aid* Powder inhaled and coughed up by a man who cannot talk. *Tuberculosis Remedy* Infusion of roots taken as an emetic for consumption. *Venereal Aid* Compound decoction used as a blood purifier and for venereal disease. (73:257) **Malecite** *Throat Aid* Roots chewed and used for hoarseness. (96:247) **Micmac** *Throat Aid* Roots used for hoarseness. (32:59)

Polystichum munitum, Western Swordfern
Cowlitz *Dermatological Aid* Infusion of stems
used as a wash for sores. (65:13) **Hesquiat** *Cancer Treatment* Young shoots or fiddleheads chewed
for cancer of the womb. (159:32) **Kwakiutl** *Gynecological Aid* Boughs placed under bed of young
girl to have as many children as plants. (157:265)
Lummi *Gynecological Aid* Leaves chewed by
women to facilitate childbirth. **Quileute** *Dermatological Aid* Poultice of chewed leaves applied to
sores and boils. **Quinault** *Burn Dressing* Poultice
of spore sacs from the leaves applied to burns.
Dermatological Aid Decoction of roots used as a
wash for dandruff. **Swinomish** *Throat Aid* Raw
plant chewed and eaten for sore throats or tonsillitis. (65:13) **Thompson** *Hunting Medicine* Plant
rubbed on the hands to bring luck in whaling and
sturgeon fishing. (161:89)

Polytaenia nuttallii, Nuttall's Prairie Parsley
Meskwaki *Antidiarrheal* and *Gynecological Aid*
Decoction of seeds taken by women for severe diarrhea. (129:249)

Polytrichum commune, Hair Moss
Nitinaht *Gynecological Aid* Plant chewed by
women in labor to speed up the process. (160:59)

Pontederia cordata, Pickerel Weed
Malecite *Contraceptive* Infusion of plant used to
prevent pregnancy. (96:259) **Micmac** *Contraceptive* Herbs used to prevent pregnancy. (32:59)
Montagnais *Panacea* "Brew" from plant used for
"illness in general." (133:315)

Populus alba, White Poplar
Iroquois *Cold Remedy* Infusion of inner bark
taken to "cleans you out after a cold." *Love Medicine* Compound decoction of branches used as a
body wash for anti-love medicine. *Tonic* Infusion
of inner bark taken as a tonic. (73:293) **Ojibwa**
Antirheumatic (*External*) Infusion of pounded
plants used as wash for rheumatism. *Blood Medicine* Infusion of bark and root or decoction of
bark taken for internal blood diseases. *Panacea*
Infusion of pounded plants used as wash for general illnesses. (112:231) *Unspecified* Roots and
bark used for medicinal purposes. (112:243)

Populus balsamifera, Balsam Poplar
Algonquin, Quebec *Dermatological Aid* Spring
buds used to make a salve. Poultice of steeped,
root scrapings applied to open sores. Buds used to
make a salve and applied to open sores. *Disinfectant* Poultice of steeped, root scrapings applied to
infected wounds. Buds used to make a salve and
applied to infected wounds. (14:148) **Bella Coola**
Analgesic Branches with leaves used in a sweat
bath for pains similar to rheumatism. Decoction of
rotten leaves used as a bath for body pain. Poultice
of compound containing buds applied for lung or
hip pains. *Antirheumatic* (*External*) Leaves used
in sweat bath for pains similar to rheumatism.
Diaphoretic Branches with leaves used in a sweat
bath for pains similar to rheumatism. *Orthopedic
Aid* Poultice of compound containing buds applied
to lung or hip pain. *Pulmonary Aid* Poultice of
compound containing buds applied for lung pains.
Carrier, Northern *Dermatological Aid* Poultice
of chewed, green roots applied to bleeding wounds.
Eye Medicine Decoction of inner bark used as an
eyewash. **Carrier, Southern** *Cough Medicine*
and *Pulmonary Aid* Decoction of buds taken for
"coughs and lung affections." (127:54) **Chippewa**
Analgesic Compound decoction of root taken for
back pain. (43:356) *Dermatological Aid* Decoction of buds used as salve for frostbite, sores, and
inflamed wounds. (59:126) *Gynecological Aid*
Compound decoction of root taken for "female
weakness." (43:356) Compound infusion of root
taken for excessive flowing during confinement.

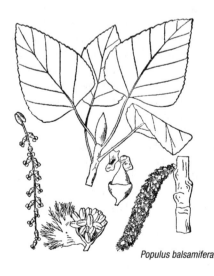

Populus balsamifera

(43:358) *Heart Medicine* Compound decoction of root, bud, and blossom prepared ceremonially and used for the heart. (43:338) *Orthopedic Aid* Poultice of infusion or decoction of used buds for sprains or strained muscles. (43:362) **Cree, Woodlands** *Disinfectant* Poultice of fresh leaves applied to a sore to draw out the infection. *Hemostat* Poultice of sticky buds applied directly to the nostril for a nosebleed. (91:52) **Malecite** *Dermatological Aid* Bud balm and burdock roots used for sores. (96:247) **Micmac** *Dermatological Aid* Buds and other parts of plant used as salve for sores. *Venereal Aid* Buds and other parts of plant used as salve for chancre. (32:59) **Ojibwa** *Antirheumatic* (*External*) Infusion of pounded plants used as wash for rheumatism. *Blood Medicine* Decoction of bark taken for internal blood diseases. (112:231) *Cold Remedy* Buds cooked in grease and rubbed in nostrils for cold. *Dermatological Aid* Buds cooked in grease and used as salve for cuts, wounds, or bruises. (130:387) *Panacea* Infusion of pounded plants used as wash for general illnesses. (112:231) *Respiratory Aid* Buds cooked in grease and rubbed in nostrils for catarrh or bronchitis. (130:387) **Paiute** *Gastrointestinal Aid* Decoction of sap taken for stomach disorders. (155:121, 122) **Potawatomi** *Dermatological Aid* Buds melted with tallow and used as ointment for sores or eczema. (131:80, 81) **Shoshoni** *Analgesic* Decoction of root used as a lotion for headaches. *Blood Medicine* Compound decoction of bark taken as a blood tonic. *Tonic* Compound decoction of bark taken as a blood tonic and for general debility. *Tuberculosis Remedy* Simple or compound decoction of bark taken for tuberculosis. *Venereal Aid* Simple or compound decoction of bark taken for venereal disease. (155:121, 122) **Tanana, Upper** *Cold Remedy* Decoction of buds taken for colds. Buds heated on top of a wood stove and the aroma inhaled for colds. Decoction of mashed buds used for colds. *Cough Medicine* Decoction of buds taken for coughs. *Dermatological Aid* Mashed buds cooked in grease or dried, powdered buds used as a salve for rashes and sores. *Panacea* Decoction of buds taken for colds, coughs, and other illnesses. (86:4)

Populus balsamifera ssp. *balsamifera*, Balsam Poplar

Anticosti *Dermatological Aid* Poultice of buds and alcohol applied to wounds. (as *P. tacamahacca* 120:65) **Cherokee** *Antirheumatic* (*Internal*) Tincture of buds used for chronic rheumatism. *Dermatological Aid* Juice of buds used on sores. *Gastrointestinal Aid* Tincture of buds used for colic and bowels. *Stimulant* Given to "persons of phlegmatic habits." *Toothache Remedy* Used for aching teeth. *Venereal Aid* Tincture of buds used for old venereal complaints. (as *P. candicans* 66:24) **Iroquois** *Anthelmintic* Compound decoction with bark taken to kill worms in adults. (73:291) *Antirheumatic* (*Internal*) Used for arthritis. *Blood Medicine* Compound with whisky taken as blood remedy and for tapeworms. (73:292) *Dermatological Aid* Compound decoction used for skin eruptions and scabs. *Laxative* Compound decoction of bark taken as a laxative. *Veterinary Aid* Decoction of bark taken by people and given to horses for worms. (73:291) **Menominee** *Cold Remedy* Decoction of resinous buds in fat used in the nostrils for a head cold. *Dermatological Aid* Decoction of resinous buds in fat used as a salve for wounds. (as *P. candicans* 128:52)

Populus balsamifera ssp. *trichocarpa*, Black Cottonwood

Bella Coola *Dermatological Aid* Buds mixed with chewed and warmed mountain goat kidney fat and used as a face cream. Infusion of buds mixed with eulachon (candlefish) grease or sockeye salmon oil and rubbed on scalp for baldness. *Orthopedic Aid* Poultice of buds applied for hip pains. *Pulmonary Aid* Infusion of buds and animal fat taken for whooping cough. Poultice of buds applied for lung and hip pains. *Throat Aid* Infusion of buds in dogfish oil taken for sore throat. *Tuberculosis Remedy* Buds mixed with balsam sap and used for tuberculosis. (as *P. trichocarpa* 158:210) **Flathead** *Cold Remedy* Bark eaten for colds. *Dermatological Aid* Poultice of leaves used for bruises, sores, and boils. *Venereal Aid* Infusion of young branches, buds, and other plants taken for syphilis. (as *P. trichocarpa* 68:68) **Haisla & Hanaksiala** *Burn Dressing* Buds cooked with mountain goat fat and rubbed on the face for sunburn. *Dermatological Aid* Buds used to make a hair dressing. Buds cooked with mountain goat fat and rubbed on the body to soften the skin. (35:284) **Hesquiat** *Dermatological Aid* Decoction of buds mixed with deer fat and used to make a fragrant salve. (159:75) **Hoh** *Unspecified* Infusion of bark used for medicine. (as *P. trichocarpa* 114:60) **Karok** *Love Medicine* Leaves used as a love medicine. (as *P. trichocarpa* 125:381) **Klallam** *Eye Medicine* Infusion of buds used as an eyewash. (as *P. trichocarpa* 65:26) **Kutenai** *Dermatological Aid* Poultice of leaves used for bruises, sores, and boils. *Respiratory Aid* Infusion of bark taken for tuberculosis. Infusion of bark taken for whooping cough. (as *P. trichocarpa* 68:68) **Kwakiutl** *Dermatological Aid* Buds and oil used as a hair tonic. Buds rubbed on the skin to prevent sunburn. (as *P. trichocarpa* 157:292) **Nez Perce** *Antirheumatic* (*External*) Leaves used for aching muscles. *Veterinary Aid* Poultice of leaves used for horses' sores. (as *P. trichocarpa* 68:68) **Nitinaht** *Dermatological Aid* Resin used as a salve for wounds and cuts. (160:126) **Okanagan-Colville** *Venereal Aid* Infusion of buds taken for gonorrhea. (162:134) **Oweekeno** *Dermatological Aid* Buds boiled with grease, strained, combined with an unknown ingredient, and used as hair dressing. (35:116) **Quileute** *Unspecified* Infusion of bark used for medicine. (as *P. trichocarpa* 114:60) **Quinault** *Dermatological Aid* and *Disinfectant* Gum of burls applied as an antiseptic to cuts and wounds. *Tuberculosis Remedy* Infusion of bark taken for tuberculosis. (as *P. trichocarpa* 65:26) **Shuswap** *Dermatological Aid* Poultice of pitch applied to sores. (as *P. trichocarpa* 102:68) **Squaxin** *Dermatological Aid* and *Disinfectant* Infusion of bruised leaves applied as an antiseptic for cuts. *Throat Aid* Infusion of bark used as a gargle for sore throats. (as *P. trichocarpa* 65:26) **Thompson** *Ceremonial Medicine* Decoction of bark taken "for your health" after childbirth if someone close had passed away. *Dermatological Aid* Poultice of mashed buds mixed with pitch used for ringworm. Infusion of white inner bark used for washing sores and especially itchy skin. *Gynecological Aid* Infusion of white inner bark taken by women after childbirth. *Orthopedic Aid* Concoction of wood, willow, soaperry branches, and "anything weeds" used for broken bones. *Unspecified* Decoction of buds taken for "some kind of disease." It was cautioned that one

should not drink too much of this decoction because it would kill you. (161:276) **Yurok** *Unspecified* Decoction of shoot tips used for medicine. (as *P. trichocarpa* 5:47)

Populus deltoides, Eastern Cottonwood
Delaware *Strengthener* Bark combined with black haw and wild plum barks and used by women for weakness and debility. (151:31) **Delaware, Oklahoma** *Gynecological Aid* Simple or compound infusion taken for "weakness and debility in women." (150:26, 78) **Flathead** *Cold Remedy* Bark eaten for colds. *Dermatological Aid* Poultice of leaves used for bruises, sores, and boils. *Venereal Aid* Infusion of young branches, buds, and other plants taken for syphilis. (68:68) **Iroquois** *Anthelmintic* Decoction of bark used for intestinal worms. *Veterinary Aid* Poultice of dried bark flour and water applied to horses with bumps containing worms. (118:39) **Kutenai** *Dermatological Aid* Poultice of leaves used for bruises, sores, and boils. *Respiratory Aid* Infusion of bark taken for whooping cough. *Tuberculosis Remedy* Infusion of bark taken for tuberculosis. (68:68) **Nanticoke** *Orthopedic Aid* Compound containing bark used as a lotion for sprains. (150:56, 84) **Nez Perce** *Antirheumatic* (*External*) Leaves used for aching muscles. *Veterinary Aid* Poultice of leaves used for horses' sores. (68:68)

Populus deltoides **ssp. *deltoides***, Eastern Cottonwood
Choctaw *Dermatological Aid* Decoction of leaves and bark steam used for wounds. (as *P. angulata* 20:24) *Herbal Steam* Steam from decoction of stems, bark, and leaves used for snakebites. *Snakebite Remedy* Steam from decoction of stems, bark, and leaves used for snakebites. (as *P. angulata* 20:23) Decoction of stems, bark, and leaves used as a steam bath for snakebites. (as *P. angulata* 152:12)

Populus deltoides **ssp. *monilifera***, Plains Cottonwood
Ojibwa, South *Dermatological Aid* Cotton down used as an absorbent on open sores. (as *P. monilifera* 77:199) **Omaha** *Ceremonial Medicine* Plant used in various rituals. (as *P. sargentii* 56:322)

Populus fremontii, Frémont's Cottonwood
Cahuilla *Analgesic* Infusion of bark and leaves used to wet a handkerchief and tie it around the head for headaches. *Antirheumatic* (*External*) Poultice of boiled bark and leaves applied to swellings caused by muscle strain. *Dermatological Aid* Infusion of bark and leaves used as a wash for cuts. *Veterinary Aid* Infusion of bark and leaves used on horses for saddle sores and swollen legs. (11:106) **Diegueño** *Dermatological Aid* Infusion of leaves used as a wash or poultice of leaves applied to bruises, wounds, or insect stings. (74:216) **Kawaiisu** *Orthopedic Aid* Decoction of inner bark used to wash broken limbs. *Poultice* Poultice of inner bark applied to injured areas. (180:53) **Mendocino Indian** *Dermatological Aid* Decoction of bark used as a wash for bruises and cuts. *Veterinary Aid* Decoction of bark used as a wash for horse sores caused by chafing. (33:330) **Pima** *Dermatological Aid* Decoction of plant used as a wash for sores. (38:109) **Yuki** *Cold Remedy* Infusion of bark or leaves taken for colds. *Dermatological Aid* Decoction of bark used as a wash for sores. Infusion of bark or leaves taken for cuts and sores. *Throat Aid* Infusion of bark or leaves taken for sore throats. (39:46)

***Populus fremontii* var. *fremontii*,**
Frémont's Cottonwood
Diegueño *Orthopedic Aid* Decoction of green leaves used as a bath or poultice of hot leaves applied to breaks or sprains. (70:30)

Populus grandidentata, Bigtooth Aspen
Cree *Abortifacient* Used to prevent childbearing. (12:485) *Gynecological Aid* Infusion of bark taken to ease and lessen menses. (12:494) **Iroquois** *Dermatological Aid* Dust from the bark applied to parts affected by itch. (73:293) **Malecite** *Dietary Aid* Infusion of bark used for stimulating the appetite. (96:253) **Ojibwa** *Hemostat* Infusion of young root used as a "hemostatic." (130:387, 388)

Populus ×jackii, Jack's Poplar
Iroquois *Oral Aid* Compound infusion used as a wash for mouth ulcers. (as *P. gileadensis* 73:292) **Malecite** *Unspecified* Used to make medicines. (as *P. gileadensis* 137:6)

Populus nigra, Lombardy Poplar
Cherokee *Antirheumatic* (*Internal*) Tincture of buds used for chronic rheumatism. *Dermatological Aid* Juice of buds used on sores. *Gastrointestinal Aid* Tincture of buds used for colic and bowels. *Stimulant* Given to "persons of phlegmatic habits." *Toothache Remedy* Used for aching teeth. *Venereal Aid* Tincture of buds used for old venereal complaints. (66:24)

Populus tremuloides, Quaking Aspen
Abnaki *Anthelmintic* Used as a vermifuge. (121:155) Infusion of bark taken as a vermifuge. (121:165) **Algonquin, Tête-de-Boule** *Antirheumatic* (*External*) Poultice of shredded roots applied to joints for rheumatism. (110:130) **Bella Coola** *Venereal Aid* Decoction of root bark taken for gonorrhea with urethral hemorrhage. (127:54) **Blackfoot** *Gastrointestinal Aid* Infusion of bark used for heartburn. (72:83) *Gynecological Aid* Infusion of bark scrapings taken by women about to give birth. (72:61) *Panacea* Infusion of bark used for general discomfort. (72:83) **Carrier, Southern** *Analgesic* and *Gastrointestinal Aid* Decoction of bark taken for stomach pain. (127:54) **Chippewa** *Dermatological Aid* Poultice of chewed bark or root applied to cuts. (43:350) *Gynecological Aid* Compound infusion of root taken for "excessive flowing" during confinement. (43:358) *Heart Medicine* Compound decoction of inner bark prepared ceremonially for heart trouble. (43:338) **Cree, Woodlands** *Dermatological Aid* Poultice of crushed leaf applied to bee stings to reduce the

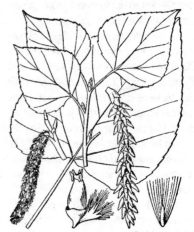

Populus tremuloides

irritation. Poultice of inner bark used as a wound dressing. *Hemostat* White, powdery substance on the outer bark surface scraped off and used as a styptic. *Venereal Aid* Bark outer surface scraped and used for venereal disease. Decoction of bark taken for venereal disease. (91:52) **Delaware, Ontario** *Cold Remedy* Compound containing bark taken for colds. (150:82) **Flathead** *Other* Infusion of bark used for ruptures. (68:37) **Gitksan** *Cathartic* Bark used as a purgative. (61:152) Decoction of bark taken as a purgative. *Dermatological Aid* Poultice of chewed or mashed root bark applied to cuts. (127:54) **Haisla** *Laxative* Decoction of bark taken as a laxative. **Haisla & Hanaksiala** *Oral Aid* Leaves used for mouth abscesses. (35: 286) **Iroquois** *Anthelmintic* Decoction of bark taken for worms. *Gastrointestinal Aid* Infusion of bark taken for cramps caused by worms. *Misc. Disease Remedy* Cold, compound infusion of bark taken for measles. Poultice of wetted bark applied for pleurisy. *Pediatric Aid* Infusion of bark from young trees given when "baby cries, but is not sick." (73:292) Infusion of bark or decoction of young shoots given to children for worms. *Urinary Aid* Compound used for bed-wetting. (73:293) *Venereal Aid* Infusion of roots or bark used internally and externally for venereal diseases. *Veterinary Aid* Decoction of bark mixed with feed for horses for worms. (73:292) Decoction of bark given to dogs and cats with fits caused by worms. (73:293) **Isleta** *Orthopedic Aid* Bark used as casts in setting broken limbs. (as *P. aurea* 85:38) **Meskwaki** *Cold Remedy, Cough Medicine,* and *Pediatric Aid* Decoction of buds used as a nasal salve by children and adults for coughs and colds. (129:245) **Micmac** *Cold Remedy* Bark used for colds. *Dietary Aid* Bark used to stimulate the appetite. (32:59) **Montagnais** *Anthelmintic* Infusion of dried bark given to children suffering from worms. (133:315) **Ojibwa** *Dermatological Aid* Poultice of bark applied to cuts and wounds. *Orthopedic Aid* Poultice of inner bark applied to sore arm or leg and used as a splint for broken limb. (130:388) **Okanagan-Colville** *Dermatological Aid* Bark powder used on the feet and underarms as a deodorant and antiperspirant. *Eye Medicine* Infusion of young growth used as a bath for bruised eyes. (162:134) **Okanagon** *Antirheumatic (External)* Decoction of stems and branches used as a wash

for rheumatism. *Antirheumatic (Internal)* Decoction of stems and branches taken for rheumatism. *Gastrointestinal Aid* Decoction of stems and branches taken for dyspepsia. (104:41) **Paiute** *Cough Medicine* Infusion of inner bark taken for coughs from pneumonia. *Febrifuge* Infusion of inner bark taken for fever with excessive perspiration. (93:61) **Penobscot** *Cold Remedy* and *Diaphoretic* Infusion of bark taken as a diaphoretic for colds. (133:310) **Potawatomi** *Veterinary Aid* Burned bark ashes mixed with lard and used as a salve for sores on horses. (131:81) **Salish** *Venereal Aid* Decoction of rootlets and stems taken for syphilis. (153:294) **Shoshoni** *Venereal Aid* Decoction of bark taken over a long period of time for venereal disease. (155:120, 121) **Sikani** *Anthelmintic* Infusion of scraped bark taken for worms and caused a stool immediately. *Dermatological Aid* Poultice of pulverized bark and water applied as paste to wounds. (127:54) **Tanana, Upper** *Cold Remedy* Decoction of inner bark, outer bark, and Hudson Bay tea used for colds. *Cough Medicine* Decoction of inner bark, outer bark, and Hudson Bay tea used for coughs. (86:5) **Tewa** *Urinary Aid* Decoction of leaves taken for urinary trouble. (115:42) **Thompson** *Antirheumatic (External)* Decoction of stems and branches used as a wash for rheumatism. *Antirheumatic (Internal)* Decoction of stems and branches taken for rheumatism. (104:41) *Dermatological Aid* Wood ash mixed with water or grease and used as a salve on swellings. (141:464) Powdery substance from bark rubbed on girls' armpits so that they would not grow underarm hair. The powder was rubbed on girls' armpits after their first menstrual period. Young men, too, rubbed the powdery substance on their arms and faces to prevent the growth of hair. Wood ashes rubbed on men's faces and arms to prevent the growth of hair. (161:277) *Disinfectant* Decoction of bark rubbed on adolescents' bodies for purification. (141:504) *Gastrointestinal Aid* Decoction of stems and branches taken for dyspepsia. (104:41) *Pediatric Aid* Decoction of bark rubbed on adolescents' bodies for purification. (141:504) *Psychological Aid* Decoction of branches taken by people suffering from insanity through excessive drinking. (161:277) *Venereal Aid* Decoction of branches or roots taken and used as a wash for syphilis. (141:464)

Porophyllum gracile, Slender Poreleaf
Havasupai *Analgesic* Decoction of pounded plant taken for pain. *Antirheumatic (External)* Decoction of pounded plant rubbed in as a liniment. *Antirheumatic (Internal)* Decoction of pounded plant taken for aches. *Dermatological Aid* Decoction of pounded plant used as a wash on sores. *Gastrointestinal Aid* Decoction of pounded plant taken for abdominal pain. (171:249) **Paiute** *Abortifacient* Decoction of root taken as "a regulator for delayed menstruation." (as *P. leucospermum* 155:122) **Shoshoni** *Abortifacient* Plant used to regulate delayed menstruation. (as *P. leucospermum* 98:46)

Porphyra abbottae, Edible Seaweed
Hanaksiala *Gastrointestinal Aid* Decoction of plant taken or poultice applied for any kind of sickness in the stomach or body. *Orthopedic Aid* Poultice of plant applied to broken collarbones. *Panacea* Decoction of plant taken or poultice applied for any kind of sickness in the stomach or body. (35:131)

Porteranthus stipulatus, Indian Physic
Cherokee *Antirheumatic (External)* Roots used for rheumatism. *Cold Remedy* Mild infusion used in slight doses for colds. *Dermatological Aid* Cold infusion of root given or root chewed "for bee and other stings." *Emetic* Mild infusion taken as an emetic. (as *Gillenia stipulata* 66:40) Decoction or strong infusion of whole plant taken a pint at a time as an emetic. (as *Gillenia stipulata* 177:74) *Kidney Aid* Infusion taken for kidneys. *Liver Aid* Compound taken for liver. *Orthopedic Aid* Poultice used for "leg swelling." *Respiratory Aid* Mild infusion used in slight doses for asthma. *Toothache Remedy* Infusion used for toothache. *Veterinary Aid* Tincture of root given for "milksick."

Porteranthus trifoliatus, Bowman's Root
Cherokee *Antirheumatic (External)* Poultice used for rheumatism. *Cold Remedy* Mild infusion used in slight doses for colds. *Dermatological Aid* Cold infusion of root given or root chewed "for bee and other stings." (as *Gillenia trifoliata* 66:40) Infusion of roots used as a wash for leg scratches. (as *Gillenia trifoliata* 152:27) *Emetic* Mild infusion taken as an emetic. (as *Gillenia trifoliata*

66:40) Decoction or strong infusion of whole plant taken a pint at a time as an emetic. (as *Gillenia trifoliata* 177:74) *Kidney Aid* Infusion taken for kidneys. *Liver Aid* Compound taken for liver. *Orthopedic Aid* Poultice used for "leg swelling." *Respiratory Aid* Mild infusion used in slight doses for asthma. *Toothache Remedy* Infusion used for toothache. *Veterinary Aid* Tincture of root given for "milksick." (as *Gillenia trifoliata* 66:40) **Iroquois** *Antidiarrheal* Compound decoction of leaves and switches taken for diarrhea. (as *Gillenia trifoliata* 73:349) *Cathartic* Plant used as a physic. *Cold Remedy* Infusion of roots taken for colds, fevers, and chills caused by fever and sore throats. *Diaphoretic* Decoction of roots taken to cause sweating. *Febrifuge* Infusion of roots taken for colds, fevers, and chills caused by fever and sore throats. *Misc. Disease Remedy* Decoction of roots taken for grippe. *Throat Aid* Infusion of roots taken for colds, fevers, and chills caused by fever and sore throats. (as *Gillenia trifoliata* 73:350)

Portulaca oleracea, Little Hogweed
Cherokee *Anthelmintic* Compound decoction taken for worms. *Ear Medicine* Juice used for earache. (66:51) **Hawaiian** *Strengthener* Plant and other plants pounded, squeezed, and resulting liquid taken to check run-down conditions. (2:24) **Iroquois** *Antidote* Good medicine to cure you if someone has given you some bad medicine. *Burn Dressing* Poultice of mashed plant used on burns. *Dermatological Aid* Poultice of entire plant used on bruises. (73:318) **Keres, Western** *Antidiarrheal* Infusion of leaf stems used for diarrhea. *Blood Medicine* Infusion of leaf stems used as an antiseptic wash for blood clots. *Oral Aid* Raw leaves rubbed in mouth for difficulty in opening the mouth. (147:62) **Navajo** *Analgesic* Plant used for pain. (45:97) *Gastrointestinal Aid* Plant taken for stomachaches. *Panacea* Plant used to "cure sick people." (45:47) **Rappahannock** *Dermatological Aid* Compound decoction of bruised leaves applied as salve for "footage" trouble. (138:28)

Portulaca oleracea ssp. oleracea, Little Hogweed
Navajo, Kayenta *Misc. Disease Remedy* Plant

used as a lotion for scarlet fever. (as _P. retusa_ 179:22)

Postelsia palmaeformis, Sea Palm
Hesquiat _Strengthener_ Whalers rubbed four or eight pieces of plant on their arms to make them as strong as the plant. (159:26) **Nitinaht** _Anticonvulsive_ Plants burned and ashes used for convulsions. _Psychological Aid_ Plants burned and ashes used for craziness. _Strengthener_ Stipes dried, burned, powdered, mixed with raccoon marrow, and salve used to strengthen young boys. **Nootka** _Strengthener_ Stipes dried, burned, powdered, mixed with raccoon marrow, and salve used to strengthen young boys. (160:54)

Potamogeton natans, Floating Pondweed
Navajo, Ramah _Ceremonial Medicine_ and _Emetic_ Decoction of plant taken as ceremonial emetic. (165:15)

Potentilla arguta, Tall Cinquefoil
Okanagan-Colville _Gynecological Aid_ Infusion of roots taken by women after childbirth. (162:126)

Potentilla arguta ssp. _arguta_, Tall Cinquefoil
Chippewa _Analgesic_ Dry, pulverized root pricked into temples or placed in nostrils for headache. (as _Drymocallis arguta_ 43:338) _Antidiarrheal_ Simple or compound decoction of root taken for dysentery. (as _Drymocallis arguta_ 43:344) _Dermatological Aid_ Poultice of moistened, dried, powdered root applied to cuts. (as _Drymocallis arguta_ 43:350)

Potentilla canadensis, Dwarf Cinquefoil
Iroquois _Antidiarrheal_ Infusion of pounded roots taken for diarrhea. (73:353) **Natchez** _Witchcraft Medicine_ Plant given to one who was bewitched. (148:667)

Potentilla crinita, Bearded Cinquefoil
Navajo, Ramah _Panacea_ Cold infusion of whole plant taken as "life medicine." (165:31)

Potentilla glandulosa, Gland Cinquefoil
Gosiute _Dermatological Aid_ Plant taken and

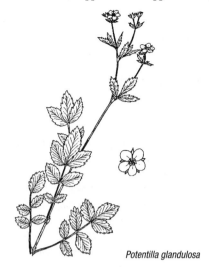

Potentilla glandulosa

poultice of plant applied to swollen parts. _Unspecified_ Root used as medicine. (31:378) **Okanagon** _Stimulant_ Infusion of whole plant taken as a stimulant. _Tonic_ Infusion of whole plant taken as a tonic. **Thompson** _Stimulant_ Infusion of whole plant taken as a stimulant. (104:42) Weak decoction of leaves taken as a stimulant. (141:469) Decoction of leaves or whole plant said to be slightly stimulant. (141:494) _Tonic_ Infusion of whole plant taken as a tonic. (104:42) Decoction of plant taken as a tonic for "general out-of-sorts feeling." (141:469)

Potentilla gracilis, Northwest Cinquefoil
Okanagan-Colville _Analgesic_ Infusion of pounded roots taken as a general tonic for pains. _Antidiarrheal_ Infusion of pounded roots taken for diarrhea. _Antirheumatic_ (_Internal_) Infusion of pounded roots taken as a general tonic for aches. _Blood Medicine_ Infusion of pounded roots taken as a blood tonic. _Dermatological Aid_ Infusion of pounded roots used to wash sores. _Venereal Aid_ Infusion of pounded roots taken for gonorrhea. (162:127) **Thompson** _Dermatological Aid_ Poultice of mashed leaves, roots, and subalpine fir pitch used on wounds, to draw out the pain. (161:263)

Potentilla hippiana var. _hippiana_, Woolly Cinquefoil
Navajo, Kayenta _Burn Dressing_ Plant used as a lotion for burns. _Dermatological Aid_ Powdered plant applied to sores caused by a bear. _Gynecological Aid_ Plant used to expedite childbirth. (179:

26) **Navajo, Ramah** *Dermatological Aid* Poultice of fresh leaves applied to injury. *Panacea* Cold infusion of root taken as "life medicine." (165:31)

Potentilla nana, Arctic Cinquefoil
Eskimo *Unspecified* Root eaten for the medicinal value. (as *P. hyparctica* 126:325)

Potentilla norvegica ssp. *monspeliensis*,
Norwegian Cinquefoil
Chippewa *Throat Aid* Decoction of root gargled or root chewed for sore throat. (as *P. monspeliensis* 43:342) **Navajo, Ramah** *Analgesic* Cold infusion of whole plant used for pain. *Venereal Aid* Fumes from plant used for sexual infection. (as *P. monspeliensis* 165:31) **Ojibwa** *Cathartic* Plant known to be a physic, even by the very young. (as *P. monspeliensis* 130:384) **Potawatomi** *Unspecified* Root used for unspecified malady. (as *P. monspeliensis* 131:77)

Potentilla pensylvanica, Pennsylvania
Cinquefoil
Navajo, Ramah *Panacea* Root used as a "life medicine." (165:31)

Potentilla recta, Sulphur Cinquefoil
Okanagan-Colville *Dermatological Aid* Poultice of pounded leaves and stems applied to open sores and wounds. *Internal Medicine* Infusion of leaves taken for all types of internal troubles. (162:127)

Potentilla simplex, Common Cinquefoil
Cherokee *Antidiarrheal* Infusion of root taken for dysentery. *Dermatological Aid* Infusion of astringent root used as a mouthwash for "thrash." *Febrifuge* Used for "fevers and acute diseases with great debility." *Oral Aid* Infusion of root used as a mouthwash for "thrash." *Pulmonary Aid* Root eaten and infusion of root used by ballplayers "for wind" and safety. (as *P. simplex* 66:29)

Prenanthes alata, Western Rattlesnakeroot
Bella Coola *Analgesic* Poultice of chewed root applied to any painful part of body. *Burn Dressing* Poultice of chewed root applied to burns. *Cold Remedy* Decoction of root taken and small dose given to babies for colds. *Pediatric Aid* Decoction

of roots taken daily and small dose given to babies for colds. (127:65)

Prenanthes alba, White Rattlesnakeroot
Chippewa *Gynecological Aid* Dried, powdered root added to food to produce postpartum milk flow. (43:360) **Iroquois** *Dermatological Aid* Poultice of roots applied to dog bites. (73:479) *Snakebite Remedy* Poultice of roots applied to rattlesnake bites. *Stimulant* Infusion of smashed roots used as wash for weakness. (73:478) **Ojibwa** *Diuretic* Milk of lettuce used, especially in female diseases, as a diuretic. *Gynecological Aid* Milk of plant used as a diuretic for female diseases and root used as a female remedy. (130:365)

Prenanthes altissima, Tall Rattlesnakeroot
Iroquois *Snakebite Remedy* Poultice of smashed roots applied to rattlesnake bites. (73:480)

Prenanthes aspera, Rough Rattlesnakeroot
Choctaw *Analgesic* Decoction of roots and plant tops used as an anodyne. *Diuretic* Decoction of roots and plant tops used as a stimulating diuretic. *Other* Plant used as a "secernant" (which induces secretion). *Stimulant* Plant used as a stimulant. (as *Nabalus asper* 23:288)

Prenanthes serpentaria, Cankerweed
Cherokee *Analgesic* Roots used in stomachache medicine. (66:35)

Prenanthes trifoliolata, Gall of the Earth
Cherokee *Analgesic* Roots used in stomachache medicine. (66:35) **Iroquois** *Dermatological Aid* Poultice of roots applied to skin swellings or bristles on a toe or foot. (73:480) *Eye Medicine* Decoction of roots used as drops for sore eyes. *Hunting Medicine* Compound infusion of root used as wash for rifles, a "deer hunting medicine." *Love Medicine* Root chewed and rubbed on hands and face as a love medicine. *Snakebite Remedy* Roots used for rattlesnake bites. (73:479)

Proboscidea althaeifolia, Devilshorn
Pima *Analgesic* and *Antirheumatic* (*External*) Plant moxa used for rheumatic pains. (as *Martynia arenaria* 38:107)

***Proboscidea parviflora* ssp. *parviflora*,**
Doubleclaw
Pima *Analgesic* and *Antirheumatic* (*External*)
Plant moxa used for rheumatic pains. (as *Martynia parviflora* 38:107)

***Prosopis glandulosa*,** Honey Mesquite
Apache, Mescalero *Eye Medicine* Juice from
leaves used for irritated eye lids. *Pediatric Aid*
and *Urinary Aid* Infusion of bark used for children
with enuresis. (10:37) **Comanche** *Gastrointestinal Aid* Leaves chewed and juice swallowed to neutralize acid stomach. (24:523) **Isleta** *Eye Medicine*
Decoction of leaves and pods without beans used
as an eye medicine. (85:39) **Keres, Western** *Eye Medicine* Leaves made into an eyewash. (147:63)

***Prosopis glandulosa* var. *torreyana*,** Western Honey Mesquite
Cahuilla *Dermatological Aid* Gum diluted with
water and used as a wash for open wounds and
sores. *Eye Medicine* Gum diluted with water and
used as a wash for sore eyes. (as *P. juliflora* var.
torreyana 11:107) **Diegueño** *Eye Medicine* Infusion of leaves used as an eyewash. *Febrifuge* Infusion of leaves taken for fevers. (as *P. juliflora* var.
torreyana 74:218)

***Prosopis pubescens*,** Screwbean Mesquite
Apache, Mescalero *Ear Medicine* Pods soaked
in water and used for earache. (as *Strombocarpa
pubescens* 10:44) **Apache, Western** *Ear Medicine* Bean placed in ear for earache. (21:178)
Cahuilla *Unspecified* Roots and bark had medicinal value. (11:118) **Paiute** *Eye Medicine* Infusion
of gummy exudate on bark used as an eyewash.
(155:123) **Pima** *Dermatological Aid* Decoction
of roots used as a wash or powdered roots applied
to sores. (as *Strombocarpa pubescens* 38:96)
Powdered root bark or decoction used to dress
wounds. (123:79) *Gynecological Aid* Infusion of
roots taken for troubles with menses. (as *Strombocarpa pubescens* 38:96) **Tewa** *Ear Medicine*
Pods twisted into the ear for an earache. (115:69)

***Prosopis velutina*,** Velvet Mesquite
Papago *Dermatological Aid* Poultice of chewed
leaves applied for red ant stings. Poultice of
chewed leaves applied to red ant stings. Poultice

of pulverized gum applied to sores and impetigo.
Poultice of pulverized plant applied to sores and
impetigo pustules. (29:65) **Pima** *Analgesic* Cold
infusion of leaves taken for headaches. Decoction
of gum held in mouth for painful gums or applied
to painful burns. *Antidiarrheal* Infusion of roots
taken for diarrhea. *Burn Dressing* Decoction of
gum applied to burns to prevent soreness. *Cathartic* Decoction of gum taken to cleanse the system.
(38:93) Decoction of inner bark taken as a cathartic. (123:79) *Dermatological Aid* Decoction of
beans used as bleach for severe sunburn. Decoction of gum applied to chapped and cracked fingers or sore lips. Poultice of dried gum applied to
prevent infection in newborn's navel. Resin used
for sores. (38:93) Decoction of black gum used as
a wash for open wounds. (123:79) *Disinfectant*
Poultice of dried gum applied to prevent infection
in newborn's navel. (38:93) *Emetic* Decoction of
inner bark taken as an emetic. (123:79) *Eye Medicine* Decoction of leaves applied as poultice to
pink eye. (38:93) Decoction of black gum used as
a wash for sore eyes. (123:79) *Gastrointestinal
Aid* Cold infusion of leaves taken for stomach troubles. *Oral Aid* Decoction of gum held in the mouth
for painful gums or sore lips. *Other* Decoction of
gum applied as a lotion for "bad disease." *Pediatric Aid* Poultice of dried gum applied to prevent
infection in newborn's navel. (38:93)

***Prunella vulgaris*,** Common Selfheal
Algonquin, Quebec *Febrifuge* Infusion of leaves
used for fevers. (14:224) **Bella Coola** *Heart Medicine* Weak decoction of roots, leaves, and blossoms taken for the heart. (127:63) **Blackfoot** *Dermatological Aid* Infusion of plant used to wash a
burst boil. Infusion of plant applied to neck sores.
(72:78) *Eye Medicine* Infusion of plant used as an
eyewash to keep the eyes moist on cold or windy
days. (72:82) *Veterinary Aid* Infusion of plant
used for saddle and back sores on horses. Infusion
of plant used as an eyewash for horses. (72:90)
Catawba *Misc. Disease Remedy* Plant used in certain diseases. (134:191) **Cherokee** *Adjuvant* Used
to flavor other medicines. *Burn Dressing* Cold infusion used as a wash for burns. *Dermatological Aid*
Infusion of root used as wash for bruises, diabetic
sores, cuts, and acne. (66:54) **Chippewa** *Cathartic* Compound decoction of root taken as a physic.

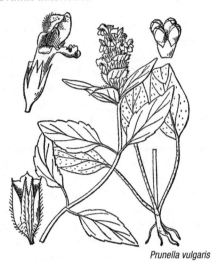

Prunella vulgaris

(43:346) **Cree**, **Hudson Bay** *Throat Aid* Plant used or herb chewed for sore throats. (78:303) **Delaware** *Febrifuge* Plant tops used to make a cooling drink and body wash for fevers. (151:37) **Delaware**, **Oklahoma** *Febrifuge* Liquid made from plant tops taken and used as a wash for fever. (150:31, 78) **Iroquois** *Analgesic* Infusion of plant taken for backaches. (73:425) *Antidiarrheal* Decoction of plants taken for diarrhea. (73:423) *Antiemetic* Decoction of plants taken for vomiting and diarrhea. *Blood Medicine* Compound decoction of roots and shoots taken as a blood purifier. (73:424) *Cold Remedy* Decoction of plants taken for colds. *Cough Medicine* Decoction of plants taken for coughs. (73:423) *Emetic* Decoction of whole plant taken as an emetic. (73:425) *Febrifuge* Decoction of plants taken for fevers and shortness of breath. (73:424) *Gastrointestinal Aid* Infusion of plants taken for stomach cramps and biliousness. (73:423) Compound infusion of roots and plants taken for upset stomachs. (73:424) Infusion of plant taken for biliousness. *Gynecological Aid* Decoction of whole plant taken to strengthen the womb. (73:425) *Hemorrhoid Remedy* Compound decoction of roots taken and used as wash for piles. (73:424) *Misc. Disease Remedy* Plant used for sugar diabetes. (73:425) *Orthopedic Aid* Compound decoction of plants used as steam bath for sore legs or stiff knees. (73:424) Infusion of plant taken for backaches. *Panacea* Infusion of plant taken for any ailment. (73:425) *Pediatric Aid* Compound infusion of plants given to babies that

cry too much. *Psychological Aid* Compound infusion of plants taken for sickness caused by grieving. *Pulmonary Aid* Decoction or infusion of roots taken for shortness of breath. *Respiratory Aid* Infusion of roots taken for heaves or shortness of breath. *Sedative* Compound infusion of plants given to babies that cry too much. *Tuberculosis Remedy* Compound decoction of roots taken for consumption. *Venereal Aid* Compound decoction of roots and shoots taken for venereal disease. (73:424) **Menominee** *Antidiarrheal* and *Pediatric Aid* Infusion of stalk used, especially good for babies, for dysentery. (44:131) **Mohegan** *Febrifuge* "Drink" made from leaves taken and used as a wash for fevers. (151:74, 130) **Ojibwa** *Gynecological Aid* Compound containing root used as a female remedy. (130:372) *Hunting Medicine* Root, sharpened the powers of observation, used to make a tea to drink before going hunting. (130: 430) **Quileute** *Dermatological Aid* Plant used for boils. **Quinault** *Dermatological Aid* Plant juice rubbed on boils. (65:45) **Salish**, **Coast** *Dermatological Aid* Leaves used for boils, cuts, bruises, and skin inflammations. (156:84) **Thompson** *Tonic* Hot or cold infusion of plant taken as a tonic for general indisposition. (141:471)

Prunus americana, American Plum
Cherokee *Cough Medicine* Bark used to make cough syrup. *Kidney Aid* Infusion of bark taken for the kidneys. *Urinary Aid* Infusion of bark taken for the bladder. (66:50) **Cheyenne** *Ceremonial Medicine* Branches used for the Sun Dance ceremony. *Oral Aid* Smashed fruits used for mouth disease. (69:35) **Chippewa** *Anthelmintic* Compound decoction of root taken for worms. (43:346) *Dermatological Aid* Compound poultice of inner bark applied to cuts and wounds. (43:352) *Disinfectant* Compound decoction of inner bark used as a disinfectant wash. (43:366) Decoction of bark used as a disinfecting wash. (43:376) **Meskwaki** *Oral Aid* Root bark used as an astringent medicine for mouth cankers. (129:242) **Mohegan** *Respiratory Aid* Infusion of twigs taken for asthma. (149:270) Infusion of twigs taken for asthma. (151:74, 130) **Ojibwa**, **South** *Antidiarrheal* Compound decoction of small rootlets taken for diarrhea. (77:200) **Omaha** *Dermatological Aid* Poultice of boiled root bark applied to skin abrasions. (58:87)

Rappahannock *Unspecified* "An ingredient of a medicine made after diagnosis." (138:31)

Prunus andersonii, Desert Peach
Paiute *Antidiarrheal* Decoction of stems, leaves, or roots taken for diarrhea. *Antirheumatic (Internal)* Weak decoction of bark taken for rheumatism. (155:123) *Cold Remedy* Infusion of branches taken for colds. (98:38) Hot infusion of leaves or decoction of branches taken for colds. *Misc. Disease Remedy* Decoction of dried bark strips taken as a winter tonic to ward off influenza. *Tonic* Decoction of dried bark strips taken as a winter tonic to ward off influenza. *Tuberculosis Remedy* Decoction of bark taken or twigs chewed for tuberculosis. (155:123)

Prunus cerasus, Sour Cherry
Cherokee *Blood Medicine* Compound used as a blood tonic. *Cold Remedy* Infusion of bark taken for colds. *Cough Medicine* Infusion of bark taken for coughs. *Dermatological Aid* Astringent root bark used in a wash for old sores and ulcers. Root bark used as a wash for old sores and ulcers. *Febrifuge* Infusion or decoction of bark used for fevers, including the "great chill." *Gastrointestinal Aid* Boiled fruit used for "blood discharged from bowels." Used in steam bath for indigestion, biliousness, and jaundice. *Gynecological Aid* Warm infusion given when labor pains begin. *Misc. Disease Remedy* Compound of barks added to corn whisky and used to break out measles. *Oral Aid* Infusion of bark used for "thrash." *Throat Aid* Decoction of inner bark used for laryngitis. (66:28, 29)

Prunus emarginata, Bitter Cherry
Bella Coola *Heart Medicine* Decoction of root and inner bark taken daily for heart trouble. (127:58) Infusion of bark used for heart trouble. *Tuberculosis Remedy* Infusion of bark used for tuberculosis. (158:209) **Cowichan** *Cold Remedy* Infusion of bark and crabapple bark used as a cure-all tonic for colds. *Panacea* Infusion of bark and crabapple bark used as a cure-all tonic for numerous ailments. (156:87) **Hoh** *Blood Medicine* Decoction of bark used as a blood remedy. (114:64) **Kwakiutl** *Cancer Treatment* Bark used to wrap lint after treating tumors. (16:383) *Dermatological Aid* Bark used to cover poultice on swellings.

(16:382) Bark ash rubbed on newborn's chest to protect against rash and sore mouth. (16:383) Bark ash rubbed on chest of baby as protection from rashes. Infusion of bark taken for eczema. (157:290) *Dietary Aid* Roots applied to nipples of mother to induce the infant to nurse. (16:386) Roots applied to the nipples of a mother to induce her infant to nurse. (157:290) *Gynecological Aid* Roots applied to nipples of mother to induce the infant to nurse. (16:386) Decoction of split roots taken for blood discharge. *Heart Medicine* Infusion of bark taken for heart trouble. (157:290) *Hemostat* Poultice of bark strips used for holding down all kinds of plasters applied to bleeding wounds. (as *P. emarginata* var. *villosa* 16:384) *Oral Aid* Bark ash rubbed on newborn's chest to protect against rash and sore mouth. Poultice of rubbed root applied to sores in child's mouth. (16:383) Bark ash rubbed on chest of baby as protection from mouth sores. Roots held in the mouth by children with canker sores. (157:290) *Pediatric Aid* Plant used as part of charm worn by children to ward off disease. (16:379) Bark ash rubbed on newborn's chest to protect against rash and sore mouth. Poultice of rubbed root applied to sores in child's mouth. (16:383) Roots applied to nipples of mother to induce the infant to nurse. (16:386) Bark ash rubbed on chest of baby as protection from rashes and mouth sores. Roots applied to the nipples of a mother to induce her infant to nurse. Roots held in the mouth by children with canker sores. (157:290) *Preventive Medicine* Plant used as part of charm worn by children to ward off disease. (16:379) *Tuberculosis Remedy* Infusion of bark taken for tuberculosis. (157:290) **Lummi** *Gynecological Aid* Bark chewed to facilitate childbirth. Infusion of rotten wood taken as a contraceptive. (65:37) **Makah** *Blood Medicine* Bark used as a blood purifier. *Laxative* Bark used as a laxative. *Tonic* Bark used as a tonic. (55:266) **Nitinaht** *Panacea* Infusion of bark taken as a general tonic for healing any sickness. (160:120) **Okanagan-Colville** *Gastrointestinal Aid* Berries eaten as a laxative for "sour stomach." (162:127) **Paiute** *Eye Medicine* Infusion of bark used as an eye medicine. (93:85) **Quileute** *Blood Medicine* Decoction of bark used as a blood remedy. (114:64) **Quinault** *Gynecological Aid* Infusion of rotten wood taken as a contraceptive. *Laxative* Decoction of bark taken as a laxative. (65:37) **Saanich** *Cold Remedy* Infusion of bark and crabapple bark used as a cure-all tonic for colds. *Panacea* Infusion of bark and crabapple bark used as a cure-all tonic for numerous ailments. *Psychological Aid* Concoction of roots and gooseberry roots used to make children intelligent and obedient. (156:87) **Skagit** *Cold Remedy* Decoction of bark taken for colds. *Gynecological Aid* Infusion of rotten wood taken as a contraceptive. **Skokomish** *Cold Remedy* Decoction of bark taken for colds. *Gynecological Aid* Infusion of rotten wood taken as a contraceptive. (65:37) **Thompson** *Orthopedic Aid* Bark used to wrap splints for broken limbs. *Unspecified* Infusion of branches taken for an unspecified illness. (161:263)

Prunus ilicifolia, Holly Leaf Cherry
Diegueño *Cough Medicine* Infusion of leaves taken as a cough medicine. (74:217) **Mahuna** *Cough Medicine* Infusion of bark or roots taken for coughs. (117:18)

Prunus nigra, Canadian Plum
Algonquin, Quebec *Cough Medicine* Infusion of inner bark taken for coughs. *Unspecified* Infusion of roots used as a medicinal tea. (14:184) **Meskwaki** *Antiemetic* Infusion of bark used to settle stomach when it will not retain food. (129:242)

Prunus pensylvanica, Pin Cherry
Algonquin, Quebec *Blood Medicine* Infusion of bark taken for blood poisoning. *Cough Medicine* Infusion of bark taken for coughs. *Disinfectant* Infusion of bark taken for infections. *Pulmonary Aid* Infusion of bark taken for bronchitis. (14:184) **Algonquin, Tête-de-Boule** *Hemostat* Poultice of boiled, shredded inner bark applied to bleeding umbilical cord. *Pediatric Aid* Poultice of boiled, shredded inner bark applied to bleeding umbilical cord. (110:130) **Cherokee** *Blood Medicine* Compound used as a blood tonic. *Cold Remedy* Infusion of bark taken for colds. *Cough Medicine* Infusion of bark taken for coughs. *Dermatological Aid* Astringent root bark used in a wash for old sores and ulcers. Root bark used as a wash for old sores and ulcers. *Febrifuge* Infusion or decoction of bark used for fevers, including the "great chill." *Gastrointestinal Aid* Boiled fruit used for "blood

discharged from bowels." Used in steam bath for indigestion, biliousness, and jaundice. *Gynecological Aid* Warm infusion given when labor pains begin. *Misc. Disease Remedy* Compound of barks added to corn whisky and used to break out measles. *Oral Aid* Infusion of bark used for "thrash." *Throat Aid* Decoction of inner bark used for laryngitis. (66:28, 29) **Cree, Woodlands** *Eye Medicine* Infusion of inner bark used for sore eyes. (91:53) **Gitksan** *Unspecified* Bark used for medicine. (61:152) **Iroquois** *Burn Dressing* Compound of roots applied as a salve to burns. (73:359) *Cough Medicine* Bark and another bark used to make cough syrup. (119:91) **Malecite** *Dermatological Aid* Outer layer of dried trees used as a powder for prickly heat. (96:250) Infusion of bark used for erysipelas. (96:256) *Pediatric Aid* Outer layer of dried trees used for chafed babies. (96:250) **Micmac** *Dermatological Aid* Wood used for chafed skin and prickly heat. *Misc. Disease Remedy* Bark used for erysipelas. (32:59) **Ojibwa** *Cough Medicine* Inner bark used as a cough remedy. (130:385) **Ojibwa, South** *Analgesic* Decoction of crushed root taken for stomach pains. *Gastrointestinal Aid* Decoction of crushed root taken for stomach disorders. (77:199) **Potawatomi** *Analgesic* and *Cough Medicine* Infusion of inner bark taken internal pain and cough. (131:77) **Wet'suwet'en** *Cough Medicine* Bark used for coughs. (61:152)

Prunus persica, Peach
Cherokee *Anthelmintic* Decoction or teaspoon of parched seed kernels taken for worms. *Antiemetic* Infusion of scraped bark taken for vomiting. *Cathartic* Infusion of any part taken as a purgative. *Dermatological Aid* Used for skin diseases and leaves wrung in cold water used to bathe swelling. *Febrifuge* Strong infusion taken for fever. *Gastrointestinal Aid* Infusion of leaves taken for sick stomach. (66:47, 48) **Delaware** *Anthelmintic* Infusion of leaves used to expel pinworms. *Antiemetic* and *Pediatric Aid* Infusion of leaves used by children for vomiting. (151:31) **Koasati** *Orthopedic Aid* Leaves rubbed on the scratches of tired legs. (152:27) **Navajo** *Cathartic* Plant used as a purgative. (45:96) Dried fruit used as a purgative. (45:54) **Rappahannock** *Kidney Aid* Infusion of fresh or dried leaves taken for kidney trouble. (138:33)

Prunus serotina, Black Cherry
Cherokee *Blood Medicine* Compound used as a blood tonic. *Cold Remedy* Infusion of bark taken for colds. *Cough Medicine* Infusion of bark taken for coughs. *Dermatological Aid* Astringent root bark used in a wash for old sores and ulcers. Root bark used as a wash for old sores and ulcers. *Febrifuge* Infusion or decoction of bark used for fevers, including the "great chill." (66:28, 29) Decoction of bark used as a wash for chills and fevers. (152:28) Infusion of bark taken for fevers. (177:74) *Gastrointestinal Aid* Boiled fruit used for "blood discharged from bowels." Used in steam bath for indigestion, biliousness, and jaundice. *Gynecological Aid* Warm infusion given when labor pains begin. (66:28, 29) Infusion of bark taken for childbirth. (152:28) *Misc. Disease Remedy* Compound of barks added to corn whisky and used to break out measles. (66:28, 29) Decoction of bark used as a wash for ague. (152:28) *Oral Aid* Infusion of bark used for "thrash." *Throat Aid* Decoction of inner bark used for laryngitis. (66:28, 29) **Chippewa** *Anthelmintic* Compound decoction of root taken for worms. (43:346) *Burn Dressing* Powder containing powdered root applied to burns. (43:354) *Dermatological Aid* Compound poultice of inner bark applied to cuts and wounds. (43:352) Poultice of fresh roots or decoction of bark used as a wash for "scrofulous neck." Powder containing powdered root applied to ulcers. (43:354) *Disinfectant* Compound decoction of inner bark used as a disinfectant wash. (43:366) *Misc. Disease Remedy* and *Pediatric Aid* Decoction of root given for "cholera infantum." (43:346) *Tuberculosis Remedy* Poultice of root applied or decoction of bark used as a wash for scrofulous, neck sores. (43:354) **Delaware** *Antidiarrheal* Bark used for diarrhea. *Cough Medicine* Fruits used to make cough syrup. *Tonic* Bark combined with other roots and used as a tonic. (151:32) **Delaware, Oklahoma** *Antidiarrheal* Bark used as a diarrhea remedy. *Cough Medicine* Fruit used to make cough syrup. *Tonic* Compound containing bark taken as a tonic. (150:27, 78) **Delaware, Ontario** *Gynecological Aid* Compound infusion of bark taken for "diseases peculiar to women." *Tonic* Compound infusion of bark taken as a tonic for general debility. (150:68, 82) **Iroquois** *Analgesic* Decoction of bark taken or poultice applied to

forehead and neck for headaches. (73:362) *Blood Medicine* Compound infusion of bark and roots taken as a blood purifier. (73:361) Infusion of roots and other roots taken by young mothers for thick blood. (118:46) *Burn Dressing* Compound of roots applied as a salve to burns. (73:362) *Cold Remedy* Infusion or decoction of bark taken or inhaled for colds or sore throats. (73:361) *Cough Medicine* Decoction of bark taken for consumption or an "old cough." (73:360) *Dermatological Aid* Compound decoction taken for "sores all over the body caused by bad blood." Compound poultice of bark applied to chancres caused by syphilis or cuts. (73:361) Compound decoction used as wash for parts affected by "Italian itch." (73:362) *Emetic* Compound decoction of plants taken to vomit for sleepiness and weakness. (73:361) *Febrifuge* Decoction of bark taken for colds and fever. (73:360) *Gynecological Aid* Compound decoction taken when a woman has a miscarriage. (73:361) *Liver Aid* Decoction of bark taken for too much gall. *Pediatric Aid* Decoction of bark used as a steam bath for babies with bronchitis. *Pulmonary Aid* Decoction of bark taken for soreness and lung inflammation. *Respiratory Aid* Decoction of bark used as a steam bath for babies with bronchitis. (73:360) *Stimulant* Compound decoction of plants taken to vomit for sleepiness and weakness. *Throat Aid* Infusion of bark taken for colds and sore throats. (73:361) *Tuberculosis Remedy* Decoction of bark or roots taken for consumption or for an "old cough." (73:360) *Venereal Aid* Compound poultice of bark applied to chancres caused by syphilis. (73:361) **Mahuna** *Cough Medicine* Infusion of bark or roots taken for coughs. (117:18) **Malecite** *Cold Remedy* Infusion of bark, "beaver castor," and gin used for colds. Castor or castorecum is a strong-smelling, brown, concrete substance from the preputial follicles of the beaver, *Castor fiber*. It has long been used in medicine as a stimulant and antispasmodic, and also in the manufacture of perfume. *Cough Medicine* Infusion of bark, beaver castor, and gin used for coughs. *Tuberculosis Remedy* Infusion of bark, beaver castor, and gin used by men for consumption. (96:249) **Micmac** *Cold Remedy* Bark used for colds. *Cough Medicine* Bark used for coughs. *Misc. Disease Remedy* Bark used for smallpox. *Tonic* Fruit used as a tonic. *Tuberculosis Remedy*

Bark used for consumption. (32:60) **Mohegan** *Antidiarrheal* Ripe fruit fermented 1 year and used for dysentery. (149:264) Liquid from fermented fruit taken for dysentery. (151:74, 130) *Cold Remedy* Compound infusion of leaves and boneset taken with molasses for colds. Infusion of buds, leaves, or bark taken with sugar for colds. (25:118) Compound infusion taken, hot at night and cold in the morning, for colds. (149:264) Compound infusion of bark taken for colds. (151:74, 13) *Gastrointestinal Aid* Fruit put in a bottle and allowed to stand, then taken for stomach trouble. (25:118) *Tonic* Complex compound infusion including wild cherry bark taken as spring tonic. (149:266) **Narraganset** *Cold Remedy* Infusion of buds, leaves, or bark taken with sugar for colds. (25:118) **Ojibwa** *Cold Remedy* Infusion of bark used for colds. *Cough Medicine* Infusion of bark used for coughs. (130:385) **Ojibwa, South** *Analgesic* Infusion of inner bark taken for chest pain and soreness. *Dermatological Aid* Poultice of boiled, bruised, or chewed inner bark applied to sores. *Pulmonary Aid* Infusion of inner bark taken for chest pain and soreness. (77:199) **Penobscot** *Cough Medicine* Infusion of bark taken for coughs. *Tonic* Infusion of berries taken as a "fine bitter tonic." (133:310) **Potawatomi** *Adjuvant* Inner bark used as a seasoner for medicines. (131:77) **Rappahannock** *Cold Remedy* Infusion of buds, leaves, or bark taken with sugar for colds. (25:118) *Cough Medicine* Infusion of bark or berries with honey used for coughs, if stale it is poisonous. *Dietary Aid* Infusion of fresh or dried bark taken as an appetizer. *Poison* Infusion of bark or berries with honey used for coughs, if stale it is poisonous. *Tonic* Infusion of fresh or dried bark taken as a tonic. (138:26) **Shinnecock** *Cold Remedy* Compound infusion of leaves and boneset taken with molasses for colds. Infusion of buds, leaves, or bark taken with sugar for colds. *Gastrointestinal Aid* Fruit put in a bottle and allowed to stand, then taken for stomach trouble. (25:118)

Prunus virginiana, Common Chokecherry **Algonquin, Quebec** *Cough Medicine* Infusion of bark and sweet flag taken for coughs. (14:185) **Blackfoot** *Antidiarrheal* Berry juice used for diarrhea. *Cathartic* Infusion of cambium and saskatoon taken as a purge. *Pediatric Aid* Infusion of cambium and saskatoon taken by nursing mothers to pass medicinal qualities to baby. *Throat Aid* Berry juice used for sore throats. (72:68) **Cherokee** *Blood Medicine* Compound used as a blood tonic. *Cold Remedy* Infusion of bark taken for colds. *Cough Medicine* Infusion of bark taken for coughs. *Dermatological Aid* Astringent root bark used in a wash for old sores and ulcers. Root bark used as a wash for old sores and ulcers. *Febrifuge* Infusion or decoction of bark used for fevers, including the "great chill." (66:28, 29) Decoction of bark used as a wash for chills and fevers. (152:28) *Gastrointestinal Aid* Boiled fruit used for "blood discharged from bowels." Used in steam bath for indigestion, biliousness, and jaundice. *Gynecological Aid* Warm infusion given when labor pains begin. *Misc. Disease Remedy* Compound of barks added to corn whisky and used to break out measles. (66:28, 29) Decoction of bark used as a wash for ague. (152:28) *Oral Aid* Infusion of bark used for "thrash." *Throat Aid* Decoction of inner bark used for laryngitis. (66:28, 29) Decoction of inner bark taken to loosen phlegm for hoarseness. (152: 28) **Cheyenne** *Antidiarrheal* Unripened berries pulverized and used for diarrhea. (68:42) Unripened fruits eaten by children for diarrhea. *Dietary Aid* and *Pediatric Aid* Dried, smashed, ripe berries given to children with loss of appetite. Unripened fruits eaten by children for diarrhea. *Unspecified* Dried, smashed, ripe berries used as an ingredient for medicines. (69:35) **Chippewa** *Analgesic* Decoction of inner bark taken for cramps. (43:344)

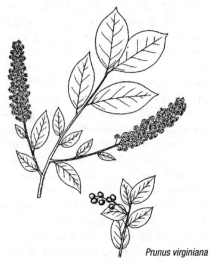

Prunus virginiana

Antihemorrhagic Compound infusion of inner bark taken for hemorrhages from the lungs. (43:340) *Blood Medicine* Compound decoction of inner bark used as cathartic blood cleanser for scrofula. *Cathartic* Compound decoction of bark used as a blood-cleansing cathartic for scrofula sores. (43:354) *Dermatological Aid* Decoction of bark used as a wash to strengthen the hair and make it grow. (43:350) *Disinfectant* Compound decoction of inner bark used as a disinfectant wash. (43:366) *Gastrointestinal Aid* Decoction of inner bark taken for stomach cramps. (43:344) *Pulmonary Aid* Compound infusion of inner bark taken for lung hemorrhage. (43:340) *Throat Aid* Decoction of inner bark gargled for sore throat. (43:342) *Tuberculosis Remedy* Compound decoction of bark used as a blood-cleansing cathartic for scrofula sores. Compound decoction of inner bark used as cathartic blood cleanser for scrofula. (43:354) **Cree**, **Hudson Bay** *Antidiarrheal* Decoction of fresh bark taken for diarrhea. (78:303) **Cree**, **Woodlands** *Antidiarrheal* Decoction of roots taken for diarrhea. (91:53) **Crow** *Antidiarrheal* Infusion of bark used for diarrhea and dysentery. *Burn Dressing* Infusion of bark used for cleansing burns. *Dermatological Aid* Infusion of bark used for cleansing sores. **Flathead** *Anthelmintic* Infusion used for intestinal worms. *Antidiarrheal* Infusion of bark used for diarrhea and dysentery. *Eye Medicine* Bark resin warmed, strained, cooled, and used for sore eyes. **Gros Ventre** *Antidiarrheal* Infusion of bark used for diarrhea and dysentery. (68:42) **Iroquois** *Antidiarrheal* Bark used for diarrhea. *Antihemorrhagic* Stalk used for hemorrhages. *Blood Medicine* Stalk used as a blood purifier. (73:359) *Cough Medicine* Decoction of plant taken as a cough syrup. (73:360) *Dermatological Aid* Inner bark used for wounds. (73:359) *Gynecological Aid* Compound decoction of stalks taken to prevent hemorrhage after childbirth. *Misc. Disease Remedy* Compound decoction of plants and bark taken for cholera. (73:360) *Pediatric Aid* Stalk used for pre-natal care. *Tuberculosis Remedy* Compound decoction of roots taken for consumption. *Veterinary Aid* Decoction of branches, leaves, and berries given to horses for diarrhea. (73:359) **Kutenai** *Antidiarrheal* Infusion of bark used for diarrhea and dysentery. (68:42) **Menominee** *Antidiar-*

rheal Infusion of inner bark or decoction of berries taken for diarrhea. *Dermatological Aid* Poultice of pounded inner bark applied to man or beast for wounds or galls. *Pediatric Aid* Sweetened infusion of inner bark given to children for diarrhea. *Veterinary Aid* Poultice of inner bark applied to heal a wound or gall on humans or beasts. (128:49, 50) **Meskwaki** *Dermatological Aid* Decoction of bark used as an astringent and spoken of as "a puckering." *Gastrointestinal Aid* Infusion of root bark used for stomach troubles and as a sedative. *Hemorrhoid Remedy* Decoction of root bark used as an astringent, rectal douche for piles. *Sedative* Infusion of root bark used as a sedative and for stomach trouble. (129:242) **Micmac** *Antidiarrheal* Bark used for diarrhea. (32:60) **Navajo**, **Ramah** *Analgesic* Cold infusion of dried fruit taken for stomachache. *Ceremonial Medicine* and *Emetic* Leaves used as an emetic in various ceremonies. *Gastrointestinal Aid* Cold infusion of dried fruit taken for stomachache. *Panacea* Dried fruit used as "life medicine." (165:31) **Ojibwa** *Pulmonary Aid* Infusion of inner bark taken for lung trouble. (130:385) **Ojibwa**, **South** *Gynecological Aid* "Branchlets" used in unspecified manner during gestation. (77:199) **Okanagan-Colville** *Antidiarrheal* Decoction of wood, branches and bark taken for diarrhea. *Cold Remedy* Decoction of wood, branches, and bark taken for colds. *Cough Medicine* Decoction of wood, branches, and bark taken for coughs. *Dermatological Aid* Poultice of wood scraped until pasty and applied to woman's stomach to eliminate the "stretch marks." *Gastrointestinal Aid* Mashed seeds taken as a stomach medicine. *Tonic* Decoction of branches and red willow roots used as a general tonic for any type of sickness. (162:127) **Penobscot** *Antidiarrheal* Infusion of bark taken for diarrhea. (133:310) **Potawatomi** *Eye Medicine* Bark used in an eyewash and berries used to make tonic drink. *Tonic* Berries used to make tonic drink and bark used in an eyewash. (131:77, 78) **Sanpoil** *Antidiarrheal* Decoction of bark taken for diarrhea. (109:221) **Thompson** *Antidiarrheal* Decoction of twigs taken for diarrhea. *Cold Remedy* Decoction of broken sticks taken for colds. Decoction of branches, sometimes with red willow branches and wild rose roots, taken for colds. *Cough Medicine* Decoction of branches, sometimes with red willow branches and wild rose roots, taken for coughs. *Laxative* Decoction of branches, sometimes with red willow branches and wild rose roots, taken as a laxative. *Misc. Disease Remedy* Decoction of branches, sometimes with red willow branches and wild rose roots, taken for influenza. *Unspecified* Decoction of broken sticks taken for a sick feeling. (161:264)

Prunus virginiana* var. *demissa, Western Chokecherry
Atsugewi *Dermatological Aid* Poultice of leaves applied to cuts, sores, bruises, and black eyes. Decoction of bark used for bathing wounds. (as *P. demissa* 50:140) **Blackfoot** *Unspecified* Decoction of bark and roots of western sweet cicely, northern valerian, and horehound taken internally. (as *P. demissa* 95:277) **Gosiute** *Blood Medicine* Decoction of bark used as a blood medicine for nose hemorrhages. (as *P. demissa* 31:378) *Gastrointestinal Aid* Decoction of wood scrapings used by children and adults for bowel troubles. (as *P. demissa* 31:350) *Hemostat* Decoction of bark used as a blood medicine for nose hemorrhages. (as *P. demissa* 31:378) *Pediatric Aid* Decoction of wood scrapings used by children and adults for bowel troubles. (as *P. demissa* 31:350) **Haisla & Hanaksiala** *Oral Aid* Poultice of mashed leaves applied to oral abscesses. (35:273) **Karok** *Cold Remedy* and *Pediatric Aid* Bark scrapings placed beside the nose of babies for colds. (as *P. demissa* 125:384) **Kawaiisu** *Laxative* Ripe berries had a laxative effect. (as *P. demissa* 180:54) **Mendocino Indian** *Antidiarrheal* Inner bark used for diarrhea. *Sedative* Inner bark used for nervous excitability. *Tonic* Inner bark used in a tonic. (as *Cerasus demissa* 33:356) **Menominee** *Pulmonary Aid* Decoction of inner bark used for lung trouble. (as *P. demissa* 44:130) **Oregon Indian** *Antidiarrheal* Pounded, dried cherries mixed with dry salmon and sugar and used for dysentery. (as *P. demissa* 98:42) **Paiute** *Analgesic* Dried, pulverized bark smoked for headache or head cold. *Cold Remedy* Decoction of peeled bark or root taken for colds and bark smoked for head colds. *Cough Medicine* Decoction of peeled bark or root taken for coughs and colds. *Dermatological Aid* Pulverized, dried bark used as a drying powder on sores. *Eye Medicine* and *Herbal Steam* Steam from boiling bark

allowed to rise into the eyes for snow-blindness. *Tuberculosis Remedy* Decoction of leaves, bark, or roots taken for tuberculosis. **Shoshoni** *Antiemetic* Decoction of bark taken for indigestion or upset stomach. *Eye Medicine* Steam from boiling bark allowed to rise into the eyes for snow-blindness. *Gastrointestinal Aid* Decoction of bark taken for indigestion or upset stomach. *Herbal Steam* Steam from boiling bark allowed to rise into the eyes for snow-blindness. (155:123, 124) **Sioux** *Adjuvant* Wood used to make "medicine-spoons" for use in ceremonial dog feasts. *Antidiarrheal* Infusion of bark used for dysentery. *Ceremonial Medicine* Wood used to make "medicine-spoons" for use in ceremonial dog feasts. *Hemostat* Dried roots chewed and placed in bleeding wounds. (as *P. demissa* 15:19) **Thompson** *Gynecological Aid* Decoction of bark taken after childbirth as a strengthening tonic. *Tonic* Decoction of bark taken as a tonic. (as *P. demissa* 141:477)

Prunus virginiana* var. *melanocarpa, Black Chokecherry
Keres, Western *Cough Medicine* Bark made into a cough medicine. (as *P. melanocarpa* 147:63) **Navajo** *Unspecified* Fruit and seeds ground raw, patted into a cake, sun dried, and used for medicinal purposes. (as *P. melanocarpa* 142:222) **Sanpoil & Nespelem** *Unspecified* Decoction of branches taken as medicine. (109:104)

Prunus virginiana* var. *virginiana, Chokecherry
Dakota *Ceremonial Medicine* Fruit prepared in unspecified way and used in old-time ceremonies. **Omaha** *Ceremonial Medicine* Fruit prepared in unspecified way and used in old-time ceremonies. **Pawnee** *Ceremonial Medicine* Fruit prepared in unspecified way and used in old-time ceremonies. **Ponca** *Antidiarrheal* Infusion of fruit or decoction of bark taken for diarrhea. *Ceremonial Medicine* Fruit prepared in unspecified way and used in old-time ceremonies. **Winnebago** *Ceremonial Medicine* Fruit prepared in unspecified way and used in old-time ceremonies. (as *Padus nana* 58:88, 89)

Psathyrotes annua, Annual Psathyrotes
Paiute *Eye Medicine* Decoction of dried plant used as an eyewash. *Toothache Remedy* Dried

leaves chewed for toothache. **Shoshoni** *Gastrointestinal Aid* and *Pediatric Aid* Decoction of entire plant used for stomachaches, especially children's. *Urinary Aid* Decoction of whole plant taken for urinary troubles. (155:124)

Psathyrotes pilifera, Hairybeast Turtleback
Navajo, Kayenta *Ceremonial Medicine* Plant used as a ceremonial emetic. *Dermatological Aid* Plant used as a lotion for chilblains. *Emetic* Plant used as a ceremonial emetic. (179:49)

Psathyrotes ramosissima, Velvet Turtleback
Paiute *Analgesic* Decoction of plant used as a head wash for headaches. *Antidiarrheal* Decoction of plant taken for diarrhea. *Cathartic* Decoction of plant taken as a physic. *Dermatological Aid* Compound poultice of crushed plants applied to draw boils and imbedded slivers. Compound poultice of plant applied to sores, cuts, swellings, and insect bites. *Emetic* Decoction of plant taken as an emetic. *Gastrointestinal Aid* Decoction of plant taken for stomachaches, bowel disorders, and biliousness. *Laxative* Decoction of plant taken for constipation. *Liver Aid* Decoction of plant taken for liver trouble. *Snakebite Remedy* Poultice of crushed, green plant or moistened dried plant used on snakebites. (155:125, 126) *Toothache Remedy* Dry bits chewed for toothache. (98:45) *Venereal Aid* Decoction of plant taken for venereal diseases. **Shoshoni** *Analgesic* Decoction of plant used as a head wash for headaches. *Antidiarrheal* Decoction of plant taken for diarrhea. *Cathartic* Decoction of plant taken as a physic. *Cough Medicine* Decoction of plant taken for tubercular cough. *Dermatological Aid* Compound poultice of crushed plants applied to draw boils and imbedded slivers. Compound poultice of plant applied to sores, cuts, swellings, and insect bites. *Emetic* Decoction of plant taken as an emetic. *Gastrointestinal Aid* Decoction of plant taken for stomachaches, bowel disorders, and biliousness. *Laxative* Decoction of plant taken for constipation. *Liver Aid* Decoction of plant taken for liver trouble. *Snakebite Remedy* Poultice of crushed, green plant applied to snakebites. *Tuberculosis Remedy* Decoction of plant taken for tubercular cough. *Venereal Aid* Decoction of plant taken for venereal diseases. (155:125, 126)

Pseudocymopterus montanus, Alpine False Springparsley
Navajo, Kayenta *Ceremonial Medicine* and *Emetic* Plant used as a ceremonial emetic. (179:35) **Navajo, Ramah** *Ceremonial Medicine* and *Emetic* Whole plant used as a ceremonial emetic. *Gastrointestinal Aid* Infusion or decoction taken after swallowing an ant. (165:38)

Pseudoroegneria spicata* ssp. *spicata, Bluebunch Wheatgrass
Okanagan-Colville *Antirheumatic (External)* Decoction of leaves used for bathing sore, swollen, crippled, or paralyzed limbs caused by arthritis. (as *Agropyron spicatum* 162:53)

Pseudostellaria jamesiana, Tuber Starwort
Navajo, Kayenta *Ceremonial Medicine* Plant chewed for corral dance. *Dermatological Aid* Poultice of plant applied to hailstone injuries. (as *Stellaria jamesiana* 179:22)

Pseudotsuga menziesii, Douglas Fir
Apache, White Mountain *Cough Medicine* Pitch used for coughs. (as *P. mucronata* 113:159) **Haisla** *Unspecified* Poultice of pitch and roasted, pounded frogs applied for unspecified serious illness. **Hanaksiala** *Gastrointestinal Aid* Infusion of green bark taken for bleeding bowels and stomach troubles. *Gynecological Aid* Infusion of green bark taken for excessive menstruation. *Throat Aid* Pitch chewed for sore throats. (35:179) **Havasupai** *Unspecified* Leaves boiled and used as medicine. (171:206) **Isleta** *Antirheumatic (External)* Infusion of leaves used for rheumatism. *Orthopedic Aid* Infusion of leaves used for paralysis. (as *P. mucronata* 85:41) **Karok** *Cold Remedy* Infusion of young sprouts used for colds. (5:48) **Kwakiutl** *Antidiarrheal* Cold, compound infusion of burned, pulverized bark taken for diarrhea. *Dermatological Aid* Poultice of bark, oil, down, and skunk cabbage leaf applied to carbuncles. *Unspecified* Pitch used as a "good medicine." (157:270) **Montana Indian** *Antirheumatic (External)* Leaves used in the sweat bath for rheumatism. *Venereal Aid* Decoction of spring buds used for certain venereal diseases. (as *P. mucronata* 15:20) **Okanagon** *Antirheumatic (External)* Moxa of ashes or ash and fat salve used for rheumatism. *Kidney Aid*

Decoction of twigs or shoots taken as a kidney remedy. *Urinary Aid* Decoction of twigs or shoots taken as a bladder remedy. (as *P. douglassii* 104:42) **Pomo**, **Little Lakes** *Antirheumatic (External)* and *Herbal Steam* Leaves used as a sweat bath for rheumatism. *Venereal Aid* Decoction of buds used for venereal disease. (as *P. mucronata* 33:309) **Thompson** *Antirheumatic (External)* Moxa of ashes or ash and fat salve used for rheumatism. (as *P. douglassii* 104:42) Heated branches or moxa of bough tips and needles used for rheumatism. (as *P. mucronata* 141:475) *Cold Remedy* Infusion of plant top used for colds. (161:107) *Dermatological Aid* Twig ashes mixed with grease and used as a general ointment or salve. (as *P. mucronata* 141:475) Shoots used in the tips of moccasins to keep the feet from perspiring and to prevent athlete's foot. Poultice of pitch used for cuts, boils, and other skin ailments. (161:107) *Disinfectant* Decoction of branches and twigs used as a purifying body wash in sweat house. (as *P. mucronata* 141:505) *Diuretic* Decoction of twigs taken as a diuretic. (as *P. mucronata* 141:475) *Kidney Aid* Decoction of twigs or shoots taken as a kidney remedy. (as *P. douglassii* 104:42) *Oral Aid* Peeled plant tops chewed, especially by young people at puberty, as a mouth freshener. *Orthopedic Aid* Poultice of pitch used for injured or dislocated bones. (161:107) *Tonic* Decoction of young twigs and leaves used for the tonic properties. (as *P. mucronata* 141:494) *Urinary Aid* Decoction of twigs or shoots taken as a bladder remedy. (as *P. douglassii* 104:42)

Pseudotsuga menziesii var. *glauca*, Rocky Mountain Douglas Fir

Okanagan-Colville *Blood Medicine* Decoction of first-year-growth shoots taken as an emetic for anemia. *Dermatological Aid* Infusion of boughs with other plants taken and used to wash the skin and hair during sweat baths. Decoction of bark used for allergies caused by touching water hemlock. *Emetic* Decoction of first-year-growth shoots taken as an emetic for high fevers and anemia. *Febrifuge* Decoction of first-year-growth shoots taken as an emetic for high fevers. (162:34)

Pseudotsuga menziesii var. *menziesii*, Douglas Fir

Bella Coola *Analgesic* Gum mixed with dogfish oil and taken as emetic and purgative for intestinal pains. *Antidiarrheal* Gum mixed with dogfish oil and taken as emetic and purgative for diarrhea. *Antirheumatic (Internal)* Gum mixed with dogfish oil and taken as emetic and purgative for rheumatism. *Cathartic* Gum and dogfish oil taken as a purgative for many ailments. *Cold Remedy* Gum mixed with dogfish oil and taken as emetic and purgative for colds. *Diuretic* Decoction of gum taken warm as a diuretic for gonorrhea. *Emetic* Gum and dogfish oil taken as an emetic for many ailments. *Gastrointestinal Aid* Gum mixed with dogfish oil and taken as emetic and purgative for intestinal pains. *Laxative* Gum mixed with dogfish oil and taken as emetic and purgative for constipation. *Venereal Aid* Decoction of gum taken warm as a diuretic for gonorrhea. Gum mixed with dogfish oil and taken as emetic and purgative for gonorrhea. (as *P. taxifolia* 127:51) **Cowlitz** *Cold Remedy* Decoction of plant taken as a cold medicine. *Dermatological Aid* Poultice of pitch applied to sores. (as *P. taxifolia* 65:19) **Karok** *Disinfectant* Boughs used as an antiseptic. *Herbal Steam* Plant used as sweat house fuel. (as *P. taxifolia* 125:379) **Navajo**, **Kayenta** *Analgesic* Plant used for headaches. *Disinfectant* Plant used for fumigation. *Gastrointestinal Aid* Plant used for stomach disease. (as *P. taxifolia* 179:15) **Navajo**, **Ramah** *Ceremonial Medicine* Needles used as a ceremonial emetic. *Emetic* Needles used as a ceremonial emetic. (as *P. taxifolia* 165:14) **Quinault** *Dermatological Aid* Poultice of pitch applied to sores. **Skagit** *Dermatological Aid* Poultice of pitch applied to sores. *Disinfectant* Decoction of bark used as an antiseptic for infections. **Squaxin** *Cold Remedy* Decoction of plant taken as a cold medicine. **Swinomish** *Analgesic* Decoction of needles applied as poultice to the chest to draw out the pain. *Cold Remedy* Decoction of root bark taken for colds. *Oral Aid* Bud tips chewed for mouth sores. *Throat Aid* Bud tips chewed for sore throats. *Tonic* Decoction of needles taken as a general tonic. (as *P. taxifolia* 65:19)

Psidium guajava, Guava

Hawaiian *Antidiarrheal* Buds chewed by mothers

and given to infants for diarrhea. Buds chewed for diarrhea. *Antihemorrhagic* Infusion of pounded roots and other plants strained and taken for bowel or intestinal hemorrhage. *Dermatological Aid* Buds and other plants pounded and resulting liquid applied to deep cuts. *Orthopedic Aid* Buds and other plants pounded and resulting liquid applied to sprains. *Pediatric Aid* Buds chewed by mothers and given to infants for diarrhea. (as *P. guayava* 2:55)

Psilostrophe sparsiflora, Greenstem Paper-flower

Hopi *Adjuvant* Plant used with other plants to make medicine stronger. (34:354) **Navajo, Kayenta** *Antidiarrheal* Plant used as a diarrhea medicine. *Blood Medicine* Plant used as a postpartum blood purifier. *Dermatological Aid* Poultice of plant applied to wounds. *Gynecological Aid* Plant used as a postpartum blood purifier. *Panacea* Plant used as a life medicine. (179:49)

Psilostrophe tagetina, Woolly Paperflower

Navajo, Ramah *Analgesic* Strong infusion taken for stomachache or as a cathartic. *Cathartic* Strong infusion of plant taken as a cathartic. *Ceremonial Medicine* Cold infusion of leaves used as ceremonial eyewash. *Dermatological Aid* Infusion of plant used as lotion for itching. *Eye Medicine* Cold infusion of leaves used as ceremonial eyewash. *Gastrointestinal Aid* Strong infusion of plant taken for stomachache. *Throat Aid* Cold infusion gargled or poultice of leaves applied for sore throat. (165:52) **Zuni** *Snakebite Remedy* Compound poultice of root applied with much ceremony to rattlesnake bite. (143:53)

Psoralidium lanceolatum, Lemon Scurfpea

Arapaho *Analgesic* Snuff of leaves and sneeze-weed blossoms inhaled for headaches. Infusion of leaves used on the head for headaches. *Dermatological Aid* Oily leaves rubbed on the skin for dryness. (100:48) *Throat Aid* Fresh leaves chewed for sore throat and voice. (98:38) Root chewed for hoarseness. (100:48) **Cheyenne** *Ceremonial Medicine* Plant used for certain ceremonies. (63:178) **Navajo, Kayenta** *Dermatological Aid* Plant used as a lotion and poultice of plant applied to itch and sores. (179:29) **Navajo, Ramah** *Anal-*

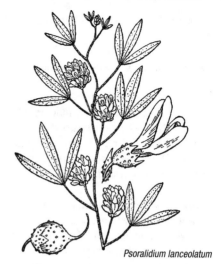

Psoralidium lanceolatum

gesic Cold infusion of plant taken for stomachache and menstrual pain. *Ceremonial Medicine* Cold infusion of plant used as ceremonial chant lotion. *Gastrointestinal Aid* Cold infusion of plant taken for stomachache. *Gynecological Aid* Cold infusion of plant taken for menstrual cramps. *Venereal Aid* Compound decoction of root used for venereal disease. *Witchcraft Medicine* Cold infusion of plant used as a lotion for protection from witches. (165:34) **Zuni** *Gastrointestinal Aid* Fresh flower eaten for stomachaches. (22:376)

Psoralidium tenuiflorum, Slimflower Scurfpea

Dakota *Tuberculosis Remedy* Decoction of plants taken for consumption. (as *Psoralea floribunda* 57:366) Compound decoction of root taken for consumption. (58:93) **Lakota** *Analgesic* Infusion of roots used for headaches. (116:48) **Navajo, Ramah** *Misc. Disease Remedy* Infusion of plant taken or leaves smoked for influenza. *Veterinary Aid* Plant used several ways for sheep with coughs. (165:34) **Zuni** *Disinfectant* Poultice of moistened leaves applied to any body part for purification. (143:58)

Psorothamnus fremontii var. **fremontii**, Frémont's Dalea

Paiute *Antihemorrhagic* Decoction of root or plant tops taken for internal hemorrhages. **Shoshoni** *Gastrointestinal Aid* Decoction of roots taken for stomach trouble. (as *Dalea fremontii* 155:64)

Psorothamnus polydenius, Nevada Smokebush

Paiute, Northern *Cathartic* Infusion of bark taken as a physic. *Cold Remedy* Infusion of bark taken for light colds. *Misc. Disease Remedy* Decoction of brush taken for the flu. *Pulmonary Aid* Decoction of brush taken for pneumonia. *Throat Aid* Decoction of brush taken for sore throats. (49:126)

Psorothamnus polydenius var. *polydenius*, Nevada Smokebush

Paiute *Analgesic* Decoction of stem taken for muscular pain and stem chewed for facial neuralgia. Decoction of stems taken for stomachaches. *Antidiarrheal* Strong infusion of plant taken for diarrhea. *Antirheumatic* (*External*) Hot decoction of plant used as a wash for rheumatism. *Cold Remedy* Plant used in a variety of ways for colds. *Cough Medicine* Plant used in a variety of ways for coughs. *Dermatological Aid* Powdered, dried stems or crushed fresh stems used for sores. *Disinfectant* Simple or compound decoction of stems and tops used as an antiseptic bath for measles. Simple or compound decoction of stems and tops used as an antiseptic bath for smallpox. *Diuretic* Decoction of plant tops taken to induce urination. *Gastrointestinal Aid* Decoction of plant taken for stomachaches. *Kidney Aid* Compound decoction of stems and tops taken for kidney ailments. *Misc. Disease Remedy* Decoction of plant taken and used as an antiseptic wash for measles. Decoction of plant used as an antiseptic wash for smallpox. Decoction of stems taken for influenza. *Orthopedic Aid* Infusion of plant taken for muscular pains. *Pulmonary Aid* Plant used in several ways for pneumonia. Sweetened decoction of stems taken for whooping cough. *Toothache Remedy* Stems chewed for toothache or face neuralgia. *Tuberculosis Remedy* Plant used in several ways for tuberculosis. *Venereal Aid* Decoction of plant taken for venereal diseases. **Shoshoni** *Analgesic* Decoction of plant tops taken for pains in the back over the kidneys. Decoction of stems taken for stomachaches. *Antidiarrheal* Strong infusion of plant taken for diarrhea. *Cold Remedy* Plant used in a variety of ways for colds. *Cough Medicine* Plant used in a variety

of ways for coughs. *Disinfectant* Simple or compound decoction of stems and tops used as an antiseptic bath for smallpox. *Gastrointestinal Aid* Decoction of plant taken for stomachaches. *Kidney Aid* Simple or compound decoction of plant tops used for kidney pain and urine incontinence. *Misc. Disease Remedy* Decoction of stems taken for influenza. Simple or compound decoction of plant taken and used as a wash for smallpox. *Pulmonary Aid* Plant used in several ways for pneumonia. *Tuberculosis Remedy* Plant used in several ways for tuberculosis. *Urinary Aid* Decoction of plant tops taken for kidney pain and urine incontinence. *Venereal Aid* Decoction of plant taken for venereal diseases. (as *Dalea polyadenia* 155:64–66)

Psorothamnus scoparius, Broom Dalea

Keres, Western *Dermatological Aid* Infusion of plant rubbed on spider bites. *Emetic* Infusion of plant used as an emetic. *Gastrointestinal Aid* Infusion of plant used for stomach trouble. (as *Parosela scoparia* 147:57)

Ptelea trifoliata, Common Hoptree

Menominee *Adjuvant* Root bark used as a seasoner and to render other medicines potent. *Panacea* Root considered a sacred medicine and credited with all sorts of cures. (128:51) **Meskwaki** *Adjuvant* Root often added to other medicines to make them potent. *Pulmonary Aid* Compound infusion of pounded root used for lung troubles, a good medicine. (129:244)

Ptelea trifoliata ssp. *pallida* var. *pallida*, Pallid Hoptree

Havasupai *Gastrointestinal Aid* and *Pediatric Aid* Decoction of leaves rubbed on a child's abdomen for stomachaches. *Poison* Leaves made into poison and used on arrow tips for hunting large game and in warfare. (as *P. pallida* 171:229)

Pteridium aquilinum, Western Brackenfern

Alaska Native *Poison* Full grown fronds poisonous to cattle. (71:51) **Cherokee** *Antiemetic* Root used as a tonic and antiemetic and given for "cholera-morbus." *Disinfectant* Root used as an antiseptic. *Misc. Disease Remedy* Root used as a tonic, antiseptic, antiemetic, and for "cholera-morbus." *Tonic* Root used as a tonic. (66:33) **Costanoan**

Dermatological Aid Decoction of root used as hair rinse or roots rubbed on scalp for hair growth. (17:5) **Hesquiat** *Cancer Treatment* Young shoots eaten as medicine for "troubles with one's insides," such as cancer of the womb. (159:32) **Iroquois** *Antidiarrheal* Decoction taken for diarrhea. *Antirheumatic* (*Internal*) Compound used for rheumatism. *Blood Medicine* Cold, compound decoction of roots taken for weak blood. *Gynecological Aid* Compound decoction taken for prolapse of uterus. Decoction taken when suffering after birth. Decoction used to make "good blood" after menses, taken after baby's birth. *Liver Aid* Used as a liver and rheumatism medicine. *Tuberculosis Remedy* Compound decoction taken during the early stages of consumption. Decoction of plant taken by women for tuberculosis. *Urinary Aid* Compound decoction taken by men to retain urine. *Venereal Aid* Compound used for infection, probably venereal disease. *Witchcraft Medicine* Ingredients placed in coffin with root shaped into a person and the person dies in 10 days. (73:259) **Koasati** *Analgesic* Decoction of ground roots taken for chest pain. (152:4) **Mendocino Indian** *Veterinary Aid* Plant used as a diuretic for horses. (33:304) **Menominee** *Gynecological Aid* Decoction of root taken for "caked breast" and a dog whisker used to pierce teat. (as *Pteris aquilina* 128:48) **Micmac** *Pediatric Aid* and *Stimulant* Fronds of plant used for weak babies and old people. (as *Pteris aquilina* 32:60) **Montagnais** *Orthopedic Aid* Fronds used as a bed to strengthen babies' backs and old people. *Pediatric Aid* Fronds used as a bed to strengthen babies' backs. (as *Pteris aquilina* 133:315) **Ojibwa** *Analgesic* Infusion of root taken by women to allay stomach cramps. Smoke from dried leaves on coals used for headaches. *Gynecological Aid* Infusion of root taken by women to allay stomach cramps. (as *Pteris aquilina* 130:382) **Okanagan-Colville** *Poison* Fronds considered poisonous when mature and known to contain carcinogenic substances. (162:18) **Thompson** *Antihemorrhagic* Infusion of rhizomes taken for vomiting blood, possibly from internal injuries. *Antirheumatic* (*External*) Leaves used in a steam bath for arthritis. The leaves were placed over red-hot rocks in a steaming pit, a little water was added, and the person laid on top of the fronds. *Cold Remedy* Decoction of rhizomes taken for colds.

Dermatological Aid Poultice of pounded fronds and leaves applied to sores of any type. Fronds, pounded with a rock, mixed with leaves and melted pine pitch, strained, and applied to sores from one to several days. *Dietary Aid* Decoction of rhizomes taken for lack of appetite. *Orthopedic Aid* Poultice of boiled, pounded fronds mixed with leaves, and used to set broken bones in place. Decoction of leaves used as a bath for broken bones or poultice of leaves used to bind broken bones. (161:90) **Yana** *Burn Dressing* Poultice of pounded, heated roots applied to burns. (as *Pteris aquilina* 124:253)

***Pteridium aquilinum* var. *latiusculum*,**
Western Brackenfern
Iroquois *Veterinary Aid* Rhizomes, raspberry leaves, and wheat flour given to cows at birthing. (as *P. latiusculum* 118:34)

***Pteridium aquilinum* var. *pubescens*,**
Hairy Brackenfern
Makah *Toothache Remedy* Fiddleheads placed on each side of the gums adjacent to the affected tooth for toothaches. (55:224) **Pomo, Kashaya** *Dermatological Aid* Young, curled frond juice used as a body deodorant. (60:44) **Tolowa** *Anticonvulsive* Poultice of pulverized leaves applied for *Toxicodendron* poisoning. (5:48)

***Pteridium caudatum*, Southern Brackenfern**
Seminole *Orthopedic Aid* Plant used for turkey sickness: permanently bent toes and fingers. Roots used for turkey sickness: permanently bent toes and fingers. (as *Pteris caudata* 145:166, 236)

***Pterocaulon virgatum*, Wand Blackroot**
Seminole *Abortifacient* Infusion of plant used "to correct irregularities and to relieve menstrual pain." (as *P. undulatum* 145:284) *Antidiarrheal* and *Antihemorrhagic* Infusion of plant taken for otter sickness: severe diarrhea, bloody stools, and severe stomachache. (as *P. undulatum* 145:223) *Cold Remedy* Infusion of plant taken for colds. *Febrifuge* Infusion of plant taken for fevers. (as *P. undulatum* 145:283) *Gastrointestinal Aid* Infusion of plant taken for otter sickness: severe diarrhea, bloody stools, and severe stomachache. (as *P. undulatum* 145:223) Plant used for water bison

sickness: digestive difficulties. (as *P. undulatum* 145:306) *Gynecological Aid* Decoction of roots used for backache and excessive bleeding following childbirth. (as *P. undulatum* 145:271) Infusion of plant used "to correct irregularities and to relieve menstrual pain." (as *P. undulatum* 145:284) Decoction of roots taken for backache and excessive bloody discharge after giving birth. (as *P. undulatum* 145:326) *Orthopedic Aid* Decoction of roots used for persistent backache. *Other* Decoction of roots used for chronic sickness. (as *P. undulatum* 145:271) Infusion of plant taken for beaver sickness. (as *P. undulatum* 145:304) *Pulmonary Aid* Plant used for pulmonary disorders. (as *P. undulatum* 145:282) *Unspecified* Plant used medicinally. (as *P. undulatum* 145:164)

Pterospora andromedea, Woodland Pinedrops
Cheyenne *Antihemorrhagic* Cold infusion of ground stems and berries taken for lung hemorrhages. (63:183) Cold infusion of stem and berries taken for "bleeding at the lungs." (63:39) *Dermatological Aid* Cold infusion of ground stems and berries used as an astringent. (63:183) Plant used as an astringent. (63:39) *Disinfectant* Infusion of ground berries and stems used as an astringent. (64:183) *Hemostat* Cold infusion of ground stems and berries used as snuff for nosebleeds. (63:183) Decoction of stem and berries snuffed and used as wash to prevent nosebleed. (63:39) *Nose Medicine* Infusion of ground berries and stems snuffed up the nose and put on the head for nosebleed. (64:183) *Pulmonary Aid* Cold infusion of ground stems and berries taken for lung hemorrhages. (63:183) Decoction of plant taken for bleeding "at the lungs." (63:39) Infusion of ground berries and stems taken for lung hemorrhage. (64:183) **Keres, Western** *Emetic* Boiled plant used as an emetic. (147:64) **Okanagan-Colville** *Venereal Aid* Infusion of roots taken for gonorrhea. (162:102)

Pteryxia terebinthina var. ***terebinthina***,
Turpentine Wavewing
Okanagan-Colville *Dermatological Aid* Poultice of dried, pounded, peeled roots, alone or with Vaseline, applied to sores. *Tonic* Infusion of dried, pounded roots taken as a general tonic. (as

Cymopteris terebinthinus var. *terebinthinus* 162:60)

Pulsatilla occidentalis, White Pasqueflower
Okanagon *Gastrointestinal Aid* Decoction of roots or plants taken for stomach and bowel troubles. (as *Anemone occidentalis* 104:40) **Thompson** *Antirheumatic* (*External*) Infusion of plant used as a wash for rheumatism. *Eye Medicine* Infusion of plant used as an eyewash. (161:249) *Gastrointestinal Aid* Decoction of roots or plants taken for stomach and bowel troubles. (as *Anemone occidentalis* 104:40) Decoction of root or whole plant taken for stomach and bowel troubles. (as *Anemone occidentalis* 141:459) *Unspecified* Plant used medicinally for unspecified purpose. (as *Anemone occidentalis* 141:466)

Pulsatilla patens, American Pasqueflower
Omaha *Analgesic* Poultice of crushed, fresh leaves applied for rheumatism and neuralgia. (58:80, 81) *Antirheumatic* (*External*) Poultice of crushed, fresh leaves applied to affected part for rheumatism. (58:80–82)

Pulsatilla patens ssp. ***multifida***, Cutleaf
Anemone
Blackfoot *Dermatological Aid* Poultice of crushed leaves applied to affected parts as a counterirritant. (as *Anemone patens* var. *wolfgangiana* 82:35) *Gynecological Aid* Decoction of plant taken to speed delivery. (as *Anemone patens* 72:60) **Cheyenne** *Poison* Plant considered poisonous. *Stimulant* Smashed root used symbolically by passing over the body to revive a person. *Unspecified* Plant used for the medicinal properties. (as *Anemone nuttalliana* 69:34) **Chippewa** *Analgesic* Dried, pulverized leaves "smelled" for headache. (as *P. hirsutissima* 43:336) *Pulmonary Aid* Compound decoction of root taken for lung trouble. (as *P. hirsutissima* 43:340) **Great Basin Indian** *Antirheumatic* (*External*) Poultice of fresh leaves used as a counterirritant for rheumatism. (as *P. hirsutissima* 100:47)

Purshia glandulosa, Desert Bitterbrush
Kawaiisu *Analgesic* Plant used for menstrual cramps. *Emetic* Decoction of inner bark and leaves used as an emetic. *Gynecological Aid* Plant

used for menstrual cramps. *Laxative* Decoction of inner bark and leaves used as a laxative. *Venereal Aid* Decoction of inner bark and leaves used for gonorrhea. (180:55)

Purshia mexicana, Mexican Cliffrose
Apache, White Mountain *Unspecified* Leaves used for medicinal purposes. (as *Cowania mexicana* 113:156) **Gosiute** *Unspecified* Leaves used as a medicine. (as *Cowania mexicana* 31:367) **Havasupai** *Cold Remedy* Decoction of green branches, sagebrush, and juniper used for colds to loosen the mucus. *Laxative* Decoction of green branches, sagebrush, and juniper used as a laxative for colds. (as *Cowania mexicana* 171:223) **Hualapai** *Antirheumatic* (*Internal*) Leaves chewed for arthritis. *Dermatological Aid* Leaves made into a tea for bathing and cleansing the skin. (as *Cowania mexicana* 169:31) **Paiute** *Cathartic* Decoction of leaves and stems or flowers taken as a physic. *Cold Remedy* Decoction of leaves and stems or flowers taken for colds. *Venereal Aid* Decoction of leaves and stem or flowers taken for venereal diseases. **Shoshoni** *Cathartic* Decoction of leaves and stems or flowers taken as a physic. *Dermatological Aid* and *Disinfectant* Decoction of plant parts used as an antiseptic wash for smallpox or measles. *Kidney Aid* Decoction of leaves and stems or flowers taken for pains over the kidneys. *Misc. Disease Remedy* Plant used in several compounds taken and used as washes for smallpox and measles. *Venereal Aid* Decoction of leaves and stem or flowers taken for venereal diseases. (as *Cowania mexicana* 155:61)

Purshia stansburiana, Stansbury Cliffrose
Hopi *Dermatological Aid* Plant used in a wash for wounds. (as *Cowania mexicana* var. *stansburiana* 34:304) Plant used in a wash for wounds. (as *Cowania stansburiana* 174:32, 78) *Emetic* Plant used as an emetic. (as *Cowania mexicana* var. *stansburiana* 34:304) Bark used as an emetic. (as *Cowania stansburiana* 174:34, 78) **Navajo, Ramah** *Ceremonial Medicine* Leaves used as an emetic in various ceremonies. *Cough Medicine* Decoction of leaves taken for bad cough. *Emetic* Leaves used as an emetic in various ceremonies. (as *Cowania stansburiana* 165:30)

Purshia tridentata, Antelope Bitterbrush
Klamath *Cough Medicine* Infusion of root taken for coughs. (as *Kunzia tridentata* 37:98) Infusion of roots taken for coughs. (as *Kunzia tridentata* 140:131) *Emetic* Ripe fruit mashed in cold water and taken as an emetic. (as *Kunzia tridentata* 37:98) Infusion of smashed, dried, ripe, bitter fruits taken as an emetic. (as *Kunzia tridentata* 140:131) *Pulmonary Aid* Infusion of root taken for lung and bronchial troubles. (as *Kunzia tridentata* 37:98) Infusion of roots taken for lung troubles. (as *Kunzia tridentata* 140:131) *Respiratory Aid* Infusion of root taken for lung and bronchial troubles. (as *Kunzia tridentata* 37:98) Infusion of roots taken for bronchial troubles. (as *Kunzia tridentata* 140:131) **Montana Indian** *Emetic* Dry, ripe fruits mashed in cold water and used as an emetic. *Pulmonary Aid* Infusion of roots taken for lung troubles. (15:20) **Navajo** *Gynecological Aid* Plant taken during confinement. (76:154) **Navajo, Ramah** *Ceremonial Medicine* Leaves used as an emetic in various ceremonies. *Disinfectant* Leaves chewed by hunters for "deer infection." *Emetic* Leaves used as an emetic in various ceremonies. *Febrifuge* Decoction of root used for fever. *Gynecological Aid* Decoction of root used to facilitate delivery of placenta. *Hunting Medicine* Leaves chewed by hunters for good luck in hunting. (165:31) **Paiute** *Analgesic* Compound infusion of twigs and leaves taken for tubercular lung pain. *Cathartic* Decoction of leaves or twigs taken as a physic. *Cold Remedy* Decoction of leaves taken for colds. *Dermatological Aid* Poultice of leaf, decoction of plant or leaf powder used for skin problems. *Emetic* Decoction of leaves or twigs taken as an emetic. *Liver Aid* Decoction of leaf taken for liver trouble. *Misc. Disease Remedy* Decoction of plant taken and used as a wash for smallpox, chickenpox, and measles. *Pulmonary Aid* Decoction of leaf taken for pneumonia. *Tonic* Decoction of leaf taken as a "blood or general tonic." *Tuberculosis Remedy* Compound decoction of bark taken for tuberculosis and tubercular lung pain. *Venereal Aid* Decoction of leaves or inner bark taken for venereal diseases. (155:126–128) **Paiute, Northern** *Anthelmintic* Decoction of sun dried leaves taken for intestinal worms. *Gastrointestinal Aid* Decoction of sun dried leaves taken to vomit and move the bowels for stomachaches and constipation.

Laxative Decoction of sun dried leaves taken to vomit and move the bowels for stomachaches and constipation. (49:126) **Sanpoil** *Antihemorrhagic* Infusion of crushed berries used for hemorrhage. *Laxative* Infusion of crushed berries used for constipation. (109:217) **Shoshoni** *Antihemorrhagic* Decoction of inner bark taken to aid the healing of an internal rupture. *Cathartic* Decoction of leaves or twigs taken as a physic. *Dermatological Aid* Decoction of leaf used as a wash for the swelling of milk leg. Poultice of leaf, decoction of plant or leaf powder used for skin problems. *Emetic* Decoction of leaves or twigs taken as an emetic. *Misc. Disease Remedy* Simple or compound decoction of plant taken and used as a wash for diseases with rashes. *Other* Bundle of inner bark strips sucked and decoction of leaf used as a wash for milk leg. *Tonic* Decoction of leaf taken as a "blood or general tonic." Decoction of leaf taken as a blood tonic or general tonic. *Venereal Aid* Compound decoction of inner bark taken specifically for gonorrhea. Decoction of leaves or roots taken for venereal diseases. **Washo** *Cathartic* Decoction of ripe, whole seeds taken as a physic. (155:126–128)

Pycnanthemum albescens, Whiteleaf Mountainmint

Choctaw *Cold Remedy* Hot decoction of leaves taken as diaphoretic for colds. (20:24) Decoction of leaves taken to cause sweating for colds. (152:54) *Diaphoretic* Hot decoction of leaves taken as diaphoretic for colds. (20:24) Decoction of leaves taken to cause sweating for colds. (152:54)

Pycnanthemum californicum, Sierra Mint

Miwok *Cold Remedy* Decoction taken for colds. (8:172)

Pycnanthemum flexuosum, Appalachian Mountainmint

Cherokee *Analgesic* Poultice of leaves used for headache. *Antidiarrheal* Infusion taken with "green corn" to prevent diarrhea. *Cold Remedy* Infusion taken for colds. *Dermatological Aid* Warm infusion used to bathe inflamed penis and infusion taken for upset stomach. *Febrifuge* Infusion taken for fevers. *Gastrointestinal Aid* Infusion used for upset stomach. *Heart Medicine* Infusion of leaves taken for "heart trouble." (66:45)

Pycnanthemum incanum, Hoary Mountainmint

Cherokee *Analgesic* Poultice of leaves used for headache. *Antidiarrheal* Infusion taken with "green corn" to prevent diarrhea. *Cold Remedy* Infusion taken for colds. *Dermatological Aid* Warm infusion used to bathe inflamed penis and infusion taken for upset stomach. *Febrifuge* Infusion taken for fevers. *Gastrointestinal Aid* Infusion used for upset stomach. *Heart Medicine* Infusion of leaves taken for "heart trouble." (66:45) **Choctaw** *Analgesic* Infusion of mashed leaves taken and used as a wash for headaches. *Panacea* Infusion of mashed leaves blown on sickly patient. **Koasati** *Analgesic* Decoction of roots taken for headaches. *Hemostat* Soaked plants put up the nose for nosebleeds. *Stimulant* Cold infusion of leaves taken and used as a bath for laziness. (152:55)

Pycnanthemum virginianum, Virginia Mountainmint

Chippewa *Abortifacient* Decoction of powdered root taken for "stoppage of periods." (as *Koellia virginiana* 43:358) *Febrifuge* Compound decoction of leaves taken for chills and fever. (as *Koellia virginiana* 43:354) **Lakota** *Cough Medicine* Infusion of plant taken for coughs. (116:50) **Meskwaki** *Alterative* Infusion of leaf used as an alterative "when a person is all run down." *Febrifuge* Infusion of plant tops taken for chills. *Misc. Disease Remedy* Infusion of plant tops taken for ague. *Stimulant* Compound containing florets applied at nostrils to rally a dying patient. (129:226, 227)

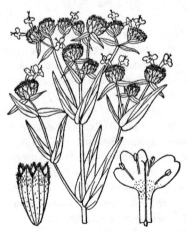

Pycnanthemum virginianum

Pyrola americana, American Wintergreen
Cherokee *Dermatological Aid* "Stick on cuts and sores to heal them." (as *P. rotundifolia* 66:55) **Ojibwa** *Hunting Medicine* Dried leaves used to make tea and drunk as good luck potion in the morning before the hunt started. (130:430)

Pyrola asarifolia, Liverleaf Wintergreen
Carrier, Southern *Eye Medicine* Decoction of leaves or leaves and roots used as an eyewash. (127:62) **Cree, Woodlands** *Antihemorrhagic* Decoction of plant taken for coughing up blood. *Eye Medicine* Infusion of leaves used for sore eyes. (91:54) **Karok** *Ceremonial Medicine, Pediatric Aid*, and *Sedative* Decoction of plant used as a steam bath for "goofy" child in the Brush Dance. (125:387) **Shoshoni** *Liver Aid* Decoction of root taken for liver trouble. (155:128)

Pyrola asarifolia ssp. **asarifolia**, Liverleaf
   Wintergreen
Micmac *Antihemorrhagic* Parts of plant used for spitting blood. *Kidney Aid* Parts of plant used for kidney trouble. *Venereal Aid* Parts of plant used for gonorrhea. (as *P. uliginosa* 32:60) **Montagnais** *Panacea* Decoction of leaves taken for any ailment. (as *P. uliginosa* 133:314) **Penobscot** *Antihemorrhagic* Compound infusion of plant taken for "spitting up blood." *Kidney Aid* Compound infusion of plant taken for kidney trouble. *Tonic* Compound infusion of plant taken as a tonic. *Venereal Aid* Compound infusion of plant taken for gonorrhea. (as *P. uliginosa* 133:311)

Pyrola chlorantha, Greenflowered Wintergreen
Navajo, Kayenta *Antidiarrheal* Plant used for infants with bloody diarrhea. *Gynecological Aid* Plant used for menorrhagia. *Hemostat* Plant used as a hemostatic. *Pediatric Aid* Plant used for infants with bloody diarrhea. (179:35)

Pyrola elliptica, Waxflower Shinleaf
Cherokee *Dermatological Aid* "Stick on cuts and sores to heal them." (66:55) **Chippewa** *Unspecified* Poultice of plant and two other plants used medicinally. (59:138) **Iroquois** *Anticonvulsive* Decoction of roots and leaves given to babies with fits or epileptic seizures. (73:408) *Antirheumatic* (*Internal*) Compound infusion of plants taken for

rheumatism. *Blood Medicine* Compound used for bad blood. *Dermatological Aid* Compound used for neck sores. *Eye Medicine* Decoction of plant used as drops for sore eyes, sties, and inflamed lids. *Gastrointestinal Aid* Compound decoction of whole plants taken for indigestion. *Orthopedic Aid* Compound infusion of smashed plants applied as poultice to sore legs. (73:409) *Pediatric Aid* Decoction of roots and leaves given to babies with fits or epileptic seizures. (73:408) **Mohegan** *Oral Aid* Infusion of leaves used as a gargle for sores or cankers in the mouth. (149:264) Infusion of leaves used as a mouthwash for canker sores. *Throat Aid* Infusion of leaves used as a wash for mouth sores and sore throat. (151:74, 130) **Montagnais** *Stimulant* Decoction of root taken for "weakness." (133:315) **Nootka** *Cancer Treatment* Poultice of bruised plant applied to "tumors." (146:79)

Pyrola picta, Whiteveined Wintergreen
Karok *Panacea* and *Pediatric Aid* Infusion of plant used as a wash for sick child. (125:387)

Pyrrhopappus carolinianus, Carolina
   Desertchicory
Cherokee *Blood Medicine* Infusion taken to purify blood. (66:31)

Pyrrhopappus pauciflorus, Desertchicory
Navajo, Ramah *Ceremonial Medicine* and *Emetic* Flower stalks used as a ceremonial emetic. (as *P. multicaulis* 165:52)

Pyrularia pubera, Buffalo Nut
Cherokee *Dermatological Aid* Used as a salve for "old sores." *Emetic* Nut chewed to "make vomit for colic." (66:27)

Pyrus sp., Service Tree
Cree, Hudson Bay *Dermatological Aid* Branch bark used for its astringent qualities. *Misc. Disease Remedy* Branch bark used for inflammatory diseases. *Pulmonary Aid* Branch bark used for pleurisy. (78:303)

Q*uercus agrifolia*, California Live Oak

Mahuna *Hemostat* and *Pediatric Aid* Plant used for newborns with bleeding navels. (117:56)

Quercus agrifolia var. *agrifolia*, California Live Oak
Diegueño *Dermatological Aid* Decoction of chipped bark used as a wash for sores. (70:33)

Quercus alba, White Oak
Cherokee *Antidiarrheal* Bark used for chronic dysentery. *Dermatological Aid* Astringent bark chewed for mouth sores. Infusion of bark applied to sore, chapped skin. *Disinfectant* Bark used as an antiseptic. *Emetic* Bark used as an emetic. (66:46) Bark used as an emetic. (177:74) *Febrifuge* Bark used after long, intermittent fevers and as a wash for chills and fevers. *Gastrointestinal Aid* Bark used for indigestion and "any debility of the system." *Oral Aid* Bark chewed for mouth sores. *Respiratory Aid* Infusion of bark taken for asthma. *Throat Aid* Decoction of inner bark used for "lost voice." *Tonic* Bark used as a tonic. *Urinary Aid* Unspecified liquid preparation taken for "milky urine." (66:46) **Delaware** *Cough Medicine* Infusion of bark used for severe coughs. *Disinfectant* Infusion of bark used as a disinfectant. *Gynecological Aid* Infusion of bark used as a douche. *Throat Aid* Infusion of bark used for sore throats. (151:30) **Delaware, Oklahoma** *Cough*

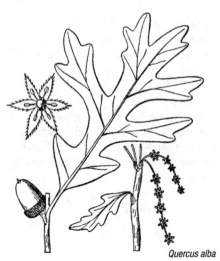

Quercus alba

Medicine Infusion of bark taken for severe cough. (150:25, 78) *Dermatological Aid* Strong infusion of bark used to cleanse bruises and ulcers. (150:25) *Disinfectant* Compound containing bark used as an antiseptic. (150:78) *Gynecological Aid* Infusion of bark used as an excellent douche. *Panacea* Bark used in many medicinal compounds. (150:25, 78) *Throat Aid* Strong infusion of bark gargled for a sore throat. (150:25) **Delaware, Ontario** *Gynecological Aid* Compound infusion of bark taken for "diseases peculiar to women." *Tonic* Compound infusion of bark taken as a tonic. (150:68, 82) **Houma** *Antirheumatic* (*External*) Crushed root mixed with whisky and used as liniment on rheumatic parts. (135:56) **Iroquois** *Psychological Aid* Compound decoction used to counteract loneliness. *Tuberculosis Remedy* Compound decoction of bark taken for consumption. *Veterinary Aid* Bark used for horses with distemper. *Witchcraft Medicine* Compound decoction used "when your woman goes off and won't come back." (73:303) **Menominee** *Unspecified* Inner bark used in compounds. (128:36) **Meskwaki** *Antidiarrheal* Compound containing bark used for diarrhea. *Pulmonary Aid* Decoction of inner bark taken to "throw up phlegm from the lungs." (129: 221) **Micmac** *Dietary Aid* Nuts used to induce thirst. *Hemorrhoid Remedy* Plant parts used for bleeding piles. (32:60) **Mohegan** *Analgesic* Infusion of bark used as liniment for muscular pains. (25:121) Infusion of inner bark used as liniment for humans and horses with pain. (151:75) *Antirheumatic* (*External*) Infusion of inner bark used as a liniment for pain. (151:75, 132) *Cold Remedy* Bark used for colds. (151:132) *Orthopedic Aid* Infusion of bark used as liniment for muscular pains. (25:121) Infusion of bark used as a liniment for people. *Veterinary Aid* Infusion of bark used as a liniment for horses. (149:266) Infusion of inner bark used as a liniment for horses with pain. (151:75, 132) **Ojibwa, South** *Antidiarrheal* Decoction of root bark and inner bark taken for diarrhea. (77:198) **Penobscot** *Dietary Aid* Acorns eaten to induce thirst and plenty of water thought to be beneficial. (133:309) *Hemorrhoid Remedy* Infusion of bark taken for bleeding piles. (133:310) **Shinnecock** *Analgesic* Infusion of bark used as liniment for muscular pains. *Orthopedic Aid* Infusion of bark used as liniment for muscular pains. (25:121)

Quercus bicolor, Swamp White Oak
Iroquois *Misc. Disease Remedy* Compound decoction of bark taken for cholera. *Orthopedic Aid* Compound decoction of bark taken for broken bones. *Respiratory Aid* Compound of leaves smoked and exhaled through the nostrils for catarrh. *Tuberculosis Remedy* Compound decoction of bark chips taken for consumption. *Witchcraft Medicine* Used "when wife runs around, takes away lonesomeness." (73:303)

Quercus chrysolepis, Canyon Live Oak
Mendocino Indian *Poison* Nuts considered poisonous. (33:342)

Quercus douglasii, Blue Oak
Kawaiisu *Burn Dressing* Poultice of ground galls and salt applied to burns. *Dermatological Aid* Poultice of ground galls and salt applied to sores and cuts. *Eye Medicine* Ground gall powder and salt wrapped in a small piece of cloth and dipped in water applied to sore eyes. (180:56) **Midoo** *Throat Aid* Leaves chewed for sore throats. (97:310)

Quercus dumosa, California Scrub Oak
Diegueño *Eye Medicine* Decoction of broken galls used as an eyewash. (70:33) **Luiseño** *Dermatological Aid* Gallnuts used for sores and wounds and as an astringent. (132:233)

Quercus ellipsoidalis, Northern Pin Oak
Menominee *Abortifacient* Compound decoction of inner bark taken for suppressed menses caused by cold. (44:133)

Quercus falcata, Southern Red Oak
Cherokee *Antidiarrheal* Bark used for chronic dysentery. *Dermatological Aid* Astringent bark chewed for mouth sores. Infusion of bark applied to sore, chapped skin. *Disinfectant* Bark used as an antiseptic. *Emetic* Bark used as an emetic. *Febrifuge* Bark used after long, intermittent fevers and as a wash for chills and fevers. *Gastrointestinal Aid* Bark used for indigestion and "any debility of the system." *Oral Aid* Bark chewed for mouth sores. *Respiratory Aid* Infusion of bark taken for asthma. *Throat Aid* Decoction of inner bark used for "lost voice." *Tonic* Bark used as a tonic. *Uri-*

nary Aid Unspecified liquid preparation taken for "milky urine." (66:46)

Quercus gambelii, Gambel's Oak
Isleta *Reproductive Aid* Acorns eaten to give greater sexual potency. (27:47) Consumption of acorns believed to give greater sexual potency. (85:41) **Navajo, Ramah** *Analgesic* Decoction of root bark used for postpartum pain. *Cathartic* Decoction of root bark used as a cathartic. *Ceremonial Medicine* and *Emetic* Leaves used as a ceremonial emetic. *Gynecological Aid* Decoction of root bark used for postpartum pain and to help in delivery of placenta. *Panacea* Root bark used as a "life medicine." (165:22)

Quercus gambelii var. *gambelii*, Gambel's Oak
Isleta *Reproductive Aid* Acorns eaten to give greater sexual potency. (as *Q. utahensis* 27:47) **Keres, Western** *Emetic* Infusion of ground leaves and oak galls used as an emetic. *Oral Aid* and *Pediatric Aid* Velvet pubescence rubbed on babies' tongues to remove milk coating. (as *Q. utahensis* 147:64)

Quercus garryana, Oregon White Oak
Cowlitz *Tuberculosis Remedy* Decoction of bark taken for tuberculosis. (65:27) **Karok** *Gynecological Aid* Infusion of plant taken by mother before her first baby comes. Pounded bark rubbed on abdomen and sides of mother before her first delivery. (125:382)

Quercus ilicifolia, Bear Oak
Iroquois *Gynecological Aid* Used as a wash and taken for "female troubles." *Other* Used as a "sugar medicine." (73:302)

Quercus imbricaria, Shingle Oak
Cherokee *Antidiarrheal* Bark used for chronic dysentery. *Dermatological Aid* Astringent bark chewed for mouth sores. Infusion of bark applied to sore, chapped skin. *Disinfectant* Bark used as an antiseptic. *Emetic* Bark used as an emetic. *Febrifuge* Bark used after long, intermittent fevers and as a wash for chills and fevers. *Gastrointestinal Aid* Bark used for indigestion and "any debility of the system." *Oral Aid* Bark chewed for mouth

sores. *Respiratory Aid* Infusion of bark taken for asthma. *Throat Aid* Decoction of inner bark used for "lost voice." *Tonic* Bark used as a tonic. *Urinary Aid* Unspecified liquid preparation taken for "milky urine." (66:46)

Quercus lobata, California White Oak
Kawaiisu *Burn Dressing* Poultice of ground galls and salt applied to burns. *Dermatological Aid* Poultice of ground galls and salt applied to sores and cuts. *Eye Medicine* Ground gall powder and salt wrapped in a small piece of cloth and dipped in water applied to sore eyes. (180:56) **Miwok** *Cough Medicine* Decoction of bark taken as a cough medicine. *Dermatological Aid* and *Pediatric Aid* Pulverized, outer bark dusted on running sores and particularly used for babies with sore umbilicus. (8:172) **Yuki** *Antidiarrheal* Bark used for diarrhea. (33:343)

Quercus macrocarpa, Bur Oak
Chippewa *Analgesic* Decoction of root or inner bark taken for cramps. *Gastrointestinal Aid* Decoction of inner bark used for cramps. (43:340) *Heart Medicine* Compound decoction of inner bark prepared ceremonially for heart trouble. (43:338) *Pulmonary Aid* Compound decoction of inner bark taken for lung trouble. (43:340) **Iroquois** *Antidiarrheal* Infusion of bark chips taken for diarrhea. *Antidote* "Plant will stop the effects of the laxative made from *V[iburnum] opulus*." *Dermatological Aid* Complex compound decoction used as wash for affected parts of "Italian itch." (73:303) **Menominee** *Abortifacient* Compound decoction of inner bark taken for suppressed menses caused by cold. (44:133) **Meskwaki** *Anthelmintic* Compound containing wood and inner bark used to expel pinworms. (129:221, 222) **Ojibwa** *Dermatological Aid* Bark used as an astringent medicine. *Orthopedic Aid* Bark used to bandage a broken foot or leg. (130:369)

Quercus marilandica, Blackjack Oak
Choctaw *Analgesic* Infusion of tree bark coal taken to remove the afterbirth and ease cramps. *Gynecological Aid* Infusion of tree bark coal taken to aid in childbirth, and to remove the afterbirth and ease cramps. (152:17)

Quercus muehlenbergii, Chinkapin Oak
Delaware, Ontario *Antiemetic* Infusion of bark taken for vomiting. (150:68, 82)

Quercus pagoda, Cherrybark Oak
Houma *Antidiarrheal* Compound decoction of bark taken for dysentery. *Orthopedic Aid* Strong decoction of root or bark applied to swollen joints. *Throat Aid* Decoction of bark and roots taken for sore throat or hoarseness. *Tonic* Decoction of bark and root taken as a tonic for "run-down health." (as *Q. pagodaefolia* 135:56)

Quercus palustris, Pin Oak
Delaware *Gastrointestinal Aid* Infusion of inner bark used for intestinal pains. (151:30) **Delaware, Oklahoma** *Analgesic* and *Gastrointestinal Aid* Infusion of inner bark taken for intestinal pains. (150:25, 78)

Quercus ×*pauciloba*, Wavyleaf Oak
Navajo, Kayenta *Sedative* Plant used for nervousness. (as *Q. undulata* 179:18) **Navajo, Ramah** *Analgesic* Decoction of root bark used for internal pains. Decoction of root bark taken for internal pains. (as *Q. undulata* 165:22)

Quercus phellos, Willow Oak
Seminole *Analgesic* Decoction of wood bits or bark applied externally as an analgesic. (169:167) *Antirheumatic (External)* Decoction of wood or bark used as a bath for aches and pains. (169:286) *Dermatological Aid* Decoction of bark used for ballgame sickness: sores, back or limb pains, and hemorrhoids. Decoction of wood or bark used as a bath for sores and cuts. (169:269, 286) *Hemorrhoid Remedy* Decoction of bark used for ballgame sickness: sores, back or limb pains, and hemorrhoids. (169:269) *Love Medicine* Decoction of wood ashes placed on the tongue to cleanse the body and strengthen the marriage. (169:250) *Orthopedic Aid* Decoction of bark used for ballgame sickness: sores, back or limb pains, and hemorrhoids. (169:269)

Quercus rubra, Northern Red Oak
Cherokee *Antidiarrheal* Bark used for chronic dysentery. *Dermatological Aid* Astringent bark chewed for mouth sores. Infusion of bark applied

to sore, chapped skin. *Disinfectant* Bark used as an antiseptic. *Emetic* Bark used as an emetic. *Febrifuge* Bark used after long, intermittent fevers and as a wash for chills and fevers. *Gastrointestinal Aid* Bark used for indigestion and "any debility of the system." *Oral Aid* Bark chewed for mouth sores. *Respiratory Aid* Infusion of bark taken for asthma. *Throat Aid* Decoction of inner bark used for "lost voice." (66:46) Decoction of inner bark taken for hoarseness. (152:17) *Tonic* Bark used as a tonic. *Urinary Aid* Unspecified liquid preparation taken for "milky urine." (66:46) **Chippewa** *Heart Medicine* Compound decoction of inner bark prepared ceremonially for heart trouble. (43:338) **Delaware** *Cough Medicine* Infusion of bark used for severe coughs. *Throat Aid* Infusion of bark used for hoarseness. (151:30) **Delaware, Oklahoma** *Cough Medicine* Infusion of bark taken for severe cough. *Throat Aid* Infusion of bark taken for hoarseness. (150:25, 78) **Mahuna** *Toothache Remedy* Plant juice used for straightening and setting loose teeth. (117:25) **Malecite** *Antidiarrheal* Infusion of plant and fir buds or cones used for diarrhea. (96:244) Infusion of bark or roots used for diarrhea. (96:255) **Micmac** *Antidiarrheal* Bark and roots used for diarrhea. (32:60) **Ojibwa** *Blood Medicine* Decoction of bark taken for internal blood diseases. (as *Q. ruba* 112:231) *Heart Medicine* and *Respiratory Aid* Bark used for "heart troubles and bronchial affections." (130:369, 370) *Unspecified* Plant used for medicinal purposes. (112:242) *Venereal Aid* Infusion of root bark taken for gonorrhea. (as *Q. ruba*

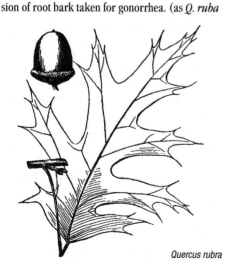

Quercus rubra

112:231) **Ojibwa, South** *Antidiarrheal* Decoction of root bark and inner bark taken for diarrhea. (77:198) **Potawatomi** *Antidiarrheal* Inner bark used for flux. (131:58) **Rappahannock** *Dietary Aid* Infusion of north side bark taken as an appetizer. *Tonic* Decoction of bark and leaves taken as a beneficial beverage (bitters). (138:26)

Quercus rubra var. *rubra*, Northern Red Oak

Alabama *Dermatological Aid* Decoction of bark used as a wash for bad smelling sores on the head or feet. *Orthopedic Aid* and *Pediatric Aid* Infusion of bark given to child old enough to walk but too weak to do so. *Pulmonary Aid* Infusion of bark taken for lung trouble. *Throat Aid* Decoction of bark taken for sore throats. **Cherokee** *Antidiarrheal* Infusion of twig juice taken for dysentery. (as *Q. borealis* var. *maxima* 152:16) **Iroquois** *Dermatological Aid* Complex compound decoction used as wash for affected parts of "Italian itch." Poultice of powdered bark bound to ruptured or improperly healed navels. (as *Q. borealis* var. *maxima* 73:304)

Quercus stellata, Post Oak

Cherokee *Antidiarrheal* Bark used for chronic dysentery. (66:46) Infusion of twig juice taken for dysentery. (152:18) *Dermatological Aid* Astringent bark chewed for mouth sores. Infusion of bark applied to sore, chapped skin. *Disinfectant* Bark used as an antiseptic. *Emetic* Bark used as an emetic. *Febrifuge* Bark used after long, intermittent fevers and as a wash for chills and fevers. *Gastrointestinal Aid* Bark used for indigestion and "any debility of the system." *Oral Aid* Bark chewed for mouth sores. *Respiratory Aid* Infusion of bark taken for asthma. *Throat Aid* Decoction of inner bark used for "lost voice." *Tonic* Bark used as a tonic. *Urinary Aid* Unspecified liquid preparation taken for "milky urine." (66:46) Infusion of inner bark taken for difficult urination with discharge. **Choctaw** *Gastrointestinal Aid* Decoction of bark taken for stomachaches. (152:18) **Creek** *Antidiarrheal* Bark used to make a drink taken for dysentery. (148:659) Infusion of bark taken for dysentery. (152:18)

Quercus velutina, Black Oak

Cherokee *Antidiarrheal* Bark used for chronic

dysentery. *Dermatological Aid* Astringent bark chewed for mouth sores. Infusion of bark applied to sore, chapped skin. *Disinfectant* Bark used as an antiseptic. *Emetic* Bark used as an emetic. *Febrifuge* Bark used after long, intermittent fevers and as a wash for chills and fevers. *Gastrointestinal Aid* Bark used for indigestion and "any debility of the system." *Gynecological Aid* Compound infusion of bark of black oak taken for "female trouble." *Oral Aid* Bark chewed for mouth sores. *Respiratory Aid* Infusion of bark taken for asthma. *Throat Aid* Decoction of inner bark used for "lost voice." *Tonic* Bark used as a tonic. *Urinary Aid* Unspecified liquid preparation taken for "milky urine." (66:46) **Delaware** *Cold Remedy* Infusion of inner bark used as a gargle for colds. *Throat Aid* Infusion of inner bark used as a gargle for hoarseness. (151:30) **Delaware, Oklahoma** *Cold Remedy* Infusion of inner bark taken and used as a gargle for colds. *Throat Aid* Decoction of inner bark taken and used as a gargle for hoarseness. (150:25, 78) **Menominee** *Eye Medicine* Decoction of crushed bark used as a wash for sore eyes. (128:36) **Meskwaki** *Pulmonary Aid* Compound containing inner bark used for lung troubles. (129:222)

Quercus virginiana, Live Oak
Houma *Antidiarrheal* Decoction of bark taken for dysentery. (135:56) **Mahuna** *Unspecified* Bark used for medicine. (117:55) **Seminole** *Analgesic* Decoction of wood bits or bark applied externally as an analgesic. (145:167) *Antirheumatic (External)* Decoction of wood or bark used as a bath for aches and pains. (145:286) *Dermatological Aid* Decoction of bark used for ballgame sickness: sores, back or limb pains, and hemorrhoids. Decoction of wood or bark used as a bath for sores and cuts. (145:269, 286) *Hemorrhoid Remedy* Decoction of bark used for ballgame sickness: sores, back or limb pains, and hemorrhoids. (145:269) *Love Medicine* Decoction of wood ashes placed on the tongue to cleanse the body and strengthen the marriage. (145:250) *Orthopedic Aid* Decoction of bark used for ballgame sickness: sores, back or limb pains, and hemorrhoids. (145:269)

Quercus wislizeni, Interior Live Oak
Miwok *Cough Medicine* Decoction of bark taken as a cough medicine. *Dermatological Aid* and *Pedi-*

atric Aid Pulverized, outer bark dusted on running sores and particularly used for babies with sore umbilicus. (8:172)

Quercus wislizeni var. *frutescens*, Interior Live Oak
Kawaiisu *Antirheumatic (Internal)* Decoction of inner bark taken for arthritis. *Burn Dressing* Ground plant applied to burns. (180:56)

Quincula lobata, Chinese Lantern
Kiowa *Misc. Disease Remedy* Decoction of roots taken or poultice of pounded roots applied for grippe. (as *Physalis lobata* 166:50)

 Ranunculus abortivus, Littleleaf Buttercup
Cherokee *Dermatological Aid* Used as poultice for abscesses. *Oral Aid* Infusion used for "thrash." *Sedative* Juice used as sedative. *Throat Aid* Infusion gargled for sore throat. (66:31) **Iroquois** *Anticonvulsive* Compound decoction of roots taken by men and women for epilepsy. (73:325) *Antidote* Decoction of smashed root taken to counteract poison. (73:320) *Blood Medicine* Compound infusion of roots taken for blood disease which caused fainting. (73:325) *Emetic* Decoction of root taken to vomit for stomach trouble and to counteract poison. (73:320) Compound decoction of plants taken to vomit after taking epilepsy medicine. *Eye Medicine* Decoction of roots and leaves used as wash for sore eyes from catching cold. (73:325) *Gastrointestinal Aid* Decoction of smashed root taken for stomach trouble. *Misc. Disease Remedy* Decoction of roots taken to dry up smallpox. (73:320) *Orthopedic Aid* Compound decoction of roots taken for stiff muscles. *Psychological Aid* Compound decoction of plants taken for "loss of senses during menses." (73:325) *Snakebite Remedy* Decoction of smashed root used as a wash for snakebites. (73:320) *Toothache Remedy* Plant used for sore teeth. (73:325) **Meskwaki** *Hemostat* Root used as a styptic for nosebleeds. (129:239)

Ranunculus acris, Tall Buttercup
Abnaki *Analgesic* Used for headaches. (121:155)

Flowers and leaves smashed and sniffed for headaches. (121:166) **Bella Coola** *Dermatological Aid* Poultice of pounded roots applied to boils. (as *R. arcis* 127:57) **Cherokee** *Dermatological Aid* Used as poultice for abscesses. *Oral Aid* Infusion used for "thrash." *Sedative* Juice used as sedative. *Throat Aid* Infusion gargled for sore throat. (66:31) **Iroquois** *Analgesic* Poultice of smashed plant applied to chest for pains. *Antidiarrheal* Infusion of roots taken for diarrhea. *Antihemorrhagic* Poultice of smashed plant applied to chest for colds. (73:320) *Blood Medicine* Poultice of plant fragments with another plant applied to the skin for excess water in the blood. (118:42) **Micmac** *Analgesic* Leaves used for headaches. (32:60) **Montagnais** *Analgesic* Crushed leaves inhaled for headaches. (133:315)

Ranunculus bulbosus, St. Anthony's Turnip
Iroquois *Toothache Remedy* Root placed in cavity to break up the tooth for a toothache. *Venereal Aid* Decoction of plants taken for venereal disease. (73:320)

Ranunculus cymbalaria, Alkali Buttercup
Kawaiisu *Dermatological Aid* Mashed leaves and flowers applied as salve to sores and cuts. (180:58) **Navajo** *Venereal Aid* Plant used for syphilis. (45:96) **Navajo**, **Kayenta** *Panacea* Plant used as a life medicine. (179:22)

Ranunculus cymbalaria var. *saximontanus*, Rocky Mountain Buttercup
Navajo, **Ramah** *Ceremonial Medicine* and *Emetic* Plant used as an emetic in various ceremonies. (165:27)

Ranunculus flabellaris, Yellow Water
    Buttercup
Meskwaki *Cold Remedy* Flower stigmas used as snuff to induce sneezing for catarrh and head colds. *Respiratory Aid* Compound containing leaves used as a snuff for catarrh and head cold. (as *R. delphinifolius* 129:239, 240)

Ranunculus glaberrimus, Sagebrush
    Buttercup
Okanagan-Colville *Analgesic* Poultice of mashed and dampened whole plants applied to pains of

any kind. *Antirheumatic* (*External*) Poultice of mashed and dampened whole plants applied to sore joints. *Poison* Dried or mashed, fresh whole plant placed on a piece of meat as poisoned bait for coyotes. (162:119) **Thompson** *Dermatological Aid* Poultice of mashed flowers used for warts. (161:249) *Poison* Flowers or whole plant rubbed on arrow points as a poison. (141:512) Plant considered a skin irritant. (161:249)

Ranunculus hispidus var. *nitidus*, Bristly
    Buttercup
Iroquois *Toothache Remedy* Root placed in cavity to break up the tooth for a toothache. (as *R. septentrionalis* 73:320)

Ranunculus inamoenus, Graceful Buttercup
Navajo, **Ramah** *Hunting Medicine* Cold infusion of plant taken and used as a lotion to protect hunters from animals. (165:27)

Ranunculus lapponicus, Lapland Buttercup
Eskimo, **Kuskokwagmiut** *Dietary Aid* Plants soaked and eaten by starving persons before eating other food. (101:23)

Ranunculus occidentalis, Western Buttercup
Aleut *Poison* Flower juice slipped into food to cause a person "to waste away to nothing." (6:428)

Ranunculus pallasii, Pallas's Buttercup
Eskimo, **Inupiat** *Poison* Young shoots poisonous, if not boiled. (83:143)

Ranunculus pensylvanicus, Pennsylvania
    Buttercup
Ojibwa *Hunting Medicine* Seeds used as a hunting medicine. (130:383) Seeds smoked in hunting medicine to lure buck deer near enough for a shot with bow and arrow. (130:431) **Potawatomi** *Dermatological Aid* Plant used as an astringent medicine for unspecified diseases. (131:75)

Ranunculus recurvatus, Blisterwort
Cherokee *Dermatological Aid* Used as poultice for abscesses. *Oral Aid* Infusion used for "thrash." *Sedative* Juice used as sedative. *Throat Aid* Infusion gargled for sore throat. (66:31) **Iroquois** *Laxative* Compound decoction of roots taken to

loosen bowels and for venereal disease. *Toothache Remedy* Decoction of roots taken to "kill the worms" in sore and hollow teeth. *Venereal Aid* Decoction of roots taken for venereal disease. (73:320)

Ranunculus repens, Creeping Buttercup
Hesquiat *Analgesic* and *Antirheumatic* (*External*) Poultice of chewed leaves used for muscular aches and rheumatic pains. *Dermatological Aid* Poultice of chewed leaves used for sores. *Gynecological Aid* Three or four leaves eaten to help heal the insides after childbirth. *Other* Chewed leaves swallowed for general sickness. (159:71) **Thompson** *Poison* Plant considered a skin irritant. (161:249)

Ranunculus sceleratus, Celeryleaf Buttercup
Thompson *Poison* Flowers or whole plant rubbed on arrow points as a poison. (141:512)

Ranunculus sceleratus var. **multifidus**, Blister Buttercup
Keres, Western *Poison* Plant considered poisonous. (as *R. eremogenes* 147:65)

Ranunculus uncinatus, Hooked Buttercup
Thompson *Antirheumatic* (*External*) Decoction of plant used as a wash or steam for stiff, sore muscles, and rheumatism. (as *R. douglasii* 141:473) *Disinfectant* Decoction of whole plant used as a body wash for purification in sweat house. (as *R. douglasii* 141:505) *Herbal Steam* Decoction of plant used as a sweat bath wash for stiff, sore muscles and bones. Decoction of plant used as a wash or steam for stiff, sore muscles and rheumatism. *Orthopedic Aid* Decoction of plant used as a sweat bath wash for stiff, sore muscles and bones. (as *R. douglasii* 141:473) *Poison* Plant considered a skin irritant. (161:249)

Ratibida columnifera, Upright Prairie Coneflower
Cheyenne *Analgesic* Infusion of leaves and stems rubbed on rattlesnake bite for pain. (as *R. columnaris* 63:188) Decoction of leaves and stems used as wash for pain. (as *R. columnaris* 64:188) *Dermatological Aid* Infusion of leaves and stems rubbed on areas affected by poison ivy. (as *R.*

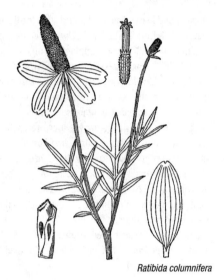

Ratibida columnifera

columnaris 63:188) Decoction of leaves and stems used for poison ivy rash. (as *R. columnaris* 64:188) *Snakebite Remedy* Infusion of leaves and stems rubbed on rattlesnake bite for pain. (as *R. columnaris* 63:188) Decoction of leaves and stems used as wash to draw out poison of a rattlesnake's bite. (as *R. columnaris* 64:188) Leaves and stems boiled and solution used for rattlesnake bites. (69:23) **Dakota** *Analgesic* Flowers used for chest pains and other ailments. *Dermatological Aid* Flowers used for wounds. *Panacea* Flowers used for chest pains and other ailments. (as *R. columnaris* 57:368) **Keres, Western** *Gynecological Aid* Crushed leaves rubbed on mothers' breast to wean child. (147:65) **Lakota** *Analgesic* Infusion of plant tops taken for headaches. *Gastrointestinal Aid* Infusion of plant tops taken for stomachaches. *Veterinary Aid* Plant given to horses for urinary problems. (116:39) **Navajo, Ramah** *Febrifuge* Cold infusion used for fever. *Veterinary Aid* Cold infusion given to sheep that are "out of their minds." (as *R. columnaris* var. *pulcherrima* 165:52) **Zuni** *Emetic* Infusion of whole plant taken as an emetic. (as *R. columnaris* 143:59)

Ratibida tagetes, Green Prairie Coneflower
Keres, Western *Hunting Medicine* Roots carried while deer hunting to prevent craziness. Chewing the root prevented craziness which occurred if a wounded deer blew his breath into one's face. *Sedative* Infusion of plant used for epileptic fits. *Un-*

specified Plant considered strong medicine. (147:65) **Navajo, Ramah** *Analgesic* Strong infusion of leaves used for stomachache or as a cathartic. *Cathartic* Strong infusion of leaves used as a cathartic. *Ceremonial Medicine* Plant used in ceremonial chant lotion. *Cough Medicine* Cold infusion of leaves taken for coughs. *Febrifuge* Cold infusion of leaves taken for fever. *Gastrointestinal Aid* Strong infusion of leaves taken for stomachache. *Panacea* Plant used as "life medicine." *Pediatric Aid* Decoction of root used for "birth injuries." *Venereal Aid* Plant used as a fumigant for sexual infection. (165:52)

Reverchonia arenaria, Sand Reverchonia
Hopi *Gynecological Aid* Plant used for postpartum hemorrhage. (174:36, 84) **Navajo, Kayenta** *Veterinary Aid* Plant used for livestock bloat. (179:31)

Rhamnus alnifolia, Alderleaf Buckthorn
Iroquois *Antidote* Infusion of plant taken and poultice applied to swelling caused by poison. *Blood Medicine* Infusion of bark given to children as a blood purifier. *Cathartic* Infusion of bark given to children as a physic. *Dermatological Aid* Infusion of plant taken and poultice applied to swelling caused by poison. *Orthopedic Aid* Infusion given and used as a wash for bad backs. *Pediatric Aid* Infusion given and used as a wash for peevish children. Infusion of bark given to children as a tonic, physic, and as blood purifier. *Sedative* Infusion given and used as a wash for peevish children. *Tonic* Infusion of bark given to children as a tonic. *Venereal Aid* Compound decoction of roots taken for gonorrhea. (73:381) **Meskwaki** *Laxative* Decoction of bark taken for constipation. (129:241) **Potawatomi** *Cathartic* Inner bark used as a physic. (131:75)

Rhamnus cathartica, Common Buckthorn
Cherokee *Cathartic* Bark and fruit used as a cathartic. *Dermatological Aid* Decoction of bark used for itch. *Eye Medicine* Used as wash for sore and inflamed eyes. (66:27)

Rhamnus crocea ssp. ***ilicifolia***, Hollyleaf Redberry
Kawaiisu *Analgesic* Decoction of roots and bark taken for internal soreness. Plant smoke inhaled for headaches. *Antirheumatic* (*Internal*) Plant smoke inhaled for rheumatism. *Blood Medicine* Infusion of roots and bark taken as a blood medicine. Plant used by women for blood shortages. *Cold Remedy* Decoction of roots and bark taken for colds. *Cough Medicine* Decoction of roots and bark taken for coughs. *Dermatological Aid* Plant used for boils and carbuncles. *Diuretic* Decoction of roots used to increase urination. *Gastrointestinal Aid* Plant used for stomach disorders and the spleen. *Gynecological Aid* Plant used by women for blood shortages. *Kidney Aid* Plant used for the kidneys. *Laxative* Decoction of roots used to loosen the bowels and as a laxative. *Liver Aid* Plant used for the liver and spleen. *Stimulant* Infusion of roots and bark taken when "one feels tired and run down." *Venereal Aid* Decoction of roots used for gonorrhea. (as *R. ilicifolia* 180:58) **Yuki** *Unspecified* Inner bark used as a "good medicine." (as *R. ilicifolia* 33:369)

Rheum rhaponticum, False Rhubarb
Cherokee *Antidiarrheal* Used for dysentery. *Cathartic* Used as a mild purgative. *Dermatological Aid* Used as an astringent. *Laxative* Infusion of plant taken for constipation. *Poison* Leaves considered poisonous. *Strengthener* Used for strengthening. (66:52)

Rhexia virginica, Handsome Harry
Micmac *Throat Aid* Leaves and stems used as a throat cleanser. (32:60) **Montagnais** *Throat Aid* "Brew" from leaves and stems used for cleaning the throat. (133:314)

Rhizomnium glabrescens, Koponen
Bella Coola *Antirheumatic* (*External*) Poultice of crushed "leaves" applied to infections and swellings. *Blood Medicine* Poultice of "leaves" used for blood blisters. *Breast Treatment* Poultice of "leaves" used for breast abscesses in women. *Dermatological Aid* Poultice of "leaves" used for boils. (158:196)

Rhododendron albiflorum, Cascade Azalea
Okanagon *Dermatological Aid* Poultice of powdered, burned wood and grease applied to swellings. *Gastrointestinal Aid* Decoction of bark taken as a stomach remedy. (104:40) **Skokomish** *Cold*

Remedy Decoction of buds taken for colds. *Dermatological Aid* Poultice of chewed buds applied to cuts. *Gastrointestinal Aid* Chewed buds eaten for an ulcerated stomach. *Throat Aid* Decoction of buds taken for sore throats. (65:43) **Thompson** *Dermatological Aid* Poultice of powdered, burned wood and grease applied to swellings. (104:40) Wood ash mixed with grease and used as a salve for swellings. (141:460) *Gastrointestinal Aid* Decoction of bark taken as a stomach remedy. (104:40)

Rhododendron calendulaceum, Flame Azalea
Cherokee *Antirheumatic* (*External*) Peeled and boiled twig rubbed on rheumatism. *Gynecological Aid* Infusion taken by women. (66:24)

Rhododendron macrophyllum, Pacific Rhododendron
Karok *Ceremonial Medicine* Plant used in the luck-getting ceremony of the sweat house. (as *R. californicum* 125:387)

Rhododendron maximum, Great Laurel
Cherokee *Analgesic* Compound used as liniment for pains and poultice of leaves used for headache. (66:52) Infusion of leaves put on scratches made over the location of the pain. (152:49) *Antirheumatic* (*Internal*) Compound decoction of leaf taken for rheumatism. *Ceremonial Medicine* "Throw clumps of leaves into a fire and dance around it to bring cold weather." *Heart Medicine* Infusion of leaf taken for heart trouble. (66:52) *Other* Decoction of leaves rubbed into scratches made on legs as preliminary treatment. (152:49)

Rhododendron occidentale var. *occidentale*, Western Azalea
Modesse *Antidote* Used for poisoning. (as *Azalea occidentalis* 97:224)

Rhus aromatica, Fragrant Sumac
Natchez *Dermatological Aid* Poultice of root applied to boils. (148:667) **Ojibwa** *Ceremonial Medicine* Bark and berries used in medicine ceremonies. *Unspecified* Bark and berries used in medicinal purposes. (112:234) **Ojibwa, South**

Antidiarrheal Compound decoction of root taken for diarrhea. (77:201)

Rhus copallinum, Flameleaf Sumac
Cherokee *Antiemetic* Red berries eaten for vomiting. *Burn Dressing* Infusion poured over sunburn blisters. (66:57) *Dermatological Aid* Decoction of bark used as a wash for blisters. (152:36) *Gynecological Aid* Infusion of bark taken "to make human milk flow abundantly." *Urinary Aid* Red berries chewed for bed-wetting. (66:57) **Creek** *Antidiarrheal* Decoction of root taken for dysentery. (148:659) Decoction of roots taken for dysentery. (152:36) **Delaware** *Dermatological Aid* Poultice of roots applied to sores and skin eruptions. Infusion of leaves used to cleanse and purify skin eruptions. *Oral Aid* Berries used to make mouthwash. *Venereal Aid* Infusion of roots used for venereal disease. (151:32) **Delaware, Oklahoma** *Ceremonial Medicine* Leaves and root used in "ceremonial tobacco mixture." *Dermatological Aid* Poultice of roots or infusion of leaves used for sores and skin eruptions. *Oral Aid* Berries used to make mouthwash. *Venereal Aid* Infusion of root taken for venereal disease. (150:26, 78) **Koasati** *Orthopedic Aid* and *Pediatric Aid* Decoction of leaves used as a bath and given to babies to make them walk. (152:36) **Ojibwa** *Ceremonial Medicine* Bark and berries used in medicine ceremonies. *Unspecified* Bark and berries used for medicinal purposes. (112:234)

Rhus copallinum var. *leucantha*, Winged Sumac
Seminole *Dermatological Aid* Poultice of plant applied for ant sickness: boils and infections. (as *R. leucantha* 145:304) *Urinary Aid* Decoction of root bark taken for urine retention. *Venereal Aid* Decoction of bark taken for gonorrhea. (as *R. leucantha* 145:274)

Rhus glabra, Smooth Sumac
Cherokee *Antiemetic* Red berries eaten for vomiting. *Burn Dressing* Infusion poured over sunburn blisters. (66:57) *Dermatological Aid* Decoction of bark used as a wash for blisters. (152:36) *Gynecological Aid* Infusion of bark taken "to make human milk flow abundantly." *Urinary Aid* Red berries chewed for bed-wetting. (66:57) **Chippewa** *Anti-*

diarrheal Decoction of "growth which sometimes appears on the tree" used for dysentery. (43:344) *Cold Remedy* Infusion of roots taken for colds. *Emetic* Infusion of roots taken as an emetic. (59:135) *Oral Aid* Compound decoction of blossoms used as mouthwash for teething children. (43:342) Blossoms chewed for sore mouth. (59:135) *Pediatric Aid* Compound decoction of flower used as a mouthwash for teething child. (43:342) *Respiratory Aid* Infusion of plants taken for asthma. (59:135) **Creek** *Antidiarrheal* Decoction of root taken for dysentery. (148:659) Decoction of roots taken for dysentery. (152:36) *Other* Leaves mixed with tobacco and smoked for "all cephalic and pectoral complaints." (148:659) **Flathead** *Cathartic* Fruits used as a purgative. *Tuberculosis Remedy* Infusion of green or dried branches taken for tuberculosis. (68:55) **Iroquois** *Alterative* Sprouts used as an alterative. (103:93) **Kiowa** *Other* Plant used to "purify" the body and mind. *Tuberculosis Remedy* Plant used for tuberculosis. (166:37) **Kutenai** *Throat Aid* Roots squeezed and juice swallowed for sore throat. (68:55) **Meskwaki** *Dermatological Aid* Root bark used as a rubefacient, to raise a blister on the patient. *Dietary Aid* Decoction of root taken as an appetizer by invalids. (129:200) **Micmac** *Ear Medicine* Parts of plant used for earaches. (32:60) **Nez Perce** *Dermatological Aid* Leaves moistened and used for skin rashes. (68:55) **Ojibwa** *Ceremonial Medicine* Bark and berries used in medicine ceremonies. (112:234) *Dermatological Aid* Inner bark of trunk or twig used in compounds as astringents. *Eye Medicine* Infusion

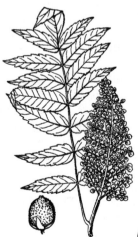

Rhus glabra

of blossoms used as a wash for sore eyes. *Hemostat* Infusion of root bark used as a "hemostatic." (130:354) *Unspecified* Bark and berries used for medicinal purposes. (112:234) Poultice of leaves used for unspecified conditions. (130:354) **Okanagan-Colville** *Dermatological Aid* Decoction of branches with seed heads used for an itchy scalp condition. Milky latex used as a salve on sores. *Gynecological Aid* Decoction of seed heads taken by women during childbirth. *Heart Medicine* Infusion of bark and/or roots taken and applied externally to the chest for a "tight chest." *Other* Decoction of branches with seed heads used as bathing water for frost-bitten limbs. *Venereal Aid* Decoction of seed heads used as bathing water for gonorrhea. (162:59) **Okanagon** *Oral Aid* Root chewed for sore mouth or tongue. (104:41) **Omaha** *Analgesic* Decoction of root taken for painful urination and retention of urine. (58:99, 100) *Antidote* Poultice of plants applied for poisoning. (56:335) *Dermatological Aid* Infusion used as wash for sores and powdered plants applied to wounds and open sores. (56:334) Poultice of leaves or fruits applied "in case of poisoning of the skin." *Diuretic* Decoction of root taken "in case of retention of urine." *Gynecological Aid* Decoction of root used as a postpartum styptic wash. *Hemostat* Decoction of fruits used as a postpartum styptic wash. *Urinary Aid* Decoction of root taken for painful urination and retention of urine. **Pawnee** *Antidiarrheal* Decoction of fruit used for "bloody flux." *Gynecological Aid* Decoction of fruit used for dysmenorrhea. (58:99, 100) **Sanpoil** *Dermatological Aid* Mashed leaves rubbed on sore lips. *Oral Aid* Leaves chewed and held in the mouth for sore gums. (109:219) **Sioux** *Antihemorrhagic* Decoction of fruits used by women for hemorrhaging after parturition. *Dermatological Aid* Poultice of bruised and wetted leaves or fruits used for poisoned skin. *Urinary Aid* Infusion of roots used for urine retention and painful urination. (68:55) **Thompson** *Gastrointestinal Aid* Decoction of shredded bark with another plant taken for ulcers. *Internal Medicine* Infusion of plant used after internal surgery, to make the wounds heal faster. (161:149) *Oral Aid* Root chewed for sore mouth or tongue. (104:41) Fresh root chewed for sore mouth or tongue. (141:466) *Poison* Decoction of plant considered poisonous if too strong or taken in large dose. (141:512) *Venereal Aid* Decoction of stems and roots taken for syphilis. (141:466)

Rhus hirta, Staghorn Sumac
Algonquin, Quebec *Antirheumatic (Internal)* Infusion of plant with chokecherry, oak, yellow birch, and dogwood used for rheumatism. *Dietary Aid* Infusion of fruits used as tonic to improve the appetite. *Unspecified* Root used as a medicine. (as *R. typhina* 14:192) **Cherokee** *Antiemetic* Red berries eaten for vomiting. *Burn Dressing* Infusion poured over sunburn blisters. *Gynecological Aid* Infusion of bark taken "to make human milk flow abundantly." *Urinary Aid* Red berries chewed for bed-wetting. (as *R. typhina* 66:57) **Chippewa** *Analgesic* Decoction of flowers taken for stomach pain. *Gastrointestinal Aid* Decoction of flowers taken for stomach pain. (43:344) **Delaware** *Venereal Aid* Roots combined with purple coneflower roots and used for venereal disease. (as *R. typhina* 151:33) **Delaware, Oklahoma** *Venereal Aid* Compound containing root used for venereal disease. (as *R. typhina* 150:28, 78) **Delaware, Ontario** *Antidiarrheal* Infusion of berries taken for diarrhea. (as *R. typhina* 150:69, 82) **Iroquois** *Dietary Aid* Wood pieces eaten by mothers to improve the milk. *Gynecological Aid* Infusion of bark, buds, and branches from another plant taken before giving birth. *Reproductive Aid* Infusion of bark and flowers taken to prevent the water from breaking too early during the pregnancy. (as *R. typhina* 118:51) **Malecite** *Blood Medicine* Infusion of roots or berries used as a blood purifier. (as *R. typhina* 96:253) *Cough Medicine* Used with blackberry roots, mountain holly, lily roots, and mountain raspberry roots for coughs. *Febrifuge* Used with blackberry roots, mountain holly, lily roots, and mountain raspberry roots for fevers. *Tuberculosis Remedy* Used with blackberry roots, mountain holly, lily roots, and mountain raspberry roots for consumption. (as *Thus typhina* 96:251) **Menominee** *Cough Medicine* Decoction of "red top" sweetened, strained, "boiled down," and used for coughs. (44:130) *Dermatological Aid* Inner bark considered astringent and used as a valuable pile remedy. *Gastrointestinal Aid* Infusion of root bark taken for "inward troubles." *Gynecological Aid* Hairy twigs of smaller shrubs used for various "female diseases." *Hemorrhoid Remedy* Astrin-

gent, inner bark of trunk considered a valuable pile remedy. *Pulmonary Aid* and *Tuberculosis Remedy* Compound containing berries used for consumption and pulmonary troubles. (as *R. typhina* 128:22) **Meskwaki** *Anthelmintic* Compound containing berries used for pinworms. (as *R. typhina* 129:201) **Micmac** *Dietary Aid* Berries and roots used for loss of appetite. *Throat Aid* Parts of plant used for sore throats. (as *R. typhina* 32:60) Used for sore throats. Used for sore throats. (as *R. typhina* 168:25) **Mohegan** *Throat Aid* Berries used to make a gargle for sore throat. (as *R. typhina* 151:75, 132) **Natchez** *Dermatological Aid* Poultice of roots applied to boils. (as *R. typhina* 152:37) **Ojibwa** *Hemostat* Root used for hemorrhages. (as *R. typhina* 130:354) *Oral Aid* Infusion of gall-infected leaves taken for mouth sores. *Throat Aid* Infusion of gall-infected leaves taken for sore throat. (as *R. typhina* 4:2244) **Potawatomi** *Anthelmintic* Compound containing berries used to expel worms. *Hemostat* Root bark used as a "hemostatic." *Misc. Disease Remedy* Infusion of leaves used as gargle for sore throat, tonsillitis, and erysipelas. *Throat Aid* Infusion of leaves gargled for sore throat, tonsillitis, and erysipelas. (as *R. typhina* 131:38) **Rappahannock** *Panacea* Decoction of stems, leaves, or berries used for complaint. (as *R. typhina* 138:30)

Rhus ovata, Sugar Sumac
Cahuilla *Cold Remedy* Infusion of leaves taken for colds. *Cough Medicine* Infusion of leaves taken for coughs. (11:131) **Coahuilla** *Analgesic* Infusion of leaves taken for chest pain. *Cough Medicine* Infusion of leaves taken for coughs. (9:78) **Diegueño** *Gynecological Aid* Infusion of leaves taken just before the birth for an easy delivery. (74:218)

Rhus trilobata, Skunkbush Sumac
Blackfoot *Misc. Disease Remedy* Dried berries ground and dusted onto smallpox pustules. (82:42) **Cheyenne** *Burn Dressing* Plant used to protect the hands when removing dog meat from a boiling pot. *Cold Remedy* Leaves used for head colds. *Diuretic* Decoction of leaves taken as a diuretic. *Hemostat* Plant used for bleeding. *Reproductive Aid* "Old man took this medicine and bore a child (an aphrodisiac?)." *Toothache Remedy* Fruit chewed for toothaches. *Veterinary Aid* Fruit used

for horses with urinary troubles and to prevent tiredness. (69:14) **Comanche** *Cold Remedy* Bark chewed and juice swallowed for colds. (24:524) **Hopi** *Ceremonial Medicine* Twigs used for ceremonial purposes. (46:16) *Dermatological Aid* Roots used as deodorant. (34:356) Buds used on the body as a medicinal deodorant or perfume. (174:84) *Tuberculosis Remedy* Compound containing root used for "consumption." (174:35, 84) *Unspecified* Roots used medicinally for unspecified purpose. (34:356) **Jemez** *Oral Aid* Bark chewed for sore gums. (36:27) **Keres**, **Western** *Emetic* Infusion of leaves used as an emetic. *Gastrointestinal Aid* Infusion of leaves used as a stomach wash. *Gynecological Aid* Infusion of bark used as a douche after childbirth. *Oral Aid* Berries used for a mouthwash. (147:66) **Kiowa** *Gastrointestinal Aid* Berries eaten for stomach troubles. *Misc. Disease Remedy* Berries eaten for grippe. (166:39) **Mahuna** *Dietary Aid* and *Gastrointestinal Aid* Plant used as appetite restorative for inactive stomach that refused food. (117:63) **Montana Indian** *Misc. Disease Remedy* Powdered fruit applied as a lotion or dusted on the affected surface in cases of smallpox. (15:21) **Navajo**, **Kayenta** *Dermatological Aid* Plant used as a lotion for poison ivy dermatitis. *Gastrointestinal Aid* Plant used for bowel troubles. (179:31) **Navajo**, **Ramah** *Analgesic* Leaves chewed for stomachache. *Contraceptive* Decoction of leaves taken to induce impotency, as a means of contraception. *Dermatological Aid* Poultice of leaves used for itch and decoction of fruits used to prevent falling hair. *Gastrointestinal Aid* Leaves chewed for stomachache. *Gynecological Aid* Decoction of root bark used to facilitate delivery of placenta. (165:35, 36) **Paiute** *Dermatological Aid* Dried, powdered fruits used as an astringent for smallpox sores. (155:129) **Round Valley Indian** *Dermatological Aid* and *Misc. Disease Remedy* Dried, powdered berries used for smallpox sores. **Yokia** *Dermatological Aid* and *Misc. Disease Remedy* Dried, powdered berries used for smallpox sores. (33:365)

Rhus trilobata var. *pilosissima*, Pubescent Squawbush
Diegueño *Eye Medicine* and *Pediatric Aid* Infusion of leaves used as a wash for babies' eyes. (70:37)

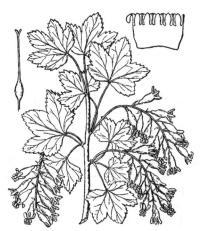

Ribes americanum

Ribes americanum, American Black Currant
Blackfoot *Gynecological Aid* Decoction of roots taken by women for uterine troubles. *Kidney Aid* Decoction of roots taken for kidney ailments. (82:37) **Iroquois** *Antidote* Compound infusion of branches taken as remedy for poison. (73:345) *Antiemetic* Compound infusion of roots and bark taken for vomiting. (73:346) *Dermatological Aid* Poultice of bark used for swellings. (73:345) *Kidney Aid* Compound infusion of roots and bark taken for kidney trouble. *Orthopedic Aid* Compound infusion of roots and bark taken for back pains. *Other* Compound decoction of bark taken for fortune-telling or divination. Decoction of leaves taken by women hurting inside from lifting. (73:346) **Meskwaki** *Anthelmintic* Root bark used to expel intestinal worms. (as *R. floridum* 129:246) **Ojibwa** *Unspecified* Root and bark used for medicinal purposes. (as *R. floridum* 112:236) **Omaha** *Kidney Aid* Strong decoction of root taken for kidney trouble. **Winnebago** *Gynecological Aid* Root used by women for "uterine trouble." (58:84)

Ribes aureum, Golden Currant
Paiute *Dermatological Aid* Dried, pulverized inner bark sprinkled on sores. *Orthopedic Aid* Decoction of inner bark taken for leg swellings. **Shoshoni** *Orthopedic Aid* Decoction of inner bark taken for leg swellings. (155:129) *Unspecified* Poultice of second bark applied medicinally. (98:43)

Ribes aureum* var. *villosum, Golden Currant
Kiowa *Snakebite Remedy* Poultice of plant parts
applied to snakebites. (as *R. odoratum* 166:29)

Ribes bracteosum, Stink Currant
Bella Coola *Unspecified* Berries and "cane" used
for medicine. (158:206) *Venereal Aid* Compound
decoction of berry taken for gonorrhea. Compound decoction taken for gonorrhea. (127:57)
Haisla *Dermatological Aid* Plant used for impetigo. *Reproductive Aid* Roots used as a birthing aid.
Hanaksiala *Unspecified* Roots used for unspecified type of medicine. (35:253) **Nitinaht** *Laxative*
Berries eaten in quantity as a laxative. (160:113)
Sanpoil *Cold Remedy* and *Pediatric Aid* Infusion
of stems given to children for colds. (109:218)

Ribes cereum, Wax Currant
Hopi *Gastrointestinal Aid* Used for stomach pains.
(164:163) **Okanagan-Colville** *Eye Medicine* Infusion of inner bark used to wash sore eyes. (162:
107) **Shoshoni** *Emetic* Fruit used as an emetic.
(100:48) **Thompson** *Antidiarrheal* Berries eaten
for diarrhea. *Pediatric Aid* and *Strengthener* Decoction of branches with many other branches used
to wash babies to make them strong. (161:226)

Ribes cereum* var. *pedicellare, Whisky
  Currant
Navajo, Kayenta *Ceremonial Medicine* Plant
used as an Evilway, Nightway, and Mountain-top-
way emetic. *Dermatological Aid* Poultice of plant
applied to sores. *Emetic* Plant used as an Evilway,
Nightway, and Mountain-top-way emetic. *Pediatric
Aid* Plant used to purify a child who has seen a for-
bidden sand painting. (as *R. inebrians* 179:26)

Ribes cynosbati, Eastern Prickly Gooseberry
Meskwaki *Gynecological Aid* Root used for uterine trouble caused by having too many children.
(129:246) **Potawatomi** *Eye Medicine* Infusion of
root used for sore eyes. *Gynecological Aid* Root
bark used by the Prairie Potawatomi as a uterine
remedy. (131:82)

Ribes divaricatum, Spreading Gooseberry
Bella Coola *Cold Remedy* Inner bark chewed and
juice swallowed for colds. (158:206) *Eye Medicine*
Simple or compound decoction of bark or root

used as an eyewash for soreness. (127:58) *Throat
Aid* Inner bark chewed and juice swallowed for
sore throats. (158:206) **Cowlitz** *Dermatological
Aid* Burned stems rubbed on neck sores. **Klallam**
Eye Medicine Infusion of bark used as an eyewash.
Makah *Eye Medicine* Infusion of bark used as an
eyewash. (65:32) **Saanich** *Psychological Aid* Roots
used with wild cherry roots to wash newborn children for intelligence and obedience. **Salish,
Coast** *Other* Infusion of roots rubbed on the skin
for a charley horse. (156:84) **Skagit, Upper**
Throat Aid Roots boiled for sore throats. (154:38)
Swinomish *Throat Aid* Infusion of roots taken for
sore throats. *Tuberculosis Remedy* Infusion of
roots taken for tuberculosis. *Venereal Aid* Infusion
of roots taken for venereal disease. (65:32)

Ribes glandulosum, Skunk Currant
Chippewa *Analgesic* Compound decoction of root
taken for back pain. *Gynecological Aid* Compound
decoction of root taken for "female weakness."
(43:356) **Cree, Woodlands** *Gynecological Aid*
Decoction of stem used alone or with wild red
raspberry to prevent blood clotting after birth.
(91:54)

Ribes hudsonianum, Northern Black Currant
Cree, Woodlands *Gynecological Aid* Decoction
of stem sections alone or with wild gooseberry
stems used for sickness after childbirth. (91:55)
Ojibwa *Unspecified* Root and bark used for medicinal purposes. (112:236) **Tanana, Upper** *Cold
Remedy* Raw currants eaten for colds. *Panacea*
Decoction of leaves and berries taken for sickness
in general. (86:11) **Thompson** *Cold Remedy* Decoction of stems and leaves taken for colds. (141:
471) Infusion of branches possibly taken for colds.
(161:227) *Gastrointestinal Aid* Decoction of stems
and leaves taken for stomach troubles. (141:471)
Panacea Roots used for any kind of sickness.
(161:227) *Pediatric Aid* and *Sedative* Sprigs
placed in baby's carrier to quiet child. (141:509)
Throat Aid Decoction of stems and leaves taken
for sore throats. (141:471) *Tuberculosis Remedy*
Roots used for tuberculosis. (161:227)

Ribes indecorum, Whiteflower Currant
Luiseño *Toothache Remedy* Roots used for toothaches. (132:232)

Ribes lacustre, Prickly Currant
Bella Coola *Dermatological Aid* Leaves or bark chewed and cud tied on sores caused by the prickers of plant. *Laxative* Decoction of root taken many times a day for constipation. **Gitksan** *Unspecified* Decoction of bark used for "some unspecified malady." (127:58) **Lummi** *Analgesic* Decoction of twigs taken for general body aches. (65:32) **Okanagan-Colville** *Antidiarrheal* Decoction of dried branches taken for diarrhea. *Cold Remedy* Decoction of dried branches taken for colds. (162:107) **Oweekeno** *Poison* Plant considered poisonous. (35:104) **Saanich** *Psychological Aid* Roots used with wild cherry roots to wash newborn children for intelligence and obedience. **Salish, Coast** *Other* Infusion of roots rubbed on the skin for a charley horse. (156:84) **Shuswap** *Panacea* Berries used for health and strength. (102:63) **Skagit** *Eye Medicine* Decoction of bark used as a wash for sore eyes. *Gynecological Aid* Decoction of bark taken during childbirth. (65:32) **Skagit, Upper** *Gynecological Aid* Decoction of bark taken by women during childbirth. (154:38) **Swinomish** *Poison* Thorns considered poisonous. (65:32) **Thompson** *Eye Medicine* Infusion of cambium layer used as a wash for sore eyes. *Gastrointestinal Aid* Decoction of wood taken as a tonic for the stomach. (141:469) *Gynecological Aid* Berries considered good medicine for women. (161:229) *Other* Decoction of roots and scraped stems taken for "general indisposition." *Tonic* Decoction of wood taken as a tonic for the stomach. (141:469)

Ribes laxiflorum, Trailing Black Currant
Bella Coola *Eye Medicine* Simple or compound decoction of root used each day as an eyewash to remove matter. (127:57) Infusion of roots and branches used as an eyewash. (158:206) **Lummi** *Tonic* Decoction of leaves and twigs taken as a general tonic. **Skagit** *Cold Remedy* Decoction of bark taken as a cold medicine. (65:32) **Skagit, Upper** *Cold Remedy* Bark boiled and used as a cold medicine. (154:38) **Skokomish** *Tuberculosis Remedy* Decoction of bark and roots taken for tuberculosis. (65:32)

Ribes lobbii, Gummy Gooseberry
Kwakiutl *Antidiarrheal* Roots used for diarrhea. *Dermatological Aid* Poultice of roots and salt

water applied to sores, blisters, and carbuncles. Root ash and oil used as salve on boils. *Oral Aid* Poultice of roots and salt water applied to mouth sores. (157:286) **Saanich** *Psychological Aid* Roots used with wild cherry roots to wash newborn children for intelligence and obedience. **Salish, Coast** *Other* Infusion of roots rubbed on the skin for a charley horse. (156:84)

Ribes malvaceum, Chaparral Currant
Luiseño *Toothache Remedy* Roots used for toothaches. (132:232)

Ribes oxyacanthoides, Canadian Gooseberry
Cree, Woodlands *Gynecological Aid* Decoction of stems and wild black currant stems used for sickness after childbirth. (91:55) **Ojibwa** *Unspecified* Root and bark used for medicinal purposes. (112:236)

Ribes oxyacanthoides ssp. *irriguum*, Idaho Gooseberry
Thompson *Gastrointestinal Aid* and *Tonic* Decoction of root taken as a tonic for the stomach. (as *Grossularia irrigua* 141:472)

Ribes oxyacanthoides ssp. *oxyacanthoides*, Canadian Gooseberry
Chippewa *Analgesic* and *Gynecological Aid* Compound decoction of berry taken for back pain and "female weakness." (as *Grossularia oxyacanthoides* 43:356)

Ribes pinetorum, Orange Gooseberry
Navajo, Ramah *Ceremonial Medicine* Leaves used as emetics in various ceremonies. *Emetic* Leaves used as a ceremonial emetic. (165:30)

Ribes rotundifolium, Appalachian Gooseberry
Cherokee *Antidiarrheal* Infusion of bark taken "to check bowels." *Misc. Disease Remedy* Infusion taken for measles. *Sedative* Infusion of leaf taken for nerves. (66:36) **Iroquois** *Other* Compound decoction of bark taken for fortune-telling or divination. (73:345)

Ribes rubrum, Cultivated Currant
Ojibwa *Unspecified* Root and bark used for medicinal purposes. (112:236)

Ribes triste, Red Currant
Chippewa *Abortifacient* Compound decoction
of stalk taken for "stoppage of periods." (43:358)
Urinary Aid Decoction of root and stalk taken for
"gravel." (43:348) **Ojibwa** *Gynecological Aid*
Leaves used as some sort of female remedy. (130:
389) **Tanana, Upper** *Eye Medicine* Decoction of
stems, without the bark, used as a wash for sore
eyes. *Unspecified* Decoction of stems, without the
bark, taken as a medicine. (86:11)

Ribes uva-crispa var. **sativum**, European
   Gooseberry
Micmac *Cathartic* Bark and roots used as a
physic. (as *R. grossularia* 32:61)

Ricinus communis, Castor Bean
Cahuilla *Dermatological Aid* Seeds crushed into
a greasy substance and used for sores. *Poison*
Seeds and leaves considered poisonous. (11:133)
Cherokee *Cathartic* Infusion of beans used as a
purgative. *Dermatological Aid* Poultice of beans
used for boils. (66:24) **Diegueño** *Dermatological
Aid* Bean nuts mashed to make an ointment, similar to cold cream, and used for acne and pimples.
(70:37) **Hawaiian** *Analgesic* Leaves used for severe headaches. *Febrifuge* Poultice of leaves applied to the head and body for strong fevers. *Pediatric Aid* Poultice of leaves applied to children's
heads and bodies for strong fevers. (2:55) **Navajo**
Contraceptive Plant used by women to become
sterile. (45:60) **Pima** *Analgesic* Beans eaten for

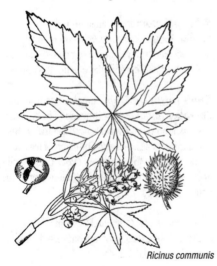

Ricinus communis

headaches. *Cathartic* Beans eaten as a purge. *Dermatological Aid* Beans dried, ground, and sprinkled on sores. *Laxative* Beans eaten for constipation. *Poison* Plant considered poisonous. (38:100)
Seminole *Cathartic* Beans used as a cathartic.
(145:167) Infusion of seeds taken as a cathartic
for constipation. (145:275)

Robinia hispida, Bristly Locust
Cherokee *Emetic* Root bark chewed as an emetic.
Toothache Remedy Beaten root held on tooth for
toothache. *Veterinary Aid* Infusion given to cows
as a "tonic." (66:43)

Robinia neomexicana, New Mexico Locust
Hopi *Emetic* Used as an emetic to purify the stomach. (174:83)

Robinia pseudoacacia, Black Locust
Cherokee *Emetic* Root bark chewed as an emetic.
Toothache Remedy Beaten root held on tooth for
toothache. *Veterinary Aid* Infusion given to cows
as a "tonic." (66:43) **Menominee** *Adjuvant*
Trunk bark used as a seasoner to give flavor to
medicines. (128:40)

Rorippa alpina, Alpine Yellowcress
Navajo *Gynecological Aid* Infusion of plants taken
as a tonic after deliverance. (as *Radicula alpina*
45:49)

Rorippa nasturtium-aquaticum, Water
   Cress
Costanoan *Febrifuge* Cold infusion of plants taken
for fevers. *Kidney Aid* Decoction of plant used as a
kidney remedy. *Liver Aid* Decoction of plant used
as a liver remedy. (as *Nasturtium officinale* 17:10)
Mahuna *Liver Aid* Plant used for torpid liver,
cirrhosis of the liver, and gallstones. (117:65)
Okanagan-Colville *Analgesic* Poultice of fresh,
whole plants applied to the forehead for headaches.
Vertigo Medicine Poultice of fresh, whole plants
applied to the forehead for dizziness. (162:92)

Rorippa palustris ssp. **hispida**, Hispid
   Yellowcress
Navajo, Ramah *Ceremonial Medicine* and *Eye
Medicine* Plant used in ceremonial eyewash. (as *R.
hispida* 165:29)

Rorippa sinuata, Spreading Yellowcress
Zuni *Eye Medicine* Infusion of plant used as a
wash and smoke from blossoms used for inflamed
eyes. (as *Radicula sinuata* 143:59)

Rorippa sylvestris, Creeping Yellowcress
Iroquois *Febrifuge* and *Pediatric Aid* Decoction
of plant taken by mother for fever in baby.
(73:342)

Rosa acicularis, Prickly Rose
Cree, Woodlands *Cough Medicine* Decoction of
roots taken as a cough remedy. *Eye Medicine* Infusion of roots used for sore eyes. (91:55) **Iroquois**
Eye Medicine Compound infusion of rose leaves
and bark used as drops for blindness. (73:358)
Gynecological Aid Cold, compound infusion of
twig bark taken for difficult birth. (73:359) *Witchcraft Medicine* Compound decoction of plants and
doll used for black magic. (73:358) **Okanagan-
Colville** *Ceremonial Medicine* Decoction of
leaves, branches, and other boughs taken and used
as body and hair wash by sweat bathers. *Dermatological Aid* Poultice of chewed leaves applied to
bee stings. (162:131) **Tanana, Upper** *Blood Medicine* Decoction of stems and branches taken for
weak blood. *Cold Remedy* Decoction of stems and
branches taken for colds. *Emetic* Infusion of bark
strained and taken to induce vomiting. *Febrifuge*
Decoction of stems and branches taken for fevers.
Gastrointestinal Aid Decoction of stems and
branches taken for stomach troubles. (86:12)
Thompson *Antidiarrheal* Decoction of branches,
chokecherry, and red willow taken for diarrhea.
Antiemetic Decoction of branches, chokecherry,
and red willow taken for vomiting. *Dermatological
Aid* Leaves placed in moccasins for athlete's foot
and possibly for protection. *Gynecological Aid*
Hips chewed by women in labor, to hasten the
delivery. Decoction of roots taken by women after
childbirth. Decoction of branches, chokecherry,
and red willow taken for women's illnesses. *Venereal Aid* Decoction of roots taken for syphilis.
(161:267)

Rosa acicularis* ssp. *sayi, Prickly Rose
Blackfoot *Antidiarrheal* and *Pediatric Aid* Root
used to make a drink given to children for diarrhea. (as *R. sayi* 95:275)

Rosa arkansana, Prairie Rose
Chippewa *Anticonvulsive* Compound infusion or
decoction of root taken for "fits." (41:63, 64) Compound decoction of root taken for convulsions.
(43:336) *Hemostat* Compound infusion or decoction of root used on bleeding wounds. (41:63, 64)
Compound decoction of root used on bleeding
wounds. (43:336) *Stimulant* Compound infusion
or decoction of root taken or used externally as
stimulant. (41:63, 64) Compound decoction of
root taken as a stimulant. *Tonic* Compound decoction of root taken as a tonic. (43:364) **Omaha** *Eye
Medicine* Roots used for eye troubles. (56:336)

Rosa arkansana* var. *suffulta, Prairie Rose
Omaha *Eye Medicine* Infusion of fruit used as a
wash for inflamed eyes. **Pawnee** *Burn Dressing*
Poultice of charred, crushed hypertrophied stem
growths applied to burns. (as *R. pratincola* 58:85)

Rosa blanda, Smooth Rose
Meskwaki *Dermatological Aid* Decoction of fruit
used for itching piles or any other itch. *Gastrointestinal Aid* Rose hip skin used for stomach troubles and decoction of fruit used for piles. *Hemorrhoid Remedy* Decoction of fruit used for itching
piles. (129:242, 243) **Ojibwa** *Gastrointestinal Aid*
Dried, powdered flowers used for heartburn. Rose
hip skin used for stomach trouble and indigestion.
(130:385) **Ojibwa, South** *Eye Medicine* Infusion
of root used as a wash for inflamed eyes. (77:200)
Potawatomi *Analgesic* Infusion of root taken for
headache or lumbago. *Orthopedic Aid* Infusion of
root taken for lumbago. *Unspecified* Rose hip skin
used as medicine by the Prairie Potawatomi.
(131:78)

Rosa californica, California Wild Rose
Cahuilla *Analgesic* and *Pediatric Aid* Infusion
of blossoms used for infant pain. (11:133) **Costanoan** *Antirheumatic* (*Internal*) Decoction of fruit
"hips" used for rheumatism. *Cold Remedy* Decoction of fruit "hips" used for colds. *Dermatological
Aid* Decoction of fruit "hips" used as a wash for
scabs and sores. *Febrifuge* Decoction of fruit
"hips" used for fevers. *Gastrointestinal Aid* Decoction of fruit "hips" used for indigestion. *Kidney
Aid* Decoction of fruit "hips" used for kidney ailments. *Throat Aid* Decoction of fruit "hips" used

for sore throats. (17:18) **Diegueño** *Febrifuge* and *Pediatric Aid* Infusion of petals given to babies with fever. (70:39) **Mahuna** *Analgesic* Infusion of seeds taken for painful congestion. *Febrifuge* Infusion of seeds taken for stomach fevers. *Gastrointestinal Aid* Infusion of seeds taken for stomach fevers and painful congestion. (117:8) **Miwok** *Analgesic* Infusion of leaves and berries taken for pains. *Gastrointestinal Aid* Infusion of leaves and berries taken for colic. (8:172)

Rosa carolina, Carolina Rose
Menominee *Gastrointestinal Aid* Fruit skin eaten for stomach troubles. (as *R. humilis* 128:50)

Rosa eglanteria, Sweetbriar Rose
Iroquois *Gastrointestinal Aid* Plant used as an intestinal astringent by forest runners. (118:47) *Urinary Aid* Compound decoction of plants taken for difficult urination. (as *R. rubiginosa* 73:358)

Rosa gallica, French Rose
Mahuna *Febrifuge* Plant used for high fevers and chills. (117:26)

Rosa gymnocarpa, Dwarf Rose
Okanagan-Colville *Ceremonial Medicine* Decoction of leaves, branches, and other boughs taken and used as body and hair wash by sweat bathers. *Dermatological Aid* Poultice of chewed leaves applied to bee stings. (162:131) **Thompson** *Eye Medicine* Decoction of bark used as a wash for sore eyes. (141:466) *Hunting Medicine* Decoction of plant poured onto hunting equipment which had "lost its luck." (141:507) *Poison* Spines considered poisonous as they caused swelling and irritation if touched. Hips considered poisonous and would give one an itchy bottom if eaten. (161:266) *Tonic* Decoction of stems taken for "general indisposition" and as a tonic. (141:466)

Rosa nutkana, Nootka Rose
Bella Coola *Diaphoretic* Roots and sprouts used in steam baths. *Eye Medicine* Infusion of roots and sprouts used as an eyewash. (158:209) **Carrier** *Eye Medicine* Decoction of roots applied to sore eyes. (26:86) **Chehalis** *Analgesic* Decoction of bark taken by women to ease labor pains in childbirth. *Gynecological Aid* Decoction of bark taken

by women to ease labor pains in childbirth. **Cowlitz** *Pediatric Aid* and *Strengthener* Decoction of leaves used as a wash to strengthen babies. (65:34) **Keres, Western** *Misc. Disease Remedy* and *Pediatric Aid* Crushed petals rubbed on children's bodies to prevent smallpox. (as *R. nelina* 147:67) **Nitinaht** *Unspecified* Infusion of leaves used for medicine. (160:123) **Okanagan-Colville** *Ceremonial Medicine* Decoction of leaves, branches, and other boughs taken and used as body and hair wash by sweat bathers. *Dermatological Aid* Poultice of chewed leaves applied to bee stings. (162:131) **Quileute** *Dermatological Aid* Poultice of haw ashes applied to "swellings." **Quinault** *Dermatological Aid* and *Venereal Aid* Poultice of twig ashes and skunk oil applied to syphilitic sores. **Skagit** *Eye Medicine* Infusion of roots used as an eyewash. *Throat Aid* Decoction of roots taken for sore throats. (65:34) **Skagit, Upper** *Throat Aid* Decoction of roots and sugar used for sore throats. (154:42) **Thompson** *Antidiarrheal* Decoction of branches, chokecherry, and red willow taken for diarrhea. *Antiemetic* Decoction of branches, chokecherry, and red willow taken for vomiting. *Dermatological Aid* Leaves placed in moccasins for athlete's foot and possibly for protection. *Gynecological Aid* Decoction of roots taken by women after childbirth. Decoction of branches, chokecherry, and red willow taken for women's illnesses. *Venereal Aid* Decoction of roots taken for syphilis. (161:267)

Rosa palustris, Swamp Rose
Cherokee *Anthelmintic* Infusion of bark and root used for worms. *Antidiarrheal* Decoction of roots taken for dysentery. (66:53)

Rosa pisocarpa, Cluster Rose
Snohomish *Throat Aid* Decoction of roots taken for sore throats. **Squaxin** *Gynecological Aid* Infusion of bark taken after childbirth. (65:34) **Thompson** *Antidiarrheal* Decoction of branches, chokecherry, and red willow taken for diarrhea. *Antiemetic* Decoction of branches, chokecherry, and red willow taken for vomiting. *Dermatological Aid* Leaves placed in moccasins for athlete's foot and possibly for protection. *Gynecological Aid* Decoction of roots taken by women after childbirth. Decoction of branches, chokecherry, and red wil-

low taken for women's illnesses. *Venereal Aid* Decoction of roots taken for syphilis. (161:267) **Yurok** *Unspecified* Fruit used to make a medicinal tea. (5:51)

Rosa virginiana, Virginia Rose

Cherokee *Anthelmintic* and *Pediatric Aid* Decoction of roots used as a bath and given to children with worms. (152:29) **Ojibwa** *Dermatological Aid* Infusion of roots taken and used as a wash for bleeding foot cuts. *Hemostat* Infusion of roots taken and used as a wash for bleeding foot cuts. (as *R. lucida* 112:231) *Unspecified* Root and bark used for medicinal purposes. (as *R. lucida* 112:236) **Ojibwa, South** *Eye Medicine* Infusion of root used as a wash for sore eyes. (as *R. lucida* 77:201)

Rosa woodsii, Woods's Rose

Arapaho *Antirheumatic* (*External*) Seeds used to produce a drawing effect for muscular pains. (100:48) **Okanagan-Colville** *Ceremonial Medicine* Decoction of leaves, branches, and other boughs taken and used as body and hair wash by sweat bathers. *Dermatological Aid* Poultice of chewed leaves applied to bee stings. (162:131) **Paiute** *Antidiarrheal* Decoction of root taken by adults and children for diarrhea. *Burn Dressing* Poultice of various plant parts applied to burns. *Cold Remedy* Decoction of root or inner bark taken for colds. *Dermatological Aid* Poultice of mashed fungus galls applied to opened boils. Poul-

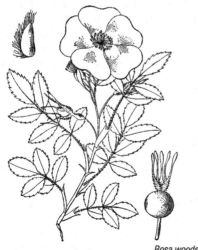

Rosa woodsii

tice of various plant parts applied to sores, cuts, swellings, and wounds. *Misc. Disease Remedy* and *Pediatric Aid* Decoction of roots given to children for intestinal influenza. *Tonic* Infusion of leaves taken as a spring tonic. **Shoshoni** *Antidiarrheal* Decoction of root taken for diarrhea. *Blood Medicine* Compound decoction of roots taken as a blood tonic and for general debility. *Burn Dressing* Poultice of various plant parts applied to burns. *Cold Remedy* Decoction of root or inner bark taken for colds. *Dermatological Aid* Poultice of various plant parts applied to sores, cuts, swellings, and wounds. *Diuretic* Decoction of root taken for "failure of urination." *Tonic* Compound decoction of roots taken as a blood tonic and for general debility. (155:129–131) **Thompson** *Antidiarrheal* Decoction of branches, chokecherry, and red willow taken for diarrhea. *Antiemetic* Decoction of branches, chokecherry, and red willow taken for vomiting. *Cough Medicine* Infusion of one handful of washed hips taken for coughs. Infusion of sticks taken for coughs. *Dermatological Aid* Leaves placed in moccasins for athlete's foot and possibly for protection. *Gynecological Aid* Hips chewed by women in labor, to hasten the delivery. Decoction of roots taken by women after childbirth. Decoction of branches, chokecherry, and red willow taken for women's illnesses. *Pediatric Aid* Infusion of one handful of washed hips taken, especially by babies, for coughs. Infusion of sticks taken for coughs, especially babies' coughs. *Throat Aid* Infusion of one handful of washed hips taken for sore, itchy throats. Infusion of sticks taken for sore, itchy throats. *Venereal Aid* Decoction of roots taken for syphilis. (161:267) **Washo** *Cold Remedy* Decoction of root or inner bark taken for colds. (155:129–131)

Rosa woodsii var. *woodsii*, Woods's Rose

Isleta *Pediatric Aid* Rose petals soaked in water and the liquid given to newborn babies before the mother's milk. (as *R. fendleri* 85:42) **Navajo, Ramah** *Ceremonial Medicine* and *Emetic* Leaves used as a ceremonial emetic. (as *R. fendleri* 165:31)

Rubus allegheniensis, Allegheny Blackberry

Cherokee *Antidiarrheal* Infusion of root or leaf used for diarrhea. *Antirheumatic* (*Internal*) Infusion given for rheumatism. (66:26) *Dermatological Aid* Compound, astringent, and tonic infusion of root used as a wash for piles. (66:25, 26) *Hemorrhoid Remedy* Compound infusion of root used for piles. *Oral Aid* Washed root chewed for coated tongue. *Stimulant* Used as a stimulant. *Throat Aid* Used with honey as a wash for sore throat. *Tonic* Used as a tonic. *Urinary Aid* Compound decoction taken to regulate urination. (66:26) Infusion of bark taken for urinary troubles. (152:29) *Venereal Aid* Used for venereal disease. (66:26) **Chippewa** *Antidiarrheal* Infusion of roots taken for diarrhea. *Gynecological Aid* Infusion of roots taken by pregnant women threatened with miscarriage. (59:133) **Iroquois** *Analgesic* Compound of plant used as a snuff for headaches. (73:357) *Antidiarrheal* Plant used as a diarrhea medicine. *Blood Medicine* Compound decoction of roots taken by all ages as blood remedy. (73:356) *Cold Remedy* Compound decoction of roots taken for colds. *Cough Medicine* Compound decoction of roots taken for coughs. *Dermatological Aid* Poultice of smashed roots applied to baby's sore navel after birth. *Other* Root used for "summer complaint." *Pediatric Aid* Poultice of smashed roots applied to baby's sore navel after birth. *Respiratory Aid* Compound of plant used as a snuff for catarrh. (73:357) *Tuberculosis Remedy* Compound decoction of roots taken for tuberculosis. *Witchcraft Medicine* Infusion of roots used to make dogs good hunters and ensure them from theft. (73:356) **Menominee** *Eye Medicine* Infusion of root used as a wash for sore eyes. *Unspecified* Poultice of infusion of root used for unspecified ailments. (128:50) **Meskwaki** *Antidote* Decoction of root used as an antidote for poison. *Eye Medicine* Root extract used for sore eyes and stomach trouble. *Gastrointestinal Aid* Root extract used for stomach trouble and sore eyes. (129:243) **Ojibwa** *Antidiarrheal* Infusion of root used to "arrest flux." *Diuretic* Decoction of canes taken as a diuretic. (130:385, 386) **Potawatomi** *Eye Medicine* Root bark used by the Prairie Potawatomi for sore eyes. (131:79)

***Rubus allegheniensis* var. *allegheniensis*,**
    Allegheny Blackberry
Delaware *Antidiarrheal* Vine combined with wild cherry bark and used for diarrhea. (as *R. nigrobaccus* 151:33) **Delaware, Oklahoma** *Antidiar-*

rheal Compound containing vine and wild cherry bark used for dysentery. (as *R. nigrobaccus* 150:28, 78)

***Rubus arcticus* ssp. *acaulis*,** Dwarf Raspberry
Shuswap *Antidiarrheal* Leaves used for diarrhea. (as *R. acaulis* 102:67)

***Rubus argutus*,** Sawtooth Blackberry
Cherokee *Antidiarrheal* Infusion of root or leaf used for diarrhea. *Antirheumatic* (*Internal*) Infusion given for rheumatism. (66:26) *Dermatological Aid* Compound, astringent, and tonic infusion of root used as a wash for piles. (66:25, 26) *Hemorrhoid Remedy* Compound infusion of root used for piles. *Oral Aid* Washed root chewed for coated tongue. *Stimulant* Used as a stimulant. *Throat Aid* Used with honey as a wash for sore throat. *Tonic* Used as a tonic. *Urinary Aid* Compound decoction taken to regulate urination. *Venereal Aid* Used for venereal disease. (66:26)

***Rubus canadensis*,** Smooth Blackberry
Delaware, Oklahoma *Antidiarrheal* Vine and berries used for dysentery. (150:78) **Iroquois** *Unspecified* Berries, maple sap, and water used to make a medicine. (170:142) **Menominee** *Antidiarrheal* Simple or compound decoction of root used for dysentery. (44:131)

***Rubus chamaemorus*,** Cloudberry
Cree, Woodlands *Gynecological Aid* Decoction of roots used as a "woman's medicine." Decoction of plant used for hard labor. *Reproductive Aid* Decoction of root and lower stem used by barren women. (91:56) **Micmac** *Cough Medicine* Roots used for cough. *Febrifuge* Roots used for fever. *Tuberculosis Remedy* Roots used for consumption. (32:61)

***Rubus cuneifolius*,** Sand Blackberry
Seminole *Other* Complex infusion of roots taken for chronic conditions. (145:272)

***Rubus flagellaris*,** Northern Dewberry
Cherokee *Antidiarrheal* Infusion of root or leaf used for diarrhea. *Antirheumatic* (*Internal*) Infusion given for rheumatism. (66:26) *Dermatologi-*

cal Aid Compound, astringent, and tonic infusion of root used as a wash for piles. (66:25, 26) *Hemorrhoid Remedy* Compound infusion of root used for piles. *Oral Aid* Washed root chewed for coated tongue. *Stimulant* Used as a stimulant. *Throat Aid* Used with honey as a wash for sore throat. *Tonic* Used as a tonic. *Urinary Aid* Compound decoction taken to regulate urination. *Venereal Aid* Used for venereal disease. (66:26)

Rubus frondosus, Yankee Blackberry
Chippewa *Abortifacient* Decoction of root taken for "stoppage of periods." (43:358) *Pulmonary Aid* Compound decoction of root taken for lung trouble. (43:340)

Rubus fruticosus, Shrubby Blackberry
Micmac *Antidiarrheal* and *Pediatric Aid* Bark and roots used for children's diarrhea. (32:61)

Rubus hawaiensis, Hawaii Blackberry
Hawaiian *Antiemetic* Plant ashes mixed with poi or potatoes and eaten for vomiting. *Dermatological Aid* Infusion of plant ashes and tobacco leaf ashes used as a wash for scaly scalps. *Gastrointestinal Aid* Plant ashes mixed with "papaia meat" and eaten for burning in the chest. (2:8)

Rubus hispidus, Bristly Dewberry
Micmac *Cough Medicine* Roots used for cough. *Febrifuge* Roots used for fever. *Tuberculosis Remedy* Roots used for consumption. (32:61) **Mohegan** *Anthelmintic* Infusion of berries taken as a vermifuge. (149:265) *Antidiarrheal* Juice of plant taken for dysentery. (149:269) Juice of berries taken for dysentery. (151:75, 132) **Rappahannock** *Antidiarrheal* Infusion taken for diarrhea. (25:119) Fermented decoction of berries or roots taken for dysentery. *Dermatological Aid* Infusion of leaves taken for boils. *Tonic* Fermented decoction of berries taken for dysentery and as a tonic. (138:32) **Shinnecock** *Antidiarrheal* Infusion taken for diarrhea and fruit used to check dysentery. (25:119)

Rubus idaeus, American Red Raspberry
Algonquin, Quebec *Antidiarrheal* Root used for diarrhea. *Unspecified* Root had medicinal value. (14:180) **Algonquin, Tête-de-Boule** *Urinary Aid*

Decoction of roots used for bloody urine. (110:130) **Cherokee** *Analgesic* Strong infusion of red raspberry leaves used for childbirth pains. *Antirheumatic (External)* Thorny branch used to scratch rheumatism. *Cathartic* Taken as a purgative. *Cough Medicine* Root chewed for cough. *Dermatological Aid* Infusion taken as a tonic for boils. Leaves highly astringent and decoction taken for bowel complaint. Used as wash for old and foul sores and infusion taken as tonic for boils. *Emetic* Taken as an emetic. *Gastrointestinal Aid* Decoction taken for bowel complaint. *Gynecological Aid* Strong infusion used for childbirth pains and decoction used for menstrual period. *Tonic* Infusion taken as a tonic for boils. *Toothache Remedy* Roots used for toothache. (66:52) **Cree, Woodlands** *Gynecological Aid* Decoction of stem and upper part of the roots used to help a woman recover after childbirth, and to slow menstrual bleeding. *Heart Medicine* Fruit used as a heart medicine. *Pediatric Aid* and *Toothache Remedy* Decoction of stem and upper part of the roots used for teething sickness. (91:57) **Iroquois** *Analgesic* Decoction of leaves taken for "burning and pain when passing water." *Blood Medicine* Compound used when the "blood is bad and sores break out on the neck." Decoction of roots taken as a blood purifier. *Cathartic* Decoction of leaves taken as a physic. *Dermatological Aid* Compound used for boils. Compound used when the "blood is bad and sores break out on the neck." *Emetic* Decoction of leaves taken as an emetic. *Gynecological Aid* Compound decoction taken by "ladies who are run

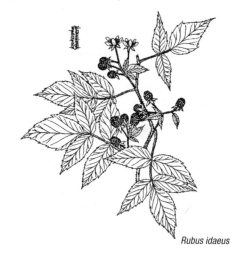

Rubus idaeus

down from period sickness." *Hypotensive* Decoction of roots taken for low or high blood pressure. *Kidney Aid* Decoction of leaves taken for the kidneys. *Liver Aid* Decoction of leaves taken for bile. *Stimulant* Compound decoction taken by "ladies who are run down from period sickness." Compound used for laziness. *Tonic* Plant used as a tonic. *Urinary Aid* Decoction of leaves taken for "burning and pain when passing water." *Venereal Aid* Compound decoction of roots taken for gonorrhea. (73:355) *Veterinary Aid* Leaves, rhizomes from another plant, and wheat flour given to cows at birthing. (118:48) **Menominee** *Adjuvant* Root used as a seasoner for medicines. (128:50) **Okanagan-Colville** *Antidiarrheal* Decoction of branches taken for diarrhea. *Cathartic* Decoction of branches taken as a physic. *Gastrointestinal Aid* Decoction of branches taken for heartburn. *Laxative* Decoction of roots taken for constipation. (162:131)

Rubus idaeus* ssp. *strigosus, Grayleaf Red
  Raspberry
Cherokee *Cathartic* Infusion of roots taken as a cathartic by women during menses. *Emetic* Infusion of roots taken as an emetic by women during menses. *Gynecological Aid* Infusion of roots taken as an emetic and cathartic by women during menses. (152:30) **Chippewa** *Antidiarrheal* Decoction of root taken for dysentery. (as *R. strigosus* 43: 344) *Eye Medicine* Infusion of root bark used as a wash for cataracts. (as *R. strigosus* 43:360) *Misc. Disease Remedy* Decoction of roots or stems taken for measles. (as *R. strigosus* 59:132) **Meskwaki** *Adjuvant* Root used as a seasoner in medicines. (as *R. idaeus-aculeatissi* 129:243) **Ojibwa** *Adjuvant* Berries used as a seasoner for medicines. *Eye Medicine* Infusion of root bark used for sore eyes. (130:386) **Ojibwa, South** *Analgesic* Decoction of crushed root taken for stomach pain. *Gastrointestinal Aid* Decoction of crushed root taken for stomach pain. (as *R. strigosus* 77:199) **Omaha** *Gastrointestinal Aid* and *Pediatric Aid* Decoction of scraped root given to children for bowel trouble. (as *R. strigosus* 58:84, 85) **Potawatomi** *Eye Medicine* Infusion of root used as an eyewash. (131:79) **Thompson** *Antihemorrhagic* Decoction of leaves taken for spitting or vomiting blood. *Gastrointes-*

tinal Aid and *Tonic* Decoction of root taken as a tonic for the stomach. (as *R. strigosus* 141:466)

Rubus leucodermis, Whitebark Raspberry
Pomo, Kashaya *Antidiarrheal* Infusion of leaves or root taken for diarrhea. *Gastrointestinal Aid* Infusion of leaves or root taken for upset stomach. *Other* Infusion of leaves or root taken for weak bowels. (60:96) **Shoshoni** *Dermatological Aid* Poultice of powdered stems applied to wounds and cuts. (155:131) **Thompson** *Misc. Disease Remedy* Mild infusion of washed roots taken for influenza. (161:269)

Rubus macraei, 'Akala
Hawaiian *Antiemetic* Plant ashes mixed with poi or potatoes and eaten for vomiting. *Dermatological Aid* Infusion of plant ashes and tobacco leaf ashes used as a wash for scaly scalps. *Gastrointestinal Aid* Plant ashes mixed with "papaia meat" and eaten for burning in the chest. (2:8)

Rubus occidentalis, Black Raspberry
Cherokee *Analgesic* Strong infusion of red raspberry leaves used for childbirth pains. *Antirheumatic (External)* Thorny branch used to scratch rheumatism. *Cathartic* Taken as a purgative. (66:52) Infusion of roots taken as a cathartic by women during menses. (152:30) *Cough Medicine* Root chewed for cough. *Dermatological Aid* Infusion taken as a tonic for boils. Leaves highly astringent and decoction taken for bowel complaint. Used as wash for old and foul sores and infusion taken as tonic for boils. *Emetic* Taken as an emetic. (66:52) Infusion of roots taken as an emetic by women during menses. (152:30) *Gastrointestinal Aid* Decoction taken for bowel complaint. *Gynecological Aid* Strong infusion used for childbirth pains and decoction used for menstrual period. (66:52) Infusion of roots taken as an emetic and cathartic by women during menses. (152:30) *Tonic* Infusion taken as a tonic for boils. *Toothache Remedy* Roots used for toothache. (66:52) **Chippewa** *Analgesic* Compound decoction of root taken for back pain. (43:356) *Eye Medicine* Decoction of roots used as a wash for sore eyes. (59:133) *Gynecological Aid* Compound decoction of root taken for "female weakness." (43:356) **Iroquois** *Antidiarrheal* Compound decoction of roots taken

for diarrhea with blood. *Cathartic* Leaves used as a physic. *Emetic* Leaves used as an emetic. *Liver Aid* Leaves used for removing bile. *Pediatric Aid* and *Pulmonary Aid* Decoction of roots, stalks, and leaves given to children with whooping cough. *Venereal Aid* Compound decoction of roots taken for gonorrhea. *Witchcraft Medicine* Decoction taken by a hunter and his wife to prevent her from fooling around. (73:356) **Menominee** *Tuberculosis Remedy* Root used with *Hypericum* sp. for consumption in the first stages. (128:50) **Ojibwa, South** *Analgesic* and *Gastrointestinal Aid* Decoction of crushed root taken for stomach pain. (77:199) **Omaha** *Gastrointestinal Aid* and *Pediatric Aid* Decoction of scraped root given to children for bowel trouble. (58:84, 85)

Rubus odoratus, Purpleflowering Raspberry
Cherokee *Analgesic* Strong infusion of red raspberry leaves used for childbirth pains. *Antirheumatic (External)* Thorny branch used to scratch rheumatism. *Cathartic* Taken as a purgative. *Cough Medicine* Root chewed for cough. *Dermatological Aid* Infusion taken as a tonic for boils. Leaves highly astringent and decoction taken for bowel complaint. Used as wash for old and foul sores and infusion taken as tonic for boils. *Emetic* Taken as an emetic. *Gastrointestinal Aid* Decoction taken for bowel complaint. *Gynecological Aid* Strong infusion used for childbirth pains and decoction used for menstrual period. *Tonic* Infusion taken as a tonic for boils. *Toothache Remedy* Roots used for toothache. (66:52) **Iroquois** *Antidiarrheal* Decoction of scraped bark or roots taken for diarrhea. *Blood Medicine* Decoction taken as blood medicine and blood purifier. (73:354) *Cold Remedy* Roots used for colds. (73:355) *Dermatological Aid* Compound decoction taken and used as wash for venereal disease chancres and sores. (73:354) *Diuretic* Berries eaten in late summer or dried in winter and used as a diuretic. (103:96) *Gastrointestinal Aid* Decoction or infusion of branches taken to settle the stomach. (73:355) *Gynecological Aid* Compound infusion of plants taken by women who have a miscarriage. *Kidney Aid* Compound decoction of stalks and leaves taken as kidney medicine. *Laxative* and *Pediatric Aid* Decoction given as blood medicine and for the bowels of newborn babies. *Venereal Aid* Com-

pound decoction taken and used as wash for venereal disease chancres and sores. (73:354)

Rubus parviflorus, Thimbleberry
Blackfoot *Pulmonary Aid* Berries given by diviners to patients to eat for chest disorders. (72:74) **Cowlitz** *Burn Dressing* Poultice of dried leaves applied to burns. (65:34) **Karok** *Dietary Aid* Infusion of roots taken by thin people as an appetizer or tonic. *Tonic* Infusion of roots taken by thin people as a tonic. (125:384) **Kwakiutl** *Antiemetic* Decoction of leaves taken for vomiting. *Antihemorrhagic* Decoction of leaves taken for blood-spitting. *Dermatological Aid* Dried, powdered leaves applied to wounds. *Gynecological Aid* Leaves used when a woman's period was unduly long. *Internal Medicine* Dried, powdered leaves eaten for internal disorders. (157:291) **Makah** *Blood Medicine* Decoction of leaves taken for anemia and to strengthen the blood. (65:34) **Montana Indian** *Alterative* Young sprouts considered a valuable alterative. *Misc. Disease Remedy* Young sprouts considered a valuable antiscorbutic. (as *R. nutkanus* 15:21) **Okanagan-Colville** *Dermatological Aid* Decoction of roots taken by young people with pimples and blackheads. Leaves rubbed on the face of young people with pimples and blackheads. *Gastrointestinal Aid* Infusion of roots taken for stomach ailments. (162:132) **Saanich** *Antidiarrheal* Leaves dried and chewed for diarrhea. *Gastrointestinal Aid* Leaves dried and chewed for stomachaches. (156:87) **Skagit** *Dermatological Aid* Poultice of leaf ashes and grease applied to swellings. (65:34) **Thompson** *Dermatological Aid* and *Pediatric Aid* Green insect galls found on stems burned and the ashes rubbed on babies' navels if they did not heal. (161:270)

Rubus procumbens, Wild Blackberry
Mahuna *Antidiarrheal* Infusion of roots taken for diarrhea. (as *R. villosus* 117:7)

Rubus pubescens, Dwarf Red Blackberry
Okanagon *Antiemetic* and *Antihemorrhagic* Decoction of leaves taken for vomiting of blood and blood-spitting. *Gastrointestinal Aid* Decoction of leaves taken as a stomach tonic. *Tonic* Decoction of leaves taken as a stomach tonic. **Thompson** *Antiemetic* Decoction of leaves taken for vomiting

of blood and blood-spitting. *Antihemorrhagic* Decoction of leaves taken for vomiting of blood and blood-spitting. (104:41) Decoction of leaves taken for spitting or vomiting blood. (141:466) *Gastrointestinal Aid* Decoction of leaves taken as a stomach tonic. (104:41) Decoction of root taken as a tonic for the stomach. (141:466) *Tonic* Decoction of leaves taken as a stomach tonic. (104:41) Decoction of root taken as a tonic for the stomach. (141:466)

Rubus pubescens var. *pubescens*, Dwarf Red Blackberry
Malecite *Abortifacient* Infusion of plant and wild strawberry used for irregular menstruation. (as *R. triflorus* 96:258) **Micmac** *Abortifacient* Parts of plant used for irregular menstruation. (as *R. triflorus* 32:61)

Rubus spectabilis, Salmon Berry
Bella Coola *Gastrointestinal Aid* Decoction of root bark taken for stomach troubles. (127:58) **Kwakiutl** *Burn Dressing* Powdered bark applied to burns. *Dermatological Aid* Powdered bark applied to sores. *Pediatric Aid* Chewed sprouts applied to the head of a child to make him grow. (157:291) **Makah** *Analgesic* and *Dermatological Aid* Poultice of bark applied to wounds for the pain. *Toothache Remedy* Poultice of bark applied to aching tooth. **Quileute** *Burn Dressing* Poultice of chewed leaves or bark applied to burns. **Quinault** *Analgesic* Decoction of bark taken to lessen labor pains. *Burn Dressing, Dermatological Aid*, and *Disinfectant* Decoction of bark used to clean infected wounds, especially burns. *Gynecological Aid* Decoction of bark taken to lessen labor pains. (65:35)

Rubus trivialis, Southern Dewberry
Cherokee *Antidiarrheal* Infusion of root or leaf used for diarrhea. *Antirheumatic (Internal)* Infusion given for rheumatism. (66:26) *Dermatological Aid* Compound, astringent, and tonic infusion of root used as a wash for piles. (66:25, 26) *Hemorrhoid Remedy* Compound infusion of root used for piles. *Oral Aid* Washed root chewed for coated tongue. *Stimulant* Used as a stimulant. *Throat Aid* Used with honey as a wash for sore throat. *Tonic* Used as a tonic. *Urinary Aid* Compound decoction

taken to regulate urination. *Venereal Aid* Used for venereal disease. (66:26) **Seminole** *Gastrointestinal Aid* Infusion of herbage used for stomach troubles. (145:276)

Rubus ursinus, California Blackberry
Diegueño *Antidiarrheal* Decoction of roots taken or fresh fruit eaten for diarrhea. (70:39) **Hesquiat** *Gastrointestinal Aid* Decoction of the entire vine taken for stomach troubles. *Other* Decoction of the entire vine taken for a general sick feeling. (159:75) **Kwakiutl** *Antidiarrheal* Compound decoction of vines taken for diarrhea. (157:264) *Antiemetic* Decoction of vines and roots taken for vomiting. *Antihemorrhagic* Decoction of vines and roots taken for blood-spitting. (157:291) **Pomo, Kashaya** *Antidiarrheal* Decoction of root taken for diarrhea. *Gynecological Aid* Berries not to be eaten by pregnant women or fathers to be; if berries eaten, the baby would be dark. (60:22)

Rubus ursinus ssp. *macropetalus*, California Blackberry
Skagit *Gastrointestinal Aid* Infusion of leaves taken for stomach trouble. (as *R. macropetalus* 65:35) **Skagit, Upper** *Gastrointestinal Aid* Infusion of leaves taken for stomach trouble. (as *R. macropetalus* 154:38)

Rubus vitifolius, Pacific Dewberry
Costanoan *Antidiarrheal* Decoction of roots used for dysentery and diarrhea. *Dermatological Aid* and *Disinfectant* Roots used for infected sores. (17:19) **Mendocino Indian** *Antidiarrheal* Infusion of roots taken for diarrhea. (33:355)

Rudbeckia fulgida, Orange Coneflower
Cherokee *Anthelmintic* Used as wash for "swelling caused by worms." *Dermatological Aid* Warm infusion of root used to bathe sores. *Ear Medicine* Root ooze used for earache. *Gynecological Aid* Taken for "flux and some private diseases." *Kidney Aid* Infusion taken for dropsy. *Snakebite Remedy* Used as wash for snakebites. *Venereal Aid* Taken for "flux and some private diseases."

Rudbeckia hirta, Black Eyed Susan
Cherokee *Anthelmintic* Used as wash for "swelling caused by worms." *Dermatological Aid* Warm

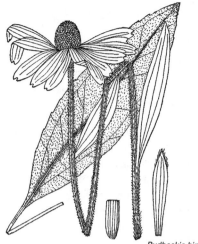

Rudbeckia hirta

infusion of root used to bathe sores. *Ear Medicine* Root ooze used for earache. *Gynecological Aid* Taken for "flux and some private diseases." *Kidney Aid* Infusion taken for dropsy. *Snakebite Remedy* Used as wash for snakebites. *Venereal Aid* Taken for "flux and some private diseases." (66:30) **Chippewa** *Pediatric Aid* Poultice of blossoms and another plant used for babies. (59:143) **Iroquois** *Anthelmintic* Infusion of roots given to children with worms. *Heart Medicine* Decoction of plants taken for the heart. *Pediatric Aid* Infusion of roots given to children with worms. (73:469) **Potawatomi** *Cold Remedy* Infusion of root taken for colds. (131:52, 53) **Shuswap** *Eye Medicine* Plant used for sore eyes. (102:59)

Rudbeckia hirta var. *angustifolia*, Black Eyed Susan
Seminole *Analgesic* Cold infusion of cone flowers used for headaches. *Febrifuge* Cold infusion of cone flowers used for fevers. (as *R. divergens* 145:283)

Rudbeckia laciniata, Cutleaf Coneflower
Cherokee *Dietary Aid* Cooked spring salad eaten to "keep well." (66:30) **Chippewa** *Burn Dressing* Compound poultice of blossoms applied to burns. (43:352) *Gastrointestinal Aid* Compound infusion of root taken for indigestion. (43:342) *Veterinary Aid* Compound infusion of root applied to chest and legs of horse as a stimulant. (43:366)

Rumex acetosa, Garden Sorrel
Apalachee *Unspecified* Plant water used for medicinal purposes. (67:98) **Eskimo, Kuskokwagmiut** *Antidiarrheal* Decoction of leaves and stems taken for diarrhea. (101:24)

Rumex acetosella, Common Sheep Sorrel
Aleut *Dermatological Aid* Poultice of steamed leaves applied to warts and bruises. (6:427) **Cherokee** *Dermatological Aid* Poultice of bruised leaves and blossoms applied to old sores. (66:56) **Mohegan** *Gastrointestinal Aid* Fresh leaves chewed as a stomach aid. (151:75, 132) **Squaxin** *Tuberculosis Remedy* Raw leaves eaten for tuberculosis. (65:29)

Rumex altissimus, Pale Dock
Dakota *Dermatological Aid* Poultice of green leaves applied to boils. (57:361) **Lakota** *Antidiarrheal* Used for diarrhea. *Antihemorrhagic* Used for hemorrhages. *Gastrointestinal Aid* Used for stomach cramps. (116:55) **Ojibwa** *Unspecified* Plant used for medicinal purposes. (112:240)

Rumex aquaticus var. *fenestratus*, Western Dock
Bella Coola *Analgesic* Leaves used in a sweat bath for pains similar to rheumatism all over body. *Antirheumatic* (*External*) Leaves used in sweat bath for pains similar to rheumatism. *Dermatological Aid* Poultice of leaves and mashed, roasted roots applied to boils and wounds. (as *R. occidentalis* 127:56) Poultice of long, yellow roots, and "klondike soap" applied to boils, cuts, and scrapes. (as *R. occidentalis* 158:207) *Herbal Steam* Leaves used in a sweat bath for pains similar to rheumatism all over body. (as *R. occidentalis* 127:56) **Haisla** *Laxative* Plant used as a laxative. **Hanaksiala** *Antirheumatic* (*External*) Poultice of pounded leaves and stems applied to sores and other painful areas. *Dermatological Aid* Roots cooked and inserted into wounds. Poultice of root paste applied to cuts and boils. Poultice of pounded leaves and stems applied to sores and other painful areas. (as *R. occidentalis* var. *procerus* 35:260) **Kwakiutl** *Dermatological Aid* Root extract used to wash sores and swellings. *Gastrointestinal Aid* Boiled roots eaten and applied as poultice for stomachaches. (as *R. occidentalis* 157:287)

Rumex arcticus, Arctic Dock
Eskimo, Inuktitut *Antidiarrheal* Leaves and stems used for diarrhea. (176:186)

Rumex conglomeratus, Clustered Dock
Karok *Herbal Steam* Decoction of plant used as a steam bath medicine. (125:383) **Miwok** *Dermatological Aid* Decoction of root taken for boils. Poultice of boiled root applied to boils. (8:172)

Rumex crispus, Curly Dock
Blackfoot *Antirheumatic* (*External*) Mashed root pulp used for swellings. *Dermatological Aid* Mashed root pulp used for sores. (98:43) **Cherokee** *Antidiarrheal* Infusion taken for dysentery. *Blood Medicine* Infusion of root taken "for blood." *Dermatological Aid* Juice and infusion of root used as poultice and salve for various skin problems. *Kidney Aid* Infusion of root taken "to correct fluids." *Laxative* Infusion of root used for constipation. *Throat Aid* Leaves rubbed in mouth for sore throat. *Veterinary Aid* Beaten roots fed to horses for "sick stomach." (66:32) **Cheyenne** *Antihemorrhagic* Infusion of dried roots taken for lung hemorrhages. *Dermatological Aid* Poultice of pounded, dried roots applied to wounds or sores. (63:172) Wet poultice of pounded, dried root applied to wounds or sores. (64:172) *Pulmonary Aid* Infusion of dried roots taken for lung hemorrhages. (63:172) Infusion of dried, pulverized root taken for lung hemorrhage. (64:172) Infusion of pulverized roots used for lung hemorrhages. (69:32)

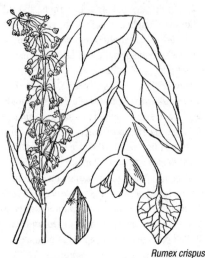

Rumex crispus

Chippewa *Dermatological Aid* Poultice of moistened, dried, powdered root applied to cuts or itches. (43:350) Poultice of dried, pounded root applied to ulcers and swellings. (43:354, 366) **Costanoan** *Urinary Aid* Decoction of plant used for urinary problems. (17:11) **Dakota** *Dermatological Aid* Poultice of crushed, green leaves applied to boils to draw out pus. (58:77) **Delaware** *Blood Medicine* Root used as a blood purifier. *Liver Aid* Root used for jaundice. (151:33) **Delaware, Oklahoma** *Blood Medicine* Root used as a blood purifier. *Liver Aid* Root used for jaundice. (150:28, 78) **Iroquois** *Antidiarrheal* Compound decoction of roots taken for diarrhea with blood. (73:311) *Antirheumatic* (*External*) Stalks cooked as greens and used for rheumatism. (103:93) *Blood Medicine* Compound decoction taken as blood medicine when "blood is bad from scrofula." *Cathartic* Decoction taken as a physic for general bowel trouble and intestinal colds. *Dermatological Aid* Infusion taken and poultice used for swellings caused by blood catching cold. (73:312) *Dietary Aid* Decoction of roots taken "when one can't eat." *Emetic* Decoction of plants taken as an emetic before running or playing lacrosse. *Gastrointestinal Aid* Decoction of roots taken for intestinal colds, cramps, or abdominal pains. Decoction of roots taken for upset stomach. Poultice used for swollen body from yellow fever, abdominal cramps, and pains. (73:311) *Hemorrhoid Remedy* Compound decoction of plant taken and used as a wash for piles. *Hemostat* Used for bleeding. (73:312) *Kidney Aid* Decoction of plants taken for kidney trouble. (73:311) *Love Medicine* Decoction used as a wash for face, hands, and clothes as love medicine. (73:312) *Misc. Disease Remedy* Decoction of roots taken and poultice applied for yellow fever. (73:311) *Orthopedic Aid* Used for strained muscles. *Panacea* "Good for all illnesses." (73:312) *Reproductive Aid* Compound decoction of roots taken to induce pregnancy. *Strengthener* Decoction taken to makes muscles strong for running or playing lacrosse. (73:311) *Tonic* Compound decoction of roots taken by women as a tonic. *Venereal Aid* Compound used for gonorrhea. (73:312) **Isleta** *Gastrointestinal Aid* Leaves eaten as greens for the beneficial effect upon the stomach. (85:42) **Micmac** *Cathartic* Roots used as a purgative. (32:61) Infusion of roots used as a purgative.

(96:259) *Urinary Aid* Roots used "cold in bladder." (32:61) Infusion of roots, hemlock, parsley, and prince's pine used for colds in the bladder. (96:259) **Mohegan** *Blood Medicine* Cooked leaves said to "purify the blood." *Tonic* Root used to make a tonic. (151:75, 132) **Navajo** *Stimulant* Plant used for fainting. (76:155) **Navajo**, **Ramah** *Ceremonial Medicine* Whole plant used as a ceremonial emetic. *Dermatological Aid* Dried, powdered leaves dusted on sores. *Emetic* Whole plant used as a ceremonial emetic. *Oral Aid* Cold infusion of leaf used on mouth sores. *Panacea* Root used as a "life medicine." (165:24) **Nevada Indian** *Veterinary Aid* Poultice of root applied to saddle sores. (98:49) **Ojibwa** *Antidiarrheal* Boiled seeds used for diarrhea. (4:2289) Seeds boiled and used for diarrhea. (4:2318) *Dermatological Aid* Root used to close and heal cuts. (130:381) *Hunting Medicine* Dried seeds smoked as a favorable lure to game when mixed with kinnikinnick. (130:431) **Ojibwa, South** *Dermatological Aid* Poultice of bruised or crushed root applied to sores and abrasions. (77:200) **Paiute** *Analgesic* Poultice of pulped root applied to rheumatic pains. *Antidiarrheal* Boiled seeds eaten alone or in a compound for diarrhea. (155:131, 132) *Antirheumatic (External)* Poultice of chewed roots used for pain and swelling of sprained or swollen areas. (93:67) Poultice of pulped root applied to rheumatic swellings. *Blood Medicine* Decoction of root taken as a blood purifier. *Burn Dressing* Poultice of pulped root applied to burns. (155:131, 132) *Dermatological Aid* Roots used for the astringent properties. (144:317) Poultice of pulped root applied to bruises and swellings. (155:131, 132) *Gastrointestinal Aid* Decoction of roots taken, or raw, peeled roots eaten for stomach disorders. *Tonic* Roots used for the tonic properties. (144:317) Decoction of root taken as a general tonic. *Venereal Aid* Decoction of root taken for venereal disease. (155:131, 132) **Paiute, Northern** *Dermatological Aid* Roots ground into a powder and used on sores and cuts. (49:128) **Rappahannock** *Blood Medicine* An ingredient of a blood medicine. (138:31) **Shoshoni** *Analgesic* Poultice of pulped root applied to rheumatic pains. *Antirheumatic (External)* Poultice of pulped root applied to rheumatic swellings. *Blood Medicine* Decoction of root taken as a blood purifier. *Burn Dressing* Poultice of

pulped root applied to burns. *Cathartic* Decoction of root taken as a physic. *Dermatological Aid* Poultice of pulped root applied to bruises and swellings. *Liver Aid* Decoction of root taken for liver complaints. *Tonic* Decoction of root taken as a general tonic. *Venereal Aid* Decoction of root taken for venereal disease. (155:131, 132) **Thompson** *Cough Medicine* Plant used as a cough medicine. (161:239) **Yavapai** *Cough Medicine* Decoction of tubers taken for coughs. *Dermatological Aid* Dried, pulverized tubers used for sores. *Gastrointestinal Aid* Decoction of tubers taken for stomachache. *Pediatric Aid* Dried, pulverized tubers used for babies with chafed skin. *Throat Aid* Decoction of tubers gargled for sore throat. *Toothache Remedy* Fresh or boiled tuber placed against gum or tooth or decoction held in mouth for toothaches. *Venereal Aid* Decoction of tuber used as wash and powder applied for gonorrhea. (53:261) **Yuki** *Antidiarrheal* Infusion of seeds taken by adults and babies for dysentery. *Dermatological Aid* Decoction of leaves and seeds applied to sores. *Pediatric Aid* Infusion of seeds taken by adults and babies for dysentery. (39:46) **Zuni** *Dermatological Aid* Poultice of powdered root applied to sores, rashes, and skin infections. Infusion of root used for athlete's foot infection. (22:378)

Rumex giganteus, Pa-wale
Hawaiian *Blood Medicine* Plant used for purifying the blood. *Heart Medicine* Plant used for heart disease. *Misc. Disease Remedy* Plant used for leprosy. *Reproductive Aid* Plant used to condition the mother for pregnancy. *Strengthener* Plant used for general body weakness. *Tuberculosis Remedy* Plant used for consumption. (as *Punex gigauteus* 2:73)

Rumex hymenosepalus, Canaigre Dock
Arapaho *Dermatological Aid* Stems and leaves used in a wash for sores. (98:44) **Hopi** *Cold Remedy* Plant used for colds. (174:34, 73) *Dermatological Aid* Plant used for ant bites and infected cuts. (34:357) **Mahuna** *Cough Medicine* Infusion of roots used as a gargle for coughs. *Throat Aid* Infusion of roots used as a gargle for sore throats. (117:17) **Navajo** *Unspecified* Plant used for medicine. (92:30) **Navajo, Kayenta** *Panacea* Plant used as a life medicine. (179:20) **Navajo, Ramah**

Ceremonial Medicine Cold infusion of root used as a ceremonial medicine. *Gynecological Aid* Cold infusion of root used as a lactagogue on breasts. *Veterinary Aid* Cold infusion of root used as a galactagogue on breasts of goats. (165:24) **Paiute** *Burn Dressing* Dried, powdered root used on burns. *Dermatological Aid* Dried, powdered root used on sores. (98:44) **Papago** *Dermatological Aid* Poultice of pulverized, dried root applied to sores. (29:64, 65) Poultice of dried and ground roots applied to sores. (29:65) *Throat Aid* Powdered root eaten or piece of root held in mouth for sore throat. (29:64, 65) Dried and pounded root taken for sore throats. (29:64) **Pawnee** *Antidiarrheal* Root used for diarrhea. (58:77) **Pima** *Cold Remedy* Root chewed for colds. *Cough Medicine* Root chewed for coughs. *Dermatological Aid* Poultice of roots applied or decoction of roots used as wash for skin sores. (38:51) Poultice of dried, powdered root applied to sores. (123:80) *Oral Aid* Root held in the mouth for sore gums. *Throat Aid* Root chewed or decoction of roots used as a gargle for sore throats. (38:51) *Unspecified* Roots used for medicine. (81:264)

Rumex maritimus, Golden Dock
Navajo, Kayenta *Gastrointestinal Aid* Infusion of plant taken for bloat. (as *R. fueginus* 179:20)

Rumex obtusifolius, Bitter Dock
Chippewa *Dermatological Aid* and *Pediatric Aid* Infusion of root applied, especially to children, for skin eruptions. (43:350) **Delaware** *Blood Medicine* Root used as a blood purifier. *Liver Aid* Root used for jaundice. (151:33) **Delaware, Oklahoma** *Blood Medicine* Root used as a blood purifier. *Liver Aid* Root used for jaundice. (150:28, 78) **Iroquois** *Blood Medicine* Compound decoction of roots taken for blood disorders and as a blood purifier. (73:313) *Contraceptive* Used as a contraceptive. (73:312) *Gynecological Aid* Used to stop menses. (73:313) *Pediatric Aid* and *Pulmonary Aid* Decoction of root given to children for whooping cough. (73:312) *Tonic* Compound decoction taken as a blood medicine and tonic. (73:313)

Rumex orbiculatus, Greater Water Dock
Cree, Woodlands *Antirheumatic (External)* Decoction of whole plant applied externally to pain-

ful joints. (91:58) **Meskwaki** *Antidote* Decoction of root taken as an antidote for poison. (as *R. britanica* 129:237) **Potawatomi** *Blood Medicine* Root used as a blood purifier. (as *R. britannica* 131:73)

Rumex patientia, Patience Dock
Cherokee *Antidiarrheal* Infusion taken for dysentery. *Blood Medicine* Infusion of root taken "for blood." *Dermatological Aid* Juice and infusion of root used as poultice and salve for various skin problems. *Kidney Aid* Infusion of root taken "to correct fluids." *Laxative* Infusion of root used for constipation. *Throat Aid* Leaves rubbed in mouth for sore throat. *Veterinary Aid* Beaten roots fed to horses for "sick stomach." (66:32)

Rumex salicifolius, Willow Dock
Blackfoot *Dermatological Aid* Boiled root used for many complaints, generally for swellings. (95:274) **Gosiute** *Blood Medicine* Roots used as a blood medicine. *Cathartic* Decoction of roots used for severe constipation. (31:380) **Kawaiisu** *Analgesic* Mashed roots used as a salve on sore limbs. *Dermatological Aid* Dried, pounded roots used as powder on sores and plant salve used on cuts. *Gastrointestinal Aid* Infusion of roots taken for stomachaches. *Misc. Disease Remedy* Mashed roots used as a salve for chickenpox. *Orthopedic Aid* Mashed roots used as a salve on sore limbs. *Unspecified* Stems, seeds, and roots used as medicine. (180:60)

Rumex salicifolius* var. *mexicanus,
    Mexican Dock
Apache, White Mountain *Gynecological Aid* Infusion of leaves taken by childless women to become pregnant. *Throat Aid* Infusion of leaves used for sore throats. (as *R. mexicanus* 113:160) **Blackfoot** *Antirheumatic (External)* Decoction of plant used for swellings. *Panacea* Decoction of plant used for many complaints. (as *R. mexicanus* 82:34) **Cree, Woodlands** *Antirheumatic (External)* Decoction of whole plant applied externally to painful joints. (as *R. mexicanus* 91:58) **Houma** *Abortifacient* Decoction of white root used to regulate menstruation. *Febrifuge* Decoction of red root taken for fever. *Gastrointestinal Aid* Decoction of plant taken for intestinal disorders. *Liver Aid* De-

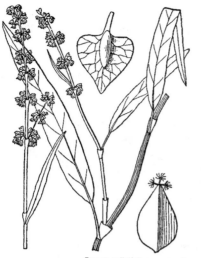

Rumex salicifolius var. mexicanus

coction of plant taken for liver trouble. Infusion of yellow root in gin taken for jaundice. (as *R. mexicana* 135:56, 57) **Keres, Western** *Burn Dressing* Poultice of crushed roots or paste of burned, ground roots and water used for burns. (as *R. mexicanus* 147:67) **Navajo, Ramah** *Ceremonial Medicine* and *Emetic* Whole plant used as a ceremonial emetic. *Panacea* Root used as a "life medicine." (as *R. mexicanus* 165:24) **Zuni** *Reproductive Aid* Strong infusion of root made and given to women by their husbands to help them to become pregnant. A strong infusion of root was made by the husband of a childless wife and given to her morning, noon, sunset, and bedtime for a month to help her to become pregnant. If the medicine did not work, it was because the wife's heart was not good. (as *R. mexicanus* 143:85) *Throat Aid* Ground root or infusion taken for sore throat, especially by sword-swallower. (as *R. mexicanus* 143:59)

Rumex venosus, Veiny Dock

Arapaho *Dermatological Aid* Stems and leaves used as a wash for sores. (100:47) **Lakota** *Gynecological Aid* Infusion of roots given to women to expel the afterbirth. (116:55) **Paiute** *Analgesic* Decoction of roots taken for stomachaches. *Antidiarrheal* Decoction of root taken for diarrhea. *Antirheumatic (Internal)* Decoction of root taken for rheumatism. *Blood Medicine* Decoction of roots taken as a blood purifier or tonic. (155:132, 133) *Burn Dressing* Powdered roots dusted on

burns. (100:47) Poultice of dried or raw roots applied and decoction used as a wash for burns. *Cold Remedy* Decoction of root taken for colds. *Cough Medicine* Decoction of root taken for coughs. (155:132, 133) *Dermatological Aid* Powdered roots dusted on impetigo. (100:47) Poultice of root applied or decoction used as a wash for wounds, sores, and swellings. *Gastrointestinal Aid* Decoction of root taken for stomachaches, stomach trouble, and gallbladder trouble. *Kidney Aid* Decoction of root taken for kidney disorders. *Misc. Disease Remedy* Decoction of roots taken for influenza. *Pulmonary Aid* Decoction of root taken for pneumonia. *Tonic* Decoction of root taken as a blood purifier or tonic. *Venereal Aid* Simple or compound decoction of root taken for venereal disease. **Shoshoni** *Blood Medicine* Decoction of roots taken as a blood purifier or tonic. *Burn Dressing* Poultice of dried or raw roots applied and decoction used as a wash for burns. (155:132, 133) *Cathartic* Decoction of whole plant taken as a physic. (98:42) *Dermatological Aid* Poultice of root applied or decoction used as a wash for wounds, sores, and swellings. *Tonic* Decoction of root taken as a blood purifier or tonic. *Venereal Aid* Decoction of root taken for venereal disease. (155:132, 133)

Rumex verticillatus, Swamp Dock

Choctaw *Misc. Disease Remedy* Decoction of leaves used in bath to prevent smallpox. (20:23) Infusion of leaves used as a bath to prevent smallpox. (152:21)

Ruta chalepensis, Fringed Rue

Costanoan *Cough Medicine* Decoction of plant used for coughs. *Ear Medicine* Heated leaves placed inside the ear for earaches. *Gastrointestinal Aid* Plant used for stomach pain. *Orthopedic Aid* Plant used for paralysis. (17:22) **Diegueño** *Ear Medicine* Mashed leaves wrapped in a piece of cotton and placed in the ear for earaches. (70:39)

Ruta graveolens, Common Rue

Cherokee *Anthelmintic* Decoction of top or leaves boiled into a syrup and taken for worms. *Orthopedic Aid* Added to whisky and taken for palsy. *Poultice* Used as poultice for gangrenous parts. *Sedative* Added to whisky and taken for hysterics. (66:53) **Diegueño** *Ear Medicine* Sprig put in the ear for an earache. *Gastrointestinal Aid* Infusion of leaves taken for stomachaches. (74:218)

Sabal minor, Dwarf Palmetto
Houma *Eye Medicine* Crushed, small root juice rubbed into sore eyes as a counterirritant. *Hypotensive* Decoction of dried root taken for high blood pressure. *Kidney Aid* Decoction of root taken for kidney trouble. (as *S. adansonii* 135:55, 56) *Stimulant* Decoction of dried root taken for "swimming in head." (as *S. adansonii* 135:55)

Sabal palmetto, Cabbage Palmetto
Seminole *Analgesic, Dietary Aid,* and *Febrifuge* Berries or seeds used for grass sickness: low fever, headache, and weight loss. (145:242)

Sabatia angularis, Rose Pink
Cherokee *Analgesic* and *Gynecological Aid* Infusion taken for periodic pains. (66:53)

Sabatia campanulata, Slender Rosegentian
Seminole *Analgesic, Antidiarrheal, Eye Medicine,* and *Febrifuge* Infusion of roots taken for sun sickness: eye disease, headache, high fever, and diarrhea. (145:206)

Sadleria cyatheoides, Amaumau Fern
Hawaiian *Dermatological Aid* Plant and other ingredients pounded, squeezed, and the resulting juice applied to boils and pimples. *Pulmonary Aid* Shoots and other ingredients used for lung troubles. *Respiratory Aid* Infusion of powdered inner bark and other ingredients taken for asthma and kindred troubles. (2:16)

Sagittaria cuneata, Arumleaf Arrowhead
Cheyenne *Unspecified* Leaves used as an ingredient in a medicinal mixture. *Veterinary Aid* Dried leaves given to horses for urinary troubles or put into sore mouth. (69:6) **Chippewa** *Unspecified* Plant characterized as having some medicinal uses. (as *S. arifolia* 59:124) **Navajo** *Analgesic* Plant used for headaches. (as *S. arifolia* 45:24) **Ojibwa** *Gastrointestinal Aid* Corms eaten for indigestion. (as *S. arifolia* 130:353) *Unspecified* Used

as a medicine for humans. *Veterinary Aid* Used as a medicine for horses. (as *S. arifolia* 130:396)

Sagittaria lancifolia, Bulltongue Arrowhead
Seminole *Dermatological Aid* Plant used for alligator bites. (145:298)

Sagittaria latifolia, Broadleaf Arrowhead
Cherokee *Febrifuge* and *Pediatric Aid* Infusion of leaves given, one sip, and used to bathe feverish baby. (66:23) **Chippewa** *Gastrointestinal Aid* Infusion of root taken for indigestion. (43:342) *Unspecified* Plant characterized as having some medicinal uses. (59:124) **Iroquois** *Antirheumatic (Internal)* Infusion of plant taken for rheumatism. *Dermatological Aid* Compound decoction taken for "boils around the abdomen of children." Compound decoction used as a wash on parts affected by "Italian itch." *Laxative* Compound decoction taken for constipation. *Pediatric Aid* Compound decoction taken for "boils around the abdomen of children." (73:273) Infusion of whole plant and rhizomes from another plant given to children who scream during the night. (118:65) **Lakota** *Unspecified* Roots used for food and eaten as medicine. (116:26) **Potawatomi** *Dermatological Aid* Poultice of pounded corms applied to wounds and sores. (131:37) **Thompson** *Love Medicine* Plant used as a love charm and for "witchcraft." (161:112)

Salicornia virginica, Virginia Glasswort
Heiltzuk *Analgesic* and *Antirheumatic (External)* Plant used for arthritic pain, rheumatism, aches, pain, and swelling. (35:91)

Salix alba, White Willow
Cherokee *Antidiarrheal* Infusion of bark taken to check bowels. *Dermatological Aid* Decoction or infusion of bark used as a wash to make the hair grow. Bark used as a poultice. *Febrifuge* Infusion taken for fever. *Respiratory Aid* Root chewed by ballplayers "for wind." *Throat Aid* Infusion of inner bark taken for lost voice and root chewed for hoarseness. (66:61) Decoction of inner bark taken for hoarseness. (152:12) *Tonic* Bark used as a tonic. (66:61)

Salix amygdaloides, Peachleaf Willow
Cheyenne *Antidiarrheal* Infusion of bark shavings used for diarrhea. (68:67) Infusion of bark taken for diarrhea. *Ceremonial Medicine* Plant used in the Sun Dance ceremony. *Dermatological Aid* Poultice of bark applied to bleeding cuts. (69:37) *Gastrointestinal Aid* Infusion of bark shavings used for stomach ailments. (68:67) *Hemostat* Poultice of bark applied to bleeding cuts. *Panacea* Infusion of bark taken for diarrhea and other ailments. (69:37) **Okanagan-Colville** *Orthopedic Aid* Decoction of branch tips used for soaking the feet and legs for cramps. (162:135)

Salix arbusculoides, Littletree Willow
Eskimo, Inuktitut *Dermatological Aid* Poultice of shredded, inner bark applied to skin sores. (176:186) **Eskimo, Kuskokwagmiut** *Dermatological Aid* Poultice of inner bark applied to sores. *Eye Medicine* Leaves placed in the corners of watery eyes. *Oral Aid* Leaves chewed for sore mouth. (101:30)

Salix babylonica, Weeping Willow
Cherokee *Antidiarrheal* Infusion of bark taken to check bowels. *Dermatological Aid* Decoction or infusion of bark used as a wash to make the hair grow. Bark used as a poultice. *Febrifuge* Infusion taken for fever. *Respiratory Aid* Root chewed by ballplayers "for wind." *Throat Aid* Infusion of inner bark taken for lost voice and root chewed for hoarseness. *Tonic* Bark used as a tonic. (66:61)

Salix bebbiana, Bebb Willow
Cree, Woodlands *Dermatological Aid* Poultice of chewed root inner bark applied to a deep cut. (91:58) **Menominee** *Unspecified* Plant used medicinally. (as *S. rostrata* 128:52) **Okanagan-Colville** *Dermatological Aid* Poultice of inner cambium and powdered tree fungus applied to serious cuts. *Gynecological Aid* Shredded inner bark used for sanitary napkins to "heal a woman's insides." Decoction of branches taken by women for several months after childbirth to increase the blood flow. *Hemostat* Poultice of bark and sap applied as a wad to bleeding wounds. *Orthopedic Aid* Poultice of damp inner bark applied to the skin over a broken bone. *Pediatric Aid* Decoction of branches taken by women after childbirth and

helped the baby through the breast milk. (162:136)

Salix bonplandiana, Red Willow
Costanoan *Febrifuge* Bark used for fevers. (as *S. laevigata* 17:21) **Kawaiisu** *Antidiarrheal* Infusion of roots taken for diarrhea. (as *S. laevigata* 180:61)

Salix candida, Sageleaf Willow
Meskwaki *Unspecified* Compound used as a medicine. (129:245) **Ojibwa** *Gastrointestinal Aid* Plant used for stomach troubles. *Sedative* Plant used for trembling. *Stimulant* Plant used for fainting. *Unspecified* Bark used for medicinal purposes. (112:243) **Ojibwa, South** *Cough Medicine* Decoction of inner bark taken for coughs. (77:200)

Salix caroliniana, Coastal Plain Willow
Houma *Blood Medicine* Decoction of roots and bark taken for "feebleness" due to thin blood. *Febrifuge* Decoction of roots and bark taken for fever. (as *S. longipes* 135:60) **Seminole** *Analgesic* Infusion of bark taken as an emetic for rainbow sickness: fever, stiff neck, and backache. (as *S. amphibia* 145:210) Infusion of bark taken as an emetic for thunder sickness: fever, dizziness, headache, and diarrhea. (as *S. amphibia* 145:213) Infusion of plant taken by men for menstruation sickness: stomachache, headache, and body soreness. (as *S. amphibia* 145:248) *Antidiarrheal* Infusion of bark taken as an emetic for thunder sickness:

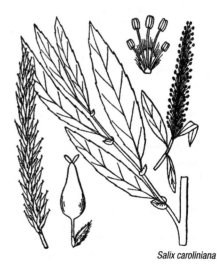

Salix caroliniana

fever, dizziness, headache, and diarrhea. (as *S. amphibia* 145:213) *Antirheumatic (External)* Plant used for fire sickness: fever and body aches. (as *S. amphibia* 145:203) Cold infusion of plant used as a bath for body aches. (as *S. amphibia* 145:215) *Antirheumatic (Internal)* Infusion of plant taken by men for menstruation sickness: stomachache, headache, and body soreness. (as *S. amphibia* 145:248) *Blood Medicine* Decoction of bark taken for menstruation sickness: yellow eyes and skin, weakness, and shaking head. (as *S. amphibia* 145:247) *Ceremonial Medicine* Plant used as a ceremonial emetic. (as *S. amphibia* 145:163) Bark used as an emetic in purification after funerals, at doctor's school, and after death of patient. (as *S. amphibia* 145:167) Roots taken by students in medical training. (as *S. amphibia* 145:95) *Dermatological Aid* Plant used for gunshot wounds. (as *S. amphibia* 145:302) *Emetic* Decoction of plant and other plants taken as an emetic by doctors to strengthen his internal medicine. (as *S. amphibia* 145:145) Bark used as an emetic to "clean the insides." (as *S. amphibia* 145:167) Infusion of bark taken as an emetic for rainbow sickness: fever, stiff neck, and backache. (as *S. amphibia* 145:210) Infusion of bark taken as an emetic for thunder sickness: fever, dizziness, headache, and diarrhea. (as *S. amphibia* 145:213) Bark used as an emetic. (as *S. amphibia* 145:288) Infusion of plant taken as an emetic to vomit the object the witch "shot" into the body. (as *S. amphibia* 145:398) Infusion of roots taken as an emetic during religious ceremonies. (as *S. amphibia* 145:408) *Eye Medicine* Infusion of inner bark taken and used as a bath for mist sickness: eye disease, fever, and chills. (as *S. amphibia* 145:209) *Febrifuge* Plant used for fire sickness: fever and body aches. (as *S. amphibia* 145:203) Plant used for dance fire sickness: fever. (as *S. amphibia* 145:206) Infusion of inner bark taken and used as a bath for mist sickness: eye disease, fever, and chills. (as *S. amphibia* 145:209) Infusion of bark taken as an emetic for rainbow sickness: fever, stiff neck, and backache. (as *S. amphibia* 145:210) Infusion of bark taken as an emetic for thunder sickness: fever, dizziness, headache, and diarrhea. (as *S. amphibia* 145:213) Plant used as a fever medicine. (as *S. amphibia* 145:283) Bark used for fevers. (as *S. amphibia* 145:288) *Gastro-*

intestinal Aid Infusion of plant taken by men for menstruation sickness: stomachache, headache, and body soreness. (as *S. amphibia* 145:248) *Hunting Medicine* Infusion of roots used as a hunting medicine to increase hunting luck. (as *S. amphibia* 145:371) *Love Medicine* Bark used as a medicine to prevent adultery. (as *S. amphibia* 145:249) *Oral Aid* Plant used for lion sickness: panting, staring, and tongue hanging out. (as *S. amphibia* 145:232) *Orthopedic Aid* Infusion of bark used as a bath for hot feet. (as *S. amphibia* 145:288) *Other* Decoction of bark taken for menstruation sickness: yellow eyes and skin, weakness, and shaking head. (as *S. amphibia* 145:247) Plant used for lightning sickness. (as *S. amphibia* 145:305) *Preventive Medicine* Plant made into medicine and used to prevent the new mother's condition from contaminating the camp. (as *S. amphibia* 145:325) *Respiratory Aid* Plant used for lion sickness: panting, staring, and tongue hanging out. *Stimulant* Plant used for lion sickness: panting, staring, and tongue hanging out. (as *S. amphibia* 145:232) Infusion of bark taken and used as a bath for menstruation sickness: lassitude, laziness, and weakness. *Strengthener* Infusion of bark taken and used as a bath for menstruation sickness: lassitude, laziness, and weakness. (as *S. amphibia* 145:244) Decoction of bark taken for menstruation sickness: yellow eyes and skin, weakness, and shaking head. (as *S. amphibia* 145:247) *Unspecified* Plant used for medicinal purposes. (as *S. amphibia* 145:161) Plant used medicinally. (as *S. amphibia* 145:164) *Vertigo Medicine* Infusion of bark taken as an emetic for thunder sickness: fever, dizziness, headache, and diarrhea. (as *S. amphibia* 145:213)

Salix cordata, Heartleaf Willow
Malecite *Dermatological Aid* Bark placed in hot water and used for blisters. (96:251) *Dietary Aid* Infusion of bark used for stimulating the appetite. (96:253) **Micmac** *Cold Remedy* Bark used for colds and to stimulate the appetite. *Dermatological Aid* Bark used for blisters. *Dietary Aid* Bark used to stimulate the appetite. (32:61) **Thompson** *Dermatological Aid* Poultice of fresh bark applied to bruises and skin eruptions. (141:471)

Salix discolor, Pussy Willow
Algonquin, Tête-de-Boule *Gynecological Aid*
Infusion of young branches used to start lactation.
Throat Aid Inner bark powdered, made into a
paste, and applied to "sick" throats. (110:130)
Blackfoot *Analgesic* Decoction of new twigs taken
as a painkiller. *Febrifuge* Decoction of new twigs
taken for fevers. (82:28) **Cree, Woodlands**
Antidiarrheal Infusion of inner bark taken for diarrhea. (91:58) **Iroquois** *Emetic* Compound decoction taken to vomit during initial stages of consumption, and to reduce loneliness. *Hemorrhoid
Remedy* Infusion of bark used for bleeding piles.
Psychological Aid Compound decoction taken to
vomit to reduce loneliness. *Tuberculosis Remedy*
Compound decoction taken to vomit during initial
stages of consumption. (73:294) **Ojibwa** *Gastrointestinal Aid* Plant used for stomach troubles.
Sedative Plant used for trembling. *Stimulant* Plant
used for fainting. *Unspecified* Bark used for medicinal purposes. (112:243) **Potawatomi** *Hemostat*
Decoction of root bark used for hemorrhages.
(131:81, 82) *Panacea* Bark used as a universal
remedy. (131:81)

Salix exigua, Sandbar Willow
Montana Indian *Adjuvant* Poles used for framework of "sweat tepee" for colds and rheumatism.
Antirheumatic (External) Poles used for framework of "sweat tepee" for rheumatism. *Cold Remedy* Poles used for framework of "sweat tepee" for
colds. *Febrifuge* Bark used for certain fevers.
(15:22) **Navajo, Ramah** *Ceremonial Medicine*
and *Emetic* Decoction of leaves used as ceremonial emetic. (165:22) **Paiute, Northern** *Venereal
Aid* Decoction of dried roots taken for venereal
diseases. (49:128) **Zuni** *Cough Medicine* Infusion
of bark taken for coughs. *Throat Aid* Infusion of
bark taken for sore throat. (22:378)

Salix fragilis, Crack Willow
Ojibwa *Dermatological Aid* Poultice of bark applied to sores as a styptic and healing aid. *Hemostat* Bark used as a styptic and poultice for sores.
(130:388)

Salix fuscescens, Alaska Bog Willow
Eskimo, Western *Eye Medicine* Cotton used by
old men in inner corner of eye for watery sore eye.

(90:60) *Oral Aid* Leaves chewed for mouth sores.
(90:17, 60)

Salix gooddingii, Goodding's Willow
Pima *Febrifuge* Decoction of leaves and bark
taken as a febrifuge. (38:108)

Salix hindsiana, Hinds's Willow
Pomo, Kashaya *Throat Aid* Decoction of bark
or leaves used for sore throats. Infusion of leaves
used for laryngitis. (60:118)

Salix hookeriana, Dune Willow
Makah *Antidote* Leaves used as an antidote for
shellfish poisoning. *Dermatological Aid* Infusion
of roots used as a hair wash. (65:27) **Quileute**
Sports Medicine Roots rubbed on bodies of athletes in training. (as *S. piperi* 65:26)

Salix humilis, Prairie Willow
Cherokee *Antidiarrheal* Infusion of bark taken
to check bowels. *Dermatological Aid* Decoction or
infusion of bark used as a wash to make the hair
grow. Bark used as a poultice. *Febrifuge* Infusion
taken for fever. *Respiratory Aid* Root chewed by
ballplayers "for wind." *Throat Aid* Infusion of inner bark taken for lost voice and root chewed for
hoarseness. *Tonic* Bark used as a tonic. (66:61)
Delaware *Venereal Aid* Infusion of roots and
other plants used for scrofula and venereal disease. (151:34) **Delaware, Oklahoma** *Tuberculosis Remedy* Compound infusion of plant used
for scrofula. *Venereal Aid* Compound infusion of
plant used for venereal disease. (150:29, 78)

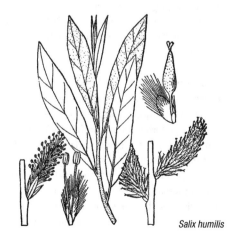

Salix humilis

Menominee *Antidiarrheal* Root taken from shrub bearing insect galls and used for dysentery and diarrhea. *Gastrointestinal Aid* Root taken only from shrub bearing insect galls and used for spasmodic colic. (128:52) *Tonic* Decoction of stalk taken as a general tonic. (44:133) **Meskwaki** *Antidiarrheal* Infusion of root used for flux and enemas. *Hemostat* Leaves used for stopping a hemorrhage. *Laxative* Infusion of root used for flux and giving enemas. (129:245)

Salix humilis var. *tristis*, Prairie Willow
Catawba *Gynecological Aid* Plant used for sore nipples. *Oral Aid* and *Pediatric Aid* Infusion of roots used as a wash for children with sore mouths. (as *S. tristis* 152:13) **Delaware** *Reproductive Aid* Infusion of roots used by women for displacement of the womb. *Venereal Aid* Infusion of plant and roots of other plants used for scrofula and venereal disease. (as *S. tristis* 151:34) **Seminole** *Analgesic*, *Antidiarrheal*, and *Eye Medicine* Infusion of plant taken for sun sickness: eye disease, headache, high fever, and diarrhea. (as *S. tristis* 145:208) *Febrifuge* Infusion of plant taken and rubbed on the body for high fevers. (as *S. tristis* 145:202) Infusion of plant taken for sun sickness: eye disease, headache, high fever, and diarrhea. (as *S. tristis* 145:208) *Hunting Medicine* Infusion of plant used as a hunting medicine to increase hunting luck. (as *S. tristis* 145:371) *Other* Plant used to make a medicine and given to students in medical training. (as *S. tristis* 145:103)

Salix interior, Sandbar Willow
Iroquois *Analgesic* Infusion of stems and other plant parts used for side pains. (118:39) **Thompson** *Unspecified* Roots used medicinally for unspecified purpose. (141:465)

Salix lasiolepis, Arroyo Willow
Costanoan *Cold Remedy* Infusion of bark or young leaves or decoction of flowers used for colds. (17:21) **Mendocino Indian** *Antidiarrheal* Infusion of leaves taken for diarrhea. *Dermatological Aid* Decoction of bark used as a wash for the itch. *Diaphoretic* Infusion of bark taken to cause sweating for any disease. *Febrifuge* Infusion of bark taken for chills and fever. *Panacea* Infusion of bark taken to cause sweating for any disease.

(33:331) **Mewuk** *Febrifuge* Decoction of bark used for fevers. *Misc. Disease Remedy* Decoction of bark used for measles. (as *S. dasiolipis* 97:366)

Salix lucida, Shining Willow
Micmac *Hemostat* Bark used for bleeding. *Respiratory Aid* Bark used for asthma. (32:61) **Montagnais** *Analgesic* Infusion of leaves taken and poultice of bark applied for headache. (133:315) **Ojibwa** *Dermatological Aid* Poultice of bark used for sores and applied to bleeding cuts. *Hemostat* Bark used on bleeding cuts. (130:388) **Penobscot** *Respiratory Aid* Bark smoked for asthma. (133:309)

Salix lucida ssp. *lasiandra*, Pacific Willow
Bella Coola *Antidiarrheal* Cold infusion of charred, pulverized sticks taken for diarrhea. *Dermatological Aid* Folded inner bark inserted in knife cuts and used for incisions. (as *S. lasiandra* 127:53) **Navajo, Ramah** *Ceremonial Medicine* Decoction of leaves used as ceremonial emetic. *Disinfectant* Painted internode of stem held by baby for "lightning infection." *Emetic* Decoction of leaves used as ceremonial emetic. *Pediatric Aid* Painted internode of stem held by baby for "lightning infection." (as *S. lasiandra* 165:22) **Okanagan-Colville** *Orthopedic Aid* Decoction of branch tips used for soaking the feet and legs for cramps. (as *S. lasiandra* 162:135) **Pomo, Kashaya** *Cold Remedy* Decoction of leaves used for colds. *Throat Aid* Decoction of leaves used for sore throats. (as *S. lasiandra* 60:118)

Salix melanopsis, Dusky Willow
Montana Indian *Adjuvant* and *Antirheumatic* (*External*) Poles used for framework of "sweat tepee" for rheumatism. *Cold Remedy* Poles used for framework of "sweat tepee" for colds. *Febrifuge* Bark used for certain fevers. (as *S. fluviatilis* 15:22)

Salix myricoides var. *myricoides*, Bayberry Willow
Iroquois *Venereal Aid* Compound used for syphilis with chancres. (as *S. glaucophylloides* 73:294)

Salix nigra, Black Willow
Cherokee *Antidiarrheal* Infusion of bark taken

to check bowels. *Dermatological Aid* Decoction or infusion of bark used as a wash to make the hair grow. Bark used as a poultice. *Febrifuge* Infusion taken for fever. *Respiratory Aid* Root chewed by ballplayers "for wind." *Throat Aid* Infusion of inner bark taken for lost voice and root chewed for hoarseness. *Tonic* Bark used as a tonic. (66:61) **Houma** *Blood Medicine* Decoction of roots and bark taken for "feebleness" due to thin blood. *Febrifuge* Decoction of roots and bark taken for fever. (135:60) **Iroquois** *Carminative* Compound decoction taken for stomach gas. *Cough Medicine* Compound decoction taken for coughs. *Throat Aid* Used for mouth and throat abscesses. (73:294) **Koasati** *Analgesic* Infusion of roots taken for headaches. *Febrifuge* Cold infusion of roots taken for fevers. *Gastrointestinal Aid* Decoction of roots taken for dyspepsia. (152:13) **Micmac** *Dermatological Aid* Poultice of bruised leaves used on sprains and bruises. Poultice of scraped root and spirits applied to bruises and sprains. *Orthopedic Aid* Poultice of bruised leaves applied to sprains and bruises. Poultice of scraped root and spirits applied to sprains and broken bones. (as *S. vulgare* 133:317)

Salix pedicellaris, Bog Willow
Ojibwa *Gastrointestinal Aid* Bark used for stomach troubles. (130:388, 389)

Salix planifolia ssp. pulchra, Tealeaf Willow
Eskimo, Alaska *Anesthetic* Bark and leaves chewed to numb the mouth and throat. *Eye Medicine* "Cotton" used to dry "moist eyes." *Oral Aid* Bark and leaves chewed for mouth sores. (1:34) **Eskimo, Inupiat** *Oral Aid* Leaves made the mouth smell good. (as *S. pulchra* 83:10) **Eskimo, Nunivak** *Analgesic* Infusion of leaves and bark used as an analgesic. *Oral Aid* Plant chewed for sore mouth. (as *S. pulchra* 126:325) **Eskimo, Western** *Oral Aid* Leaves chewed for mouth sores. (as *S. pulchra* 90:17)

Salix pyrifolia, Balsam Willow
Ojibwa *Gastrointestinal Aid* Plant used for stomach troubles. *Sedative* Plant used for trembling. *Stimulant* Plant used for fainting. *Unspecified* Bark used for medicinal purposes. (as *S. balsamifera* 112:243)

Salix rotundifolia, Least Willow
Eskimo, Nunivak *Analgesic* Infusion of leaves and bark used as an analgesic. *Oral Aid* Plant chewed for sore mouth. (126:325)

Salix scouleriana, Scouler's Willow
Bella Coola *Dermatological Aid* Folded inner bark inserted in knife cuts and used for incisions. (127:54) **Okanagan-Colville** *Dermatological Aid* Poultice of inner cambium and powdered tree fungus applied to serious cuts. *Gynecological Aid* Shredded inner bark used for sanitary napkins to "heal a woman's insides." Decoction of branches taken by women for several months after childbirth to increase the blood flow. *Hemostat* Poultice of bark and sap applied as a wad to bleeding wounds. *Orthopedic Aid* Poultice of damp inner bark applied to the skin over a broken bone. *Pediatric Aid* Decoction of branches taken by women after childbirth and helped the baby through the breast milk. (162:136) **Sanpoil** *Antidiarrheal* Decoction of roots taken to counteract diarrhea. (109:220)

Salix sericea, Silky Willow
Iroquois *Oral Aid* Used for mouth and throat abscesses. (73:294)

Salix sitchensis, Sitka Willow
Eskimo, Alaska *Dermatological Aid* Poultice of pounded bark applied to wounds. (126:331) **Karok** *Ceremonial Medicine* Roots and branches used in the World Renewal ceremony fire. (125:381) **Klallam** *Tonic* Decoction of peeled bark taken as a tonic. (65:26) **Okanagan-Colville** *Gastrointestinal Aid* Infusion of stalks taken for stomach ailments. (162:136) **Skagit** *Tonic* Decoction of peeled bark taken as a tonic. (65:26)

Salix washingtonia, American Willow
Mahuna *Blood Medicine* Infusion of pounded leaves taken as a blood tonic. (117:32)

Salsola australis, Prickly Russian Thistle
Navajo *Dermatological Aid* Poultice of chewed plants applied to ant, bee, and wasp stings. (as *S. kali* var. *tragus* 45:44) **Navajo, Ramah** *Dermatological Aid* Infusion of plant ashes used internally and externally for smallpox. *Misc. Disease Remedy*

Infusion of plant ashes taken and used externally for smallpox and influenza. (as *S. pestifer* 165:25)

Salvia apiana, White Sage

Cahuilla *Cold Remedy* Leaves eaten, smoked, and used in the sweat house for colds. *Dermatological Aid* Crushed leaves and water used as a hair shampoo, dye, and hair straightener. Poultice of fresh, crushed leaves applied before retiring to the armpits for body odors. *Eye Medicine* Seeds used as eye cleansers. *Hunting Medicine* Leaves used to prevent bad luck if a menstruating woman accidentally touched hunting equipment. (11:136) **Diegueño** *Blood Medicine* Infusion of leaves taken as a tonic for the blood. (74:219) *Cold Remedy* Decoction of leaves taken for colds. (70:39) *Cough Medicine* Infusion of leaves taken as a cough medicine. (74:219) *Misc. Disease Remedy* Leaves burned in hot coals to fumigate the house after a case of sickness such as measles. *Other* Decoction of leaves taken for a serious case of poison oak that "has entered the blood." (70:39) **Mahuna** *Gynecological Aid* Infusion of roots taken to heal internally and remove particles of afterbirth. (as *Ramona polystachya* 117:14)

Salvia columbariae, Chia

Cahuilla *Disinfectant* Poultice of seed mush applied to infections. *Eye Medicine* Seeds used to cleanse the eyes or remove foreign matter from the eyes. (11:136) **Costanoan** *Eye Medicine* Gelatinous seeds placed in the eye to remove foreign objects. *Febrifuge* Infusion of seeds taken for fevers. (17:16) **Diegueño** *Strengthener* Seeds kept in the mouth and chewed during long journeys on foot, to give strength. (70:41) **Kawaiisu** *Eye Medicine* Seeds placed in the eye for irritation and inflammation. (180:62) **Mahuna** *Eye Medicine* Seeds placed under the eyelids while sleeping to remove sand particles. (117:54)

Salvia dorrii, Grayball Sage

Kawaiisu *Analgesic* Decoction of leaves used as a wash for headaches. *Gastrointestinal Aid* Infusion of leaves taken for stomachaches. *Witchcraft Medicine* Plant thrown into the fire to keep away the ghosts. (180:62) **Paiute** *Pediatric Aid* Infusion of leaves taken by children for colds and sore throat. (as *Ramona incana* 98:38) **Paiute, Northern**

Analgesic Decoction of leaves taken and used as a wash for headaches. *Cold Remedy* Decoction of leaves taken for colds. (49:129) *Venereal Aid* Decoction of leaves taken for gonorrhea. (49:125)

Salvia dorrii ssp. *dorrii* var. *incana*, Purple Sage

Hopi *Anticonvulsive* Smoke blown in face or plant taken in a drink for epilepsy or faintness. (as *S. carnosa* 174:33, 91) *Other* Plant used as a "deer medicine." *Stimulant* Plant used as a medicine for an epileptic or faint person. (as *S. carnosa* 174:91) **Okanagan-Colville** *Cold Remedy* Decoction or infusion of leaves used for colds. *Panacea* Decoction or infusion of leaves used for any illness of a general nature. (162:110) **Paiute** *Analgesic* Decoction of leaf or stem taken, used as a wash, and fumes inhaled for headaches. Decoction of leaf and sometimes stem taken for stomachaches. *Cold Remedy* Compound of dried plant smoked for colds. Compound poultice of crushed leaves applied for chest congestion from colds. Decoction of leaf or stem taken and poultice applied for colds. Infusion or simple or compound decoction of leaf and sometimes stem used for colds. *Cough Medicine* Decoction of leaf or stem taken and poultice applied for coughs. *Ear Medicine* Decoction of leaf used as drops and poultice of leaf and stem used for earaches. *Eye Medicine* Decoction of leaves used as an eyewash. *Febrifuge* Decoction of leaf or stem taken and poultice applied for fever. *Gastrointestinal Aid* Decoction of leaf and sometimes stem taken for stomachaches or indigestion. *Herbal Steam* Decoction of leaf and sometimes stem used as herbal steam for headaches. *Misc. Disease Remedy* Decoction of leaf and sometimes stem taken for fevers and influenza. *Poultice* Poultice of boiled plant tops applied to swollen leg veins. *Pulmonary Aid* Compound poultice of crushed leaves applied for chest congestion from colds. Decoction of leaves and sometimes stems taken for pneumonia. *Venereal Aid* Decoction of leaf and sometimes stem taken for venereal disease. **Shoshoni** *Analgesic* Decoction of leaf and sometimes stem taken for stomachaches. *Cold Remedy* Infusion or decoction of leaves, and sometimes stems, taken for colds. *Gastrointestinal Aid* Decoction of leaf and sometimes stem taken for stomachaches or indigestion. *Other* Decoction of plant tops used as a wash for swollen leg veins. *Pediatric Aid* and *Throat Aid* Decoction of leaf or stem given and used as a wash for children's sore throat. **Washo Cold Remedy** Infusion or decoction of leaves, and sometimes stems, taken for colds. *Respiratory Aid* Dried leaves smoked in a pipe to clear congested nasal passages. (as *S. carnosa* 155:136, 137)

Salvia lyrata, Lyreleaf Sage
Catawba *Dermatological Aid* Roots used as a salve for sores. (134:191) Root salve applied to sores. (152:55) **Cherokee** *Antidiarrheal* Infusion taken to check bowels. *Cold Remedy* Infusion taken for colds. *Cough Medicine* Infusion taken for coughs. *Diaphoretic* Used as a mild diaphoretic. *Gynecological Aid* Taken by weakly females. *Laxative* Infusion taken as a laxative. *Respiratory Aid* Syrup of leaves and honey taken for asthma. *Sedative* Infusion taken for nervous debility. *Stimulant* Taken by persons of phlegmatic habits. (66:53)

Salvia mellifera, Black Sage
Costanoan *Analgesic* Green leaves chewed for gas pains. Poultice of heated leaves applied to the ear for earache pain. *Carminative* Green leaves chewed for gas pains. *Cough Medicine* Decoction of plant taken for coughs. *Ear Medicine* Poultice of heated leaves applied to the ear for earache pain. *Heart Medicine* Infusion of green leaves taken for heart disorders. *Orthopedic Aid* Decoction of plant used as a bath for paralysis. *Throat Aid* Poultice of heated leaves applied to the neck for sore throats. (17:16) **Mahuna** *Cough Medicine* Infusion of plant taken for chronic bronchial coughs. *Respiratory Aid* Infusion of plant taken for chronic bronchial coughs. (as *Audibertias stachyoides* 117:19)

Salvia officinalis, Kitchen Sage
Cherokee *Antidiarrheal* Infusion taken to check bowels. *Cold Remedy* Infusion taken for colds. *Cough Medicine* Infusion taken for coughs. *Diaphoretic* Used as a mild diaphoretic. *Gynecological Aid* Taken by weakly females. *Laxative* Infusion taken as a laxative. *Respiratory Aid* Syrup of leaves and honey taken for asthma. *Sedative* Infusion taken for nervous debility. *Stimulant* Taken by persons of phlegmatic habits. (66:53) **Mohegan** *Anthelmintic* "Sage tea" taken as a vermifuge. *Panacea* Fresh leaves chewed to benefit the entire body. (151:75, 132) *Tonic* Green or dried leaves used to make a tonic. (151:132)

Sambucus canadensis, American Elder
Algonquin, Quebec *Emetic* Infusion of bark scraped upward and used as an emetic. *Laxative* Infusion of bark scraped downward and used as a laxative. (14:236) **Cherokee** *Antirheumatic (Internal)* Infusion of berry used for rheumatism. *Burn Dressing* Salve used for burns. *Cathartic* Used as a cathartic. *Dermatological Aid* Salve used for skin eruptions and infusion taken as tonic for boils. *Diaphoretic* Infusion of flowers taken to "sweat out fever." *Disinfectant* Leaves used to wash sores to prevent infection. *Diuretic* Used as a diuretic. *Emetic* Used as an emetic. *Kidney Aid* Taken for "dropsy." *Other* Decoction taken for "summer complaint." *Pediatric Aid* Given for "light sickness among children" and taken for "dropsy." (66:33) **Chickasaw** *Analgesic* Infusion of branches applied to head for severe headaches. (152:58) **Chippewa** *Emetic* Infusion of roots taken as an emetic. (59:142) **Choctaw** *Liver Aid* Decoction of seeds and roots taken for liver troubles. **Creek** *Breast Treatment* Poultice of pounded roots applied to swollen breasts. (152:58) *Gynecological Aid* Poultice of pounded root or stalk skin applied to women for swollen breast. (148:661) **Delaware** *Blood Medicine* Leaves and stems used as a blood purifier. *Dermatological Aid* Poultice of bark scrapings applied to sores, swellings, and wounds. *Liver Aid* Leaves and stems used for jaundice. *Pedi-*

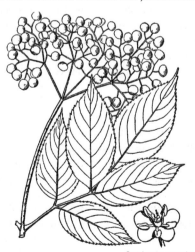

Sambucus canadensis

atric Aid Infusion of flowers used for infants with colic. (151:31) **Delaware, Oklahoma** *Blood Medicine* Leaves and stems used as a blood purifier. *Dermatological Aid* Poultice or salve of bark scrapings applied to wounds, sores, and swellings. *Gastrointestinal Aid* Infusion of flowers given to infants for colic. (150:26, 78) *Liver Aid* Leaves and stems used for jaundice. *Pediatric Aid* Infusion of flower given to infants for colic. (150:26) **Houma** *Analgesic* Decoction of bark used as a wash for pain. *Dermatological Aid* Decoction of bark used as a wash for swelling. *Tonic* Wine made from berries taken as a tonic. (135:60) **Iroquois** *Analgesic* Poultice of bark applied for headaches. (73:448) *Cathartic* Decoction of bark taken as a physic. Infusion of blossoms given to babies as a physic. (73:449) *Ceremonial Medicine* Decoction of flowers with other plants used as medicine to soak corn seeds before planting. (170:19) *Dermatological Aid* Compound poultice of plants and leaves applied to swellings of all kinds. Compound poultice of powdered roots and bark applied to baby's unhealed navel. (73:448) Poultice of bark applied to cuts. *Emetic* Infusion of bark taken as a spring emetic and to vomit up gall. (73:449) *Febrifuge* Berries used for fevers. (103:96) *Gastrointestinal Aid* Plant used for stomach troubles. *Heart Medicine* Infusion of pith taken for heart disease. (73:450) *Kidney Aid* Decoction of bark taken for the kidneys. (73:449) *Laxative* Compound decoction of twigs given to children as a laxative. (73:448) Infusion of bark taken as a laxative. (73:449) *Liver Aid* Infusion of bark taken to vomit up gall. (73:450) *Misc. Disease Remedy* Infusion of bark taken for the measles. (73:448) Compound decoction of plants taken for diphtheria. Infusion of berries taken and poultice applied to swellings caused by mumps. (73:450) *Pediatric Aid* Compound decoction of twigs given to children as a laxative. Compound poultice of powdered roots and bark applied to baby's unhealed navel. (73:448) Infusion of blossoms given to babies as a physic. (73:449) *Unspecified* Berries used for convalescents. (103:96) *Venereal Aid* Compound infusion used as wash on parts affected by venereal disease. (73:448) Decoction of pith taken for gonorrhea. (73:449) **Menominee** *Febrifuge* Infusion of dried flowers used as a febrifuge. (128:27) **Meskwaki** *Cathartic* Inner bark of young shoots used as a

purgative. *Diuretic* Inner bark of young shoots used as a diuretic. *Gynecological Aid* Infusion of bark used in extremely difficult cases of parturition. *Pulmonary Aid* Root bark used to free lungs of phlegm. (129:207) **Micmac** *Cathartic* Berries, bark, and flower used as a purgative and bark used as a physic. *Emetic* Berries, bark, and flower used as a purgative and bark used as an emetic. *Sedative* Berries, bark, and flower used as a soporific and purgative. (32:61) **Mohegan** *Cathartic* Infusion of bark scraped downward and used as a physic. *Emetic* Infusion of bark scraped upward and used as an emetic. (149:265) Inner bark, scraped upward, used as an emetic. (151:75, 132) *Gastrointestinal Aid* Infusion of flowers given to babies with colic. (149:265) Infusion of dried flowers given to infants for colic. *Laxative* Inner bark, scraped downward, used as a laxative. *Pediatric Aid* Infusion of dried flowers given to infants for colic. (151:75, 132) **Rappahannock** *Antirheumatic (Internal)* Fermented decoction of berries taken for "rheumatism" (neuritis). (138:33) *Dermatological Aid* Compound infusion with bark used for swellings and sores. (138:34) **Seminole** *Ceremonial Medicine* Root bark used as a purification emetic after funerals, at doctor's school, and after death of patient. (as *S. simpsonii* 145:167) *Emetic* Decoction of root bark taken as an emetic for stomachaches. (as *S. simpsoni* 145:276) Root bark used as an emetic to "clean the insides." (as *S. simpsonii* 145:167) *Gastrointestinal Aid* Decoction of root bark taken as an emetic for stomachaches. (as *S. simpsoni* 145:276) **Thompson** *Toothache Remedy* Fresh bark used in hollow tooth for toothaches. (141:474)

Sambucus cerulea, Blue Elderberry
Choctaw *Dermatological Aid* Poultice of beaten leaves applied to swollen hands. *Gastrointestinal Aid* Decoction of root taken for dyspepsia. *Urinary Aid* Decoction of root taken for bladder troubles. (as *S. intermedia* 152:59) **Clallam** *Antidiarrheal* Infusion of bark used for diarrhea. (47:198) **Costanoan** *Cathartic* Decoction of leaves used as a purgative. *Cold Remedy* Decoction of leaves used for new colds. (17:24) **Houma** *Analgesic* Decoction of bark used as a wash for pain. *Dermatological Aid* Decoction of bark used as a wash for swelling. *Tonic* Wine made from berries taken as

a tonic. (as *S. intermedia* 135:60) **Kawaiisu** *Analgesic* Infusion of leaves and flowers used as steam bath for headaches. *Blood Medicine* Decoction of leaves used as a wash on limb affected by blood poisoning. *Cold Remedy* Infusion of leaves and flowers used as steam bath for colds. *Diaphoretic* Infusion of leaves and flowers used as steam bath to cause perspiration. *Febrifuge* Infusion of flowers taken for fevers. *Herbal Steam* Infusion of leaves and flowers used as steam bath for headaches and colds. Infusion of leaves and flowers used as steam bath to cause perspiration. *Misc. Disease Remedy* Infusion of flowers taken for measles. (180:62) **Okanagan-Colville** *Antirheumatic* (*External*) Dead stalks used to make a steam bath for arthritis or rheumatism. (162:94) **Pomo, Kashaya** *Febrifuge* Infusion of dried flowers taken to break a fever. (60:42) **Thompson** *Antirheumatic* (*Internal*) Decoction of finely chopped bark taken for arthritis. One informant cautioned that this decoction must be boiled in a nonmetal pot or it would become poisonous. (161:199) *Toothache Remedy* Fresh bark used in hollow tooth for toothaches. (141:474) *Venereal Aid* Decoction of dried flowers taken for syphilis. (161:199) **Yuki** *Febrifuge* Infusion of flowers taken for fevers. (39:46)

***Sambucus cerulea* var. *cerulea*, Blue Elderberry**

Karok *Ceremonial Medicine, Panacea,* and *Pediatric Aid* Infusion of branches used as a wash for sick child in the Brush Dance. (as *S. glauca* 125:389) **Klallam** *Antidiarrheal* Infusion of bark taken for diarrhea. (as *S. glauca* 65:47) **Luiseño** *Gynecological Aid* Flowers used for female complaints. (as *S. glauca* 132:229) **Mendocino Indian** *Dermatological Aid* Decoction of plant rubbed on bruises. *Febrifuge* Decoction of plant rubbed on the body for fevers. *Orthopedic Aid* Decoction of plant rubbed on sprains. *Veterinary Aid* Decoction of plant used as an antiseptic wash for itch and sores on animals. (as *S. glauca* 33:388) **Mewuk** *Unspecified* Flowers and roots used for medicine. (as *S. glauca* 97:366) **Miwok** *Misc. Disease Remedy* Decoction of blossoms taken for ague. (as *S. glauca* 8:172) **Montana Indian** *Antirheumatic* (*External*) Decoction of dried flowers applied externally for sprains and bruises. *Derma-*

tological Aid Decoction of dried flowers used as an antiseptic wash for open sores and itch. *Emetic* Inner bark used as a strong emetic. *Febrifuge* Decoction of dried flowers applied externally for fevers. *Gastrointestinal Aid* Decoction of dried flowers used internally for stomach troubles. *Pulmonary Aid* Decoction of dried flowers used internally for lung troubles. (as *S. glauca* 15:23) **Paiute** *Antirheumatic* (*External*) Poultice of heated stems applied to the body that ached from rheumatism and similar disorders. *Gastrointestinal Aid* Decoction of root scrapings taken for stomachaches. (as *S. glauca* 93:111) **Pomo, Little Lakes** *Antihemorrhagic* and *Tuberculosis Remedy* Decoction of plant taken for bleeding lungs from consumption. **Pomo, Potter Valley** *Disinfectant* Decoction of leaves used as an antiseptic wash. *Emetic* Inner bark used as a strong emetic. *Gastrointestinal Aid* Decoction of plant taken for stomachaches. (as *S. glauca* 33:388) **Quinault** *Emetic* Infusion of bark taken as an emetic. (as *S. glauca* 65:47) **Yokia** *Disinfectant* Decoction of leaves used as an antiseptic wash. *Emetic* Inner bark used as a strong emetic. *Gastrointestinal Aid* Decoction of plant taken for stomachaches. (as *S. glauca* 33:388) **Yokut** *Burn Dressing* Poultice of bruised leaves applied to burns. *Cathartic* Infusion of pith used as a purge. *Emetic* Infusion of flowers used as an emetic. (as *S. glauca* 97:436)

***Sambucus cerulea* var. *mexicana*, Blue Elder**

Cahuilla *Cold Remedy* Infusion of blossoms taken for colds. *Febrifuge* Infusion of blossoms taken for fevers. *Gastrointestinal Aid* Infusion of blossoms taken for upset stomachs. *Laxative* Decoction of roots used for constipation. *Misc. Disease Remedy* Infusion of blossoms taken for flu. *Pediatric Aid* Infusion of blossoms given to newborn babies. *Toothache Remedy* Infusion of blossoms used for the teeth. (as *S. mexicana* 11:138) **Diegueño** *Febrifuge* Infusion of fresh or dried blossoms given to babies with fever. *Laxative* Infusion of fresh or dried blossoms used as an enema. *Pediatric Aid* Infusion of fresh or dried blossoms given to babies with fever. (as *S. mexicana* 70:41) **Pima** *Cold Remedy* Decoction of flowers taken for colds. *Febrifuge* Infusion of dried flowers taken to break a fever. *Gastrointestinal Aid* Decoction of flowers taken for stomachaches. *Throat Aid* Decoction of flowers taken for sore throats. (as *S. mexicana* 38:75)

Sambucus cerulea var. **neomexicana**, New Mexican Elderberry
Navajo, Kayenta *Disinfectant* Plant used for lightning infection. *Veterinary Aid* Plant used for livestock with lightning infection. (as *S. neomexicana* 179:43)

Sambucus cerulea var. **velutina**, Blue Elderberry
Paiute *Antidiarrheal* Infusion of dried flowers taken for diarrhea. (as *S. velutina* 155:138)

Sambucus nigra, European Black Elder
Cherokee *Antirheumatic (Internal)* Infusion of berry used for rheumatism. *Burn Dressing* Salve used for burns. *Cathartic* Used as a cathartic. *Dermatological Aid* Salve used for skin eruptions and infusion taken as tonic for boils. *Diaphoretic* Infusion of flowers taken to "sweat out fever." *Disinfectant* Leaves used to wash sores to prevent infection. *Diuretic* Used as a diuretic. *Emetic* Used as an emetic. *Kidney Aid* Taken for "dropsy." *Other* Decoction taken for "summer complaint." *Pediatric Aid* Given for "light sickness among children" and taken for "dropsy." (66:33)

Sambucus racemosa, Scarlet Elderberry
Bella Coola *Analgesic* Infusion of roots used as an emetic and purgative for stomach pain. *Cathar-*

tic Infusion of root bark used or root bark chewed as a purgative. *Emetic* Infusion of root bark used or root bark chewed as an emetic. *Gastrointestinal Aid* Infusion of roots used as an emetic and purgative for stomach pain. **Carrier, Northern** *Cathartic* Decoction of root, second brewing only, taken as a purgative. **Carrier, Southern** *Cathartic* Decoction of root taken twice a day as a purgative. **Gitksan** *Cathartic* Infusion of root bark taken as a purgative. (127:64) *Emetic* Bark used as an emetic. (61:152) Infusion of root bark taken as an emetic. (127:64) *Witchcraft Medicine* Bark, juniper roots, and cow parsnip roots used for evil witchcraft victims. (62:24) **Hesquiat** *Analgesic* Roots rubbed on the skin for aching, tired muscles. *Antirheumatic (External)* Roots rubbed on the skin for aching, tired muscles. *Emetic* Raw roots chewed as an emetic. *Gastrointestinal Aid* Raw roots chewed to clean out the stomach. *Laxative* Raw roots chewed as a laxative. *Poison* Berries should always be eaten cooked, as they are potentially poisonous when raw. (159:63) **Kwakiutl** *Emetic* Root extract taken to induce vomiting. *Gynecological Aid* and *Herbal Steam* Infusion of bark used as steam bath to relax body of woman after childbirth. *Orthopedic Aid* Compound infusion of bark used as a foot bath for aching legs and feet. (157:280) **Malecite** *Emetic* Infusion of plant strips used with round wood as an emetic. (96:254) **Menominee** *Antidote* Decoction of scraped inner bark used as a quick emetic in cases of poisoning. (44:131) *Cathartic* Decoction of peeled twigs, a drastic purgative, taken for severe constipation. (128:27, 28) *Emetic* Decoction of scraped inner bark used as a quick emetic in cases of poisoning. (44:131) Decoction of inner bark and rind taken as a powerful emetic. (128:27, 28) **Micmac** *Emetic* Herbs used as an "emetic (with round wood)." (32:61) **Nitinaht** *Emetic* Bark soaked in water and taken as an emetic and purge. *Laxative* Bark used as a very strong laxative. *Strengthener* Bark used by athletes to "draw out all the slime in the system," for better wind and endurance. (55:318) **Ojibwa** *Cathartic* Decoction of inner bark, considered dangerous, taken as a cathartic. *Emetic* Decoction of inner bark, considered dangerous, taken as an emetic. (130:360, 361) *Unspecified* Infusion of roots used as a medicine. (112:237) **Okanagon** *Antirheumatic (Internal)*

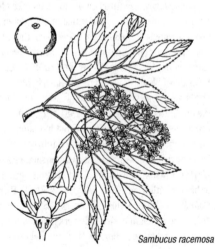
Sambucus racemosa

Plant used for rheumatism. *Dermatological Aid* Plant used for erysipelas. *Toothache Remedy* Bark placed in the hollow of a tooth for toothaches. (104:42) **Pomo** *Dermatological Aid* Decoction of roots used as a lotion on open sores and cuts. (54:15) **Potawatomi** *Cathartic* Infusion of inner bark taken as a physic and emetic. *Emetic* Infusion of stem bark taken as a strong emetic. (131:46) **Sikani** *Cathartic* Decoction of bark taken as a purgative. (127:64) **Thompson** *Antirheumatic (Internal)* Plant used for rheumatism. *Dermatological Aid* Plant used for erysipelas. (104:42) *Liver Aid* Infusion of white roots and cascara bark taken for liver diseases. (161:199) *Toothache Remedy* Bark placed in the hollow of a tooth for toothaches. (104:42) **Wet'suwet'en** *Unspecified* Bark used for medicine. (61:152)

Sambucus racemosa ssp. *pubens* var. *arborescens*, Pacific Red Elder

Cowlitz *Orthopedic Aid* Poultice of leaves or bark applied to sore joints for the swelling. (as *S. calliocarpa* 65:47) **Haisla & Hanaksiala** *Abortifacient* Leaves boiled and used to shorten pregnancy. *Gastrointestinal Aid* Berries cooked and eaten for stomach problems. *Reproductive Aid* Leaves boiled and used in aiding childbirth. **Hanaksiala** *Analgesic* Poultice of cooked shoots applied for pain. Cooked shoots put in bath water and used as a soak for pain. *Antirheumatic (External)* Poultice of cooked shoots applied to sore, arthritic areas. Cooked shoots put in bath water and used as a soak for sore, arthritic areas. *Dermatological Aid* Root slivers inserted into boil eruptions. (35:229) **Hoh** *Cold Remedy* Infusion of roots or bark used for colds. *Cough Medicine* Infusion of roots or bark used for coughs. *Gynecological Aid* Infusion of roots or bark used by women during confinement. (as *S. calliocarpa* 114:69) **Makah** *Dermatological Aid* Poultice of pounded leaves applied to an abscess or boil. (as *S. callicarpa* 65:47) **Nitinaht** *Cathartic* Infusion of bark and roots taken by boys and girls as a purgative to cleanse the system. *Psychological Aid* Bark used with black twinberry bark for nervous breakdowns. (160:100) **Quileute** *Cold Remedy* Infusion of roots or bark used for colds. *Cough Medicine* Infusion of roots or bark used for coughs. *Gynecological Aid* Infusion of roots or bark used by women during con-

finement. (as *S. calliocarpa* 114:69) **Quinault** *Gynecological Aid* Decoction of bark applied to breast after childbirth to start milk flow. **Squaxin** *Blood Medicine* Infusion of leaves used as a wash on area infected with blood poisoning. *Disinfectant* Infusion of leaves used as a wash on area infected with blood poisoning. (as *S. callicarpa* 65:47)

Sambucus racemosa ssp. *pubens* var. *leucocarpa*, European Red Elderberry

Mahuna *Misc. Disease Remedy* Blossoms used for measles. (as *S. pubens* 117:10)

Sambucus racemosa ssp. *pubens* var. *melanocarpa*, Black Elderberry

Paiute *Antidiarrheal* Dried ripe berries eaten or decoction of root taken for diarrhea. *Cold Remedy* Decoction of flowers taken for colds. *Cough Medicine* Decoction of flowers taken for coughs. *Dermatological Aid* Poultice of boiled, mashed root applied to cuts and wounds. Poultice of leaves applied to bruises. *Gynecological Aid* Poultice of boiled, mashed root applied to caked breasts. *Hemostat* Poultice of bruised leaves applied to bleeding wounds. *Pediatric Aid* and *Tonic* Decoction of flowers given to children as a spring tonic. **Shoshoni** *Antidiarrheal* Decoction of root taken for dysentery. *Blood Medicine* Decoction of root taken as a blood tonic. *Cold Remedy* Decoction of blossoms taken for colds. *Cough Medicine* Decoction of blossoms taken for coughs. *Tuberculosis Remedy* Decoction of blossoms taken for tuberculosis. (as *S. melanocarpa* 155:137, 138)

Sambucus tridentata, Antelope Brush

Paiute *Emetic* Infusion of leaves taken as an emetic. *Laxative* Infusion of leaves taken as a laxative. (144:317)

Sanguinaria canadensis, Blood Root

Abnaki *Abortifacient* Used as an abortifacient. (121:154) *Veterinary Aid* Used as an abortifacient for horses. (121:167) **Algonquin** *Love Medicine* Used as a love charm and red dye for skin, clothing, and weapons. (18:142) **Algonquin, Quebec** *Heart Medicine* Root chewed for heart trouble. *Tonic* Rhizomes used to make a medicinal tonic. (14:171) **Cherokee** *Cough Medicine* Decoction of

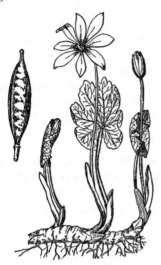

Sanguinaria canadensis

root in small doses and infusion with broomsedge used for coughs. *Dermatological Aid* Used as wash for ulcers and sores and infusion with vinegar used for tetterworm. *Nose Medicine* Used as "snuff for polypus." *Pulmonary Aid* Decoction of root taken in small doses for lung inflammations and croup. *Respiratory Aid* Pulverized root sniffed for catarrh. (66:26) **Chippewa** *Analgesic* Compound decoction of root taken for cramps. *Gastrointestinal Aid* Compound decoction of root taken for stomach cramps. (43:344) *Unspecified* Plant used medicinally. (59:131) **Delaware** *Gastrointestinal Aid* Combined with other roots and used as a stomach remedy. *Strengthener* Pea-sized piece of roots taken every morning for 30 days for general debility. (151:38) **Delaware, Oklahoma** *Gastrointestinal Aid* Compound containing root used as a "stomach remedy." *Panacea* Piece of root eaten daily "for general debility." (150:32, 80) *Tonic* Root used in a tonic. (150:80) **Delaware, Ontario** *Antiemetic* Infusion of powdered root taken for vomiting. *Blood Medicine* Compound containing root taken as a blood purifier. (150:68, 82) **Iroquois** *Analgesic* Infusion of roots taken for inside pain. (73:335) *Anthelmintic* Compound infusion of roots and whisky taken as blood remedy and for tapeworms. (73:338) *Antidiarrheal* Compound infusion of plants taken for diarrhea. *Antiemetic* Compound infusion of plants taken for vomiting. (73:336) *Antihemorrhagic* Infusion of roots taken for stomach and lump hemorrhages. (73:335)

Blood Medicine Compound infusion of roots taken to purify the blood and loosen the bowels. Infusion of branches taken as a blood tonic, "don't vomit." (73:336) Compound infusion of roots taken as a blood purifier. (73:337) *Carminative* Compound decoction of roots taken for stomach gas. (73:336) *Cold Remedy* Dried plant used as a snuff for head colds. (73:335) Decoction or infusion of roots taken for colds. (73:337) Plant chewed for colds. (73:338) *Cough Medicine* Compound infusion of roots and liquor taken as consumption cough medicine. (73:336) Decoction of powdered roots or infusion of roots taken for coughs. (73:337) *Dermatological Aid* Infusion of mashed roots taken or poultice applied to cuts or poison ivy. Plant juice taken as a wound medicine. Poultice of plants applied for drawing thorns and slivers or on leg sores. (73:336) Infusion of split root used as a wash for cuts and boils. Poultice of cooked roots applied to cuts and wounds. (73:337) Decoction of roots taken for swellings above the waist, wounds, and sores. Plant chewed for sores and cuts. (73:338) *Ear Medicine* Infusion of dried root fragments used as ear drops for earaches. (118:44) *Emetic* Decoction of branches or infusion of roots taken as a spring emetic. (73:336) *Eye Medicine* Decoction of powdered root used as a wash for sore eyes. *Febrifuge* Infusion of plants or decoction of roots or powdered roots taken for fevers. (73:337) *Gastrointestinal Aid* Infusion of roots taken for stomach hemorrhages. (73:335) Compound infusion of plants taken for upset stomach. Decoction of smashed roots taken for stomach cramps. (73:336) Compound decoction of bark taken to clean the stomach and for ulcers. Compound taken for intestinal trouble. Decoction of dried roots taken for ulcers or by women who are ugly. (73:338) Decoction of rhizomes taken for stomachaches after a big meal. (118:44) *Gynecological Aid* Infusion of plant taken for menses. (73:335) *Heart Medicine* Compound decoction of roots taken to regulate the heart and make blood redder. *Hemorrhoid Remedy* Decoction of roots used to push piles back into intestines. (73:337) *Hemostat* Decoction of roots applied to bleeding axe cuts on the foot. (73:336) *Kidney Aid* Compound decoction of roots taken for fevers or the kidneys. (73:337) *Laxative* Compound infusion or decoction of roots taken to loosen the bowels. (73:

336) *Liver Aid* Compound infusion of roots taken as a gall medicine. (73:337) *Other* Cold infusion of roots taken for sickness caught from a menstruating girl. (73:335) Decoction of smashed roots taken for hiccups. (73:336) *Panacea* Compound decoction of roots taken as a panacea. *Pediatric Aid* Compound infusion of roots taken for prenatal strength or as blood purifier. (73:337) *Pulmonary Aid* Infusion of plant taken for bleeding lungs. *Respiratory Aid* Dried plant used as a snuff for catarrh. (73:335) Decoction of roots taken for asthma. *Throat Aid* Plant chewed or poultice applied for sore throats. (73:338) *Tuberculosis Remedy* Compound infusion of roots and liquor taken as consumption cough medicine. Infusion or decoction of mashed roots taken for tuberculosis. (73:336) *Venereal Aid* Cold infusion or decoction of smashed roots taken for gonorrhea and syphilis. (73:335) *Witchcraft Medicine* Smoke from plant used as a wash for a person who has seen a dead person. (73:336) **Malecite** *Antihemorrhagic* Infusion of plant used for hemorrhages in patients suffering from consumption. (96:252) *Dermatological Aid* Decoction of plant used for black, infected cuts. (96:246) Roots used for infected cuts. *Hemorrhoid Remedy* Roots boiled and used for bleeding piles. *Tuberculosis Remedy* Roots used for consumption. (96:250) **Menominee** *Abortifacient* Compound decoction of root used for irregular periods. (44:133) *Adjuvant* Root often added to medicines to strengthen their effect. (128:44) *Dermatological Aid* Fresh root used to paint the face of a warrior. (128:78) **Meskwaki** *Adjuvant* Added to other medicines to strengthen their effect. *Analgesic* Root chewed and spittle applied to burn pains. *Burn Dressing* Infusion of root used as a wash for burns and chewed root spittle applied to burn pain. (129:234) **Micmac** *Abortifacient* Used as an abortifacient. *Cold Remedy* Infusion of roots used for colds. (122:56) *Dermatological Aid* Roots used for infected cuts. *Hemostat* Roots used for hemorrhages and to prevent bleeding. (32:61) *Love Medicine* Used as an aphrodisiac. *Throat Aid* Infusion of roots used for sore throats. (122:56) *Tuberculosis Remedy* Roots used for consumption with hemorrhage. (32:61) **Mohegan** *Blood Medicine* Infusion of plant used as a blood medicine. (149:264) Infusion of inner bark of dried root taken as a blood purifier. (151:75, 132) *Emetic* In-

fusion of plant used as an emetic. (149:264) *Tonic* Leaves used to make a tonic. (151:132) **Ojibwa** *Analgesic* Plant used for stomach pain, fainting, and trembling in fits. *Anticonvulsive* Plant used for trembling in fits or infusion of leaves taken for fits. *Antirheumatic* (*External*) Infusion of pounded plants used as wash for general illnesses and rheumatism. *Blood Medicine* Leaf infusion taken as blood medicine and bark decoction used for blood disease. (112:231) *Ceremonial Medicine* Juice used as face paint for the medicine lodge ceremony or when on warpath. (130:377) *Dermatological Aid* Poultice of plant applied or root infusion taken and used as a wash for sores and cuts. *Gastrointestinal Aid* Decoction or infusion of plants taken for stomach or bowel troubles. *Hemostat* Infusion of roots taken and used as a wash for bleeding foot cuts. *Laxative* Decoction of plants taken for sick stomach, bowels, or for constipation. *Panacea* Infusion of pounded plants used as a wash for general illnesses. *Stimulant* Infusion of leaves taken for fainting, fits, and as a blood medicine. (112:231) *Throat Aid* Root juice on maple sugar used for sore throat. (130:377, 378) *Venereal Aid* Infusion of root bark taken for gonorrhea. (112:231) **Penobscot** *Preventive Medicine* Bits of dried root worn as a necklace to prevent bleeding. (133:311) **Ponca** *Love Medicine* Root rubbed on palm of bachelor as a love charm. (58:83) **Potawatomi** *Misc. Disease Remedy* Infusion of root used for diphtheria, considered a throat disease. *Throat Aid* Root juice squeezed on maple sugar as throat lozenge for mild sore throat. (131:68)

Sanicula bipinnata, Poison Sanicle
Miwok *Snakebite Remedy* Poultice of boiled plant applied to snakebites. (8:172)

Sanicula bipinnatifida, Purple Sanicle
Miwok *Panacea* Decoction of root taken as a cure-all. *Snakebite Remedy* Infusion of leaves applied to snakebites. (8:172)

Sanicula canadensis, Canadian Blacksnakeroot
Chippewa *Abortifacient* Decoction of powdered root taken for "stoppage of periods." (43:358) *Gynecological Aid* Compound decoction of root taken during confinement. (43:360) **Houma**

Heart Medicine Hot decoction of root taken for heart trouble. (135:64)

Sanicula crassicaulis, Pacific Blacksnakeroot **Miwok** *Dermatological Aid* Poultice of leaves used for rattlesnake bites and other wounds. *Snakebite Remedy* Poultice of leaves used for rattlesnake bites and other wounds. (as *S. menziesii* 8:173)

Sanicula marilandica, Maryland Sanicle **Iroquois** *Antidote* Compound decoction of plants taken to vomit to counteract a poison. (73:397) *Dermatological Aid* Decoction of roots used as a wash and given to children with sore navels. (73:396) *Emetic* Compound decoction of plants taken to vomit to counteract a poison. (73:397) *Kidney Aid* Decoction of plants taken for dropsy. *Laxative* Compound decoction of roots taken to loosen the bowels. *Pediatric Aid* Decoction of roots used as a wash and given to children with sore navels. *Venereal Aid* Compound decoction of roots taken for venereal disease. (73:396) **Malecite** *Abortifacient* Infusion of bulb roots used for irregular menstruation. (96:258) **Menominee** *Witchcraft Medicine* Root thought to be used by sorcerers for evil purposes. (128:55) **Micmac** *Abortifacient* Roots used for irregular menstruation. *Analgesic* Roots used for menstrual pain. *Antirheumatic (Internal)* Roots used for rheumatism. *Gynecological Aid* Roots used for menstrual pain and slow parturition. *Kidney Aid* Roots used for kidney trouble. *Snakebite Remedy* Roots used as a snakebite remedy and for rheumatism. (32:61) **Ojibwa** *Febrifuge* Infusion of root used for various fevers. *Snakebite Remedy* Poultice of pounded root applied to rattlesnake bite or any snakebite. (130:391)

Sanicula odorata, Clustered Blacksnakeroot **Malecite** *Analgesic* Infusion of plant and spikenard used by women with back and side pain. *Kidney Aid* Infusion of plant and spikenard used for kidney trouble. (as *S. gregaria* 96:257) **Menominee** *Witchcraft Medicine* Root thought to be used by sorcerers for evil purpose. (as *S. gregaria* 128:56) **Meskwaki** *Dermatological Aid* Plant used as an astringent and for nosebleeds. *Hemostat* Steam of burning plant on hot stones inhaled for nosebleed. (as *S. gregaria* 129:250)

Sanicula smallii, Small's Blacksnakeroot **Cherokee** *Analgesic* and *Gastrointestinal Aid* Infusion with pink lady's slipper taken for stomach cramps and colic. *Orthopedic Aid* Used as a liniment and infusion taken for colic. (66:55)

Sanvitalia abertii, Albert's Creeping Zinnia **Navajo** *Diaphoretic* Plant used to increase perspiration. *Oral Aid* Plant chewed for mouth sores. (45:88) **Navajo, Ramah** *Analgesic* Cold infusion of leaves taken and used as lotion for headache. Compound decoction used for menstrual pain. *Cold Remedy* Chewed leaves swallowed for cold. *Dermatological Aid* Poultice of chewed leaves or infusion of leaves applied to skin sores. *Febrifuge* Cold infusion of leaves taken and used as lotion for fever. *Gynecological Aid* Compound decoction of plant used for menstrual pain. *Oral Aid* Warm infusion used as mouthwash and leaves chewed for canker sores. *Panacea* Plant used as "life medicine." *Snakebite Remedy* Compound decoction of plant used for snakebite. *Throat Aid* Chewed leaves swallowed for sore throat. *Toothache Remedy* Leaves chewed for toothache. (165:53)

Sapindus saponaria var. **drummondii**, Western Soapberry **Kiowa** *Dermatological Aid* Poultice of sap applied to wounds. (as *S. drummondii* 166:41)

Sapium biloculare, Mexican Jumpingbean **Seri** *Poison* Juice used for arrow poison. (40:138)

Saponaria officinalis, Bouncing Bet **Cherokee** *Dermatological Aid* Used as a poultice for boils. (66:26) **Mahuna** *Analgesic* Poultice of leaves applied to spleen pain. *Dermatological Aid* Root juice used as a hair tonic. (117:40)

Sarcobatus vermiculatus, Greasewood **Cheyenne** *Blood Medicine* Sharpened stick used to draw out bad blood. *Ceremonial Medicine* Sharpened stick used in acupuncture ceremony. *Veterinary Aid* Stick used to make holes in horse's shoulder for sprained or bruised legs. (69:17) **Hopi** *Ceremonial Medicine* Plant used for kiva fuel. (46:18) **Keres, Western** *Dermatological Aid* Crushed leaves used for insect bites. *Emetic* Infusion of leaves used as an emetic for lightning shock. (147:68) **Navajo** *Dermatological Aid* Plant used for insect bites. (45:97) **Navajo**, **Ramah** *Gastrointestinal Aid* Warm infusion of leaves taken to kill a swallowed red ant. (165:25) **Paiute** *Antidiarrheal* Infusion of burned plant taken for diarrhea. *Antihemorrhagic* Infusion of burned plant taken for rectal bleeding. (155:138, 139) **Paiute, Northern** *Toothache Remedy* Wood or roots heated until burned or blackened and used on aching and decayed teeth. (49:129)

Sarracenia purpurea, Purple Pitcherplant
Algonquin, Quebec *Gynecological Aid* Infusion of leaves taken to make childbirth easier. *Urinary Aid* Decoction of root tops taken for urinary difficulties. (14:173) **Algonquin, Tête-de-Boule** *Diuretic* Roots used as a diuretic. *Urinary Aid* Roots mixed with beaver kidneys and used for urinary tract diseases. (110:131) **Cree, Woodlands** *Abortifacient* Decoction or infusion of leaves taken for sickness associated with absence of menstrual period. *Gynecological Aid* Decoction of root given to women to prevent sickness after childbirth. Decoction of root and other herbs taken to expel the afterbirth. *Orthopedic Aid* Decoction taken for lower back pain. *Venereal Aid* Decoction of roots taken for venereal disease. (91:59) **Iroquois** *Basket Medicine* Used as a "basket medicine." *Dietary Aid* Plant used as a medicine for thirst. *Febrifuge* Compound decoction of leaves taken for recurring chills followed by fever. Infusion of dried leaves taken for high fever and shakiness. (73:342) Infusion of leaves and other plant fragments used for chills. (118:43) *Liver Aid* Compound infusion of whole roots taken for liver sickness. *Love Medicine* Powdered plant sprinkled on person for a love medicine. *Pulmonary Aid* Cold decoction of whole plant taken for whooping cough. Plant used for pneumonia. *Sports Medicine* Powdered plant sprinkled on person for a lacrosse medicine. (73:343) **Malecite** *Tuberculosis Remedy* Infusion of plants used for consumption. (96:251) **Menominee** *Witchcraft Medicine* Plant thought to be used by sorcerers. (128:52, 53) **Micmac** *Antihemorrhagic* Herbs used for spitting blood. (32:61) Strong decoction of root taken for "spitting blood" and pulmonary complaints. (133:316) *Kidney Aid* Herbs used for kidney trouble and consumption. *Misc. Disease Remedy* Roots used for

smallpox and herbs used for consumption. (32:61) *Pulmonary Aid* Decoction of root taken for "spitting blood and other pulmonary complaints." *Throat Aid* Infusion of root taken for sore throat. (133:316) *Tuberculosis Remedy* Herbs used for consumption. (32:61) **Montagnais** *Misc. Disease Remedy* Infusion of leaves used as medicine for smallpox. (133:314) **Ojibwa** *Gynecological Aid* Infusion of root used "to help a woman accomplish parturition." (130:389) **Penobscot** *Antihemorrhagic* Infusion of plant taken for "spitting up blood." *Kidney Aid* Infusion of plant "supposedly" taken for kidney trouble. (133:310) **Potawatomi** *Gynecological Aid* Foliage used to make a "squaw remedy." (131:82)

Sassafras albidum, Sassafras
Cherokee *Anthelmintic* Compound taken for worms. (66:54) Infusion of bark used as a wash or given to children with worms. (152:24) *Antidiarrheal* Infusion of root bark taken for diarrhea. *Antirheumatic* (*Internal*) Infusion taken for rheumatism. *Blood Medicine* Infusion taken to purify blood. *Cold Remedy* Infusion of root bark taken for colds. *Dermatological Aid* Taken for skin diseases and used to poultice wounds and sores. *Dietary Aid* Infusion of bark taken for "overfatness." *Eye Medicine* Used as a wash for sore eyes. *Misc. Disease Remedy* Taken for ague. (66:54) *Oral Aid* Roots chewed to remove odor caused by eating ramps (*Allium tricoccum*?). (105:44) *Pediatric Aid* Infusion of bark used as a wash or given to children with worms. (152:24) *Venereal Aid* Taken

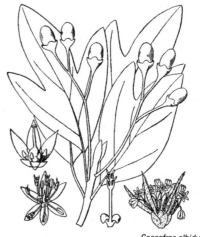

Sassafras albidum

for venereal diseases. (66:54) **Chippewa** *Blood Medicine* Infusion of root bark taken to thin the blood. (as *S. variifolium* 59:130) **Choctaw** *Blood Medicine* Decoction of roots taken to thin the blood. *Misc. Disease Remedy* Decoction of roots taken for measles. (152:24) **Creek** *Unspecified* Plant used for unspecified medicinal purpose. (as *S. variifolium* 148:661) **Delaware** *Blood Medicine* Root bark used as a blood purifier. (151:30) **Delaware, Oklahoma** *Blood Medicine* Compound containing root bark used as a blood purifier. (150:25, 80) *Tonic* Bark used in a tonic. (150:80) **Houma** *Misc. Disease Remedy* Decoction of fresh or dried root taken for measles and scarlet fever. (135:60) **Iroquois** *Anthelmintic* Compound infusion of roots and whisky taken as blood remedy and for tapeworms. (73:334) *Antirheumatic* (*Internal*) Compound infusion of plant with whisky taken for rheumatism. *Blood Medicine* Decoction of pith from new sprouts used as blood medicine. (73:333) Decoction or infusion of bark taken as a blood purifier and for watery blood. Decoction or infusion of roots taken for watery blood or to clear the blood. Plant taken to thin the blood. (73:334) *Cold Remedy* Infusion of roots taken by women for colds. *Dermatological Aid* Leaves used as a poultice for wounds, cuts, and bruises. (73:333) *Eye Medicine* Infusion or decoction of plant used as a wash for sore eyes or cataracts. (73:334) *Febrifuge* and *Gynecological Aid* Infusion of roots taken by women with fevers after childbirth. *Hemostat* Decoction of pith from new sprouts used for nosebleed. *Hypotensive* Decoction of pith from new sprouts or roots taken for high blood pressure. (73:333) Plant taken for blood pressure. *Orthopedic Aid* Compound decoction of roots taken for swellings on the shins and calves. *Tonic* Taken as a tonic. (73:334) **Koasati** *Dermatological Aid* Poultice of mashed leaves applied to bee stings. *Heart Medicine* Decoction of roots taken for heart troubles. (152:24) **Mohegan** *Eye Medicine* Infusion of young shoots used as a wash for sore eyes. (as *S. officinale* 151:75, 132) *Tonic* Complex compound infusion including sassafras root taken as spring tonic. (as *S. sassafras* 149:266) Root, leaves, and bark mixed with other herbs to make a tonic. (as *S. officinale* 151:75, 132) **Nanticoke** *Febrifuge* Infusion of root taken to ward off "fever and ague." (150:56, 84) *Misc. Disease Rem-*

edy Infusion of plant taken to prevent fever and ague. (150:56) **Rappahannock** *Burn Dressing* Decoction of branch pith used as wash for burns. *Dermatological Aid* Infusion of roots taken for the rash of measles. *Eye Medicine* Decoction of branch pith used as wash for sore eyes. *Febrifuge* Infusion of roots taken for the fever of measles. *Misc. Disease Remedy* Infusion of roots taken for the rash and fever of measles. *Sedative* Infusion of root taken as a nerve medicine. *Stimulant* Raw buds chewed to "increase vigor in males." *Tonic* Infusion of root taken as a spring tonic. (as *S. molle* 138:26) **Seminole** *Analgesic* Bark used for cow sickness: lower chest pain, digestive disturbances, and diarrhea. (145:188) Infusion of plant taken for wolf sickness: vomiting, stomach pain, diarrhea, and frequent urination. (145:227) Plant used for gallstones and bladder pain. (145:275) *Antidiarrheal* Bark used for cow sickness: lower chest pain, digestive disturbances, and diarrhea. (145: 188) Infusion of plant taken by small children for raccoon sickness: diarrhea. (145:218) Infusion of bark taken by babies and adults for otter sickness: diarrhea and vomiting. (145:222) Infusion of plant taken for wolf sickness: vomiting, stomach pain, diarrhea, and frequent urination. (145:227) Decoction of plant taken for wolf ghost sickness: diarrhea and painful defecation. (145:228) *Antiemetic* Decoction of bark used for horse sickness: nausea, constipation, and blocked urination. (145:188) Infusion of bark taken by babies and adults for otter sickness: diarrhea and vomiting. (145:222) Infusion of bark taken as an emetic and rubbed on the body for cat sickness: nausea. (145:224) Infusion of plant taken for wolf sickness: vomiting, stomach pain, diarrhea, and frequent urination. (145:227) Decoction of roots taken and rubbed on the stomach for continuous vomiting. (145:307) *Cathartic* Decoction of plant taken for wolf ghost sickness: diarrhea and painful defecation. (145:228) *Ceremonial Medicine* Bark used as an emetic in purification after funerals, at doctor's school, and after death of patient. (145:167) *Cold Remedy* Infusion of plant used as a mouthwash and gargle for colds. *Cough Medicine* Plant used as a cough medicine. (145:281) *Dermatological Aid* Infusion of bark taken and used as bath for babies with monkey sickness: fever, itch, and enlarged eyes. (145:219) *Dietary Aid* Infusion of bark taken by babies for opossum sickness: appetite loss and drooling. (145:220) Infusion of bark taken as an emetic by children and adults for dog sickness: appetite loss and drooling. (145:225) *Emetic* Bark used as an emetic to "clean the insides." (145:167) Infusion of bark taken as an emetic and rubbed on the body for cat sickness: nausea. (145:224) *Eye Medicine* Infusion of bark taken and used as bath for babies with monkey sickness: fever, itch, and enlarged eyes. *Febrifuge* Infusion of bark taken and used as bath for babies with monkey sickness: fever, itch, and enlarged eyes. (145:219) *Gastrointestinal Aid* Bark used for cow sickness: lower chest pain, digestive disturbances, and diarrhea. (145:188) Infusion of plant taken for wolf sickness: vomiting, stomach pain, diarrhea, and frequent urination. (145:227) *Laxative* Decoction of bark used for horse sickness: nausea, constipation, and blocked urination. (145:188) *Oral Aid* Infusion of bark taken by babies for opossum sickness: appetite loss and drooling. (145:220) Infusion of bark taken as an emetic by children and adults for dog sickness: appetite loss and drooling. (145:225) *Other* Infusion of plant taken and rubbed on the body for "mythical wolf" sickness. (145:306) *Pediatric Aid* Infusion of plant taken by small children for raccoon sickness: diarrhea. (145:218) Infusion of bark taken and used as bath for babies with monkey sickness: fever, itch, and enlarged eyes. (145:219) Infusion of bark taken by babies for opossum sickness: appetite loss and drooling. (145:220) Infusion of bark taken by babies and adults for otter sickness: diarrhea and vomiting. (145:222) Infusion of bark taken as an emetic by children and adults for dog sickness: appetite loss and drooling. (145:225) *Throat Aid* Infusion of plant used as a mouthwash and gargle for sore throats. (145:281) *Unspecified* Plant used for medicinal purposes. (145:161) Plant used as medicine. (145:158) Plant used medicinally. (145:164) *Urinary Aid* Decoction of bark used for horse sickness: nausea, constipation, and blocked urination. (145:188) Infusion of plant taken for wolf sickness: vomiting, stomach pain, diarrhea, and frequent urination. (145:227) Plant used for gallstones and bladder pain. (145:275)

Satureja douglasii, Yerba Buena
Cahuilla *Cold Remedy* Decoction of plant parts

taken for colds. *Febrifuge* Decoction of plant parts taken for fevers. (11:139) **Costanoan** *Anthelmintic* Decoction of plant used for pinworms. *Toothache Remedy* Poultice of warm leaves applied to jaw or plant held in mouth for toothaches. (17:17) **Karok** *Kidney Aid* Infusion of leaves taken for the kidneys. *Love Medicine* Infusion of leaves taken as an aphrodisiac. (5:54) **Luiseño** *Cold Remedy* Decoction of plant parts taken for colds. *Febrifuge* Decoction of plant parts taken for fevers. (11:139) *Unspecified* Infusion of plant used for medicinal purposes. (as *Micromeria douglasii* 132:229) **Mahuna** *Sedative* Infusion of plant taken as a sedative for insomnia. (as *Micromeria douglasii* 117:23) **Mendocino Indian** *Blood Medicine* Infusion of dried, leafy vines taken to purify the blood. *Gastrointestinal Aid* Infusion of dried, leafy vines taken for colic. (as *Micromeria chamissonis* 33:383) **Pomo** *Blood Medicine* Infusion of plant taken to purify the blood. *Dietary Aid* Decoction of plant taken for becoming thin. *Gastrointestinal Aid* Decoction of plant taken for upset stomach. (as *Micromeria chamissonis* 54:15) **Pomo, Kashaya** *Blood Medicine* Decoction of crawling stems and leaves used to purify the blood. *Cold Remedy* Decoction of crawling stems and leaves used for chest colds. *Gastrointestinal Aid* Decoction of crawling stems and leaves used for an upset stomach and thinness. *Sedative* Decoction of crawling stems and leaves used to make you sleepy. (60:121) **Saanich** *Blood Medicine* Infusion of leaves taken for the blood. (156:84) **Yurok** *Blood Medicine* Infusion of leaves taken for the blood. (5:54)

Satureja hortensis, Summer Savory
Cherokee *Analgesic* Snuff of leaves used for headache. (66:54)

Saururus cernuus, Lizard's Tail
Cherokee *Dermatological Aid* Roasted and mashed roots used as poultice. (66:43) *Poultice* Roasted and mashed roots used as poultices. (177:74) **Choctaw** *Dermatological Aid* Poultice of boiled, mashed roots applied to wounds. (20:23) **Ojibwa** *Antirheumatic* (*External*) Infusion of pounded plants used as wash for rheumatism. *Gastrointestinal Aid* Infusion of plant taken for stomach troubles and plant used as stomach medi-

cine. *Panacea* Infusion of pounded plants used as wash for general illnesses. (112:231) **Seminole** *Antirheumatic* (*External*) Plant used for fire sickness: fever and body aches. (145:204) Roots used for rheumatism. (145:286) *Dermatological Aid* Poultice of plant applied to spider bites. (145:307) *Emetic* Plant used as an emetic during religious ceremonies. (145:409) *Febrifuge* Plant used for fire sickness: fever and body aches. (145:204) *Other* Complex infusion of whole plant taken for chronic conditions. (145:272) *Unspecified* Plant used for medicinal purposes. (145:161)

Saxifraga ferruginea, Rustyhair Saxifrage
Bella Coola *Urinary Aid* Decoction of root and leaf taken for "strangulation of the bladder." (as *S. bongardi* 127:58)

Saxifraga pensylvanica, Eastern Swamp Saxifrage
Cherokee *Dermatological Aid* Poultice of root used for sore, swollen muscles. (66:26) **Iroquois** *Blood Medicine* Compound infusion of roots and leaves taken as a blood purifier. *Ceremonial Medicine* Ingredient in "Little Water Medicine" ritual. *Kidney Aid* Infusion of roots taken for weak kidneys or dropsy. Compound used for dropsy. *Panacea* Compound infusion taken or placed on injured part, a "Little Water Medicine." (73:344) **Menominee** *Unspecified* Remedy known as "the rabbit's ear," less famous than *Valeriana uliginosa*. (128:53)

Scaevola sericea, Beach Naupaka
Hawaiian *Dermatological Aid* Root bark pounded, mixed with salt, and used for cuts and skin diseases. (as *Scaevolo frutescens* 2:72)

Schizachyrium scoparium* ssp. *scoparium, Little Bluestem
Comanche *Venereal Aid* Stem ashes used for syphilitic sores. (as *Andropogon scoparius* 24:520)

Schkuhria multiflora, Manyflower False Threadleaf
Navajo, **Ramah** *Oral Aid* Plant chewed 10 minutes for mouth sores. (as *Bahia neomexicana* 165:49)

Schoenocrambe linearifolia, Slimleaf Plainsmustard
Navajo, **Ramah** *Ceremonial Medicine* and *Eye Medicine* Infusion of leaves used as a ceremonial eyewash. *Oral Aid* Cold infusion of leaves used as a mouthwash for sore gums. (as *Hesperidanthus linearifolius* 165:29)

Scirpus acutus, Hardstem Bulrush
Clallam *Other* Used to suck out the cause of an illness. (47:201) **Cree**, **Woodlands** *Hemostat* Poultice of stem pith applied under the dressing to stop bleeding. (91:59) **Montana Indian** *Dietary Aid* Roots chewed "as a preventative to thirst." (as *S. lacustris occid.* 15:23) **Navajo**, **Ramah** *Ceremonial Medicine* and *Emetic* Plant used as a ceremonial emetic. (165:19) **Thompson** *Hemostat* and *Pediatric Aid* Burned stalk ashes used on baby's bleeding navel. (161:115)

Scirpus americanus, American Bulrush
Kwakiutl *Dermatological Aid* and *Pediatric Aid* Grass and oil used on child's head to make the hair grow long and thick. (157:272)

Scirpus microcarpus, Panicled Bulrush
Malecite *Dermatological Aid* Poultice of pounded roots used for abscesses. (as *S. rubrotinctus* 96:247) *Throat Aid* Infusion of plants and blue flag used as a gargle for sore throats. (as *S. rubrotinctus* 96:248) **Micmac** *Dermatological Aid* Roots used for abscesses. *Throat Aid* Herbs used for sore throats. (as *S. rubrotinctus* 32:61)

Scirpus nevadensis, Nevada Bulrush
Cheyenne *Ceremonial Medicine* Plant used in the Sun Dance ceremony. (69:8)

Scirpus pallidus, Cloaked Bulrush
Navajo, **Ramah** *Ceremonial Medicine* and *Emetic* Plant used as a ceremonial emetic. (165:19)

Scirpus tabernaemontani, Softstem Bulrush
Cherokee *Emetic* Decoction used as emetic. (as *S. validus* 66:27) Decoction of plant taken as an emetic. (as *S. validus* 152:6) *Oral Aid* Compound used as medicine for "spoiled saliva." (as *S. validus* 66:27) **Cree**, **Woodlands** *Hemostat* Poultice of stem pith applied under the dressing to stop

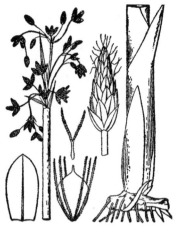

Scirpus tabernaemontani

bleeding. (as *S. validus* 91:60) **Iroquois** *Snake-bite Remedy* Compound decoction of roots and stems used as a poultice for snakebite. *Tuberculosis Remedy* Compound taken for consumption caused by *Nuphar lutea*. (as *S. validus* 73:275) **Potawatomi** *Love Medicine* Flowers used by women as a love medicine. (as *S. validus* 131:118)

Scrophularia californica, California Figwort
Costanoan *Dermatological Aid* Poultice of heated twigs applied to swollen sores. Poultice of leaves applied to boils or swellings. *Disinfectant* Decoction of twigs used as a wash for infections. *Eye Medicine* Plant juice used as an eyewash for poor vision. Poultice of leaves applied to sore eyes. (17:15) **Pomo** *Dermatological Aid* Poultice of heated leaves applied to boils. (54:15) **Pomo, Kashaya** *Dermatological Aid* Poultice of fresh, warm leaves used to draw a boil to a head. Leaves used to draw the pus out of a burst boil. (60:49)

Scrophularia californica ssp. *floribunda*, California Figwort
Diegueño *Febrifuge* Infusion of roots taken for fevers. (74:219)

Scrophularia lanceolata, Lanceleaf Figwort
Iroquois *Antihemorrhagic* Decoction of roots taken for hemorrhage after childbirth. *Blood Medicine* Decoction of roots taken by women for the blood after childbirth. *Cold Remedy* Infusion of roots taken to prevent cramps and colds after birth. (73:434) *Dermatological Aid* Poultice applied for

the soreness of sunburns, sunstroke, and frostbite. *Gynecological Aid* Compound decoction of leaves and roots taken for a "sick womb." (73:433) Infusion of roots taken to prevent cramps and colds after birth. *Kidney Aid* Compound taken for dropsy. (73:434)

Scrophularia marilandica, Carpenter's Square
Iroquois *Gynecological Aid* Infusion of roots taken by women who are weak due to irregular menses. (73:433) **Meskwaki** *Unspecified* Roots used as a medicine. (129:247)

Scutellaria angustifolia, Narrowleaf Skullcap
Miwok *Eye Medicine* Decoction used as wash for sore eyes. (8:173)

Scutellaria californica, California Skullcap
Mendocino Indian *Febrifuge* Plant used for chills and fevers. (33:385)

Scutellaria elliptica, Hairy Skullcap
Cherokee *Abortifacient* Infusion of root used for monthly period. *Antidiarrheal* Infusion of root taken for monthly period and diarrhea. *Breast Treatment* Decoction taken for nerves and compound used for breast pains. *Gynecological Aid* Compound used for expelling afterbirth. *Kidney Aid* Root compound used as a kidney medicine. (66:55)

Scutellaria galericulata, Marsh Skullcap
Delaware *Gastrointestinal Aid* Plant tops used as a stomach stimulant. *Laxative* Plant tops used as a laxative. (151:37) **Delaware, Oklahoma** *Laxative* Plant top used as a laxative and "stomach stimulant." (150:31, 80) **Ojibwa** *Heart Medicine* Plant used for heart trouble. (130:372)

Scutellaria incana, Hoary Skullcap
Cherokee *Abortifacient* Infusion of root used for monthly period. *Antidiarrheal* Infusion of root taken for monthly period and diarrhea. *Breast Treatment* Decoction taken for nerves and compound used for breast pains. *Gynecological Aid* Compound used for expelling afterbirth. *Kidney*

Aid Root compound used as a kidney medicine. (66:55)

Scutellaria lateriflora, Blue Skullcap
Cherokee *Abortifacient* Infusion of root used for monthly period. *Antidiarrheal* Infusion of root taken for monthly period and diarrhea. *Breast Treatment* Decoction taken for nerves and compound used for breast pains. (66:55) *Emetic* Decoction of roots taken as an emetic to expel the afterbirth. (152:56) *Gynecological Aid* Compound used for expelling afterbirth. (66:55) Decoction of roots taken as an emetic to expel the afterbirth. (152:56) *Kidney Aid* Root compound used as a kidney medicine. (66:55) **Iroquois** *Misc. Disease Remedy* Infusion of powdered roots taken to prevent smallpox. *Throat Aid* Infusion of powdered roots taken to keep throat clean. (73:422)

Scutellaria parvula, Small Skullcap
Meskwaki *Antidiarrheal* Plant used for flux. (129:227)

Sebastiania fruticosa, Gulf Sebastiana
Alabama *Laxative* Roots chewed "to produce a movement of the bowels." (as *S. ligustrina* 148:665)

Sedum divergens, Pacific Stonecrop
Okanagon *Hemorrhoid Remedy* Plant used for piles. *Laxative* and *Pediatric Aid* Plant given to children as a laxative. **Thompson** *Hemorrhoid Remedy* Plant used for piles. *Laxative* and *Pediatric Aid* Plant given to children as a laxative. (104:41) Decoction of whole plant given to children for constipation. (141:463)

Sedum integrifolium ssp. ***integrifolium***, Entireleaf Stonecrop
Eskimo, Alaska *Oral Aid* Roots chewed and the juice spat out for sores in the mouth. (as *S. rosea* ssp. *integrifolium* 1:36)

Sedum lanceolatum, Spearleaf Stonecrop
Okanagan-Colville *Gynecological Aid* Infusion of stems, leaves, and flowers taken to clean out the womb after childbirth. *Laxative* Infusion of stems, leaves, and flowers taken or raw leaves chewed as a laxative. (162:98)

Sedum rosea, Roseroot Stonecrop
Eskimo, Nunivak *Unspecified* Infusion of flowers used for its medicinal value. (126:325) **Eskimo, Western** *Analgesic* and *Gastrointestinal Aid* Compound decoction of flowers taken for stomachache and intestinal discomfort. (as *S. roseum* 90:5) *Tuberculosis Remedy* Raw flowers eaten for tuberculosis. (as *S. roseum* 90:24, 60)

Sedum spathulifolium, Broadleaf Stonecrop
Bella Coola *Gynecological Aid* Leaves eaten or poultice of warmed leaves used to start maternal milk flow. (127:57) Decoction of stalks taken for easy deliveries. (158:204) **Kuper Island Indian** *Hemostat* Leaves and stems squeezed and juice rubbed over bleeding wounds. (156:81) **Okanagon** *Hemorrhoid Remedy* Plant used for piles. *Pediatric Aid* and *Sedative* Infusion of whole plant used as a wash for babies with extreme nervousness. (104:41) **Songish** *Gynecological Aid* Leaves chewed by women in their ninth month of pregnancy to facilitate childbearing. (156:81) **Thompson** *Hemorrhoid Remedy* Plant used for piles. (104:41) *Laxative* Decoction of whole plant given to children for constipation. (141:463) *Oral Aid* Plant used for sore gums. (161:205) *Pediatric Aid* Infusion of whole plant used as a wash for babies with extreme nervousness. (104:41) Decoction of whole plant used as a wash to soothe cross babies. (141:462) Decoction of whole plant given to children for constipation. (141:463) *Sedative* Infusion of whole plant used as a wash for babies with extreme nervousness. (104:41) Decoction of whole plant used as a wash to soothe cross babies. (141:462)

Sedum stenopetalum, Wormleaf Stonecrop
Okanagan-Colville *Venereal Aid* Infusion of whole plant taken for venereal disease. (162:98)

Sedum telphioides, Allegheny Stonecrop
Delaware, Ontario *Dermatological Aid* Poultice of crushed leaves applied to wounds as a disinfectant. *Disinfectant* Poultice of crushed leaves applied to infected wounds. (150:66)

Sedum telephium ssp. ***telephium***, Witch's Moneybags
Iroquois *Dermatological Aid* Plant used when

babies cry or for bruises. Poultice of stalks and leaves applied to injuries resulting from witching. *Liver Aid* Compound infusion of whole roots taken for liver sickness. *Other* Rubbed on paralyzed face. *Pediatric Aid* Used for crying babies or bruises. *Veterinary Aid* Infusion of plant given to horses as a diuretic. *Witchcraft Medicine* Poultice of stalks and leaves applied to injuries resulting from witching. (73:343) **Malecite** *Dermatological Aid* Poultice of pounded leaves used for boils and carbuncles. (as *S. purpureum* 96:247) **Micmac** *Dermatological Aid* Leaves used for boils and carbuncles. (as *S. purpureum* 32:62)

Selaginella densa, Lesser Spikemoss
Blackfoot *Antihemorrhagic* Infusion of plant taken for spitting up blood. (72:74) *Gynecological Aid* Decoction of plant used to induce labor and expel the afterbirth. (72:61) *Narcotic* Plant eaten by a starving person for its doping effect and to make one feel unusually strong. (72:105) *Veterinary Aid* Powdered roots applied to the mouth of racehorses to make them hyperactive. (72:90)

Sempervivum tectorum, Common Houseleek
Cherokee *Dermatological Aid* Poultice of wilted plant applied to remove corns. *Ear Medicine* Juice warmed and used for earache. (66:42)

Senecio anonymus, Small's Ragwort
Catawba *Tuberculosis Remedy* Plant used for consumption. (as *S. smallii* 134:191)

Senecio aureus, Golden Ragwort
Cherokee *Gynecological Aid* Infusion taken to prevent pregnancy. *Heart Medicine* Infusion taken for heart trouble. (66:52) **Iroquois** *Blood Medicine* Decoction of plants taken for the blood. *Diaphoretic* Roots used as a diaphoretic. *Febrifuge* Infusion of rosettes given to children with fevers. *Kidney Aid* Decoction of plants taken for the kidneys. *Orthopedic Aid* Decoction of plants taken for broken bones. *Pediatric Aid* Infusion of rosettes given to children with fevers. (73:473)

Senecio congestus, Marsh Fleabane
Eskimo, Inuktitut *Poison* Plant considered poisonous. (176:187) **Eskimo, Western** *Poison* Roots considered poisonous. (90:17)

Senecio fendleri, Fendler's Ragwort
Keres, Western *Psychological Aid* Infusion of plant used for homesickness. (147:68) **Navajo, Ramah** *Ceremonial Medicine* Plant used in ceremonial chant lotion. *Dermatological Aid* Plant used for frozen feet. Poultice of moistened, crushed leaves and flowers applied to pimples or sores. *Gastrointestinal Aid* Decoction taken after swallowing an ant. *Panacea* Plant used as "life medicine." *Pediatric Aid* Strong decoction used for "birth injury." (165:53)

Senecio flaccidus var. *douglasii*, Douglas's Groundsel
Costanoan *Dermatological Aid* Infusion of plant used externally for infected sores or cuts. *Disinfectant* Infusion of plant used externally for infected sores. *Gynecological Aid* Infusion of plant taken by women for "lockjaw" after childbirth. *Kidney Aid* Infusion of plant taken for a "cold in the kidneys." *Other* Infusion of plant taken by women for "lockjaw" after childbirth. (as *S. douglasii* 17:27) **Kawaiisu** *Laxative* Infusion of leaves taken as a strong laxative and could cause death. *Unspecified* Infusion of leaves used as a very strong medicine. (as *S. douglasii* 180:63)

Senecio flaccidus var. *flaccidus*, Threadleaf Groundsel
Hopi *Antirheumatic* (*External*) Poultice of flowers and leaves used for sore muscles. *Dermatological Aid* Poultice of ground leaf used for pimples and skin diseases. (as *S. longilobus* 34:359) Ground leaves applied to pimples. *Orthopedic Aid* Pounded plant smeared over sore muscles. (as *S. longilobus* 174:32, 98) **Jemez** *Stimulant* Plant placed on hot coals and smoke stimulated faint and sick person. (as *S. filifolius* 36:27) **Keres, Western** *Dermatological Aid* Leaves used in shoes to prevent sweaty feet. Plant mixed with artemisia and deer marrow to make a salve. *Gastrointestinal Aid* Infusion of 6-inch piece of twig used for stomach trouble. (as *Seneci filifolius* 147:69) **Navajo, Kayenta** *Dermatological Aid* Poultice of plant applied to boils. (as *Senecio longilobus* 179:49)

Senecio jacobaea, Stinking Willie
Makah *Unspecified* Infusion of plant used as a medicinal tea. (55:327)

Senecio multicapitatus, Ragwort Groundsel
Navajo *Dermatological Aid* Decoction of plants used as a steam bath for sores. (76:156) **Navajo, Ramah** *Cathartic* Decoction of root taken as a cathartic. *Gynecological Aid* Decoction of root used to facilitate delivery of placenta. (165:53) **Zuni** *Analgesic* Cold infusion of pulverized root rubbed over limbs for "aching bones." (143:59, 60) *Ceremonial Medicine* Infusion of powdered root ceremonially rubbed on limbs for "aching bones." (143:59) *Eye Medicine* Infusion of blossoms used as drops for inflamed eyes. (143:59, 60) *Orthopedic Aid* Infusion of powdered root ceremonially rubbed on limbs for "aching bones." (143:59)

Senecio multilobatus, Lobeleaf Groundsel
Navajo, Ramah *Analgesic* Decoction of plant used for menstrual pain. *Ceremonial Medicine* Plant rubbed on body as ceremonial medicine. *Gynecological Aid* Decoction of plant taken for menstrual pain. (165:53) **Yavapai** *Cold Remedy* Decoction of leaf stem inhaled for colds. *Dermatological Aid* Boiled or dried and powdered leaves used for sores. *Gastrointestinal Aid* Decoction of root taken for stomachache. *Nose Medicine* Decoction of leaf steam inhaled for sore nose. *Venereal Aid* Decoction of root used as a wash for gonorrheal sores. (53:261)

Senecio neomexicanus, New Mexico Groundsel
Navajo, Kayenta *Antidote* Plant used as an antidote for narcotics. *Burn Dressing* Powdered plant, poultice of plant applied and plant used as lotion for burns. *Disinfectant* Plant used for bear infections. (179:49) **Navajo, Ramah** *Hunting Medicine* Cold infusion used as lotion for good luck in hunting. (165:53)

Senecio pseudoarnica, Seaside Ragwort
Aleut *Dermatological Aid* Poultice of leaves applied to drain cuts and boils. (6:427)

Senecio spartioides, Broom Groundsel
Hopi *Antirheumatic* (*External*) Poultice of flowers and leaves used for sore muscles. *Dermatological Aid* Poultice of ground leaf used for pimples and skin diseases. (34:360) **Keres, Western**

Gynecological Aid Infusion of leaves used as a tonic after childbirth. (147:68)

Senecio triangularis, Arrowleaf Groundsel
Cheyenne *Analgesic* Infusion of leaves or roots taken as a sedative for chest pains. (63:190) Infusion of pulverized leaves or roots taken for chest pains. (64:190) *Sedative* Infusion of leaves or roots taken as a sedative for chest pains. (63:190) Infusion of pulverized leaves or roots taken as a sedative. (64:190)

Senna hebecarpa, American Wild Sensitive Plant
Cherokee *Analgesic* Infusion taken for cramps. *Cathartic* Infusion given to children and adults as a purgative. *Dermatological Aid* Poultice of root used for sores. *Febrifuge* Infusion taken for fever and infusion of root given to children for fever. *Heart Medicine* Infusion of root taken for heart trouble. *Misc. Disease Remedy* Infusion taken for "blacks" (hands and eye sockets turn black). *Pediatric Aid* Infusion given to children as a purgative and for fever. *Pulmonary Aid* Compound taken for pneumonia. *Stimulant* Compound infusion given for fainting spells. (as *Cassia hebecarpa* 66:54) **Iroquois** *Anthelmintic* Plant used as a worm remedy. *Laxative* Compound decoction of flowers taken as a laxative. (as *Cassia hebecarpa* 73:362)

Senna marilandica, Maryland Wild Sensitive Plant
Cherokee *Analgesic* Infusion taken for cramps.

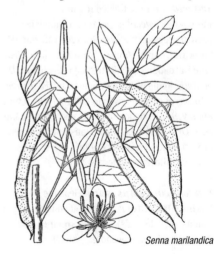

Senna marilandica

Cathartic Infusion given to children and adults as a purgative. *Dermatological Aid* Poultice of root used for sores. *Febrifuge* Infusion taken for fever and infusion of root given to children for fever. *Heart Medicine* Infusion of root taken for heart trouble. *Misc. Disease Remedy* Infusion taken for "blacks" (hands and eye sockets turn black). *Pediatric Aid* Infusion given to children as a purgative and for fever. *Pulmonary Aid* Compound taken for pneumonia. *Stimulant* Compound infusion given for fainting spells. (as *Cassia marilandica* 66:54) **Iroquois** *Anthelmintic* Compound infusion taken for tapeworms. *Blood Medicine* Compound infusion taken as a blood remedy. (as *Cassia marilandica* 73:362) **Meskwaki** *Throat Aid* Seeds soaked until mucilaginous, then eaten for sore throat. (as *Cassia marilandica* 129:228)

Senna occidentalis, Septicweed
Hawaiian *Dermatological Aid* Plant and other ingredients pounded, mixed, squeezed, and resulting juice used as wash for skin diseases. (as *Cassis occidentalis* 2:4)

Senna tora, Senna
Houma *Misc. Disease Remedy* Compound decoction of root taken for typhoid. (as *Cassia tora* 135:65)

Sequoia sempervirens, Redwood
Houma *Blood Medicine* Scraped "knees" or inner bark mixed with whisky and taken as a blood purifier. *Liver Aid* Infusion of inner bark in whisky taken for jaundice and to purify the blood. (as *Taxodium sempervirens* 135:61) **Pomo** *Ear Medicine* Poultice of heated leaves applied for earaches. *Stimulant* Gummy sap taken for rundown conditions. *Tonic* Infusion of gummy sap taken as a tonic. (54:11) **Pomo, Kashaya** *Ear Medicine* Poultice of warmed, new foliage used for earaches. *Stimulant* Gummy sap and water taken as medicine for rundown condition. (60:97) **Tlingit** *Venereal Aid* Compound poultice of bark applied for syphilis. (as *Taxodium sempervirens* 89:283)

Sesamum orientale, Sesame
Cherokee *Antidiarrheal* Decoction of leaves and seeds given for dysentery. *Cathartic* Oil of seed used as a cathartic. *Gynecological Aid* Decoction

of leaves and seeds given for flux. *Misc. Disease Remedy* and *Pediatric Aid* Decoction of leaves and seeds given for cholera infantum. (as *Sesamum indicum* 66:25)

Shepherdia argentea, Silver Buffalo Berry
Blackfoot *Gastrointestinal Aid* Berries eaten for stomach troubles. *Laxative* Berries eaten as a mild laxative. (72:68) **Cheyenne** *Unspecified* Dried, smashed berries used as an ingredient in medicinal mixtures. (69:24) **Dakota** *Ceremonial Medicine* Fruit used occasionally in ceremonial feasts at female puberty rites. (as *Lepargyrea argentea* 58:106) **Navajo** *Febrifuge* Berries taken for fevers. (76:156)

Shepherdia canadensis, Russet Buffalo Berry
Algonquin, Quebec *Orthopedic Aid* Poultice of hot-water-softened bark and pin cherry bark used to make broken bone plaster or bandage. *Unspecified* Infusion of bark used for a medicinal tea. (14:203) **Carrier** *Dermatological Aid* Berries, froth, or jelly eaten to reduce injury from mosquito bites. The berries were ripe in June and were eaten at this time to reduce injury from mosquito bites: they seem apparently to feel that the occurrence of berries and mosquitoes simultaneously was a divine indication that one was an antidote for the other. Decoction of branches used as a hair tonic for dyeing and curling the hair. The branches were taken in July, broken up, and boiled for 2 to 3 hours in water, until the liquid looked like brown

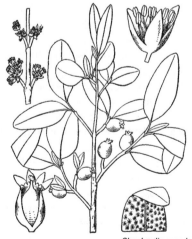

Shepherdia canadensis

coffee. The liquid was decanted off and bottled without further treatment but did not deteriorate over a long period of time. To use, the decoction was rubbed into the hair, which was simultaneously curled and dyed a brownish color. *Gynecological Aid* Infusion of roots used in childbirth. (75:12) *Laxative* Decoction of stems taken for constipation. (26:76) *Tuberculosis Remedy* Roots used for tuberculosis. (75:12) **Carrier, Northern** *Cathartic* Decoction of root taken as a purgative. (127:60) **Cree, Woodlands** *Antihemorrhagic* Infusion of roots taken for coughing up blood. *Antirheumatic* (*External*) Decoction of plant applied externally for aching limbs and arthritis. *Dermatological Aid* Decoction of plant applied externally to head and face sores. *Laxative* Infusion of inner bark, scraped from the stem with a downward motion, used as a laxative. *Venereal Aid* Decoction of stems taken for venereal disease. (91:60) **Eskimo, Inupiat** *Poison* Berries poisonous in great quantities. (83:111) **Flathead** *Eye Medicine* Bark solution used for sore eyes. (68:53) *Tuberculosis Remedy* Roots used for tuberculosis. *Unspecified* Wood used for drug purposes. (75:12) **Gitksan** *Antirheumatic* (*Internal*) Compound decoction of root taken three times a day for rheumatism. *Cough Medicine* Decoction of bark, branches, and leaves taken for chronic cough. *Venereal Aid* Decoction of roots, stem, and branches used as a wash for gonorrhea. (127:60) **Haisla & Hanaksiala** *Reproductive Aid* Berries given to women in labor to ease the birth. (35:236) **Kutenai** *Eye Medicine* Bark solution used for sore eyes. (68:53) **Okanagan-Colville** *Dermatological Aid* Decoction of branches used as a shampoo. *Hunting Medicine* Leaves chewed and spit out by hunter to stop a wounded deer from running. (162:99) **Salish** *Cathartic* Decoction of twigs taken as a mild physic. *Gastrointestinal Aid* Decoction of twigs taken as a tonic for the stomach. *Tonic* Decoction of twigs taken as a tonic for the stomach. (153:294) **Shuswap** *Cathartic* Decoction of plants taken by young men in training to purge themselves. *Gastrointestinal Aid* Decoction of berries taken for stomach. (102:61) *Tuberculosis Remedy* Roots used for tuberculosis. *Unspecified* Wood used for drug purposes. (75:12) **Sioux** *Antidiarrheal* Bark used for diarrhea. *Cathartic* Root used as a cathartic. *Poison* Fruit very acrid and considered poisonous.

(15:24) **Tanana, Upper** *Antirheumatic* (*External*) Decoction of stems and leaves used as a wash for swellings. *Dermatological Aid* Decoction of stems and leaves used as a wash for cuts. Decoction of whole plant above the ground used as a wash for sores. *Panacea* Decoction of berries taken for sickness. *Tuberculosis Remedy* Decoction of stems and leaves taken for tuberculosis. (86:13) **Thompson** *Cancer Treatment* Decoction of branches and leaves taken in a 1-cupful dose for stomach cancer. (161:209) *Cathartic* Decoction of root or decoction of dried stem and leaves taken as a physic. (as *Lepargyrea canadensis* 141:472) *Dermatological Aid* Berry juice used for acne and boils. (161:209) *Disinfectant* Decoction of stem and leaf taken by hunters and warriors in sweat house to purify. (141:505) *Gastrointestinal Aid* Decoction of bark taken as a tonic for the stomach. (as *Lepargyrea canadensis* 141:472) Berry juice and whip taken in a 1-teaspoon dose for indigestion. Berry juice used for digestive problems. Infusion of fruits and leaves used for ulcers. Berries eaten for stomach cancer. *Heart Medicine* Berry juice and whip taken in a 1-teaspoon dose for heart attacks. *Hypotensive* Decoction of branches and leaves taken in a 1-cupful dose for high blood pressure. Berries eaten for high blood pressure. *Laxative* Decoction of twigs and sticks used as a laxative. *Liver Aid* Berry juice used for gallstones. *Sedative* Infusion of fruits and leaves considered a good sedative. Berry whip said to make one sleepy. (161:209) *Tonic* Decoction of bark taken as a tonic for the stomach. (as *Lepargyrea canadensis* 141:472) Berry jam taken as a tonic. (161:209) *Tuberculosis Remedy* Roots used for tuberculosis. **Umatilla** *Gynecological Aid* Infusion of roots used in childbirth. (75:12)

Shepherdia rotundifolia, Roundleaf Buffalo Berry

Havasupai *Poison* Dust from the underside of the leaves said to make the eyes sore and to cause blindness. (171:234) **Navajo, Kayenta** *Analgesic* Ash used as lotion for headaches. *Ceremonial Medicine* Plant used as a Plumeway emetic. *Dermatological Aid* Ash used as lotion to heal navels. *Emetic* Plant used as a Plumeway emetic. *Pediatric Aid* Ash used as lotion to heal navels. *Throat Aid*

Ash used as lotion for sore throat. *Toothache Remedy* Ash used as lotion for toothaches. (179:32)

Shinnersoseris rostrata, Beaked Skeletonweed
Navajo *Sedative* Plant smoked as a sedative. (as *Lygodesmia rostrata* 45:88)

Sicyos angulatus, Oneseed Burr Cucumber
Iroquois *Venereal Aid* Decoction of vine taken for venereal disease. *Veterinary Aid* Compound plants mixed with cow's feed for difficult birth of a calf. (73:451)

Sida sp., Ilima
Hawaiian *Gynecological Aid* Flowers and other plants chewed, squeezed, and resulting liquid placed in the vagina for womb troubles. *Laxative* and *Pediatric Aid* Chewed flowers given to infants and children as a laxative. *Respiratory Aid* Flowers, shoots, root bark, and other plants pounded, squeezed, and resulting liquid taken for asthma. *Strengthener* Bark and other plants pounded, squeezed, and resulting liquid taken for general debility. (2:26)

Sidalcea neomexicana, New Mexico Checkermallow
Navajo, **Ramah** *Internal Medicine* Cold infusion of plant taken for internal injury. (165:36)

Sideroxylon foetidissimum, False Mastic
Seminole *Love Medicine* Decoction of wood ashes placed on the tongue to cleanse the body and strengthen the marriage. (145:250)

Silene acaulis, Moss Campion
Gosiute *Gastrointestinal Aid* and *Pediatric Aid* Plant used for children with colic. (31:381)

Silene campanulata, Red Mountain Catchfly
Karok *Pediatric Aid* and *Unspecified* Plant used as medicine for babies. (125:383)

Silene douglasii var. douglasii, Douglas's Campion
Gosiute *Analgesic*, *Emetic*, and *Gastrointestinal Aid* Infusion of roots taken as an emetic for stomach trouble pain. (as *S. multicaulis* 31:350) Warm

infusion of pounded plant used as an emetic for stomach pain. *Veterinary Aid* Plant used as a horse medicine. (as *S. multicaulis* 31:381) **Navajo**, **Ramah** *Dermatological Aid* and *Veterinary Aid* Cold infusion of plant used as a lotion for coyote bite on humans, sheep, or horses. (as *S. pringlei* 165:27)

Silene drummondii var. drummondii, Drummond's Campion
Navajo, **Ramah** *Panacea* Root used as a "life medicine." (as *Lychnis drummondii* 165:27)

Silene laciniata, Mexican Campion
Keres, **Western** *Dermatological Aid* Crushed plant rubbed on ant bites. *Other* Infusion of plant used as a reducing medicine. (147:69)

Silene laciniata ssp. greggii, Gregg's Campion
Navajo, **Ramah** *Burn Dressing* Poultice of leaves applied to burns. *Dermatological Aid* Decoction of root taken for mad dog or mad coyote bite. (165:27)

Silene latifolia ssp. alba, Bladder Campion
Ojibwa *Cathartic* Infusion of root used as a physic. (as *Lychnis alba* 130:361)

Silene menziesii, Menzies's Campion
Okanagan-Colville *Eye Medicine* Infusion of pounded roots used as eye drops for cataracts. (162:95)

Silene noctiflora, Nightflowering Silene
Menominee *Unspecified* Plant used as a medicine. (128:28) **Navajo**, **Ramah** *Dermatological Aid* Poultice of leaves applied to prairie dog bite. (165:27)

Silene scouleri, Scouler's Campion
Gosiute *Analgesic*, *Emetic*, and *Gastrointestinal Aid* Warm infusion of pounded plant used as an emetic for stomach pain. *Veterinary Aid* Plant used as a horse medicine. (31:381)

Silene stellata, Widowsfrill
Meskwaki *Dermatological Aid* Poultice of root

applied to dry up swellings that discharge pus. (129:208)

Silphium compositum, Kidneyleaf Rosinweed
Cherokee *Gynecological Aid* and *Stimulant* Used as a strong stimulant for whites and taken by weakly females. (66:53)

Silphium integrifolium, Wholeleaf Rosinweed
Meskwaki *Analgesic* and *Herbal Steam* Root steam directed to crippled area and used for pain. *Kidney Aid* Root used for "one with kidney trouble or who was crippled." *Orthopedic Aid* Root steam directed to crippled area and used for pain. *Urinary Aid* Infusion of leaves used for bladder troubles. (129:216)

Silphium laciniatum, Compass Plant
Dakota *Veterinary Aid* Decoction of pounded root used as a vermifuge for horses. *Witchcraft Medicine* Dried root burned during storms to act as a charm against lightning. (58:132) **Meskwaki** *Emetic* Decoction of smaller roots taken as an emetic. (129:216, 217) **Omaha** *Veterinary Aid* Roots given to horses as a tonic. (56:335) Decoction of root given to horses as a tonic. *Witchcraft Medicine* Dried root burned during storms to act as a charm against lightning. **Pawnee** *Tonic* Decoction of root taken for general debility. *Witchcraft Medicine* Dried root burned during storms to act as a charm against lightning. **Ponca** *Veteri-*

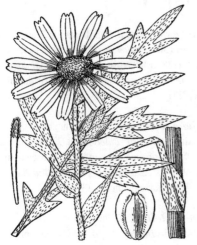

Silphium laciniatum

nary Aid Decoction of root given to horses as a tonic. *Witchcraft Medicine* Dried root burned during storms to act as a charm against lightning. **Winnebago** *Witchcraft Medicine* Dried root burned during storms to act as a charm against lightning. (58:132)

Silphium perfoliatum, Cup Plant
Chippewa *Abortifacient* Simple or compound decoction of root taken for "stoppage of periods." (43:358) *Analgesic* Decoction of root taken for back and chest pain. *Antihemorrhagic* Decoction of root taken for lung hemorrhage. (43:340) *Hemostat* Poultice of moistened, dried root applied to wounds as a styptic. (43:356) *Orthopedic Aid* Decoction of root taken for back pain. *Pulmonary Aid* Decoction of root taken for chest pain. (43:340) **Iroquois** *Emetic* Decoction of roots taken as an emetic. *Orthopedic Aid* Decoction of roots used as face wash for paralysis. *Pediatric Aid* Burned root soot placed on child's cheek to prevent them from seeing ghosts. *Witchcraft Medicine* Burned root soot placed on cheek to prevent sickness caused by the dead. (73:468) **Meskwaki** *Antiemetic* Root used to "alleviate the vomiting of pregnancy." *Gynecological Aid* Infusion of root taken by women to prevent premature birth. Root used to reduce profuse menstruation and as an antiemetic during pregnancy. (129:217) **Ojibwa** *Antirheumatic* (*Internal*) Infusion of root taken for lumbago and other rheumatic back pains. *Gastrointestinal Aid* Plant used for stomach trouble. *Hemostat* Plant used for hemorrhage. (130:365) **Omaha** *Analgesic* Smoke from burning plant inhaled for pain. (56:334) Root used in smoke treatment for neuralgia. *Antirheumatic* (*Internal*) Root used in smoke treatment for rheumatism. (58:132) *Cold Remedy* Smoke from burning plant inhaled for head colds. (56:334) Root used in smoke treatment for head cold. *Herbal Steam* Rootstock used in the vapor bath. **Ponca** *Analgesic* Root used in smoke treatment for neuralgia. *Antirheumatic* (*Internal*) Root used in smoke treatment for rheumatism. *Cold Remedy* Root used in smoke treatment for head cold. *Herbal Steam* Rootstock used in the vapor bath. **Winnebago** *Analgesic* Root used in smoke treatment for neuralgia. *Antirheumatic* (*Internal*) Root used in smoke treatment for rheumatism. *Ceremonial Medicine*

Decoction of root used as a ceremonial emetic. *Cold Remedy* Root used in smoke treatment for head cold. *Emetic* Decoction of root used as a ceremonial emetic. *Herbal Steam* Rootstock used in the vapor bath. (58:132)

Simmondsia chinensis, Jojoba
Papago *Dermatological Aid* Poultice of dried and pulverized nuts applied to sores. Poultice of parched, pulverized nuts applied to sores. (as *S. californica* 29:65) **Yavapai** *Cathartic* Plant yielded oily food with cathartic qualities. *Dermatological Aid* Parched, charred berry charcoal rubbed on sores. (as *S. californica* 51:211)

Sinapis alba, White Mustard
Cherokee *Dietary Aid* Taken to increase appetite. *Febrifuge* Taken for fever and "nervous fever." *Kidney Aid* Taken for "dropsy." *Misc. Disease Remedy* Taken for "ague." *Orthopedic Aid* Taken for palsy. *Pulmonary Aid* Given for "phthisic" or asthma. *Respiratory Aid* Used as a poultice for croup. *Stimulant* Taken as a stimulant. *Tonic* Taken as a tonic. (as *Brassica hirta* 66:46) **Hoh** *Unspecified* Plants used for medicine. (as *Brassica alba* 114:62) **Micmac** *Tuberculosis Remedy* Parts of plant used for tuberculosis of lungs. (32:62) **Quileute** *Unspecified* Plants used for medicine. (as *Brassica alba* 114:62)

Sinapis arvensis, Charlock Mustard
Navajo, Ramah *Ceremonial Medicine, Disinfectant*, and *Emetic* Plant used as a ceremonial emetic for "deer infection." (as *Brassica kaber* 165:28)

Sisymbrium altissimum, Tall Tumblemustard
Navajo, Ramah Plant probably used in emetics. (165:29)

Sisymbrium irio, London Rocket
Pima *Eye Medicine* Dried seeds placed under the lids of sore eyes to cause weeping. (38:84)

Sisymbrium officinale, Hedge Mustard
Cherokee *Pulmonary Aid* Used as a poultice for croup. (66:46) **Iroquois** *Veterinary Aid* Compound decoction of plants mixed with feed for horses with cramps. (73:341)

Sisyrinchium albidum, White Blueeyed Grass
Menominee *Antidote* Root used for poisonous bite inflicted by horse which has eaten root. *Veterinary Aid* Roots mixed with horse feed to make horse sleek, vicious, and bite poisonous. *Witchcraft Medicine* Plant kept in house or pocket as a charm to ward off snakes. (128:38)

Sisyrinchium angustifolium, Narrowleaf Blueeyed Grass
Cherokee *Antidiarrheal* Infusion of root given to children for diarrhea. *Gastrointestinal Aid* Eaten as cooked greens for "regular bowels." *Pediatric Aid* Infusion of root given to children for diarrhea. (as *S. augustifolium* 66:26) **Iroquois** *Laxative* Decoction of roots and stalks taken before morning meals for constipation. *Other* Compound with plant used for "summer complaint." (as *S. graminoides* 73:288) **Mahuna** *Anthelmintic* Infusion of plant taken for stomach worms. *Gastrointestinal Aid* Infusion of plant taken for stomach troubles and stomach worms. (117:6)

Sisyrinchium atlanticum, Eastern Blueeyed Grass
Menominee *Gynecological Aid* Compound decoction of plant taken to help expel afterbirth. (44:133)

Sisyrinchium bellum, Western Blueeyed Grass
Costanoan *Febrifuge* Decoction of plant taken for chills. *Gastrointestinal Aid* Decoction of plant taken for stomachaches. (17:29) **Luiseño** *Cathartic* Roots used as a purgative. (132:233) **Pomo, Kashaya** *Gastrointestinal Aid* Infusion of washed roots taken for upset stomach, heartburn, and ulcers. *Respiratory Aid* Infusion of washed roots taken for asthma. (60:24)

Sisyrinchium campestre, Prairie Blueeyed Grass
Meskwaki *Analgesic* Plant used for cramps and decoction used for hay fever. *Gynecological Aid* Compound decoction of plant base taken by women for injured womb. *Respiratory Aid* Decoction of whole plant used for hay fever. (129:224)

Sisyrinchium montanum, Mountain
  Blueeyed Grass
Iroquois *Cathartic* Used as a physic for old people. *Misc. Disease Remedy* Decoction taken for
fevers such as malaria and scarlet fever but not
typhoid. *Poison* "Feared it was poison." (73:288)

Sisyrinchium mucronatum, Needletip
  Blueeyed Grass
Navajo *Nose Medicine* Plant used for nose troubles. *Throat Aid* Plant used for throat troubles.
(45:37)

Sisyrinchium nashii, Nash's Blueeyed Grass
Seminole *Analgesic* Roots used with a song or
spell as an analgesic. (as *S. fibrosum* 145:167)
Infusion of roots used for moving sickness: moving pain in the waist region. (as *S. fibrosum*
145:285)

Sitanion sp., Wild Rye
Miwok *Witchcraft Medicine* Used dry or green to
strike patient with, before and after the shaman
sucks the cause of the illness out of the patient.
(8:173)

Sium suave, Hemlock Waterparsnip
Iroquois *Analgesic* Infusion of smashed roots applied as poultice for pain from broken limb. *Anticonvulsive* Compound decoction of roots taken by
women for epilepsy. *Orthopedic Aid* Infusion of
smashed roots applied as poultice for pain from
broken limb. Poultice of fried turnips applied to
sprained muscles or out of joint limbs. (73:399)
Lakota *Gastrointestinal Aid* Roots used for the
stomach. (116:33) **Ojibwa** *Hunting Medicine*
Seeds smoked over a fire to drive away and blind
evil spirit that steals away one's hunting luck. (as
S. cicutaefolium 130:432) **Shuswap** *Poison* White
flowers considered poisonous. (102:57)

Smallanthus uvedalia, Hairy Leafcup
Cherokee *Burn Dressing* Bruised root used on
burns. *Dermatological Aid* Bruised root used as a
salve for cuts. Poultice of root used for "inflammations," and bruised root in hog's lard used for itch.
(as *Polymnia uvedalia* 66:42) *Emetic* Decoction
of roots taken to vomit to expel the afterbirth. (as
Polymnia uvedalia 152:63) *Gynecological Aid*

Compound decoction used "for expelling afterbirth." (as *Polymnia uvedalia* 66:42) Decoction
of roots taken to vomit to expel the afterbirth. (as
Polymnia uvedalia 152:63) *Other* Plant used for
rheumatism and "white swelling." (as *Polymnia
uvedalia* 66:42) **Iroquois** *Analgesic* Compound
infusion of stalks and roots taken for back pain.
Antiemetic Compound infusion of stalks and roots
taken for vomiting. (as *Polymnia uvedalia* 73:467)
Disinfectant Dried roots used as fumigant for
ghosts. (as *Polymnia uvedalia* 73:468) *Febrifuge*
Infusion of roots taken for fevers. *Kidney Aid* Compound infusion of stalks and roots taken for kidney troubles. *Orthopedic Aid* Compound infusion
of stalks and roots taken for back pain. *Sedative*
Dried root smoke used as rub to sleep without being disturbed by ghosts. (as *Polymnia uvedalia*
73:467)

Smilacina sp., False Solomon's Seal
Yana *Dermatological Aid* Poultice of pounded
roots applied to swellings or boils. (124:253)

Smilax auriculata, Earleaf Greenbrier
Seminole *Other* Complex infusion of buds, or buds
and leaves, taken for chronic conditions. (145:272)

Smilax bona-nox, Saw Greenbrier
Choctaw *Tonic* Decoction of stems taken as a general tonic. (152:8) **Creek** *Other* Plant moistened
and rubbed on face to make one young. (148:667)
Houma *Urinary Aid* Decoction of root taken for
urinary disturbances. (135:58, 59)

Smilax glauca, Cat Greenbrier
Cherokee *Analgesic* Rubbed in brier scratches
for local pains. *Antirheumatic* (*Internal*) Used
for rheumatism. *Burn Dressing* Parched and powdered leaves used for "scalds." *Dermatological
Aid* Powdered and beaten leaves put on "galled
places" and wilted leaves put on boils. *Gastrointestinal Aid* Infusion taken for stomach trouble. *Gynecological Aid* Compound decoction used to aid in
expelling afterbirth. (66:37) Decoction of roots
taken to cause discharge of the afterbirth. (152:8)
Orthopedic Aid Rubbed in brier scratches for muscular cramps and twitching. *Other* Compound infusion of bark taken for "bad disease." (66:37)

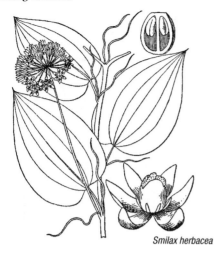

Smilax herbacea

Smilax herbacea, Smooth Carrionflower **Cherokee** *Analgesic* Rubbed in brier scratches for local pains. *Antirheumatic* (*Internal*) Used for rheumatism. *Burn Dressing* Parched and powdered leaves used for "scalds." *Dermatological Aid* Powdered and beaten leaves put on "galled places" and wilted leaves put on boils. *Gastrointestinal Aid* Infusion taken for stomach trouble. *Gynecological Aid* Compound decoction used to aid in expelling afterbirth. *Orthopedic Aid* Rubbed in brier scratches for muscular cramps and twitching. *Other* Compound infusion of bark taken for "bad disease." (66:37) **Chippewa** *Analgesic* Decoction of root taken for back pain. *Cathartic* Compound decoction of root taken as a physic. *Kidney Aid* and *Orthopedic Aid* Decoction of root taken for kidney trouble. (43:346) **Iroquois** *Antirheumatic* (*External*) Compound decoction used as a wash and steam bath for rheumatism. *Dermatological Aid* Powdered root used as a "deodorant." (73:287) *Gastrointestinal Aid* Decoction of roots taken by the elderly for stomach troubles. *Psychological Aid* Compound decoction of plant taken for "loss of senses during menses." (73:286) **Ojibwa** *Pulmonary Aid* Root used for lung troubles. (130: 374) **Omaha** *Throat Aid* Fruits used for hoarseness. (58:71)

Smilax laurifolia, Laurel Greenbrier **Cherokee** *Burn Dressing* Compound of root bark used as a wash for burns. *Dermatological Aid* Astringent and slightly tonic root bark used as a wash for burns and sores. Compound of root bark

used for pox and as a wash for sores. *Tonic* Root bark astringent and slightly tonic. (66:24) **Houma** *Urinary Aid* Decoction of root taken for urinary disturbances. (135:58, 59)

Smilax pseudochina, Bamboovine **Cherokee** *Analgesic* Rubbed in brier scratches for local pains. *Antirheumatic* (*Internal*) Used for rheumatism. *Burn Dressing* Parched and powdered leaves used for "scalds." *Dermatological Aid* Powdered and beaten leaves put on "galled places" and wilted leaves put on boils. *Gastrointestinal Aid* Infusion taken for stomach trouble. *Gynecological Aid* Compound decoction used to aid in expelling afterbirth. *Orthopedic Aid* Rubbed in brier scratches for muscular cramps and twitching. *Other* Compound infusion of bark taken for "bad disease." (as *S. tamnifolia* 66:37)

Smilax rotundifolia, Roundleaf Greenbrier **Cherokee** *Analgesic* Rubbed in brier scratches for local pains. *Antirheumatic* (*Internal*) Used for rheumatism. *Burn Dressing* Parched and powdered leaves used for "scalds." *Dermatological Aid* Powdered and beaten leaves put on "galled places" and wilted leaves put on boils. *Gastrointestinal Aid* Infusion taken for stomach trouble. *Gynecological Aid* Compound decoction used to aid in expelling afterbirth. *Orthopedic Aid* Rubbed in brier scratches for muscular cramps and twitching. *Other* Compound infusion of bark taken for "bad disease." (66:37) **Koasati** *Analgesic* Plant splints used to scratch the back for headaches. (152:8)

Smilax tamnoides, Bristly Greenbrier **Choctaw** *Tonic* Decoction of stems taken as a general tonic. (20:23) **Iroquois** *Eye Medicine* Poultice of bark applied to eyes to "draw out foreign substances." *Witchcraft Medicine* Plant used to make doll to be used "to kill a woman who is using you badly." (as *S. hispida* 73:287)

Solanum carolinense, Carolina Horsenettle **Cherokee** *Anthelmintic* Infusion of leaf used for worms. *Dermatological Aid* Used "for ulcers and proud flesh" and wilted plant used on poison ivy. *Oral Aid* and *Pediatric Aid* Roots strung around baby's neck for teething. *Throat Aid* Infusion of seed gargled for sore throat and taken for goiter.

Veterinary Aid Cut berries fried in grease and grease used for dogs with mange. (66:46)

Solanum donianum, Mullein Nightshade
Seminole *Analgesic* Decoction of root bark poured onto the head for headaches. (as *S. verbascifolium* 145:278)

Solanum douglasii, Greenspot Nightshade
Cahuilla *Eye Medicine* Berry juice used for sore or infected eyes, pink eye, and eye strain, and to improve vision in older people. *Poison* Whole plant considered poisonous. (11:140) **Luiseño** *Eye Medicine* Berry juice used for inflamed eyes. (132:229)

Solanum dulcamara, Climbing Nightshade
Delaware, **Oklahoma** *Dermatological Aid* Plant used to make a salve for unspecified use. *Febrifuge* Compound containing root used for fever. (150:80) **Iroquois** *Gastrointestinal Aid* Compound decoction of plants taken for biliousness. (73:431) **Malecite** *Antiemetic* Infusion of roots used for nausea. (96:253) **Micmac** *Antiemetic* Roots used for nausea. (32:62) **Nootka** *Gastrointestinal Aid* Plant used for "derangement" of stomach and bowels. (146:81)

Solanum elaeagnifolium, Silverleaf Nightshade
Apache, **White Mountain** *Unspecified* Plant used for medicinal purposes. (113:160) **Isleta** *Laxative* Raw seedpods eaten or boiled into a syrup and taken as a laxative. (85:43) **Keresan** *Gynecological Aid* Infusion of plant taken by nursing mothers to sustain milk flow. (172:562) **Navajo** *Eye Medicine* Plant used for sore eyes. (45:75) *Nose Medicine* Plant used for nose troubles. *Throat Aid* Plant used for throat troubles. (45:97) **Pima** *Cold Remedy* Crushed, dried berries used for colds. (38:88) **Zuni** *Snakebite Remedy* Fresh or dried root chewed by medicine man before sucking snakebite and poultice applied to wound. *Toothache Remedy* Fruit chewed over sore tooth. (22:378) Chewed root placed in cavity of aching tooth. (143:60)

Solanum fendleri, Fendler's Horsenettle
Navajo *Carminative* and *Gastrointestinal Aid* Raw tubers taken for gastric distress from hyperacidity. (76:163)

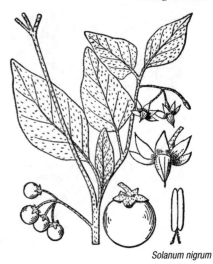

Solanum nigrum

Solanum nigrum, Black Nightshade
Cherokee *Emetic* Taken as an emetic and to relieve loneliness because of death in family. *Psychological Aid* Infusion of leaves and stem taken "if lonesome because of death in family." (66:51) **Costanoan** *Dermatological Aid* Poultice of heated leaves applied to boils. *Misc. Disease Remedy* Decoction of plant used for scarlet fever. *Toothache Remedy* Plant smoke inhaled for toothaches. (17:14) **Delaware**, **Oklahoma** *Venereal Aid* Compound containing root used for venereal disease. (150:29, 80) **Houma** *Anthelmintic* Decoction of root given to babies for worms. *Dermatological Aid* Poultice of crushed, green leaves, and grease applied to sores. *Pediatric Aid* Decoction of root given to babies for worms. (135:65) **Iroquois** *Other* Plant used for injured person who had relapse. (73:431) **Karok** *Poison* Plant considered poisonous. (125:389) **Mendocino Indian** *Poison* Berries considered poisonous. (33:387) **Miwok** *Eye Medicine* Decoction used as wash for sore eyes. (8:173) **Ojibwa** *Ceremonial Medicine* Plant used for medicinal purposes or medicine ceremonies. (112:239) **Rappahannock** *Poison* and *Sedative* Weak infusion of dried leaves, poisonous, taken for sleeplessness. (138:34)

Solanum physalifolium, Hoe Nightshade
Paiute *Antidiarrheal* Ripe fruit eaten or decoction of dried fruit taken for diarrhea. (as *S. villosum* 155:140)

Solanum rostratum, Buffalobur Nightshade
Zuni *Gastrointestinal Aid* Infusion of powdered root, not an emetic, taken for "sick stomach." (143:60)

Solanum triflorum, Cutleaf Nightshade
Blackfoot *Antidiarrheal* and *Pediatric Aid* Decotion of berries given to children for diarrhea. (82:53) Decoction of berries given to children for diarrhea. (95:275) **Lakota** *Gastrointestinal Aid* Berries used for stomachaches. (116:60) **Navajo, Ramah** *Veterinary Aid* Cold infusion used as lotion on horses' sores. (165:43)

Solanum tuberosum, Irish Potato
Cherokee *Emetic* Taken as an emetic and to relieve loneliness because of death in family. *Psychological Aid* Infusion of leaves and stem taken "if lonesome because of death in family." (66:51) **Iroquois** *Eye Medicine* Poultice of scraped potato applied to eye for inflammation. (73:431) **Rappahannock** *Dermatological Aid* Bruised tuber rubbed on warts. (138:27)

Solanum xantii, Purple Nightshade
Kawaiisu *Dermatological Aid* Poultice of heated plant applied to sores. *Orthopedic Aid* Poultice of heated plant applied to swollen leg and shoulder. (180:64)

Solidago californica, California Goldenrod
Cahuilla *Dermatological Aid* Used in making a hair rinse. *Gynecological Aid* Used as a medicine for feminine hygiene. (11:140) **Costanoan** *Burn Dressing* Decoction of leaves used as a wash for burns. *Dermatological Aid* Decoction of leaves used as a wash for sores. Toasted, crumbled leaves applied to wounds. (17:27) **Diegueño** *Dermatological Aid* Decoction of leaves and stems used to wash the hair to prevent falling hair. (70:43) **Kawaiisu** *Dermatological Aid* Infusion of leaves and flowers used as wash for boils and "holes" in neck and limbs, and for open sores and skin irritations. (180:64) **Miwok** *Antirheumatic* (*External*) Leaf powder dusted on sores. (8:170) *Dermatological Aid* Leaf powder applied to open sores. *Toothache Remedy* Decoction held in mouth for toothaches. (8:173)

Solidago canadensis, Canada Goldenrod
Iroquois *Analgesic* Infusion of roots and flowers used for side pains. (118:65) *Emetic* Compound infusion of roots taken as an emetic. Infusion of flowers taken as an emetic for too much gall. *Gastrointestinal Aid* and *Liver Aid* Infusion of flowers taken as an emetic for too much gall. *Love Medicine* Compound infusion of roots taken to kill a love medicine. *Other* Plant used as a "gambling medicine." *Pediatric Aid* and *Sedative* Compound infusion of tubers given to babies that start suddenly during sleep. (73:461) **Meskwaki** *Psychological Aid* Compound decoction used as wash for child who does not talk or laugh. (129:217) **Okanagan-Colville** *Antidiarrheal* Infusion of flower heads taken for diarrhea. *Febrifuge* Infusion of shoots given to children with fevers. *Misc. Disease Remedy* Decoction of flower heads taken for the flu. *Pediatric Aid* Infusion of shoots given to children with fevers. (162:84) **Potawatomi** *Febrifuge* Infusion of blossoms used for special kinds of fevers. (131:53) **Shuswap** *Gynecological Aid* Infusion of plant used as a bath for the mother at childbirth. (102:59) **Thompson** *Antidiarrheal* Decoction of plant used as a bath for babies with diarrhea. Decoction of plant tops taken for diarrhea. *Orthopedic Aid* Plant used to make a steam bath for crippled, paralyzed people. *Pediatric Aid* Decoction of plant used as a bath for babies with diarrhea, sleeplessness, or excessive crying. *Sedative* Decoction of plant used as a bath for babies with sleeplessness or excessive crying. *Veterinary Aid* Decoction of plant and wild tarragon used as a wash for horses with cuts and sores. (161:184) **Zuni** *Analgesic* Crushed blossoms chewed for sore throat. Infusion of crushed blossoms taken for body pain. (143:60)

Solidago canadensis var. *scabra*, Canada Goldenrod
Chippewa *Burn Dressing* Compound poultice of flowers applied to burns. (as *S. altissima* 43:352) *Dermatological Aid* Poultice of moistened, pulverized root applied to boils. (as *S. altissima* 43:348) Poultice of moistened, dry flowers applied to ulcers. (as *S. altissima* 43:354)

Solidago confinis, Southern California
Goldenrod
Kawaiisu *Dermatological Aid* Infusion of leaves
and flowers used as wash for boils and "holes" in
neck and limbs, and for open sores and skin irritations. (180:64)

Solidago flexicaulis, Zigzag Goldenrod
Chippewa *Throat Aid* Root chewed for sore throat.
(43:342) **Iroquois** *Gastrointestinal Aid* Compound decoction of plants taken for biliousness.
(73:459) **Menominee** *Analgesic* Snuff of dried,
powdered leaves used for headache. (44:129)
Hemostat Compound of powdered, dried leaves
inserted in nostrils to check nosebleed. (44:132)
Potawatomi *Febrifuge* Infusion of whole plant
used for certain fevers. (as *S. latifolia* 131:53)

Solidago gigantea, Giant Goldenrod
Keres, **Western** *Cathartic* Infusion of leaves used
as a strong physic. (as *Salidago pitcheri* 147:67)
Menominee *Unspecified* Plant used in medicine.
(as *Solidago serotina* 128:31) **Potawatomi** *Febrifuge* Infusion of blossoms used for various fevers.
(as *S. serotina* 131:53)

Solidago juncea, Early Goldenrod
Chippewa *Anticonvulsive* Decoction of root taken
for convulsions. (43:336) **Delaware** *Antidiarrheal*
Infusion of green leaves used or green leaves
chewed for diarrhea. *Febrifuge* Infusion of green
leaves used or green leaves chewed for fever. (151:
33) **Delaware**, **Oklahoma** *Antidiarrheal* Leaves
chewed or infusion taken for diarrhea. *Febrifuge*
Leaves chewed or infusion taken for fever. (150:28,
80) **Iroquois** *Antiemetic* Infusion of plants taken
for nausea. *Emetic* Decoction of flowers taken as
an emetic. *Febrifuge* Decoction of roots taken for
fevers. *Gastrointestinal Aid* Decoction or infusion
of flowers taken for biliousness and upset stomach.
Liver Aid Infusion of plants taken for jaundice.
(73:460)

Solidago multiradiata, Mountain Goldenrod
Cree, **Hudson Bay** *Tonic* Plant used as a tonic.
(as *S. virgaurea* 78:303)

Solidago nemoralis, Dyersweed Goldenrod
Houma *Liver Aid* Decoction of root taken for "yel-

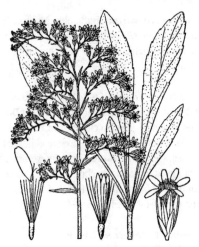

Solidago nemoralis

low jaundice." (135:66) **Iroquois** *Kidney Aid*
Decoction of roots taken for the kidneys. (73:460)
Mahuna *Burn Dressing* Decoction of leaves used
as a wash or poultice of leaves applied to burns.
Dermatological Aid Decoction of leaves used as a
wash or poultice of leaves applied to skin ulcers.
Decoction of plant used as a bath for the 7-year
itch. *Disinfectant* Decoction of leaves used as a disinfecting wash for burns or skin ulcers. (117:12)

Solidago odora, Anisescented Goldenrod
Cherokee *Abortifacient* Used for "female obstructions." *Antidiarrheal* Infusion taken for bloody discharge from bowels. *Cold Remedy* Infusion taken
for cold. *Cough Medicine* Infusion taken for
coughs. *Diaphoretic* Infusion taken as a diaphoretic. *Febrifuge* Infusion taken for fever. *Misc.
Disease Remedy* Infusion taken for nerves and
measles. *Oral Aid* Root chewed for sore mouth.
Sedative Infusion taken for "nerves" and infusion
of root held in mouth for neuralgia. *Stimulant*
Used as a stimulant. *Tonic* Used as a tonic. *Tuberculosis Remedy* Infusion of leaf taken for tuberculosis. (66:36)

Solidago rigida, Stiff Goldenrod
Chippewa *Cathartic* Decoction of root used as an
enema. (43:364) *Diuretic* Infusion of root taken
for "stoppage of urine." (43:348) **Meskwaki**
Dermatological Aid Flowers made into a lotion
and used on bee stings and for swollen faces.
(129:217, 218)

Solidago rugosa, Wrinkleleaf Goldenrod
Iroquois *Liver Aid* Whole plant used for biliousness and as liver medicine. *Other* Decoction of
flowers and leaves taken for dizziness, weakness,
or sunstroke. (73:461)

Solidago simplex ssp. **simplex** var. **nana**,
 Dwarf Goldenrod
Thompson *Dietary Aid* and *Tonic* Decoction of
plant taken as a tonic to restore appetite. (as *S.
decumbens* 141:468) *Venereal Aid* Decoction of
whole plant taken for syphilis. (as *S. decumbens*
141:472)

Solidago spathulata, Coast Goldenrod
Thompson *Misc. Disease Remedy* Poultice of
toasted, powdered leaves mixed with grease and
used for mumps. (161:184)

Solidago speciosa, Showy Goldenrod
Meskwaki *Burn Dressing* Infusion of root used
for burns or steam scalds. (129:218)

Solidago speciosa var. **rigidiuscula**, Showy
 Goldenrod
Chippewa *Antihemorrhagic* Decoction of root
taken for hemorrhaging from the mouth after being wounded. (as *S. rigidiuscula* 43:352) *Dermatological Aid* Root or stalk combined with bear
grease used as an ointment for the hair. (as *S.
rigidiuscula* 43:350) *Gynecological Aid* Infusion
of root taken to ease difficult labor. (as *S. rigidiuscula* 43:358) *Orthopedic Aid* Warm poultice of
boiled stalk or root applied to sprains or strained
muscles. (as *S. rigidiuscula* 43:362) *Pulmonary
Aid* Cold decoction of root taken for lung hemorrhages. Compound decoction of root taken for lung
trouble. *Stimulant* Decoction of root and stalk
taken as a stimulant. (as *S. rigidiuscula* 43:340)
Tonic Decoction of root and stalk taken as a tonic.
(as *S. rigidiuscula* 43:364)

Solidago squarrosa, Downy Ragged Goldenrod
Iroquois *Burn Dressing* Compound infusion of
dried leaves and roots used as wash for scalds and
burns. *Emetic* Compound infusion of dried leaves
and roots taken as an emetic. *Gastrointestinal Aid*
Compound infusion of dried leaves and roots used
as wash for bad stomach. *Venereal Aid* Compound

infusion of dried leaves and roots used as wash for
venereal disease. (73:459)

Solidago uliginosa, Bog Goldenrod
Potawatomi *Dermatological Aid* Poultice of root
used to bring a boil to a head. (131:53, 54)

Solidago ulmifolia, Elmleaf Goldenrod
Meskwaki *Stimulant* Smoke of smudged plant
directed up nostrils to revive unconscious patient.
(129:218)

Solidago velutina, Threenerve Goldenrod
Navajo, **Kayenta** *Pediatric Aid* and *Psychological
Aid* Plant used as a lotion to bathe an infant her-
maphrodite to become sensible. (as *S. sparsiflora*
179:50) **Navajo**, **Ramah** *Witchcraft Medicine*
Cold infusion taken and used as lotion in witchcraft. (as *S. sparsiflora* 165:53)

Sonchus arvensis, Field Sowthistle
Cherokee *Sedative* Infusion taken to calm nerves.
(66:59) **Potawatomi** *Gynecological Aid* Infusion
of leaves used for caked breast. (131:54)

Sonchus asper, Spiny Sowthistle
Iroquois *Pediatric Aid* and *Sedative* Compound
infusion given to babies "who cry until they hold
their breath." (73:478) **Navajo**, **Kayenta** *Heart
Medicine* Plant smoked or taken for palpitations.
Poison Plant considered poisonous. (179:50)

Sonchus oleraceus, Common Sowthistle
Houma *Abortifacient* Infusion of plant taken to
"make tardy menstruation come." *Antidiarrheal*
Infusion of whole plant taken to "correct looseness
of bowels." *Pediatric Aid* and *Toothache Remedy*
Infusion of plant given to children for teething.
(135:64) **Pima** *Cathartic* Gum used as a cathartic.
Other Gum used as a cure for the opium habit.
(38:106)

Sophora secundiflora, Mescal Bean
Comanche *Ear Medicine* Decoction of ground
beans used for earaches and ear sores. (as *S.
seundiflora* 84:3)

Sorbus americana, American Mountainash
Algonquin, **Quebec** *Cold Remedy* Infusion of

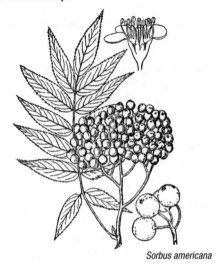

Sorbus americana

inner bark taken for colds. Infusion of terminal buds and inner bark taken for colds. *Tonic* Infusion of inner bark and sweet flag used as a tonic. (as *Pyrus americana* 14:177) **Algonquin, Tête-de-Boule** *Psychological Aid* Buds and inner bark fibers boiled and used for moral depression. *Strengthener* Buds and inner bark fibers boiled and used for general weakness. (110:131) **Iroquois** *Gastrointestinal Aid* Fruit used to facilitate digestion. (119:91) **Malecite** *Analgesic* Infusion of bark used for pain after childbirth. (as *Pyrus americana* 96:258) *Dermatological Aid* Poultice of burned bark used for boils. (as *Pyrus americana* 96:247) **Micmac** *Analgesic* Bark used for "mother pains." *Dermatological Aid* Bark used for boils. *Emetic* Parts of plant used as an emetic. (as *Pyrus americana* 32:60) *Gastrointestinal Aid* Infusion of root taken for colic. (133:317) *Gynecological Aid* Bark used for "mother pains." (as *Pyrus americana* 32:60) *Unspecified* Infusion of bark taken for unspecified purpose. (133:317) **Montagnais** *Blood Medicine* Decoction of bark taken to purify the blood and to stimulate the appetite. *Dietary Aid* Decoction of bark taken to stimulate the appetite and to purify the blood. (133:313) **Ojibwa** *Unspecified* Root bark used for medicinal purposes. (as *Pyrus americana* 112:236) *Venereal Aid* Infusion of root bark taken for gonorrhea. (as *Pyrus americana* 112:231) **Penobscot** *Emetic* Plant used as an emetic. (133:309) **Potawatomi** *Unspecified* Inner bark used as a medicine. (as *Pyrus americana* 131:78) **Tlingit** *Pulmonary Aid*

Plant used for pleurisy. (as *Pyrus sambucifolius* 89:283)

Sorbus aucuparia, European Mountainash
Potawatomi *Cold Remedy* Infusion of leaves taken as a cold medicine. *Emetic* Infusion of leaves taken as an emetic for pneumonia, diphtheria, and croup. *Misc. Disease Remedy* Infusion of leaves taken as an emetic for diphtheria. *Pulmonary Aid* Infusion of leaves taken as an emetic for pneumonia and croup. (as *Pyrus aucuparia* 131:78)

Sorbus decora, Northern Mountainash
Cree, Woodlands *Antirheumatic (External)* Decoction of inner bark from the stem base used for rheumatism. *Orthopedic Aid* Decoction of peeled sticks taken for back pain. Decoction of inner bark from the stem base used for backaches. (91:61)

Sorbus scopulina, Greene Mountainash
Okanagan-Colville *Pediatric Aid* and *Urinary Aid* Infusion of branches given to young children with bed-wetting problems. (162:133) **Wet'suwet'en** *Febrifuge* Bark used for fevers. *Tonic* Bark used as a tonic. *Unspecified* Bark used for general sickness. (61:152)

Sorbus sitchensis, Western Mountainash
Bella Coola *Antirheumatic (Internal)* Infusion of root and branch bark taken for rheumatism. *Gastrointestinal Aid* Infusion of root and branch bark taken for stomach troubles. (158:210) **Carrier** *Unspecified* Scraped bark used for medicine. (26:70) **Okanagan-Colville** *Pediatric Aid* and *Urinary Aid* Infusion of branches given to young children with bed-wetting problems. (162:133) **Thompson** *Ear Medicine* Warmed stick used in the ear for earache. *Kidney Aid* Infusion of branches taken for weak kidneys, to stop frequent urination. (161:273)

Sorbus sitchensis* var. *grayi, Gray's Mountainash
Heiltzuk *Dermatological Aid* Berries mashed and rubbed on the head for lice. (35:116)

Sorbus sitchensis* var. *sitchensis, Sitka Mountainash
Bella Coola *Antirheumatic (Internal)* Decoction

of root bark or stem bark taken or used as bath for rheumatism. *Eye Medicine* Decoction of root bark or inner bark of stem used as eyewash. *Gastrointestinal Aid* Decoction of root bark or inner bark of stem taken "for the stomach." **Carrier, Southern** *Cold Remedy* Bark chewed for colds. **Gitksan** *Cathartic* Crushed fresh fruit eaten raw as a strong purgative. (as *Pyrus sitchensis* 127:59)

Sparganium eurycarpum, Broadfruit Burreed
Iroquois *Febrifuge* Infusion of whole plant and other plant leaves used for chills. (118:71) *Veterinary Aid* Compound of chopped plants mixed with cows feed for difficult birth of calf. *Witchcraft Medicine* Compound poultice bound to "soreness all over in men from being witched." (73:272)

Sphaeralcea ambigua, Desert Globemallow
Shoshoni *Antiemetic* Decoction of root taken for upset stomach. (155:141, 142) *Antirheumatic* (*External*) Poultice of mashed root used for swollen feet. (98:43) Poultice of wilted plants bound onto rheumatic or swollen areas. *Cathartic* Decoction of root or whole plant taken as a physic. *Cold Remedy* Decoction of leaves taken for colds. (155:141, 142) *Contraceptive* Infusion of root taken as birth control. (98:46) Decoction of root taken as a contraceptive, "uncertain report." *Dermatological Aid* Poultice of crushed, raw root applied to swellings. Poultice of wilted plants applied for rheumatism or swellings. *Emetic* Decoction of root or whole plant taken as an emetic. *Eye Medicine* Decoction of leaves used as an eyewash. (155:141, 142) *Unspecified* Poultices of cooked root applied medicinally. (98:43) *Venereal Aid* Decoction of root or whole plant taken for venereal disease. *Veterinary Aid* Poultice of boiled plant applied to wire cuts on horses. (155:141, 142)

Sphaeralcea angustifolia, Copper Globemallow
Navajo *Cold Remedy* Plant used for colds. *Cough Medicine* Plant used for coughs. *Misc. Disease Remedy* Plant used for influenza. (76:163) **Pima** *Antidiarrheal* Decoction of leaves used for diarrhea. *Gastrointestinal Aid* Decoction of root used for biliousness. (123:79)

Sphaeralcea angustifolia ssp. **lobata**, Copper Globemallow
Keres, Western *Gynecological Aid* Roots used for medicine by pregnant women. (as *S. lobata* 147:71) **Navajo** *Ceremonial Medicine* Roots used as a ceremonial medicine. (as *S. lobata* 45:63) **Tewa** *Dermatological Aid* and *Disinfectant* Poultice of pulverized roots applied to purulent sores. *Snakebite Remedy* Poultice of pulverized roots applied to snakebites. (as *S. lobata* 115:60, 61)

Sphaeralcea coccinea, Scarlet Globemallow
Cheyenne *Ceremonial Medicine* Plant used in ceremonies. (69:30) **Lakota** *Dermatological Aid* Poultice of chewed roots applied to sores. (116:51) **Navajo, Kayenta** *Ceremonial Medicine* Plant used as a ceremonial fumigant ingredient. *Dermatological Aid* Dried plant used as a dusting powder for sores. Plant used as a lotion for skin diseases. *Dietary Aid* Plant used as a tonic to improve appetite. *Disinfectant* Plant used as a ceremonial fumigant ingredient. *Other* Plant used for hydrophobia. *Strengthener* Plant used as a medicine to give singer strength. (179:31) **Navajo, Ramah** *Panacea* Plant used as "life medicine." (165:36)

Sphaeralcea coccinea ssp. **coccinea**, Scarlet Globemallow
Cheyenne *Adjuvant* Infusion of ground leaves, stems, and roots added to sweeten medicines. (as *Malvastrum coccineum* 63:180) Infusion of ground leaves, stems, and roots mixed with other

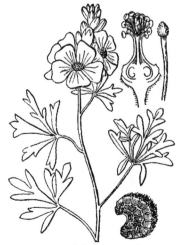

Sphaeralcea coccinea ssp. *coccinea*

medicine to render it more palatable. (as *Malvastrum coccineum* 64:180) **Comanche** *Dermatological Aid* Infusion of plant used for swellings. (as *Malvastrum coccineum* 24:522) **Dakota** *Analgesic* Plant used for pain. (as *Malvastrum coccineum* 57:362) *Burn Dressing* Chewed plant rubbed on skin to protect against boiling water in ceremony. *Dermatological Aid* Chewed plant applied as a cooling and healing salve to sores and wounds. (as *Malvastrum coccineum* 58:103) **Keres**, **Western** *Gynecological Aid* Roots used by women when they become pregnant. (as *Malvastrum coccineum* 147:53) **Navajo** *Hemostat* Infusion of plants used to stop bleeding. *Witchcraft Medicine* Infusion of plants taken for diseases produced by witchcraft. (as *Malvastrum coccineum* 45:62)

Sphaeralcea digitata, Slippery Globemallow
Navajo, **Ramah** *Gastrointestinal Aid* Infusion of whole plant taken for stomachache. *Panacea* Root used as a "life medicine." (165:36)

Sphaeralcea emoryi ssp. variabilis, Emory's Globemallow
Pima *Antidiarrheal* Decoction of root taken for diarrhea. (38:80)

Sphaeralcea fendleri, Fendler's Globemallow
Navajo, **Kayenta** *Dermatological Aid* Plant used for sand cricket bites. *Oral Aid* Infusion of plant taken for sore mouth. (179:32) **Navajo**, **Ramah** *Antihemorrhagic* Cold, compound infusion of plant taken for internal injury and hemorrhage. *Dermatological Aid* Infusion of plant used as lotion for external injury. (165:36)

Sphaeralcea grossulariifolia, Gooseberry-leaf Globemallow
Hopi *Antihemorrhagic* Roots chewed or boiled with cactus root and used for difficult defecation. *Diuretic* Plant used for babies with bowel trouble. *Orthopedic Aid* Root chewed or boiled for broken bones. *Pediatric Aid* Plant used for babies with bowel trouble. (34:362)

Sphaeralcea incana, Gray Globemallow
Hopi *Antidiarrheal* Plant used as a diarrhea medicine. (46:16)

Sphaeralcea parvifolia, Smallflower Globemallow
Hopi *Antihemorrhagic* Root chewed or boiled with cactus root and used for difficult defecation. *Dermatological Aid* Plant used for sores, cuts, and wounds. *Diuretic* Plant used for babies with bowel trouble. *Orthopedic Aid* Chewed or boiled root used for broken bones. *Pediatric Aid* Plant used for babies with bowel trouble. (34:363)

Sphagnum sp., Diaper Moss
Carrier *Dermatological Aid* Berries rubbed on children's sores. *Pediatric Aid* Berries rubbed on children's sores. (diaper moss 26:87) **Nitinaht** *Disinfectant* Used as a good disinfectant. (sphagnum moss 160:59)

Sphenosciadium capitellatum, Woollyhead Parsnip
Paiute *Venereal Aid* Decoction of roots applied to venereal sores. (144:317)

Spigelia anthelmia, West Indian Pinkroot
Creek *Anthelmintic* Plant considered a "well-known remedy" for children with worms. (148:669) Plant used as a worm remedy. (152:51) *Pediatric Aid* Plant considered a "well-known remedy" for children with worms. (148:669)

Spigelia marilandica, Woodland Pinkroot
Cherokee *Anthelmintic* Infusion taken for worms. (66:40) Decoction of roots taken for worms. (152:51) Used as a general vermifuge. **Creek** *Anthelmintic* Used as a general vermifuge. (177:74)

Spiraea alba, White Meadowsweet
Algonquin, **Quebec** *Unspecified* Infusion of leaves and stems used as a medicinal tea. (14:176) **Iroquois** *Analgesic* Compound decoction of mashed and powdered dried roots taken for side pain. (73:349)

Spiraea alba var. latifolia, White Meadowsweet
Algonquin, **Quebec** *Unspecified* Infusion of leaves and stems used as a medicinal tea. (as *Spirea latifolia* 14:176) **Iroquois** *Antiemetic* Decoction of plant with other leaves and branches

taken for nausea and vomiting. (as *Spiraea latifolia* 118:47)

Spiraea betulifolia, White Spirea
Okanagan-Colville *Analgesic* Decoction of branches used for menstrual pains. Infusion of branches taken for abdominal pains. *Cold Remedy* Infusion of branches taken for colds. *Gastrointestinal Aid* Infusion of branches taken for abdominal pains. *Gynecological Aid* Decoction of branches used for menstrual pains or heavy or prolonged menstruation. *Kidney Aid* Infusion of branches taken for poor kidneys. *Other* Infusion of branches taken for ruptures. (162:133) **Shuswap** *Antidiarrheal* Decoction of roots and leaves taken for diarrhea. *Gastrointestinal Aid* Decoction of roots and leaves taken for the stomach. (102:67) **Thompson** *Cold Remedy* Infusion of whole plant taken for colds. *Gastrointestinal Aid* Infusion of whole plant taken for internal stomach problems. *Venereal Aid* Decoction of leaves and branches taken or used as a bath for venereal diseases. (161:274)

Spiraea douglasii, Douglas's Spirea
Lummi *Antidiarrheal* Infusion of seeds taken for diarrhea. (65:33)

Spiraea ×pyramidata, Pyramid Spirea
Thompson *Tonic* Decoction of plant taken as a tonic. (141:471)

Spiraea salicifolia, Willowleaf Meadowsweet
Mahuna *Cold Remedy* Roots used for chest colds. *Cough Medicine* Roots used for coughs. (117:18) **Meskwaki** *Antidiarrheal* Immature seeds used for bloody flux. (129:243) **Ojibwa** *Hunting Medicine* Root used as a trapping medicine. (130:386) **Potawatomi** *Unspecified* Bark used for unspecified ailments. (131:79, 80)

Spiraea splendens var. **splendens**, Mountain Spirea
Blackfoot *Laxative* Infusion of root used as an enema. (as *S. densiflora* 72:68) *Venereal Aid* Infusion of roots taken for venereal complaints. (as *S. densiflora* 72:70)

Spiraea tomentosa, Steeple Bush
Algonquin, **Quebec** *Unspecified* Infusion of leaves and stems used as a medicinal tea. (14:177) **Mohegan** *Antidiarrheal* Infusion of leaves taken for dysentery. (149:266) **Ojibwa** *Antiemetic* Infusion of leaves and flowers taken for the sickness of pregnancy. *Gynecological Aid* Infusion of leaves and flowers taken for the sickness of pregnancy. Infusion of leaves and flowers used to ease childbirth. (130:386)

Spiranthes lacera var. **gracilis**, Northern Slender Ladiestresses
Ojibwa *Hunting Medicine* Roots used as an ingredient of the hunting charm to bring game to the hunter. (as *S. gracilis* 130:431)

Spiranthes lucida, Shining Ladiestresses
Cherokee *Pediatric Aid* Warm infusion used as a wash for infants "to insure fast, healthy growth." *Urinary Aid* Roots with "twayblade" used "for urinary trouble." (66:42)

Spiranthes romanzoffiana, Hooded Ladiestresses
Gosiute *Venereal Aid* Plant used for venereal disease. (31:383)

Sporobolus cryptandrus, Sand Dropseed
Navajo, **Ramah** *Veterinary Aid* Cold infusion of plant applied to sores or bruises on horse's leg. (165:17)

Sporobolus heterolepis, Prairie Dropseed
Ojibwa, **South** *Dermatological Aid* Poultice of crushed root applied to sores. *Emetic* and *Liver Aid* Decoction of root taken as an emetic "to remove bile." (77:200)

Stachys bullata, California Hedgenettle
Costanoan *Dermatological Aid* Poultice of plant applied or decoction taken for swollen sores. *Disinfectant* Poultice of plant applied or decoction taken for infected sores. *Ear Medicine* Poultice of heated leaves applied for earaches. *Gastrointestinal Aid* Poultice of plant applied or decoction of plant taken for stomachaches. *Throat Aid* Poultice of leaves applied or decoction of roots used as a gargle for sore throats. (17:17) **Pomo**, **Kashaya** *Dermatological Aid* Poultice of heated leaves used on boils to bring them to a head. (60:77)

Stachys ciliata, Great Hedgenettle
Saanich *Tonic* Infusion of pounded roots used as a spring tonic. (as *S. cooleyae* 156:84)

Stachys mexicana, Emerson Betony
Green River Group *Dermatological Aid* Plant used for boils. **Puyallup** *Dermatological Aid* Plant used for boils. (as *S. ciliata* 65:45)

Stachys palustris, Marsh Hedgenettle
Chippewa *Gastrointestinal Aid* Infusion of fresh or dried leaves taken for "sudden colic." (43:344) **Delaware** *Venereal Aid* Used with common nightshade, "pretty flower," and button snakeroot for venereal disease. (151:35) **Delaware, Oklahoma** *Venereal Aid* Compound containing root used for venereal disease. (150:29, 80)

Stachys rothrockii, Rothrock's Hedgenettle
Navajo, Ramah *Ceremonial Medicine* Dried leaves used as a ceremonial medicine and plant used in chant lotion. *Dermatological Aid* Decoction of plant used as foot deodorant. *Disinfectant* Dried leaves used for "deer infection." (165:42)

Stachys tenuifolia var. **tenuifolia**, Smooth
    Hedgenettle
Meskwaki *Cold Remedy* Infusion of leaves taken for bad colds. *Emetic* Infusion of leaves given as an emetic. (129:227)

Stanleya pinnata, Desert Princesplume
Havasupai *Poison* Fresh leaves considered poisonous. (171:220) **Navajo** *Gland Medicine* Poultice of plants applied to glandular swellings. (45:50) **Paiute** *Analgesic* Poultice of mashed root applied for throat pain. *Misc. Disease Remedy* Poultice of mashed root applied for congestion of diphtheria. *Throat Aid* Poultice of mashed root applied for throat pain. *Tonic* Decoction of root taken as a tonic for general debility after an illness. **Shoshoni** *Analgesic* Poultice of pulped root applied for rheumatic pains. *Antirheumatic (External)* Poultice of hot, pulped root applied for rheumatic pains. *Ear Medicine* Poultice of hot, pulped root applied for an earache. *Toothache Remedy* Poultice of root applied to gums or placed in cavity for toothache. (155:142) **Zuni** *Dermatological Aid* Poultice of fresh, chewed pods used for itching.

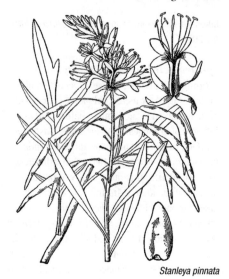

Stanleya pinnata

(22:375) *Venereal Aid* Powdered plant applied, as a specific, to scraped syphilitic sores. (143:60)

Staphylea trifolia, American Bladdernut
Iroquois *Antirheumatic (Internal)* Compound infusion of plants taken for rheumatism. *Dermatological Aid* Infusion of powdered bark used as a wash for sore faces. *Gynecological Aid* Compound poultice of bark applied when a woman swells after copulation. *Pediatric Aid* and *Sedative* Infusion of bark used as a wash to keep children from crying. (73:377) **Meskwaki** *Ceremonial Medicine* Seeds used in gourd rattles for dream and medicine dances. (129:248)

Stellaria media, Common Chickweed
Chippewa *Eye Medicine* Decoction of leaves strained and used as a wash for sore eyes. (43:360) **Iroquois** *Antirheumatic (External)* Poultice of plant fragments with other plants applied for swellings. (118:41) *Dermatological Aid* Raw, compound poultice applied to cuts and wounds. (73:317)

Stenandrium dulce, Sweet Shaggytuft
Seminole *Pediatric Aid* and *Sedative* Plant and other plants used as a baby's charm for fear from dreams about raccoons or opossums. (as *S. floridanum* 145:221) *Stimulant* Decoction of whole plant used as a bath for hog sickness: unconsciousness. (as *S. floridanum* 145:229)

Stenanthium occidentale, Western
    Stenanthium
Thompson *Unspecified* Plant used medicinally.
(161:129)

Stenotaphrum secundatum, St. Augustine
    Grass
Hawaiian *Dermatological Aid* Leaf ash used for
sores and navel sores on babies. Leaf ash used for
skin ulcers. *Gynecological Aid* Leaves and stems
pounded, resulting juice mixed with other ingredients and taken for excessive menses. Leaf ash used
on the vagina and neighboring parts after giving
birth. *Oral Aid* Leaf ash used for excessive saliva
from babies' mouths. *Pediatric Aid* Leaf ash used
for sores and navel sores on babies. Leaf ash used
for excessive saliva from babies' mouths. (as *S.
americanum* 2:10)

Stenotus lanuginosus* var. *lanuginosus,
    Cespitose Goldenweed
Navajo *Gastrointestinal Aid* Plant used for indigestion. *Nose Medicine* Plant used for nose troubles. (as *Aplopappus lanuginosus* 45:96) *Oral Aid*
Plant used for sore gums. (as *Aplopappus lanuginosus* 45:97) *Throat Aid* Plant used for throat
troubles. (as *Aplopappus lanuginosus* 45:96)
Toothache Remedy Plant used as a toothache medicine. (as *Aplopappus lanuginosus* 45:80)

Stephanomeria exigua, Small Wirelettuce
Hopi *Diuretic* and *Venereal Aid* Plant used as a
diuretic for venereal disease. (as *Ptiloria exigua*
174:35, 97) **Navajo, Kayenta** *Misc. Disease Remedy* Plant used for measles. (179:50)

Stephanomeria pauciflora, Brownplume
    Wirelettuce
Hopi *Gynecological Aid* Root used in various
ways to increase mother's milk supply. (as *Ptiloria
pauciflora* 174:36, 98) **Navajo, Kayenta** *Narcotic*
Roots used as a narcotic. (179:50) **Navajo, Ramah**
Gynecological Aid Strong infusion of root used to
hasten delivery of placenta. *Panacea* Root used as
a "life medicine." (165:53)

Stephanomeria runcinata, Desert Wire-
    lettuce
Keres, Western *Eye Medicine* Milky sap used for
sore eyes. (as *S. ramosa* 147:72)

Stephanomeria spinosa, Thorn Skeletonweed
Cheyenne *Cold Remedy, Diaphoretic*, and *Herbal
Steam* Decoction of smashed roots taken and used
as a steam bath to cause sweating for colds. *Misc.
Disease Remedy* Decoction of smashed roots used
as a steam bath for mumps. *Panacea* Plant used
for almost every ailment. *Tuberculosis Remedy*
Decoction of smashed roots used as a steam bath
for tuberculosis. (as *Lygodesmia spinosa* 69:22)
Paiute *Antidiarrheal* Decoction of plant tops taken
for diarrhea. *Cathartic* Decoction of plant tops
taken as a physic. *Dermatological Aid* Compound
decoction of root used as a wash for swellings. Poultice of cottony fuzz applied to boils or sores to promote healing. *Emetic* Decoction of plant tops taken
as an emetic. *Toothache Remedy* Cottony fuzz
placed in cavity of aching tooth. **Shoshoni** *Antiemetic* Decoction of plant tops taken for vomiting.
Eye Medicine Decoction of plant tops used as an
eyewash. *Tonic* Compound decoction of root taken
as a tonic. (as *Lygodesmia spinosa* 155:102, 103)

Stephanomeria tenuifolia, Narrowleaf Wire-
    lettuce
Apache, White Mountain *Snakebite Remedy*
Poultice of powdered plants applied to rattlesnake
bites. (as *Ptiloria tenuifolia* 113:160) **Shoshoni**
Venereal Aid Decoction of plant taken for venereal
diseases. (155:143) **Thompson** *Unspecified* Plant
used medicinally for unspecified purpose. (as *Ptiloria tenuifolia* 141:468) **Zuni** *Snakebite Remedy*
Poultice of pulverized plant applied and infusion
taken for rattlesnake bite. (as *Ptiloria tenuifolia*
143:58)

Stephanomeria virgata, Rod Wirelettuce
Kawaiisu *Eye Medicine* Milky plant juice used as
an eye medicine. (180:65)

Stillingia sylvatica, Queen's Delight
Cherokee *Venereal Aid* Decoction or tincture of
root used for the worst forms of venereal disease
or "clap." (66:51)

Stillingia sylvatica* ssp. *sylvatica, Queen's
Delight
Seminole *Antidiarrheal* Plant used as an astringent for diarrhea. (as *S. angustifolia* 145:168)
Decoction of roots taken by babies and adults for
bird sickness: diarrhea, vomiting, and appetite
loss. (as *S. angustifolia* 145:234) Plant used as a
diarrhea medicine. (as *S. angustifolia* 145:275)
Antiemetic Decoction of roots taken by babies and
adults for bird sickness: diarrhea, vomiting, and
appetite loss. (as *S. angustifolia* 145:234) *Blood
Medicine* Decoction of roots taken for menstruation sickness: yellow eyes and skin, weakness, and
shaking head. (as *S. angustifolia* 145:247) *Dietary Aid* Decoction of roots taken by babies and
adults for bird sickness: diarrhea, vomiting, and
appetite loss. (as *S. angustifolia* 145:234) *Other*
Decoction of roots taken for menstruation sickness: yellow eyes and skin, weakness, and shaking
head. (as *S. angustifolia* 145:247) *Pediatric Aid*
Decoction of roots taken by babies and adults for
bird sickness: diarrhea, vomiting, and appetite
loss. (as *S. angustifolia* 145:234) *Strengthener*
Decoction of roots taken for menstruation sickness: yellow eyes and skin, weakness, and shaking
head. (as *S. angustifolia* 145:247)

Streptanthus cordatus, Heartleaf Twistflower
Navajo, **Kayenta** *Eye Medicine* Root juice used as
eye drops for sore eyes. (179:25)

Streptopus amplexifolius, Claspleaf Twistedstalk
Makah *Gynecological Aid* Chewed roots taken to
produce labor in case of protracted delay. (65:25)
Micmac *Antihemorrhagic* Parts of plant used for
spitting blood. *Kidney Aid* Parts of plant used for
kidney trouble. *Venereal Aid* Parts of plant used
for gonorrhea. (32:62) **Montagnais** *Panacea* Infusion of stems and berries taken "for sickness in
general." (133:314) **Penobscot** *Antihemorrhagic*
Compound infusion of plant taken for "spitting up
blood." *Kidney Aid* Compound infusion of plant
taken for kidney trouble. *Tonic* Compound infusion
of plant taken as a tonic. *Venereal Aid* Compound
infusion of plant taken for gonorrhea. (133:311)
Thompson *Analgesic* Compound decoction of
roots taken for internal pains. (141:459) *Dietary
Aid* Infusion of whole plant taken for loss of appe-

tite. *Gastrointestinal Aid* Infusion of whole plant
taken for stomachache. (161:130)

Streptopus roseus, Rosy Twistedstalk
Chippewa *Eye Medicine* Poultice of steeped root
applied to sties. (43:360) **Iroquois** *Gynecological Aid* Infusion of roots taken for fallen womb.
(73:284) **Montagnais** *Diaphoretic* Infusion of
blossoms taken to cause sweating. (133:314)
Ojibwa *Cathartic* Plant used as a physic and infusion taken as a cough remedy. *Cough Medicine* Infusion of plant taken as a cough remedy and used
as a physic. (130:374) **Okanagon** *Tonic* Plant
used as a tonic medicine. (104:42) **Potawatomi**
Cough Medicine Root used to make a cough syrup
or tea. (131:63) **Thompson** *Tonic* Plant used as a
tonic medicine. (104:42) *Unspecified* Decoction
of root used medicinally. (141:467)

Strophostyles helvula, Trailing Fuzzybean
Houma *Misc. Disease Remedy* Compound decoction of bean taken for typhoid. (135:65) **Iroquois**
Dermatological Aid Leaves rubbed on parts affected by poison ivy and warts. (73:365)

Stylosanthes biflora, Sidebeak Pencilflower
Cherokee *Abortifacient* Compound used to promote menstruation. *Gynecological Aid* Infusion of
root used for female complaint. (66:57)

Styphelia tameiameiae, Pukiawe
Hawaiian *Dermatological Aid* and *Tuberculosis
Remedy* Flowers and other plants dried, pounded
into a powder, and applied to scrofulous sores.
(2:49)

Suaeda moquinii , Mojave Seablite
Hopi *Analgesic* Poultice of dried leaves used on
sore places. (as *S. intermedia* 164:161) *Ceremonial Medicine* Plant used to bathe the doctor before
administering to patients. (as *Dondia fruticosa*
174:31, 74) **Navajo**, **Kayenta** *Gastrointestinal Aid*
Plant used for bleeding bowels. (as *S. torreyana*
179:21) **Paiute** *Dermatological Aid* Crushed fresh
plants rubbed on chickenpox to stop itching and to
dry sores. *Kidney Aid* Decoction of plant taken for
kidney trouble. *Misc. Disease Remedy* Crushed
fresh plants rubbed on chickenpox to stop itching
and to dry sores. *Urinary Aid* Decoction of plant

taken for bladder trouble. **Shoshoni** *Kidney Aid* Decoction of plant taken for kidney trouble. *Urinary Aid* Decoction of plant taken for bladder trouble. (as *S. torreyana* var. *ramosissima* 155:143)

Symphoricarpos albus, Common Snowberry **Chehalis** *Dermatological Aid* Berries used for the hair. Poultice of chewed leaves applied or infusion of leaves used as a wash for injuries. *Venereal Aid* Decoction of root bark taken for venereal disease. (65:47) **Chippewa** *Diuretic* Compound decoction of root taken for "stoppage of urine." (43:348) **Cowichan** *Burn Dressing* Berries rubbed on skin for burns. *Dermatological Aid* Berries rubbed on skin for rashes and sores. (156:80) **Cree, Woodlands** *Dermatological Aid* Infusion of whole plant taken and applied externally for skin rash. *Eye Medicine* Infusion of fruit used for sore eyes. *Febrifuge* and *Pediatric Aid* Decoction of roots and stems taken for fever associated with teething sickness. *Venereal Aid* Decoction of roots and stems used for venereal disease. (91:62) **Crow** *Veterinary Aid* Decoction of crushed roots used for horses failing to void. **Flathead** *Burn Dressing* Poultice of crushed leaves, fruits, and bark used for burns. *Dermatological Aid* Poultice of crushed leaves, fruits, and bark used for sores, cuts, and chapped and injured skin. *Eye Medicine* Bark and wild rose used to make an eyewash. Fruit chewed and the juice used for injured eyes. (68:59) **Green River Group** *Dermatological Aid* and *Disinfectant* Plant used to disinfect a festering sore. (65:47) **Hesquiat** *Dermatological Aid* Berry juice rubbed on warts or sores. (159:63) **Klallam** *Cold Remedy* Decoction of leaves taken for colds. (65:47) **Kutenai** *Abortifacient* Infusion of cut branches taken for menstrual disorders. (68:59) **Kwakiutl** *Eye Medicine* Burned berries and oil rubbed on inflamed eyes. (157:280) **Makah** *Witchcraft Medicine* Leaves chewed and swallowed to counteract evil charms. (160:102) **Miwok** *Cold Remedy* Infusion of root taken for colds. *Gastrointestinal Aid* Infusion of root taken for stomachache. (8:173) **Nez Perce** *Febrifuge* Infusion of twigs used for fevers. Infusion of twigs used for young children with fevers. *Pediatric Aid* Infusion of twigs used for young children with fevers. (68:59) **Nitinaht** *Diuretic* Infusion of bark taken for inability to urinate. (160:102) **Okanagan-Colville** *Cathartic*

Decoction of branches, leaves, and berries taken as a physic to clean out the system. *Dermatological Aid* Poultice of mashed berries applied to children's skin sores. Poultice of mashed berries applied to itchy skin. Berries mashed and rubbed in the armpits as an antiperspirant. *Eye Medicine* Berries mashed, mixed with small amount of warm water, and put into the eyes for sore, running eyes. Infusion of roots used as an eyewash. *Pediatric Aid* Poultice of mashed berries applied to children's skin sores. *Poison* Berries considered poisonous. (162:95) **Saanich** *Burn Dressing* Berries rubbed on skin for burns. *Dermatological Aid* Berries rubbed on skin for rashes and sores. (156:80) **Sanpoil** *Dermatological Aid* Crushed berries rubbed in the armpits as an antiperspirant. *Diuretic* Decoction of leaves used by men for urine retention. *Eye Medicine* Mashed berries mixed with water and used as a wash for sore eyes. *Unspecified* Decoction of roots used "for illness of an indefinite character." *Veterinary Aid* Decoction of leaves used for animals with urine retention. (109:220) **Sioux** *Diuretic* Decoction of berries used as a diuretic. *Eye Medicine* Infusion used for sore eyes. (68:59) **Skagit** *Antidote* Berries eaten as an antidote for poisoning. *Oral Aid* and *Pediatric Aid* Infusion of plant given to babies with coated tongues. *Tuberculosis Remedy* Bark used for tuberculosis. (65:47) **Thompson** *Antidiarrheal* Chewed berry juice swallowed, infusion of berries taken, or mashed berries eaten for diarrhea. (161:200) *Dermatological Aid* Strong decoction of wood used to cleanse sores. (141:455) Strong decoction of wood used as a wash for sores. (141:458) Decoction of berries, bark, or leaves, sometimes mixed with bear grease, used as a wash for sores. *Eye Medicine* Strained decoction of scraped bark or leaves used as a wash for sore eyes or impending blindness. Crushed berries or decoction of berries used as a wash for sore eyes or impending blindness. (161:200) *Gastrointestinal Aid* Decoction of stems or roots taken for stomach trouble. (141:458) Sap from young shoots used for stomachache. *Gynecological Aid* Decoction of berries, bark, or leaves used as an antiseptic wash for breasts before nursing. Decoction of berries, bark, or leaves taken after a birth "to clean you out." *Laxative* Sap from young shoots used as a laxative. (161:200) *Pediatric Aid* Mild decoction of wood used as a wash to keep babies healthy. (141:458) *Poison* Berries considered "deadly poisonous" if more than two or three eaten. (141:511) Berries considered poisonous, even fatal. (141:489) Berries considered very poisonous. An antidote for poisoning from the berries was to eat a large quantity of lard. (161:200) **Wet'suwet'en** *Eye Medicine* Bark used to make an eye medicine. (61:152)

Symphoricarpos albus var. albus, Common
  Snowberry
Bella Coola *Diuretic* Decoction of branches taken as a diuretic and for gonorrhea. *Venereal Aid* Decoction of branches taken as "the best cure for gonorrhea." **Carrier, Southern** *Eye Medicine* Juice of ripe berries used in sore eyes. (as *Symphoricarpus racemosa* 127:64) **Kwakiutl** *Analgesic* Moxa of tips while still on plant used for headache. (as *Symphoricarpor racemosus* 16:386) **Ojibwa** *Gynecological Aid* Infusion of root taken "to clear up the afterbirth" and hasten convalescence. (as *Symphoricarpos racemosus* 130:361)

Symphoricarpos albus var. laevigatus,
  Common Snowberry
Yuki *Dermatological Aid* Infusion of plant used as a wash for sores. (as *S. rivularis* 39:47)

Symphoricarpos longiflorus, Desert Snowberry
Paiute *Analgesic* Decoction of plant taken for stomach pains. *Gastrointestinal Aid* Decoction of plant taken for indigestion or stomach pains. (155:143)

Symphoricarpos mollis, Creeping Snowberry
Shuswap *Eye Medicine* Infusion of berries used as a wash for sore and tired eyes. (102:61)

Symphoricarpos occidentalis, Western
  Snowberry
Blackfoot *Veterinary Aid* Decoction of berries given to horses for water retention. (82:55) **Dakota** *Eye Medicine* Infusion of leaves used as wash for weak or inflamed eyes. (58:116) **Meskwaki** *Gynecological Aid* Infusion of root taken to cleanse the afterbirth and aid in convalescence. (129:207) **Omaha** *Eye Medicine* Infusion of leaves used as wash for weak or inflamed eyes. **Ponca** *Eye Medi-*

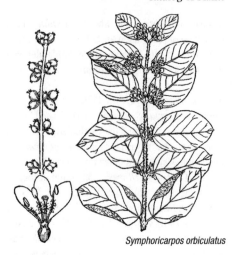

Symphoricarpos orbiculatus

cine Infusion of leaves used as wash for weak or inflamed eyes. (58:116)

Symphoricarpos orbiculatus, Coralberry
Dakota *Eye Medicine* Decoction of inner bark or leaves used for sore eyes. (as *S. symphoricarpos* 57:367) Infusion of leaves used as wash for weak or inflamed eyes. (as *S. symphoricarpos* 58:116) **Ojibwa, South** *Eye Medicine* Cold decoction of root bark applied to sore eyes. (as *Symphoricarpus vulgaris* 77:200) **Omaha** *Eye Medicine* Infusion of leaves used as wash for weak or inflamed eyes. **Ponca** *Eye Medicine* Infusion of leaves used as wash for weak or inflamed eyes. (as *Symphoricarpos symphoricarpos* 58:116)

Symphoricarpos oreophilus, Whortleleaf
  Snowberry
Navajo, Ramah *Ceremonial Medicine* and *Emetic* Leaves used as a ceremonial emetic. (165:45)

Symphoricarpos oreophilus var. parishii,
  Parish's Snowberry
Navajo, Kayenta *Throat Aid* Plant used for sore throat. (as *S. parishii* 179:44)

Symphytum officinale, Common Comfrey
Cherokee *Antidiarrheal* Taken for "flux" or dysentery. *Gastrointestinal Aid* Infusion taken for heartburn. *Gynecological Aid* Infusion taken for heartburn in pregnancy and for flooding after birth. *Laxative* Infusion taken for "costiveness" in pregnancy. *Orthopedic Aid* Used for sprains and

bruises. *Venereal Aid* Infusion of roots in water used for gonorrhea. (66:30)

Symplocarpus foetidus, Skunk Cabbage

Abnaki *Antirheumatic* (*External*) Used for swellings. (121:153) **Chippewa** *Cough Medicine* Infusion of roots taken as a cough medicine. (59:124) **Delaware** *Analgesic* Poultice of crushed leaves applied for pain. *Misc. Disease Remedy* Small portions of leaves chewed for epilepsy. *Pulmonary Aid* Infusion of roots used for whooping cough. (151:37) **Delaware, Oklahoma** *Analgesic* Poultice of crushed leaves applied for pain. *Anticonvulsive* Leaves chewed by epileptics. *Cough Medicine* Infusion of root taken for whooping cough. (150:31, 80) **Iroquois** *Anthelmintic* Plant used for children with worms. (73:278) *Antirheumatic* (*External*) Steam from compound decoction of roots used for rheumatism. *Dermatological Aid* Poultice used on bite from a fight or dog and caused the biter's teeth to fall out. (73:277) Plant used for bad wounds. (73:278) *Gynecological Aid* Compound decoction of upper parts and seeds taken for "falling of the womb." Decoction of crushed stalks used as a douche for displacement of womb. (73:277) "Pass seed over female genitals to bring about childbirth." *Pediatric Aid* Used for children with worms. (73:278) *Tuberculosis Remedy* Infusion of powdered root taken for consumption. *Witchcraft Medicine* Poultice used on bite from a fight or dog and caused the biter's teeth to fall out. (73:277) **Malecite** *Unspecified* Used for medicines. (137:6) **Menominee** *Adjuvant* Root used as a seasoner

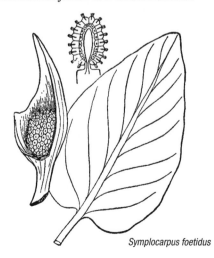

Symplocarpus foetidus

with medicines. *Analgesic* Root used for cramps. (as *Spatheyma foetida* 128:23, 24) *Anticonvulsive* Compound infusion of dried, powdered root used by children and adults for convulsions. (as *Spathyema foetida* 44:128, 129) *Dermatological Aid* Poultice of dried root applied to wounds. (as *Spatheyma foetida* 128:23, 24) *Heart Medicine* Decoction of root used for "weak heart." (as *Spathyema foetida* 44:128, 129) *Hemostat* Root hairs used for hemorrhages. (as *Spatheyma foetida* 128:23, 24) *Pediatric Aid* Compound infusion used by children or adults for convulsions. (as *Spathyema foetida* 44:128) *Witchcraft Medicine* Root used in tattooing, as a talisman against the return of diseases. (as *Spatheyma foetida* 128:23, 24) **Meskwaki** *Dermatological Aid* Poultice of leaf bases applied to swellings. *Toothache Remedy* Fine rootlets or root hairs used for toothache. *Unspecified* Seeds used as medicine. (129:203) **Micmac** *Analgesic* Herbs used for headache. (32:62) **Mohegan** *Anticonvulsive* Raw leaves rolled and chewed for fits. (as *Spathyema foetida* 149:268) Small piece of leaf eaten for epileptic seizures. (as *Spathyema foetida* 151:75, 132) **Nanticoke** *Cold Remedy* Infusion of leaves taken as a cold medicine. (150:55, 84)

Symplocos tinctoria, Common Sweetleaf

Choctaw *Febrifuge* Decoction of scraped roots taken for fevers. (152:50)

Syringa vulgaris, Common Lilac

Iroquois *Oral Aid* Bark or leaves chewed by children for sore mouths. Bark or leaves chewed for sore mouth caused by kissing a girl with menses, or caused by smoking someone else's pipe. *Pediatric Aid* Bark or leaves chewed by children for sore mouths. (73:413)

Syzygium malaccense, Malaysian Apple

Hawaiian *Dermatological Aid* Bark pounded, mixed with salt and coconut fibers, squeezed, and resulting liquid used on deep cuts. *Emetic* Bark chewed to cause vomiting and bring out the tough phlegm from the throat and lungs. *Gastrointestinal Aid* Bark and other plants pounded, squeezed, and the resulting liquid given to children for stomach weakness. *Oral Aid* Bark and other plants pounded, squeezed, and the resulting liquid taken for bad breath and mouth sores. *Pediatric Aid* Bark and other plants pounded, squeezed, and the resulting liquid given to children for general debility or for stomach weakness. *Strengthener* Bark and other plants pounded, squeezed, and the resulting liquid given to children for general debility. (as *Jambosa malaecensis* 2:31)

Taenidia integerrima, Yellow Pimpernel **Menominee** *Adjuvant* Plant used as a seasoner to make various female remedies taste good. *Pulmonary Aid* Infusion of root taken for pulmonary troubles. *Respiratory Aid* Steeped root chewed for "bronchial affections." (128:56) **Meskwaki** *Adjuvant* Root used as a seasoner for other medicines because of the good smell. (129:250) **Ojibwa** *Hunting Medicine* Seeds smoked in a pipe when one goes hunting for they will bring him luck. (130:432)

Tagetes erecta, Aztec Marigold **Cherokee** *Dermatological Aid* Infusion used as wash for "eczema." (66:44)

Tagetes micrantha, Licorice Marigold **Navajo** *Cold Remedy* Plants used for colds. *Febrifuge* Plants used for fevers. *Gastrointestinal Aid* Plants used for stomach troubles. *Other* Plants used for "summer complaint." (45:89)

Talinum parviflorum, Sunbright **Navajo, Ramah** *Dermatological Aid* Poultice of root bark applied to sores and infusion of root bark used as lotion. *Veterinary Aid* Cold simple or compound infusion given to livestock as an aphrodisiac. (165:26)

Tanacetum parthenium, Feverfew **Cherokee** *Orthopedic Aid* Infusion used to bathe swollen feet. (as *Chrysanthemum parthenium* 66:34) **Mahuna** *Antirheumatic* (*Internal*) Plant used for rheumatism. (as *Crysanthemum parthenium* 117:60)

Tanacetum vulgare, Common Tansy **Cherokee** *Analgesic* Infusion used for backache. *Anthelmintic* Given to children for worms. *Gyne-*

cological Aid Worn around waist and in shoes to prevent miscarriages and abortions. *Orthopedic Aid* Infusion used for backache. *Pediatric Aid* Given to children for worms. *Tonic* Taken as a tonic. (66:58) **Cheyenne** *Other* Infusion of leaves and blossoms taken for weakness and dizziness. (63:190) *Strengthener* Infusion of pulverized leaves and blossoms taken for weakness. *Vertigo Medicine* Infusion of pulverized leaves and blossoms taken for dizziness. (64:190) **Chippewa** *Abortifacient* Decoction of leaf taken, especially by young girls, for "stoppage of period." (43:358) *Diaphoretic* Compound infusion of leaves taken to "produce profuse perspiration." (43:354) *Ear Medicine* Weak decoction of root used as drops for sore ear. (43:362) *Febrifuge* Compound infusion of leaves taken to "break up a fever." (43:354) *Throat Aid* Decoction of root gargled or dried root chewed for sore throat. (43:342) **Delaware, Ontario** *Gastrointestinal Aid* Whole plant used for stomach disorders. (150:66, 82) **Iroquois** *Analgesic* Poultice of leaves applied to the head for headaches. Poultice of smashed leaves applied to body pains caused by too much gall. (as *Chrysanthemum vulgare* 73:472) *Cold Remedy* Poultice of plants applied for colds. *Dermatological Aid* Plant used for bruises and cuts. (as *Chrysanthemum vulgare* 73:473) *Liver Aid* Poultice of smashed leaves applied to body pains caused by too much gall. (as *Chrysanthemum vulgare* 73:472) *Orthopedic Aid* Plant used for bone decay and headaches. *Panacea* Poultice of plants applied for any

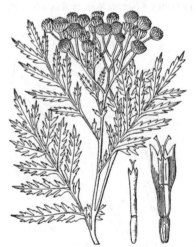

Tanacetum vulgare

ailment. (as *Chrysanthemum vulgare* 73:473) **Malecite** *Contraceptive* Infusion of plant used to prevent pregnancy. (96:259) *Kidney Aid* Infusion of dried leaves used for kidney troubles. *Veterinary Aid* Infusion of dried leaves used for horses with colic. (96:243) **Micmac** *Contraceptive* Herbs used to prevent pregnancy. *Kidney Aid* Leaves used for kidney trouble. (32:62) **Mohegan** *Dietary Aid* Cold, compound infusion taken as an appetizer. *Gastrointestinal Aid* Cold, compound infusion taken for the stomach. (149:266) Compound infusion of leaves taken as a stomach aid and to improve the appetite. (151:75, 132) **Nanticoke** *Diaphoretic* Whole plant used as a sudorific. (150:58, 84) **Ojibwa** *Febrifuge* Plant used as a fever medicine. (130:366) **Paiute** *Emetic* Decoction of leaves taken as an emetic. (155:143, 144) **Shinnecock** *Analgesic* Infusion of leaves taken for "inside pains." (25:119) **Shoshoni** *Antidiarrheal* Decoction of leaves taken for bloody diarrhea. *Dermatological Aid* Decoction of leaves used as an antiseptic wash. *Disinfectant* Decoction of leaves and sometimes stems used as a warm antiseptic wash. (155:143, 144)

Taraxacum officinale, Common Dandelion
Aleut *Dermatological Aid* Poultice of steamed or wilted leaves applied to indolent ulcers. *Gastrointestinal Aid* Poultice of steamed or wilted leaves applied to stomachaches. *Throat Aid* Poultice of steamed or wilted leaves applied to sore throats. (126:327) **Algonquin, Quebec** *Blood Medicine* Greens eaten to purify the blood. *Poultice* Leaves used for plasters or poultices. (14:242) **Bella Coola** *Analgesic* and *Gastrointestinal Aid* Decoction of root taken for stomach pain. (127:65) **Cherokee** *Blood Medicine* Infusion of root used for blood. *Sedative* Infusion of herb used to "calm nerves." *Toothache Remedy* Chewed for toothache. (66:31) *Unspecified* Leaves and stems used as medicine. (105:35) **Chippewa** *Gynecological Aid* Compound infusion of root taken to produce postpartum milk flow. (43:360) **Delaware** *Laxative* Plant used to make a "laxative-tonic." (151:39) **Delaware, Oklahoma** *Laxative* and *Tonic* Plant used to make a "laxative-tonic." (150:32, 80) **Hoh** *Unspecified* Used for medicine. (114:69) **Iroquois** *Analgesic* Compound decoction of dried plants taken for pain. Compound infusion of roots

and bark taken for back pain. (73:477) Infusion of flowers, roots, and roots from another plant taken for lower back pain. (118:61) *Blood Medicine* Decoction of plants taken for anemia. (73:478) *Dermatological Aid* Compound infusion of plants and roots taken and used as wash for liver spots. (73:476) Compound decoction of bark and roots taken for sores caused by bad blood. (73:478) *Emetic* Infusion of roots taken as an emetic. (73:476) *Eye Medicine* Compound infusion of roots and bark taken for dark circles and puffy eyes. *Kidney Aid* Compound infusion of roots and bark taken for kidney trouble and dropsy. *Laxative* Compound decoction of flowers and leaves taken as a laxative. *Love Medicine* Decoction of roots used as wash for a love medicine. *Orthopedic Aid* Compound infusion of roots and bark taken for back pain. *Pulmonary Aid* Compound decoction of dried plants taken for swollen lungs. (73:477) *Toothache Remedy* Flower stem chewed for worms in the teeth that cause decay. *Urinary Aid* Poultice of smashed flowers applied to swollen testicles. (73:476) Decoction of plants used as wash on parts affected by smashed testicles. *Witchcraft Medicine* Decoction of roots used as a wash for an anti-witch medicine. (73:477) **Kiowa** *Gynecological Aid* Decoction of young leaves taken by women for menstrual cramps. (166:62) **Meskwaki** *Pulmonary Aid* Infusion of root taken for chest pain when other remedies fail. (129:218) **Mohegan** *Cathartic* Infusion of plant taken as a physic. (149:266) Strong infusion of dried leaves taken as a physic. (151:76, 132) *Tonic* Dandelion and white daisy used to make wines and taken as tonics. (25:121) Compound decoction or infusion of plants taken as a spring tonic. (149:266) Compound infusion of root taken as a tonic. (151:76, 132) **Ojibwa** *Blood Medicine* Roots used as a blood medicine. (112:238) *Gastrointestinal Aid* Infusion of root taken for heartburn. (130:366) **Papago** *Analgesic* Infusion of blossoms taken for menstrual cramps. *Gynecological Aid* Infusion of blossoms taken for menstrual cramps. (29:65) **Potawatomi** *Tonic* Root used as a bitter tonic. (131:54) **Quileute** *Unspecified* Used for medicine. (114:69) **Rappahannock** *Blood Medicine* Infusion of root taken as a blood tonic. *Gastrointestinal Aid* Infusion of root taken for dyspepsia. (138:34) **Shinnecock** *Tonic* Dandelion and white daisy used to make wines and taken as tonics. (25:121)

Taraxacum officinale ssp. *vulgare*,
Common Dandelion

Navajo, Ramah *Dermatological Aid* Poultice of crushed plant applied to swellings. *Gynecological Aid* Cold infusion of plant used to speed delivery of baby. (as *T. palustre* var. *vulgare* 165:53) **Tewa** *Dermatological Aid* Poultice of pulverized leaves mixed with dough applied to a bad bruise. *Orthopedic Aid* Poultice of pulverized fresh leaves used to dress bone fractures. (as *T. taraxacum* 115:61)

Tauschia arguta, Southern Umbrellawort
Luiseño *Unspecified* Root used for medicinal purposes. (as *Deweya arguta* 132:230)

Tauschia parishii, Parish's Umbrellawort
Kawaiisu *Analgesic* Dried root smoke inhaled for head pains. Dried root smoke used for eye pains. Ground root applied as a salve for aching limbs. Infusion of roots taken for inside pain. *Cold Remedy* Dried root smoke inhaled for head colds. *Dermatological Aid* Infusion of pounded roots used as a bath for swollen limbs. *Eye Medicine* Dried root smoke used for eye pains. *Orthopedic Aid* Ground root applied as a salve for aching limbs. Infusion of pounded roots used as a bath for swollen limbs. *Toothache Remedy* Mashed, ground root placed on hot rock, and cheek laid on rock for toothache. (180:66)

Taxus baccata, English Yew
Iroquois *Abortifacient* Compound taken for menstruation when stopped by a cold. *Adjuvant* "Put in all medicines to give them strength." *Antirheumatic (External)* Steam from compound decoction used for rheumatism. *Antirheumatic (Internal)* Compound decoction taken for rheumatism. *Cold Remedy* Compound decoction taken for colds. Compound taken for menstruation when stopped by a cold. *Cough Medicine* Compound decoction taken for coughs. *Diaphoretic* Used for colds and sweating. *Orthopedic Aid* Decoction of twigs used for finger or leg numbness. *Respiratory Aid* Steam from decoction used for chest colds. *Tuberculosis Remedy* Compound decoction taken during the early stages of consumption. (73:264)

Taxus brevifolia, Pacific Yew
Bella Coola *Pulmonary Aid* Decoction of branches with leaves taken "for the lungs." (127:48) **Chehalis** *Diaphoretic* Infusion of crushed leaves used as a wash to cause perspiring. *Panacea* Infusion of crushed leaves used as a wash to improve general health. **Cowlitz** *Dermatological Aid* Poultice of ground leaves applied to wounds. (65:16) **Haihais** *Gastrointestinal Aid* Decoction of wood and bark used for stomach pains. *Internal Medicine* Decoction of wood and bark used for internal ailments. (35:319) **Hanaksiala** *Urinary Aid* Cooled decoction of small wood pieces taken for bloody urine. (35:187) **Karok** *Blood Medicine* Decoction of bark taken as a "blood medicine." (5:57) *Gastrointestinal Aid* Decoction of twig bark taken for stomachaches. (125:379) **Kitasoo** *Gastrointestinal Aid* Decoction of wood and bark used for stomach pains. *Internal Medicine* Decoction of wood and bark used for internal ailments. (35:319) **Klallam** *Analgesic* Decoction of leaves taken for internal injury or pain. (65:16) **Mendocino Indian** *Poison* Seeds considered poisonous. (33:305) **Okanagan-Colville** *Burn Dressing* Wood scrapings and Vaseline used as a sunburn ointment. (162:35) **Quinault** *Dermatological Aid* Poultice of chewed leaves applied to wounds. *Pulmonary Aid* Decoction of dried bark taken as lung medicine. **Swinomish** *Strengthener* Smooth twigs of plant rubbed on the body to gain strength. (65:16) **Thompson** *Panacea* Decoction of bark taken for any illness. (161:111) **Tsimshian** *Cancer Treatment* Plant used for cancer. *Internal Medicine* Plant used for internal ailments. (35:187) **Yurok** *Blood Medicine* Decoction of bark taken to "purify the blood." (5:57)

Taxus canadensis, Canada Yew
Abnaki *Antirheumatic (External)* Leaves used for rheumatism. (121:155) *Antirheumatic (Internal)* Infusion of leaves taken for rheumatism. (121:163) **Algonquin, Quebec** *Antirheumatic (Internal)* Decoction of needles used for rheumatism. *Gynecological Aid* Used in a sudatory taken by women experiencing complications after childbirth and other complaints. *Poultice* Needles used for poultices. *Unspecified* Used in a sudatory taken by women experiencing complications after childbirth and other complaints. (14:123) **Algonquin,**

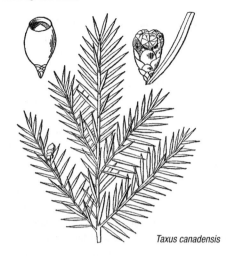

Taxus canadensis

Tête-de-Boule *Abortifacient* Infusion of young branches, alone or with other plants, used for stomachaches and irregular menses. (110:132) **Chippewa** *Antirheumatic* (*External*) Compound decoction of twigs used as herbal steam for rheumatism. *Antirheumatic* (*Internal*) Compound decoction of twigs taken for rheumatism. *Herbal Steam* Compound decoction of twigs taken or used as herbal steam for rheumatism. (43:362) *Other* Plant used as one of the ingredients of "the thirty-two medicine." (59:122) **Malecite** *Unspecified* Bark used as medicine. (137:6) **Menominee** *Antirheumatic* (*External*) Herbal steam from branches used in sudatory for rheumatism and numbness. *Herbal Steam* Branches used in herbal steam for rheumatism, numbness, and paralysis. (128:54) **Micmac** *Analgesic* and *Blood Medicine* Parts of plant used for afterbirth pain and blood clots. *Febrifuge* Parts of plant used for fever. *Gastrointestinal Aid* Bark used for bowel and internal troubles. *Gynecological Aid* Parts of plant used for afterbirth pain and clots. *Misc. Disease Remedy* Parts of plant used for scurvy. (as *T. minor* 32:62) **Montagnais** *Febrifuge* "Brew" from plant used for weakness and fever. *Stimulant* Compound containing plant used for weakness and fever. (as *T. minor* 133:315) **Penobscot** *Cold Remedy* Infusion of twigs taken for colds. (as *T. minor* 133:309) **Potawatomi** *Diuretic* Infusion of leaves used as a diuretic. *Venereal Aid* Compound containing leaves used for gonorrhea. (131:84, 85)

Tellima grandiflora, Bigflower Tellima
Nitinaht *Psychological Aid* Plants chewed as medicine to stop dreams of having sexual intercourse with the dead. *Unspecified* Used as a "special medicine." (160:127) **Skagit** *Dietary Aid* Decoction of pounded plants taken to restore the appetite. *Panacea* Decoction of pounded plants taken for any kind of sickness. (65:31)

Tephrosia florida, Florida Hoarypea
Choctaw *Dermatological Aid* Decoction of beaten roots applied to sores. **Koasati** *Snakebite Remedy* Infusion of roots applied to snakebites. (as *T. ambigua* 152:33)

Tephrosia hispidula, Sprawling Hoarypea
Choctaw *Cough Medicine* Root chewed and juice swallowed, too much would loosen the bowels, for bad coughs. (as *T. elegans* 23:287)

Tephrosia purpurea, Fishpoison
Hawaiian *Dermatological Aid* Leaves or buds, salt, baked coconut, water, and child's urine applied to skin diseases and cuts. *Poison* Poisonous herb. (as *T. piscatoria* 2:4) **Seminole** *Hemostat* Decoction of plant used for nosebleeds. (as *Cracca purpurea* 145:304)

Tephrosia virginiana, Virginia Tephrosia
Catawba *Analgesic* Leaves put in shoes for pain in the flesh of the body (fever). (134:187) *Antirheumatic* (*External*) Leaves placed in shoe for rheumatism. (152:33) *Antirheumatic* (*Internal*) Plant used for rheumatism. *Febrifuge* Leaves put in shoes for pain in the flesh of the body (fever). (134:187) **Cherokee** *Anthelmintic* Infusion taken for worms. *Dermatological Aid* Decoction of roots used as shampoo by women to prevent hair loss. *Kidney Aid* Compound used for kidneys. *Orthopedic Aid* Compound rubbed on limbs of ballplayers to toughen them. (66:31) Decoction of roots given to children to make them strong and muscular. (152:33) *Pediatric Aid* Infusion of root given to children to make them strong and muscular. (66:31) Decoction of roots given to children to make them strong and muscular. (152:33) *Stimulant* Decoction taken for "lassitude." (66:31) **Creek** *Abortifacient* Compound decoction of plant taken and used as wash for irregular menstrua-

tion. *Reproductive Aid* Compound infusion of root used in "cases of loss of manhood." (as *Cracca virginiana* 148:658) Cold infusion of roots taken by men to regain potency. (152:33) *Tuberculosis Remedy* Roots, a very strong medicine, used in cases of "pulmonary consumption." (as *Cracca virginiana* 148:658) Plant used for pulmonary tuberculosis. (152:33) *Urinary Aid* Cold, compound infusion of root taken for bladder trouble. (as *Cracca virginiana* 148:658) Cold infusion of mashed roots taken for bladder troubles. (152:33) **Mahuna** *Gynecological Aid* Infusion of plant taken for women's diseases. (as *Cracca virginiana* 117:15) **Natchez** *Cough Medicine* Plant used as a cough medicine. (152:33)

Tetraclea coulteri, Coulter's Wrinklefruit
Navajo, Ramah *Ceremonial Medicine* Plant used in a ceremonial chant lotion. *Febrifuge* Plant used as a fever medicine. (165:42)

Tetradymia canescens, Spineless Horsebrush
Hopi *Gynecological Aid* Decoction of leaf and root taken after birth to shrink uterus and stop discharge. (174:35, 98) *Tonic* Plant used as a tonic. (174:98) **Navajo** *Abortifacient* Infusion of plant used as bath for (inducing?) menstruation. (76:156) **Navajo, Ramah** *Analgesic* Cold simple or compound infusion of leaves taken for various aches and pain. *Ceremonial Medicine* Plant used as a ceremonial emetic. *Cold Remedy* Cold simple or compound infusion of leaf used for colds. *Cough Medicine* Cold simple or compound infusion of leaves taken for cough. *Disinfectant* Cold simple or compound infusion of leaf used for "ghost infection." *Emetic* Plant used as a ceremonial emetic. *Febrifuge* Cold simple or compound infusion of leaves taken for fever. *Gastrointestinal Aid* Cold simple or compound infusion of leaves taken for stomachache. *Herbal Steam* Leaves used as sweat bath medicine. *Orthopedic Aid* Cold simple or compound infusion of leaves taken for backache. *Witchcraft Medicine* Leaves used as for protection from witches. (165:53) **Shoshoni** *Cathartic* Infusion or decoction of dried plant taken as a physic. *Venereal Aid* Decoction of plant taken for venereal diseases. (155:144)

Tetradymia comosa, Hairy Horsebrush
Paiute *Cold Remedy* Simple or compound decoction of stems and leaves taken for colds. *Cough Medicine* Simple or compound decoction of stems and leaves taken for coughs. *Gastrointestinal Aid* Decoction of stems and leaves used for stomachaches. *Misc. Disease Remedy* Compound decoction of stems taken for influenza. *Pulmonary Aid* Compound decoction of stems taken for pneumonia. **Shoshoni** *Antidiarrheal* Decoction of bark or root taken for diarrhea. *Cold Remedy* Decoction of stems and leaves taken for colds. *Cough Medicine* Decoction of stems and leaves taken for coughs. *Dermatological Aid* Decoction of stems and turpentine used as a wash for swellings from cuts or bruises. *Gastrointestinal Aid* Decoction of stems and leaves used for stomachaches. (155:144, 145)

Tetradymia stenolepis, Mojave Cottonthorn
Kawaiisu *Dermatological Aid* Spines used for warts. (180:66)

Tetraneuris acaulis* var. *arizonica, Arizona Hymenoxys
Hopi *Analgesic* Poultice of plant applied for hip and back pain, especially in pregnancy. (as *Actinea acaulis* 174:33, 94) *Antirheumatic (External)* Used for severe pains in hips and back. *Gynecological Aid* Used for severe pains in hips and back, especially in pregnant state. (as *Hymenoxys aculis* var. *arizonica* 34:327) Poultice of plant applied for hip and back pain, especially in pregnancy. (as *Actinea acaulis* 174:35, 94) *Orthopedic Aid* Poultice of plant applied to hip and back pain, especially during pregnancy. (as *Actinea acaulis* 174:94) *Stimulant* Used as a stimulant. (as *Hymenoxys aculis* var. *arizonica* 34:327) Plant used to make a stimulating drink. (as *Actinea acaulis* 174:31, 94)

Tetraneuris argentea, Perkysue
Navajo, Kayenta *Ceremonial Medicine* Plant used in special ceremony for illness caused by lunar eclipse. *Dermatological Aid* Plant used as a lotion for eczema. *Psychological Aid* Plant used for dreaming of being bitten by an "alligator." (as *Actinea argentea* 179:44) **Navajo, Ramah** *Disinfectant* Plant used for "coyote infection." *Gastrointestinal Aid* Plant used for heartburn. *Other*

Cold infusion taken and used as lotion for emergency treatment of injuries. *Panacea* Plant used as "life medicine." *Witchcraft Medicine* Plant used for protection from witches. (as *Actinea argentea* 165:47)

Tetraneuris scaposa, Stemmy Hymenoxys
Zuni *Eye Medicine* Infusion of plant used as an eyewash, not for persons with "bad heart." (143:60, 61)

Thalictrum dasycarpum, Purple Meadowrue
Lakota *Dermatological Aid* Seeds chewed and rubbed on the hands as a lotion. *Veterinary Aid* Seeds given to horses to make them lively. (116:56) **Meskwaki** *Love Medicine* Used as a love medicine to reconcile a quarrelsome couple. (129:240) **Ojibwa** *Febrifuge* Infusion of root used for fevers. (130:383) **Pawnee** *Veterinary Aid* Plant mixed with clay and rubbed on muzzle of horses as a stimulant. **Ponca** *Love Medicine* Plant tops rubbed in hands of bachelors as a love charm. (58:80) **Potawatomi** *Dermatological Aid* Seeds peppered on surface of poultices to make them more effective. *Gastrointestinal Aid* Compound containing leaves and seeds used for cramps. (131:75) *Hunting Medicine* Dried seeds smoked while hunting to bring good luck. *Love Medicine* Seeds mixed with tobacco and smoked when going to call upon a favorite lady friend. (131:123) Seeds used as a love medicine by the Prairie Potawatomi. (131:75)

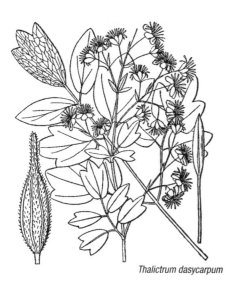

Thalictrum dasycarpum

Thalictrum dioicum, Early Meadowrue
Cherokee *Antidiarrheal* Infusion of root taken for diarrhea. *Antiemetic* Infusion of root taken for vomiting. (66:53) **Iroquois** *Eye Medicine* Decoction of roots used as a wash for sore eyes from a head cold. *Heart Medicine* Decoction of roots taken for heart palpitations. *Other* Plant used to "make you crazy." (73:327)

Thalictrum fendleri, Fendler's Meadowrue
Keres, Western *Cold Remedy* Infusion of plant used for colds. (147:72) **Navajo, Ramah** *Ceremonial Medicine* Decoction of plant taken as ceremonial medicine. (165:28) **Shoshoni** *Venereal Aid* Decoction of root used for gonorrhea. **Washo** *Cold Remedy* Decoction of root taken as a cold remedy. (155:145)

Thalictrum occidentale, Western Meadowrue
Blackfoot *Dermatological Aid* Powdered fruits mixed with water and used as cosmetic on the hair and body. (72:125) *Pulmonary Aid* Infusion of seeds used for chest pains. (72:74) **Gitksan** *Analgesic* Root chewed and juice swallowed for headache. *Blood Medicine* Root chewed and juice swallowed to improve blood circulation. *Eye Medicine* Root chewed and juice swallowed for eye trouble. *Orthopedic Aid* Root chewed and juice swallowed for sore legs. *Pulmonary Aid* Root chewed and juice swallowed to loosen phlegm. (127:57) **Thompson** *Dermatological Aid* Poultice of mashed roots applied to open wounds. (161:250)

Thalictrum polycarpum, Fendler's
 Meadowrue
Kawaiisu *Poison* Root caused death when eaten by cows and horses. (180:67) **Mendocino Indian** *Panacea* Root used as a universal charm and panacea. *Poison* Stems considered poisonous. **Wailaki** *Analgesic* Crushed stem and leaf juice used as a wash for headaches. (33:348) **Yuki** *Orthopedic Aid* Poultice of pounded plant applied to sprains. (39:47)

Thalictrum pubescens, King of the Meadow
Iroquois *Hemostat* Infusion of smashed plant used to wash the head and neck for nosebleeds. *Liver Aid* Compound infusion of roots taken as a gall medicine. (73:327)

Thalictrum sparsiflorum, Fewflower
  Meadowrue
Blackfoot *Veterinary Aid* Dried leaves ground
into powder and given to horses to make them
long-winded, spirited, and enduring. (82:35)
Cheyenne *Veterinary Aid* Dried, ground plant
used to make a horse spirited, long-winded and
enduring. (63:173) Dried, powdered plant used to
make a horse spirited, long-winded, and enduring.
(64:173) Flower used for horses as perfume and
medicine for long-windedness and endurance.
(69:34) **Great Basin Indian** *Dermatological Aid*
Dried seeds and roots used as a perfume. Powdered root used as a shampoo. (100:47)

Thalictrum thalictroides, Rue Anemone
Cherokee *Antidiarrheal* Infusion of root taken
for diarrhea. *Antiemetic* Infusion of root taken for
vomiting. (66:53)

Thamnosma montana, Turpentine Broom
Havasupai *Emetic* Decoction of leaves taken one
to three times a day to cause vomiting. *Gastrointestinal Aid* Pounded leaves rubbed onto a hurting
abdomen. *Laxative* Decoction of leaves taken one
to three times a day to act as a laxative. (171:229)
Kawaiisu *Analgesic* Decoction of stems taken for
chest pains. *Cold Remedy* Decoction of stems
taken for colds. *Dermatological Aid* Crushed stems
rubbed into open wounds. *Diaphoretic* Powdered
plant caused men to sweat. *Hallucinogen* Infusion
of plant taken by medicine men "to go crazy like
coyotes." *Hunting Medicine* Powdered plant used
as an aid in hunting. Powdered plant put in deer
tracks as an aid in hunting. This procedure would
slow down the deer so that it could be overtaken.
Snakebite Remedy Powdered plant used to keep
snakes away. *Veterinary Aid* Powdered plant caused
horses to sweat. (180:67) **Paiute** *Gynecological
Aid* Decoction of stems used as a wash or douche
for female complaints. *Misc. Disease Remedy*
Decoction of stems taken for smallpox. (155:145,
146) **Pima** *Venereal Aid* Decoction of plant taken
for gonorrhea. (123:80) **Shoshoni** *Cold Remedy*
Decoction of stems taken or dried stems smoked
with tobacco for colds. *Tonic* Decoction of stems
taken as a tonic. (155:145, 146)

Thaspium barbinode, Hairyjoint Meadowparsnip
Chippewa *Gastrointestinal Aid* and *Pediatric Aid*
Decoction of root given to children for colic.
(43:344)

Thelesperma filifolium* var. *filifolium,
  Stiff Greenthread
Keres, **Western** *Pediatric Aid* and *Tuberculosis
Remedy* Plant formerly used for children with tu-
berculosis. (as *Theleosperma trifidum* 147:72)

Thelesperma megapotamicum, Hopi Tea
  Greenthread
Keres, **Western** *Pediatric Aid* and *Tuberculosis
Remedy* Plant formerly used for children with tuberculosis. (as *Theleosperma gracile* 147:72)
Navajo *Stimulant* Infusion of leaves and stems
taken as a "nervous stimulant." *Toothache Remedy* Infusion of leaves and stems taken for the teeth.
(as *Thelesperma gracile* 45:89)

Thelypodiopsis elegans, Westwater Tumblemustard
Navajo, **Kayenta** *Veterinary Aid* Plant used as a
charm to make a horse run fast. (as *Sisymbrium
elegans* 179:24)

Thelypodium wrightii, Wright's Thelypody
Navajo *Dermatological Aid* Plant used for swellings. (45:97)

Thelypodium wrightii* ssp. *wrightii,
  Wright's Thelypody
Navajo, **Kayenta** *Eye Medicine* Ashes rubbed on
lids for eye disease. *Pediatric Aid* and *Sedative*
Plant tied to cradle bow to make baby sleep. (as
Stanleyella wrightii 179:25)

Thelypteris kunthii, Kunth's Maiden Fern
Seminole *Orthopedic Aid* and *Psychological Aid*
Leaves used for old paint woman sickness: insanity
and weakness of the limbs and neck. (as *Dryopteris normalis* 145:267)

Thelypteris palustris, Eastern Marsh Fern
Iroquois *Gynecological Aid* Roots used for woman's troubles. (73:256)

Thermopsis macrophylla, California Golden-
banner
Pomo *Eye Medicine* Cold decoction of leaves used
as a wash for sore eyes. (54:13) **Pomo, Kashaya**
Eye Medicine Cooled decoction of leaves used as
an eyewash for sore eyes and vision difficulties.
Gynecological Aid Infusion of leaves or root and
bark used to slow down menstrual flow. (60:66)

Thermopsis rhombifolia, Prairie Thermopsis
Cheyenne *Analgesic* Dried leaves burned and
smoke inhaled for headaches. *Cold Remedy* Dried
leaves burned and smoke inhaled for colds.
(69:30)

Thermopsis rhombifolia* var. *montana,
    Mountain Thermopsis
Navajo, **Ramah** *Analgesic* Compound containing
plant used as fumigant for headache. *Cough Medicine* Decoction of plant taken as cough medicine.
Eye Medicine Compound containing plant used as
fumigant for sore eyes. *Hunting Medicine* Compound containing plant used as fumigant for sickness caused by hunting. *Witchcraft Medicine* Plant
used as a lotion for protection from witches. (as *T.
pinetorum* 165:34)

Thlaspi arvense, Field Pennycress
Iroquois *Throat Aid* Infusion of plant taken for
sore throats. (73:341)

Thlaspi montanum* var. *fendleri, Fendler's
    Pennycress
Navajo, **Ramah** *Ceremonial Medicine* Plant used
in ceremonial chant lotion. *Dermatological Aid*
Cold infusion used internally and externally for
itch. *Preventive Medicine* Cold infusion taken and
used as lotion to prevent injury from deer. *Witchcraft Medicine* Cold infusion taken and used as
lotion to protect from witches. (as *T. fendleri*
165:29)

Thuja excelsa, Cedar
Tlingit *Venereal Aid* Compound infusion of
sprouts and bark taken for syphilis. (89:283)

Thuja occidentalis, Eastern Arborvitae
Abnaki *Antirheumatic* (*External*) Used for swellings. (121:155) Poultice of powdered leaves applied

to swellings. (121:163) *Panacea* Leaves made into
pillows and used as a panacea. (121:155) **Algonquin, Quebec** *Antirheumatic* (*Internal*) Decoction of branches taken for rheumatism. *Cold Remedy* Branches used in the steam bath for colds.
Dermatological Aid Poultice of powdered, rotten
wood used for rashes and skin irritations. *Febrifuge* Branches used in the steam bath for fevers.
Gastrointestinal Aid Infusion of cones used for
babies with colic. *Gynecological Aid* Branches
used in the steam bath for women after childbirth.
Infusion of plant taken for menstrual disorders.
Pediatric Aid Infusion of cones used for babies
with colic. *Toothache Remedy* Decoction of
crushed branches used as a steam for toothache.
(14:130) **Chippewa** *Analgesic* Compound containing charcoal pricked into temples with needles
for headache. (43:338) *Ceremonial Medicine*
Twigs burned for incense in religious ceremonies.
(59:123) *Cough Medicine* Compound containing
leaves taken as a cough syrup. (43:340) *Dermatological Aid* Plant used as a deodorant. *Disinfectant*
and *Misc. Disease Remedy* Twigs burned as a disinfectant to fumigate a house for smallpox. *Unspecified* Leaves combined with ground hemlock
for medicinal purposes. (59:123) **Cree, Woodlands** *Panacea* Powdered branches and many
herbs used for various ailments. *Pulmonary Aid*
Decoction of branches taken for pneumonia. *Urinary Aid* Decoction of needle covered branches
or juice taken for urine retention or sore bladder.
(91:62) **Iroquois** *Antirheumatic* (*External*)

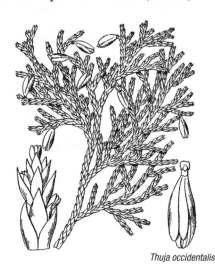

Thuja occidentalis

Decoction of plant tips used as a foot bath for rheumatism. Steam from compound decoction used as a bath for rheumatism. *Blood Medicine* Fermented compound decoction taken when "blood gets bad and cold." *Cold Remedy* Steam from decoction of leaves inhaled for colds. *Dermatological Aid* Decoction used as a wash or poultice applied to cuts, bruises, and sores. *Febrifuge* Fermented compound decoction taken for fever. *Gynecological Aid* Infusion used by "women during confinement." Steam from compound decoction used as a bath for parturition. (73:270) Infusion of leaves taken by women as a tonic and diaphoretic to increase the milk flow. *Hunting Medicine* Branches, without fruit, used in the vapor baths by hunters. (118:35) *Orthopedic Aid* Decoction used as a wash for weakness in the hips due to untreated broken coccyx. Decoction of plant used as a wash or poultice of leaves applied to sprains. Fermented compound decoction taken for soreness. (73:270) Poultice of bough and milk decoction mixed with grease and applied for paralysis. (118:35) *Stimulant* Fermented compound decoction taken when a "person is tired." (73:270) **Malecite** *Burn Dressing* Dried under bark pounded, mixed with grease, and used for burns. (as *Thuya occidentalis* 96:247) *Cough Medicine* Infusion of boughs used for coughs. (96:249) *Toothache Remedy* Gum used to fill cavities and for tooth pain. (as *Thuya occidentalis* 96:248) *Tuberculosis Remedy* Infusion of bark used for consumption. (96:251) **Menominee** *Abortifacient* Infusion of dried inner bark taken during a cold to treat suppressed menses. *Adjuvant* Inner bark used as a seasoner for enhancing medicines. (128:46) *Dermatological Aid* Compound poultice of dried, powdered leaves applied to swellings. (44:134) *Diaphoretic* Plant used in the sudatory. *Stimulant* Smudge of leaves used to revive "lost consciousness." (128:46) **Micmac** *Analgesic* Stems used for headaches. *Burn Dressing* Inner bark, bark, and stems used for burns. *Cough Medicine* Inner bark, bark, and stems used for cough. *Orthopedic Aid* Leaves used for swollen feet and hands and stems used for headaches. *Toothache Remedy* Gum used for toothache. *Tuberculosis Remedy* Inner bark, bark, and stems used for consumption. (32:62) **Montagnais** *Diaphoretic* Infusion of bruised twigs taken to cause sweating. (as *Arbor vitae* 133:315) **Ojibwa**

Analgesic Infusion of leaves used for headache. *Blood Medicine* Decoction of leaves taken as a blood purifier. *Ceremonial Medicine* Smoke used to purify sacred objects, hands, and bodies of participants. *Cough Medicine* Decoction of leaves taken for coughs. *Diaphoretic* Compound containing leaves used in the sweat bath. (130:380) **Penobscot** *Analgesic* Compound poultice of bark used on cuts made in painful area to treat pain. (as *Arbor vitae* 133:311) *Dermatological Aid* Poultice of leaves applied to swollen hands or feet. (as *Arbor vitae* 133:309) *Panacea* Compound poultice of bark applied "for all kinds of trouble." (as *Arbor vitae* 133:311) **Potawatomi** *Adjuvant* Plant used as a seasoner for medicines. *Unspecified* Poultice of leaves used for unspecified ailments. *Witchcraft Medicine* Leaves burned on coals to purify patient and exorcise evil spirits. (131:70, 71)

Thuja plicata, Western Red Cedar
Bella Coola *Analgesic* Decoction of powdered leaves used externally for various internal pains. *Antirheumatic* (*External*) Infusion of leaves used externally for rheumatism. (127:49) Poultice of pounded bough tips and eulachon (candlefish) grease applied to the back and chest for rheumatism. Poultice of pounded bough tips and eulachon grease applied to the back and chest for a swollen neck. (158:197) *Cough Medicine* Infusion of leaves used externally for coughs. *Dermatological Aid* Very soft bark used to bind wounds and cover poultices. *Gastrointestinal Aid* Simple decoction, compound decoction or infusion of leaf taken and used externally for stomach pain. (127:49) Poultice of pounded bough tips and eulachon (candlefish) grease applied to the back and chest for stomach pains. (158:197) *Heart Medicine* Infusion of leaves used externally for heart trouble. (127:49) Poultice of pounded bough tips and eulachon (candlefish) grease applied to the back and chest for heart trouble. (158:197) *Other* Infusion of leaves used externally for swollen neck. (127:49) *Respiratory Aid* Poultice of pounded bough tips and eulachon (candlefish) grease applied to the back and chest for bronchitis. (158:197) **Chehalis** *Abortifacient* Chewed bark or decoction of bark taken to induce menstruation. (65:19) **Clallam** *Tuberculosis Remedy* Decoction of small limbs used for tuberculosis. (47:195) **Cowlitz** *Cold*

Remedy Decoction of plant tips and roots taken as a cold medicine. *Toothache Remedy* Buds chewed for toothaches. (65:19) **Haisla** *Dermatological Aid* Moxa of inner bark used as a counter irritant for the skin. **Hanaksiala** *Antidiarrheal* Infusion of pounded, bough tip leaves in cold water taken for diarrhea. (35:162) **Hoh** *Unspecified* Infusion of green bark juice used for medicine. (114:57) **Klallam** *Tuberculosis Remedy* Decoction of branches taken as a tuberculosis medicine. (65:19) **Kwakiutl** *Dermatological Aid* Poultice of inner bark applied to carbuncles. Shredded bark used to cauterize sores and swellings. *Eye Medicine* Sticks broken in front of the eye for sties. *Hemostat* Shredded bark used to cauterize sores and swellings. *Orthopedic Aid* Compound poultice of leaves applied to sore backs. (157:266) **Lummi** *Antiemetic* Tips chewed by men to avoid nausea while burying a corpse. *Pulmonary Aid* Chewed buds taken for sore lungs. (65:19) **Makah** *Cough Medicine* Infusion of boughs taken for coughs. *Dermatological Aid* Bark pounded until soft as cotton and used to rub the face. (55:228) **Nez Perce** *Antidiarrheal* Leaves used for diarrhea. *Cold Remedy* Infusion of boughs used for colds. *Cough Medicine* Infusion of boughs used for coughs. *Pediatric Aid* Infusion of boughs sweetened and used for children with colds or coughs. (68:54) **Okanagan-Colville** *Antirheumatic (External)* Infusion of boughs used to soak painful joints from arthritis and rheumatism. Weak infusion of boughs taken for painful joints from arthritis and rheumatism. *Dermatological Aid* Decoction of boughs and three plants used for washing the skin and hair during sweat bathing. Infusion of boughs used as a hair wash for dandruff and scalp "germs." *Poison* Infusion of boughs considered toxic in large doses. *Tonic* Decoction of boughs and three plants taken as a sweat house tonic. Weak infusion of boughs taken as a sweat house tonic. (162:20) **Oweekeno** *Ceremonial Medicine* Wood made into shamanistic soul catchers to use in ritual healing. (35:66) **Quileute** *Unspecified* Infusion of green bark juice used for medicine. (114:57) **Quinault** *Dermatological Aid* Infusion of twigs used as a wash for venereal disease sores. *Febrifuge* Infusion of seeds and twigs taken for fevers. *Kidney Aid* Infusion of bark and twigs taken for kidney trouble. *Venereal Aid* Infusion of twigs used as a wash for venereal

disease sores. **Skagit** *Cough Medicine* Decoction of leaves taken for coughs. **Skokomish** *Oral Aid* Decoction of buds used as a gargle. (65:19) **Thompson** *Gynecological Aid* Compound decoction of twigs taken after childbirth. (141:461) *Misc. Disease Remedy* Decoction of old or green cones taken for leprosy. *Psychological Aid* Tree or spruce tree said to cause vivid dreams for those who slept under them. (161:94)

Thymophylla acerosa, Pricklyleaf Dogweed
Isleta *Febrifuge* Decoction of leaves used as a body bath for fevers. (as *Aciphyllaea acerosa* 85:20)

Thymophylla pentachaeta var.
     belenidium, Fiveneedle Pricklyleaf
Paiute *Cathartic* Decoction of root taken as a physic. (as *Dyssodia thurberi* 155:67)

Thymophylla pentachaeta var. *pentachaeta*, Fiveneedle Pricklyleaf
Navajo, Kayenta *Psychological Aid* Plant used for dreaming of being pursued by a deer. (as *Dyssodia pentachaeta* 179:46)

Thymus praecox ssp. *arcticus*, Creeping Thyme
Delaware, Ontario *Febrifuge* Compound infusion of plant taken for chills and fever. (as *T. serpyllum* 150:56, 84)

Thysanocarpus curvipes, Sand Fringepod
Mendocino Indian *Gastrointestinal Aid* Decoction of whole plant taken for stomachaches. (as *T. elegans* 33:352)

Tiarella cordifolia, Heartleaf Foamflower
Cherokee *Oral Aid* Infusion held in mouth to "remove white coat from tongue." (66:34) **Iroquois** *Dermatological Aid* Poultice of smashed roots applied to wounds. *Dietary Aid* Infusion of roots and leaves given to fatten little children. (73:344) *Eye Medicine* Infusion of dried leaves used as drops for sore eyes. (73:345) *Hunting Medicine* Decoction of whole plant used as a wash for the rifle, a "hunting medicine." *Oral Aid* Infusion of smashed roots given to babies with sore mouths. *Orthopedic Aid* Compound poultice of smashed plants applied to sore backs of babies. (73:344) *Other*

Compound decoction of dried roots given to children with "summer complaint." (73:345) *Pediatric Aid* Compound poultice of smashed plants applied to sore backs of babies. Infusion of roots and leaves given to fatten little children. (73:344) Compound decoction of dried roots given to children with "summer complaint." (73:345) *Tonic* Infusion of roots and leaves taken as a tonic. (73:344) **Malecite** *Antidiarrheal* and *Pediatric Aid* Infusion of roots used by children for diarrhea. (96:255) **Micmac** *Antidiarrheal* Roots used for diarrhea. (32:62)

Tiarella trifoliata, Threeleaf Foamflower
Quileute *Cough Medicine* Raw leaves chewed as a cough medicine. (65:31)

Tilia americana, American Basswood
Algonquin, Quebec *Eye Medicine* Infusion of leaves used as an eyewash. *Unspecified* Poultice of leaves used for medicinal purposes. (14:200) **Cherokee** *Antidiarrheal* Compound of inner bark used for dysentery. (66:24) Infusion of inner bark taken for dysentery. (152:42) *Cough Medicine* Jelly used for coughs. *Dermatological Aid* Decoction of bark mixed with cornmeal and used as poultice for boils. *Gastrointestinal Aid* Inside bark and twigs used during pregnancy for heartburn, weak stomach, and bowels. Used "when stomach has been overheated by too free use of spirituous liquors." *Snakebite Remedy* Bark from tree struck by lightning chewed and spit on snakebite. *Tuber-*

culosis Remedy Jelly used for consumption. (66:24) **Iroquois** *Antihemorrhagic* Compound decoction of roots and bark taken for internal hemorrhage. *Burn Dressing* Compound decoction of leaves applied as poultice to burns or scalds. *Diuretic* Infusion of bark taken to increase urination. *Emetic* Compound decoction taken to vomit during initial stages of consumption. (73:384) *Gynecological Aid* Infusion of branches and bark and buds from another plant taken before giving birth. (118:51) *Orthopedic Aid* Decoction of branches used as wash for babies that do not walk but should. (73:383) Compound poultice of leaves applied to broken bones and swollen areas. *Other* Infusion of plant used for severe injuries. *Panacea* Compound infusion of twigs and roots taken as a panacea. (73:384) *Pediatric Aid* Decoction of branches used as wash for babies that do not walk but should. (73:383) *Stimulant* Infusion of shoots taken when feeling worn out. *Tuberculosis Remedy* Compound decoction taken to vomit during initial stages of consumption. (73:384) **Malecite** *Anthelmintic* Infusion of roots or bark used for worms. (96:255) **Meskwaki** *Dermatological Aid* Poultice of boiled inner bark applied to cause boils to open. *Pulmonary Aid* Decoction of twigs taken for lung trouble. (129:248) **Micmac** *Anthelmintic* Roots used for worms. *Dermatological Aid* Bark used for suppurating wounds. (32:62)

Tilia americana* var. *heterophylla, American Basswood
Cherokee *Antidiarrheal* Compound of inner bark used for dysentery. *Cough Medicine* Jelly used for coughs. *Dermatological Aid* Decoction of bark mixed with cornmeal and used as poultice for boils. *Gastrointestinal Aid* Inside bark and twigs used during pregnancy for heartburn, weak stomach, and bowels. Used "when stomach has been overheated by too free use of spirituous liquors." *Snakebite Remedy* Bark from tree struck by lightning chewed and spit on snakebite. *Tuberculosis Remedy* Jelly used for consumption. (as *T. heterophylla* 66:24)

Tillandsia usneoides, Spanish Moss
Houma *Febrifuge* Decoction of moss taken for chills and fever. (135:59)

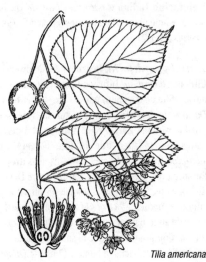

Tilia americana

Tiquilia latior, Matted Crinklemat
Navajo, **Kayenta** *Gastrointestinal Aid* Plant used for gastrointestinal disease. (as *Coldenia hispidissima* var. *latior* 179:39)

Tolmiea menziesii, Youth on Age
Cowlitz *Dermatological Aid* Poultice of fresh leaves applied to boils. (65:31)

Torreya californica, California Nutmeg
Costanoan *Analgesic* Smashed nuts and fat rubbed on temples for headaches. *Diaphoretic* Smashed nuts and fat rubbed on body to cause sweating. *Febrifuge* Smashed nuts and fat rubbed on body for chills. *Gastrointestinal Aid* Nuts chewed for indigestion. (as *Tumion californica* 17:6) **Pomo** *Tuberculosis Remedy* Decoction of nuts taken for tuberculosis. (54:11) **Pomo, Kashaya** *Tuberculosis Remedy* Decoction of cracked, soaked nut taken for tuberculosis. (60:78)

Touchardia latifolia, Olona
Hawaiian *Laxative* Slimy substance, water, plant milk, and watermelon juice mixed, strained, and taken as a laxative. *Pediatric Aid* Shoots chewed and given to infants for bodily ailments or weaknesses. *Strengthener* Shoots chewed and given to infants for bodily ailments or weaknesses. Shoots chewed for bodily ailments or weaknesses. (2:71)

Townsendia exscapa, Stemless Townsendia
Blackfoot *Veterinary Aid* Decoction of roots given to tired horses to relieve them. (as *T. sericea* 82:61) **Navajo** *Ceremonial Medicine* Chewed and spit upon ceremonial knots to unravel them, "untying medicine." (45:89) **Navajo, Ramah** *Gynecological Aid* Plant chewed or infusion taken to ease delivery. (165:54)

Townsendia incana, Hoary Townsendia
Hopi *Reproductive Aid* Plant taken to induce pregnancy and insure male child. *Throat Aid* Plant used to clear the throat. (as *T. arizonica* 174:35, 99) **Navajo** *Gynecological Aid* Plant used in labor to facilitate delivery of the baby. (76:156) **Navajo, Kayenta** *Gynecological Aid* Plant used to expedite labor. *Unspecified* Plant used as a strong medicine. (as *T. arizonica* 179:50)

Townsendia strigosa, Hairy Townsendia
Hopi *Throat Aid* Plant used to clear the throat. (34:368) **Keres, Western** *Gynecological Aid* Dried leaves ground into a powder and used on lacerations at childbirth. Infusion of plant used as a wash or douche. (147:73) **Navajo** *Gastrointestinal Aid* Decoction of crushed, dried leaves taken for stomach troubles. *Gynecological Aid* Decoction of crushed, dried leaves taken to accelerate deliverance. *Nose Medicine* Dried, pulverized plants used as a snuff for nose troubles. *Throat Aid* Dried, pulverized plants used as a snuff for throat troubles. (45:89)

Toxicodendron diversilobum, Pacific Poison Oak
Diegueño *Eye Medicine* Decoction of roots used in the eyes for tiny sores inside the lids and to improve vision. (70:43) **Karok** *Contraceptive* Leaf swallowed in the spring as a prophylactic. (as *Rhus diversiloba* 125:385) *Poison* Plant considered poisonous. (5:58) **Mahuna** *Preventive Medicine* Infusion of dried roots taken as an immunity against any further poisoning. (as *Rhus diversiloba* 117:11) **Mendocino Indian** *Dermatological Aid* Moxa of plant used for warts and ringworms. (as *Rhus diversiloba* 33:364) **Tolowa** *Antidote* Buds eaten in the spring to obtain immunity from the plant poisons. *Poison* Plant considered poisonous. (5:58) **Wailaki** *Snakebite Remedy* Poultice of fresh leaves applied to rattlesnake bites. (as *Rhus diversiloba* 33:364) **Yuki** *Dermatological Aid* Plant juice used on warts. (as *Rhus diversiloba* 39:46) **Yurok** *Poison* Plant considered poisonous. (5:58)

Toxicodendron pubescens, Atlantic Poison Oak
Cherokee *Emetic* Decoction given as an emetic. (as *Rhus toxicodendron* 66:41) Decoction of bark taken as an emetic. (as *Rhus toxicodendron* 152:37) **Delaware** *Unspecified* Poultice of roasted, crushed roots regarded as medicinally valuable. (as *Rhus toxicodendron* 151:33) **Delaware, Oklahoma** *Dermatological Aid* Poultice and salve containing root used on chronic sores and swollen glands. (as *Rhus toxicondendron* 150:27, 78) **Iroquois** *Oral Aid* Poultice of plant applied to infectious sores on lips. *Pediatric Aid* Given to nervous boys and girls. *Sedative* Given to nervous

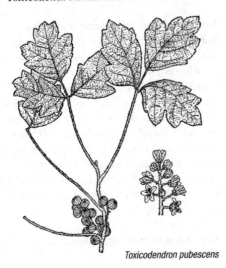

Toxicodendron pubescens

boys and girls. (as *Rhus toxicodendron* ssp. *radicans* 73:373) **Meskwaki** *Dermatological Aid* Poultice of pounded root applied to swelling "to make it open," dangerous. (as *Rhus toxicodendron* 129:201) **Omaha** *Poison* Plant considered poisonous. (as *T. toxicodendron* 58:100) **Paiute** *Poison* Plant considered poisonous. (as *Rhus toxicodendron* 93:88) **Ponca** *Poison* Plant considered poisonous. (as *T. toxicodendron* 58:100) **Potawatomi** *Dermatological Aid* Poultice of pounded root applied to swellings by skilled medicine men. *Poison* Plant considered poisonous. (as *Rhus toxicodendron* 131:38)

Toxicodendron radicans, Eastern Poison Ivy
Houma *Tonic* Decoction of leaves taken as a tonic and "rejuvenator." (135:59)

Toxicodendron radicans ssp. *radicans*,
Eastern Poison Ivy
Algonquin, Quebec *Dermatological Aid* Leaves rubbed on the skin affected by a poison ivy reaction. (as *Rhus radicans* 14:194) **Cherokee** *Emetic* Decoction given as an emetic. (as *Rhus radicans* 66:41) **Kiowa** *Dermatological Aid* Plant used for running or nonhealing sores. Whole or broken leaves rubbed over boils or skin eruptions. (as *Rhus radicans* 166:38) **Navajo, Ramah** *Poison* Compound containing plant used to poison arrows. (as *Rhus radicans* 165:35) **Thompson** *Poison* Plant considered poisonous because it caused skin irritations. One informant said that it affected her

eyes, causing temporary blindness. (as *Rhus radicans* 161:149)

Toxicodendron rydbergii, Western Poison Ivy
Iroquois *Blood Medicine* Poultice of plant applied to the skin as a vesicant for water in the blood. Poultice of plant applied to the skin as a vesicant for water in the blood. (as *Rhus radicans* var. *rydbergii* 118:52) **Lakota** *Poison* Poisonous plant caused a rash resembling venereal disease. (116:33)

Toxicodendron vernix, Poison Sumac
Cherokee *Dermatological Aid* Plant considered poison and used in some form as a wash for foul ulcers. *Febrifuge* Plant considered poison and taken in some form for fever. *Misc. Disease Remedy* Plant considered poison and taken in some form for ague. *Poison* Plant considered poison and taken in some form for clap and "gleet" or ulcerated bladder. *Respiratory Aid* Plant considered poison and taken in some form for asthma and phthisic. *Urinary Aid* Plant considered poison and taken in some form for ulcerated bladder. *Venereal Aid* Plant considered poison and taken in some form for clap and "gleet." (as *Rhus vernix* 66:57) **Chippewa** *Poison* Plant considered poisonous. (as *Rhus vernix* 59:135)

Tradescantia occidentalis, Prairie
Spiderwort
Meskwaki *Diuretic* Infusion of root used as a "urinary." *Psychological Aid* Root gum inserted in cut on head "to stop craziness." (129:209) **Navajo, Kayenta** *Love Medicine* Plant used as an aphrodisiac. (179:16) **Navajo, Ramah** *Disinfectant* Cold infusion of root used internally and externally for "deer infection." *Internal Medicine* Decoction of root taken for internal injury. *Veterinary Aid* Cold simple or compound infusion given to livestock as an aphrodisiac. (165:20)

Tradescantia pinetorum, Pinewoods
Spiderwort
Navajo, Ramah *Veterinary Aid* Cold simple or compound infusion given to livestock as an aphrodisiac. (165:20)

Tradescantia virginiana, Virginia Spiderwort
Cherokee *Analgesic* Infusion used for stomach-

ache from overeating. *Antihemorrhagic* Compound infusion taken for "female ailments or rupture." *Cancer Treatment* Poultice of root used for cancer. *Dermatological Aid* Plant mashed and rubbed on insect bites. *Gastrointestinal Aid* Infusion used for stomachache from overeating. *Gynecological Aid* Compound infusion taken for "female ailments or rupture." *Kidney Aid* Compound used for kidney trouble. *Laxative* Infusion taken as a laxative and plant mashed and rubbed on insect bites. (66:56, 57)

Tragia nepetifolia, Catnip Noseburn
Navajo, **Kayenta** *Snakebite Remedy* Plant used as a lotion to keep snakes away. (179:31) **Navajo**, **Ramah** *Panacea* Plant used as "life medicine." (165:35)

Tragia ramosa, Branched Noseburn
Keres, **Western** *Dermatological Aid* Infusion of plant used on ant bites. *Pediatric Aid* Nettle used to strike male infants, to increase pain threshold during battle. *Strengthener* Nettle used to strike male infants, to increase pain threshold during battle. (147:73)

Tragopogon porrifolius, Salsify
Navajo, **Ramah** *Ceremonial Medicine* Plant used as a ceremonial emetic. *Dermatological Aid* Cold infusion taken or used as lotion for mad coyote bite on humans or livestock. *Emetic* Plant used as a ceremonial emetic. *Veterinary Aid* Cold infusion taken or used as lotion for mad coyote bite on humans or livestock. (165:54)

Tragopogon pratensis, Meadow Salsify
Navajo, **Ramah** *Ceremonial Medicine* Cold infusion gargled as ceremonial treatment for throat trouble. *Dermatological Aid* Cold infusion used as lotion for boils. *Throat Aid* Cold infusion gargled as ceremonial treatment for throat trouble. *Veterinary Aid* Cold infusion used in large amounts for internal injury to horses. (165:54)

Trautvetteria caroliniensis, Carolina
   Bugbane
Bella Coola *Dermatological Aid* Poultice of pounded roots, too strong for children, applied to boils. (as *T. grandis* 127:57)

Trema micranthum, Trema
Seminole *Reproductive Aid* Bark used for difficult deliveries. (as *T. floridanus* 145:323)

Triadenum virginicum, Virginia Marsh St.
   Johnswort
Potawatomi *Febrifuge* Infusion of leaves used for fevers. (as *Hypericum virginicum* 131:60)

Tribulus terrestris, Puncturevine
Navajo *Ceremonial Medicine* Plant used as a traditional ceremonial medicine. (76:163)

Trichostema lanatum, Woolly Bluecurls
Cahuilla *Gastrointestinal Aid* Decoction of leaves and flowers taken for stomach ailments. (11:141)
Mahuna *Panacea* Plant used for many ailments. (117:48)

Trichostema lanceolatum, Vinegar Weed
Concow *Analgesic* Infusion of leaves used as a wash for feverish headaches. *Febrifuge* Infusion of leaves used as a wash for feverish headaches. *Misc. Disease Remedy* Infusion of leaves used as a wash for typhoid fever. (33:385) **Costanoan** *Analgesic* Ground leaves rubbed on the skin for pain. *Cold Remedy* Cold infusion of leaves used for colds. Ground leaves rubbed on the face and chest for colds. *Dermatological Aid* and *Disinfectant* Decoction of plant used for infected sores. *Gastrointestinal Aid* Decoction of plant used for stomachaches. (17:17) **Kawaiisu** *Cold Remedy* Infusion of plants taken for colds. *Gastrointestinal Aid* Infusion of plants taken for stomachaches. (180:67) **Miwok** *Analgesic* Decoction of leaves and flowers taken for headaches. *Cold Remedy* Decoction of leaves and flowers taken for colds. (8:173) *Dermatological Aid* Decoction of flat leaves used as bath for pustules and prevented skin eruptions caused by smallpox. *Gynecological Aid* Decoction steam used for uterine trouble. (8:173, 174) *Misc. Disease Remedy* Decoction of leaves and flowers taken for malaria. Decoction of leaves and flowers taken for ague. (8:173) Decoction of leaves and flowers used as a bath for ague, and smallpox. (8:173, 174) *Stimulant* Decoction of leaves and flowers taken for general debility. (8:173) *Toothache Remedy* Leaves chewed and placed in cavity or around aching tooth. (8:173, 174) *Urinary Aid* Decoction of

leaves and flowers taken for stricture of the bladder. (8:173) **Tubatulabal** *Analgesic* Infusion of entire plant snuffed up the nose for headaches. *Hemostat* Infusion of entire plant snuffed up the nose for nosebleeds. (167:59)

Trientalis borealis* ssp. *borealis, Maystar
Montagnais *Panacea* Infusion of plant used for "general sickness." *Tuberculosis Remedy* Infusion of plant taken for consumption. (as *T. americana* 133:314)

Trientalis borealis* ssp. *latifolia, Broadleaf
Starflower
Cowlitz *Eye Medicine* Infusion of plant juice used as an eyewash. (as *T. latifolia* 65:45) **Paiute** *Eye Medicine* Plant used as an eye medicine. (as *T. latifolia* 93:105)

Trifolium dubium, Suckling Clover
Navajo, Ramah *Ceremonial Medicine* and *Emetic* Plant used as a ceremonial emetic. (165:34) *Hemostat* Poultice of chopped plant applied to cut as hemostat. (165:33)

Trifolium hybridum, Alsike Clover
Iroquois *Gynecological Aid* Cold infusion of plant used as a wash for breasts to increase milk flow. *Veterinary Aid* Cold infusion of plant used as a wash for cow's teats to increase milk flow. (73:364)

Trifolium pratense, Red Clover
Algonquin, Quebec *Pulmonary Aid* Infusion of plant taken for whooping cough. (14:188) **Cherokee** *Febrifuge* Infusion taken for fevers. *Gynecological Aid* Infusion taken for fevers and leukorrhea. *Kidney Aid* Infusion taken for "Bright's disease." (66:29) **Iroquois** *Blood Medicine* Decoction of flowers taken as a blood medicine. *Gynecological Aid* Cold infusion of blossoms taken by women for the change of life. (73:363) **Rappahannock** *Blood Medicine* Infusion of stems and leaves used as an ingredient of a blood medicine. (138:31) **Shinnecock** *Cancer Treatment* Teaspoonful of powder mixed in boiling water and taken for cancer. (25:119) **Thompson** *Cancer Treatment* Infusion of heads taken for stomach cancer. (161:224)

Trifolium repens, White Clover
Cherokee *Febrifuge* Infusion taken for fevers. *Gynecological Aid* Infusion taken for fevers and leukorrhea. *Kidney Aid* Infusion taken for "Bright's disease." (66:29) **Iroquois** *Dermatological Aid* Compound infusion of whole plant used as a wash for liver spots. *Eye Medicine* Poultice of plant applied to eyes for paralysis. (73:363) Infusion of flowers used as an eyewash. *Respiratory Aid* Infusion of flowers, leaves, and roots of another plant used for asthma. (118:50) **Mohegan** *Cold Remedy* Infusion of plant taken for colds. (149:270) Infusion of dried leaves taken for colds. (151:76, 132) *Cough Medicine* Infusion of plant taken for coughs. (149:270) Infusion of dried leaves taken for coughs. (151:76, 132)

Trifolium wormskioldii, Cow Clover
Makah *Unspecified* Used for medicine. (55:281)

Triglochin maritimum, Seaside Arrowgrass
Blackfoot *Poison* Leaves known to be poisonous to stock. (82:19)

Trillium chloropetalum, Giant Wakerobin
Costanoan *Analgesic* Poultice of heated plant applied to the chest for chest pains. (17:28) **Yurok** *Burn Dressing* Poultice of bulb scrapings applied to burns. (5:59)

Trillium erectum, Red Trillium
Abnaki *Panacea* Used by children for maladies.

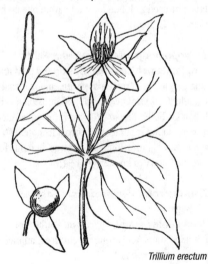

Trillium erectum

(121:155) Bulbs ground and given to sick children with unidentified illnesses. (121:174) *Pediatric Aid* Used by children for maladies. (121:155) Bulbs ground and given to sick children with unidentified illnesses. (121:174) **Cherokee** *Cancer Treatment* Poultice used for "putrid ulcers, tumors and inflamed parts." *Cough Medicine* Taken for coughs. *Dermatological Aid* Poultice used for "putrid ulcers, tumors and inflamed parts." *Gastrointestinal Aid* Taken for bowel complaints. *Gynecological Aid* Infusion used for profuse menstruation, hemorrhages, and the change of life. *Respiratory Aid* Taken for asthma. (66:59) **Iroquois** *Dermatological Aid* Infusion of rhizomes and flowers from another plant used for pimples and sunburn. (118:66)

Trillium grandiflorum, Snow Trillium
Chippewa *Antirheumatic* (*External*) Decoction of root "pricked in with needles" near sore joints. *Ear Medicine* Decoction of root bark used as drops for sore ear. (43:362) **Menominee** *Abortifacient* Decoction of root taken for "irregularity of the menses." *Analgesic* Infusion of grated root taken for cramps. *Disinfectant* Decoction of root purified man after intercourse with menstruating woman. (128:41) *Diuretic* Infusion of root used as a diuretic. (44:131) *Eye Medicine* Poultice of grated, raw root applied to eye swellings. (128:41) **Potawatomi** *Gynecological Aid* Infusion of root taken for sore nipples and, to hasten the effect, the teats are pierced with a dog whisker. (131:63)

Trillium ovatum, Pacific Trillium
Karok *Dermatological Aid* Plant juice applied to boils. (125:381) **Lummi** *Eye Medicine* Juice from smashed plants used as drops for sore eyes. **Makah** *Love Medicine* Poultice of pounded bulbs applied as a love medicine. (65:25) **Paiute** *Eye Medicine* Decoction of fresh or dried corms used as an eyewash. Fresh root juice dripped into an afflicted eye. (93:58) **Quileute** *Dermatological Aid* Poultice of scraped bulbs applied to boils. **Skagit** *Eye Medicine* Infusion of roots used as a wash for sore eyes. *Poison* Plant considered poisonous. (65:25) **Thompson** *Eye Medicine* Powdered root dropped or blown into sore eyes. (141:472) Infusion of roots placed in the eyes with an eye dropper. (161:130)

Trillium sessile, Toadshade
Concow *Poison* Plant considered poisonous. **Wailaki** *Dermatological Aid* Poultice of bruised leaves and crushed roots applied to boils. *Other* Decoction of plant taken to prevent deep and lasting sleep. *Panacea* Decoction of plants taken for any kind of sickness. **Yuki** *Dermatological Aid* Poultice of bruised leaves and crushed roots applied to boils. *Other* Decoction of plant taken to prevent deep and lasting sleep. *Panacea* Decoction of plants taken for any kind of sickness. (33:329)

Trillium undulatum, Painted Trillium
Algonquin, Tête-de-Boule *Gynecological Aid* Flowers, sepals, and leaves eaten to accelerate the delivery. (110:133)

Triodanis perfoliata* var. *perfoliata, Clasping Venus's Lookingglass
Cherokee *Gastrointestinal Aid* Liquid compound of root taken for dyspepsia from overeating. (as *Specularia perfoliata* 66:60) Infusion of roots taken and used as a bath for dyspepsia. (as *Specularia perfoliata* 152:60) **Meskwaki** *Emetic* Used as an emetic and "will make one sick all day long." (as *Specularia perfoliata* 129:206)

Triosteum perfoliatum, Feverwort
Cherokee *Dermatological Aid* Infusion used for soaking sore feet and ooze used as a wash for leg swelling. *Emetic* Plant used as an emetic. *Febrifuge* Plant used as a febrifuge. *Orthopedic Aid* Infusion used for soaking sore feet and ooze used as a wash for leg swelling. (66:39) **Creek** *Unspecified* Plant used medicinally for unspecified purpose. (148:667) **Iroquois** *Abortifacient* Infusion of roots taken for irregular or profuse menses. (73:444) *Analgesic* Compound decoction of roots taken for urinating pain. *Cold Remedy* Cold infusion of roots taken for bad colds. *Diaphoretic* Root used to cause sweating. (73:445) *Dietary Aid* Infusion of roots given to babies and adults to fatten them. (73:444) *Diuretic* Root used as a diuretic. *Gastrointestinal Aid* Decoction or poultice of roots used for stomach trouble caused by witchcraft. (73:445) *Gynecological Aid* Decoction or infusion of roots taken for irregular or profuse menses. (73:444) *Laxative* Compound decoction of roots taken as a laxative. (73:445) *Pediatric Aid*

Infusion of roots given to babies to fatten them. (73:444) *Pulmonary Aid* Root used for pneumonia. *Throat Aid* Cold infusion of roots taken for dry throats. *Urinary Aid* Compound decoction of roots taken for urinating pain. *Venereal Aid* Root used for venereal disease. *Witchcraft Medicine* Decoction of roots taken for stomach trouble caused by witchcraft. Poultice of smashed roots applied for stomach trouble caused by witchcraft. (73:445) **Meskwaki** *Analgesic* Root used on a newborn infant with a sore head. *Cathartic* Decoction of root used as a "drink for cleansing the system." *Dermatological Aid* Poultice of root applied to old, raw sores and root used for snakebite. *Pediatric Aid* Root used on a newborn infant with a sore head. *Snakebite Remedy* Root used for snakebite and poultice used for old, raw sores. (129:207, 208)

Tripterocalyx carnea var. *wootonii*, Wooton's Sandpuffs

Hopi *Pediatric Aid* and *Sedative* Plant placed on child's head to induce sleep. (as *T. wootoni* 174:36, 75) **Navajo**, **Ramah** *Other* Cold infusion of plant used for injury from falling off a horse. *Witchcraft Medicine* Cold infusion of plant taken to give protection from witches. (as *T. wootonii* 165:26) **Zuni** *Diaphoretic* Crushed leaves used in sweat bath for snakebite. *Snakebite Remedy* Infusion of powdered root taken for snakebite. *Throat Aid* Infusion of powdered root taken for swollen glands, especially in the throat. (as *T. wootonii* 143:61) *Witchcraft Medicine* Poultice of powdered seeds and water applied to swellings caused by being witched by a bullsnake. (as *T. wootonii* 22:377)

Triteleia grandiflora, Wild Hyacinth

Okanagan-Colville *Poison* Plant considered poisonous. (as *Brodiaea douglasii* 162:41) **Thompson** *Adjuvant* Bulb used in medicine bag "to make the bag more potent." (141:508) *Unspecified* Bulbs eaten and used medicinally. (161:131)

Triticum aestivum, Common Wheat

Iroquois *Veterinary Aid* Wheat flour, rhizomes from another plant, and raspberry leaves given to cows at birthing. (118:67)

Trollius laxus, American Globeflower

Cherokee *Oral Aid* Infusion of leaves and stem used for "thrash." (66:36)

Tsuga canadensis, Eastern Hemlock

Abnaki *Antirheumatic* (*External*) Used as a medicine for rheumatism. (121:155) *Antirheumatic* (*Internal*) Infusion of leaves taken for rheumatism. (121:163) Decoction of leaves taken for rheumatism. (121:164) *Dermatological Aid* Used for "slight" itches. (121:155) **Algonquin**, **Quebec** *Antirheumatic* (*External*) Decoction of branches boiled down to a thick syrup or paste and used as a poultice for arthritis. *Cold Remedy* Infusion of inner bark taken for colds. *Dermatological Aid* Decoction of inner bark applied externally to eczema and other similar skin conditions. *Disinfectant* Poultice of crushed branch tips applied to the infected navel of an infant. *Gynecological Aid* Used in the sudatory by women experiencing complications in childbirth and for other complaints. *Pediatric Aid* Poultice of crushed branch tips applied to the infected navel of an infant. *Unspecified* Used in the sudatory by women experiencing complications in childbirth and for other complaints. Decoction of branches used as a medicinal tea. (14:125) **Cherokee** *Antidiarrheal* Root chewed "to check bowels." *Dermatological Aid* Poultice of bark used for itching armpits. *Gynecological Aid* Compound decoction used to aid in expelling afterbirth. *Kidney Aid* Infusion of stem tips taken for kidneys. (66:38) **Chippewa** *Anti-*

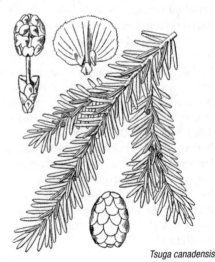

Tsuga canadensis

diarrheal Infusion of twigs taken for dysentery. (59:123) *Hemostat* Pulverized inner bark applied to wounds as a styptic. (43:356) **Delaware** *Antirheumatic (External)* Hot infusion of roots or twigs used as a steam treatment for muscular swellings and stiff joints. (151:36) **Delaware, Oklahoma** *Antirheumatic (External)* Decoction of roots or twigs used as herbal steam for rheumatism. (150:30, 80) *Herbal Steam* Infusion of roots or twigs used as herbal steam for rheumatism. (150:30) **Iroquois** *Antirheumatic (External)* Steam from decoction of leaves and bark used for rheumatism and as a foot soak. (73:268) *Antirheumatic (Internal)* Compound decoction taken for rheumatism. (73:269) *Blood Medicine* Fermented compound decoction taken when "blood gets bad and cold." (73:268) *Cold Remedy* Cold infusion of twigs and bark taken for mild colds with fever. Decoction of smashed needles taken for colds. Infusion of twigs and bark taken for colds. *Cough Medicine* Compound decoction taken for coughs. *Diaphoretic* Infusion of twigs and bark taken to induce sweating. (73:269) *Febrifuge* Fermented compound decoction taken for fever. (73:268) Cold infusion of twigs and bark taken for mild colds with fever. *Misc. Disease Remedy* Compound decoction taken for cholera. (73:269) *Orthopedic Aid* Fermented compound decoction taken for soreness. *Stimulant* Fermented compound decoction taken when a "person is tired." (73:268) *Tuberculosis Remedy* Compound decoction taken during early stages of consumption. *Venereal Aid* Compound powder poultice "put in bag, place penis in bag and tie around waist." (73:269) **Malecite** *Antidiarrheal* Infusion of young bark and fir buds or cones used for diarrhea. (96:244) Infusion of inside bark used for diarrhea. (96:255) *Cold Remedy* Infusion of boughs used for colds. (96:249) *Dermatological Aid* Outer layer of dried trees used as a powder for prickly heat. (96:250) *Kidney Aid* Infusion of boughs used for cold in the kidneys. (96:249) *Pediatric Aid* Outer layer of dried trees used for chafed babies. (96:250) *Unspecified* Bark used as medicine. (137:6) **Menominee** *Analgesic* Infusion of inner bark taken for abdominal pains. *Cold Remedy* Infusion of inner bark taken, 1 quart required, for cold. (128:46) *Dermatological Aid* Compound containing branches steamed for swellings. (44:134) *Diaphoretic* Leaves used in the sudatory. *Gastrointestinal Aid* Infusion of inner bark used for abdominal pains. (128:46) *Herbal Steam* Herbal steam from compound containing branches used for swellings. (44:134) **Micmac** *Antidiarrheal* Inner bark used for diarrhea. (32:62, 63) *Cold Remedy* Bark and stems used for colds. (32:62) *Cough Medicine* Bark used as cough medicine and for grippe. *Dermatological Aid* Inner bark used for chapped skin. (32:62, 63) *Gastrointestinal Aid* Parts of plant used for bowel, stomach, and internal troubles. *Kidney Aid* Roots and stems used for "cold in kidney." (32:62) *Misc. Disease Remedy* Bark used for grippe and inner bark used for scurvy. (32:62, 63) *Urinary Aid* Roots and stems used for "cold in bladder." (32:62) **Ojibwa** *Adjuvant* Leaves used to flavor medicinal tea. (130:380) Leaves made into a tea and used as a beverage and to disguise medicine. (130:408) *Dermatological Aid* Bark used for cuts, wounds, and bleeding wounds. *Hemostat* Bark used for bleeding wounds. (130:380) **Potawatomi** *Antidiarrheal* Compound of inner bark used for flux. *Cold Remedy* Infusion of leaves taken to cause perspiration, which broke up a cold. *Diaphoretic* Infusion of leaves taken to cause perspiration, which broke up a cold. (131:71)

***Tsuga caroliniana*, Carolina Hemlock**
Cherokee *Antidiarrheal* Root chewed "to check bowels." *Dermatological Aid* Poultice of bark used for itching armpits. *Gynecological Aid* Compound decoction used to aid in expelling afterbirth. (66:38) Decoction of roots taken to cause discharge of the afterbirth. (152:5) *Kidney Aid* Infusion of stem tips taken for kidneys. (66:38)

***Tsuga heterophylla*, Western Hemlock**
Bella Coola *Antirheumatic (External)* Poultice of compound containing gum applied to the arms for rheumatism. *Burn Dressing* Poultice of chewed leaves applied to burns. (127:51) Leaves chewed and used for burns. (158:198) *Dermatological Aid* Warm gum applied to cuts. *Heart Medicine* Poultice of compound containing gum applied to the chest for heart trouble. *Internal Medicine* Moxa of twigs applied to the skin for "various internal ailments." (127:51) Twigs burned and used to cauterize the skin for internal ailments. (158:198) **Che-**

halis *Tuberculosis Remedy* Decoction of pounded bark taken for tuberculosis. *Venereal Aid* Decoction of pounded bark taken for syphilis. (65:17) **Clallam** *Antihemorrhagic* Bark boiled, added to licorice ferns, and used for hemorrhages. (47:195) **Cowlitz** *Antihemorrhagic* Infusion of bark taken for hemorrhage. *Dermatological Aid* Infusion of plants used as wash for skin sores. Pitch used to prevent chapping. *Eye Medicine* Infusion of plants used as wash for sore eyes. (65:17) **Gitksan** *Gastrointestinal Aid* Cambium used as a "cleanser." *Liver Aid* Cambium used for the gallbladder. *Other* Inner bark used for elimination of hard or sharp swallowed objects. (61:152) **Hesquiat** *Antirheumatic (Internal)* Decoction or infusion of bark, from inside of a crevice, taken for rheumatic fever. *Dermatological Aid* Gum and deer grease used on fur seal hunters faces to prevent skin from cracking and peeling in the sun. Gum and deer grease used for healing sores on the face. Poultice of chewed needles used for burns. Pitch and deer fat used on faces to heal abrasions cause by rubbing on hunting camouflage. Pitch and deer fat used as salve to prevent and soothe sunburn. *Eye Medicine* Boughs used by girls, at puberty ceremony, to prevent eye disease to herself and future children. *Other* Decoction or infusion of bark, from inside of a crevice, taken for phlebitis. *Tuberculosis Remedy* Decoction or infusion of bark, from inside of a crevice, taken for tuberculosis and rheumatic fever. (159:44) **Hoh** *Emetic* Bark used as an emetic. (114:58) **Klallam** *Antihemorrhagic* Compound infusion of bark taken for hemorrhage. *Dietary Aid* Infusion of plant tips taken to stimulate appetite. *Tuberculosis Remedy* Infusion of plant tips taken for tuberculosis. (65:17) **Kwakiutl** *Antidiarrheal* Compound decoction of plants or bark taken for diarrhea. (157:264) *Burn Dressing* Cold infusion of scraped, pounded bark applied to burns. *Dermatological Aid* Cold infusion of scraped, pounded bark applied to sores. Moxa of twigs used to cauterize warts and moles. *Eye Medicine* Infusion of boughs used as a wash for upper lids of inflamed eyes. *Gynecological Aid* Hemlock used as wash and tree tips prayed to by pregnant women to aid delivery. *Hunting Medicine* Branches rubbed on hunters and fishermen to purify them. (157:270) **Kwakwaka'wakw** *Ceremonial Medicine* Plant considered to have special powers to

purify and cure. (35:71) **Makah** *Dermatological Aid* Pitch used to prevent sunburn. Poultice of bark applied to obstinate sores. (65:17) Pitch used as a sunburn preventative and rubbed on hair to remove lice. (160:74) *Hemostat* Poultice of plant applied to bleeding wounds. *Internal Medicine* Decoction of plant taken for internal injury. (65:17) **Nitinaht** *Dermatological Aid* Infusion of bark, grand fir and red alder barks taken for bruises. *Internal Medicine* Infusion of bark, grand fir and red alder barks taken for internal injuries. *Orthopedic Aid* Infusion of bark, grand fir and red alder barks taken for broken bones. (160:74) **Oweekeno** *Ceremonial Medicine* Plant considered to have special powers to purify and cure. (35:71) **Quileute** *Dermatological Aid* Poultice of chewed plants applied to swellings. (65:17) *Emetic* Bark used as an emetic. (114:58) **Quinault** *Cold Remedy* Poultice of pitch and ground bark applied to child's chest for a cold. *Laxative* Infusion of plants taken as a laxative. *Pediatric Aid* Poultice of pitch and ground bark applied to child's chest for a cold. (65:17) **Shuswap** *Tuberculosis Remedy* Decoction of bark taken for tuberculosis. (102:53) **Skagit** *Dermatological Aid* and *Eye Medicine* Infusion of plants used as wash for sore eyes. *Throat Aid* Infusion of bark taken for sore throats. (65:17) **Thompson** *Cold Remedy* Infusion of bark used for colds. *Disinfectant* Boughs considered an important disinfectant. One informant noted that those desiring to cleanse themselves would scrub their bodies with the branches. *Misc. Disease Remedy* Infusion of bark used for influenza. (161:111)

Tsuga mertensiana, Mountain Hemlock
Bella Coola *Burn Dressing* Poultice of chewed leaves applied to burns. *Dermatological Aid* Warm gum applied to cuts. *Internal Medicine* Moxa of twigs applied to the skin for "various internal ailments." (127:51) **Hoh** *Emetic* Bark used as an emetic. (114:58) **Kwakiutl** *Ceremonial Medicine*, *Dermatological Aid*, and *Pediatric Aid* Bark used in ritual to make children as light-skinned as the inner bark. (157:271) **Quileute** *Emetic* Bark used as an emetic. (114:58) **Thompson** *Cold Remedy* Infusion of bark used for colds. *Disinfectant* Boughs steamed or rubbed on furniture and used as a room deodorizer and disinfectant. *Misc. Disease Remedy* Infusion of bark used for influenza.

(161:111) **Tlingit** *Toothache Remedy* Compound containing warmed seeds used for toothache. *Venereal Aid* Compound poultice of sap applied for syphilis. (as *Pinus mertensiana* 89:284)

Turricula parryi, Common Turricula
Kawaiisu *Antirheumatic* (*External*) Infusion of leaves used as a wash for rheumatism. *Dermatological Aid* Infusion of leaves used as a wash for swellings. (180:68) **Luiseño** *Unspecified* Plant used for medicinal purposes. (as *Eriodictyon parryi* 132:230)

Tussilago farfara, Coltsfoot
Iroquois *Cough Medicine* and *Tuberculosis Remedy* Compound infusion of roots taken as a consumption cough medicine. (73:473)

Typha angustifolia, Narrowleaf Cattail
Malecite *Kidney Aid* Infusion of one root used for gravel. (96:257) **Micmac** *Urinary Aid* Roots used for gravel. (32:63)

Typha latifolia, Broadleaf Cattail
Algonquin, Quebec *Dermatological Aid* Poultice of crushed roots applied to wounds. *Disinfectant* Poultice of crushed roots applied to infections. (14:132) **Apache, Mescalero** *Unspecified* Pollen used as medicine. (10:46) **Cahuilla** *Dermatological Aid* Roots used for bleeding wounds. (11:142) **Cheyenne** *Ceremonial Medicine* Leaves used in the Sun Dance ceremony. (69:13) *Gastrointesti-*

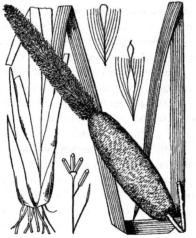
Typha latifolia

nal Aid Infusion of dried roots and white base of leaves taken for abdominal cramps. (63:170) Infusion of dried, pulverized root and white base of the leaves taken for abdominal cramps. (64:170) **Dakota** *Burn Dressing* Down used as a dressing for burns and scalds. *Dermatological Aid* and *Pediatric Aid* Down used on infants to prevent chafing. (58:64, 65) **Delaware** *Kidney Aid* Roots used for kidney stones. (151:36) **Delaware, Oklahoma** *Kidney Aid* Root used to dissolve kidney stones. (150:30, 80) **Houma** *Pulmonary Aid* Decoction of stalks taken for whooping cough. (135:60) **Iroquois** *Gynecological Aid* "Patient sleeps on mattress made of plant" for cysts of breast. *Hemostat* Infusion of roots used as a wash for bleeding cuts. *Misc. Disease Remedy* "Patient sleeps on mattress made of plant" for cysts of yellow fever. *Orthopedic Aid* Decoction of smashed root applied as poultice for sprains. *Venereal Aid* Root chewed by women for gonorrhea. *Veterinary Aid* Infusion of roots used as a wash for horses with bleeding cuts. (73:271) **Mahuna** *Hemostat* and *Pediatric Aid* Plant used for newborns with bleeding navels. (117:56) **Malecite** *Dermatological Aid* Greased leaves used for sores. (96:246) **Meskwaki** *Dermatological Aid* Poultice of fuzz applied to old sores on neck. (129:248) **Micmac** *Dermatological Aid* Leaves used for sores. (32:63) **Montana Indian** *Burn Dressing* Poultice of fruit spikes' "down" applied to burns and scalds. (15:25) **Navajo, Ramah** *Ceremonial Medicine* and *Emetic* Whole plant used as a ceremonial emetic. (165:14, 15) **Ojibwa** *Dermatological Aid* Poultice of root inner skin applied to carbuncles and boils. (4:2306) **Other** Fruit fuzz used as a war medicine. (130:390) **Ojibwa, South** *Dermatological Aid* Poultice of crushed root applied to sores. (77:200) **Okanagan-Colville** *Dermatological Aid* Cottony fluff used as dressing for wounds. (162:57) **Omaha** *Burn Dressing* Down used as a dressing for burns and scalds. (58:64, 65) *Ceremonial Medicine* Plant used in various rituals. (56:322) *Dermatological Aid* and *Pediatric Aid* Down used on infants to prevent chafing. **Pawnee** *Burn Dressing* Down used as a dressing for burns and scalds. *Dermatological Aid* and *Pediatric Aid* Down used on infants to prevent chafing. (58:64, 65) **Plains Indian** *Dermatological Aid* and *Pediatric Aid* Down used on infants to prevent chafing.

(68:60) **Ponca** *Burn Dressing* Down used as a dressing for burns and scalds. *Dermatological Aid* and *Pediatric Aid* Down used on infants to prevent chafing. (58:64, 65) **Potawatomi** *Dermatological Aid* Poultice of pounded root applied to inflammations. (131:85) **Sioux** *Burn Dressing* Poultice of fruit spikes' "down" applied to burns and scalds. *Dermatological Aid* and *Misc. Disease Remedy* Poultice of fruit spikes, down, and coyote fat applied to smallpox pustules. (15:25) **Washo** *Antidiarrheal* Young flowering heads eaten for diarrhea. (155:146) **Winnebago** *Burn Dressing* Down used as a dressing for burns and scalds. *Dermatological Aid* and *Pediatric Aid* Down used on infants to prevent chafing. (58:64, 65)

Ulmus americana, American Elm
Cheyenne *Gynecological Aid* and *Pediatric Aid* Infusion of bark taken by pregnant women to insure stability of children. (69:39) **Choctaw** *Analgesic* and *Gynecological Aid* Decoction of inner bark taken for menstrual cramps. (152:18) **Delaware** *Cold Remedy* Infusion of inner bark used for colds. *Cough Medicine* Infusion of inner bark used for severe coughs. (151:31) **Delaware, Oklahoma** *Cold Remedy* Infusion of inner bark taken for colds. *Cough Medicine* Infusion of inner bark taken for severe coughs. (150:26, 80) **Houma** *Antidiarrheal* Compound decoction of bark taken for dysentery. (135:56) **Iroquois** *Antidiarrheal* and *Antiemetic* Compound decoction taken for "summer disease—vomiting, diarrhea and cramps." *Antihemorrhagic* Compound decoction with smashed twigs taken for internal hemorrhage. *Gastrointestinal Aid* Compound decoction taken for "summer disease": vomiting, diarrhea, and cramps. *Gynecological Aid* Compound decoction of bark taken to facilitate childbirth and for parturition. Infusion of root bark taken for excessive menstruation. *Hemorrhoid Remedy* Infusion taken for piles caused by contact with menstruating woman. *Orthopedic Aid* Compound decoction of bark taken for broken bones. (73:304) *Other* Infusion of bark used for ruptures caused by exaggerated efforts. (118:40) **Koasati** *Dermatological Aid* Decoction of bark taken and used as a wash for gun wounds. *Gastrointestinal Aid* Infusion of inner bark taken

and used as a bath for appendicitis. (152:18) **Meskwaki** *Eye Medicine* Decoction of root bark applied to sore eyes as an eye lotion. (129:251) **Mohegan** *Cold Remedy* Infusion of bark taken for colds. (149:266) Infusion of inner bark taken for colds. (151:76, 132) *Cough Medicine* Infusion of bark taken for coughs. (149:266) Infusion of inner bark taken for coughs. (151:76, 132) **Montana Indian** *Cancer Treatment* Inner bark used as an emollient for tumors. (15:25) **Ojibwa** *Venereal Aid* Infusion of root bark taken for gonorrhea. (112:231) **Penobscot** *Antihemorrhagic* Infusion of bark taken for "bleeding at the lungs." *Pulmonary Aid* Infusion of bark taken for pulmonary hemorrhage. (133:311) **Potawatomi** *Analgesic* Bark used for cramps. *Antidiarrheal* Bark used for diarrhea. (131:86)

Ulmus rubra, Slippery Elm
Alabama *Gynecological Aid* Decoction of bark and gunpowder taken as sympathetic magic for delayed labor. (as *U. fulva* 148:665) Decoction of bark taken for prolonged labor. **Catawba** *Tuberculosis Remedy* Bark used for consumption. (as *U. fulva* 152:19) **Cherokee** *Antidiarrheal* Taken to soothe stomach and bowels and for dysentery and bowels of pregnant women. (66:33) Decoction of inner bark taken for dysentery. (as *U. fulva* 152:19) *Burn Dressing* Poultice of inside bark used for burns. *Cold Remedy* Used for colds. *Cough Medicine* Used for coughs. *Dermatological Aid* Poultice of inside bark used for old sores and wounds. *Eye Medicine* Decoction of bark used to wash eyes. *Gastrointestinal Aid* Taken to soothe stomach and bowels and for heartburn and bowels of pregnant women. *Gynecological Aid* Taken to soothe stomach and bowels and for heartburn and bowels of pregnant women. (66:33) Decoction of bark taken to ease labor. (as *U. fulva* 152:19) *Laxative* Used as a mild laxative and "soothes stomach and bowels." *Respiratory Aid* Used for catarrh. *Throat Aid* Used for "quinsies." *Tuberculosis Remedy* Used for "quinsies," coughs, "consumptions and breast complaints." (66:33) **Chippewa** *Throat Aid* Decoction of bark gargled or dried root chewed for sore throat. (as *U. fulva* 43:342) **Creek** *Witchcraft Medicine* Decoction of bark with gunpowder taken to speed delivery, sympathetic magic. (as *U. fulva* 148:665) **Dakota** *Laxative* Decoction of in-

ner bark taken as a laxative. (as _U. fulva_ 58:76)
Iroquois _Blood Medicine_ Complex compound
used as a blood purifier. _Emetic_ Compound decoction taken to vomit for sleepiness and weakness.
Eye Medicine Infusion of bark used as drops and
as a wash for sore eyes. (73:305) _Gastrointestinal
Aid_ Decoction of bark taken to clean stomach and
used for biliousness. (73:306) _Gynecological Aid_
Compound decoction of bark taken to facilitate
childbirth and for parturition. Infusion of bark
taken for dry birth. (73:305) _Kidney Aid_ Decoction of bark taken for kidneys. (73:306) _Respira-
tory Aid_ Compound of leaves smoked and exhaled
through the nostrils for catarrh. _Stimulant_ Compound decoction with black center of tree taken
when feeling drowsy. (73:305) _Throat Aid_ Raw
bark chewed for sore throats. (73:306) _Tubercu-
losis Remedy_ Compound decoction used as a poultice for infected and swollen tubercular glands.
(73:304) **Kiowa** _Oral Aid_ Fresh, inner bark used
as a masticatory. (as _U. fulva_ 166:23) **Mahuna**
Orthopedic Aid Poultice of bark applied to broken
and fractured arms or legs. (as _U. pubescens_
117:27) **Menominee** _Cathartic_ Infusion of inner
bark taken as a physic. _Dermatological Aid_ Poultice of inner bark applied to draw pus from a
wound. (as _U. fulva_ 128:56, 57) **Meskwaki** _Der-
matological Aid_ Poultice of bark applied to old
sores. _Gynecological Aid_ Decoction of root taken
by women to ease childbirth. (as _U. fulva_ 129:251)
Micmac _Dermatological Aid_ Bark used for suppurating wounds. _Pulmonary Aid_ Bark used for
bleeding lungs. (as _U. fulva_ 32:63) **Mohegan**

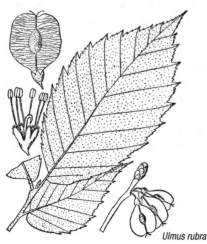

Ulmus rubra

Cough Medicine Bark used for coughs. (151:132)
Pulmonary Aid Inner bark chewed to soothe the
lungs. (151:76) _Throat Aid_ Inner bark chewed for
sore throat. (151:76, 132) **Ojibwa** _Dermatological
Aid_ Infusion of roots taken and used as a wash for
bleeding foot cuts. _Gastrointestinal Aid_ Infusion
of plants taken for stomach troubles. _Hemostat_ Infusion of roots taken and used as a wash for bleeding foot cuts. (as _U. fluva_ 112:231) _Throat Aid_
Inner bark used for dry, sore throat. (as _U. fulva_
130:392) _Venereal Aid_ Plant used for gonorrhea.
(as _U. fluva_ 112:240) **Omaha** _Laxative_ Decoction
of inner bark taken as a laxative. **Pawnee** _Laxative_
Decoction of inner bark taken as a laxative. **Ponca**
Laxative Decoction of inner bark taken as a laxative. (as _U. fulva_ 58:76) **Potawatomi** _Dermatolog-
ical Aid_ Inner bark used for boils. _Eye Medicine_
Poultice of chewed inner bark applied to eye inflammations. _Throat Aid_ Inner bark used to lubricate throat for removal of lodged bone. (as _U. fulva_
131:86, 87) **Winnebago** _Laxative_ Decoction of
inner bark taken as a laxative. (as _U. fulva_ 58:76)

Umbellularia californica, California Laurel
Cahuilla _Analgesic_ Leaves used for headaches.
(11:143) **Karok** _Analgesic_ Infusion of plant taken
by women for the pains of afterbirth. _Cold Remedy_
Plant used as steam bath or burning boughs used
to fumigate house for colds. (125:383) _Dermato-
logical Aid_ Poultice of ground seeds applied to
sores. (5:59) _Disinfectant_ Boughs used in fire to
fumigate the house for colds and other sicknesses.
Gynecological Aid Infusion of plant taken by wom-
en for the pains of afterbirth. _Panacea_ Plant used
as steam bath or burning bough to fumigate house
for any sickness. (125:383) **Mendocino Indian**
Analgesic Decoction taken, used as wash, or poultice of leaves applied for headaches. _Antirheumat-
ic (External)_ Infusion of leaves used as a bath for
rheumatism. _Dermatological Aid_ Decoction of
leaves used as wash for vermin on the head. _Gas-
trointestinal Aid_ Decoction of plant taken for
stomachaches and headaches. Poultice of leaves
applied as counterirritant for chronic stomach
complaints. _Panacea_ Burning leaf vapor used for
many diseases. _Stimulant_ Nuts eaten as a stimulant. (33:349) **Miwok** _Analgesic_ Poultice of leaves
and twigs bound to forehead for headaches. (8:174)
Pomo _Analgesic_ Poultice of heated leaves applied

for rheumatic and neuralgic pains. *Antirheumatic (External)* Poultice of heated leaves applied for rheumatic pains. (54:13) **Pomo, Kashaya** *Analgesic* Poultice of leaves used for rheumatic and neuralgic pains. Indian doctor would sing and hit you with little branches for pain or headache. *Antirheumatic (External)* Poultice of leaves used for rheumatic pains. *Cold Remedy* Decoction of leaves taken for colds. Indian doctor would sing and hit you with little branches for a cold. *Dermatological Aid* Decoction of leaves used to wash sores. Peppernut charcoal rubbed into a man's mustache to groom it. *Gynecological Aid* Decoction of leaves taken for menstrual cramps and clotting. *Respiratory Aid* Decoction of leaves taken to clear up "slime" in the chest. *Throat Aid* Decoction of leaves taken for sore throats. (60:90) **Yuki** *Analgesic* Crushed leaves inhaled for headaches. (39:47) Poultice of crushed leaves applied as compress for headaches. *Antirheumatic (External)* Decoction of leaves used as wash for rheumatism. (98:43) *Respiratory Aid* Crushed leaves inhaled to open the nasal passages. (39:47) **Yurok** *Unspecified* Plant used for medicinal purposes. (5:59)

Urtica dioica, Stinging Nettle
Cherokee *Gastrointestinal Aid* Taken for upset stomach. *Misc. Disease Remedy* Infusion taken for "ague." (66:46) **Cree, Woodlands** *Gynecological Aid* Decoction of plant taken to keep blood flowing after childbirth. (91:63) **Hesquiat** *Analgesic* Nettles rubbed on body for aches, pains, and back-

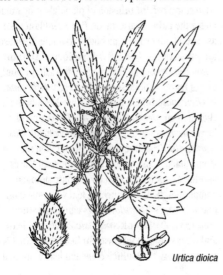

Urtica dioica

aches. *Antirheumatic (External)* Poultice of steamed leaves and roots used on swollen, sore, arthritic legs, ankles, and joints. *Gastrointestinal Aid* Nettles rubbed on stomach when sore. (159:76) **Iroquois** *Witchcraft Medicine* Compound of plant and dried snake's blood used as a "witching medicine." (73:307) **Kwakiutl** *Analgesic* Plant rubbed on the skin for chest pains. *Dermatological Aid* Plant juice rubbed into the scalp to prevent hair from falling out. *Gynecological Aid* Plant juice taken by overdue, pregnant women. *Other* Moxa of plant fiber used to cauterize the skin for various ailments. *Venereal Aid* Plant used for locomotor ataxia. (157:292) **Kwakiutl, Southern** *Analgesic* Fiber used to cauterize headaches. *Antirheumatic (External)* Fiber used to cauterize swellings. (157:297) **Lakota** *Gastrointestinal Aid* Infusion of roots taken for stomach pains. (116:61) **Makah** *Hunting Medicine* Used to rub the whale hunters' bodies in order to be strong. Leaves rubbed on fishing line to give it a green color or used as medicine for good fishing. *Oral Aid* Stems put under splints to hasten the healing process. *Reproductive Aid* Infusion of roots given to expectant mothers. *Stimulant* Used to rub down after the morning bath. (55:246) **Nitinaht** *Antirheumatic (External)* Plants whipped over body for arthritis and rheumatism. *Tonic* Young shoots chewed and swallowed as a tonic to prevent sickness. *Unspecified* Plants whipped over body by married persons for affection and faithfulness of spouses. (160:128) **Okanagan-Colville** *Antirheumatic (External)* Fresh plants used to beat the skin after "sweathousing" and for rheumatic and arthritic pain. (162:140) **Paiute, Northern** *Antirheumatic (External)* Leaves and stalks used to whip aching arms and legs for rheumatism. *Dermatological Aid* Decoction of roots taken for hives and itches. (49:126) **Shuswap** *Analgesic* and *Antirheumatic (External)* Decoction of stems and roots used as a sweat bath for rheumatism pain. *Dermatological Aid* Used for bathing and drinking. *Herbal Steam* Decoction of stems and roots used as a sweat bath for rheumatism pain. (102:70) **Thompson** *Antirheumatic (External)* Nettles used for arthritis. One informant said that a neighboring woman who had arthritis hit her skin all over with nettles and within 2 months, she was getting strong and healthy again. *Dermatological Aid* Decoction of roots used as a hair tonic for growing long, silky hair. Plant tops used for skin disease. *Hemorrhoid Remedy* Decoction of roots used as a soaking solution for bleeding hemorrhoids. *Orthopedic Aid* Poultice of leaves and stalks used for paralyzed limbs. *Unspecified* Infusion of leaves and tops used as medicine. (161:289)

***Urtica dioica* ssp. *gracilis*,** California Nettle **Abnaki** *Hemostat* Used for bloody noses. (as *U. procera* 121:154) Powdered leaves used as a snuff for nosebleeds. (as *U. procera* 121:166) **Bella Coola** *Analgesic* and *Antirheumatic* (*External*) Used in a sweat bath for pains similar to rheumatism all over the body. (as *U. lyallii* 127:55) *Hemostat* Burning stem fibers used to cauterize sores and swellings. (158:211) *Herbal Steam* Used in a sweat bath for pains similar to rheumatism all over the body. *Orthopedic Aid* Used to sting paralyzed limbs daily to cause sores and revive sensation. (as *U. lyallii* 127:55) **Carrier** *Analgesic* Used as whip for pain. *Dermatological Aid* Rubbed on the skin for rashes. (as *U. gracilis* 26:83) **Chehalis** *Antirheumatic* (*External*) Whole stalk used as a whip on a person with rheumatism. *Dermatological Aid* Decoction of roots used as a hair wash. (as *U. lyallii* 65:28) **Chippewa** *Antidiarrheal* Infusion of root taken for dysentery. (as *U. gracilis* 43:344) *Diuretic* Compound decoction of root taken for "stoppage of urine." (as *U. gracilis* 43:348) **Cowlitz** *Gynecological Aid* Infusion of nettles taken by women about to deliver a child. *Orthopedic Aid* Poultice of sprouts applied or person whipped with stalk for paralysis. (as *U. lyallii* 65:28) **Gitksan** *Antihemorrhagic* Decoction of plant taken for hemorrhage and many illnesses. *Unspecified* Decoction of entire plant taken for many illnesses. *Urinary Aid* Decoction of plant taken for bladder trouble and many illnesses. (as *U. lyallii* 127:55) **Haisla & Hanaksiala** *Antirheumatic* (*External*) Poultice of roots applied to aches and swollen joints. (35:294) **Klallam** *Analgesic* Infusion of stalks rubbed on the body for soreness or stiffness. *Orthopedic Aid* Infusion of stalks rubbed on the body for soreness or stiffness. *Panacea* Infusion of nettles taken for many ailments. **Lummi** *Gynecological Aid* Infusion of nettles taken by women to relax the muscles during childbirth. (as *U. lyallii* 65:28) **Miwok** *Antirheumatic*

(*External*) Decoction of root used as a bath for rheumatism. Leaf powder rubbed on affected rheumatic body parts. (as *U. gracilis* 8:174) **Navajo, Ramah** *Poison* Plant considered poisonous. (as *U. gracilis* 165:23) **Ojibwa** *Dermatological Aid* Poultice of soaked leaves applied to heat rash. (as *U. lyallii* 130:392) **Paiute** *Antirheumatic* (*External*) Decoction of root used as a wash for rheumatism. *Cold Remedy* Decoction of leaves taken for colds. *Diaphoretic, Herbal Steam,* and *Misc. Disease Remedy* Plant used as an inhalant in the sweat bath for grippe or pneumonia. *Pulmonary Aid* Plant fumes inhaled in the sweat bath for pneumonia or grippe. *Unspecified* Plant used as switch on body as a counterirritant for unspecified purposes. (as *U. gracilis* 155:146) **Pomo, Kashaya** *Analgesic* Nettle used to strike the skin as a counterirritant for rheumatism and other such pains. *Antirheumatic* (*External*) Nettle used to strike the skin as a counterirritant for rheumatism. (as *U. lyallii* 60:77) **Potawatomi** *Febrifuge* Infusion of root used for intermittent fevers. *Unspecified* Infusion of leaves used medicinally for unspecified purposes. (as *U. lyallii* 131:87) **Quileute** *Antirheumatic* (*External*) Whole stalk used as a whip on a person with rheumatism. *Antirheumatic* (*Internal*) Infusion of pounded roots taken for rheumatism. **Quinault** *Analgesic* Decoction of peeled bark taken for headaches. *Gynecological Aid* Plant tips chewed by women during labor. *Hemostat* Decoction of peeled bark taken for nosebleeds. *Orthopedic Aid* Whole stalk used as a whip on a person with paralysis. **Samish** *Tonic* Decoction of plant taken as a general tonic. (as *U. lyallii* 65:28) **Shoshoni** *Antirheumatic* (*External*) Hot poultice of mashed leaves applied for rheumatism. *Blood Medicine* Compound decoction of roots taken as a blood tonic and for general debility. *Cold Remedy* Decoction of leaves taken for colds. *Tonic* Compound decoction of root taken as a blood tonic and for general debility. (as *U. gracilis* 155:146) **Sioux** *Diuretic* Root used for urine retention. (as *U. gracilis* 15:25) **Skagit** *Cold Remedy* Decoction of plant taken for colds. **Skokomish** *Dermatological Aid* Decoction of roots used as a hair wash. **Snohomish** *Cold Remedy* Infusion of nettles taken or nettles rubbed on the body for colds. **Squaxin** *Gynecological Aid* Infusion of crushed leaves taken by women having difficulties in childbirth. **Swinomish** *Tonic* Decoction of plant taken as a general tonic. (as *U. lyallii* 65:28) **Tanaina** *Antirheumatic (Internal)* Plant used for diseases from rheumatism to tuberculosis. *Misc. Disease Remedy* Plant used for diseases from rheumatism to tuberculosis. *Tuberculosis Remedy* Plant used for diseases from rheumatism to tuberculosis. (as *U. lyallii* 126:329) **Thompson** *Orthopedic Aid* Plant dipped in water and rubbed on stiff, sore joints and muscles. (as *U. lyallii* 141:471, 472) **Tolowa** *Dermatological Aid* Poultice of fresh, pounded leaves applied to skin inflammations. (as *U. lyallii* 5:60)

Urtica dioica ssp. *holosericea*, Stinging Nettle

Cahuilla *Analgesic* Used for headaches and sore backs. *Antirheumatic (External)* Used for rheumatism and muscular stiffness. (as *U. holosericea* 11:143) **Diegueño** *Antirheumatic (External)* Nettles used to whip rheumatic or arthritic joints. (as *U. holosericea* 70:43) **Kawaiisu** *Analgesic* Poultice of leaves applied for headaches. Poultice of mashed plant applied to the neck for pain. Stems and leaves used as a counterirritant for sore limbs and back. *Dermatological Aid* "Children walk through nettles to toughen their skin." Poultice of leaves applied for sores. *Orthopedic Aid* Stems and leaves used as a counterirritant for sore limbs and back. *Pediatric Aid* "Children walk through nettles to prepare them for practice of witchcraft." "Children walk through nettles to toughen their skin." "Younger people walk through nettles to procure dreams." *Psychological Aid* "Younger people walk through nettles to procure dreams." *Witchcraft Medicine* "Children walk through nettles to prepare them for practice of witchcraft." (as *U. holosericea* 180:68) **Mahuna** *Antirheumatic (External)* Leaves rubbed on parts ailing from inflammatory rheumatism. (as *U. holosericea* 117:59) **Miwok** *Analgesic* Branch used to strike affected parts for certain pains. (as *U. gracilis* var. *holosericea* 8:174) **Pomo** *Analgesic* and *Antirheumatic (External)* Nettle used to strike skin as a counterirritant for rheumatic pains. (as *U. gracilis* var. *holosericea* 54:13)

Urtica urens, Dwarf Nettle

Shuswap *Analgesic* and *Antirheumatic (External)* Decoction of stems and roots used as a sweat bath for rheumatism pain. *Dermatological Aid* Used for bathing and drinking. *Herbal Steam* Decoction of stems and roots used as a sweat bath for rheumatism pain. (102:70)

Usnea longissima

Nitinaht *Dermatological Aid* Used for wound dressing material and as bandages. (maidenhair moss 160:55)

Uvularia grandiflora, Largeflower Bellwort

Menominee *Dermatological Aid* Plant used for swellings. (128:41) **Ojibwa** *Analgesic* and *Gastrointestinal Aid* Root used for stomach pain, perhaps pleurisy. *Pulmonary Aid* Root used for "pain in the solar plexus, which may mean pleurisy." (130:374) **Potawatomi** *Analgesic* Infusion of root used for backache or with lard as a salve for sore muscles. (131:56, 57) *Orthopedic Aid* Infusion of root mixed with lard and used as salve to massage sore muscles and tendons. Infusion of root used for backaches. (131:64)

Uvularia perfoliata, Perfoliate Bellwort

Iroquois *Cough Medicine* Infusion of roots given to children as cough medicine. *Eye Medicine* Infusion of smashed roots used as a wash for sore eyes of any degree. *Orthopedic Aid* Plant used several ways, internally and externally, for broken bones. *Pediatric Aid* Infusion of roots given to children as cough medicine. (73:280)

Uvularia sessilifolia, Sessileleaf Bellwort

Cherokee *Antidiarrheal* Infusion of root taken for diarrhea. *Dermatological Aid* Used as poultice for boils. (66:25) **Iroquois** *Blood Medicine* Infusion of roots taken as a blood purifier. *Orthopedic Aid* Infusion of roots taken and roots used as a poultice for broken bones. (73:281) **Ojibwa** *Hunting Medicine* Root used as a part of the hunting medicine to bring a buck deer near the hunter. (as *Oakesia sessilifolia* 130:430)

V *Vaccinium angustifolium*,
　　Lowbush Blueberry
Algonquin, **Quebec** *Gastrointestinal Aid* Infusion of leaves given to infants for colic. *Gynecological Aid* Infusion of leaves used by women after a miscarriage. Infusion of roots used by women to induce labor. *Pediatric Aid* Infusion of leaves given to infants for colic. (14:217) **Chippewa** *Psychological Aid* Dried flowers placed on hot stones as inhalant for "craziness." (43:338) **Iroquois** *Ceremonial Medicine* Berries used ceremonially by those desiring health and prosperity for the coming season. (as *V. pennsylvanicum* 170:142) **Ojibwa** *Blood Medicine* Infusion of leaves taken as a blood purifier. (as *V. pennsylvanicum* 130:369)

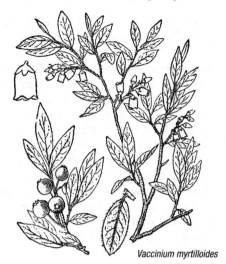

Vaccinium myrtilloides

Vaccinium macrocarpon, Cranberry
Montagnais *Pulmonary Aid* Infusion of branches used as a medicine for pleurisy. (as *Oxycoccus macrocarpus* 133:316)

Vaccinium membranaceum, Blue Huckleberry
Flathead *Antirheumatic* (*Internal*) Infusion of roots and stems taken for rheumatism and arthritis. *Heart Medicine* Infusion of roots and stems taken for heart trouble. (as *V. globulare* 68:63)

Vaccinium myrsinites, Shiny Blueberry
Seminole *Analgesic* and *Antidiarrheal* Infusion of leaves taken for sun sickness: eye disease, headache, high fever and diarrhea. (145:208) *Ceremonial Medicine* Infusion of plant added to food after a recent death. (145:342) *Cold Remedy* Infusion of plant taken for colds. (145:283) *Emetic* Plant used as an emetic during religious ceremonies. (145:409) *Eye Medicine* and *Febrifuge* Infusion of leaves taken for sun sickness: eye disease, headache, high fever, and diarrhea. (145:208) Infusion of plant taken for fevers. (145:283) *Pediatric Aid* Plant used for chronically ill babies. (145:328) *Stimulant* Decoction of roots used as a bath for hog sickness: unconsciousness. (145:229) *Unspecified* Plant used for medicinal purposes. (145:162)

Vaccinium myrtilloides, Velvetleaf Huckleberry
Cree, **Woodlands** *Abortifacient* Decoction of leafy stems, or of plant, used to bring menstruation. *Contraceptive* Decoction of stems used to prevent pregnancy. *Diaphoretic* Decoction of leafy stem, or of plant, used to make a person sweat. *Gynecological Aid* Decoction of leafy stems, or of plant, used as a "woman's medicine," used to bring blood after childbirth, and used to slow excessive menstrual bleeding. *Reproductive Aid* Decoction of leafy stems taken to prevent miscarriage. Decoction of plant taken to prevent miscarriage. (91:63) **Potawatomi** *Unspecified* Root bark used for unspecified ailment. (as *V. canadense* 131:57)

Vaccinium ovalifolium, Ovalleaf Blueberry
Makah *Gynecological Aid* Infusion of leaves and sugar given to mothers after childbirth. (55:305)

Vaccinium ovatum, Evergreen Huckleberry
Makah *Gynecological Aid* Infusion of leaves and sugar given to mothers after childbirth to gain their strength. (55:306) **Pomo**, **Kashaya** *Misc. Disease Remedy* Decoction of leaves taken for diabetes. (60:60)

Vaccinium oxycoccos, Small Cranberry
Mohegan *Unspecified* Plant used medicinally for unspecified purpose. (as *Oxycoccus microcarpus* 151:130) **Ojibwa** *Antiemetic* Infusion of plant taken by person with slight nausea. (130:369)

Vaccinium parvifolium, Red Huckleberry
Skagit *Cold Remedy* Decoction of bark taken for

colds. (65:44) **Skagit**, **Upper** *Cold Remedy* Decoction of bark taken for colds. (154:38)

Vaccinium scoparium, Grouse Whortleberry **Cheyenne** *Antiemetic* Infusion of dried leaves and stems taken for nausea. (63:183) Infusion of dried, pulverized leaves and stems taken for nausea. (64:183) *Dietary Aid* Dried berries given to children for poor appetites. (63:183) Dried, pulverized berries given to children with poor appetites. Infusion of dried, pulverized leaves and stems taken to increase appetite. (64:183) *Pediatric Aid* Dried berries given to children for poor appetites. (63:183) Dried, pulverized berries given to children with poor appetites. (64:183)

Vaccinium uliginosum, Bog Blueberry **Makah** *Gynecological Aid* Infusion of leaves and sugar given to mothers a few days after childbirth to gain their strength. (55:309)

Vaccinium vitis-idaea, Lingonberry **Tanana**, **Upper** *Cold Remedy* Berries eaten raw or juice used for colds. *Cough Medicine* Berries eaten raw or juice used for coughs. *Throat Aid* Raw berries chewed or juice gargled for sore throat. (86:9)

Valeriana acutiloba, Sharpleaf Valerian **Navajo**, **Ramah** *Cough Medicine* Plant used for cough. *Hunting Medicine* Plant rubbed on hunter's body for good luck in hunting. *Misc. Disease Remedy* Plant used for influenza. *Tuberculosis Remedy* Plant used for tuberculosis. *Witchcraft Medicine* Plant used for protection from witches. (165:45)

Valeriana capitata, Capitate Valerian **Eskimo** *Gastrointestinal Aid* Plant used for stomach troubles. (126:325) **Eskimo**, **Inuktitut** *Gastrointestinal Aid* Used for "stomach troubles." (176:182)

Valeriana dioica var. *sylvatica*, Woods Valerian **Blackfoot** *Gastrointestinal Aid* Decoction of roots taken for stomach troubles. (as *V. septentrionalis* 82:56) Hot drink made from root taken for stomach trouble. (as *V. septentrionalis* 95:275) Infusion of roots taken for stomach trouble. (as *V.*

septentrionalis 98:45) *Veterinary Aid* Decoction of roots given to horses for colic or distemper. (as *V. septentrionalis* 82:56) **Carrier**, **Northern** *Dermatological Aid* Oil of blossoms mixed with bear fat and used as a hair tonic to help growth. (as *V. septentrionalis* 127:64) **Cree**, **Woodlands** *Analgesic* Chewed roots rubbed on the head and temples for headaches. *Anticonvulsive* Poultice of roots applied externally, especially to babies, for seizures. *Cold Remedy* Roots used in a smoking mixture for colds. *Ear Medicine* Poultice of chewed roots applied to the ear for earaches. *Gynecological Aid* Powdered roots and many other herbs used for menstrual troubles. *Love Medicine* Roots used as a love medicine to attract a person whose affections were desired. It was a kind of bad medicine and viewed as a curse. The root of this plant was said by some to be an ingredient in love medicine; others denied this. *Panacea* Powdered roots and many other herbs used for various ailments. Infusion of roots used as an all purpose medicine. *Pediatric Aid* Poultice of roots applied externally, especially to babies, for seizures. *Pulmonary Aid* Decoction of roots used for pneumonia. (as *V. septentrionalis* 91:64) **Gosiute** *Poison* Roots used for arrow poison. (as *V. sylvatica* 31:384) **Thompson** *Adjuvant* Dried, powdered roots and leaves mixed with tobacco as a flavoring. (as *V. sylvatica* 141:495) *Analgesic* Decoction of roots taken for pains. (as *V. sylvatica* 141:460) *Antidiarrheal* Decoction of roots taken for diarrhea. (161:290) *Ceremonial Medicine* Root used as ceremonial medicine for unspecified purpose. *Cold Remedy* Decoction of roots taken for colds. (as *V. sylvatica* 141:460) Bitter infusion of roots used for colds. Decoction of roots taken for colds. (161:290) *Dermatological Aid* Poultice of various plant parts used on cuts, wounds, bruises, or inflammations. (as *V. sylvatica* 141:460) Chewed leaves spat on cuts and bruises. *Gastrointestinal Aid* Decoction of roots, leaves, stems, and flowers taken for ulcers and stomach trouble. (161:290) *Hunting Medicine* Decoction of whole plant taken and used as a wash by hunters for good luck. (as *V. sylvatica* 141:506) *Misc. Disease Remedy* Decoction of roots, leaves, stems, and flowers taken for influenza. *Tuberculosis Remedy* Decoction of roots taken for "shadow on your lung." (161:290) *Veterinary Aid* Decoction of roots used as a lotion or wash for swellings or sores on horses. (as *V. sylvatica* 141:513)

Valeriana edulis, Edible Valerian

Blackfoot *Poison* Raw roots considered poisonous. (82:56) **Gosiute** *Antirheumatic* (*External*) Pounded roots rubbed on parts affected by rheumatism. (31:350, 384) *Dermatological Aid* Pounded roots rubbed on skin for swollen bruises. (31:349) Pounded roots rubbed on swollen and bruised parts. (31:384) **Menominee** *Analgesic* Poultice of pulverized root applied to painful, bleeding cuts and wounds. *Anthelmintic* Root used as a tapeworm medicine. *Dermatological Aid* Poultice of pulverized root applied to draw out inflammation of boils. Poultice of pulverized root applied to painful, bleeding cuts and wounds. *Hemostat* Pulverized root placed on painful and bleeding cuts. (128:57) **Meskwaki** *Hemostat* Root used for hemorrhages. (129:251) **Snake** *Poison* Raw root poisonous and cooked root used for food. (15:26)

Valeriana sitchensis, Sitka Valerian

Okanagon *Analgesic* Decoction of roots taken for pains. *Cold Remedy* Decoction of roots taken for colds. *Dermatological Aid* Poultice of roots applied to cuts, wounds, bruises, and inflamed regions. (104:40) **Thompson** *Adjuvant* Dried, powdered roots and leaves mixed with tobacco as a flavoring. (141:495) *Analgesic* Decoction of roots taken for pains. (104:40) Decoction of root taken for pains. (141:460) *Antidiarrheal* Decoction of roots taken for diarrhea. (161:290) *Ceremonial Medicine* Root used as ceremonial medicine for unspecified purpose. (141:460) *Cold Remedy* Decoction of roots taken for colds. (104:40) Decoction of root taken as a cold remedy. (141:460) Decoction of roots taken for colds. Bitter infusion of roots used for colds. (161:290) *Dermatological Aid* Poultice of roots applied to cuts, wounds, bruises, and inflamed regions. (104:40) Poultice of various plant parts used on cuts, wounds, bruises, or inflammations. (141:460) Chewed leaves spat on cuts and bruises. *Gastrointestinal Aid* Decoction of roots, leaves, stems, and flowers taken for ulcers or stomach trouble. (161:290) *Hunting Medicine* Decoction of whole plant taken and used as a wash by hunters for good luck. (141:506) *Misc. Disease Remedy* Decoction of roots, leaves, stems, and

flowers taken for influenza. *Tuberculosis Remedy* Decoction of roots taken for "shadow on your lung." (161:290) *Veterinary Aid* Decoction of roots used as a lotion or wash for swellings or sores on horses. (141:513)

Valeriana uliginosa, Mountain Valerian

Menominee *Analgesic* Infusion of root taken for cramps and "disorders of the head." *Cathartic* Large doses of plant produced purging. *Dermatological Aid* Poultice of pulverized root applied to cuts and wounds. *Hunting Medicine* Root chewed and spit on fishhook to lure fish to Indian, but not to white man. *Psychological Aid* Large doses of plant produced mental stupor. *Pulmonary Aid* Infusion of root taken for "disorders of the throat and lungs." *Sedative* Plant used as a "feeble sedative to the nervous system." *Throat Aid* Infusion of root taken for "disorders of the throat and lungs." (128:57)

Vanclevea stylosa, Pillar False Gumweed

Navajo, Kayenta *Dermatological Aid* Compound poultice of plants applied to tarantula or solpugid (wind scorpion) bites. (179:51)

Vancouveria chrysantha, Golden Insideout Flower

Tolowa *Unspecified* Used for medicine. (5:61)

Vancouveria hexandra, White Insideout Flower

Yurok *Cough Medicine* Leaves eaten for coughs. (5:61)

Veratrum californicum, California False Hellebore

Paiute *Antirheumatic* (*External*) Poultice of root applied for rheumatism. Pulped root or decoction of root applied with friction as a liniment. (155:147, 14) *Burn Dressing* Plant used for burns. (87:196) *Contraceptive* Decoction of root taken as a contraceptive "to insure permanent sterility." Decoction of root taken by both men and women as a contraceptive. (155:147, 148) *Dermatological Aid* Poultice of dried, pounded roots applied to bruises. (87:196) Dry, powdered root sprinkled on sores to promote healing. Poultice of mashed, raw root applied to boils, sores, cuts, or swellings. *Disinfec-*

tant Poultice of root applied for infections. (155: 147, 148) *Febrifuge* Infusion of plant used as a febrifuge. (87:197) *Gland Medicine* Poultice of root applied for enlarged throat glands and blood poisoning. *Gynecological Aid* Poultice of root applied for sore nipples. (155:147, 148) *Panacea* Plant used for a variety of maladies. *Snakebite Remedy* Poultice of chewed roots applied to snakebites. (87:195) Poultice of pulped root applied to snakebites. *Throat Aid* Poultice of root applied for sore throats and enlarged glands from tonsillitis. (155:147, 148) *Toothache Remedy* Powdered roots rubbed on the face for toothaches. (87:197) *Venereal Aid* Decoction of roots taken for venereal disease. (87:198) Decoction of root taken for venereal disease. (155:147, 148) *Veterinary Aid* Poultice of mashed roots applied to saddle sores on horses. (93:54) **Paiute, Northern** *Antirheumatic (External)* Poultice of mashed roots applied to swollen arms and legs. *Cold Remedy* Roots grated, chewed, and the juice swallowed for colds. *Dermatological Aid* Poultice of mashed roots applied to rattlesnake bites to draw out the poison. Poultice of grated roots applied to cuts, sores, and snakebites. *Orthopedic Aid* Poultice of mashed plant applied to sprains and broken bones. (49:127) **Shoshoni** *Antirheumatic (External)* Poultice of root applied for rheumatism. Pulped root applied with friction as a liniment. *Cold Remedy* Raw root chewed and juice swallowed for "heavy colds." (155:147, 148) *Contraceptive* Infusion of fresh or cured root taken for birth control to ensure sterility for life. (98:46) Decoction of root taken as a contraceptive "to insure permanent sterility." Decoction of root taken by both men and women as a contraceptive. *Dermatological Aid* Poultice of mashed, raw root applied to boils, sores, cuts, or swellings. *Disinfectant* Poultice of root applied for infections. *Gland Medicine* Poultice of root applied for enlarged throat glands and blood poisoning. *Gynecological Aid* Poultice of root applied for sore nipples. *Snakebite Remedy* Poultice of pulped root applied to snakebites. *Throat Aid* Poultice of root applied for sore throats and enlarged glands from tonsillitis. Raw root chewed and juice swallowed for sore throats or inflamed tonsils. (155:147, 148) **Thompson** *Blood Medicine* Decoction of root ashes taken for blood disorders. (141:460) *Poison* Plant considered poisonous if

eaten in large quantities. (141:512) *Respiratory Aid* Dried, powdered root used as snuff to cause sneezing to clear a head cold. *Venereal Aid* Decoction of root ashes taken for blood disorders, especially syphilis. (141:460) **Washo** *Antirheumatic (External)* Pulped root applied with friction as a liniment. (155:147, 148) *Contraceptive* Infusion of fresh or cured root taken for birth control to ensure sterility for life. (98:46) *Dermatological Aid* Dry, powdered root sprinkled on sores to promote healing. *Emetic* Decoction of root taken as an emetic. (155:147, 148)

Veratrum californicum var. *californicum*, California False Hellebore

Blackfoot *Analgesic* Small piece of root snuffed up nose for headache. *Poison* Root poisonous to eat. (as *V. speciosum* 95:275)

Veratrum viride, American False Hellebore

Alaska Native *Poison* Plant considered poisonous. (as *V. eschscholtzii* 71:161) **Bella Coola** *Analgesic* Decoction of bulbs taken or pieces of root swallowed for stomach pain. *Antirheumatic (External)* Poultice of compound containing bulb applied to arms for rheumatism. *Cough Medicine* Decoction of bulb taken for chronic cough. (127:53) *Dermatological Aid* Roots used for skin washes and compresses for bruises. (62:26) *Emetic* Decoction of bulb taken or raw root eaten as an emetic for stomach pains. (127:53) Outer roots used as an emetic. (as *V. eschscholtzii* 158:199)

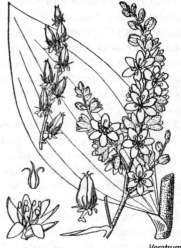

Veratrum viride

Gastrointestinal Aid Decoction of bulb taken or raw root eaten for stomach pain. *Heart Medicine* Poultice of compound containing bulb applied to chest for heart trouble. *Laxative* Decoction of bulb taken for constipation and cough. (127:53) *Orthopedic Aid* Roots used as compresses for sprains and fractures. (62:26) *Poison* Overdose of raw root considered fatal. *Venereal Aid* Decoction of bulb taken for gonorrhea and chronic cough. (127:53) **Blackfoot** *Analgesic* Poisonous roots dried, crushed, and snuffed for headaches. (as *V. eschscholtzii* 82:25) *Gastrointestinal Aid* Infusion of plant taken for indigestion. (72:69) *Nose Medicine* Stems scraped and the powder snuffed to induce sneezing. (72:74) *Oral Aid* Leaves chewed by children for drooling. (72:105) *Poison* Poisonous roots ingested for suicide. (as *V. eschscholtzii* 82:25) **Carrier, Southern** *Emetic* Infusion of dried, powdered root taken as "an emetic for sickness." *Poison* Infusion of powdered root, strong infusion fatal, taken as an emetic. (127:53) **Cherokee** *Analgesic* Compound used as liniment for pains. (66:40) Infusion of leaves used as wash for aches and pains. *Antirheumatic (External)* Infusion of roots rubbed on "leg scratches" for rheumatism. (152:8) *Orthopedic Aid* Compound used as a liniment for pains or sore muscles. Compound used as liniment for sore muscles. (66:40) *Panacea* Infusion of roots rubbed on "leg scratches" for kindred ailments. *Stimulant* Infusion of roots rubbed on "leg scratches" for languor. (152:8) **Cowlitz** *Analgesic* Poultice of leaves applied for pain. *Poison* Plant considered poisonous. (as *V. eschscholtzii* 65:24) **Flathead** *Nose Medicine* Snuff of dried, powdered rootstocks used to clear the nasal passages. (68:73) **Gitksan** *Hunting Medicine* Roots used in purification rituals for hunting and trapping. *Other* Smoke used to assist the spirits of sleepwalkers to return to their bodies. (62:26) **Haisla** *Antirheumatic (External)* Decoction of cleaned, sliced, dried, and boiled roots used for rheumatism. *Cold Remedy* Plant used as a snuff for colds. *Emetic* Plant used as an emetic. *Hemostat* Poultice of roots applied to stop flow of blood from areas cut to release disease-causing objects. *Laxative* Decoction of cleaned, sliced, dried, and boiled roots used as a laxative. *Sedative* Decoction of cleaned, sliced, dried, and boiled roots used as a sedative. **Haisla & Hanaksiala** *Ceremonial*

Medicine Roots put on the ends of arrows by the shaman to shoot towards "disease spirits." *Poison* Plant considered highly toxic. **Hanaksiala** *Antirheumatic (External)* Poultice of roots, rhizomes, and Sitka spruce pitch applied to sore areas. *Antirheumatic (Internal)* Infusion of roots taken for various types of swellings. *Blood Medicine* Plant used for any blood-related disorder. *Hypotensive* Plant used for high blood pressure. *Respiratory Aid* Poultice of roots, rhizomes, and Sitka spruce pitch paste applied to chest for respiratory afflictions. *Unspecified* Decoction of roots used as an internal medicine for unspecified purposes. (35:201) **Iroquois** *Analgesic* Compound of dried plants used as snuff for catarrh, headaches, and colds. *Cold Remedy* Dried plants or powdered roots used as snuff for catarrh, headaches, and colds. *Dermatological Aid* Compound infusion of roots used as a poultice to break open boils. *Respiratory Aid* Dried plants or dried roots used as snuff for catarrh, headaches, and colds. *Tuberculosis Remedy* Dried root used as snuff for tuberculosis. (73:280) **Kitasoo** *Antirheumatic (External)* Decoction of roots and rhizomes applied externally for arthritis. (35:323) **Kutenai** *Nose Medicine* Snuff of dried, powdered rootstocks used to clear the nasal passages. (68:73) **Kwakiutl** *Abortifacient* Juice taken by women to bring about an abortion. *Analgesic* Infusion of scraped roots taken to induce vomiting for internal pains. Poultice of roots or leaves applied to the chest for chest pains. Roots and oil rubbed on bloody back for back pains. *Cold Remedy* Powdered leaves used as snuff for bad colds. *Dermatological Aid* Cold infusion of roots rubbed on the scalp for dandruff. Poultice of scraped roots applied to swellings. *Emetic* Infusion of scraped roots taken to induce vomiting for internal pains. *Hunting Medicine* Leaves rubbed on body to purify hunter. *Laxative* Large, fleshy roots held in the mouth as a laxative. (157:273) *Orthopedic Aid* Compound poultice of roots applied to sore backs. (157:267) Roots and oil rubbed on bloody back for back pains. *Panacea* Braided leaves with the root suspended worn around the neck by sick people. *Pediatric Aid* Root hung around child's neck to ward off disease-causing spirits. *Poison* Secondary roots considered poisonous. (157:273) **Okanagan-Colville** *Antirheumatic (External)* Roots used for rheumatism or arthritis. (62:26) Poultice of raw roots applied carefully to the skin for rheumatic and arthritic pains. *Cold Remedy* Roots dried, powdered, and used as a snuff to cause sneezing and clear the sinuses for colds. *Hunting Medicine* Roots rubbed in each eye and the tip of the nose of hunting dogs during "training." *Orthopedic Aid* Poultice of leaves applied to the skin by hunters for backaches. *Poison* Plant considered poisonous. *Witchcraft Medicine* Plant used in "witchcraft" or "plhax" to jinx people. (162:50) **Okanagon** *Blood Medicine* Decoction of dried, burned roots taken for blood disorders. (104:40) **Oweekeno** *Antirheumatic (External)* Dried roots used in bath water for arthritis or rheumatism. *Poison* Plant poisonous to animals. (35:79) **Quinault** *Antirheumatic (Internal)* Decoction of whole plant taken for rheumatism. *Poison* Plant considered poisonous. (as *V. eschscholtzii* 65:24) **Salish** *Cold Remedy* Dried, powdered roots used as a snuff for colds. *Poison* Plant considered poisonous. (153:294) **Salish, Coast** *Analgesic* Roots used in small doses for internal pains. *Antirheumatic (External)* Roots used in small doses for rheumatism. *Diaphoretic* Roots used in medicinal sweat baths. (156:76) **Shuswap** *Dermatological Aid* Plant used to make hair grow on a bald head. *Poison* Plant considered poisonous. (102:55) **Thompson** *Antirheumatic (External)* Plant used externally for arthritis. Washed, mashed roots rubbed on body parts with water or mixed with snowbrush for arthritis. The informants cautioned never to use this medicine internally or to let it get near the eyes, mouth, or open sores because of its extreme toxicity. Decoction of plant used for sore feet. (161:131) *Blood Medicine* Decoction of dried, burned roots taken for blood disorders. (104:40) *Misc. Disease Remedy* Poultice of root used for phlebitis. *Orthopedic Aid* Decoction of plant considered good for broken bones. *Pediatric Aid* Burned leaf ashes and Vaseline used as a diaper ointment to prevent babies from messing diapers. The ashes were probably originally mixed with deer or bear fat. The ointment was very strong and had to be used with extreme caution. One informant cautioned that it should not be taken internally because of its extreme toxicity. *Throat Aid* Poultice of boiled roots used for sore throat. (161:131) **Tsimshian** *Antirheumatic (External)* Leaves used for arthri-tis. *Dermatological Aid* Roots used for scalp disease. *Psychological Aid* Roots used for insanity. *Respiratory Aid* Roots used as a snuff for sinus infections. (62:26)

***Verbascum thapsus*, Common Mullein**
Abnaki *Pediatric Aid* Roots used to make a necklace worn by teething babies. (121:171) Used by children for teething. (121:155) *Toothache Remedy* Plant made into a magical necklace and worn by children for teething. (121:154) Roots used to make a necklace worn by teething babies. (121:171) Used by children for teething. (121:155) **Atsugewi** *Antirheumatic (Internal)* Decoction of leaves taken for rheumatism. *Cold Remedy* Decoction of leaves taken for colds. *Dermatological Aid* Poultice of pounded, raw leaves applied to cuts. Poultice of raw leaves applied to cuts. *Diaphoretic* and *Unspecified* Crushed leaves rubbed over the body during a sweat bath. (50:140) **Catawba** *Analgesic* Poultice of smashed leaves applied to pain. *Dermatological Aid* Poultice of smashed leaves applied to swellings, bruises, and wounds. *Orthopedic Aid* Poultice of smashed leaves applied to sprains. *Pediatric Aid* Decoction of roots given to children with croup. *Pulmonary Aid* Decoction of roots given to children with croup. (134:190) **Cherokee** *Analgesic* Compound taken for "pains." *Cough Medicine* Compound decoction of leaf taken with brown sugar or honey as a cough syrup. *Dermatological Aid* Leaves rubbed under armpits for "prickly rash" and flowers used on sores. *Gland Medicine*

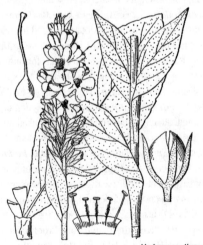

Verbascum thapsus

Scalded leaves used on swollen glands. *Gynecological Aid* Infusion of root or leaf taken for "female trouble." *Kidney Aid* Infusion of root taken "for kidneys" and used to bathe legs for "dropsy." *Misc. Disease Remedy* Leaves wrapped around neck for mumps and scalded leaves used on swollen glands. (66:45) Poultice of beaten leaves applied to the throat for diphtheria. (152:57) **Creek** *Cough Medicine* Compound decoction of root taken for coughs. (148:660, 661) Decoction of roots taken as a cough remedy. (152:57) **Delaware** *Antirheumatic (External)* Poultice of heated leaves applied to the joints and body for rheumatism pain and swelling. *Cough Medicine* Leaves combined with coltsfoot, plum root, and glycerin and used as a syrup for coughs. *Pulmonary Aid* Leaves combined with coltsfoot, plum root, and glycerin and used as a syrup for lung trouble. *Respiratory Aid* Leaves combined with coltsfoot, plum root, and glycerin and used as a syrup for catarrh. (151:36) **Delaware, Oklahoma** *Analgesic* Poultice of heated leaves applied for rheumatic pain. (150:30, 31) *Antirheumatic (External)* Poultice of heated leaves used for rheumatism. (150:30, 80) *Cold Remedy* Leaves used for colds. (150:80) *Cough Medicine* Compound containing leaves taken for catarrh, coughs, and lung trouble. (150:30, 31) *Pulmonary Aid* Compound decoction of leaves taken for lung trouble. *Respiratory Aid* Compound decoction of leaves taken for catarrh. (150:30, 80) **Delaware, Ontario** *Analgesic* Poultice of crushed leaves applied to bruises for pain and swelling. (150:66, 82) *Dermatological Aid* Poultice of crushed leaves applied to bruises for swelling and pain. (150:66) **Hopi** *Anticonvulsive* Leaves smoked with *Onosmodium* for "fits," craziness, and witchcraft. (174:33, 92) *Psychological Aid* Compound of plant smoked by persons not in their "right mind." *Witchcraft Medicine* Compound of plant smoked as cure for persons "with power to charm." (174:92) **Iroquois** *Anticonvulsive* Dried leaves smoked for bad hiccups. *Antidiarrheal* Compound decoction of roots and leaves taken for diarrhea with blood. *Blood Medicine* Complex compound taken as blood purifier. *Dermatological Aid* Decoction of whole plant given to babies with a rash. Poultice of leaves applied to swellings, abscesses, sores, and erysipelas. *Ear Medicine* Poultice of heated leaves applied for earaches. (73:432)

Febrifuge Decoction of leaves taken for fevers. *Hemorrhoid Remedy* Poultice of leaves applied to piles. (73:433) *Laxative* Infusion of leaves given to babies to regulate their bowels. (73:431) *Misc. Disease Remedy* Poultice of leaves applied to face for mumps. *Orthopedic Aid* Compound decoction given and applied as poultice to baby's broken coccyx. (73:432) *Pediatric Aid* Infusion of leaves given to babies to regulate their bowels. (73:431) Compound decoction given and applied as poultice to baby's broken coccyx. Decoction of whole plant given to babies with a rash. (73:432) *Respiratory Aid* Dried leaves smoked for catarrh and asthma. (73:431) Infusion of leaves, roots, and flowers from another plant used for asthma. (118:57) *Toothache Remedy* Poultice of leaves applied to face for toothaches. (73:431) *Tuberculosis Remedy* Dried leaves smoked for consumption. (73:432) **Malecite** *Dermatological Aid* Leaves used for sores and cuts. (96:246) *Respiratory Aid* Plants smoked and used for catarrh. (96:248) **Menominee** *Pulmonary Aid* Root used for pulmonary disease. (128:53) **Micmac** *Dermatological Aid* Parts of plant used for sores and cuts. *Respiratory Aid* Parts of plant used for catarrh and leaves used for asthma. (32:63) **Mohegan** *Cold Remedy* Infusion of leaves taken with sugar for colds. (25:118) *Cough Medicine* Compound infusion of leaves taken for coughs. (149:270) Infusion of leaves mixed with molasses and taken for coughs. (151:77, 132) *Respiratory Aid* Leaves smoked for asthma. (149:265) Dried leaves smoked for asthma. (151:77, 132) *Throat Aid* Leaves smoked for sore throat. (149:265) Dried leaves smoked for sore throat. (151:77, 13) **Nanticoke** *Febrifuge* Poultice of leaves in vinegar bound to neck, head, wrists, and feet for fever. (150:56, 84) **Navajo** *Veterinary Aid* Plants "lighted and smoked for worms in sheep's nose." (76:156) **Navajo, Ramah** *Cough Medicine* Leaves smoked for cough. *Febrifuge* Leaves smoked for fever. *Psychological Aid* Dried leaves smoked in corn husk "to clear the mind if lost." *Strengthener* Cold infusion of leaves rubbed on bodies of hunters for strength. *Veterinary Aid* Cold infusion of leaves rubbed on bodies of horses for strength. (165:45) **Ojibwa** *Heart Medicine* Peeled roots used as a heart stimulant. (4:2304) **Penobscot** *Respiratory Aid* Dried, powdered leaves smoked for asthma. (133:310) **Potawatomi**

Respiratory Aid Dried leaves smoked in a pipe for asthma and smudged leaves inhaled for catarrh. *Stimulant* Leaves smudged to revive unconscious person. (131:83, 84) **Rappahannock** *Dermatological Aid* Decoction of leaves rubbed on human or cattle swellings. *Orthopedic Aid* Decoction of leaves used as a hot poultice for human or animal sprains. *Veterinary Aid* Decoction of leaves rubbed or poultice applied to cattle swellings and sprains. (138:28) **Salish** *Tuberculosis Remedy* Decoction of plants taken for consumption. (153:293) **Shinnecock** *Cold Remedy* Infusion of leaves taken with sugar for colds. (25:118) **Thompson** *Cold Remedy* Decoction of leaves taken for colds. *Cough Medicine* Decoction of leaves taken for coughs. *Dermatological Aid* Juice rubbed on warts. (161:287) **Zuni** *Dermatological Aid* Poultice of powdered root applied to sores, rashes, and skin infections. Infusion of root used for athlete's foot infection. (22:378)

Verbena hastata, Swamp Verbena
Cherokee *Abortifacient* Used for female obstructions. *Analgesic* Used for afterpains and taken as a tonic. *Antidiarrheal* Compound taken for flux, old bowel complaints, and dysentery. *Breast Treatment* Taken as a tonic for breast complaints. *Cold Remedy* Taken for colds. *Cough Medicine* Taken for coughs. *Dermatological Aid* Astringent root compound taken for flux. *Diaphoretic* Used as a sudorific. *Emetic* Leaves, seeds, and roots used as an emetic. *Febrifuge* Leaves, seeds, and roots used for early stages of fever. *Gastrointestinal Aid* Compound used for flux and old bowel complaints. Taken to strengthen stomach. *Kidney Aid* One quart proof spirits and one handful of roots used for dropsy. *Tonic* Taken as a general or breast complaint tonic. (66:60) **Chippewa** *Hemostat* Snuff of dried flowers used for nosebleed. (43:356) **Dakota** *Analgesic* and *Gastrointestinal Aid* Decoction of leaves taken for stomachache. (58:111) **Delaware, Oklahoma** *Febrifuge* Compound containing root used for "chills." (150:80) **Iroquois** *Anthelmintic* Compound decoction of roots taken for worms. *Ear Medicine* Compound infusion of roots used as drops for earaches. *Gastrointestinal Aid* Compound decoction of roots taken for stomach cramps. *Other* Decoction of whole plant taken for "summer complaint." (73:422) *Poultice* Poul-

tice of cut, wetted root applied to the head to cool off. (118:58) *Witchcraft Medicine* Cold infusion of smashed leaves used to make an obnoxious person leave. (73:422) **Mahuna** *Febrifuge* and *Gastrointestinal Aid* Roots used for complicated stomach fevers. (117:9) **Menominee** *Urinary Aid* Infusion of root taken to "clear up cloudy urine." (128:58)

Verbena lasiostachys, Western Vervain
Costanoan *Febrifuge* Infusion of plant used for fevers. *Gastrointestinal Aid* Infusion of plant used for "fever of the stomach." *Misc. Disease Remedy* Infusion of plant used for typhoid fever. (17:15)

Verbena macdougalii, Macdougal Verbena
Navajo, Ramah *Ceremonial Medicine* Plant used in various ceremonial ways as a lotion and fumigant. *Febrifuge* Cold infusion taken and used as lotion for fever. (165:41)

Verbena officinalis, Herb of the Cross
Houma *Kidney Aid* and *Liver Aid* Decoction of root taken for kidney and liver trouble. (135:65)

Verbena stricta, Hoary Verbena
Dakota *Gastrointestinal Aid* Infusion of leaves taken for stomachaches. (57:363)

Verbena urticifolia, White Vervain
Meskwaki *Gynecological Aid* Infusion of root used for profuse menstruation. *Stimulant* Root eaten to revive patient and restore him to health. (129:251, 252)

Verbesina encelioides, Golden Crownbeard
Hopi *Dermatological Aid* Infusion of plant used as a wash for fever or itch from spider bites. (174:32, 99) Infusion of plant said to remove fever and itch from a spider bite. *Febrifuge* Infusion of plant said to remove fever and itch from a spider bite. (174:99) **Navajo, Kayenta** *Dermatological Aid* Infusion of plant taken and plant used as a lotion for spider bites. (179:51)

Verbesina encelioides ssp. exauriculata, Golden Crownbeard
Navajo *Gastrointestinal Aid* Infusion of dried, crushed leaves taken for stomach troubles. (45:90) **Navajo, Ramah** *Hunting Medicine* Petals

chewed for good luck in hunting. (165:54) **Zuni** *Analgesic*, *Emetic*, and *Gastrointestinal Aid* Blossoms chewed and swallowed with water as an emetic for stomach cramps. (as *Ximenesia exauriculata* 143:63) *Snakebite Remedy* Compound poultice of root applied with much ceremony to rattlesnake bite. (as *Ximinesia exauriculata* 143:53, 54)

Verbesina virginica, White Crownbeard
Chickasaw *Abortifacient* Plant used as a "deobstruant." *Diuretic* Plant used as a diuretic. *Gynecological Aid* Infusion of root used for "Fluor Albus" and uterine weakness. *Stimulant* Plant used as a stimulant. *Venereal Aid* Plant used to treat venereal disease. (23:289) **Choctaw** *Febrifuge* Infusion of root taken "during attacks of fever." (20:23) Cold infusion of pounded roots taken for fevers. (152:64) **Seminole** *Analgesic* Infusion of leaf taken for bear sickness: fever, headache, thirst, constipation, and blocked urination. (145:198) *Antirheumatic* (*External*) Plant used for fire sickness: fever and body aches. (145:203) *Ceremonial Medicine* Root bark used as a purification emetic after funerals, at doctor's school, and after death of patient. *Emetic* Root bark used as an emetic to "clean the insides." (145:167) Decoction of root bark taken as an emetic for stomachaches. (145:276) *Eye Medicine* Infusion of plant taken and used as a bath for mist sickness: eye disease, fever, and chills. (145:209) *Febrifuge* Infusion of leaf taken for bear sickness: fever, headache, thirst, constipation, and blocked urination. (145:198) Plant used for fire sickness: fever and body aches. (145:203) Infusion of plant taken and used as a bath for mist sickness: eye disease, fever, and chills. (145:209) Plant used as a fever medicine. (145:283) *Gastrointestinal Aid* Decoction of root bark taken as an emetic for stomachaches. (145:276) *Laxative* and *Oral Aid* Infusion of leaf taken for bear sickness: fever, headache, thirst, constipation, and blocked urination. (145:198) *Unspecified* Plant used for medicinal purposes. (145:162) *Urinary Aid* Infusion of leaf taken for bear sickness: fever, headache, thirst, constipation, and blocked urination. (145:198)

Vernonia glauca, Broadleaf Ironweed
Cherokee *Analgesic* Infusion of root given for pains after childbirth. *Blood Medicine* Infusion taken for blood. *Gastrointestinal Aid* Infusion of root given "for stomach ulcers or hemorrhage." *Gynecological Aid* Infusion of root given for pains after childbirth. Various infusions given "for monthly period" and to "prevent menstruation." *Toothache Remedy* Infusion of root used for loose teeth. (66:41)

Vernonia missurica, Missouri Ironweed
Kiowa *Dermatological Aid* Decoction of plants used as a wash for dandruff. (166:62)

Vernonia noveboracensis, New York Ironweed
Cherokee *Analgesic* Infusion of root given for pains after childbirth. *Blood Medicine* Infusion taken for blood. *Gastrointestinal Aid* Infusion of root given "for stomach ulcers or hemorrhage." *Gynecological Aid* Infusion of root given for pains after childbirth. Various infusions given "for monthly period" and to "prevent menstruation." *Toothache Remedy* Infusion of root used for loose teeth. (66:41)

Veronica americana, American Speedwell
Navajo, **Ramah** *Ceremonial Medicine* and *Emetic* Plant used as a ceremonial emetic. (165:45)

Veronica officinalis, Common Gypsyweed
Cherokee *Cough Medicine* Taken with sugar for coughs. *Dermatological Aid* Used to poultice boils. *Ear Medicine* Warm juice used for earaches. *Febrifuge* Taken by thirsty patient for chills. (66:56) *Gynecological Aid* Decoction of roots taken to ease childbirth. (152:57) **Iroquois** *Emetic* Decoction of plants taken as an emetic to neutralize witchcraft and spoil hunting. *Veterinary Aid* Infusion of plants mixed with feed and used as wash for dried up cow's udders. *Witchcraft Medicine* Decoction of plants taken as an emetic to neutralize witchcraft and spoil hunting. (73:436)

Veronica peregrina ssp. **xalapensis**, Hairy Purslane Speedwell
Navajo, **Ramah** *Ceremonial Medicine* Plant used as a ceremonial emetic and fumigant. *Disinfectant* Decoction taken for "deer infection" from overeating venison. *Emetic* Plant used as a ceremonial

emetic. *Gastrointestinal Aid* Decoction taken for "deer infection" from overeating venison. *Hunting Medicine* Plant chewed and blown toward deer for good luck in hunting. (165:45)

Veronica serpyllifolia, Thymeleaf Speedwell **Cherokee** *Cough Medicine* Taken with sugar for coughs. *Dermatological Aid* Used to poultice boils. *Ear Medicine* Warm juice used for earaches. *Febrifuge* Taken by thirsty patient for chills. (66:56)

Veronicastrum virginicum, Culver's Root **Cherokee** *Analgesic* Infusion used for backache. *Cathartic* Used as a purgative. *Diaphoretic* Root used as a diaphoretic. *Disinfectant* Used as an antiseptic. *Febrifuge* "Good for typhus and bilious fevers." *Gastrointestinal Aid* Chewed for colic. *Liver Aid* Compound taken for "inactive liver." *Misc. Disease Remedy* "Good for typhus and bilious fevers." *Tonic* Used as a tonic. (66:31) **Chippewa** *Blood Medicine* Decoction of root taken "to cleanse the blood." (as *Leptandra virginica* 43:346) Compound decoction of root used as cathartic to cleanse blood in scrofula cases. (as *Leptandra virginica* 43:354) *Cathartic* Decoction of root taken as a physic. (as *Leptandra virginica* 43:346) Compound decoction of root used as a blood-cleansing cathartic for scrofula sores. *Tuberculosis Remedy* Compound decoction of root used as a blood-cleansing cathartic for scrofula sores, and to cleanse blood in scrofula cases. (as *Leptandra virginica* 43:354) **Iroquois** *Antidiarrheal*

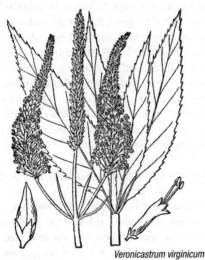

Veronicastrum virginicum

Infusion of roots taken for chills or diarrhea. *Antirheumatic (Internal)* Plant used for rheumatism. *Cathartic* Decoction or infusion of roots taken as a physic. *Cough Medicine* Infusion of roots taken for coughs and as a physic. *Emetic* Infusion of roots taken as an emetic. *Febrifuge* Infusion of roots taken for chills and fevers. *Gastrointestinal Aid* Infusion of smashed roots taken for biliousness and gallstones. (73:435) *Heart Medicine* Decoction of roots taken as a physic or for a bad heart. (73:436) *Panacea* Infusion of roots taken for all ailments and fevers. (73:435) *Poison* Plant considered poisonous. (73:436) *Pulmonary Aid* Infusion of smashed roots taken for chest lumps caused by a cold drink. *Witchcraft Medicine* Infusion of roots taken as a witch medicine. (73:435) **Menominee** *Cathartic* Strong decoction of root taken as powerful cathartic. (as *Leptandra virginica* 44:131) Root used as a strong physic. *Ceremonial Medicine* Used as a "reviver" to purify whoever had been defiled by touch of bereaved. (128:53, 54) *Emetic* Strong decoction of root taken as powerful emetic. *Laxative* Infusion of root taken as a mild laxative. (as *Leptandra virginica* 44:131) **Meskwaki** *Anticonvulsive* Root used for fits and constipation. *Gynecological Aid* Root used by women in labor. *Kidney Aid* Root used to dissolve gravel in the kidneys and for fits. *Laxative* Root used for constipation and fits. *Misc. Disease Remedy* Infusion of root taken for "ague of long standing." *Stimulant* Root used by women for weakness. (129:247) **Ojibwa, South** *Cathartic* Decoction of crushed root taken as a cathartic. (77:200)

Viburnum acerifolium, Mapleleaf Viburnum **Cherokee** *Anticonvulsive* Infusion taken to prevent recurrent spasms. *Diaphoretic* Root bark taken as a diaphoretic. *Febrifuge* Compound infusion taken for fever. *Misc. Disease Remedy* Compound infusion taken for smallpox and ague. *Oral Aid* Infusion of bark used as a wash for sore tongue. *Tonic* Root bark taken as a tonic. (as *Virburnum acerifolium* 66:62) **Chippewa** *Analgesic* Decoction of inner bark taken for cramps. (43:344) *Emetic* Compound decoction of scraped inner bark taken as an emetic. Cool infusion of bark taken as an emetic. (43:346) *Gastrointestinal Aid* Decoction of inner bark taken for stomach cramps. (43:344) **Iroquois** *Analgesic* Infusion of bark taken and applied as poultice for pain caused by witchcraft. *Gynecological Aid* Infusion of plants taken to suppress excessive menses. *Urinary Aid* Infusion of plants taken by men for stricture and painful urination. *Witchcraft Medicine* Infusion of bark taken and applied as poultice for pain caused by witchcraft. (73:447) **Menominee** *Analgesic* Infusion of inner bark taken for cramps. (128:29) *Gastrointestinal Aid* Infusion of inner bark taken for colic. (128:28)

Viburnum dentatum var. *lucidum*,
Southern Arrowwood
Iroquois *Contraceptive* Decoction of twigs taken by women to prevent conception. (as *V. recognitum* 73:447) *Orthopedic Aid* Compound poultice applied to swollen legs of woman after birth of the baby. (as *V. recognitum* 73:448)

Viburnum edule, Mooseberry Viburnum
Bella Coola *Cold Remedy* Bark chewed and juice swallowed for "cold on the lungs." *Pulmonary Aid* Bark chewed and juice swallowed for whooping cough and "cold on the lungs." (as *V. pauciflorum* 127:64) **Carrier** *Cough Medicine* Decoction of stems taken for coughs. (26:77) **Carrier, Northern** *Antidiarrheal* Infusion of crushed inner bark taken for dysentery. *Cathartic* Infusion of crushed inner bark taken as a purgative. (as *V. pauciflorum* 127:64) **Cree, Woodlands** *Dermatological Aid* Poultice of chewed, unopened flower buds applied to lip sores. *Pediatric Aid* Decoction of roots taken for sickness associated with teething. *Throat Aid* Twig tips chewed and swallowed for sore throats. Plant used in a gargle taken for sore throats. Infusion of leaves and stems taken for sore throats. *Toothache Remedy* Decoction of roots taken for sickness associated with teething. (91:65) **Eskimo, Chugach** *Throat Aid* Decoction of leaves used as a gargle for sore throats. (as *V. pauciflorum* 126:326) **Gitksan** *Analgesic* Compound decoction taken for headache. *Cough Medicine* Compound decoction of twigs and bark taken for coughs. *Eye Medicine* Compound decoction taken for weak eyes. *Tuberculosis Remedy* Compound decoction of twigs and bark taken for consumption. (as *V. pauciflorum* 127:64) **Tanana, Upper** *Cold Remedy* Berries eaten for colds. *Gastrointestinal Aid* Decoction of bark taken for

stomach troubles. *Throat Aid* Berries eaten for sore throats. (86:11)

Viburnum lantanoides, Hobble Bush
Algonquin, Tête-de-Boule *Analgesic* Leaves mashed and rubbed on the head for migraines. (110:134) **Iroquois** *Anthelmintic* Compound decoction of plants taken for worms caused by venereal disease. *Blood Medicine* Decoction of roots taken as a blood medicine. *Gynecological Aid* Decoction of roots taken as fertility drug by women. *Love Medicine* Plant used as a love medicine. *Pulmonary Aid* Decoction of plants taken for a sore chest and loss of breath. *Venereal Aid* Compound decoction of plants taken for worms caused by venereal disease. (73:446)

Viburnum lentago, Nannyberry
Chippewa *Urinary Aid* Infusion of leaves taken or poultice of leaves applied for dysuria. (59:142) **Delaware, Ontario** *Misc. Disease Remedy* Compound infusion of leaves taken for measles. (150:66, 82) **Iroquois** *Antihemorrhagic* Decoction of roots taken for spitting blood. *Emetic* and *Tuberculosis Remedy* Compound decoction taken to vomit during initial stages of consumption. (73:448) **Malecite** *Abortifacient* Infusion of roots used for irregular menstruation. (96:258) **Micmac** *Abortifacient* Roots used for irregular menstruation. (32:63) **Ojibwa** *Diuretic* Infusion of inner bark used as a diuretic. (130:361)

Viburnum nudum var. *cassinoides*,
Possumhaw
Cherokee *Anticonvulsive* Infusion taken to prevent recurrent spasms. *Diaphoretic* Root bark used as a diaphoretic. *Febrifuge* Compound infusion taken for fever. *Misc. Disease Remedy* Compound infusion taken for smallpox and ague. *Oral Aid* Infusion of bark used as a wash for sore tongue. *Tonic* Root bark used as a tonic. (as *Virburnum cassinoides* 66:62)

Viburnum opulus, European Cranberrybush
Viburnum
Iroquois *Blood Medicine* Berries considered "good" for the blood. *Liver Aid* Berries considered "good" for the liver. (103:96) **Meskwaki** *Analgesic* Decoction of root taken by "one who feels pain

over his entire body." (129:208) **Micmac** *Misc. Disease Remedy* Bark used for swollen glands and mumps. (32:63) **Montagnais** *Eye Medicine* Decoction of plant used as a salve for sore eyes. (133:316) **Penobscot** *Misc. Disease Remedy* Infusion of berries taken for swollen glands and mumps. (133:310)

Viburnum opulus var. americanum,
    American Cranberry Viburnum
Chippewa *Gynecological Aid* Infusion of roots taken for prolapse of the uterus. (as *V. americanum* 59:141) **Iroquois** *Blood Medicine* Decoction of plants taken as a blood purifier and blood medicine. Infusion of bark taken to vomit for bad blood. (73:446) *Cold Remedy* Compound infusion of plants taken for colds and fevers. (73:447) *Emetic* Infusion of bark taken to vomit for bad blood and fever. *Febrifuge* Decoction of roots given to babies with fevers. Infusion of bark taken to vomit for fever. *Gynecological Aid* Decoction of branches taken for fallen womb after birth. (73:446) Compound decoction of stalks taken to prevent hemorrhage after childbirth. *Heart Medicine* Compound decoction of root taken to regulate the heart and as blood medicine. *Kidney Aid* Compound decoction of roots taken for fevers and kidneys. (73:447) *Laxative* Infusion of bark taken as a laxative. *Pediatric Aid* Decoction of roots given to babies with fevers. (73:446) Compound infusion of roots taken as blood purifier or for prenatal strength. (73:447) *Pulmonary Aid* Compound decoction of bark taken by fat people who have difficulty breathing. (73:446) *Strengthener* Compound infusion of roots taken as blood purifier or for prenatal strength. (73:447) **Ojibwa** *Analgesic* Infusion of inner bark taken for stomach cramps. *Cathartic* Infusion of inner bark taken as a physic. *Gastrointestinal Aid* Infusion of inner bark taken for stomach cramps. (130:361)

Viburnum prunifolium, Black Haw
Cherokee *Anticonvulsive* Infusion taken to prevent recurrent spasms. *Diaphoretic* Root bark taken as a diaphoretic. *Febrifuge* Compound infusion taken for fever. *Misc. Disease Remedy* Compound infusion taken for smallpox and ague. *Oral Aid* Infusion of bark used as a wash for sore tongue. *Tonic* Root bark taken as a tonic. (as *Virburnum*

prunifolium 66:62) **Delaware** *Reproductive Aid* Root bark combined with leaves of other plants and used to strengthen female generative organs. (151:31) **Delaware, Oklahoma** *Gynecological Aid* Compound containing root bark used as a tonic for the "female generative organs." (150:26, 80) **Micmac** *Gynecological Aid* Infusion of plant taken before and during parturition. (as *Viburnum pomifolium* 168:28)

Vicia americana, American Vetch
Iroquois *Love Medicine* Infusion of roots used by women as a love medicine. (73:365) **Keres, Western** *Dermatological Aid* Leaves rubbed in hands and applied to spider bites. (147:74) **Navajo, Kayenta** *Veterinary Aid* Plant smoked by horse to increase the horse's endurance. (179:29) **Navajo, Ramah** *Eye Medicine* Infusion of plant used as an eyewash. *Panacea* Plant used as "life medicine." (165:33) **Okanagan-Colville** *Ceremonial Medicine* Infusion of tops used as a bathing solution in the sweat house. (162:106) **Squaxin** *Analgesic* Infusion of crushed leaves used as a bath for soreness. (65:39)

Vicia caroliniana, Carolina Vetch
Cherokee *Analgesic* Used for back pains, local pains, and rubbed on stomach cramps. (66:60) Infusion of plant rubbed into scratches made over location of muscle pain. (152:34) *Antirheumatic (Internal)* Compound used for rheumatism. (66:60) *Emetic* Infusion of plant taken as an emetic. (152:34) *Gastrointestinal Aid* Decoction taken for dyspepsia. *Misc. Disease Remedy* Used for "blacks" and compound used for rheumatism. *Orthopedic Aid* Used for back pains, to toughen muscles, for muscular cramps and twitching. (66:60) Infusion of plant rubbed into scratches made over location of muscle pain. (152:34) *Respiratory Aid* Compound taken by ballplayers for wind during game. (66:60)

Vicia faba, Horsebean
Navajo *Ceremonial Medicine* Plant used in the Coyote Chant for medicine. *Poison* Plant considered poisonous. (45:59)

Vicia nigricans ssp. gigantea, Giant Vetch
Costanoan *Laxative* Decoction of roots used as a

laxative. (as *V. gigantea* 17:19) **Makah** *Dermatological Aid* Infusion of roots used as a hair wash. (as *V. gigantea* 65:39) *Love Medicine* Used as a "love medicine." If you want your girlfriend to love you, take the plant and rub down with it after bathing, and she will love you forever. (as *V. gigantea* 55:283) **Quinault** *Love Medicine* Roots rubbed on woman and placed under pillow to bring back husband. (as *V. gigantea* 65:39) **Saanich** *Dermatological Aid* Infusion of pounded roots used as a hair tonic for falling hair and dandruff. (as *Vicea gigantea* 156:85)

Vicia sativa ssp. *nigra*, Common Vetch
Iroquois *Abortifacient* Decoction of plant taken by women with suppressed menses. *Gynecological Aid* Decoction of plant taken by women with swollen external sexual organs. *Love Medicine* Cold infusion of plant used as a love medicine. (as *V. angustifolia* 73:365) **Snohomish** *Analgesic* Infusion of plant used on the hair for headaches. (as *V. angustifolia* 65:39)

Vicia villosa, Winter Vetch
Rappahannock *Dermatological Aid* Compound infusion with dried leaves taken for sores. *Gastrointestinal Aid* Compound infusion with dried leaves taken for stomach pain. (138:35)

Vigna luteola, Hairypod Cowpea
Hawaiian *Dermatological Aid* Whole plant and other plants pounded, squeezed, and resulting liquid applied to boils and ruptured skin. *Pediatric Aid* Flowers and buds chewed by the mother and given to infants for general body weakness. *Respiratory Aid* Whole plant and other plants pounded, squeezed, the resulting liquid heated and taken for asthma. *Strengthener* Flowers and buds chewed by the mother and given to infants for general body weakness. (as *V. luta* 2:33)

Viola adunca, Hookedspur Violet
Blackfoot *Antirheumatic* (*External*) Infusion of roots and leaves applied to sore and swollen joints. (72:79) *Pediatric Aid* and *Respiratory Aid* Infusion of leaves and roots given to asthmatic children. (72:74) **Carrier**, **Southern** *Analgesic* and *Gastrointestinal Aid* Decoction of entire plant taken for stomach pain. (127:60) **Klallam** *Analgesic* Poul-

tice of smashed flowers applied to the chest or side for pain. **Makah** *Gynecological Aid* Roots and leaves chewed by women during labor. (65:40) **Tolowa** *Eye Medicine* Poultice of chewed leaves applied to sore eyes. (5:62)

Viola bicolor, Field Pansy
Cherokee *Analgesic* Poultice of leaves used for headache. *Antidiarrheal* Infusion taken for dysentery. *Blood Medicine* Infusion taken for blood. *Cold Remedy* Infusion taken for colds. *Cough Medicine* Infusion with sugar taken for cough. *Dermatological Aid* Poultice of crushed root applied to boils. *Respiratory Aid* Infusion sprayed up nose for catarrh. *Tonic* Infusion taken as spring tonic. (as *V. rafinesquil* 66:60)

Viola canadensis, Canadian White Violet
Ojibwa, **South** *Analgesic* Decoction of root used for pains near the bladder. (77:201)

Viola conspersa, American Dog Violet
Ojibwa *Heart Medicine* Infusion of whole plant taken for heart trouble. (130:392)

Viola cucullata, Marsh Blue Violet
Cherokee *Analgesic* Poultice of leaves used for headache. *Antidiarrheal* Infusion taken for dysentery. *Blood Medicine* Infusion taken for blood. *Cold Remedy* Infusion taken for colds. *Cough Medicine* Infusion with sugar taken for cough. *Dermatological Aid* Poultice of crushed root applied to boils. *Respiratory Aid* Infusion sprayed up nose for catarrh. *Tonic* Infusion taken as spring tonic. (66:60) **Ute** *Unspecified* Roots used as medicine. (30:37)

Viola nephrophylla, Northern Bog Violet
Navajo, **Ramah** *Ceremonial Medicine* and *Emetic* Plant used as a ceremonial emetic. (165:36)

Viola pedata, Birdfoot Violet
Cherokee *Analgesic* Poultice of leaves used for headache. *Antidiarrheal* Infusion taken for dysentery. *Blood Medicine* Infusion taken for blood. *Cold Remedy* Infusion taken for colds. *Cough Medicine* Infusion with sugar taken for cough. *Dermatological Aid* Poultice of crushed root applied to boils. *Respiratory Aid* Infusion sprayed up

nose for catarrh. *Tonic* Infusion taken as spring tonic. (66:60)

Viola pubescens, Downy Yellow Violet
Cherokee *Analgesic* Poultice of leaves used for headache. *Antidiarrheal* Infusion taken for dysentery. *Blood Medicine* Infusion taken for blood. *Cold Remedy* Infusion taken for colds. *Cough Medicine* Infusion with sugar taken for cough. *Dermatological Aid* Poultice of crushed root applied to boils. *Respiratory Aid* Infusion sprayed up nose for catarrh. *Tonic* Infusion taken as spring tonic. (66:60) **Iroquois** *Dermatological Aid* Decoction of plant taken and used as wash for facial eruptions. (73:387) **Ojibwa, South** *Throat Aid* Decoction of root taken in small doses for sore throat. (77:201) **Potawatomi** *Heart Medicine* Root used for various heart diseases. (131:87, 88)

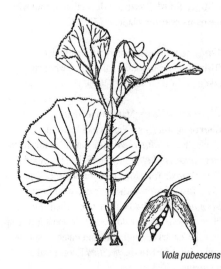

Viola pubescens

Viola pubescens* var. *pubescens, Smooth Yellow Violet
Iroquois *Gastrointestinal Aid* Compound decoction of plants taken for indigestion. (as *V. eriocarpa* 73:387)

Viola rotundifolia, Roundleaf Yellow Violet
Cherokee *Analgesic* Poultice of leaves used for headache. *Antidiarrheal* Infusion taken for dysentery. *Blood Medicine* Infusion taken for blood. *Cold Remedy* Infusion taken for colds. *Cough Medicine* Infusion with sugar taken for cough. *Dermatological Aid* Poultice of crushed root ap-

plied to boils. *Respiratory Aid* Infusion sprayed up nose for catarrh. *Tonic* Infusion taken as spring tonic. (66:60)

Viola sagittata, Arrowleaf Violet
Iroquois *Witchcraft Medicine* Compound used to detect bewitchment. (73:386)

Viola sororia, Common Blue Violet
Cherokee *Analgesic* Poultice of leaves used for headache. *Antidiarrheal* Infusion taken for dysentery. *Blood Medicine* Infusion taken for blood. *Cold Remedy* Infusion taken for colds. *Cough Medicine* Infusion with sugar taken for cough. *Dermatological Aid* Poultice of crushed root applied to boils. *Respiratory Aid* Infusion sprayed up nose for catarrh. *Tonic* Infusion taken as spring tonic. (as *V. papilionacea* 66:60)

Viola striata, Striped Cream Violet
Iroquois *Witchcraft Medicine* Plant used to make a girl sick and crazy by her rejected suitor after he has been refused by her parents. (73:387)

Vitex trifolia* var. *unifoliolata, Simpleleaf Chastetree
Hawaiian *Unspecified* Leaves and wood thoroughly pounded and used to make a good bath. (2:72)

Vitis aestivalis, Summer Grape
Cherokee *Antidiarrheal* Compound taken for diarrhea. *Blood Medicine* Infusion of leaf taken "for blood." *Gastrointestinal Aid* Taken as a "fall tonic" and infusion taken "for stomach." *Gynecological Aid* Wilted leaves used to draw soreness from breast after birth of a child. *Liver Aid* Infusion of leaf taken for liver. *Oral Aid* Compound decoction used to wash child's mouth for thrush. *Other* Compound infusion of bark taken for "bad disease." *Pediatric Aid* Compound decoction used to wash child's mouth for thrush. *Tonic* Taken as a "fall tonic." *Urinary Aid* Compound taken for "irregular urination." (66:37) Infusion of bark taken for urinary troubles. (152:41) **Choctaw** *Febrifuge* Used as a "refrigerant." *Gynecological Aid* "Water of the grape vine" taken and used as a wash to induce lactation. *Tonic* Used as a tonic. (23:287)

Vitis aestivalis var. *aestivalis*, Summer
  Grape
Seminole *Analgesic* Decoction of leaves and
stems taken for headaches. (as *V. rufotomentosa*
145:282) *Ceremonial Medicine* Infusion of plant
added to food after a recent death. (as *V. rufotomentosa* 145:342) *Emetic* Plant used as an
emetic during religious ceremonies. (as *V. rufotomentosa* 145:409) *Febrifuge* Decoction of leaves
and stems taken for fevers. *Gastrointestinal Aid*
Decoction of leaves and stems taken for stomachaches. (as *V. rufotomentosa* 145:282) *Pediatric
Aid* Plant used for chronically ill babies. (as *V.
rufotomentosa* 145:328)

Vitis arizonica, Canyon Grape
Navajo *Love Medicine* Vine used to make a cross
and put on top of the basket of cornmeal and paper
bread (flat bread), offered in courtship. (45:62)

Vitis girdiana, Valley Grape
Diegueño *Dermatological Aid* Sap rubbed on
falling or thin hair to keep it healthy and make it
grow. (70:43)

Vitis labrusca, Fox Grape
Cherokee *Antidiarrheal* Compound taken for
diarrhea. *Blood Medicine* Infusion of leaf taken
"for blood." *Gastrointestinal Aid* Taken as a "fall
tonic" and infusion taken "for stomach." *Gynecological Aid* Wilted leaves used to draw soreness
from breast after birth of a child. *Liver Aid* Infusion of leaf taken for liver. *Oral Aid* Compound
decoction used to wash child's mouth for thrush.
Other Compound infusion of bark taken for "bad
disease." *Pediatric Aid* Compound decoction used
to wash child's mouth for thrush. *Tonic* Taken as
a "fall tonic." *Urinary Aid* Compound taken for
"irregular urination." (66:37) Infusion of bark
taken for urinary troubles. (152:41) **Iroquois**
Veterinary Aid Decoction of roots mixed with feed
to assist horse conception. (73:383) **Mohegan**
Analgesic Poultice of leaves bound to the head for
headache. (149:264) Poultice of leaves applied to
painful area. (151:77, 132) *Febrifuge* Poultice of
leaves bound to the head for fever. (149:264)

Vitis munsoniana, Munson's Grape
Seminole *Ceremonial Medicine* Infusion of plant

added to food after a recent death. (145:342)
Emetic Plant used as an emetic during religious
ceremonies. (145:409) *Pediatric Aid* Plant used
for chronically ill babies. (145:328) *Snakebite
Remedy* Infusion of plant used to wash snakebites.
(145:297)

Vitis rupestris, Sand Grape
Delaware *Reproductive Aid* Vine mixed with other
plants and used to increase fertility. *Strengthener*
Vine mixed with other plants and used as a tonic
for frail women. (151:31) **Delaware, Oklahoma**
Reproductive Aid Compound containing vine used
as a tonic by frail women and increases fertility.
(150:26, 80) *Tonic* Compound containing vine
used as a tonic by frail women and increases fertility. (150:26)

Vitis vulpina, Frost Grape
Cherokee *Antidiarrheal* Compound taken for
diarrhea. *Blood Medicine* Infusion of leaf taken
"for blood." *Gastrointestinal Aid* Taken as a "fall
tonic" and infusion taken for stomach. *Gynecological Aid* Wilted leaves used to draw soreness from
breast after birth of a child. *Liver Aid* Infusion of
leaf taken for liver. *Oral Aid* Compound decoction
used to wash child's mouth for thrush. *Other* Compound infusion of bark taken for "bad disease."
Pediatric Aid Compound decoction used to wash
child's mouth for thrush. *Tonic* Taken as a "fall
tonic." *Urinary Aid* Compound taken for "irregular urination." (66:37) **Chippewa** *Antirheumatic*
(*Internal*) Infusion of root taken for rheumatism.
(as *V. cordifolia* 43:362) *Misc. Disease Remedy*
Infusion of root taken for diabetes. (as *V. cordifolia* 43:364) **Delaware, Oklahoma** *Dermatological Aid* Sap considered beneficial to the hair.
(150:26) *Gynecological Aid* Vine sap used for leukorrhea. (150:26, 80) **Iroquois** *Blood Medicine*
Compound decoction of plants taken to make
blood. (73:383) Infusion of plant with root bark
from another plant and wine taken for anemia.
(118:54) *Gastrointestinal Aid* Infusion of plant
given to children with stomach troubles. *Kidney
Aid* Decoction of plant taken for kidney trouble.
Other Vines chewed for hiccups. *Pediatric Aid*
Infusion of plant given to children with urinating
or stomach troubles. *Urinary Aid* Decoction of
plant taken for burning urination. Infusion of plant

given to children with urinating troubles. (73:383) **Menominee** *Eye Medicine* Ripe grape squeezed into eye to remove rice husk at rice-making camp. (44:134) Seed or juice used to remove foreign matter from eyes. (as *V. cordifolia* 128:58) **Meskwaki** *Analgesic* Infusion of twigs held in child's mouth for pain of Indian turnip poisoning. *Antidote* Infusion of twigs held in mouth by children as antidote for poisoning. *Psychological Aid* Decoction of twigs taken for insanity. (as *V. cordifolia* 129:252) **Ojibwa** *Gastrointestinal Aid* Sap used for stomach and bowel troubles. *Gynecological Aid* Decoction of twigs taken to facilitate passing of afterbirth. (130:392)

Vittaria lineata, Appalachian Shoestring Fern **Seminole** *Other* Complex infusion of leaves taken for chronic conditions. (145:272) *Pediatric Aid* Plant used for chronically ill babies. (145:329) *Psychological Aid* Infusion of plant used to steam and bathe the body for insanity. (145:292) *Unspecified* Plant used for medicinal purposes. (145:162)

Waldsteinia fragarioides, Barren Strawberry **Iroquois** *Blood Medicine* Compound decoction of plants taken as a blood remedy. *Snakebite Remedy* Poultice of smashed plants applied to snakebites. (73:352)

Waltheria indica, Uhaloa **Hawaiian** *Dietary Aid* Root bark, buds, leaves, and other plants pounded and resulting liquid taken for losing weight. *Laxative* and *Pediatric Aid* Buds chewed by the mother and given to infants as a laxative. *Pulmonary Aid* Whole plant and other plants pounded, squeezed, and resulting liquid taken for pulmonary complications. (as *W. americana* 2:37) *Respiratory Aid* Buds and leaves pounded, mixed with water, and taken for asthma. (as *W. americana* 2:12) Whole plant and other plants pounded, squeezed, resulting liquid heated and taken for chronic asthma. Root bark, buds, leaves, and other plants pounded and resulting liquid taken for asthma. *Strengthener* Root bark, buds, leaves, and other plants pounded and resulting liquid taken for run-down condition. *Throat*

Aid Root bark chewed and the juice swallowed for sore throats. (as *W. americana* 2:37)

Wikstroemia sp., Akia Launui **Hawaiian** *Laxative* Plant pounded, squeezed, the resulting liquid poured into a sweet potato and eaten as a laxative. *Respiratory Aid* Plant and other ingredients pounded, squeezed, and the resulting liquid taken for asthma. (2:8)

Woodsia neomexicana, New Mexico Cliff Fern **Keres**, **Western** *Gynecological Aid* Infusion of plant used as a douche at childbirth. (as *W. mexicana* 147:74) **Navajo**, **Ramah** *Dermatological Aid* Cold, compound infusion taken and used as a lotion for injury, a "life medicine." (as *W. mexicana* 165:11)

Woodwardia radicans, Rooting Chainfern **Luiseño** *Analgesic* Decoction of roots used externally and internally for pain from injuries. (132:234)

Wyethia amplexicaulis, Mulesears Wyethia **Gosiute** *Dermatological Aid* Infusion of roots used for bruise swellings. (31:349) Poultice of roots applied to bruised limbs. *Orthopedic Aid* Poultice of roots applied to swollen limbs. (31:384) **Okanagan-Colville** *Antirheumatic* (*External*) Poultice of warmed, pounded roots applied for arthritic or rheumatic pain. (162:85) **Paiute** *Emetic* Infusion or decoction of pulverized root taken as an emetic. **Shoshoni** *Dermatological Aid* Poultice of pulped root applied to swellings. *Emetic* Infusion or decoction of pulverized root taken as an emetic. *Misc. Disease Remedy* Decoction of root used as a wash for measles. *Venereal Aid* Compound decoction of root taken as an "unfailing cure for syphilis." (155:148)

Wyethia angustifolia, California Compassplant **Costanoan** *Dermatological Aid* Poultice of pounded root lather used to draw blisters. *Pulmonary Aid* Poultice of pounded root lather used for lung problems. (17:27) **Miwok** *Diaphoretic* Decoction of leaves used as a bath for fever and produced perspiration. *Febrifuge* Decoction of leaves

used as a bath for fever. (8:174) **Yuki** *Emetic*
Decoction of roots taken as an emetic. (39:47)

Wyethia longicaulis, Humboldt Mulesears
Mendocino Indian *Analgesic* Decoction of roots
used as a wash for headaches. *Antirheumatic*
(*External*) Poultice of baked roots applied for
rheumatism. *Burn Dressing* Poultice of dried,
powdered roots applied to burns. *Dermatological
Aid* Poultice of dried, powdered roots applied to
running sores. *Emetic* Decoction of roots taken as
an emetic. *Eye Medicine* Decoction of roots used
as a wash for inflamed and sore eyes. *Gastrointestinal Aid* Decoction of roots taken for stomach
complaints. (33:396)

Wyethia mollis, Woolly Wyethia
Klamath *Antirheumatic* (*External*) Poultice of
root used for swellings. (37:106) *Dermatological
Aid* Poultice of smashed roots applied to swellings.
(140:131) **Paiute** *Blood Medicine* Decoction of
root taken as a blood tonic. *Cathartic* Decoction
of root taken as a physic or emetic. *Cold Remedy*
Simple or compound decoction of chopped roots
taken for colds. (155:148, 149) *Dermatological
Aid* Poultice of crushed leaves applied to swellings.
(87:196) *Febrifuge* Compound decoction of
chopped roots taken for colds and fevers. (155:148,
149) *Orthopedic Aid* Poultice of crushed leaves
applied to broken bones and sprains. (87:196)
Tonic Decoction of root taken as a blood tonic and
for colds. *Tuberculosis Remedy* Decoction of root
taken for tuberculosis. *Venereal Aid* Decoction
of root taken for venereal diseases. **Shoshoni**
Cathartic Decoction of root taken as a physic or
emetic. **Washo** *Cathartic* Decoction of root taken
as a physic. *Emetic* Decoction of root taken as an
emetic. (155:148, 149)

Wyethia scabra, Badlands Wyethia
Hopi *Emetic* Plant said to be a very strong, potentially lethal emetic. (174:34, 99) *Poison* Plant
sometimes used as an emetic, but if not vomited it
would kill the person. (174:99) **Navajo**, **Kayenta**
Emetic and *Gastrointestinal Aid* Plant used as an
emetic for stomachaches. (179:51)

Xanthium spinosum, Spiny
   Cockleburr
Cherokee *Emetic* Infusion of root
   given to induce vomiting. *Gastrointestinal Aid* Taken for cramps. *Pulmonary Aid*
Infusion given for croup. *Snakebite Remedy* Roots
chewed for rattlesnake bite. *Throat Aid* Infusion of
bur used "to unstick object in throat." (66:29, 30)
Mahuna *Kidney Aid* Plant used for the kidneys.
(117:69)

Xanthium strumarium, Rough Cockleburr
Costanoan *Urinary Aid* Decoction of seeds used
for bladder ailments. (17:28) **Lakota** *Ceremonial
Medicine* Used as a medicine in ceremonies.
(116:40) **Paiute**, **Northern** *Oral Aid* Burs rubbed
on sore gums to take the pain, poison, and blood
out. (as *Zanthium strumarium* 49:130)

Xanthium strumarium var. *canadense*,
   Canada Cockleburr
Apache, **White Mountain** *Blood Medicine* Roots
and leaves used as a blood medicine. (as *X. commune* 113:161) **Houma** *Febrifuge* Decoction of
root taken for high fever. (as *X. commune* 135:60)
Keres, **Western** *Dermatological Aid* Poultice of
ground seed powder used on open sores or saddle
galls. (as *X. commune* 147:74) **Koasati** *Gynecological Aid* Decoction of roots taken to remove the
afterbirth. (as *X. commune* 152:64) **Mahuna** *Antirheumatic* (*Internal*) Plant used for rheumatism.
Kidney Aid Plant used for diseased kidneys. *Ortho-*

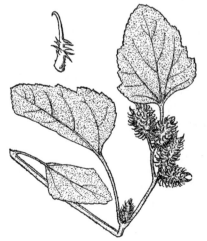

Xanthium strumarium var. canadense

pedic Aid Plant used for total paralysis. *Tuberculosis Remedy* Plant used for tuberculosis. *Venereal Aid* Plant used for gonorrhea. (as *X. canadense* 117:69) **Navajo** *Dermatological Aid* Plant used as a liniment for the armpit to remove excessive perspiration. (as *X. canadense* 45:90) Plant used to decrease perspiration. (as *X. canadense* 76:164) **Pima** *Antidiarrheal* Decoction of burs taken for diarrhea. *Eye Medicine* Pulp used for sore eyes. (as *X. saccharatum* 38:97) Pulp mixed with soot and used for sore eyes. (as *X. canadense* 123:80) *Laxative* Decoction of burs taken for constipation. *Veterinary Aid* Poultice of leaves applied to screwworm sores in livestock. (as *X. saccharatum* 38:97) **Rappahannock** *Dermatological Aid* Decoction of seeds used as salve for sores. (as *X. canadense* 138:31) *Panacea* Compound decoction used for complaint. (as *X. canadense* 138:30) **Tewa** *Antidiarrheal* Plant used for diarrhea. *Antiemetic* Plant used for vomiting. *Pediatric Aid* and *Urinary Aid* Plant used as fumigant for children with urinary disorders. (as *X. commune* 115:49) **Zuni** *Ceremonial Medicine* Chewed seeds rubbed on body prior to cactus ceremony to protect from spines. *Dermatological Aid* Compound poultice of seeds applied to wounds or used to remove splinters. (as *X. commune* 143:62, 63)

Xanthium strumarium var. *glabratum*, Rough Cockleburr

Iroquois *Witchcraft Medicine* Plant used in a witching medicine. (as *X. orientale* 73:469)

Xanthorhiza simplicissima, Yellow Root

Catawba *Cold Remedy* Decoction of roots taken for colds. *Gastrointestinal Aid* Decoction of roots taken for ulcerated stomachs. (as *Xanthorrhiza apiifolia* 134:188) Decoction of plant taken for ulcerated stomach. (as *Zanthorhiza apiifolia* 152:22) *Liver Aid* Decoction of roots taken for jaundice. (as *Xanthorrhiza apiifolia* 134:188) Decoction of plant taken for jaundice. (as *Zanthorhiza apiifolia* 152:22) **Cherokee** *Analgesic* Infusion of root taken for cramps. *Blood Medicine* Compound decoction taken as a blood tonic. *Cancer Treatment* Ashes "burnt from greenswitch" used for cancer. *Dermatological Aid* Astringent and tonic infusion of root used for piles. *Eye Medicine* Poultice used for sore eyes. *Hemorrhoid*

Remedy Infusion of root used for piles. *Oral Aid* Stem chewed for sore mouth. *Sedative* Infusion taken for nerves. *Throat Aid* Stem chewed for sore throat. *Tonic* Taken as a tonic. (66:62)

Xerophyllum tenax, Common Beargrass

Blackfoot *Dermatological Aid* Poultice of chewed roots applied to wounds. *Hemostat* Grated roots used for bleeding. *Orthopedic Aid* Decoction of grated roots used for breaks and sprains. (82:25) **Pomo, Kashaya** *Dermatological Aid* Roots washed, rubbed to make a lather and used to wash sores. (60:52)

Ximenia americana, Tallow Wood

Seminole *Antirheumatic* (*External*) Decoction of inner bark or "beans" used as a body rub and steam for deer sickness: numb, painful limbs and joints. (145:192) Decoction of inner bark used as a body rub and steam for joint swellings. (145:193) *Oral Aid* Decoction of roots used as a mouthwash for sore mouth and gums. *Orthopedic Aid* Infusion of roots used as a steam and rubbed on the legs for soreness. (145:307) *Unspecified* Plant used medicinally. (145:164)

Xyris ambigua, Coastalplain Yelloweyed Grass

Seminole *Cold Remedy* Infusion of herbage rubbed on the chest for colds. *Pulmonary Aid* Infusion of herbage rubbed on the chest for pulmonary disorders. (145:281)

Xyris caroliniana, Carolina Yelloweyed Grass

Cherokee *Antidiarrheal* Infusion of root taken for diarrhea. *Pediatric Aid* Infusion of root taken for diarrhea and "good for children." (66:62)

Yucca aloifolia, Aloe Yucca

Choctaw *Dermatological Aid* Boiled mashed root with grease or tallow used as salve for various purposes. (20:24) *Unspecified* Decoction of roots used as a salve for various purposes. (152:9)

Yucca angustissima, Narrowleaf Yucca

Apache *Snakebite Remedy* Emulsion used in cases of snake or insect bites. (13:51) **Hopi** *Ceremonial Medicine* Crushed root used in purification ceremony. *Dermatological Aid* Crushed root used as shampoo for baldness. *Disinfectant* Crushed root used in purification ceremony. (174:71) *Laxative* Root used as a strong laxative. (174:34, 71)

Yucca baccata, Banana Yucca
Keresan *Dermatological Aid* Used for washing hair. (172:564) **Navajo** *Antiemetic* Infusion of pulverized leaves taken for vomiting. *Gastrointestinal Aid* Plant used for heartburn. (45:32) **Navajo, Ramah** *Ceremonial Medicine* Suds made from root used for ceremonial purification baths. *Gynecological Aid* Juice used to lubricate midwife's hand while removing retained placenta. (165:21) **Pima** *Cathartic* Fruits eaten raw as a cathartic. (123:72) **Tewa** *Ceremonial Medicine* Infusion of root used as a wash in adoption and name-giving ceremonies. *Emetic* Unspecified plant part chewed as ritual emetic. *Gynecological Aid* Fruit eaten to promote easy childbirth. (115:49, 50)

Yucca baileyi var. *navajoa*, Navajo Yucca
Hopi *Laxative* Plant used as a laxative. (as *Y. navaja* 34:370)

Yucca elata, Soaptree Yucca
Apache, Western *Ceremonial Medicine* Peeled stalk shaped like a short snake, heated, eaten by a practitioner and spit at the sick. (21:182)

Yucca filamentosa, Adam's Needle
Catawba *Dermatological Aid* Root rubbed on the body for skin disease. (134:188) Roots rubbed on body or decoction of roots taken for skin disease. (152:9) **Cherokee** *Ceremonial Medicine* Used as an ingredient with broom sedge and amaranth in green corn medicine. *Dermatological Aid* Beaten root used as salve for sores. *Misc. Disease Remedy* Infusion taken for diabetes. (66:25) *Sedative* Used as a soporific. (177:75) **Nanticoke** *Orthopedic Aid* Poultice of roots applied to sprains. (150:56)

Yucca glauca, Small Soapweed
Blackfoot *Antirheumatic* (*External*) Decoction of grated roots used for sprains. (72:80) *Dermatological Aid* Decoction of root used as a tonic for falling hair. Poultice of roots applied to inflamed and bleeding cuts. (95:274) *Hemostat* Poultice of grated roots applied to bleeding cuts. (82:25)

Poultice of roots applied to inflamed and bleeding cuts. *Herbal Steam* Decoction of grated roots used as herbal steam for breaks and sprains. (95:274) *Orthopedic Aid* Decoction of grated roots used for breaks. (72:80) Decoction of grated roots used as herbal steam for breaks and sprains. (95:274) *Veterinary Aid* Decoction of roots applied to saddle sores. (82:25) **Cheyenne** *Dermatological Aid* Decoction of dried root used as hair wash for dandruff and to prevent baldness. Smashed root applied as powder or used as a wash for sores, scabs, and skin outbreaks. (69:12) **Dakota** *Dermatological Aid* Root used to wash the scalp to make the hair grow. (57:358) **Isleta** *Dermatological Aid* Root mixed with ground stolons from vine mesquite grass and used as a hair wash to make the hair grow. (85:45) **Keres, Western** *Herbal Steam* Tender heart shoots used in the sweat bath. *Strengthener* Infusion of tender heart shoots used for weakness. (147:76) **Kiowa** *Dermatological Aid* Plant used for dandruff, baldness, and skin irritations. (166:18) **Lakota** *Abortifacient* Roots and prickly pear cactus roots used as "medicine for not give birth." *Dermatological Aid* Infusion of roots used to soak the hair as a vermin killer and to make the hair grow. *Gastrointestinal Aid* Infusion of pulverized roots taken for stomachaches. *Gynecological Aid* Roots and prickly pear cactus roots used by mothers when they cannot give birth. *Veterinary Aid* Burning root fumes used to allow a horse to be caught and haltered easily. (116:28) **Navajo** *Dermatological Aid* Roots used to wash hair. (45:33) *Laxative* Plant used as a laxative. *Stimulant* Plant used as a delirifacient, a drug that causes delirium. (76:164) **Navajo, Ramah** *Contraceptive* Rotten root used to make suds taken to induce menopause. *Gynecological Aid* Cold infusion of root used to expedite delivery of baby or placenta. *Poison* Compound containing leaf juice used to poison arrows. (165:21) **Omaha** *Unspecified* Root used in smoke treatment for unspecified illnesses. **Pawnee** *Herbal Steam* Root used in smoke treatment for unspecified illnesses. (58:71)

Yucca glauca var. *glauca*, Soapweed Yucca
Montana Indian *Dermatological Aid* Root used as a substitute for soap and as a wash for the hair. (as *Y. angustifolia* 15:27)

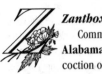

Zanthoxylum americanum, Common Prickly Ash

Alabama *Dermatological Aid* Decoction of bark used as a wash for itching. (148:663) Infusion of inner bark rubbed on itchy area. (as *Xanthoxylum americanum* 152:35) *Toothache Remedy* Pounded inner bark used for toothache. (148:663) Inner bark put into cavity and packed around the tooth for toothaches. (as *Xanthoxylum americanum* 152:35) **Cherokee** *Antirheumatic* (*External*) Infusion used as a wash for swollen joints. (66:51) **Chippewa** *Cold Remedy* Infusion of bark taken for colds. *Cough Medicine* Infusion of bark taken for coughs. (as *Xanthoxylum americanum* 59:134) *Orthopedic Aid* Decoction of root used as a wash for paralysis and to strengthen child's legs and feet. *Pediatric Aid* Decoction of root used as a wash to strengthen legs and feet of weak children. (43:364) *Pulmonary Aid* Infusion of bark taken for all pulmonary troubles. (as *Xanthoxylum americanum* 59:134) *Throat Aid* Decoction of root gargled or taken for sore throat. (43:342) **Comanche** *Burn Dressing* Roots pulverized and powder used for burns. (84:6) *Febrifuge* Infusion of bark taken for fever. (24:524) Infusion of pulverized roots used for fever. (84:6) *Throat Aid* Inner bark placed in throat for sore throat. *Toothache Remedy* Root bark held against tooth for toothache. (24:524) Roots pulverized and used for toothache. (84:6) **Creek** *Veterinary Aid* Infusion of bark used to rub on dog's nose to improve his scent. (148:663) **Delaware** *Heart Medicine* Infusion of inner bark used for heart trouble. (as *Xanthoxylum americanum* 151:35) **Delaware, Oklahoma** *Heart Medicine* Infusion of inner bark taken sparingly for heart trouble. (as *Xanthoxylum americanum* 150:30, 80) *Tonic* Bark used alone and in compound as a tonic. (as *Xanthoxylum americanum* 150:80) **Iroquois** *Abortifacient* Decoction of bark taken to promote miscarriage. (73:368) *Analgesic* Bark smoked for toothaches or neuralgia. (73:367) Compound infusion taken for back pain. Infusion of bark taken for pain after confinement. *Anthelmintic* Decoction of bark taken for worms. *Antiemetic* Compound infusion taken for vomiting. *Diuretic* Infusion of roots taken when water stops because of gonorrhea. *Emetic* Compound decoction taken to vomit during initial stages of con-

sumption. *Gastrointestinal Aid* Decoction of bark taken for cramps. *Gynecological Aid* Infusion of bark taken for pain after confinement. *Kidney Aid* Compound infusion taken for kidney trouble. *Orthopedic Aid* Compound infusion taken for back pain. *Toothache Remedy* Bark smoked, chewed, or placed into the tooth for toothaches. *Tuberculosis Remedy* Compound decoction taken to vomit during initial stages of consumption. *Venereal Aid* Infusion of roots taken when water stops because of gonorrhea. (73:368) **Menominee** *Adjuvant* Infusion of berries used as a seasoner in medicines. (128:51) *Analgesic* Poultice of pounded inner bark used for rheumatism and sharp pains. *Antirheumatic* (*External*) Poultice of pounded inner bark applied for rheumatism and sharp pains. (44:133) *Cold Remedy* Decoction of inner bark used for cold settled in the chest. (44:130) *Dermatological Aid* Infusion of berries sprayed from mouth onto sores. Poultice of root bark applied to swellings in special rite. *Other* Infusion of berries taken for minor maladies. *Pulmonary Aid* Infusion of berries sprayed on the chest or throat for bronchial diseases. (128:51, 52) *Sedative* Compound infusion taken and rubbed on body to quiet person near convulsions. (44:128) **Meskwaki** *Cough Medicine* Bark and berries used to make cough syrup. *Expectorant* Bark and berries used as an expectorant. *Hemostat* Bark and berry medicine used for hemorrhages. *Kidney Aid* Compound infusion of root used for kidney trouble.

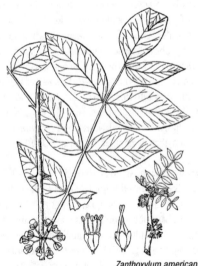

Zanthoxylum americanum

Strengthener Compound decoction of inner bark given to strengthen convalescent patient. *Toothache Remedy* Powdered inner bark used for toothache. *Tuberculosis Remedy* Bark and berries used for hemorrhages and tuberculosis. (129:244, 245) **Mohegan** *Heart Medicine* Infusion of bark taken for heart, 3 days on, 3 days off, before resuming. (as *Xanthoxylum americanum* 149:269) Infusion of inner bark taken in small doses for heart trouble. (as *Xanthoxylum americanum* 151:77, 132) **Ojibwa** *Respiratory Aid* Infusion of berries sprayed on chest for congestion from bronchitis. *Throat Aid* Bark or berries used for sore throat and tonsillitis. (130:387) **Pawnee** *Veterinary Aid* Fruits used as diuretic for horses. (58:98) **Potawatomi** *Venereal Aid* Root bark used for gonorrhea, an historic reference (1796) (131:80)

Zanthoxylum clava-herculis, Hercules's Club
Houma *Orthopedic Aid* Salve of grated root mixed with whisky rubbed on swollen limbs. *Toothache Remedy* Poultice of grated root and bark applied to aching teeth. (as *Xanthoxylum clava-hercules* 135:61)

Zea mays, Corn
Cherokee *Dermatological Aid* "Smut" from plant used as salve. *Kidney Aid* Infusion taken for "gravel." *Pulmonary Aid* Parched grains eaten for "long wind." (66:30) **Keres**, **Western** *Panacea* Pollen eaten for almost any kind of medicine. (147:77) **Mohegan** *Dermatological Aid* Decoction of dried cobs used as a wash for poison ivy rash. (151:77) **Navajo** *Ceremonial Medicine* Poultice of plant applied as ceremonial medicine for sore throats. Leaves used in mixture for the Night Chant medicine. One part of the Night Chant medicine consists of a mixture of "blue pollen," wild plants, and tobacco to which was added the leaves from corn plants gathered in the east, south, west, and north corners of the field, squash from the southeast side, bean leaves from the southwest, watermelon leaves from the northwest, and muskmelon leaves from the northeast. *Throat Aid* Poultice of plant applied as ceremonial medicine for sore throats. (45:27) **Tewa** *Analgesic* Blue cornmeal and water used for "palpitations or pains." *Dermatological Aid* Warm ear of corn rubbed with foot

for child's glandular swelling in neck. *Gynecological Aid* Black corn with red streaks good for menstruating woman. *Heart Medicine* Blue cornmeal and water used for "heart-sickness," "palpitations or pains." *Pediatric Aid* Warm ear of corn rubbed with foot for child's glandular swelling in neck. (115:97)

Zephyranthes sp., Zephyr Lily
Seminole *Toothache Remedy* Infusion of bulbs used for toothaches. (145:304)

Zeuxine strateumatica, Soldier's Orchid
Seminole *Gynecological Aid* Decoction of whole plant taken and used as a wash for barrenness. *Reproductive Aid* Decoction of whole plant used as a wash for impotency. (145:318)

Zigadenus elegans, Mountain Deathcamas
Alaska Native *Poison* Plant considered poisonous. (71:163) **Eskimo**, **Inupiat** *Poison* Whole plant considered poisonous. (83:139) **Keres**, **Western** *Antirheumatic* (*External*) Infusion of 11 plants used as an athletic rubdown. *Diaphoretic* Eleven plants used in sweat bath. An infusion of 11 plants was sprinkled on hot rocks to form dense steam. Men stayed in the sweat bath for 3 to 5 minutes for several successive evenings before the deer hunt or race. *Poison* Plant considered poisonous. *Strengthener* Root rubbed on muscles as a strengthener. Infusion of 11 plants used as an emetic before breakfast prior to athletic events or deer hunts. Infusion of 11 plants used during athletic training every morning prior to breakfast until the brew had been depleted, to give long endurance, a keen eye, and so that the deer could not smell you. (147:78) **Navajo**, **Ramah** *Dermatological Aid* Cold infusion of plant used as a lotion for mad coyote bite. (165:21) **Thompson** *Analgesic* Pulverized, baked root used as salve on painful areas, especially back and feet. (141:463) *Poison* Bulb caused "human poisoning" and leaves usually fatal to cattle. *Veterinary Aid* Leaves usually fatal to cattle. (141:512)

Zigadenus nuttallii, Nuttall's Deathcamas
Gosiute *Emetic* Plant used as an emetic. *Venereal Aid* Plant used for venereal affections. (31:384) **Ute** *Poison* Bulbs considered poisonous. (30:37)

Zigadenus paniculatus, Foothill Deathcamas
Navajo, Kayenta *Veterinary Aid* Infusion of plant
given to sheep with bloat. (179:17) **Paiute** *Analgesic* Poultice of bulb used for neuralgia. *Antirheumatic (External)* Poultice of root, sometimes
mixed with tobacco, applied for rheumatism. *Dermatological Aid* Poultice of bulb used for swellings. *Emetic* Decoction of root taken as an emetic,
in spite of poisonous nature of plant. *Orthopedic
Aid* Poultice of bulb used for sprains and lameness. *Toothache Remedy* Poultice of bulb used for
toothache. (155:149) **Paiute, Northern** *Antirheumatic (External)* Poultice of roasted, mashed
bulbs applied to swollen parts or used for rheumatism. (49:128) **Shoshoni** *Analgesic* Poultice of
bulb used for neuralgia. *Antirheumatic (External)*
Poultice of crushed raw or roasted root applied for
rheumatism. *Dermatological Aid* Poultice of bulb
used for swellings. *Emetic* Decoction of root taken
as an emetic, in spite of poisonous nature of plant.
Orthopedic Aid Poultice of bulb used for sprains
and lameness. *Toothache Remedy* Poultice of bulb
used for toothache. **Washo** *Analgesic* Poultice of
bulb used for neuralgia. *Antirheumatic (External)* Poultice of crushed, raw root applied for
rheumatism. *Dermatological Aid* Poultice of bulb
used for swellings. *Orthopedic Aid* Poultice of bulb
used for sprains and lameness. *Toothache Remedy*
Poultice of bulb used for toothache. (155:149)

Zigadenus venenosus, Meadow Deathcamas
Chehalis *Emetic* Plant sometimes used as a violent emetic. (65:23) **Haisla & Hanaksiala** *Poison* Roots considered highly toxic. (35:203)
Klamath *Emetic* Roots mixed with rootstocks of
blue flag and used for vomiting. (37:93) **Lakota**
Poison Plant poisonous to humans. (116:28)
Mendocino Indian *Analgesic* Poultice of mashed
bulbs applied to painful bruises and sprains. *Antirheumatic (External)* Poultice of mashed bulbs
applied to rheumatism. *Dermatological Aid* Poultice of mashed bulbs applied for boils and painful
bruises. *Orthopedic Aid* Poultice of mashed bulbs
applied to painful bruises and sprains. *Poison*
Root considered poisonous. (33:321) **Montana
Indian** *Analgesic* Poultice of cooked, mashed
bulbs applied to strain and bruise pains. *Antirheumatic (External)* Poultice of mashed bulbs
applied for rheumatism. *Dermatological Aid* Poul-

tice of cooked, mashed bulbs applied to boils.
(15:27) **Okanagan-Colville** *Poison* Bulbs considered extremely poisonous. (162:50) **Okanagon**
Antirheumatic (External) Bulbs mashed and
used for rheumatism. (104:37) **Paiute** *Analgesic*
Poultice of bulb used for rheumatic pains. *Antirheumatic (External)* Poultice of bulb used for
rheumatic pains. *Burn Dressing* Poultice of bulb
used for burns. *Dermatological Aid* Poultice of
bulb used for swellings. (155:149, 150) *Poison*
Seeds and roots considered a deadly poison if eaten by humans or horses. (93:54) *Snakebite Remedy* Poultice of bulb used for rattlesnake bites.
(155:149, 150) **Paiute, Northern** *Antirheumatic
(External)* Poultice of roasted, mashed bulbs
applied to swollen parts or used for rheumatism.
(49:128) **Pomo, Kashaya** *Poison* Plant considered poisonous. (60:30) **Shuswap** *Orthopedic
Aid* Poultice of plant applied to sore legs. *Poison*
Plant considered poisonous. (102:55) **Squaxin**
Emetic Plant sometimes used as a violent emetic.
(65:23) **Thompson** *Antirheumatic (External)*
Bulbs mashed and used for rheumatism. (104:37)
Orthopedic Aid Mashed bulbs rubbed on broken
bones to help them heal more quickly. (161:133)
Yuki *Poison* Bulbs considered poisonous. (39:94)

Zingiber zerumbet, Bitter Ginger
Hawaiian *Analgesic* Roots or bulbs pounded with
salt and the resulting juice used as a head wash for
headaches. *Dermatological Aid* Juice used for hair
dressing. Leaf ashes, other ashes, and nut juice
used for cuts and skin sores. Roots and other roots
pounded with salt, mixed with urine, and used for
ringworm and white skin blotches. Roots and other
roots pounded with salt and used for itch and kindred afflictions of the skin. Flowers and roots
and other plants pounded, mixed with water, and
rubbed on the body during massages. Roots with
other plant parts mixed with water and used as a
bath for bruises. *Orthopedic Aid* Roots with other
plant parts mixed with water and used as a bath
for slight sprains. *Toothache Remedy* Roots
cooked and used in the tooth hollow for toothaches. (2:19)

Zinnia acerosa, Desert Zinnia
Keres, Western *Antirheumatic (External)*
Crushed plant paste mixed with salt and used on

swellings or aches. *Psychological Aid* Plant given to children to quickly learn to talk. (as *Crassina pulmila* 147:39)

Zinnia grandiflora, Rocky Mountain Zinnia
Keres, Western *Kidney Aid* Hot infusion of plant drunk for kidney trouble. *Other* Infusion of plant used as a bath for excessive sweating. (as *Crassina grandiflora* 147:38) **Navajo** *Nose Medicine* Plant used for nose troubles. *Throat Aid* Plant used for throat troubles. (45:97) **Navajo, Ramah** *Analgesic* Decoction of plant taken for stomachache, heartburn, and as a cathartic. *Cathartic* Decoction of plant taken as a cathartic. *Ceremonial Medicine* Plant used as a ceremonial emetic. *Emetic* Plant used as a ceremonial emetic. *Gastrointestinal Aid* Decoction of plant taken for stomachache or heartburn. (165:54) **Zuni** *Dermatological Aid* Poultice of powdered plant applied to bruises. *Diaphoretic* Plant used in a sweat bath for fever. *Eye Medicine* Cold infusion of blossoms used as an eyewash. *Febrifuge* Smoke from powdered plant inhaled in sweat bath for fever. (as *Crassina grandiflora* 143:45)

Zizia aurea, Golden Zizia
Meskwaki *Analgesic* Compound containing flower stalks used as snuff for sick headache. *Febrifuge* Root used for fevers and compound containing flower stalks used for headache. (129:250)

Ziziphus obtusifolia, Lote Bush
Pima *Eye Medicine* Decoction of pounded root used as a wash for sore eyes. (as *Zizyphus lycioides* 123:79)

Ziziphus obtusifolia var. **canescens**, Lote Bush
Pima *Analgesic* and *Antirheumatic* (*External*) Thorns used to prick the skin over rheumatic pains. *Dermatological Aid* Infusion of roots used as a shampoo. *Eye Medicine* Decoction of roots used as a wash for sore eyes. (as *Condalia lycioides* var. *canescens* 38:50)

Bibliography

1. Ager, Thomas A., and Lynn Price Ager. 1980. Ethnobotany of the Eskimos of Nelson Island, Alaska. Arctic Anthropology 27:26–48.

2. Akana, Akaiko. 1922. Hawaiian Herbs of Medicinal Value. Honolulu: Pacific Book House.

3. Anderson, J. P. 1939. Plants Used by the Eskimo of the Northern Bering Sea and Arctic Regions of Alaska. American Journal of Botany 26:714–716.

4. Arnason, Thor, Richard J. Hebda and Timothy Johns. 1981. Use of Plants for Food and Medicine by Native Peoples of Eastern Canada. Canadian Journal of Botany 59(11):2189–2325.

5. Baker, Marc A. 1981. The Ethnobotany of the Yurok, Tolowa and Karok Indians of Northwest California. M.A. Thesis, Humboldt State University, Arcata, California.

6. Bank, Theodore P., II. 1953. Botanical and Ethnobotanical Studies in the Aleutian Islands II. Health and Medical Lore of the Aleuts. Botanical and Ethnobotanical Studies Papers, Michigan Academy of Science, Arts and Letters, 38:415–431.

7. Barrett, S. A. 1952. Material Aspects of Pomo Culture. Bulletin of the Public Museum of the City of Milwaukee, Number 20.

8. Barrett, S. A., and E. W. Gifford. 1933. Miwok Material Culture. Bulletin of the Public Museum of the City of Milwaukee 2(4):11.

9. Barrows, David Prescott. 1967. The Ethno-Botany of the Coahuilla Indians of Southern California. Banning, California: Malki Museum Press. Originally published in 1900.

10. Basehart, Harry W. 1974. Apache Indians XII. Mescalero Apache Subsistence Patterns and Socio-Political Organization. New York: Garland Publishing.

11. Bean, Lowell John, and Katherine Siva Saubel. 1972. Temalpakh (From the Earth); Cahuilla Indian Knowledge and Usage of Plants. Banning, California: Malki Museum Press.

12. Beardsley, Gretchen 1941. Notes on Cree Medicines, Based on Collections Made by I. Cowie in 1892. Papers of the Michigan Academy of Science, Arts and Letters 28: 483–496.

13. Bell, Willis H., and Edward F. Castetter. 1941. Ethnobiological Studies in the Southwest VII. The Utilization of Yucca, Sotol and Beargrass by the Aborigines in the American Southwest. University of New Mexico Bulletin 5(5):1–74.

14. Black, Meredith Jean. 1980. Algonquin Ethnobotany: An Interpretation of Aboriginal Adaptation in South Western Quebec. Ottawa: National Museums of Canada. Mercury Series, Number 65.

15. Blankinship, J. W. 1905. Native Economic Plants of Montana. Bozeman: Montana Agricultural College Experimental Station, Bulletin 56.

16. Boas, Franz 1966. Kwakiutl Ethnography. Chicago: University of Chicago Press.

17. Bocek, Barbara R. 1984. Ethnobotany of Costanoan Indians, California, Based on Collections by John P. Harrington. Economic Botany 38(2):240–255.

18. Bradley, Will T. 1936. Medical Practices of the New England Aborigines. Journal of the American Pharmaceutical Association 25(2):138–147.

19. Burgesse, J. Allen 1944. The Woman and the Child among the Lac-St.-Jean Montagnais. Primitive Man 17:1–18.

20. Bushnell, David I., Jr. 1909. The Choctaw of Bayou Lacomb, St. Tammany Parish, Louisiana. Smithsonian Institution–Bureau of American Ethnology Bulletin, Number 48.

21. Buskirk, Winfred. 1986. The Western Apache: Living with the Land before 1950. Norman: University of Oklahoma Press.

22. Camazine, Scott, and Robert A. Bye 1980. A Study of the Medical Ethnobotany of the Zuni Indians of New Mexico. Journal of Ethnopharmacology 2:365–388.

23. Campbell, T. N. 1951. Medicinal Plants Used by Choctaw, Chickasaw, and Creek Indians in the Early Nineteenth Century. Journal of the Washington Academy of Sciences 41(9): 285–290.

24. Carlson, Gustav G., and Volney H. Jones. 1940. Some Notes on Uses of Plants by the Comanche

Indians. Papers of the Michigan Academy of Science, Arts and Letters 25:517–542.

25. Carr, Lloyd G., and Carlos Westey. 1945. Surviving Folktales and Herbal Lore among the Shinnecock Indians. Journal of American Folklore 58:113–123.

26. Carrier Linguistic Committee. 1973. Plants of Carrier Country. Fort St. James, British Columbia: Carrier Linguistic Committee.

27. Castetter, Edward F. 1935. Ethnobiological Studies in the American Southwest I. Uncultivated Native Plants Used as Sources of Food. University of New Mexico Bulletin 4(1):1–44.

28. Castetter, Edward F., and M. E. Opler. 1936. Ethnobiological Studies in the American Southwest III. The Ethnobiology of the Chiricahua and Mescalero Apache. University of New Mexico Bulletin 4(5):1–63.

29. Castetter, Edward F., and Ruth M. Underhill. 1935. Ethnobiological Studies in the American Southwest II. The Ethnobiology of the Papago Indians. University of New Mexico Bulletin 4(3):1–84.

30. Chamberlin, Ralph V. 1909. Some Plant Names of the Ute Indians. American Anthropologist 11:27–40.

31. Chamberlin, Ralph V. 1911. The Ethno-Botany of the Gosiute Indians of Utah. Memoirs of the American Anthropological Association 2(5):331–405.

32. Chandler, R. Frank, Lois Freeman, and Shirley N. Hooper. 1979. Herbal Remedies of the Maritime Indians. Journal of Ethnopharmacology 1:49–68.

33. Chesnut, V. K. 1902. Plants Used by the Indians of Mendocino County, California. Contributions from the U.S. National Herbarium 7:295–408.

34. Colton, Harold S. 1974. Hopi History and Ethnobotany. Pages 279–373 in D. A. Horr (editor), Hopi Indians. New York: Garland Publishing.

35. Compton, Brian Douglas. 1993. Upper North Wakashan and Southern Tsimshian Ethnobotany: The Knowledge and Usage of Plants . . . Ph.D. Dissertation, University of British Columbia, Vancouver.

36. Cook, Sarah Louise. 1930. The Ethnobotany of Jemez Indians. M.A. Thesis, University of New Mexico, Albuquerque.

37. Coville, Frederick V. 1897. Notes on the Plants Used by the Klamath Indians of Oregon. Contributions from the U.S. National Herbarium 5(2):87–110.

38. Curtin, L. S. M. 1949. By the Prophet of the Earth. Sante Fe, New Mexico: San Vicente Foundation.

39. Curtin, L. S. M. 1957. Some Plants Used by the Yuki Indians . . . II. Food Plants. Masterkey 31:85–94.

40. Dawson, E. Yale. 1944. Some Ethnobotanical Notes on the Seri Indians. Desert Plant Life 9:133–138.

41. Densmore, Frances. 1913. Chippewa Music. II. Smithsonian Institution–Bureau of American Ethnology Bulletin, Number 53.

42. Densmore, Frances. 1918. Teton Sioux Music. Smithsonian Institution–Bureau of American Ethnology Bulletin, Number 61.

43. Densmore, Frances. 1928. Uses of Plants by the Chippewa Indians. Smithsonian Institution–Bureau of American Ethnology Annual Report 44:273–379.

44. Densmore, Francis. 1932. Menominee Music. Smithsonian Institution–Bureau of American Ethnology Bulletin, Number 102.

45. Elmore, Francis H. 1944. Ethnobotany of the Navajo. Sante Fe, New Mexico: School of American Research.

46. Fewkes, J. Walter. 1896. A Contribution to Ethnobotany. American Anthropologist 9:14–21.

47. Fleisher, Mark S. 1980. The Ethnobotany of the Clallam Indians of Western Washington. Northwest Anthropological Research Notes 14(2):192–210.

48. Fletcher, Alice C., and Francis la Flesche. 1911. The Omaha Tribe. Smithsonian Institution–Bureau of American Ethnology Annual Report, Number 27.

49. Fowler, Catherine S. 1989. Willard Z. Park's Ethnographic Notes on the Northern Paiute of Western Nevada 1933–1940. Salt Lake City: University of Utah Press.

50. Garth, Thomas R. 1953. Atsugewi Ethnography. Anthropological Records 14(2):140–141.

51. Gifford, E. W. 1932. The Southeastern Yavapai. University of California Publications in American Archaeology and Ethnology 29:177–252.

52. Gifford, E. W. 1933. The Cocopa. University of California Publications in American Archaeology and Ethnology 31:263–270.

53. Gifford, E. W. 1936. Northeastern and Western Yavapai. University of California Publications in American Archaeology and Ethnology 34:247–345.

54. Gifford, E. W. 1967. Ethnographic Notes on the Southwestern Pomo. Anthropological Records 25:10–15.

55. Gill, Steven J. 1983. Ethnobotany of the Makah and Ozette People, Olympic Peninsula, Washington (USA). Ph.D. Thesis, Washington State University, Pullman.

56. Gilmore, Melvin R. 1913. A Study in the Ethnobotany of the Omaha Indians. Nebraska State Historical Society Collections 17:314–357.

57. Gilmore, Melvin R. 1913. Some Native Nebraska Plants with Their Uses by the Dakota. Collections of the Nebraska State Historical Society 17:358–370.

58. Gilmore, Melvin R. 1919. Uses of Plants by the Indians of the Missouri River Region. Smithsonian Institution–Bureau of American Ethnology Annual Report, Number 33.

59. Gilmore, Melvin R. 1933. Some Chippewa Uses of Plants. Ann Arbor: University of Michigan Press.

60. Goodrich, Jennie, and Claudia Lawson. 1980. Kashaya Pomo Plants. Los Angeles: American Indian Studies Center, University of California, Los Angeles.

61. Gottesfeld, Leslie M. J. 1992. The Importance of Bark Products in the Aboriginal Economies of Northwestern British Columbia, Canada. Economic Botany 46(2):148–157.

62. Gottesfeld, Leslie M. J., and Beverley Anderson. 1988. Gitksan Traditional Medicine: Herbs And Healing. Journal of Ethnobiology 8(1):13–33.

63. Grinnell, George Bird. 1905. Some Cheyenne Plant Medicines. American Anthropologist 7:37–43.

64. Grinnell, George Bird. 1972. The Cheyenne Indians: Their History and Ways of Life, Volume 2. Lincoln: University of Nebraska Press.

65. Gunther, Erna. 1973. Ethnobotany of Western Washington. Revised edition. Seattle: University of Washington Press.

66. Hamel, Paul B., and Mary U. Chiltoskey. 1975. Cherokee Plants and Their Uses: A 400 Year History. Sylva, North Carolina: Herald Publishing.

67. Hann, John H. 1986. The Use and Processing of Plants by Indians of Spanish Florida. Southeastern Archaeology 5(2):1–102.

68. Hart, Jeff. 1992. Montana Native Plants and Early Peoples. Helena: Montana Historical Society Press.

69. Hart, Jeffrey A. 1981. The Ethnobotany of the Northern Cheyenne Indians of Montana. Journal of Ethnopharmacology 4:1–55.

70. Hedges, Ken. 1986. Santa Ysabel Ethnobotany. San Diego Museum of Man Ethnic Technology Notes, Number 20.

71. Heller, Christine A. 1953. Edible and Poisonous Plants of Alaska. College, Alaska: Cooperative Agricultural Extension Service.

72. Hellson, John C. 1974. Ethnobotany of the Blackfoot Indians. Ottawa: National Museums of Canada. Mercury Series, Number 19.

73. Herrick, James William. 1977. Iroquois Medical Botany. Ph.D. Thesis, State University of New York, Albany.

74. Hinton, Leanne. 1975. Notes on La Huerta Diegueno Ethnobotany. Journal of California Anthropology 2:214–222.

75. Hocking, George M. 1949. From Pokeroot to Penicillin. Rocky Mountain Druggist, November 1949, pages 12, 38.

76. Hocking, George M. 1956. Some Plant Materials Used Medicinally and Otherwise by the Navaho Indians in the Chaco Canyon, New Mexico. Palacio 56:146–165.

77. Hoffman, W. J. 1891. The Midewiwin or "Grand Medicine Society" of the Ojibwa. Smithsonian Institution–Bureau of American Ethnology Annual Report, Number 7.

78. Holmes, E. M. 1884. Medicinal Plants Used by Cree Indians, Hudson's Bay Territory. Pharmaceutical Journal and Transactions 15:302–304.

79. Holt, Catharine. 1946. Shasta Ethnography. Anthropological Records 3(4):308.

80. Howard, James. 1965. The Ponca Tribe. Smithsonian Institution–Bureau of American Ethnology Bulletin, Number 195.

81. Hrdlicka, Ales. 1908. Physiological and Medical Observations among the Indians of Southwestern United States and Northern Mexico. Smithsonian Institution–Bureau of American Ethnology Bulletin 34:1–427.

82. Johnston, Alex. 1987. Plants and the Blackfoot. Lethbridge, Alberta: Lethbridge Historical Society.

83. Jones, Anore. 1983. Nauriat Niginaqtuat = Plants That We Eat. Kotzebue, Alaska: Maniilaq Association Traditional Nutrition Program.

84. Jones, David E. 1968. Comanche Plant Medicine. Papers in Anthropology 9:1–13.

85. Jones, Volney H. 1931. The Ethnobotany of the Isleta Indians. M.A. Thesis, University of New Mexico, Albuquerque.

86. Kari, Priscilla Russe. 1985. Upper Tanana Ethnobotany. Anchorage: Alaska Historical Commission.

87. Kelly, Isabel T. 1932. Ethnography of the Sur-

prise Valley Paiute. University of California Publications in American Archaeology and Ethnology 31(3):67–210.

88. Kraft, Shelly Katherene. 1990. Recent Changes in the Ethnobotany of Standing Rock Indian Reservation. M.A. Thesis, University of North Dakota, Grand Forks.

89. Krause, Aurel. 1956. The Tlingit Indians. Translated by Erna Gunther. Seattle: University of Washington Press.

90. Lantis, Margaret. 1959. Folk Medicine and Hygiene. Anthropological Papers of the University of Alaska 8:1–75.

91. Leighton, Anna L. 1985. Wild Plant Use by the Woods Cree (Nihithawak) of East-Central Saskatchewan. Ottawa. National Museums of Canada. Mercury Series, Number 101.

92. Lynch, Regina H. 1986. Cookbook. Chinle, Arizona: Navajo Curriculum Center, Rough Rock Demonstration School.

93. Mahar, James Michael. 1953. Ethnobotany of the Oregon Paiutes of the Warm Springs Indian Reservation. B.A. Thesis, Reed College, Portland, Oregon.

94. Malo, David. 1903. Hawaiian Antiquities. Honolulu: Hawaiian Gazette Co., Ltd.

95. McClintock, Walter. 1909. Medizinal- und Nutzpflanzen der Schwarzfuss Indianer. Zeitschrift für Ethnologie 41:273–279.

96. Mechling, W. H. 1959. The Malecite Indians with Notes on the Micmacs. Anthropologica 8:239–263.

97. Merriam, C. Hart. 1966. Ethnographic Notes on California Indian Tribes. Berkeley: University of California Archaeological Research Facility.

98. Murphey, Edith Van Allen. 1990. Indian Uses of Native Plants. Glenwood, Illinois: Meyerbooks. Originally published in 1959.

99. Nelson, Richard K. 1983. Make Prayers to the Raven: A Koyukon View of the Northern Forest. Chicago: University of Chicago Press.

100. Nickerson, Gifford S. 1966. Some Data on Plains and Great Basin Indian Uses of Certain Native Plants. Tebiwa 9(1):45–51.

101. Oswalt, W. H. 1957. A Western Eskimo Ethnobotany. Anthropological Papers of the University of Alaska 6:17–36.

102. Palmer, Gary. 1975. Shuswap Indian Ethnobotany. Syesis 8:29–51.

103. Parker, Arthur Caswell. 1910. Iroquois Uses of Maize and Other Food Plants. Albany, New York: University of the State of New York.

104. Perry, F. 1952. Ethno-Botany of the Indians in the Interior of British Columbia. Museum and Art Notes 2(2):36–43.

105. Perry, Myra Jean. 1975. Food Use of "Wild" Plants by Cherokee Indians. M.S. Thesis, University of Tennessee, Knoxville.

106. Porsild, A. E. 1953. Edible Plants of the Arctic. Arctic 6:15–34.

107. Powers, Stephen. 1874. Aboriginal Botany. Proceedings of the California Academy of Science 5:373–379.

108. Radin, Paul. 1923. The Winnebago Tribe. Smithsonian Institution–Bureau of American Ethnology Annual Report, Number 37.

109. Ray, Verne F. 1932. The Sanpoil and Nespelem: Salishan Peoples of Northeastern Washington. University of Washington Publications in Anthropology, Volume 5.

110. Raymond, Marcel. 1945. Notes Ethnobotaniques sur les Tête-de-Boule de Manouan. Contributions de l'Institut Botanique de l'Université de Montréal 55:113–134.

111. Reagan, Albert. 1934. Various Uses of Plants by West Coast Indians. Washington Historical Quarterly 25:133–137.

112. Reagan, Albert B. 1928. Plants Used by the Bois Fort Chippewa (Ojibwa) Indians of Minnesota. Wisconsin Archeologist 7(4):230–248.

113. Reagan, Albert B. 1929. Plants Used by the White Mountain Apache Indians of Arizona. Wisconsin Archeologist 8:143–161.

114. Reagan, Albert B. 1936. Plants Used by the Hoh and Quileute Indians. Kansas Academy of Science 37:55–70.

115. Robbins, W. W., J. P. Harrington, and B. Freire-Marreco 1916. Ethnobotany of the Tewa Indians. Smithsonian Institution–Bureau of American Ethnology Bulletin, Number 55.

116. Rogers, Dilwyn J. 1980. Lakota Names and Traditional Uses of Native Plants by Sicangu (Brule) People in the Rosebud Area, South Dakota. St. Francis, South Dakota: Rosebud Educational Society.

117. Romero, John Bruno. 1954. The Botanical Lore of the California Indians. New York: Vantage Press.

118. Rousseau, Jacques. 1945. Le Folklore Botanique de Caughnawaga. Contributions de l'Institut Botanique de l'Université de Montréal 55:7–72.

119. Rousseau, Jacques. 1945. Le Folklore Botanique de l'Ile aux Coudres. Contributions de l'Institut Botanique de l'Université de Montréal 55:75–111.

120. Rousseau, Jacques. 1946. Notes Sur l'Ethno-botanique d'Anticosti. Archives de Folklore 1:60–71.

121. Rousseau, Jacques. 1947. Ethnobotanique Abénakise. Archives de Folklore 11:145–182.

122. Rousseau, Jacques. 1948. Ethnobotanique et Ethnozoologie Gaspésiennes. Archives de Folklore 3:51–64.

123. Russell, Frank. 1908. The Pima Indians. Smithsonian Institution–Bureau of American Ethnology Annual Report 26:1–390.

124. Sapir, Edward, and Leslie Spier. 1943. Notes on the Culture of the Yana. Anthropological Records 3(3):252–253.

125. Schenck, Sara M., and E. W. Gifford. 1952. Karok Ethnobotany. Anthropological Records 13(6):377–392.

126. Smith, G. Warren. 1973. Arctic Pharmacognosia. Arctic 26:324–333.

127. Smith, Harlan I. 1929. Materia Medica of the Bella Coola and Neighboring Tribes of British Columbia. National Museum of Canada Bulletin 56:47–68.

128. Smith, Huron H. 1923. Ethnobotany of the Menomini Indians. Bulletin of the Public Museum of the City of Milwaukee 4:1–174.

129. Smith, Huron H. 1928. Ethnobotany of the Meskwaki Indians. Bulletin of the Public Museum of the City of Milwaukee 4:175–326.

130. Smith, Huron H. 1932. Ethnobotany of the Ojibwe Indians. Bulletin of the Public Museum of Milwaukee 4:327–525.

131. Smith, Huron H. 1933. Ethnobotany of the Forest Potawatomi Indians. Bulletin of the Public Museum of the City of Milwaukee 7:1–230.

132. Sparkman, Philip S. 1908. The Culture of the Luiseno Indians. University of California Publications in American Archaeology and Ethnology 8(4):187–234.

133. Speck, Frank G. 1917. Medicine Practices of the Northeastern Algonquians. Proceedings of the 19th International Congress of Americanists, pages 303–321.

134. Speck, Frank G. 1937. Catawba Medicines and Curative Practices. Publications of the Philadelphia Anthropological Society 1:179–197.

135. Speck, Frank G. 1941. A List of Plant Curatives Obtained from the Houma Indians of Louisiana. Primitive Man 14:49–75.

136. Speck, Frank G., and R. W. Dexter. 1951. Utilization of Animals and Plants by the Micmac Indians of New Brunswick. Journal of the Washington Academy of Sciences 41:250–259.

137. Speck, Frank G., and R. W. Dexter. 1952. Utilization of Animals and Plants by the Malecite Indians of New Brunswick. Journal of the Washington Academy of Sciences 42:1–7.

138. Speck, Frank G., R. B. Hassrick, and E. S. Carpenter. 1942. Rappahannock Herbals, Folk-Lore and Science of Cures. Proceedings of the Delaware County Institute of Science 10:7–55.

139. Spier, Leslie. 1928. Havasupai Ethnography. Anthropological Papers of the American Museum of Natural History 29(3):101–123, 284–285.

140. Spier, Leslie. 1930. Klamath Ethnography. University of California Publications in American Archaeology and Ethnology 30:1–338.

141. Steedman, E. V. 1928. The Ethnobotany of the Thompson Indians of British Columbia. Smithsonian Institution–Bureau of American Ethnology Annual Report 45:441–522.

142. Steggerda, Morris. 1941. Navajo Foods and Their Preparation. Journal of the American Dietetic Association 17(3):217–225.

143. Stevenson, Matilda Coxe. 1915. Ethnobotany of the Zuni Indians. Smithsonian Institution–Bureau of American Ethnology Annual Report, Number 30.

144. Steward, Julian H. 1933. Ethnography of the Owens Valley Paiute. University of California Publications in American Archaeology and Ethnology 33(3):233–250.

145. Sturtevant, William Curtis. 1955. The Mikasuki Seminole: Medical Beliefs and Practices. Ph.D. Thesis, Yale University, New Haven, Connecticut. Ann Arbor: University Microfilms.

146. Swan, James Gilchrist. 1869. The Indians of Cape Flattery . . . Washington Territory. Washington, D.C.: Smithsonian Institution.

147. Swank, George R. 1932. The Ethnobotany of the Acoma and Laguna Indians. M.A. Thesis, University of New Mexico, Albuquerque.

148. Swanton, John R 1928. Religious Beliefs and Medical Practices of the Creek Indians. Smithsonian Institution–Bureau of American Ethnology Annual Report 42:473–672.

149. Tantaquidgeon, Gladys. 1928. Mohegan Medicinal Practices, Weather-Lore and Superstitions. Smithsonian Institution–Bureau of American Ethnology Annual Report 43:264–270.

150. Tantaquidgeon, Gladys. 1942. A Study of Delaware Indian Medicine Practice and Folk Beliefs. Harrisburg: Pennsylvania Historical Commission.

151. Tantaquidgeon, Gladys. 1972. Folk Medicine of the Delaware and Related Algonkian Indians.

Harrisburg: Pennsylvania Historical Commission Anthropological Papers, Number 3.

152. Taylor, Linda Averill. 1940. Plants Used as Curatives by Certain Southeastern Tribes. Cambridge, Massachusetts: Botanical Museum of Harvard University.

153. Teit, James A. 1928. The Salishan Tribes of the Western Plateaus. Smithsonian Institution–Bureau of American Ethnology Annual Report, Number 45.

154. Theodoratus, Robert J. 1989. Loss, Transfer, and Reintroduction in the Use of Wild Plant Foods in the Upper Skagit Valley. Northwest Anthropological Research Notes 23(1):35–52.

155. Train, Percy, James R. Henrichs, and W. Andrew Archer. 1941. Medicinal Uses of Plants by Indian Tribes of Nevada. Washington, D.C.: U.S. Department of Agriculture.

156. Turner, Nancy Chapman, and Marcus A. M. Bell. 1971. The Ethnobotany of the Coast Salish Indians of Vancouver Island, I and II. Economic Botany 25(1):63–104, 335–339.

157. Turner, Nancy Chapman, and Marcus A. M. Bell. 1973. The Ethnobotany of the Southern Kwakiutl Indians of British Columbia. Economic Botany 27:257–310.

158. Turner, Nancy J. 1973. The Ethnobotany of the Bella Coola Indians of British Columbia. Syesis 6:193–220.

159. Turner, Nancy J., and Barbara S. Efrat 1982. Ethnobotany of the Hesquiat Indians of Vancouver Island. Victoria: British Columbia Provincial Museum.

160. Turner, Nancy J., John Thomas, Barry F. Carlson, and Robert T. Ogilvie. 1983. Ethnobotany of the Nitinaht Indians of Vancouver Island. Victoria: British Columbia Provincial Museum.

161. Turner, Nancy J., Laurence C. Thompson, M. Terry Thompson, and Annie Z. York. 1990. Thompson Ethnobotany: Knowledge and Usage of Plants by the Thompson Indians of British Columbia. Victoria: Royal British Columbia Museum.

162. Turner, Nancy J., R. Bouchard, and Dorothy I. D. Kennedy. 1980. Ethnobotany of the Okanagan-Colville Indians of British Columbia and Washington. Victoria: British Columbia Provincial Museum.

163. Veniamenov, I. 1840. Notes on the Islands in the Unalaska District. Translated by Human Relations Area Files, New Haven, Connecticut.

164. Vestal, Paul A. 1940. Notes on a Collection of Plants from the Hopi Indian Region of Arizona Made by J. G. Owens in 1891. Botanical Museum Leaflets (Harvard University) 8(8):153–168.

165. Vestal, Paul A. 1952. The Ethnobotany of the Ramah Navaho. Papers of the Peabody Museum of American Archaeology and Ethnology 40(4):1–94.

166. Vestal, Paul A., and Richard Evans Schultes. 1939. The Economic Botany of the Kiowa Indians. Cambridge, Massachusetts: Botanical Museum of Harvard University.

167. Voegelin, Ermine W. 1938. Tubatulabal Ethnography. Anthropological Records 2(1):1–84.

168. Wallis, Wilson D. 1922. Medicines Used by the Micmac Indians. American Anthropologist 24:24–30.

169. Watahomigie, Lucille J. 1982. Hualapai Ethnobotany. Peach Springs, Arizona: Hualapai Bilingual Program, Peach Springs School District Number 8.

170. Waugh, F. W. 1916. Iroquois Foods and Food Preparation. Ottawa: Canada Department of Mines.

171. Weber, Steven A., and P. David Seaman. 1985. Havasupai Habitat: A. F. Whiting's Ethnography of a Traditional Indian Culture. Tucson: University of Arizona Press.

172. White, Leslie A. 1945. Notes on the Ethnobotany of the Keres. Papers of the Michigan Academy of Arts, Sciences and Letters 30:557–568.

173. White, Leslie A. 1962. The Pueblo of Sia, New Mexico. Smithsonian Institution–Bureau of American Ethnology Bulletin, Number 184.

174. Whiting, Alfred F. 1939. Ethnobotany of the Hopi. Museum of Northern Arizona Bulletin, Number 15.

175. Willoughby, C. 1889. Indians of the Quinaielt Agency, Washington Territory. Smithsonian Institution Annual Report for 1886.

176. Wilson, Michael R. 1978. Notes on Ethnobotany in Inuktitut. Western Canadian Journal of Anthropology 8:180–196.

177. Witthoft, John. 1947. An Early Cherokee Ethnobotanical Note. Journal of the Washington Academy of Sciences 37(3):73–75.

178. Witthoft, John. 1977. Cherokee Indian Use of Potherbs. Journal of Cherokee Studies 2(2):250–255.

179. Wyman, Leland C., and Stuart K. Harris. 1951. The Ethnobotany of the Kayenta Navaho. Albuquerque: University of New Mexico Press.

180. Zigmond, Maurice L. 1981. Kawaiisu Ethnobotany. Salt Lake City: University of Utah Press.

Index of Tribes

Plant usages are listed under the names of Native American groups, which are arranged alphabetically. Usages are listed alphabetically. Plants are identified below to the level of species. If subspecies or varieties appear in the Catalog of Plants, check under those names, too, for all usages given below. For example, one may find Comanche below and under Cold Remedy see that *Rhus trilobata* was used. The specific ethnobotanical information and the sources from which the information was obtained may be found by turning to *Rhus trilobata* and *R. trilobata* var. *pilosissima* in the Catalog of Plants.

Abnaki

Abortifacient: *Fraxinus americana, Sanguinaria canadensis*

Analgesic: *Arctium minus, Carum carvi, Cornus canadensis, Plantago major, Ranunculus acris*

Anthelmintic: *Cirsium arvense, Populus tremuloides*

Antihemorrhagic: *Maianthemum racemosum, Polygonatum pubescens*

Antirheumatic (External): *Arctium minus, Mitchella repens, Plantago major, Symplocarpus foetidus, Taxus canadensis, Thuja occidentalis, Tsuga canadensis*

Antirheumatic (Internal): *Arctium minus, Taxus canadensis, Tsuga canadensis*

Blood Medicine: *Aralia nudicaulis*

Carminative: *Acorus calamus*

Cold Remedy: *Achillea millefolium, Asarum canadense, Chimaphila umbellata, Coptis trifolia, Kalmia angustifolia, Ledum groenlandicum*

Cough Medicine: *Asarum canadense, Coptis trifolia, Epilobium angustifolium, Larix laricina, Pinus strobus*

Dermatological Aid: *Abies balsamea, Alnus incana, Tsuga canadensis*

Disinfectant: *Abies balsamea*

Eye Medicine: *Cornus sericea, Corylus cornuta*

Febrifuge: *Achillea millefolium, Arctium minus*

Gastrointestinal Aid: *Polypodium virginianum*

Hemostat: *Urtica dioica*

Misc. Disease Remedy: *Achillea millefolium, Arctium minus*

Nose Medicine: *Chimaphila umbellata, Kalmia angustifolia, Ledum groenlandicum*

Orthopedic Aid: *Eupatorium perfoliatum*

Other: *Botrychium virginianum, Gymnocarpium disjunctum*

Panacea: *Abies balsamea, Mentha canadensis, Thuja occidentalis, Trillium erectum*

Pediatric Aid: *Achillea millefolium, Botrychium virginianum, Cirsium arvense, Mentha canadensis, Trillium erectum, Verbascum thapsus*

Poison: *Caltha palustris, Iris versicolor*

Respiratory Aid: *Acer pensylvanicum*

Sedative: *Mentha canadensis*

Toothache Remedy: *Verbascum thapsus*

Unspecified: *Abies balsamea, Botrychium virginianum*

Urinary Aid: *Picea glauca*

Veterinary Aid: *Sanguinaria canadensis*

Alabama

Antidiarrheal: *Hypericum hypericoides, H. multicaule*

Antirheumatic (External): *Callicarpa americana*

Ceremonial Medicine: *Ilex vomitoria*

Dermatological Aid: *Quercus rubra, Zanthoxylum americanum*

Diaphoretic: *Callicarpa americana*

Emetic: *Eryngium aquaticum, Ilex vomitoria*

Eye Medicine: *Hypericum hypericoides, H. multicaule, Ilex opaca*

Febrifuge: *Callicarpa americana, Cercis canadensis*

Gastrointestinal Aid: *Erythrina herbacea*

Gynecological Aid: *Ulmus rubra*

Herbal Steam: *Callicarpa americana*

Laxative: *Sebastiania fruticosa*

Orthopedic Aid: *Ceanothus americanus, Hypericum hypericoides, Quercus rubra*

Pediatric Aid: *Hypericum hypericoides, Quercus rubra*

Pulmonary Aid: *Cercis canadensis, Quercus rubra*

Respiratory Aid: *Cercis canadensis*

Sedative: *Gnaphalium obtusifolium*

Throat Aid: *Quercus rubra*

Toothache Remedy: *Zanthoxylum americanum*

Urinary Aid: *Morus rubra*

Alaska Native

Poison: *Actaea rubra, Caltha palustris, Cicuta douglasii, C. maculata, C. virosa, Hedysarum boreale, Lupinus nootkatensis, Pteridium aquilinum, Veratrum viride, Zigadenus elegans*

Aleut

Analgesic: *Achillea millefolium, Angelica lucida, Lycopodium clavatum, Matricaria discoidea, Menyanthes trifoliata*

Antihemorrhagic: *Anemone narcissiflora*

Antirheumatic (External): *Artemisia vulgaris*

Antirheumatic (Internal): *Menyanthes trifoliata*

Carminative: *Matricaria discoidea, Menyanthes trifoliata*

Cold Remedy: *Achillea millefolium, Angelica lucida, Conioselinum gmelinii, Geum calthifolium, Heracleum maximum*

Dermatological Aid: *Artemisia vulgaris, Geum calthifolium, Heracleum maximum, Rumex acetosella, Senecio pseudoarnica, Taraxacum officinale*

Gastrointestinal Aid: *Achillea millefolium, Matricaria discoidea, Taraxacum officinale*

Gynecological Aid: *Lycopodium clavatum*

Hemostat: *Achillea millefolium*

Laxative: *Iris setosa, Matricaria discoidea, Menyanthes trifoliata*

Misc. Disease Remedy: *Leptarrhena pyrolifolia*

Orthopedic Aid: *Artemisia vulgaris, Heracleum maximum*

Panacea: *Matricaria discoidea*

Poison: *Aconitum maximum, Ranunculus occidentalis*

Throat Aid: *Achillea millefolium, Angelica lucida, Conioselinum gmelinii, Geranium erianthum, Geum calthifolium, Heracleum maximum, Taraxacum officinale*

Tonic: *Angelica lucida, Artemisia vulgaris, Geum calthifolium, Matricaria discoidea, Menyanthes trifoliata, Plantago macrocarpa, Polygonum bistorta*

Tuberculosis Remedy: *Achillea millefolium*

Algonquin

Analgesic: *Actaea rubra*

Love Medicine: *Sanguinaria canadensis*

Other: *Juniperus communis*

Algonquin, Quebec

Analgesic: *Achillea millefolium, Comptonia peregrina, Gaultheria procumbens, Ledum groenlandicum*

Anticonvulsive: *Asarum canadense*

Antidiarrheal: *Coptis trifolia, Rubus idaeus*

Antirheumatic (External): *Tsuga canadensis*

Antirheumatic (Internal): *Maianthemum racemosum, Rhus hirta, Taxus canadensis, Thuja occidentalis*

Blood Medicine: *Prunus pensylvanica, Taraxacum officinale*

Cathartic: *Cornus canadensis, Lonicera dioica*

Ceremonial Medicine: *Ledum groenlandicum*

Cold Remedy: *Achillea millefolium, Acorus calamus, Cornus sericea, Gaultheria procumbens, Kalmia angustifolia, Sorbus americana, Thuja occidentalis, Tsuga canadensis*

Cough Medicine: *Acorus calamus, Larix laricina, Picea glauca, Prunus nigra, P. pensylvanica, P. virginiana*

Dermatological Aid: *Abies balsamea, Betula papyrifera, Clintonia borealis, Nuphar lutea, Picea glauca, P. mariana, Populus balsamifera, Thuja occidentalis, Toxicodendron radicans, Tsuga canadensis, Typha latifolia*

Dietary Aid: *Rhus hirta*

Disinfectant: *Clintonia borealis, Larix laricina, Nuphar lutea, Populus balsamifera, Prunus pensylvanica, Tsuga canadensis, Typha latifolia*

Emetic: *Alnus incana, Sambucus canadensis*

Eye Medicine: *Coptis trifolia, Tilia americana*

Febrifuge: *Asarum canadense, Cardamine diphylla, Prunella vulgaris, Thuja occidentalis*

Gastrointestinal Aid: *Corylus cornuta, Gaultheria hispidula, Lilium canadense, L. philadelphicum, Thuja occidentalis, Vaccinium angustifolium*

Gynecological Aid: *Abies balsamea, Acorus calamus, Cypripedium acaule, Eupatorium maculatum, Linnaea borealis, Lonicera dioica, Picea glauca, Sarracenia purpurea, Taxus canadensis, Thuja occidentalis, Tsuga canadensis, Vaccinium angustifolium*

Heart Medicine: *Abies balsamea, Acorus calamus, Aralia hispida, Cardamine diphylla, Coptis trifolia, Corylus cornuta, Polypodium virginianum, Sanguinaria canadensis*

Hemorrhoid Remedy: *Cornus sericea*

Internal Medicine: *Picea glauca, P. mariana*

Kidney Aid: *Aralia nudicaulis, Epigaea repens, Lonicera dioica*

Laxative: *Abies balsamea, Alnus incana, Dirca palustris, Picea glauca, Sambucus canadensis*

Misc. Disease Remedy: *Aralia racemosa*

Orthopedic Aid: *Shepherdia canadensis*

Pediatric Aid: *Aralia nudicaulis, Asarum canadense, Betula papyrifera, Cardamine diphylla,*

Thuja occidentalis, Tsuga canadensis, Vaccinium angustifolium
Poison: *Kalmia angustifolia*
Poultice: *Abies balsamea, Achillea millefolium, Plantago major, Taraxacum officinale, Taxus canadensis*
Preventive Medicine: *Acorus calamus*
Pulmonary Aid: *Prunus pensylvanica, Trifolium pratense*
Respiratory Aid: *Achillea millefolium*
Tonic: *Ledum groenlandicum, Sanguinaria canadensis, Sorbus americana*
Toothache Remedy: *Alnus incana, Coptis trifolia, Thuja occidentalis*
Tuberculosis Remedy: *Aralia racemosa*
Unspecified: *Abies balsamea, Acer pensylvanicum, Aralia hispida, Betula lenta, Chelone glabra, Gaultheria procumbens, Larix laricina, Ledum groenlandicum, Picea glauca, P. mariana, Prunus nigra, Rhus hirta, Rubus idaeus, Shepherdia canadensis, Spiraea alba, S. tomentosa, Taxus canadensis, Tilia americana, Tsuga canadensis*
Urinary Aid: *Sarracenia purpurea*
Venereal Aid: *Cypripedium acaule, Eupatorium maculatum*
Veterinary Aid: *Acer pensylvanicum*

Algonquin, Tête-de-Boule

Abortifacient: *Taxus canadensis*
Analgesic: *Achillea millefolium, Kalmia angustifolia, Viburnum lantanoides*
Antihemorrhagic: *Geum rivale*
Antirheumatic (External): *Populus tremuloides*
Burn Dressing: *Anaphalis margaritacea, Iris versicolor, Plantago major*
Cold Remedy: *Abies balsamea, Coptis trifolia, Cornus canadensis, Gaultheria procumbens, Pinus resinosa, P. strobus*
Dermatological Aid: *Acer spicatum, Clintonia borealis, Epilobium angustifolium, Iris versicolor, Plantago major*
Diuretic: *Diervilla lonicera, Sarracenia purpurea*
Ear Medicine: *Aralia nudicaulis*
Febrifuge: *Mentha canadensis*
Gastrointestinal Aid: *Cypripedium acaule, Gaultheria procumbens*
Gynecological Aid: *Cornus canadensis, Salix discolor, Trillium undulatum*
Heart Medicine: *Corylus cornuta*
Hemostat: *Prunus pensylvanica*
Kidney Aid: *Cypripedium acaule*
Laxative: *Larix laricina*
Misc. Disease Remedy: *Gaultheria procumbens*

Pediatric Aid: *Cypripedium acaule, Prunus pensylvanica*
Poison: *Kalmia angustifolia*
Psychological Aid: *Fraxinus pennsylvanica, Sorbus americana*
Respiratory Aid: *Coptis trifolia*
Stimulant: *Fraxinus pennsylvanica*
Strengthener: *Sorbus americana*
Throat Aid: *Salix discolor*
Urinary Aid: *Cypripedium acaule, Rubus idaeus, Sarracenia purpurea*

Anticosti

Dermatological Aid: *Populus balsamifera*
Kidney Aid: *Abies balsamea, Larix laricina*
Sedative: *Gaultheria hispidula*
Throat Aid: *Abies balsamea*
Unspecified: *Ledum groenlandicum*

Apache

Snakebite Remedy: *Yucca angustissima*
Unspecified: *Frasera speciosa*

Apache, Chiricahua & Mescalero

Narcotic: *Broussonetia papyrifera, Opuntia leptocaulis*

Apache, Mescalero

Cold Remedy: *Pinus edulis*
Ear Medicine: *Prosopis pubescens*
Eye Medicine: *Mahonia haematocarpa, Prosopis glandulosa*
Pediatric Aid: *Prosopis glandulosa*
Unspecified: *Typha latifolia*
Urinary Aid: *Prosopis glandulosa*

Apache, Western

Ceremonial Medicine: *Yucca elata*
Dermatological Aid: *Pinus edulis, P. monophylla*
Ear Medicine: *Prosopis pubescens*
Veterinary Aid: *Cucurbita foetidissima*

Apache, White Mountain

Anticonvulsive: *Juniperus californica, J. monosperma, J. occidentalis*
Antidiarrheal: *Phragmites australis*
Blood Medicine: *Malacothrix glabrata, Xanthium strumarium*
Burn Dressing: *Cercocarpus montanus*
Cathartic: *Croton texensis*
Ceremonial Medicine: *Cornus sericea, Datura wrightii, Dimorphocarpa wislizeni, Eriogonum jamesii, Mahonia fremontii, Nicotiana attenuata*

Cold Remedy: *Juniperus californica, J. monosperma, J. occidentalis*
Cough Medicine: *Juniperus californica, J. monosperma, J. occidentalis, Pseudotsuga menziesii*
Dermatological Aid: *Dimorphocarpa wislizeni*
Disinfectant: *Datura wrightii*
Eye Medicine: *Linum puberulum*
Gastrointestinal Aid: *Croton texensis, Phragmites australis*
Gynecological Aid: *Juniperus californica, J. monosperma, J. occidentalis, Rumex salicifolius*
Laxative: *Mentzelia pumila*
Narcotic: *Datura wrightii*
Oral Aid: *Chamaesyce serpyllifolia, Eriogonum jamesii*
Snakebite Remedy: *Helianthus annuus, Stephanomeria tenuifolia*
Throat Aid: *Dimorphocarpa wislizeni, Rumex salicifolius*
Unspecified: *Berula erecta, Eriogonum jamesii, Polygonum lapathifolium, Purshia mexicana, Solanum elaeagnifolium*
Venereal Aid: *Ephedra nevadensis, Pinus edulis*
Witchcraft Medicine: *Penstemon barbatus*

Apalachee

Unspecified: *Cuminum cyminum, Rumex acetosa*

Arapaho

Analgesic: *Psoralidium lanceolatum*
Antirheumatic (External): *Rosa woodsii*
Cough Medicine: *Artemisia frigida*
Dermatological Aid: *Psoralidium lanceolatum, Rumex hymenosepalus, R. venosus*
Disinfectant: *Juniperus communis*
Gastrointestinal Aid: *Juniperus communis*
Misc. Disease Remedy: *Juniperus communis*
Throat Aid: *Psoralidium lanceolatum*
Tonic: *Ivesia gordonii*
Unspecified: *Heuchera cylindrica*

Atsugewi

Analgesic: *Ligusticum grayi*
Antirheumatic (External): *Eriodictyon californicum*
Antirheumatic (Internal): *Verbascum thapsus*
Burn Dressing: *Arctostaphylos patula*
Cold Remedy: *Eriodictyon californicum, Ligusticum grayi, Verbascum thapsus*
Cough Medicine: *Ligusticum grayi*
Dermatological Aid: *Arctostaphylos patula, Prunus virginiana, Verbascum thapsus*
Diaphoretic: *Verbascum thapsus*
Gastrointestinal Aid: *Ligusticum grayi*

Herbal Steam: *Eriodictyon californicum*
Panacea: *Ligusticum grayi*
Pediatric Aid: *Ligusticum grayi*
Pulmonary Aid: *Eriodictyon californicum*
Unspecified: *Verbascum thapsus*

Bannock

Throat Aid: *Glycyrrhiza lepidota*

Bella Coola

Adjuvant: *Chamaecyparis nootkatensis*
Analgesic: *Alnus incana, Antennaria howellii, Aralia nudicaulis, Aruncus dioicus, Asarum caudatum, Geum macrophyllum, Heracleum maximum, Juniperus communis, Lactuca biennis, Ledum groenlandicum, Mentha canadensis, Nuphar lutea, Physocarpus opulifolius, Picea sitchensis, Polypodium virginianum, Populus balsamifera, Prenanthes alata, Pseudotsuga menziesii, Rumex aquaticus, Sambucus racemosa, Taraxacum officinale, Thuja plicata, Urtica dioica, Veratrum viride*
Antidiarrheal: *Aruncus dioicus, Lactuca biennis, Pseudotsuga menziesii, Salix lucida*
Antidote: *Dryopteris carthusiana, D. filix-mas*
Antiemetic: *Lactuca biennis*
Antihemorrhagic: *Arceuthobium americanum, Lactuca biennis*
Antirheumatic (External): *Alnus incana, Asarum caudatum, Heracleum maximum, Picea sitchensis, Pinus contorta, Plagiomnium insigne, Populus balsamifera, Rhizomnium glabrescens, Rumex aquaticus, Thuja plicata, Tsuga heterophylla, Urtica dioica, Veratrum viride*
Antirheumatic (Internal): *Nuphar lutea, Oplopanax horridus, Pseudotsuga menziesii, Sorbus sitchensis*
Blood Medicine: *Nuphar lutea, Plagiomnium insigne, Rhizomnium glabrescens*
Breast Treatment: *Achillea millefolium, Plagiomnium insigne, Rhizomnium glabrescens*
Burn Dressing: *Achillea millefolium, Picea sitchensis, Prenanthes alata, Tsuga heterophylla, T. mertensiana*
Cathartic: *Alnus rubra, Angelica genuflexa, Cicuta douglasii, Empetrum nigrum, Oplopanax horridus, Osmorhiza berteroi, Pseudotsuga menziesii, Sambucus racemosa*
Ceremonial Medicine: *Picea sitchensis*
Cold Remedy: *Prenanthes alata, Pseudotsuga menziesii, Ribes divaricatum, Viburnum edule*
Cough Medicine: *Juniperus communis, Lonicera involucrata, Thuja plicata, Veratrum viride*

Dermatological Aid: *Achillea millefolium, Clintonia uniflora, Epilobium angustifolium, Gaultheria shallon, Geum macrophyllum, Heracleum maximum, Lonicera involucrata, Picea sitchensis, Pinus contorta, Plagiomnium insigne, Populus balsamifera, Ranunculus acris, Rhizomnium glabrescens, Ribes lacustre, Rumex aquaticus, Salix lucida, S. scouleriana, Thuja plicata, Trautvetteria caroliniensis, Tsuga heterophylla, T. mertensiana, Veratrum viride*

Diaphoretic: *Populus balsamifera, Rosa nutkana*

Disinfectant: *Picea sitchensis*

Diuretic: *Aruncus dioicus, Myrica gale, Picea sitchensis, Pseudotsuga menziesii, Symphoricarpos albus*

Emetic: *Cicuta douglasii, Oplopanax horridus, Osmorhiza berteroi, Physocarpus capitatus, P. opulifolius, Pseudotsuga menziesii, Sambucus racemosa, Veratrum viride*

Eye Medicine: *Abies amabilis, A. grandis, Athyrium filix-femina, Clintonia uniflora, Cornus sericea, Malus fusca, Ribes divaricatum, R. laxiflorum, Rosa nutkana, Sorbus sitchensis*

Gastrointestinal Aid: *Abies amabilis, A. grandis, Aralia nudicaulis, Aruncus dioicus, Asarum caudatum, Geum macrophyllum, Juniperus communis, Ledum groenlandicum, Lysichiton americanus, Mentha canadensis, Picea sitchensis, Polypodium virginianum, Pseudotsuga menziesii, Rubus spectabilis, Sambucus racemosa, Sorbus sitchensis, Taraxacum officinale, Thuja plicata, Veratrum viride*

Gynecological Aid: *Sedum spathulifolium*

Heart Medicine: *Lactuca biennis, Nuphar lutea, Picea sitchensis, Pinus contorta, Prunella vulgaris, Prunus emarginata, Thuja plicata, Tsuga heterophylla, Veratrum viride*

Hemostat: *Urtica dioica*

Herbal Steam: *Rumex aquaticus, Urtica dioica*

Internal Medicine: *Tsuga heterophylla, T. mertensiana*

Laxative: *Frangula purshiana, Physocarpus opulifolius, Picea sitchensis, Pseudotsuga menziesii, Ribes lacustre, Veratrum viride*

Misc. Disease Remedy: *Aruncus dioicus*

Oral Aid: *Polypodium glycyrrhiza*

Orthopedic Aid: *Heracleum maximum, Populus balsamifera, Urtica dioica, Veratrum viride*

Other: *Thuja plicata*

Pediatric Aid: *Achillea millefolium, Prenanthes alata*

Poison: *Veratrum viride*

Pulmonary Aid: *Alnus incana, Arceuthobium americanum, Heracleum maximum, Juniperus communis, Populus balsamifera, Taxus brevifolia, Viburnum edule*

Respiratory Aid: *Achillea millefolium, Thuja plicata*

Throat Aid: *Abies amabilis, A. grandis, Polypodium glycyrrhiza, P. virginianum, Populus balsamifera, Ribes divaricatum*

Tuberculosis Remedy: *Abies amabilis, A. grandis, Anaphalis margaritacea, Nuphar lutea, Physocarpus opulifolius, Pinus contorta, Populus balsamifera, Prunus emarginata*

Unspecified: *Alnus incana, A. viridis, Artemisia ludoviciana, Ligusticum scothicum, Paxistima myrsinites, Ribes bracteosum*

Urinary Aid: *Saxifraga ferruginea*

Venereal Aid: *Amelanchier alnifolia, Aruncus dioicus, Lonicera involucrata, Myrica gale, Nuphar lutea, Physocarpus opulifolius, Picea sitchensis, Populus tremuloides, Pseudotsuga menziesii, Ribes bracteosum, Symphoricarpos albus, Veratrum viride*

Blackfoot

Abortifacient: *Anemone multifida, Artemisia campestris, Betula occidentalis, Draba incerta, Physaria didymocarpa*

Analgesic: *Abies lasiocarpa, Achillea millefolium, Acorus calamus, Anemone multifida, Glycyrrhiza lepidota, Liatris punctata, Mentha canadensis, Penstemon acuminatus, Physaria didymocarpa, Salix discolor, Veratrum californicum, V. viride*

Antidiarrheal: *Argentina anserina, Conyza canadensis, Delphinium bicolor, Erigeron philadelphicus, Escobaria vivipara, Fragaria virginiana, Heracleum maximum, Heuchera cylindrica, H. richardsonii, Matricaria discoidea, Perideridia gairdneri, Polyporus sp., Prunus virginiana, Rosa acicularis, Solanum triflorum*

Antiemetic: *Juniperus scopulorum, Penstemon acuminatus, Perideridia gairdneri*

Antihemorrhagic: *Angelica dawsonii, Astragalus canadensis, Conyza canadensis, Erigeron philadelphicus, Lycoperdon sp., Mahonia aquifolium, M. repens, Selaginella densa*

Antirheumatic (External): *Achillea millefolium, Angelica dawsonii, Artemisia campestris, Asclepias viridiflora, Glycyrrhiza lepidota, Heuchera parvifolia, Juniperus scopulorum, Pediomelum esculentum, Physaria didymocarpa, Rumex crispus, R. salicifolius, Viola adunca, Yucca glauca*

Antirheumatic (Internal): *Balsamorhiza sagittata*

Blood Medicine: *Geum triflorum*

Breast Treatment: *Gaillardia aristata, Osmorhiza occidentalis, Perideridia gairdneri*

Cathartic: *Acer glabrum, Amelanchier alnifolia, Lonicera involucrata, Prunus virginiana*

Ceremonial Medicine: *Abies lasiocarpa, Angelica dawsonii, Hierochloe odorata, Lithospermum incisum, Lomatium dissectum*

Cold Remedy: *Abies lasiocarpa, Actaea pachypoda, A. rubra, Artemisia frigida, Cornus sericea, Geranium viscosissimum, Hierochloe odorata, Osmorhiza berteroi*

Cough Medicine: *Actaea pachypoda, A. rubra, Artemisia campestris, A. frigida, Geum triflorum, Glycyrrhiza lepidota, Hierochloe odorata, Lygodesmia juncea, Monarda fistulosa, Osmorhiza occidentalis, Perideridia gairdneri*

Dermatological Aid: *Abies lasiocarpa, Achillea millefolium, Angelica dawsonii, Apocynum cannabinum, Arctostaphylos uva-ursi, Argentina anserina, Artemisia campestris, A. frigida, A. ludoviciana, Asclepias viridiflora, Astragalus canadensis, Balsamorhiza sagittata, Delphinium bicolor, Elaeagnus commutata, Epilobium angustifolium, Equisetum arvense, Evernia vulpina, Gaillardia aristata, Geum triflorum, Heracleum maximum, Heuchera cylindrica, H. parviflora, H. parvifolia, Hierochloe odorata, Liatris punctata, Lycopodium complanatum, Lygodesmia juncea, Mahonia repens, Monarda fistulosa, Oenothera cespitosa, Orobanche fasciculata, O. ludoviciana, Osmorhiza occidentalis, Oxytropis lagopus, O. sericea, Perideridia gairdneri, Physaria didymocarpa, Prunella vulgaris, Pulsatilla patens, Rumex crispus, R. salicifolius, Thalictrum occidentale, Xerophyllum tenax, Yucca glauca*

Dietary Aid: *Angelica dawsonii, Lomatium dissectum, Physaria didymocarpa*

Disinfectant: *Mahonia repens*

Diuretic: *Achillea millefolium, Equisetum arvense, Lygodesmia juncea, Perideridia gairdneri*

Ear Medicine: *Amelanchier alnifolia, Oxytropis sericea, Pediomelum esculentum, Physaria didymocarpa*

Emetic: *Abies lasiocarpa, Argentina anserina, Lonicera involucrata, Monarda fistulosa, Phragmites australis*

Eye Medicine: *Amelanchier alnifolia, Artemisia campestris, Asclepias viridiflora, Disporum trachycarpum, Dodecatheon pulchellum, Escobaria vivipara, Gaillardia aristata, Geranium viscosissimum, Geum triflorum, Heuchera cylindrica, H. parvifolia, Hierochloe odorata, Monarda fistulosa, Osmorhiza occidentalis,*

Pediomelum esculentum, Physaria didymocarpa, Prunella vulgaris

Febrifuge: *Abies lasiocarpa, Artemisia frigida, Salix discolor*

Gastrointestinal Aid: *Acorus calamus, Amelanchier alnifolia, Angelica dawsonii, Artemisia campestris, A. frigida, Evernia vulpina, Gaillardia aristata, Heuchera flabellifolia, Liatris punctata, Lonicera involucrata, Lygodesmia juncea, Mahonia aquifolium, M. repens, Pediomelum esculentum, Penstemon acuminatus, Physaria didymocarpa, Populus tremuloides, Shepherdia argentea, Valeriana dioica, Veratrum viride*

Gynecological Aid: *Achillea millefolium, Artemisia frigida, Camassia quamash, Lygodesmia juncea, Osmorhiza occidentalis, Populus tremuloides, Pulsatilla patens, Ribes americanum, Selaginella densa*

Heart Medicine: *Mentha canadensis*

Hemostat: *Artemisia frigida, Heuchera parvifolia, Lycoperdon sp., Lycopodium complanatum, Xerophyllum tenax, Yucca glauca*

Herbal Steam: *Gutierrezia sarothrae, Yucca glauca*

Kidney Aid: *Juniperus horizontalis, Lygodesmia juncea, Mahonia repens, Monarda fistulosa, Ribes americanum*

Laxative: *Amelanchier alnifolia, Apocynum cannabinum, Crataegus chrysocarpa, Epilobium angustifolium, Perideridia gairdneri, Phlox hoodii, Shepherdia argentea, Spiraea splendens*

Liver Aid: *Achillea millefolium, Cornus sericea, Grindelia squarrosa*

Misc. Disease Remedy: *Angelica dawsonii, Artemisia frigida, Rhus trilobata*

Narcotic: *Selaginella densa*

Nose Medicine: *Draba incerta, Gaillardia aristata, Osmorhiza occidentalis, Veratrum viride*

Oral Aid: *Abies lasiocarpa, Arctostaphylos uva-ursi, Artemisia campestris, Asclepias viridiflora, Delphinium bicolor, Dodecatheon pulchellum, Geum triflorum, Glycyrrhiza lepidota, Heuchera parvifolia, Veratrum viride*

Orthopedic Aid: *Equisetum arvense, Gaillardia aristata, Lygodesmia juncea, Pediomelum esculentum, Physaria didymocarpa, Xerophyllum tenax, Yucca glauca*

Other: *Angelica dawsonii, Geranium viscosissimum*

Panacea: *Achillea millefolium, Lomatium triternatum, Perideridia gairdneri, Populus tremuloides, Rumex salicifolius*

Pediatric Aid: *Amelanchier alnifolia, Angelica dawsonii, Arctostaphylos uva-ursi, Artemisia campestris, A. ludoviciana, Asclepias viridiflora,*

Astragalus canadensis, Delphinium bicolor, Dodecatheon pulchellum, Elaeagnus commutata, Epilobium angustifolium, Heuchera parvifolia, Lygodesmia juncea, Pediomelum esculentum, Phlox hoodii, Physaria didymocarpa, Prunus virginiana, Rosa acicularis, Solanum triflorum, Viola adunca

Poison: *Cornus sericea, Triglochin maritimum, Valeriana edulis, Veratrum californicum, V. viride*

Pulmonary Aid: *Abies lasiocarpa, Acorus calamus, Artemisia ludoviciana, Astragalus canadensis, Juniperus communis, Lomatium triternatum, Lonicera involucrata, Lycopodium complanatum, Pediomelum esculentum, Phlox hoodii, Rubus parviflorus, Thalictrum occidentale*

Respiratory Aid: *Artemisia ludoviciana, Geum triflorum, Gutierrezia sarothrae, Perideridia gairdneri, Polygala senega, Viola adunca*

Snakebite Remedy: *Heuchera cylindrica*

Stimulant: *Abies lasiocarpa, Artemisia frigida, Delphinium bicolor, Lomatium dissectum*

Strengthener: *Hierochloe odorata, Lomatium macrocarpum, L. triternatum, Perideridia gairdneri*

Throat Aid: *Achillea millefolium, Acorus calamus, Artemisia ludoviciana, Asclepias viridiflora, Geum triflorum, Glycyrrhiza lepidota, Hierochloe odorata, Lewisia rediviva, Monarda fistulosa, Osmorhiza berteroi, Oxytropis lagopus, Pediomelum esculentum, Perideridia gairdneri, Physaria didymocarpa, Prunus virginiana*

Tonic: *Geum triflorum, Lomatium dissectum, Lygodesmia juncea*

Toothache Remedy: *Acorus calamus, Echinacea angustifolia, Pediomelum esculentum, Physaria didymocarpa*

Tuberculosis Remedy: *Abies lasiocarpa, Alnus incana, Pinus contorta*

Unspecified: *Angelica dawsonii, Pediomelum esculentum, Prunus virginiana*

Venereal Aid: *Abies lasiocarpa, Hierochloe odorata, Juniperus communis, Lycopodium complanatum, Spiraea splendens*

Veterinary Aid: *Abies lasiocarpa, Achillea millefolium, Actaea rubra, Angelica dawsonii, Artemisia campestris, A. frigida, A. ludoviciana, Clematis occidentalis, Equisetum arvense, E. hyemale, Gaillardia aristata, Geum triflorum, Glycyrrhiza lepidota, Heuchera cylindrica, H. parvifolia, Hierochloe odorata, Juniperus horizontalis, Lomatium dissectum, L. macrocarpum, Lycoperdon sp., Lygodesmia juncea, Mahonia repens, Muhlenbergia richardsonis, Osmorhiza berteroi, Perideridia gairdneri, Physaria didymocarpa,*

Prunella vulgaris, Selaginella densa, Symphoricarpos occidentalis, Thalictrum sparsiflorum, Townsendia exscapa, Valeriana dioica, Yucca glauca

Cahuilla

Analgesic: *Datura wrightii, Populus fremontii, Rosa californica, Umbellularia californica, Urtica dioica*

Antidiarrheal: *Arctostaphylos glandulosa, A. glauca, A. pungens, Conyza canadensis, Matricaria discoidea*

Antidote: *Datura wrightii*

Antihemorrhagic: *Hyptis emoryi*

Antirheumatic (External): *Adenostoma fasciculatum, A. sparsifolium, Datura wrightii, Eriodictyon trichocalyx, Larrea tridentata, Populus fremontii, Urtica dioica*

Antirheumatic (Internal): *Eriodictyon trichocalyx*

Blood Medicine: *Ephedra nevadensis, Eriodictyon trichocalyx*

Burn Dressing: *Opuntia acanthocarpa*

Cancer Treatment: *Larrea tridentata*

Cathartic: *Cucurbita foetidissima, Opuntia ficus-indica*

Cold Remedy: *Adenostoma sparsifolium, Anemopsis californica, Artemisia californica, Atriplex lentiformis, Eriodictyon trichocalyx, Eucalyptus sp., Larrea tridentata, Rhus ovata, Salvia apiana, Sambucus cerulea, Satureja douglasii*

Cough Medicine: *Eriodictyon trichocalyx, Rhus ovata*

Dermatological Aid: *Anemopsis californica, Arctostaphylos glandulosa, A. glauca, A. pungens, Baccharis salicifolia, Bursera microphylla, Chamaesyce melanadenia, Chlorogalum pomeridianum, Cucurbita foetidissima, Ericameria palmeri, Isocoma acradenia, Larrea tridentata, Lepidium nitidum, Nicotiana clevelandii, N. glauca, N. trigonophylla, Opuntia acanthocarpa, O. ficus-indica, Pinus monophylla, P. quadrifolia, Populus fremontii, Prosopis glandulosa, Ricinus communis, Salvia apiana, Solidago california, Typha latifolia*

Disinfectant: *Adenostoma fasciculatum, Artemisia tridentata, Larrea tridentata, Salvia columbariae*

Ear Medicine: *Chamaesyce melanadenia, Croton californicus, Nicotiana clevelandii, N. glauca, N. trigonophylla*

Emetic: *Adenostoma sparsifolium, Cucurbita foetidissima, Larrea tridentata, Nicotiana clevelandii, N. glauca, N. trigonophylla*

Eye Medicine: *Prosopis glandulosa, Salvia apiana, S. columbariae, Solanum douglasii*
Febrifuge: *Eriodictyon trichocalyx, Sambucus cerulea, Satureja douglasii*
Gastrointestinal Aid: *Adenostoma sparsifolium, Anemopsis californica, Arbutus menziesii, Chenopodium californicum, Descurainia pinnata, Larrea tridentata, Matricaria discoidea, Monardella villosa, Sambucus cerulea, Trichostema lanatum*
Gynecological Aid: *Artemisia californica, Baccharis salicifolia, Larrea tridentata, Solidago californica*
Hallucinogen: *Datura wrightii*
Hunting Medicine: *Datura wrightii, Nicotiana clevelandii, N. glauca, N. trigonophylla, Salvia apiana*
Kidney Aid: *Marrubium vulgare*
Laxative: *Adenostoma sparsifolium, Frangula californica, Opuntia ficus-indica, Sambucus cerulea*
Misc. Disease Remedy: *Sambucus cerulea*
Nose Medicine: *Atriplex lentiformis*
Oral Aid: *Eriodictyon trichocalyx*
Orthopedic Aid: *Arundo donax, Phragmites australis*
Other: *Cucurbita foetidissima, Datura wrightii, Ephedra nevadensis*
Panacea: *Bursera microphylla*
Pediatric Aid: *Artemisia californica, Croton californicus, Rosa californica, Sambucus cerulea*
Poison: *Croton californicus, Datura wrightii, Ricinus communis, Solanum douglasii*
Pulmonary Aid: *Adenostoma sparsifolium, Anemopsis californica, Larrea tridentata*
Respiratory Aid: *Anemopsis californica, Artemisia tridentata, Croton californicus, Datura wrightii, Eriodictyon trichocalyx, Larrea tridentata*
Snakebite Remedy: *Datura wrightii*
Sports Medicine: *Datura wrightii*
Throat Aid: *Ericameria palmeri, Eriodictyon trichocalyx, Isocoma acradenia*
Tonic: *Frangula californica, Larrea tridentata*
Toothache Remedy: *Chrysothamnus nauseosus, Datura wrightii, Encelia farinosa, Gutierrezia microcephala, Sambucus cerulea*
Tuberculosis Remedy: *Eriodictyon trichocalyx*
Unspecified: *Apocynum cannabinum, Artemisia californica, Datura wrightii, Prosopis pubescens*
Veterinary Aid: *Adenostoma sparsifolium, Anemopsis californica, Cucurbita foetidissima, Datura wrightii, Populus fremontii*

California Indian

Antirheumatic (Internal): *Heracleum maximum*
Kidney Aid: *Mentha arvensis*
Snakebite Remedy: *Asclepias fascicularis*
Toothache Remedy: *Eschscholzia californica*

Carrier

Analgesic: *Cornus sericea, Oplopanax horridus, Urtica dioica*
Antirheumatic (External): *Achillea millefolium, Heracleum maximum*
Blood Medicine: *Chenopodium album*
Cough Medicine: *Plantago major, Viburnum edule*
Dermatological Aid: *Arctostaphylos uva-ursi, Lonicera involucrata, Shepherdia canadensis, Sphagnum sp., Urtica dioica*
Eye Medicine: *Lonicera involucrata, Rosa nutkana*
Gastrointestinal Aid: *Plantago major*
Gynecological Aid: *Shepherdia canadensis*
Kidney Aid: *Equisetum hyemale*
Laxative: *Plantago major, Shepherdia canadensis*
Pediatric Aid: *Sphagnum sp.*
Pulmonary Aid: *Cornus sericea*
Toothache Remedy: *Achillea millefolium*
Tuberculosis Remedy: *Juniperus communis, Shepherdia canadensis*
Unspecified: *Sorbus sitchensis*
Urinary Aid: *Equisetum hyemale*

Carrier, Northern

Analgesic: *Artemisia ludoviciana, Oplopanax horridus*
Antidiarrheal: *Viburnum edule*
Cathartic: *Juniperus communis, Oplopanax horridus, Sambucus racemosa, Shepherdia canadensis, Viburnum edule*
Cough Medicine: *Juniperus communis*
Dermatological Aid: *Cornus sericea, Heracleum maximum, Lonicera involucrata, Pinus contorta, Populus balsamifera, Valeriana dioica*
Eye Medicine: *Pinus contorta, Populus balsamifera*
Gastrointestinal Aid: *Alnus rubra, Oplopanax horridus*
Orthopedic Aid: *Cornus sericea, Lonicera involucrata, Pinus contorta* Stimulant: *Cornus sericea, Lonicera involucrata, Pinus contorta*
Unspecified: *Cornus canadensis*

Carrier, Southern

Analgesic: *Juniperus communis, Lycopodium clavatum, Picea sitchensis, Pinus contorta, Populus tremuloides, Viola adunca*
Antihemorrhagic: *Arceuthobium americanum*
Antirheumatic (External): *Mnium affine*

Cathartic: *Oplopanax horridus, Physocarpus opuli-folius, Sambucus racemosa*

Cold Remedy: *Achillea millefolium, Anemone multifida, Mentha canadensis, Sorbus sitchensis*

Cough Medicine: *Populus balsamifera*

Dermatological Aid: *Achillea millefolium, Alnus rubra, Artemisia ludoviciana, Geum macrophyllum*

Dietary Aid: *Arceuthobium americanum*

Emetic: *Physocarpus opulifolius, Veratrum viride*

Eye Medicine: *Cornus canadensis, Lonicera involucrata, Orthilia secunda, Picea sitchensis, Pyrola asarifolia, Symphoricarpos albus*

Gastrointestinal Aid: *Mentha canadensis, Picea sitchensis, Pinus contorta, Populus tremuloides, Viola adunca*

Gynecological Aid: *Oplopanax horridus*

Orthopedic Aid: *Achillea millefolium, Artemisia ludoviciana*

Panacea: *Anemone multifida, Geum macrophyllum*

Poison: *Veratrum viride*

Pulmonary Aid: *Mentha canadensis, Populus balsamifera*

Tuberculosis Remedy: *Arceuthobium americanum*

Unspecified: *Abies grandis*

Catawba

Analgesic: *Andropogon glomeratus, Aplectrum hyemale, Arnica acaulis, Chimaphila umbellata, Glyceria obtusa, Hexastylis arifolia, Pedicularis canadensis, Tephrosia virginiana, Verbascum thapsus*

Antidiarrheal: *Aletris farinosa*

Antirheumatic (External): *Tephrosia virginiana*

Antirheumatic (Internal): *Tephrosia virginiana*

Burn Dressing: *Parthenium integrifolium*

Cold Remedy: *Hedeoma pulegioides, Xanthorhiza simplicissima*

Dermatological Aid: *Aplectrum hyemale, Ilex opaca, Orbexilum pedunculatum, Salvia lyrata, Verbascum thapsus, Yucca filamentosa*

Febrifuge: *Tephrosia virginiana*

Gastrointestinal Aid: *Aletris farinosa, Hexastylis arifolia, Pedicularis canadensis, Xanthorhiza simplicissima*

Gynecological Aid: *Oxydendrum arboreum, Salix humilis*

Heart Medicine: *Erigeron strigosus, Hexastylis arifolia*

Kidney Aid: *Manfreda virginica*

Liver Aid: *Xanthorhiza simplicissima*

Misc. Disease Remedy: *Ilex opaca, Marshallia obovata, Prunella vulgaris*

Oral Aid: *Salix humilis*

Orthopedic Aid: *Andropogon glomeratus, Arnica acaulis, Chimaphila umbellata, Glyceria obtusa, Hexastylis arifolia, Orbexilum pedunculatum, Verbascum thapsus*

Pediatric Aid: *Salix humilis, Verbascum thapsus*

Pulmonary Aid: *Verbascum thapsus*

Snakebite Remedy: *Manfreda virginica*

Tuberculosis Remedy: *Senecio anonymus, Ulmus rubra*

Veterinary Aid: *Lachnanthes caroliana, Parthenium integrifolium*

Chehalis

Abortifacient: *Thuja plicata*

Analgesic: *Rosa nutkana*

Antidiarrheal: *Achillea millefolium*

Antirheumatic (External): *Urtica dioica*

Cold Remedy: *Abies grandis*

Contraceptive: *Geum macrophyllum, Lonicera ciliosa*

Dermatological Aid: *Delphinium menziesii, Lonicera ciliosa, Marah oreganus, Symphoricarpos albus, Urtica dioica*

Diaphoretic: *Taxus brevifolia*

Emetic: *Zigadenus venenosus*

Gynecological Aid: *Rosa nutkana*

Love Medicine: *Eriophyllum lanatum*

Misc. Disease Remedy: *Holodiscus discolor*

Panacea: *Taxus brevifolia*

Poison: *Delphinium menziesii*

Tuberculosis Remedy: *Marah oreganus, Tsuga heterophylla*

Venereal Aid: *Symphoricarpos albus, Tsuga heterophylla*

Cherokee

Abortifacient: *Angelica atropurpurea, Apocynum cannabinum, Aristolochia serpentaria, Armoracia rusticana, Asarum canadense, Asplenium trichomanes, Carya alba, C. laciniosa, C. pallida, Chamaemelum nobile, Cimicifuga racemosa, Echinocystis lobata, Erigeron philadelphicus, E. pulchellus, Hedeoma pulegioides, Hydrangea arborescens, Hypericum gentianoides, H. hypericoides, H. perforatum, Hyssopus officinalis, Juniperus virginiana, Lindera benzoin, Monarda didyma, M. fistulosa, Nepeta cataria, Orbexilum pedunculatum, Petroselinum crispum, Platanus occidentalis, Polygala senega, Scutellaria elliptica, S. incana, S. lateriflora, Solidago odora, Stylosanthes biflora, Verbena hastata*

Adjuvant: *Eupatorium maculatum, E. purpureum,*

Gleditsia triacanthos, Mentha ×piperita, M. spicata, Prunella vulgaris

Analgesic: *Acer rubrum, A. saccharinum, Acorus calamus, Alnus serrulata, Anaphalis margaritacea, Anthemis cotula, Arisaema triphyllum, Aristolochia serpentaria, Artemisia biennis, Asarum canadense, Asclepias perennis, A. quadrifolia, A. syriaca, A. tuberosa, Aster linariifolius, A. novae-angliae, Blephilia ciliata, Cardamine diphylla, Carya alba, C. laciniosa, C. pallida, Castanea pumila, Celastrus scandens, Chenopodium botrys, Chimaphila maculata, Cimicifuga racemosa, Cirsium altissimum, C. vulgare, Clematis virginiana, Cornus alternifolia, C. florida, Cunila marina, Cypripedium acaule, C. parviflorum, Daphne mezereum, Desmodium nudiflorum, D. perplexum, Epigaea repens, Erigeron philadelphicus, E. pulchellus, Euonymus americana, Gnaphalium obtusifolium, Hamamelis virginiana, Hedeoma pulegioides, Hepatica nobilis, Humulus lupulus, Kalmia latifolia, Lactuca canadensis, Leucothoe axillaris, Liatris spicata, Lobelia cardinalis, L. inflata, L. siphilitica, Magnolia acuminata, M. macrophylla, Mentha ×piperita, M. spicata, Mitchella repens, Monarda didyma, M. fistulosa, Nicotiana rustica, N. tabacum, Panax quinquefolius, P. trifolius, Papaver somniferum, Pastinaca sativa, Phoradendron leucarpum, Plantago aristata, P. lanceolata, P. major, Platanthera ciliaris, Polygonum aviculare, P. hydropiper, P. persicaria, Prenanthes serpentaria, P. trifoliolata, Pycnanthemum flexuosum, P. incanum, Rhododendron maximum, Rubus idaeus, R. occidentalis, R. odoratus, Sabatia angularis, Sanicula smallii, Satureja hortensis, Senna hebecarpa, S. marilandica, Smilax glauca, S. herbacea, S. pseudochina, S. rotundifolia, Tanacetum vulgare, Tradescantia virginiana, Veratrum viride, Verbascum thapsus, Verbena hastata, Vernonia glauca, V. noveboracensis, Veronicastrum virginicum, Vicia caroliniana, Viola bicolor, V. cucullata, V. pedata, V. pubescens, V. rotundifolia, V. sororia, Xanthorhiza simplicissima*

Anthelmintic: *Acorus calamus, Amelanchier arborea, A. canadensis, Artemisia biennis, Asarum canadense, Bidens bipinnata, Cerastium fontanum, Chelone glabra, Chenopodium botrys, Comptonia peregrina, Cornus alternifolia, C. florida, Cucurbita pepo, Cypripedium acaule, C. parviflorum, C. pubescens, Dryopteris filix-mas, Fagus grandifolia, Gleditsia triacanthos, Juniperus virginiana, Liriodendron tulipifera, Lobelia cardinalis, L. siphilitica, Manfreda virginica,*

Melia azedarach, Morus alba, M. rubra, Nepeta cataria, Nicotiana rustica, N. tabacum, Nyssa sylvatica, Oxalis corniculata, O. violacea, Pinus glabra, P. virginiana, Podophyllum peltatum, Portulaca oleracea, Prunus persica, Rosa palustris, R. virginiana, Rudbeckia fulgida, R. hirta, Ruta graveolens, Sassafras albidum, Solanum carolinense, Spigelia marilandica, Tanacetum vulgare, Tephrosia virginiana

Anticonvulsive: *Acorus calamus, Anthemis cotula, Caulophyllum thalictroides, Cypripedium acaule, C. parviflorum, Erigeron philadelphicus, E. pulchellus, Monotropa uniflora, Nepeta cataria, Nicotiana rustica, N. tabacum, Panax quinquefolius, Papaver somniferum, Phoradendron leucarpum, Viburnum acerifolium, V. nudum, V. prunifolium*

Antidiarrheal: *Acer rubrum, A. saccharinum, Acorus calamus, Ageratina altissima, Agrimonia gryposepala, A. parviflora, Amelanchier arborea, Amphicarpaea bracteata, Andropogon virginicus, Asarum canadense, Asclepias tuberosa, Aster linariifolius, A. novae-angliae, Aureolaria flava, A. laevigata, A. pedicularia, A. virginica, Berberis canadensis, Betula lenta, B. nigra, Campanula divaricata, Carpinus caroliniana, Coreopsis tinctoria, Cornus alternifolia, C. florida, Diospyros virginiana, Epigaea repens, Fragaria virginiana, Frasera caroliniensis, Gaultheria procumbens, Gaylussacia baccata, Hedeoma pulegioides, Heuchera americana, Hypericum gentianoides, H. hypericoides, H. perforatum, Juglans cinerea, Lilium canadense, Liquidambar styraciflua, Liriodendron tulipifera, Magnolia acuminata, M. macrophylla, Manfreda virginica, Menispermum canadense, Mitchella repens, Morus alba, M. rubra, Nyssa sylvatica, Oxydendrum arboreum, Pedicularis canadensis, Pinus glabra, P. virginiana, Plantago aristata, P. lanceolata, P. major, Platanthera ciliaris, Platanus occidentalis, Polygonatum biflorum, Polygonum aviculare, P. hydropiper, Potentilla simplex, Pycnanthemum flexuosum, P. incanum, Quercus alba, Q. falcata, Q. imbricaria, Q. rubra, Q. stellata, Q. velutina, Rheum rhaponticum, Ribes rotundifolium, Rosa palustris, Rubus allegheniensis, R. argutus, R. flagellaris, R. trivialis, Rumex crispus, R. patientia, Salix alba, S. babylonica, S. humilis, S. nigra, Salvia lyrata, S. officinalis, Sassafras albidum, Scutellaria elliptica, S. incana, S. lateriflora, Sesamum orientale, Sisyrinchium angustifolium, Solidago odora, Symphytum officinale, Thalictrum dioicum, T.*

thalictroides, Tilia americana, Tsuga canadensis, T. caroliniana, Ulmus rubra, Uvularia sessilifolia, Verbena bastata, Viola bicolor, V. cucullata, V. pedata, V. pubescens, V. rotundifolia, V. sororia, Vitis aestivalis, V. labrusca, V. vulpina, Xyris caroliniana

Antidote: *Cornus alternifolia, C. florida, Plantago aristata, P. lanceolata, P. major*

Antiemetic: *Baptisia australis, B. tinctoria, Chamaemelum nobile, Clethra acuminata, Frasera caroliniensis, Hydrangea arborescens, H. cinerea, Lupinus perennis, Mentha ×piperita, M. spicata, Oxalis corniculata, O. violacea, Prunus persica, Pteridium aquilinum, Rhus copallinum, R. glabra, R. birta, Thalictrum dioicum, T. thalictroides*

Antihemorrhagic: *Achillea millefolium, Allium tricoccum, Erigeron philadelphicus, E. pulchellus, Euonymus americana, Hosta lancifolia, Lachnanthes caroliana, Lupinus perennis, Tradescantia virginiana*

Antirheumatic (External): *Adiantum pedatum, Aesculus pavia, Celastrus scandens, Coronilla varia, Ipomoea pandurata, Kalmia latifolia, Leucothoe axillaris, Osmunda cinnamomea, Phacelia purshii, Pinus glabra, P. virginiana, Polystichum acrostichoides, Porteranthus stipulatus, P. trifoliatus, Rhododendron calendulaceum, Rubus idaeus, R. occidentalis, R. odoratus, Veratrum viride, Zanthoxylum americanum*

Antirheumatic (Internal): *Adiantum pedatum, Aletris farinosa, Anthemis cotula, Apocynum cannabinum, Aralia spinosa, Arctium lappa, Aristolochia serpentaria, Armoracia rusticana, Caulophyllum thalictroides, Chimaphila maculata, Cimicifuga racemosa, Dryopteris marginalis, Echinocystis lobata, Eupatorium maculatum, E. purpureum, Gnaphalium obtusifolium, Humulus lupulus, Juniperus virginiana, Leucothoe axillaris, Lilium canadense, Liriodendron tulipifera, Lobelia cardinalis, L. siphilitica, Panax trifolius, Phytolacca americana, Pinus glabra, P. virginiana, Podophyllum peltatum, Polygala senega, Polystichum acrostichoides, Populus balsamifera, P. nigra, Rhododendron maximum, Rubus alleghaniensis, R. argutus, R. flagellaris, R. trivialis, Sambucus canadensis, S. nigra, Sassafras albidum, Smilax glauca, S. herbacea, S. pseudochina, S. rotundifolia, Vicia caroliniana*

Blood Medicine: *Agrimonia gryposepala, A. parviflora, Alnus serrulata, Aralia nudicaulis, Arctium lappa, Asarum canadense, Barbarea vulgaris, Bignonia capreolata, Cornus alternifolia, C. florida, Goodyera pubescens, G. repens, Lindera benzoin, Ostrya virginiana, Oxalis corniculata, O. violacea, Phytolacca americana, Prunus cerasus, P. pensylvanica, P. serotina, P. virginiana, Pyrrhopappus carolinianus, Rumex crispus, R. patientia, Sassafras albidum, Taraxacum officinale, Vernonia glauca, V. noveboracensis, Viola bicolor, V. cucullata, V. pedata, V. pubescens, V. rotundifolia, V. sororia, Vitis aestivalis, V. labrusca, V. vulpina, Xanthorhiza simplicissima*

Breast Treatment: *Asarum canadense, Asplenium rhizophyllum, A. trichomanes, Collinsonia canadensis, Eupatorium pilosum, Hepatica nobilis, Humulus lupulus, Marrubium vulgare, Panax trifolius, Polygonatum biflorum, Scutellaria elliptica, S. incana, S. lateriflora, Verbena bastata*

Burn Dressing: *Aralia racemosa, Goodyera pubescens, G. repens, Hydrangea arborescens, Plantago aristata, P. lanceolata, P. major, Prunella vulgaris, Rhus copallinum, R. glabra, R. birta, Sambucus canadensis, S. nigra, Smallanthus uvedalia, Smilax glauca, S. herbacea, S. laurifolia, S. pseudochina, S. rotundifolia, Ulmus rubra*

Cancer Treatment: *Aesculus pavia, Arnoglossum atriplicifolium, Chamaesyce maculata, Chimaphila maculata, Cynoglossum virginianum, Euphorbia corollata, Hackelia virginiana, Hydrangea arborescens, Hydrastis canadensis, Lachnanthes caroliana, Oxalis corniculata, O. violacea, Tradescantia virginiana, Trillium erectum, Xanthorhiza simplicissima*

Carminative: *Acorus calamus, Aletris farinosa, Allium canadense, A. sativum, A. vineale, Angelica atropurpurea, Aralia spinosa, Arisaema triphyllum, Foeniculum vulgare, Liatris spicata, Mentha ×piperita, M. spicata, Monarda didyma, M. fistulosa*

Cathartic: *Allium canadense, A. sativum, A. vineale, Alnus incana, A. serrulata, Baptisia australis, B. tinctoria, Chamaesyce maculata, Eupatorium perfoliatum, Euphorbia corollata, Gentianella quinquefolia, Hydrangea arborescens, H. cinerea, Juglans cinerea, Morus alba, M. rubra, Nicotiana rustica, N. tabacum, Platanus occidentalis, Podophyllum peltatum, Polygala senega, Prunus persica, Rhamnus cathartica, Rheum rhaponticum, Ricinus communis, Rubus idaeus, R. occidentalis, R. odoratus, Sambucus canadensis, S. nigra, Senna hebe-*

carpa, *S. marilandica, Sesamum orientale, Veronicastrum virginicum*

Ceremonial Medicine: *Amaranthus hybridus, A. retroflexus, A. spinosus, Ambrosia artemisiifolia, A. trifida, Andropogon virginicus, Cicuta maculata, Clematis virginiana, Cucurbita pepo, Cynoglossum virginianum, Impatiens capensis, I. pallida, Lactuca canadensis, Lycopus virginicus, Nicotiana rustica, N. tabacum, Pinus virginiana, Rhododendron maximum, Yucca filamentosa*

Cold Remedy: *Acorus calamus, Allium cernuum, A. tricoccum, Anaphalis margaritacea, Angelica atropurpurea, Arisaema triphyllum, Aristolochia serpentaria, Armoracia rusticana, Asarum canadense, Betula lenta, B. nigra, Capsicum annuum, Cardamine diphylla, Carya alba, C. laciniosa, C. pallida, Chenopodium botrys, Chimaphila maculata, Cimicifuga racemosa, Cunila marina, Cypripedium acaule, C. parviflorum, Erigeron philadelphicus, E. pulchellus, Eupatorium perfoliatum, E. pilosum, Foeniculum vulgare, Gaultheria procumbens, Glechoma hederacea, Gnaphalium obtusifolium, Goodyera pubescens, G. repens, Hamamelis virginiana, Hedeoma pulegioides, Hyssopus officinalis, Juniperus virginiana, Lindera benzoin, Linum usitatissimum, Lobelia cardinalis, L. siphilitica, Marrubium vulgare, Melissa officinalis, Mentha ×piperita, M. spicata, Monarda didyma, M. fistulosa, Nepeta cataria, Obolaria virginica, Picea rubens, Pinus glabra, P. virginiana, Polygala senega, Porteranthus stipulatus, P. trifoliatus, Prunus cerasus, P. pensylvanica, P. serotina, P. virginiana, Pycnanthemum flexuosum, P. incanum, Salvia lyrata, S. officinalis, Sassafras albidum, Solidago odora, Ulmus rubra, Verbena hastata, Viola bicolor, V. cucullata, V. pedata, V. pubescens, V. rotundifolia, V. sororia*

Contraceptive: *Cicuta maculata*

Cough Medicine: *Aletris farinosa, Alnus serrulata, Anaphalis margaritacea, Apocynum cannabinum, Aralia racemosa, Arisaema triphyllum, Aristolochia serpentaria, Asarum canadense, Asplenium trichomanes, Castanea dentata, Celastrus scandens, Cimicifuga racemosa, Erigeron philadelphicus, E. pulchellus, Galium circaezans, Glycyrrhiza glabra, Gnaphalium obtusifolium, Hedeoma pulegioides, Hosta lancifolia, Hyssopus officinalis, Inula helenium, Ipomoea pandurata, Lindera benzoin, Linum usitatissimum, Liriodendron tulipifera, Marrubium vulgare, Nepeta cataria, Obolaria virgi-*

nica, *Pedicularis canadensis, Pinus glabra, P. virginiana, Platanus occidentalis, Prunus americana, P. cerasus, P. pensylvanica, P. serotina, P. virginiana, Rubus idaeus, R. occidentalis, R. odoratus, Salvia lyrata, S. officinalis, Sanguinaria canadensis, Solidago odora, Tilia americana, Trillium erectum, Ulmus rubra, Verbascum thapsus, Verbena hastata, Veronica officinalis, V. serpyllifolia, Viola bicolor, V. cucullata, V. pedata, V. pubescens, V. rotundifolia, V. sororia*

Dermatological Aid: *Abies fraseri, Acer rubrum, A. saccharinum, Achillea millefolium, Acorus calamus, Actaea pachypoda, Aesculus pavia, Agrimonia gryposepala, A. parviflora, Alisma subcordatum, Allium cernuum, Alnus serrulata, Amaranthus hybridus, A. retroflexus, A. spinosus, Ambrosia artemisiifolia, A. trifida, Amianthium muscitoxicum, Andropogon virginicus, Anthemis cotula, Apocynum cannabinum, Aralia racemosa, A. spinosa, Arctium minus, Arisaema triphyllum, Aristolochia macrophylla, Arnoglossum atriplicifolium, Artemisia biennis, Aruncus dioicus, Asarum canadense, Asclepias perennis, A. quadrifolia, A. syriaca, Brassica oleracea, Calycanthus floridus, Carpinus caroliniana, Carya alba, C. laciniosa, C. pallida, Castanea dentata, C. pumila, Caulophyllum thalictroides, Celastrus scandens, Chamaemelum nobile, Chamaesyce maculata, Chelone glabra, Chimaphila maculata, Cimicifuga racemosa, Collinsonia canadensis, Comandra umbellata, Cornus alternifolia, C. florida, Corylus americana, Cuscuta gronovii, Cynoglossum virginianum, Datura stramonium, Daucus carota, Diospyros virginiana, Erigeron philadelphicus, E. pulchellus, Erythronium americanum, Euonymus americana, Euphorbia corollata, Geranium maculatum, Glechoma hederacea, Hackelia virginiana, Hamamelis virginiana, Heteranthera reniformis, Heuchera americana, Hosta lancifolia, Hydrangea arborescens, Hydrastis canadensis, Hypericum gentianoides, H. hypericoides, H. perforatum, Impatiens capensis, I. pallida, Iris cristata, I. verna, I. virginica, Jeffersonia diphylla, Juglans nigra, Juniperus virginiana, Kalmia latifolia, Lachnanthes caroliana, Lagenaria siceraria, Lepidium virginicum, Leucothoe axillaris, Lindera benzoin, Liquidambar styraciflua, Liriodendron tulipifera, Lobelia cardinalis, L. inflata, L. siphilitica, Lyonia mariana, Malva neglecta, Melia azedarach, Menispermum canadense, Mirabilis nyctaginea, Mitchella repens,*

Monotropa uniflora, Nepeta cataria, Nicotiana rustica, N. tabacum, Oxalis corniculata, O. violacea, Oxydendrum arboreum, Panax trifolius, Passiflora incarnata, Pedicularis canadensis, Phytolacca americana, Pilea pumila, Pinus glabra, P. virginiana, Piper nigrum, Plantago aristata, P. lanceolata, P. major, Platanus occidentalis, Podophyllum peltatum, Polygonatum biflorum, Polygonum aviculare, P. hydropiper, P. persicaria, Polypodium virginianum, Populus balsamifera, P. nigra, Porteranthus stipulatus, P. trifoliatus, Potentilla simplex, Prunella vulgaris, Prunus cerasus, P. pensylvanica, P. persica, P. serotina, P. virginiana, Pycnanthemum flexuosum, P. incanum, Pyrola americana, P. elliptica, Pyrularia pubera, Quercus alba, Q. falcata, Q. imbricaria, Q. rubra, Q. stellata, Q. velutina, Ranunculus abortivus, R. acris, R. recurvatus, Rhamnus cathartica, Rheum rhaponticum, Rhus copallinum, R. glabra, Ricinus communis, Rubus alleghaniensis, R. argutus, R. flagellaris, R. idaeus, R. occidentalis, R. odoratus, R. trivialis, Rudbeckia fulgida, R. hirta, Rumex acetosella, R. crispus, R. patientia, Salix alba, S. babylonica, S. humilis, S. nigra, Sambucus canadensis, S. nigra, Sanguinaria canadensis, Saponaria officinalis, Sassafras albidum, Saururus cernuus, Saxifraga pensylvanica, Sempervivum tectorum, Senna hebecarpa, S. marilandica, Smallanthus uvedalia, Smilax glauca, S. herbacea, S. laurifolia, S. pseudochina, S. rotundifolia, Solanum carolinense, Tagetes erecta, Tephrosia virginiana, Tilia americana, Toxicodendron vernix, Tradescantia virginiana, Trillium erectum, Triosteum perfoliatum, Tsuga canadensis, T. caroliniana, Ulmus rubra, Uvularia sessilifolia, Verbascum thapsus, Verbena hastata, Veronica officinalis, V. serpyllifolia, Viola bicolor, V. cucullata, V. pedata, V. pubescens, V. rotundifolia, V. sororia, Xanthorhiza simplicissima, Yucca filamentosa, Zea mays

Diaphoretic: *Acorus calamus, Anthemis cotula, Aralia racemosa, A. spinosa, Arisaema triphyllum, Carya alba, C. laciniosa, C. pallida, Cornus alternifolia, C. florida, Cunila marina, Daphne mezereum, Diphylleia cymosa, Erigeron philadelphicus, E. pulchellus, Eupatorium perfoliatum, Euphorbia ipecacuanhae, Hedeoma pulegioides, Ilex cassine, Juniperus virginiana, Liatris spicata, Lindera benzoin, Mitchella repens, Monarda didyma, M. fistulosa, Nicotiana rustica, N. tabacum, Obolaria virginica, Orbexilum pedunculatum, Polygala senega,*

Salvia lyrata, S. officinalis, Sambucus canadensis, S. nigra, Solidago odora, Verbena hastata, Veronicastrum virginicum, Viburnum acerifolium, V. nudum, V. prunifolium

Dietary Aid: *Agrimonia gryposepala, A. parviflora, Aplectrum hyemale, Arctium lappa, Armoracia rusticana, Asparagus officinalis, Brassica napus, B. nigra, Chelone glabra, Chenopodium album, Crataegus spathulata, Frasera caroliniensis, Goodyera pubescens, G. repens, Hydrastis canadensis, Lilium canadense, Mitchella repens, Oenothera biennis, Passiflora incarnata, Phlox maculata, Pilea pumila, Rudbeckia laciniata, Sassafras albidum, Sinapis alba*

Disinfectant: *Ambrosia artemisiifolia, A. trifida, Aralia racemosa, Aristolochia serpentaria, Cornus alternifolia, C. florida, Diphylleia cymosa, Euonymus americana, Eupatorium perfoliatum, Frasera caroliniensis, Hydrangea arborescens, Kalmia latifolia, Pteridium aquilinum, Quercus alba, Q. falcata, Q. imbricaria, Q. rubra, Q. stellata, Q. velutina, Sambucus canadensis, S. nigra, Veronicastrum virginicum*

Diuretic: *Acorus calamus, Ageratina altissima, Allium canadense, A. sativum, A. vineale, Aristolochia serpentaria, Armoracia rusticana, Cimicifuga racemosa, Cucurbita pepo, Diphylleia cymosa, Erigeron philadelphicus, E. pulchellus, Eupatorium maculatum, E. perfoliatum, E. purpureum, Ipomoea pandurata, Liatris spicata, Mitchella repens, Monarda didyma, M. fistulosa, Nicotiana rustica, N. tabacum, Polygala senega, Sambucus canadensis, S. nigra*

Ear Medicine: *Allium canadense, A. sativum, A. tricoccum, A. vineale, Passiflora incarnata, Podophyllum peltatum, Portulaca oleracea, Rudbeckia fulgida, R. hirta, Sempervivum tectorum, Veronica officinalis, V. serpyllifolia*

Emetic: *Adiantum pedatum, Alnus incana, A. serrulata, Anthemis cotula, Aralia spinosa, Asarum canadense, Asplenium rhizophyllum, Baptisia australis, B. tinctoria, Botrychium virginianum, Calycanthus floridus, Carya alba, C. laciniosa, C. pallida, Chimaphila maculata, Clethra acuminata, Collinsonia canadensis, Coronilla varia, Corylus americana, Dryopteris marginalis, Epigaea repens, Eryngium aquaticum, Eupatorium perfoliatum, Euphorbia ipecacuanhae, Goodyera pubescens, G. repens, Hepatica nobilis, Hydrangea arborescens, H. cinerea, Ilex cassine, I. vomitoria, Juncus effusus, Lobelia inflata, Nicotiana rustica, N. tabacum, Nyssa sylvatica, Platanus occidentalis, Polystichum acrostichoides, Porteranthus stipu-*

latis, *P. trifoliatus, Pyrularia pubera, Quercus alba, Q. falcata, Q. imbricaria, Q. rubra, Q. stellata, Q. velutina, Robinia bispida, R. pseudoacacia, Rubus idaeus, R. occidentalis, R. odoratus, Sambucus canadensis, S. nigra, Scirpus tabernaemontani, Scutellaria lateriflora, Smallanthus uvedalia, Solanum nigrum, S. tuberosum, Toxicodendron pubescens, T. radicans, Triosteum perfoliatum, Verbena bastata, Vicia caroliniana, Xanthium spinosum*

Expectorant: *Allium canadense, A. sativum, A. vineale, Aralia racemosa, Arisaema triphyllum, Asclepias tuberosa, Euonymus americana, Euphorbia ipecacuanbae, Galium circaezans, Glycyrrhiza glabra, Hedeoma pulegioides, Ipomoea pandurata, Liatris spicata, Nicotiana rustica, N. tabacum, Panax quinquefolius, Polygala senega*

Eye Medicine: *Acer rubrum, A. saccharinum, Alnus incana, A. serrulata, Anaphalis margaritacea, Aruncus dioicus, Asarum canadense, Calycanthus floridus, Erigeron philadelphicus, E. pulchellus, Goodyera pubescens, G. repens, Maianthemum racemosum, Monotropa uniflora, Nyssa sylvatica, Plantago aristata, P. lanceolata, P. major, Rhamnus cathartica, Sassafras albidum, Ulmus rubra, Xanthorhiza simplicissima*

Febrifuge: *Achillea millefolium, Adiantum pedatum, Ageratina altissima, Agrimonia gryposepala, A. parviflora, Aletris farinosa, Allium cernuum, Alnus serrulata, Ambrosia artemisiifolia, A. trifida, Angelica atropurpurea, Anthemis cotula, Aristolochia serpentaria, Asarum canadense, Aster linariifolius, A. novae-angliae, Brassica napus, B. nigra, Capsicum annuum, Castanea pumila, Chelone glabra, Chimaphila maculata, Clethra acuminata, Cornus alternifolia, C. florida, Cunila marina, Cystopteris protrusa, Dennstaedtia punctilobula, Echinocystis lobata, Erythronium americanum, Eupatorium perfoliatum, Hamamelis virginiana, Hedeoma pulegioides, Hypericum gentianoides, H. hypericoides, H. perforatum, Hyssopus officinalis, Linum usitatissimum, Liriodendron tulipifera, Lobelia cardinalis, L. siphilitica, Melissa officinalis, Mentha arvensis, M. ×piperita, M. spicata, Monarda didyma, M. fistulosa, Nepeta cataria, Osmunda cinnamomea, Phytolacca americana, Pinus glabra, P. virginiana, Polystichum acrostichoides, Potentilla simplex, Prunus cerasus, P. pensylvanica, P. persica, P. serotina, P. virginiana, Pycnanthemum flexuosum, P. incanum, Quercus alba, Q. falcata, Q. imbricaria, Q. rubra, Q. stellata, Q. velutina, Sagittaria latifolia,*

Salix alba, S. babylonica, S. humilis, S. nigra, Senna hebecarpa, S. marilandica, Sinapis alba, Solidago odora, Toxicodendron vernix, Trifolium pratense, T. repens, Triosteum perfoliatum, Verbena hastata, Veronica officinalis, V. serpyllifolia, Veronicastrum virginicum, Viburnum acerifolium, V. nudum, V. prunifolium

Gastrointestinal Aid: *Abies fraseri, Achillea millefolium, Acorus calamus, Aesculus pavia, Agrimonia gryposepala, A. parviflora, Alisma subcordatum, Allium cernuum, Alnus incana, A. serrulata, Antennaria plantaginifolia, Aristolochia serpentaria, Armoracia rusticana, Artemisia biennis, Asarum canadense, Betula lenta, B. nigra, Capsicum annuum, Carya alba, C. laciniosa, C. pallida, Castanea dentata, Caulophyllum thalictroides, Ceanothus americanus, Celastrus scandens, Chamaemelum nobile, Cirsium altissimum, C. vulgare, Clematis virginiana, Clethra acuminata, Cornus alternifolia, C. florida, Cypripedium acaule, C. parviflorum, Diospyros virginiana, Epigaea repens, Eryngium aquaticum, Eupatorium perfoliatum, Foeniculum vulgare, Fragaria virginiana, Frasera caroliniensis, Fraxinus americana, F. nigra, Galium triflorum, Gaultheria procumbens, Gentianella quinquefolia, Gleditsia triacanthos, Hepatica nobilis, Heuchera americana, Hexastylis virginica, Hieracium venosum, Hydrangea arborescens, Hydrastis canadensis, Hypericum gentianoides, H. hypericoides, H. perforatum, Ilex opaca, Impatiens capensis, I. pallida, Lachnanthes caroliana, Leonurus cardiaca, Liatris spicata, Ligusticum canadense, Liriodendron tulipifera, Lobelia cardinalis, L. inflata, L. siphilitica, Lysimachia quadrifolia, Magnolia acuminata, M. macrophylla, Malus coronaria, M. pumila, Matricaria discoidea, Menispermum canadense, Mentha ×piperita, M. spicata, Mitchella repens, Monarda didyma, M. fistulosa, Nepeta cataria, Nicotiana rustica, N. tabacum, Nyssa sylvatica, Obolaria virginica, Orbexilum pedunculatum, Oxydendrum arboreum, Panax quinquefolius, P. trifolius, Pedicularis canadensis, Penstemon laevigatus, Pinus glabra, P. virginiana, Plantago aristata, P. lanceolata, P. major, Platanus occidentalis, Polygonatum biflorum, Polystichum acrostichoides, Populus balsamifera, P. nigra, Prunus cerasus, P. pensylvanica, P. persica, P. serotina, P. virginiana, Pycnanthemum flexuosum, P. incanum, Quercus alba, Q. falcata, Q. imbricaria, Q. rubra, Q. stellata, Q. velutina, Rubus idaeus, R. occidentalis, R. odoratus, Sanicula smallii,*

Sisyrinchium angustifolium, Smilax glauca, S. herbacea, S. pseudochina, S. rotundifolia, Symphytum officinale, Tilia americana, Tradescantia virginiana, Trillium erectum, Triodanis perfoliata, Ulmus rubra, Urtica dioica, Verbena hastata, Vernonia glauca, V. noveboracensis, Veronicastrum virginicum, Vicia caroliniana, Vitis aestivalis, V. labrusca, V. vulpina, Xanthium spinosum

Gland Medicine: *Verbascum thapsus*

Gynecological Aid: *Abies fraseri, Acer rubrum, A. saccharinum, Achillea millefolium, Aesculus pavia, Agrimonia gryposepala, A. parviflora, Aletris farinosa, Alnus incana, A. serrulata, Amaranthus hybridus, A. retroflexus, A. spinosus, Antennaria plantaginifolia, Aquilegia canadensis, Aralia racemosa, Arctium lappa, Artemisia biennis, Aruncus dioicus, Asarum canadense, Asclepias tuberosa, Baptisia australis, B. tinctoria, Castanea dentata, Caulophyllum thalictroides, Celastrus scandens, Chamaesyce maculata, Cornus alternifolia, C. florida, Cunila marina, Cypripedium acaule, C. parviflorum, Euonymus americana, Eupatorium maculatum, E. purpureum, Euphorbia corollata, E. ipecacuanhae, Foeniculum vulgare, Fraxinus americana, F. nigra, Hamamelis virginiana, Helenium autumnale, Heuchera americana, Humulus lupulus, Hydrangea cinerea, Impatiens capensis, I. pallida, Inula helenium, Lachnanthes caroliana, Liquidambar styraciflua, Lysimachia quadrifolia, Menispermum canadense, Mitchella repens, Nyssa sylvatica, Orbexilum pedunculatum, Panax quinquefolius, Petroselinum crispum, Phoradendron leucarpum, Pinus glabra, P. virginiana, Plantago aristata, P. lanceolata, P. major, Platanus occidentalis, Polygonatum biflorum, Prunus cerasus, P. pensylvanica, P. serotina, P. virginiana, Quercus velutina, Rhododendron calendulaceum, Rhus copallinum, R. glabra, R. hirta, Rubus idaeus, R. occidentalis, R. odoratus, Rudbeckia fulgida, R. hirta, Sabatia angularis, Salvia lyrata, S. officinalis, Scutellaria elliptica, S. incana, S. lateriflora, Senecio aureus, Sesamum orientale, Silphium compositum, Smallanthus uvedalia, Smilax glauca, S. herbacea, S. pseudochina, S. rotundifolia, Stylosanthes biflora, Symphytum officinale, Tanacetum vulgare, Tradescantia virginiana, Trifolium pratense, T. repens, Trillium erectum, Tsuga canadensis, T. caroliniana, Ulmus rubra, Verbascum thapsus, Vernonia glauca, V. noveboracensis, Veronica officinalis, Vitis aestivalis, V. labrusca, V. vulpina*

Hallucinogen: *Ilex vomitoria*

Heart Medicine: *Adiantum pedatum, Alnus serrulata, Aquilegia canadensis, Asarum canadense, Asclepias tuberosa, Castanea dentata, Consolida ajacis, Crataegus spathulata, Delphinium tricorne, Hypoxis hirsuta, Monarda didyma, M. fistulosa, Pycnanthemum flexuosum, P. incanum, Rhododendron maximum, Senecio aureus, Senna hebecarpa, S. marilandica*

Hemorrhoid Remedy: *Achillea millefolium, Aesculus pavia, Alnus serrulata, Diospyros virginiana, Heuchera americana, Lachnanthes caroliana, Malus coronaria, M. pumila, Mentha ×piperita, M. spicata, Mitchella repens, Oenothera biennis, Pinus glabra, P. virginiana, Rubus allegheniensis, R. argutus, R. flagellaris, R. trivialis, Xanthorhiza simplicissima*

Hemostat: *Geranium maculatum, Hypericum gentianoides, H. hypericoides, H. perforatum, Lobelia cardinalis, L. siphilitica, Monarda didyma, M. fistulosa*

Hunting Medicine: *Erythronium americanum*

Hypotensive: *Alnus serrulata, Hydrangea arborescens, Phoradendron leucarpum*

Kidney Aid: *Abies fraseri, Acalypha virginica, Acorus calamus, Allium canadense, A. cernuum, A. sativum, A. vineale, Alnus serrulata, Anthemis cotula, Apocynum cannabinum, Arctostaphylos uva-ursi, Asclepias perennis, A. quadrifolia, A. syriaca, Brassica napus, B. nigra, Citrullus lanatus, Clematis virginiana, Comandra umbellata, Cucurbita pepo, Cypripedium acaule, C. parviflorum, Echinocystis lobata, Epigaea repens, Equisetum arvense, E. hyemale, Erigeron philadelphicus, E. pulchellus, Eupatorium maculatum, E. purpureum, Fragaria virginiana, Galax urceolata, Gaylussacia baccata, Goodyera pubescens, G. repens, Hackelia virginiana, Helianthemum canadense, Humulus lupulus, Ilex cassine, Ipomoea pandurata, Jeffersonia diphylla, Liatris spicata, Lysimachia quadrifolia, Lythrum alatum, Nicotiana rustica, N. tabacum, Panax trifolius, Petroselinum crispum, Phytolacca americana, Pinus glabra, P. virginiana, Polygala senega, Porteranthus stipulatus, P. trifoliatus, Prunus americana, Rudbeckia fulgida, R. hirta, Rumex crispus, R. patientia, Sambucus canadensis, S. nigra, Scutellaria elliptica, S. incana, S. lateriflora, Sinapis alba, Tephrosia virginiana, Tradescantia virginiana, Trifolium pratense, T. repens, Tsuga canadensis, T. caroliniana, Verbascum thapsus, Verbena hastata, Zea mays*

Laxative: *Abies fraseri, Asclepias perennis, A.*

quadrifolia, A. syriaca, A. tuberosa, Chelone glabra, Cimicifuga racemosa, Equisetum arvense, E. hyemale, Eupatorium pilosum, Galium aparine, Gentianella quinquefolia, Hepatica nobilis, Ipomoea pandurata, Menispermum canadense, Morus alba, M. rubra, Phytolacca americana, Pinus glabra, P. virginiana, Podophyllum peltatum, Rheum rhaponticum, Rumex crispus, R. patientia, Salvia lyrata, S. officinalis, Symphytum officinale, Tradescantia virginiana, Ulmus rubra

Liver Aid: *Aletris farinosa, Allium cernuum, Asplenium trichomanes, Carya alba, C. laciniosa, C. pallida, Clethra acuminata, Diospyros virginiana, Fragaria virginiana, Hepatica nobilis, Hydrangea arborescens, H. cinerea, Iris cristata, I. verna, I. virginica, Manfreda virginica, Panax trifolius, Parthenocissus quinquefolia, Passiflora incarnata, Porteranthus stipulatus, P. trifoliatus, Veronicastrum virginicum, Vitis aestivalis, V. labrusca, V. vulpina*

Love Medicine: *Hackelia virginiana, Phoradendron leucarpum*

Misc. Disease Remedy: *Acalypha virginica, Acer rubrum, A. saccharinum, Adiantum pedatum, Ageratina altissima, Allium canadense, A. sativum, A. vineale, Angelica atropurpurea, Aristolochia serpentaria, Asarum canadense, Brassica napus, B. nigra, Carya alba, C. laciniosa, C. pallida, Castanea dentata, Chenopodium botrys, Cornus alternifolia, C. florida, Cypripedium acaule, C. parviflorum, Diphylleia cymosa, Eupatorium maculatum, E. perfoliatum, E. purpureum, Fragaria virginiana, Glechoma hederacea, Gleditsia triacanthos, Gnaphalium obtusifolium, Impatiens capensis, I. pallida, Ipomoea pandurata, Juglans nigra, Juniperus virginiana, Lindera benzoin, Liriodendron tulipifera, Melissa officinalis, Mentha ×piperita, M. spicata, Monarda didyma, M. fistulosa, Nicotiana rustica, N. tabacum, Panax trifolius, Picea rubens, Pinus glabra, P. virginiana, Platanus occidentalis, Prunus cerasus, P. pensylvanica, P. serotina, P. virginiana, Pteridium aquilinum, Ribes rotundifolium, Sassafras albidum, Senna hebecarpa, S. marilandica, Sesamum orientale, Sinapis alba, Solidago odora, Toxicodendron vernix, Urtica dioica, Verbascum thapsus, Veronicastrum virginicum, Viburnum acerifolium, V. nudum, V. prunifolium, Vicia caroliniana, Yucca filamentosa*

Nose Medicine: *Aristolochia serpentaria, Helenium autumnale, Helianthus giganteus, Sanguinaria canadensis*

Oral Aid: *Alnus serrulata, Angelica atropurpurea, Armoracia rusticana, Carya alba, C. laciniosa, C. pallida, Clitoria mariana, Desmodium nudiflorum, D. perplexum, Diospyros virginiana, Gaultheria procumbens, Geranium maculatum, Gnaphalium obtusifolium, Heuchera americana, Juncus effusus, J. tenuis, Lachnanthes caroliana, Malus coronaria, Oxalis corniculata, O. violacea, Oxydendrum arboreum, Panax quinquefolius, Potentilla simplex, Prunus cerasus, P. pensylvanica, P. serotina, P. virginiana, Quercus alba, Q. falcata, Q. imbricaria, Q. rubra, Q. stellata, Q. velutina, Ranunculus abortivus, R. acris, R. recurvatus, Rubus allegheniensis, R. argutus, R. flagellaris, R. trivialis, Sassafras albidum, Scirpus tabernaemontani, Solanum carolinense, Solidago odora, Tiarella cordifolia, Trollius laxus, Viburnum acerifolium, V. nudum, V. prunifolium, Vitis aestivalis, V. labrusca, V. vulpina, Xanthorhiza simplicissima*

Orthopedic Aid: *Aesculus pavia, Alnus serrulata, Aralia racemosa, A. spinosa, Arisaema triphyllum, Aruncus dioicus, Brassica napus, B. nigra, Carya alba, C. laciniosa, C. pallida, Clematis virginiana, Coronilla varia, Elytrigia repens, Euonymus americana, Gnaphalium obtusifolium, Hydrangea arborescens, Ilex opaca, Juncus effusus, J. tenuis, Kalmia latifolia, Liriodendron tulipifera, Lobelia inflata, L. spicata, Ostrya virginiana, Pinus glabra, P. virginiana, Plantago aristata, P. lanceolata, P. major, Porteranthus stipulatus, P. trifoliatus, Ruta graveolens, Sanicula smallii, Sinapis alba, Smilax glauca, S. herbacea, S. pseudochina, S. rotundifolia, Symphytum officinale, Tanacetum parthenium, T. vulgare, Tephrosia virginiana, Triosteum perfoliatum, Veratrum viride, Vicia caroliniana*

Other: *Adiantum pedatum, Aureolaria flava, A. laevigata, A. pedicularia, Euonymus americana, Eupatorium maculatum, E. purpureum, Leucothoe axillaris, Liquidambar styraciflua, Lobelia inflata, Lycopus virginicus, Nicotiana rustica, N. tabacum, Nyssa sylvatica, Panax quinquefolius, P. trifolius, Phytolacca americana, Pinus glabra, P. virginiana, Platanus occidentalis, Polygala senega, P. verticillata, Rhododendron maximum, Sambucus canadensis, S. nigra, Smallanthus uvedalia, Smilax glauca, S. herbacea, S. pseudochina, S. rotundifolia, Vitis aestivalis, V. labrusca, V. vulpina*

Panacea: *Kalmia latifolia, Veratrum viride*

Pediatric Aid: *Agrimonia gryposepala, A. parviflora, Allium canadense, A. cernuum, A. sati-*

vum, *A. vineale, Alnus serrulata, Amelanchier canadensis, Antennaria plantaginifolia, Aplectrum hyemale, Calycanthus floridus, Castanea dentata, Cerastium fontanum, Chamaesyce maculata, Chimaphila maculata, Cimicifuga racemosa, Citrullus lanatus, Coix lacryma-jobi, Cornus alternifolia, C. florida, Epigaea repens, Euphorbia corollata, Foeniculum vulgare, Geranium maculatum, Glechoma hederacea, Hydrangea arborescens, Impatiens capensis, I. pallida, Juncus effusus, J. tenuis, Lilium canadense, Liriodendron tulipifera, Lycopus virginicus, Marrubium vulgare, Mentha ×piperita, M. spicata, Mitchella repens, Monotropa uniflora, Nepeta cataria, Nyssa sylvatica, Oxalis corniculata, O. violacea, Panax trifolius, Passiflora incarnata, Phlox maculata, Pilea pumila, Plantago aristata, P. lanceolata, P. major, Platanus occidentalis, Polygonum aviculare, P. hydropiper, Rosa virginiana, Sagittaria latifolia, Sambucus canadensis, S. nigra, Sassafras albidum, Senna hebecarpa, S. marilandica, Sesamum orientale, Sisyrinchium angustifolium, Solanum carolinense, Spiranthes lucida, Tanacetum vulgare, Tephrosia virginiana, Vitis aestivalis, V. labrusca, V. vulpina, Xyris caroliniana*

Poison: *Amianthium muscitoxicum, Aralia spinosa, Calycanthus floridus, Castilleja coccinea, Chimaphila maculata, Consolida ajacis, Delphinium tricorne, Juglans nigra, Phytolacca americana, Podophyllum peltatum, Polygonum aviculare, P. hydropiper, Rheum rhaponticum, Toxicodendron vernix*

Poultice: *Capsicum annuum, Cirsium altissimum, C. vulgare, Cornus florida, Liriodendron tulipifera, Polygonum aviculare, P. hydropiper, Ruta graveolens, Saururus cernuus*

Preventive Medicine: *Crataegus spathulata*

Psychological Aid: *Cynoglossum virginianum, Fragaria virginiana, Hackelia virginiana, Solanum nigrum, S. tuberosum*

Pulmonary Aid: *Abies fraseri, Aletris farinosa, Allium canadense, A. cernuum, A. sativum, A. tricoccum, A. vineale, Ambrosia artemisiifolia, A. trifida, Anemone virginiana, Apocynum cannabinum, Aralia racemosa, Aristolochia serpentaria, Asclepias tuberosa, Brassica napus, B. nigra, Cercis canadensis, Epigaea repens, Eryngium yuccifolium, Euphorbia ipecacuanhae, Gleditsia triacanthos, Hedeoma pulegioides, Hyssopus officinalis, Inula helenium, Lepidium virginicum, Lindera benzoin, Linum usitatissimum, Lobelia cardinalis, L. inflata, L. siphilitica, Malus pumila, Mertensia virginica, Oxyden-*

drum arboreum, Panax trifolius, Polygala senega, Polygonatum biflorum, Polygonum virginianum, Polystichum acrostichoides, Potentilla simplex, Sanguinaria canadensis, Senna hebecarpa, S. marilandica, Sinapis alba, Sisymbrium officinale, Xanthium spinosum, Zea mays*

Reproductive Aid: *Cinchona calisaya*

Respiratory Aid: *Achillea millefolium, Adiantum pedatum, Allium canadense, A. cernuum, A. sativum, A. vineale, Anaphalis margaritacea, Anthemis cotula, Apocynum cannabinum, Aralia racemosa, Armoracia rusticana, Aster linariifolius, A. novae-angliae, Brassica napus, B. nigra, Datura stramonium, Euonymus americana, Eupatorium pilosum, Galium circaezans, Glycyrrhiza glabra, Gnaphalium obtusifolium, Hyssopus officinalis, Inula helenium, Ipomoea pandurata, Lindera benzoin, Lobelia inflata, Magnolia acuminata, M. macrophylla, Oxydendrum arboreum, Pimpinella anisum, Pinus glabra, P. virginiana, Porteranthus stipulatus, P. trifoliatus, Quercus alba, Q. falcata, Q. imbricaria, Q. rubra, Q. stellata, Q. velutina, Salix alba, S. babylonica, S. humilis, S. nigra, Salvia lyrata, S. officinalis, Sanguinaria canadensis, Sinapis alba, Toxicodendron vernix, Trillium erectum, Ulmus rubra, Vicia caroliniana, Viola bicolor, V. cucullata, V. pedata, V. pubescens, V. rotundifolia, V. sororia*

Sedative: *Achillea millefolium, Angelica atropurpurea, Anthemis cotula, Asarum canadense, Caulophyllum thalictroides, Chamaemelum nobile, Cimicifuga racemosa, Cypripedium acaule, C. parviflorum, Fragaria virginiana, Galax urceolata, Gentianella quinquefolia, Humulus lupulus, Lactuca canadensis, Leonurus cardiaca, Liquidambar styraciflua, Liriodendron tulipifera, Mentha ×piperita, M. spicata, Monarda didyma, M. fistulosa, Nepeta cataria, Oxydendrum arboreum, Papaver somniferum, Pinus glabra, P. virginiana, Ranunculus abortivus, R. acris, R. recurvatus, Ribes rotundifolium, Ruta graveolens, Salvia lyrata, S. officinalis, Solidago odora, Sonchus arvensis, Taraxacum officinale, Xanthorhiza simplicissima, Yucca filamentosa*

Snakebite Remedy: *Amphicarpaea bracteata, Aristolochia serpentaria, Botrychium virginianum, Cunila marina, Eryngium yuccifolium, Hypericum gentianoides, H. hypericoides, H. perforatum, Liriodendron tulipifera, Lycopus virginicus, Nicotiana rustica, N. tabacum, Osmunda cinnamomea, Plantago aristata, P. lanceolata,*

P. major, Polygala senega, Rudbeckia fulgida, R. hirta, Tilia americana, Xanthium spinosum

Sports Medicine: *Chamaecrista fasciculata, C. nictitans*

Stimulant: *Acorus calamus, Actaea pachypoda, Aesculus pavia, Ageratina altissima, Allium canadense, A. sativum, A. vineale, Arisaema triphyllum, Aristolochia serpentaria, Asarum canadense, Brassica napus, B. nigra, Capsicum annuum, Chamaecrista fasciculata, C. nictitans, Cimicifuga racemosa, Cornus alternifolia, C. florida, Cunila marina, Daphne mezereum, Erythronium americanum, Eupatorium perfoliatum, Gentianella quinquefolia, Hedeoma pulegioides, Hydrangea arborescens, Hydrastis canadensis, Lactuca canadensis, Leonurus cardiaca, Leucothoe axillaris, Liatris spicata, Liriodendron tulipifera, Melissa officinalis, Menispermum canadense, Mentha ×piperita, M. spicata, Nepeta cataria, Panax trifolius, Papaver somniferum, Pinus glabra, P. virginiana, Piper nigrum, Populus balsamifera, P. nigra, Rubus allegheniensis, R. argutus, R. flagellaris, R. trivialis, Salvia lyrata, S. officinalis, Senna hebecarpa, S. marilandica, Silphium compositum, Sinapis alba, Solidago odora, Tephrosia virginiana, Veratrum viride*

Strengthener: *Hypericum gentianoides, H. hypericoides, H. perforatum, Juncus effusus, J. tenuis, Rheum rhaponticum*

Throat Aid: *Acorus calamus, Actaea pachypoda, Allium cernuum, Anaphalis margaritacea, Angelica atropurpurea, Arisaema triphyllum, Aristolochia serpentaria, Armoracia rusticana, Bidens bipinnata, Cardamine diphylla, Cornus alternifolia, C. florida, C. foemina, Diospyros virginiana, Eupatorium perfoliatum, Galium circaezans, Glycyrrhiza glabra, Gnaphalium obtusifolium, Hamamelis virginiana, Lachnanthes caroliana, Lobelia inflata, Malus pumila, M. sylvestris, Marrubium vulgare, Oxalis corniculata, O. violacea, Prunus cerasus, P. pensylvanica, P. serotina, P. virginiana, Quercus alba, Q. falcata, Q. imbricaria, Q. rubra, Q. stellata, Q. velutina, Ranunculus abortivus, R. acris, R. recurvatus, Rubus allegheniensis, R. argutus, R. flagellaris, R. trivialis, Rumex crispus, R. patientia, Salix alba, S. babylonica, S. humilis, S. nigra, Solanum carolinense, Ulmus rubra, Xanthium spinosum, Xanthorhiza simplicissima*

Tonic: *Ageratina altissima, Aletris farinosa, Amelanchier arborea, Anthemis cotula, Aralia racemosa, A. spinosa, Aristolochia serpentaria, Armoracia rusticana, Brassica napus, B. nigra,*

Cichorium intybus, Cimicifuga racemosa, Cinchona calisaya, Cornus alternifolia, C. florida, Cunila marina, Euonymus americana, Eupatorium maculatum, E. perfoliatum, E. pilosum, E. purpureum, Foeniculum vulgare, Frasera caroliniensis, Gentianella quinquefolia, Hydrastis canadensis, Lindera benzoin, Melissa officinalis, Nepeta cataria, Orbexilum pedunculatum, Osmunda cinnamomea, Panax quinquefolius, Polygonatum biflorum, Pteridium aquilinum, Quercus alba, Q. falcata, Q. imbricaria, Q. rubra, Q. stellata, Q. velutina, Rubus allegheniensis, R. argutus, R. flagellaris, R. idaeus, R. occidentalis, R. odoratus, R. trivialis, Salix alba, S. babylonica, S. humilis, S. nigra, Sinapis alba, Smilax laurifolia, Solidago odora, Tanacetum vulgare, Verbena hastata, Veronicastrum virginicum, Viburnum acerifolium, V. nudum, V. prunifolium, Viola bicolor, V. cucullata, V. pedata, V. pubescens, V. rotundifolia, V. sororia, Vitis aestivalis, V. labrusca, V. vulpina, Xanthorhiza simplicissima

Toothache Remedy: *Actaea pachypoda, Alnus serrulata, Aralia spinosa, Aristolochia serpentaria, Baptisia australis, B. tinctoria, Caulophyllum thalictroides, Ceanothus americanus, Chamaesyce maculata, Coix lacryma-jobi, Diospyros virginiana, Dryopteris marginalis, Erigenia bulbosa, Eryngium yuccifolium, Euphorbia corollata, Fragaria virginiana, Goodyera pubescens, G. repens, Hedeoma pulegioides, Juglans cinerea, J. nigra, Magnolia acuminata, M. macrophylla, Nicotiana rustica, N. tabacum, Ostrya virginiana, Polystichum acrostichoides, Populus balsamifera, P. nigra, Porteranthus stipulatus, P. trifoliatus, Robinia hispida, R. pseudoacacia, Rubus idaeus, R. occidentalis, R. odoratus, Taraxacum officinale, Vernonia glauca, V. noveboracensis*

Tuberculosis Remedy: *Aletris farinosa, Arisaema triphyllum, Chimaphila maculata, Cimicifuga racemosa, Hamamelis virginiana, Inula helenium, Ipomoea pandurata, Mertensia virginica, Panax trifolius, Pinus glabra, P. virginiana, Solidago odora, Tilia americana, Ulmus rubra*

Unspecified: *Coix lacryma-jobi, Phytolacca americana, Taraxacum officinale*

Urinary Aid: *Abies fraseri, Acalypha virginica, Achillea millefolium, Acorus calamus, Ageratina altissima, Aletris farinosa, Allium cernuum, Alnus serrulata, Ampelopsis cordata, Arctium lappa, Arctostaphylos uva-ursi, Aristolochia macrophylla, Armoracia rusticana, Aruncus dioicus, Asclepias perennis, A. quadrifolia, A.*

syriaca, Betula lenta, B. nigra, Calycanthus floridus, Carpinus caroliniana, Chamaesyce hypericifolia, C. maculata, Chimaphila maculata, Citrullus lanatus, Cucurbita pepo, Cynoglossum virginianum, Echium vulgare, Elytrigia repens, Euonymus americana, Eupatorium maculatum, E. pilosum, E. purpureum, Euphorbia corollata, Fragaria virginiana, Houstonia caerulea, Humulus lupulus, Ilex cassine, Ipomoea pandurata, Iris cristata, I. verna, I. virginica, Jeffersonia diphylla, Linum usitatissimum, Liparis loeselii, Lysimachia quadrifolia, Mentha ×piperita, M. spicata, Nyssa sylvatica, Petroselinum crispum, Pinus glabra, P. virginiana, Plantago aristata, P. lanceolata, P. major, Platanus occidentalis, Polygonum aviculare, P. hydropiper, P. persicaria, Prunus americana, Quercus alba, Q. falcata, Q. imbricaria, Q. rubra, Q. stellata, Q. velutina, Rhus copallinum, R. glabra, R. hirta, Rubus allegheniensis, R. argutus, R. flagellaris, R. trivialis, Spiranthes lucida, Toxicodendron vernix, Vitis aestivalis, V. labrusca, V. vulpina

Venereal Aid: Abies fraseri, Aralia spinosa, Arctium lappa, Asclepias perennis, A. quadrifolia, A. syriaca, Chamaesyce maculata, Daphne mezereum, Diospyros virginiana, Euonymus americana, Euphorbia corollata, Hypericum gentianoides, H. hypericoides, H. perforatum, Lachnanthes caroliana, Lobelia cardinalis, L. siphilitica, Menispermum canadense, Panax trifolius, Pinus glabra, P. virginiana, Populus balsamifera, P. nigra, Rubus allegheniensis, R. argutus, R. flagellaris, R. trivialis, Rudbeckia fulgida, R. hirta, Sassafras albidum, Stillingia sylvatica, Symphytum officinale, Toxicodendron vernix

Vertigo Medicine: Nicotiana rustica, N. tabacum

Veterinary Aid: Apocynum androsaemifolium, Asclepias perennis, A. quadrifolia, A. syriaca, Chimaphila maculata, Collinsonia canadensis, Lactuca canadensis, Lepidium virginicum, Leucothoe axillaris, Lycopus virginicus, Mitchella repens, Pedicularis canadensis, Porteranthus stipulatus, P. trifoliatus, Robinia hispida, R. pseudoacacia, Rumex crispus, R. patientia, Solanum carolinense

Cheyenne

Adjuvant: Osmorhiza berteroi, Sphaeralcea coccinea

Analgesic: Achillea millefolium, Acorus calamus, Agastache foeniculum, Ambrosia psilostachya, Arctostaphylos uva-ursi, Artemisia ludoviciana,

Balsamorhiza incana, B. sagittata, Capsella bursa-pastoris, Echinacea angustifolia, Erigeron peregrinus, Lithospermum ruderale, Lomatium dissectum, L. orientale, Oplopanax horridus, Ratibida columnifera, Senecio triangularis, Thermopsis rhombifolia

Antidiarrheal: Ambrosia psilostachya, Frasera speciosa, Glycyrrhiza lepidota, Lomatium orientale, Pediomelum esculentum, Prunus virginiana, Salix amygdaloides

Antiemetic: Achillea millefolium, Mentha arvensis, M. canadensis, Vaccinium scoparium

Antihemorrhagic: Ambrosia psilostachya, Boykinia jamesii, Epilobium angustifolium, Pterospora andromedea, Rumex crispus

Antirheumatic (External): Heuchera cylindrica, Lithospermum ruderale, Onosmodium molle

Antirheumatic (Internal): Echinacea pallida, Heuchera cylindrica, Mentzelia laevicaulis

Blood Medicine: Actaea rubra, Sarcobatus vermiculatus

Breast Treatment: Lygodesmia juncea, Mertensia ciliata

Burn Dressing: Echinacea pallida, Pediomelum esculentum, Rhus trilobata

Ceremonial Medicine: Abies lasiocarpa, Acer negundo, Acorus calamus, Actaea rubra, Anaphalis margaritacea, Artemisia frigida, A. ludoviciana, Carex nebrascensis, Glycyrrhiza lepidota, Hierochloe odorata, Juniperus communis, J. horizontalis, J. scopulorum, Koeleria macrantha, Madia glomerata, Matricaria discoidea, Mentha arvensis, Monarda fistulosa, Pentaphylloides floribunda, Prunus americana, Psoralidium lanceolatum, Salix amygdaloides, Sarcobatus vermiculatus, Scirpus nevadensis, Sphaeralcea coccinea, Typha latifolia

Cold Remedy: Achillea millefolium, Acorus calamus, Agastache foeniculum, Ambrosia psilostachya, Arabis glabra, Arctostaphylos uva-ursi, Balsamorhiza incana, B. sagittata, Chrysothamnus nauseosus, Echinacea pallida, Juniperus communis, J. horizontalis, J. scopulorum, Osmorhiza berteroi, Rhus trilobata, Stephanomeria spinosa, Thermopsis rhombifolia

Cough Medicine: Achillea millefolium, Arctostaphylos uva-ursi, Chrysothamnus nauseosus, Juniperus communis, J. horizontalis, J. scopulorum, Pedicularis groenlandica

Dermatological Aid: Actaea rubra, Allium brevistylum, Astragalus adsurgens, Chrysothamnus nauseosus, Echinacea pallida, Grindelia squarrosa, Heuchera cylindrica, Koeleria macrantha, Matricaria discoidea, Mentha arvensis, Merten-

Venereal Aid: *Madia glomerata*

Vertigo Medicine: *Tanacetum vulgare*

Veterinary Aid: *Anaphalis margaritacea, Calochortus gunnisonii, Equisetum arvense, E. hyemale, Monarda fistulosa, Rhus trilobata, Sagittaria cuneata, Sarcobatus vermiculatus, Thalictrum sparsiflorum*

Witchcraft Medicine: *Abies lasiocarpa, Acorus calamus, Hierochloe odorata*

Cheyenne, Northern

Disinfectant: *Grindelia squarrosa*

Eye Medicine: *Grindelia squarrosa*

Chickasaw

Abortifacient: *Verbesina virginica*

Analgesic: *Sambucus canadensis*

Dermatological Aid: *Heuchera americana*

Diaphoretic: *Botrychium virginianum*

Diuretic: *Verbesina virginica*

Emetic: *Aureolaria pedicularia, Botrychium virginianum, Chaerophyllum procumbens*

Expectorant: *Botrychium virginianum*

Eye Medicine: *Cephalanthus occidentalis, Hedeoma pulegioides*

Gynecological Aid: *Verbesina virginica*

Misc. Disease Remedy: *Aureolaria pedicularia*

Poison: *Chaerophyllum procumbens*

Stimulant: *Verbesina virginica*

Tonic: *Heuchera americana*

Toothache Remedy: *Ageratina altissima*

Urinary Aid: *Citrullus lanatus*

Venereal Aid: *Verbesina virginica*

Chippewa

Abortifacient: *Aralia nudicaulis, A. racemosa, Artemisia dracunculus, Eupatorium perfoliatum, Hepatica nobilis, Pycnanthemum virginianum, Ribes triste, Rubus frondosus, Sanicula canadensis, Silphium perfoliatum, Tanacetum vulgare*

Adjuvant: *Asarum canadense*

Analgesic: *Abies balsamea, Achillea millefolium, Agastache foeniculum, Andropogon gerardii, Apocynum androsaemifolium, Arctostaphylos uva-ursi, Betula nigra, Capsella bursa-pastoris, Carya ovata, Caulophyllum thalictroides, Conyza canadensis, Corylus americana, Diervilla lonicera, Euthamia graminifolia, Heuchera americana, Maianthemum racemosum, Monarda fistulosa, Polygonatum biflorum, Polygonum persicaria, P. punctatum, Populus balsamifera, Potentilla arguta, Prunus virginiana, Pulsatilla patens, Quercus macrocarpa, Rhus hirta, Ribes glandulosum, R. oxyacanthoides, Rubus occidentalis, Sanguinaria canadensis, Silphium perfoliatum, Smilax herbacea, Thuja occidentalis, Viburnum acerifolium*

Anthelmintic: *Monarda fistulosa, Prunus americana, P. serotina*

Anticonvulsive: *Actaea pachypoda, Apocynum androsaemifolium, Artemisia frigida, Astragalus crassicarpus, Hepatica nobilis, Lathyrus venosus, Polygala senega, Polygonum pensylvanicum, Rosa arkansana, Solidago juncea*

Antidiarrheal: *Amelanchier canadensis, Artemisia dracunculus, Betula lenta, Capsella bursa-pastoris, Comarum palustre, Cornus sericea, Geranium maculatum, Potentilla arguta, Rhus glabra, Rubus allegheniensis, R. idaeus, Tsuga canadensis, Urtica dioica*

Antidote: *Artemisia ludoviciana*

Antihemorrhagic: *Caulophyllum thalictroides, Ostrya virginiana, Prunus virginiana, Silphium perfoliatum, Solidago speciosa*

Antirheumatic (External): *Abies balsamea, Anaphalis margaritacea, Eupatorium maculatum, E. perfoliatum, Juniperus virginiana, Lycopodium obscurum, Ostrya virginiana, Picea glauca, Plantago major, Taxus canadensis, Trillium grandiflorum*

Antirheumatic (Internal): *Juniperus virginiana, Taxus canadensis, Vitis vulpina*

Blood Medicine: *Alnus incana, Aralia nudicaulis, Gaultheria procumbens, Larix laricina, Pedicularis canadensis, Prunus virginiana, Sassafras albidum, Veronicastrum virginicum*

Burn Dressing: *Agastache foeniculum, Clintonia borealis, Larix laricina, Ledum groenlandicum, Monarda fistulosa, Prunus serotina, Rudbeckia laciniata, Solidago canadensis*

Cancer Treatment: *Celastrus scandens*

Carminative: *Mentha canadensis*

Cathartic: *Acorus calamus, Amphicarpaea bracteata, Betula papyrifera, Celastrus scandens, Dirca palustris, Juglans cinerea, Prunella vulgaris, Prunus virginiana, Smilax herbacea, Solidago rigida, Veronicastrum virginicum*

Ceremonial Medicine: *Comptonia peregrina, Thuja occidentalis*

Cold Remedy: *Acorus calamus, Allium stellatum, Apocynum androsaemifolium, Caltha palustris, Castilleja coccinea, Eupatorium purpureum, Gaultheria procumbens, Monarda fistulosa, Rhus glabra, Zanthoxylum americanum*

Cough Medicine: *Acorus calamus, Agastache foeniculum, Aralia racemosa, Arctium minus, Ceanothus herbaceus, Cornus alternifolia,*

Ostrya virginiana, Symplocarpus foetidus, Thuja occidentalis, Zanthoxylum americanum

Dermatological Aid: *Abies balsamea, Acer saccharinum, Achillea millefolium, Anemone canadensis, Aralia nudicaulis, A. racemosa, Artemisia dracunculus, Asarum canadense, Caltha palustris, Celastrus scandens, Clintonia borealis, Cornus sericea, Cypripedium pubescens, Dirca palustris, Epilobium angustifolium, Erysimum cheiranthoides, Galium aparine, Hamamelis virginiana, Hepatica nobilis, Heracleum maximum, Impatiens capensis, Iris versicolor, Lactuca canadensis, Ledum groenlandicum, Lilium philadelphicum, Monarda fistulosa, Osmorhiza claytonii, Pinus strobus, Plantago major, Populus balsamifera, P. tremuloides, Potentilla arguta, Prunus americana, P. serotina, P. virginiana, Rumex crispus, R. obtusifolius, Solidago canadensis, S. speciosa, Thuja occidentalis*

Diaphoretic: *Caltha palustris, Tanacetum vulgare*

Disinfectant: *Amelanchier canadensis, Artemisia frigida, Equisetum hyemale, Prunus americana, P. serotina, P. virginiana, Thuja occidentalis*

Diuretic: *Andropogon gerardii, Athyrium filix-femina, Caltha palustris, Celastrus scandens, Lonicera dioica, Solidago rigida, Symphoricarpos albus, Urtica dioica*

Ear Medicine: *Apocynum androsaemifolium, Aster nemoralis, Campanula rotundifolia, Tanacetum vulgare, Trillium grandiflorum*

Emetic: *Allium tricoccum, Alnus incana, Caltha palustris, Caulophyllum thalictroides, Hamamelis virginiana, Lathyrus venosus, Physocarpus opulifolius, Rhus glabra, Sambucus canadensis, Viburnum acerifolium*

Eye Medicine: *Alnus incana, Arisaema triphyllum, Chimaphila umbellata, Cornus alternifolia, C. sericea, Diervilla lonicera, Hamamelis virginiana, Heuchera americana, Hordeum jubatum, Rubus idaeus, R. occidentalis, Stellaria media, Streptopus roseus*

Febrifuge: *Comptonia peregrina, Nepeta cataria, Pycnanthemum virginianum, Tanacetum vulgare*

Gastrointestinal Aid: *Andropogon gerardii, Artemisia frigida, Asarum canadense, Betula nigra, Capsella bursa-pastoris, Caulophyllum thalictroides, Ceanothus americanus, Conyza canadensis, Cypripedium pubescens, Diervilla lonicera, Geum triflorum, Heuchera americana, Polygonum persicaria, P. punctatum, Prunus virginiana, Quercus macrocarpa, Rhus hirta, Rudbeckia laciniata, Sagittaria latifolia,*

Sanguinaria canadensis, Stachys palustris, Thaspium barbinode, Viburnum acerifolium

Gynecological Aid: *Actaea rubra, Alnus incana, Amelanchier canadensis, Artemisia dracunculus, Asclepias syriaca, Caltha palustris, Conyza canadensis, Eupatorium purpureum, Geum canadense, Maianthemum racemosum, Osmorhiza longistylis, Populus balsamifera, P. tremuloides, Prenanthes alba, Ribes glandulosum, R. oxyacanthoides, Rubus allegheniensis, R. occidentalis, Sanicula canadensis, Solidago speciosa, Taraxacum officinale, Viburnum opulus*

Heart Medicine: *Apocynum androsaemifolium, Artemisia dracunculus, Dalea purpurea, Polygala senega, Populus balsamifera, P. tremuloides, Quercus macrocarpa, Q. rubra*

Hemostat: *Anemone canadensis, Apocynum androsaemifolium, Aralia nudicaulis, Artemisia frigida, Astragalus crassicarpus, Lathyrus venosus, Polygala senega, Rosa arkansana, Silphium perfoliatum, Tsuga canadensis, Verbena hastata*

Herbal Steam: *Abies balsamea, Achillea millefolium, Anaphalis margaritacea, Artemisia dracunculus, Carya ovata, Juniperus virginiana, Polygonatum biflorum, Taxus canadensis*

Hunting Medicine: *Acorus calamus, Arctostaphylos uva-ursi, Aster novae-angliae, A. puniceus, Cornus alternifolia, Eupatorium perfoliatum, Hepatica nobilis*

Kidney Aid: *Ostrya virginiana, Smilax herbacea*

Laxative: *Ceanothus americanus, Diervilla lonicera*

Liver Aid: *Hepatica nobilis*

Misc. Disease Remedy: *Fragaria virginiana, Polygonatum biflorum, Prunus serotina, Rubus idaeus, Thuja occidentalis, Vitis vulpina*

Oral Aid: *Geranium maculatum, Nymphaea odorata, Rhus glabra*

Orthopedic Aid: *Anaphalis margaritacea, Aralia racemosa, Artemisia absinthium, Asarum canadense, Castilleja coccinea, Mirabilis nyctaginea, Populus balsamifera, Silphium perfoliatum, Smilax herbacea, Solidago speciosa, Zanthoxylum americanum*

Other: *Taxus canadensis*

Pediatric Aid: *Acorus calamus, Actaea pachypoda, Allium stellatum, Apocynum androsaemifolium, Artemisia dracunculus, Asclepias incarnata, Celastrus scandens, Eupatorium maculatum, Fragaria virginiana, Geranium maculatum, Hepatica nobilis, Prunus serotina, Rhus glabra, Rudbeckia hirta, Rumex obtusifolius, Thaspium barbinode, Zanthoxylum americanum*

Poison: *Toxicodendron vernix*

Psychological Aid: *Apocynum androsaemifolium, Vaccinium angustifolium*

Pulmonary Aid: *Betula lenta, Caulophyllum thalictroides, Ceanothus americanus, Dirca palustris, Euthamia graminifolia, Fagus grandifolia, Ostrya virginiana, Prunus virginiana, Pulsatilla patens, Quercus macrocarpa, Rubus frondosus, Silphium perfoliatum, Solidago speciosa, Zanthoxylum americanum*

Respiratory Aid: *Acorus calamus, Ceanothus americanus, Juniperus communis, Rhus glabra*

Sedative: *Eupatorium maculatum, Polygonatum biflorum*

Snakebite Remedy: *Botrychium virginianum, Eupatorium perfoliatum, Lilium canadense, Plantago major*

Stimulant: *Achillea millefolium, Artemisia frigida, Astragalus crassicarpus, Geum triflorum, Heliopsis helianthoides, Lathyrus venosus, Polygala senega, Rosa arkansana, Solidago speciosa*

Strengthener: *Artemisia dracunculus, Asclepias incarnata*

Throat Aid: *Acorus calamus, Heracleum maximum, Osmorhiza claytonii, Phryma leptostachya, Potentilla norvegica, Prunus virginiana, Solidago flexicaulis, Tanacetum vulgare, Ulmus rubra, Zanthoxylum americanum*

Tonic: *Artemisia frigida, Astragalus crassicarpus, Gaultheria procumbens, Lathyrus venosus, Polygala senega, Rosa arkansana, Solidago speciosa*

Toothache Remedy: *Acorus calamus, Cypripedium pubescens*

Tuberculosis Remedy: *Caltha palustris, Iris versicolor, Prunus serotina, P. virginiana, Veronicastrum virginicum*

Unspecified: *Comptonia peregrina, Lindera benzoin, Mitchella repens, Polygala senega, Pyrola elliptica, Sagittaria cuneata, S. latifolia, Sanguinaria canadensis, Thuja occidentalis*

Urinary Aid: *Equisetum arvense, Lonicera dioica, Ribes triste, Viburnum lentago*

Venereal Aid: *Chimaphila umbellata*

Vertigo Medicine: *Apocynum androsaemifolium*

Veterinary Aid: *Achillea millefolium, Aralia nudicaulis, Geum triflorum, Liatris scariosa, Osmorhiza longistylis, Pediomelum argophyllum, Rudbeckia laciniata*

Witchcraft Medicine: *Lilium philadelphicum*

Choctaw

Abortifacient: *Galium boreale*

Analgesic: *Aralia racemosa, Aristolochia serpentaria, Arundinaria gigantea, Gnaphalium obtusifolium, Hypericum crux-andreae, Monarda fistulosa, Prenanthes aspera, Pycnanthemum incanum, Quercus marilandica, Ulmus americana*

Anthelmintic: *Pinus echinata, P. virginiana*

Antidiarrheal: *Callicarpa americana, Cephalanthus occidentalis, Malvella leprosa*

Antidote: *Eryngium aquaticum*

Blood Medicine: *Arisaema triphyllum, Berchemia scandens, Sassafras albidum*

Burn Dressing: *Malvella leprosa*

Cathartic: *Monarda fistulosa*

Cold Remedy: *Gnaphalium obtusifolium, Pycnanthemum albescens*

Contraceptive: *Galium boreale*

Cough Medicine: *Echinacea purpurea, Tephrosia hispidula*

Dermatological Aid: *Aralia spinosa, Baptisia alba, Chionanthus virginicus, Galium uniflorum, Geranium maculatum, Heuchera americana, Liquidambar styraciflua, Magnolia grandiflora, Obolaria virginica, Polygala lutea, Populus deltoides, Sambucus cerulea, Saururus cernuus, Tephrosia florida, Yucca aloifolia*

Diaphoretic: *Asclepias verticillata, Galium asprellum, G. boreale, G. uniflorum, Pycnanthemum albescens*

Disinfectant: *Chionanthus virginicus*

Diuretic: *Eryngium aquaticum, Galium asprellum, G. boreale, G. uniflorum, Prenanthes aspera*

Expectorant: *Aralia racemosa, Eryngium aquaticum*

Eye Medicine: *Aralia racemosa, Cephalanthus occidentalis, Hypericum crux-andreae, H. hypericoides, Ilex opaca*

Febrifuge: *Cephalanthus occidentalis, Myrica cerifera, Pluchea foetida, Symplocos tinctoria, Verbesina virginica, Vitis aestivalis*

Gastrointestinal Aid: *Aralia racemosa, Aristolochia serpentaria, Callicarpa americana, Echinacea purpurea, Hypericum hypericoides, Malvella leprosa, Quercus stellata, Sambucus cerulea*

Gynecological Aid: *Polygonum aviculare, Quercus marilandica, Ulmus americana, Vitis aestivalis*

Herbal Steam: *Populus deltoides*

Kidney Aid: *Bignonia capreolata, Magnolia grandiflora*

Liver Aid: *Sambucus canadensis*

Misc. Disease Remedy: *Galium asprellum, Rumex verticillatus, Sassafras albidum*

Oral Aid: *Pityopsis graminifolia*

Other: *Callicarpa americana, Prenanthes aspera*

Panacea: *Pycnanthemum incanum*

Pediatric Aid: *Aralia racemosa, Monarda fistulosa*

Poultice: *Aralia spinosa*

Pulmonary Aid: *Gnaphalium obtusifolium*
Snakebite Remedy: *Asclepias verticillata, Eryngium aquaticum, Populus deltoides*
Stimulant: *Ageratina altissima, Aralia racemosa, Asclepias verticillata, Eryngium aquaticum, Prenanthes aspera*
Throat Aid: *Myrica cerifera*
Tonic: *Ageratina altissima, Cephalanthus occidentalis, Erythrina herbacea, Heuchera americana, Smilax bona-nox, S. tamnoides, Vitis aestivalis*
Toothache Remedy: *Ageratina altissima, Cephalanthus occidentalis*
Unspecified: *Yucca aloifolia*
Urinary Aid: *Sambucus cerulea*
Venereal Aid: *Eryngium aquaticum, Geranium maculatum*

Chumash
Hallucinogen: *Datura wrightii*
Unspecified: *Datura wrightii*

Clallam
Antidiarrheal: *Sambucus cerulea*
Antihemorrhagic: *Tsuga heterophylla*
Cold Remedy: *Achillea millefolium*
Dermatological Aid: *Alnus rubra, Frangula purshiana, Geum macrophyllum, Lysichiton americanus*
Gastrointestinal Aid: *Alnus rubra*
Gynecological Aid: *Achillea millefolium*
Other: *Scirpus acutus*
Pulmonary Aid: *Alnus rubra*
Tuberculosis Remedy: *Thuja plicata*

Coahuilla
Analgesic: *Adenostoma sparsifolium, Chrysothamnus nauseosus, Ericameria palmeri, Eriodictyon californicum, Eriogonum fasciculatum, Rhus ovata*
Cathartic: *Acourtia microcephala, Adenostoma sparsifolium*
Cough Medicine: *Chrysothamnus nauseosus, Rhus ovata*
Dermatological Aid: *Adenostoma sparsifolium, Eriodictyon californicum*
Emetic: *Adenostoma sparsifolium*
Eye Medicine: *Baccharis salicifolia, Eriogonum fasciculatum*
Gastrointestinal Aid: *Adenostoma sparsifolium, Artemisia tridentata, Eriogonum fasciculatum, Larrea tridentata*
Hallucinogen: *Datura wrightii*
Orthopedic Aid: *Ericameria palmeri, Eriodictyon californicum*

Poison: *Datura wrightii*
Tuberculosis Remedy: *Larrea tridentata*
Unspecified: *Ephedra nevadensis*
Veterinary Aid: *Adenostoma fasciculatum, Cucurbita foetidissima, Datura wrightii, Eriodictyon californicum, Larrea tridentata*

Cocopa
Dermatological Aid: *Ephedra trifurca*

Comanche
Adjuvant: *Poliomintha incana*
Analgesic: *Juniperus pinchotii*
Burn Dressing: *Zanthoxylum americanum*
Ceremonial Medicine: *Juniperus pinchotii, Lophophora williamsii, Matelea biflora, M. cynanchoides*
Cold Remedy: *Rhus trilobata*
Dermatological Aid: *Amphiachyris dracunculoides, Artemisia ludoviciana, Carya illinoinensis, Juglans nigra, Matelea biflora, M. cynanchoides, Sphaeralcea coccinea*
Disinfectant: *Juniperus virginiana*
Ear Medicine: *Sophora secundiflora*
Eye Medicine: *Argemone polyanthemos, Maclura pomifera*
Febrifuge: *Helenium autumnale, Zanthoxylum americanum*
Gastrointestinal Aid: *Eriogonum longifolium, Matelea biflora, M. cynanchoides, Prosopis glandulosa*
Gynecological Aid: *Artemisia filifolia, Helenium microcephalum, Juniperus pinchotii, Matelea biflora, M. cynanchoides*
Heart Medicine: *Helenium microcephalum*
Hypotensive: *Helenium microcephalum*
Misc. Disease Remedy: *Matelea biflora, M. cynanchoides*
Narcotic: *Lophophora williamsii*
Orthopedic Aid: *Matelea biflora, M. cynanchoides*
Other: *Juniperus pinchotii*
Pediatric Aid: *Matelea biflora, M. cynanchoides*
Pulmonary Aid: *Gutierrezia sarothrae*
Respiratory Aid: *Helenium microcephalum*
Throat Aid: *Zanthoxylum americanum*
Toothache Remedy: *Zanthoxylum americanum*
Urinary Aid: *Liatris punctata*
Venereal Aid: *Cirsium undulatum, Schizachyrium scoparium*

Concow
Analgesic: *Croton setigerus, Pogogyne douglasii, Trichostema lanceolatum*
Burn Dressing: *Cynoglossum grande*

Dermatological Aid: *Arctostaphylos manzanita,*
Petasites frigidus*
Emetic: *Arbutus menziesii*
Febrifuge: *Croton setigerus, Trichostema lanceo-
latum*
Gastrointestinal Aid: *Pogogyne douglasii*
Misc. Disease Remedy: *Croton setigerus, Petasites
frigidus, Trichostema lanceolatum*
Poison: *Trillium sessile*
Tuberculosis Remedy: *Petasites frigidus*
Veterinary Aid: *Arctostaphylos manzanita*

Costanoan

Abortifacient: *Equisetum laevigatum*
Analgesic: *Adiantum jordanii, Anemopsis californica, Artemisia californica, A. douglasiana,
Clematis ligusticifolia, Datura wrightii, Eriodic-
tyon californicum, Gnaphalium californicum,
Juniperus californica, Malva nicaeensis, Matri-
caria discoidea, Salvia mellifera, Torreya cali-
fornica, Trichostema lanceolatum, Trillium
chloropetalum*
Anthelmintic: *Satureja douglasii*
Anticonvulsive: *Matricaria discoidea*
Antidiarrheal: *Artemisia dracunculus, Capsella
bursa-pastoris, Croton setigerus, Rubus viti-
folius*
Antihemorrhagic: *Pellaea mucronata*
Antirheumatic (External): *Artemisia californica,
A. douglasiana, Eriodictyon californicum*
Antirheumatic (Internal): *Cupressus macrocarpa,
Pinus sabiniana, Rosa californica*
Blood Medicine: *Adiantum jordanii, A. pedatum,
Chamaesyce maculata, Daucus pusillus, Erio-
dictyon californicum, Hoita orbicularis, Juglans
californica, Limonium californicum, Monardel-
la villosa, Pellaea mucronata*
Burn Dressing: *Navarretia atractyloides, Solidago
californica*
Carminative: *Salvia mellifera*
Cathartic: *Datura wrightii, Frangula californica,
Nicotiana quadrivalvis, Sambucus cerulea*
Ceremonial Medicine: *Nicotiana quadrivalvis*
Cold Remedy: *Artemisia californica, Asclepias
eriocarpa, Daucus pusillus, Eriodictyon californicum, Eriogonum latifolium, Gnaphalium californicum, Helenium puberulum, Rosa californica, Salix lasiolepis, Sambucus cerulea,
Trichostema lanceolatum*
Contraceptive: *Equisetum laevigatum, Maianthemum racemosum*
Cough Medicine: *Artemisia californica, Eriogonum
latifolium, Lotus scoparius, Marrubium vulgare, Ruta chalepensis, Salvia mellifera*

Dermatological Aid: *Achillea millefolium, Anemopsis californica, Artemisia californica, A. douglasiana, Asclepias eriocarpa, Baccharis douglasii, B. salicifolia, Castilleja affinis, Chamaesyce
maculata, Chlorogalum pomeridianum, Datura
wrightii, Daucus pusillus, Dryopteris arguta,
Epilobium canum, Equisetum laevigatum, Eriodictyon californicum, Frangula californica,
Grindelia camporum, Helenium puberulum,
Lithocarpus densiflorus, Malva nicaeensis,
Marah macrocarpus, Marrubium vulgare, Matricaria discoidea, Pellaea mucronata, Penstemon centranthifolius, Pteridium aquilinum,
Rosa californica, Rubus vitifolius, Scrophularia
californica, Senecio flaccidus, Solanum nigrum,
Solidago californica, Stachys bullata, Tricho-
stema lanceolatum, Wyethia angustifolia*
Diaphoretic: *Juniperus californica, Torreya cali-
fornica*
Disinfectant: *Anemopsis californica, Baccharis
douglasii, Castilleja affinis, Epilobium canum,
Eriodictyon californicum, Matricaria discoidea,
Penstemon centranthifolius, Rubus vitifolius,
Scrophularia californica, Senecio flaccidus,
Stachys bullata, Trichostema lanceolatum*
Ear Medicine: *Artemisia douglasiana, Medicago
sativa, Nicotiana quadrivalvis, Ruta chalepen-
sis, Salvia mellifera, Stachys bullata*
Emetic: *Lathyrus vestitus, Malva nicaeensis, Nicotiana quadrivalvis, Pellaea mucronata*
Eye Medicine: *Chamaesyce maculata, Datura
wrightii, Eriodictyon californicum, Salvia
columbariae, Scrophularia californica*
Febrifuge: *Cornus sericea, Daucus pusillus, Epilobium canum, Fraxinus latifolia, Hoita orbicularis, Malva nicaeensis, Matricaria discoidea,
Pellaea mucronata, Phacelia californica, Plantago major, Rorippa nasturtium-aquaticum,
Rosa californica, Salix bonplandiana, Salvia
columbariae, Sisyrinchium bellum, Torreya
californica, Verbena lasiostachys*
Gastrointestinal Aid: *Achillea millefolium, Adiantum jordanii, A. pedatum, Artemisia dracunculus, Gnaphalium californicum, Malva nicaeen-
sis, Matricaria discoidea, Melissa officinalis,
Paeonia brownii, Rosa californica, Ruta cha-
lepensis, Sisyrinchium bellum, Stachys bullata,
Torreya californica, Trichostema lanceolatum,
Verbena lasiostachys*
Gynecological Aid: *Adiantum jordanii, Anemopsis
californica, Senecio flaccidus*
Hallucinogen: *Datura wrightii*
Heart Medicine: *Salvia mellifera*
Hemorrhoid Remedy: *Aesculus californica*

Kidney Aid: *Baccharis douglasii, Diplacus aurantiacus, Disporum hookeri, Rorippa nasturtium-aquaticum, Rosa californica, Senecio flaccidus*

Laxative: *Frangula californica, Paeonia brownii, Plantago major, Vicia nigricans*

Liver Aid: *Rorippa nasturtium-aquaticum*

Love Medicine: *Datura wrightii*

Misc. Disease Remedy: *Erodium cicutarium, Solanum nigrum, Verbena lasiostachys*

Orthopedic Aid: *Ambrosia psilostachya, Chenopodium californicum, Ruta chalepensis, Salvia mellifera*

Other: *Asclepias eriocarpa, Malva nicaeensis, Senecio flaccidus*

Panacea: *Baccharis pilularis, Epilobium canum, Lathyrus vestitus, Platanus racemosa*

Pediatric Aid: *Artemisia dracunculus, Epilobium canum, Eschscholzia californica, Malva nicaeensis, Matricaria discoidea, Melissa officinalis*

Poison: *Aesculus californica, Chlorogalum pomeridianum, Eschscholzia californica*

Pulmonary Aid: *Marrubium vulgare, Monardella villosa, Paeonia brownii, Wyethia angustifolia*

Respiratory Aid: *Artemisia californica, A. douglasiana, Asclepias eriocarpa, Datura wrightii, Eriodictyon californicum, Limonium californicum, Monardella villosa*

Sedative: *Eschscholzia californica*

Snakebite Remedy: *Daucus pusillus, Fraxinus latifolia*

Throat Aid: *Datisca glomerata, Rosa californica, Salvia mellifera, Stachys bullata*

Toothache Remedy: *Achillea millefolium, Aesculus californica, Artemisia californica, Lithocarpus densiflorus, Satureja douglasii, Solanum nigrum*

Tuberculosis Remedy: *Eriodictyon californicum*

Unspecified: *Amsinckia douglasiana*

Urinary Aid: *Artemisia douglasiana, A. dracunculus, Diplacus aurantiacus, Epilobium canum, Equisetum laevigatum, Eriogonum fasciculatum, Hordeum murinum, Limonium californicum, Rumex crispus, Xanthium strumarium*

Venereal Aid: *Limonium californicum*

Costanoan (Olhonean)

Abortifacient: *Heteromeles arbutifolia*

Antihemorrhagic: *Arctostaphylos tomentosa*

Cowichan

Burn Dressing: *Arbutus menziesii, Symphoricarpos albus*

Cold Remedy: *Lomatium nudicaule, Polypodium virginianum, Prunus emarginata*

Dermatological Aid: *Arbutus menziesii, Moneses uniflora, Symphoricarpos albus*

Gastrointestinal Aid: *Polypodium virginianum*

Misc. Disease Remedy: *Arbutus menziesii*

Panacea: *Malus fusca, Prunus emarginata*

Throat Aid: *Lomatium nudicaule, Polypodium virginianum*

Unspecified: *Lonicera ciliosa*

Cowlitz

Analgesic: *Alnus rubra, Athyrium filix-femina, Veratrum viride*

Anthelmintic: *Fraxinus latifolia*

Antihemorrhagic: *Tsuga heterophylla*

Antirheumatic (External): *Lysichiton americanus, Oplopanax horridus*

Burn Dressing: *Rubus parviflorus*

Cold Remedy: *Oplopanax horridus, Pseudotsuga menziesii, Thuja plicata*

Dermatological Aid: *Achillea millefolium, Adenocaulon bicolor, Claytonia sibirica, Clintonia uniflora, Polystichum munitum, Pseudotsuga menziesii, Ribes divaricatum, Taxus brevifolia, Tolmiea menziesii, Tsuga heterophylla*

Eye Medicine: *Clintonia uniflora, Oxalis oregana, Trientalis borealis, Tsuga heterophylla*

Gastrointestinal Aid: *Achillea millefolium*

Gynecological Aid: *Urtica dioica*

Laxative: *Frangula purshiana*

Love Medicine: *Galium aparine*

Misc. Disease Remedy: *Polypodium virginianum*

Orthopedic Aid: *Alnus rubra, Sambucus racemosa, Urtica dioica*

Pediatric Aid: *Rosa nutkana*

Poison: *Galium aparine, Oplopanax horridus, Veratrum viride*

Pulmonary Aid: *Arctium minus*

Strengthener: *Rosa nutkana*

Tonic: *Goodyera oblongifolia*

Toothache Remedy: *Thuja plicata*

Tuberculosis Remedy: *Achlys triphylla, Quercus garryana*

Cree

Abortifacient: *Equisetum hyemale, Grindelia squarrosa, Populus grandidentata*

Burn Dressing: *Ledum groenlandicum*

Ceremonial Medicine: *Agastache foeniculum*

Dermatological Aid: *Cirsium discolor, Heracleum maximum*

Diuretic: *Ledum groenlandicum*

Emetic: *Ledum groenlandicum*

Gastrointestinal Aid: *Acorus calamus*

Gynecological Aid: *Grindelia squarrosa, Populus grandidentata*
Heart Medicine: *Ligusticum canbyi*
Kidney Aid: *Grindelia squarrosa*
Poison: *Heracleum maximum*
Throat Aid: *Acorus calamus*
Toothache Remedy: *Heracleum maximum*
Venereal Aid: *Grindelia squarrosa, Heracleum maximum*

Cree, Alberta

Hallucinogen: *Acorus calamus*
Stimulant: *Acorus calamus*
Unspecified: *Acorus calamus*

Cree, Hudson Bay

Analgesic: *Ledum groenlandicum*
Antidiarrheal: *Conyza canadensis, Kalmia latifolia, Prunus virginiana*
Antirheumatic (External): *Ledum groenlandicum*
Cathartic: *Actaea rubra, Apocynum cannabinum, Geocaulon lividum, Iris versicolor*
Cold Remedy: *Cornus sericea*
Cough Medicine: *Cornus sericea*
Dermatological Aid: *Alnus viridis, Apocynum cannabinum, Betula pubescens, Geocaulon lividum, Juniperus communis, Ledum groenlandicum, Pyrus* sp.
Disinfectant: *Juniperus communis*
Diuretic: *Galium boreale, Juniperus virginiana*
Emetic: *Apocynum cannabinum, Cornus sericea, Geocaulon lividum, Lobelia kalmii*
Febrifuge: *Cornus sericea*
Gastrointestinal Aid: *Kalmia angustifolia, Mentha canadensis*
Kidney Aid: *Alnus viridis*
Liver Aid: *Iris versicolor*
Misc. Disease Remedy: *Pyrus* sp.
Orthopedic Aid: *Ledum groenlandicum*
Poison: *Aconitum heterophyllum, Kalmia latifolia*
Pulmonary Aid: *Pyrus* sp.
Throat Aid: *Prunella vulgaris*
Tonic: *Kalmia angustifolia, Solidago multiradiata*
Unspecified: *Apocynum cannabinum, Geocaulon lividum*

Cree, Woodlands

Abortifacient: *Abies balsamea, Alnus viridis, Arctostaphylos uva-ursi, Aster puniceus, Sarracenia purpurea, Vaccinium myrtilloides*
Adjuvant: *Acorus calamus*
Analgesic: *Achillea millefolium, Acorus calamus, Artemisia frigida, Heracleum maximum, Mentha canadensis, Nuphar lutea, Valeriana dioica*

Anticonvulsive: *Valeriana dioica*
Antidiarrheal: *Arctostaphylos uva-ursi, Heuchera richardsonii, Juniperus communis, Picea mariana, Prunus virginiana, Salix discolor*
Antiemetic: *Larix laricina*
Antihemorrhagic: *Achillea millefolium, Acorus calamus, Agastache foeniculum, Chimaphila umbellata, Mentha canadensis, Pyrola asarifolia, Shepherdia canadensis*
Antirheumatic (External): *Acorus calamus, Chenopodium album, Cicuta maculata, Heracleum maximum, Nuphar lutea, Rumex orbiculatus, R. salicifolius, Shepherdia canadensis, Sorbus decora*
Antirheumatic (Internal): *Chenopodium album, Picea glauca*
Blood Medicine: *Picea glauca, Polygala senega*
Breast Treatment: *Ledum groenlandicum*
Burn Dressing: *Betula papyrifera, Ledum groenlandicum, Picea mariana*
Cold Remedy: *Abies balsamea, Acorus calamus, Amelanchier alnifolia, Mentha canadensis, Valeriana dioica*
Contraceptive: *Vaccinium myrtilloides*
Cough Medicine: *Abies balsamea, Acorus calamus, Amelanchier alnifolia, Juniperus communis, Rosa acicularis*
Dermatological Aid: *Abies balsamea, Acorus calamus, Aralia nudicaulis, Betula papyrifera, Epilobium angustifolium, Heracleum maximum, Larix laricina, Ledum groenlandicum, Nuphar lutea, Petasites sagittatus, Picea glauca, P. mariana, Pinus banksiana, Populus tremuloides, Salix bebbiana, Shepherdia canadensis, Symphoricarpos albus, Viburnum edule*
Diaphoretic: *Amelanchier alnifolia, Aster puniceus, Betula papyrifera, Geum aleppicum, Vaccinium myrtilloides*
Disinfectant: *Populus balsamifera*
Diuretic: *Empetrum nigrum, Ledum groenlandicum, Lonicera dioica*
Ear Medicine: *Acorus calamus, Mitella nuda, Valeriana dioica*
Eye Medicine: *Alnus incana, Apocynum androsaemifolium, Cornus sericea, Diervilla lonicera, Heuchera richardsonii, Prunus pensylvanica, Pyrola asarifolia, Rosa acicularis, Symphoricarpos albus*
Febrifuge: *Achillea millefolium, Acorus calamus, Amelanchier alnifolia, Artemisia frigida, Aster puniceus, Juniperus communis, Mentha canadensis, Symphoricarpos albus*
Gastrointestinal Aid: *Acorus calamus, Alisma plantago-aquatica, Astragalus americanus*

Gynecological Aid: *Actaea rubra, Apocynum andro-saemifolium, Aralia nudicaulis, Arctostaphylos uva-ursi, Aster puniceus, Betula papyrifera, Diervilla lonicera, Juniperus communis, Lonicera dioica, Matteuccia struthiopteris, Ribes glandulosum, R. hudsonianum, R. oxyacanthoides, Rubus chamaemorus, R. idaeus, Sarracenia purpurea, Urtica dioica, Vaccinium myrtilloides, Valeriana dioica*

Heart Medicine: *Alisma plantago-aquatica, Campanula rotundifolia, Chimaphila umbellata, Rubus idaeus*

Hemostat: *Acorus calamus, Mentha canadensis, Populus balsamifera, P. tremuloides, Scirpus acutus, S. tabernaemontani*

Kidney Aid: *Juniperus communis*

Laxative: *Alisma plantago-aquatica, Alnus incana, Shepherdia canadensis*

Love Medicine: *Valeriana dioica*

Misc. Disease Remedy: *Alisma plantago-aquatica, Amelanchier alnifolia, Astragalus americanus, Lonicera dioica*

Oral Aid: *Achillea sibirica, Aralia nudicaulis, Mentha canadensis, Picea mariana, Polygala senega, Polygonum amphibium*

Orthopedic Aid: *Acorus calamus, Aster puniceus, Betula papyrifera, Calla palustris, Chimaphila umbellata, Matteuccia struthiopteris, Sarracenia purpurea, Sorbus decora*

Panacea: *Acorus calamus, Alisma plantago-aquatica, Aralia nudicaulis, Geum aleppicum, Nuphar lutea, Polygala senega, Polygonum amphibium, Thuja occidentalis, Valeriana dioica*

Pediatric Aid: *Achillea millefolium, A. sibirica, Acorus calamus, Amelanchier alnifolia, Aralia nudicaulis, Arctostaphylos uva-ursi, Aster puniceus, Betula papyrifera, Carum carvi, Empetrum nigrum, Geum aleppicum, G. macrophyllum, Juniperus communis, Ledum groenlandicum, Picea glauca, Rubus idaeus, Symphoricarpos albus, Valeriana dioica, Viburnum edule*

Poison: *Calla palustris*

Pulmonary Aid: *Acorus calamus, Amelanchier alnifolia, Aralia nudicaulis, Chimaphila umbellata, Juniperus communis, Ledum groenlandicum, Thuja occidentalis, Valeriana dioica*

Reproductive Aid: *Rubus chamaemorus, Vaccinium myrtilloides*

Respiratory Aid: *Juniperus communis*

Sedative: *Carum carvi*

Stimulant: *Alisma plantago-aquatica*

Throat Aid: *Acorus calamus, Geum aleppicum, Picea mariana, Polygala senega, Viburnum edule*

Toothache Remedy: *Achillea millefolium, A. sibirica, Acorus calamus, Amelanchier alnifolia, Aralia nudicaulis, Aster puniceus, Betula papyrifera, Geum aleppicum, G. macrophyllum, Juniperus communis, Mentha canadensis, Monotropa uniflora, Picea mariana, Polygala senega, Rubus idaeus, Viburnum edule*

Tuberculosis Remedy: *Abies balsamea, Polypodium virginianum*

Urinary Aid: *Thuja occidentalis*

Venereal Aid: *Acorus calamus, Betula papyrifera, Lonicera dioica, Picea mariana, Populus tremuloides, Sarracenia purpurea, Shepherdia canadensis, Symphoricarpos albus*

Creek

Abortifacient: *Tephrosia virginiana*

Adjuvant: *Gnaphalium obtusifolium*

Alterative: *Persea palustris*

Analgesic: *Celastrus scandens, Eryngium yuccifolium, Erythrina herbacea, Lindera benzoin*

Anthelmintic: *Spigelia anthelmia, S. marilandica*

Antidiarrheal: *Quercus stellata, Rhus copallinum, R. glabra*

Antiemetic: *Gnaphalium obtusifolium*

Antirheumatic (Internal): *Eryngium yuccifolium, Lindera benzoin*

Blood Medicine: *Eryngium yuccifolium, Lindera benzoin*

Breast Treatment: *Sambucus canadensis*

Cathartic: *Eryngium yuccifolium, Ilex vomitoria, Iris verna, I. versicolor*

Cold Remedy: *Gnaphalium obtusifolium*

Cough Medicine: *Verbascum thapsus*

Dermatological Aid: *Heuchera americana, Panax quinquefolius*

Diaphoretic: *Lindera benzoin, Panax quinquefolius, Persea palustris*

Diuretic: *Ipomoea pandurata*

Emetic: *Ilex vomitoria, Lindera benzoin, Morus rubra*

Febrifuge: *Chenopodium ambrosioides, Panax quinquefolius, Persea palustris*

Gastrointestinal Aid: *Eryngium yuccifolium, Ligusticum canadense*

Gynecological Aid: *Celastrus scandens, Sambucus canadensis*

Hemostat: *Panax quinquefolius*

Herbal Steam: *Lindera benzoin*

Kidney Aid: *Eryngium yuccifolium, Ipomoea pandurata, Persea palustris*

Liver Aid: *Frangula caroliniana*

Misc. Disease Remedy: *Gleditsia triacanthos, Gnaphalium obtusifolium*

Orthopedic Aid: *Celastrus scandens*
Other: *Rhus glabra, Smilax bona-nox*
Panacea: *Chenopodium ambrosioides, Eryngium yuccifolium, Gleditsia triacanthos*
Pediatric Aid: *Gleditsia triacanthos, Spigelia anthelmia*
Poison: *Lomatium nuttallii*
Psychological Aid: *Gnaphalium obtusifolium*
Pulmonary Aid: *Panax quinquefolius, Phoradendron leucarpum*
Reproductive Aid: *Tephrosia virginiana*
Sedative: *Eryngium yuccifolium, Gnaphalium obtusifolium*
Snakebite Remedy: *Eryngium yuccifolium, Manfreda virginica*
Stimulant: *Morus rubra*
Tonic: *Chenopodium ambrosioides, Heuchera americana*
Toothache Remedy: *Achillea millefolium*
Tuberculosis Remedy: *Collinsia violacea, Nyssa sylvatica, Phoradendron leucarpum, Platanus occidentalis, Tephrosia virginiana*
Unspecified: *Bignonia capreolata, Camassia scilloides, Lomatium nuttallii, Sassafras albidum, Triosteum perfoliatum*
Urinary Aid: *Celastrus scandens, Morus rubra, Tephrosia virginiana*
Venereal Aid: *Eryngium yuccifolium*
Veterinary Aid: *Zanthoxylum americanum*
Witchcraft Medicine: *Gnaphalium obtusifolium, Ulmus rubra*

Crow

Analgesic: *Equisetum hyemale, Oplopanax horridus*
Antidiarrheal: *Juniperus scopulorum, Prunus virginiana*
Antihemorrhagic: *Juniperus scopulorum*
Antirheumatic (External): *Lomatium macrocarpum*
Burn Dressing: *Achillea millefolium, Prunus virginiana*
Ceremonial Medicine: *Abies lasiocarpa, Catabrosa aquatica, Glyceria fluitans, Juniperus chinense, Lobelia inflata, Madia glomerata*
Cold Remedy: *Abies lasiocarpa, Echinacea pallida, Grindelia squarrosa, Ligusticum canbyi, Lomatium macrocarpum*
Cough Medicine: *Abies lasiocarpa, Grindelia squarrosa, Ligusticum canbyi*
Dermatological Aid: *Achillea millefolium, Artemisia ludoviciana, Prunus virginiana*
Dietary Aid: *Juniperus scopulorum*
Diuretic: *Equisetum hyemale*

Ear Medicine: *Ligusticum canbyi*
Eye Medicine: *Artemisia dracunculus*
Gastrointestinal Aid: *Echinacea pallida, Juniperus scopulorum*
Gynecological Aid: *Juniperus scopulorum*
Laxative: *Abies lasiocarpa*
Oral Aid: *Arctostaphylos uva-ursi*
Pulmonary Aid: *Grindelia squarrosa*
Respiratory Aid: *Grindelia squarrosa, Ligusticum canbyi, Monarda fistulosa*
Throat Aid: *Lomatium macrocarpum*
Toothache Remedy: *Echinacea pallida*
Veterinary Aid: *Symphoricarpos albus*

Dakota

Abortifacient: *Artemisia frigida*
Analgesic: *Callirhoe involucrata, Echinacea angustifolia, Helianthus annuus, Humulus lupulus, Monarda fistulosa, Penstemon grandiflorus, Ratibida columnifera, Sphaeralcea coccinea, Verbena hastata*
Anthelmintic: *Echinacea pallida, Mirabilis nyctaginea*
Antidiarrheal: *Ambrosia artemisiifolia, Dalea aurea*
Antidote: *Echinacea angustifolia*
Antiemetic: *Ambrosia artemisiifolia*
Burn Dressing: *Echinacea angustifolia, Sphaeralcea coccinea, Typha latifolia*
Carminative: *Acorus calamus, Mentha canadensis*
Ceremonial Medicine: *Acorus calamus, Hierochloe odorata, Prunus virginiana, Shepherdia argentea*
Cold Remedy: *Acorus calamus, Callirhoe involucrata, Hedeoma hispida, Juniperus virginiana*
Cough Medicine: *Acorus calamus, Juniperus virginiana*
Dermatological Aid: *Echinacea pallida, Humulus lupulus, Lilium philadelphicum, Mirabilis nyctaginea, Opuntia humifusa, Ratibida columnifera, Rumex altissimus, R. crispus, Sphaeralcea coccinea, Typha latifolia, Yucca glauca*
Dietary Aid: *Hedeoma hispida*Ear Medicine: *Glycyrrhiza lepidota*
Eye Medicine: *Echinacea pallida, Symphoricarpos occidentalis, S. orbiculatus*
Febrifuge: *Acorus calamus, Astragalus canadensis, Glycyrrhiza lepidota, Humulus lupulus, Mentzelia nuda, Mirabilis nyctaginea*
Gastrointestinal Aid: *Acorus calamus, Dalea aurea, Grindelia squarrosa, Humulus lupulus, Monarda fistulosa, Verbena hastata, V. stricta*
Laxative: *Gymnocladus dioicus, Ulmus rubra*
Love Medicine: *Lomatium foeniculaceum*

Misc. Disease Remedy: *Echinacea angustifolia, Juniperus virginiana*

Other: *Echinacea angustifolia*

Panacea: *Acorus calamus, Cucurbita foetidissima, Ratibida columnifera*

Pediatric Aid: *Astragalus canadensis, Glycyrrhiza lepidota, Grindelia squarrosa, Typha latifolia*

Poison: *Dalea enneandra*

Psychological Aid: *Acorus calamus*

Pulmonary Aid: *Helianthus annuus*

Snakebite Remedy: *Echinacea angustifolia, E. pallida*

Stimulant: *Gymnocladus dioicus*

Tonic: *Gentiana saponaria*

Toothache Remedy: *Acorus calamus, Echinacea angustifolia, Glycyrrhiza lepidota*

Tuberculosis Remedy: *Psoralidium tenuiflorum*

Veterinary Aid: *Clematis ligusticifolia, Dyssodia papposa, Echinacea angustifolia, Glycyrrhiza lepidota, Gutierrezia sarothrae, Juniperus virginiana, Silphium laciniatum*

Witchcraft Medicine: *Silphium laciniatum*

Delaware

Abortifacient: *Acorus calamus, Mitchella repens*

Analgesic: *Cornus canadensis, Symplocarpus foetidus*

Anthelmintic: *Eryngium aquaticum, Juglans nigra, Prunus persica*

Antidiarrheal: *Prunus serotina, Rubus allegheniensis, Solidago juncea*

Antiemetic: *Cercis canadensis, Prunus persica*

Antirheumatic (External): *Aesculus glabra, Asclepias tuberosa, Cirsium vulgare, Gaultheria procumbens, Goodyera pubescens, Iris versicolor, Mitchella repens, Phytolacca americana, Tsuga canadensis, Verbascum thapsus*

Antirheumatic (Internal): *Arctium minus*

Blood Medicine: *Ambrosia artemisiifolia, Arctium minus, Chimaphila umbellata, Comptonia peregrina, Gelsemium sempervirens, Gentianopsis crinita, Gleditsia triacanthos, Phytolacca americana, Rumex crispus, R. obtusifolius, Sambucus canadensis, Sassafras albidum*

Cathartic: *Maianthemum stellatum, Pimpinella anisum*

Cold Remedy: *Acorus calamus, Platanus occidentalis, Quercus velutina, Ulmus americana*

Cough Medicine: *Acorus calamus, Gleditsia triacanthos, Petasites frigidus, Prunus serotina, Quercus alba, Q. rubra, Ulmus americana, Verbascum thapsus*

Dermatological Aid: *Baptisia tinctoria, Celastrus scandens, Chimaphila umbellata, Comptonia*

peregrina, Datura stramonium, Juglans nigra, Monarda punctata, Phytolacca americana, Rhus copallinum, Sambucus canadensis

Disinfectant: *Quercus alba*

Ear Medicine: *Aesculus glabra, Humulus lupulus*

Febrifuge: *Cercis canadensis, Eupatorium perfoliatum, Monarda punctata, Prunella vulgaris, Solidago juncea*

Gastrointestinal Aid: *Acorus calamus, Angelica atropurpurea, Cardamine diphylla, Gentianopsis crinita, Hedeoma pulegioides, Inula helenium, Juglans nigra, Maianthemum stellatum, Pimpinella anisum, Quercus palustris, Sanguinaria canadensis, Scutellaria galericulata*

Gland Medicine: *Phytolacca americana*

Gynecological Aid: *Asclepias tuberosa, Baptisia tinctoria, Goodyera pubescens, Leonurus cardiaca, Maianthemum stellatum, Plantago major, Quercus alba*

Heart Medicine: *Zanthoxylum americanum*

Hemorrhoid Remedy: *Datura stramonium*

Kidney Aid: *Achillea millefolium, Gaultheria procumbens, Hydrangea arborescens, Iris versicolor, Typha latifolia*

Laxative: *Podophyllum peltatum, Scutellaria galericulata, Taraxacum officinale*

Liver Aid: *Achillea millefolium, Celastrus scandens, Iris versicolor, Rumex crispus, R. obtusifolius, Sambucus canadensis*

Misc. Disease Remedy: *Daucus carota, Lobelia cardinalis, Symplocarpus foetidus*

Narcotic: *Crotalaria sagittalis*

Oral Aid: *Rhus copallinum*

Panacea: *Lophophora williamsii*

Pediatric Aid: *Chrysopsis mariana, Nepeta cataria, Prunus persica, Sambucus canadensis*

Poison: *Aesculus glabra*

Pulmonary Aid: *Asclepias tuberosa, Chimaphila umbellata, Comptonia peregrina, Goodyera pubescens, Petasites frigidus, Symplocarpus foetidus, Verbascum thapsus*

Reproductive Aid: *Salix humilis, Viburnum prunifolium, Vitis rupestris*

Respiratory Aid: *Petasites frigidus, Verbascum thapsus*

Sedative: *Chrysopsis mariana, Humulus lupulus*

Stimulant: *Arctium minus, Humulus lupulus, Phytolacca americana*

Strengthener: *Populus deltoides, Sanguinaria canadensis, Vitis rupestris*

Throat Aid: *Helianthemum canadense, Platanus occidentalis, Quercus alba, Q. rubra, Q. velutina*

Tonic: *Aristolochia serpentaria, Chrysopsis mari-*

ana, Cimicifuga racemosa, Cornus florida, Gaultheria procumbens, Inula helenium, Panax quinquefolius, Podophyllum peltatum, Prunus serotina

Toothache Remedy: *Humulus lupulus*

Tuberculosis Remedy: *Lophophora williamsii*

Unspecified: *Panax quinquefolius, Plantago major, Toxicodendron pubescens*

Urinary Aid: *Chimaphila umbellata, Comptonia peregrina*

Venereal Aid: *Cardamine diphylla, Chimaphila umbellata, Comptonia peregrina, Crotalaria sagittalis, Echinacea purpurea, Iris versicolor, Rhus copallinum, R. hirta, Salix humilis, Stachys palustris*

Delaware, Oklahoma

Abortifacient: *Acorus calamus, Mitchella repens*

Analgesic: *Acorus calamus, Cornus canadensis, Hedeoma pulegioides, Helianthemum canadense, Quercus palustris, Symplocarpus foetidus, Verbascum thapsus*

Anthelmintic: *Eryngium aquaticum*

Anticonvulsive: *Symplocarpus foetidus*

Antidiarrheal: *Prunus serotina, Rubus alleghaniensis, R. canadensis, Solidago juncea*

Antiemetic: *Cercis canadensis*

Antirheumatic (External): *Cirsium vulgare, Juniperus virginiana, Mitchella repens, Phytolacca americana, Tsuga canadensis, Verbascum thapsus*

Antirheumatic (Internal): *Arctium minus, Asclepias tuberosa, Gaultheria procumbens, Goodyera pubescens, Iris versicolor, Phytolacca americana*

Blood Medicine: *Ambrosia artemisiifolia, Arctium minus, Chimaphila umbellata, Comptonia peregrina, Gelsemium sempervirens, Gentianopsis crinita, Gleditsia triacanthos, Phytolacca americana, Rumex crispus, R. obtusifolius, Sambucus canadensis, Sassafras albidum*

Cathartic: *Betula alleghaniensis, Frangula caroliniana, Fraxinus americana, Juglans nigra, Maianthemum stellatum, Morus nigra, Pimpinella anisum*

Ceremonial Medicine: *Artemisia frigida, Rhus copallinum*

Cold Remedy: *Acorus calamus, Platanus occidentalis, Quercus velutina, Ulmus americana, Verbascum thapsus*

Cough Medicine: *Acorus calamus, Gleditsia triacanthos, Petasites frigidus, Prunus serotina, Quercus alba, Q. rubra, Symplocarpus foetidus, Ulmus americana, Verbascum thapsus*

Dermatological Aid: *Ambrosia artemisiifolia, Baptisia tinctoria, Chimaphila umbellata, Comptonia peregrina, Datura stramonium, Gelsemium sempervirens, Juglans nigra, Menispermum canadense, Quercus alba, Rhus copallinum, Sambucus canadensis, Solanum dulcamara, Toxicodendron pubescens, Vitis vulpina*

Disinfectant: *Quercus alba*

Ear Medicine: *Aesculus glabra, Humulus lupulus*

Emetic: *Betula alleghaniensis, Frangula caroliniana, Fraxinus americana, Juglans nigra, Morus nigra*

Expectorant: *Chimaphila umbellata, Comptonia peregrina*

Febrifuge: *Cercis canadensis, Eupatorium perfoliatum, Monarda punctata, Prunella vulgaris, Solanum dulcamara, Solidago juncea, Verbena hastata*

Gastrointestinal Aid: *Angelica atropurpurea, Betula alleghaniensis, Cardamine diphylla, Frangula caroliniana, Fraxinus americana, Gentianopsis crinita, Hedeoma pulegioides, Inula helenium, Juglans nigra, Maianthemum stellatum, Morus nigra, Pimpinella anisum, Quercus palustris, Sambucus canadensis, Sanguinaria canadensis*

Gynecological Aid: *Asclepias tuberosa, Baptisia tinctoria, Goodyera pubescens, Leonurus cardiaca, Maianthemum stellatum, Mitchella repens, Plantago major, Populus deltoides, Quercus alba, Viburnum prunifolium, Vitis vulpina*

Heart Medicine: *Zanthoxylum americanum*

Hemorrhoid Remedy: *Datura stramonium*

Herbal Steam: *Cirsium vulgare, Juniperus virginiana, Mitchella repens, Phytolacca americana, Tsuga canadensis*

Kidney Aid: *Achillea millefolium, Iris versicolor, Typha latifolia*

Laxative: *Inula helenium, Podophyllum peltatum, Scutellaria galericulata, Taraxacum officinale*

Liver Aid: *Achillea millefolium, Betula alleghaniensis, Frangula caroliniana, Fraxinus americana, Hydrangea arborescens, Iris versicolor, Juglans nigra, Morus nigra, Rumex crispus, R. obtusifolius, Sambucus canadensis*

Love Medicine: *Podophyllum peltatum*

Misc. Disease Remedy: *Daucus carota, Lobelia cardinalis*

Narcotic: *Crotalaria sagittalis*

Oral Aid: *Rhus copallinum*

Panacea: *Panax quinquefolius, Quercus alba, Sanguinaria canadensis*

Pediatric Aid: *Nepeta cataria, Sambucus canadensis*

Poison: *Aesculus glabra*

Pulmonary Aid: *Asclepias tuberosa, Goodyera pubescens, Petasites frigidus, Verbascum thapsus*
Reproductive Aid: *Vitis rupestris*
Respiratory Aid: *Petasites frigidus, Verbascum thapsus*
Sedative: *Chrysopsis mariana, Humulus lupulus*
Stimulant: *Arctium minus, Humulus lupulus, Maianthemum stellatum, Phytolacca americana*
Throat Aid: *Platanus occidentalis, Quercus alba, Q. rubra, Q. velutina*
Tonic: *Anaphalis margaritacea, Aralia nudicaulis, Aristolochia serpentaria, Chrysopsis mariana, Cimicifuga racemosa, Cornus florida, Gaultheria procumbens, Gleditsia triacanthos, Helianthemum canadense, Humulus lupulus, Inula helenium, Maianthemum racemosum, Mentha ×piperita, Nepeta cataria, Panax quinquefolius, Pimpinella anisum, Podophyllum peltatum, Prunus serotina, Sanguinaria canadensis, Sassafras albidum, Taraxacum officinale, Vitis rupestris, Zanthoxylum americanum*
Toothache Remedy: *Humulus lupulus*
Tuberculosis Remedy: *Cardamine diphylla, Chimaphila umbellata, Comptonia peregrina, Iris versicolor, Maianthemum stellatum, Salix humilis*
Unspecified: *Goodyera pubescens, Plantago major*
Urinary Aid: *Chimaphila umbellata, Comptonia peregrina*
Venereal Aid: *Cardamine diphylla, Crotalaria sagittalis, Echinacea purpurea, Eryngium aquaticum, Maianthemum stellatum, Rhus copallinum, R. hirta, Salix humilis, Solanum nigrum, Stachys palustris*

Delaware, Ontario

Analgesic: *Arctium minus, Armoracia rusticana, Pinus strobus, Verbascum thapsus*
Antidiarrheal: *Rhus hirta*
Antiemetic: *Quercus muehlenbergii, Sanguinaria canadensis*
Blood Medicine: *Arctium minus, Sanguinaria canadensis*
Cold Remedy: *Acorus calamus, Inula helenium, Populus tremuloides*
Dermatological Aid: *Pinus strobus, Plantago major, Sedum telephioides, Verbascum thapsus*
Disinfectant: *Sedum telephioides*
Febrifuge: *Thymus praecox*
Gastrointestinal Aid: *Eupatorium perfoliatum, Tanacetum vulgare*
Gynecological Aid: *Carpinus caroliniana, Carya alba, C. ovata, Juniperus communis, Ostrya virginiana, Prunus serotina, Quercus alba*
Kidney Aid: *Pinus strobus*

Misc. Disease Remedy: *Viburnum lentago*
Pediatric Aid: *Nepeta cataria, Pinus strobus*
Pulmonary Aid: *Pinus strobus*
Sedative: *Nepeta cataria*
Tonic: *Carpinus caroliniana, Carya alba, C. ovata, Juniperus communis, Ostrya virginiana, Prunus serotina, Quercus alba*
Tuberculosis Remedy: *Celastrus scandens*
Unspecified: *Pinus strobus*

Diegueño

Analgesic: *Juniperus californica, Lamarckia aurea*
Antidiarrheal: *Eriogonum fasciculatum, Fragaria vesca, Gutierrezia sarothrae, Rubus ursinus*
Antidote: *Cuscuta californica*
Antihemorrhagic: *Pellaea mucronata*
Antirheumatic (External): *Hazardia squarrosa, Larrea tridentata, Urtica dioica*
Blood Medicine: *Ephedra californica, Grindelia hallii, Platanus racemosa, Salvia apiana*
Cathartic: *Frangula californica*
Cold Remedy: *Artemisia tridentata, Eriodictyon lanatum, Marrubium vulgare, Salvia apiana*
Cough Medicine: *Artemisia tridentata, Baccharis sarothroides, Croton californicus, Eriodictyon lanatum, Prunus ilicifolia, Salvia apiana*
Dermatological Aid: *Ambrosia psilostachya, Baccharis salicifolia, Ceanothus leucodermis, Chamaesyce albomarginata, Dudleya pulverulenta, Ericameria brachylepis, Frangula californica, Heteromeles arbutifolia, Malva parviflora, Phoradendron macrophyllum, Populus fremontii, Quercus agrifolia, Ricinus communis, Solidago californica, Vitis girdiana*
Dietary Aid: *Ephedra californica*
Ear Medicine: *Ruta chalepensis, R. graveolens*
Emetic: *Eriogonum fasciculatum*
Eye Medicine: *Physalis philadelphica, Prosopis glandulosa, Quercus dumosa, Rhus trilobata, Toxicodendron diversilobum*
Febrifuge: *Brickellia californica, Malva parviflora, Matricaria discoidea, Prosopis glandulosa, Rosa californica, Sambucus cerulea, Scrophularia californica*
Gastrointestinal Aid: *Adenostoma sparsifolium, Ambrosia psilostachya, Baccharis sarothroides, Ephedra californica, Lepidium nitidum, Paeonia californica, Ruta graveolens*
Gynecological Aid: *Matricaria discoidea, Rhus ovata*
Hallucinogen: *Datura wrightii*
Heart Medicine: *Eriogonum fasciculatum*
Hypotensive: *Equisetum laevigatum, Juniperus californica*

Kidney Aid: *Ephedra californica*
Laxative: *Sambucus cerulea*
Misc. Disease Remedy: *Ericameria brachylepis,*
Salvia apiana
Orthopedic Aid: *Larrea tridentata, Populus fre-*
montii
Other: *Salvia apiana*
Pediatric Aid: *Eriogonum fasciculatum, Marru-*
bium vulgare, Matricaria discoidea, Rhus tri-
lobata, Rosa californica, Sambucus cerulea
Poison: *Datura wrightii*
Pulmonary Aid: *Marrubium vulgare*
Respiratory Aid: *Artemisia tridentata, Dudleya*
pulverulenta, Platanus racemosa
Strengthener: *Salvia columbariae*
Toothache Remedy: *Adenostoma sparsifolium*
Unspecified: *Anemopsis californica, Datura*
wrightii, Monardella lanceolata
Veterinary Aid: *Croton setigerus, Lonicera sub-*
spicata

Eskimo

Cancer Treatment: *Artemisia tilesii*
Disinfectant: *Artemisia tilesii*
Febrifuge: *Artemisia tilesii*
Gastrointestinal Aid: *Valeriana capitata*
Panacea: *Angelica lucida*
Preventive Medicine: *Angelica lucida*
Psychological Aid: *Angelica lucida*
Unspecified: *Potentilla nana*

Eskimo, Alaska

Anesthetic: *Salix planifolia*
Antihemorrhagic: *Equisetum sylvaticum, Ledum*
palustre, Matricaria discoidea
Antirheumatic (External): *Artemisia tilesii*
Cold Remedy: *Moneses uniflora, Pinus contorta*
Cough Medicine: *Moneses uniflora, Pinus contorta*
Dermatological Aid: *Alnus viridis, Picea glauca,*
Salix sitchensis
Eye Medicine: *Salix planifolia*
Gastrointestinal Aid: *Ledum palustre*
Hemostat: *Artemisia tilesii*
Laxative: *Artemisia tilesii, Epilobium angusti-*
folium
Oral Aid: *Salix planifolia, Sedum integrifolium*
Respiratory Aid: *Artemisia tilesii*
Tonic: *Artemisia tilesii*
Unspecified: *Achillea millefolium, Ledum palustre,*
Picea glauca, Pinus contorta

Eskimo, Arctic

Poison: *Actaea rubra*

Eskimo, Chugach

Throat Aid: *Viburnum edule*

Eskimo, Inuktitut

Antidiarrheal: *Rumex arcticus*
Antirheumatic (Internal): *Alnus viridis*
Dermatological Aid: *Artemisia tilesii, Picea glauca,*
P. mariana, Salix arbusculoides
Gastrointestinal Aid: *Valeriana capitata*
Laxative: *Fomes igniarius*
Poison: *Senecio congestus*
Respiratory Aid: *Picea glauca, P. mariana*
Strengthener: *Nephroma arcticum*
Unspecified: *Angelica lucida, Eriophorum angusti-*
folium, Matricaria discoidea

Eskimo, Inupiat

Carminative: *Chenopodium album*
Cold Remedy: *Juniperus communis, Petasites*
frigidus
Cough Medicine: *Juniperus communis*
Dermatological Aid: *Epilobium latifolium*
Eye Medicine: *Epilobium latifolium*
Misc. Disease Remedy: *Juniperus communis*
Oral Aid: *Salix planifolia*
Poison: *Aconitum delphiniifolium, Caltha palus-*
tris, Cicuta virosa, Hedysarum boreale, Iris
setosa, Lathyrus japonicus, Ledum palustre,
Lupinus arcticus, Ranunculus pallasii, Shep-
herdia canadensis, Zigadenus elegans
Respiratory Aid: *Juniperus communis, Petasites*
frigidus
Unspecified: *Ledum palustre*

Eskimo, Kuskokwagmiut

Adjuvant: *Matricaria discoidea*
Antidiarrheal: *Rumex acetosa*
Cold Remedy: *Matricaria discoidea*
Cough Medicine: *Picea glauca*
Dermatological Aid: *Artemisia tilesii, Salix arbus-*
culoides
Dietary Aid: *Ranunculus lapponicus*
Disinfectant: *Angelica lucida*
Eye Medicine: *Salix arbusculoides*
Gastrointestinal Aid: *Matricaria discoidea*
Oral Aid: *Salix arbusculoides*
Orthopedic Aid: *Artemisia tilesii*
Panacea: *Eriophorum angustifolium*
Pediatric Aid: *Ledum palustre*
Poison: *Cicuta virosa*

Eskimo, Nunivak

Analgesic: *Salix planifolia, S. rotundifolia*
Dermatological Aid: *Picea glauca*

Oral Aid: *Salix planifolia, S. rotundifolia*
Panacea: *Picea glauca*
Unspecified: *Achillea millefolium, Ledum palustre, Sedum rosea*

Eskimo, Western

Adjuvant: *Matricaria discoidea*
Analgesic: *Betula nana, Dryopteris campyloptera, Epilobium angustifolium, Ledum palustre, Sedum rosea*
Cold Remedy: *Matricaria discoidea*
Cough Medicine: *Picea glauca*
Dermatological Aid: *Eriophorum russeolum, E. scheuchzeri*
Eye Medicine: *Eriophorum russeolum, Salix fuscescens*
Gastrointestinal Aid: *Artemisia tilesii, Betula nana, Dryopteris campyloptera, Epilobium angustifolium, Ledum palustre, Matricaria discoidea, Sedum rosea*
Laxative: *Caltha palustris*
Oral Aid: *Salix fuscescens, S. planifolia*
Orthopedic Aid: *Artemisia tilesii*
Poison: *Cicuta virosa, Ligusticum scothicum, Senecio congestus*
Tuberculosis Remedy: *Sedum rosea*

Flathead

Analgesic: *Hierochloe odorata, Opuntia polyacantha, Pinus ponderosa*
Anthelmintic: *Prunus virginiana*
Anticonvulsive: *Ligusticum canbyi*
Antidiarrheal: *Heuchera cylindrica, Matricaria discoidea, Opuntia polyacantha, Prunus virginiana*
Antirheumatic (External): *Achillea millefolium, Artemisia dracunculus, Mahonia repens, Nuphar lutea, Pinus ponderosa*
Antirheumatic (Internal): *Vaccinium membranaceum*
Breast Treatment: *Lewisia rediviva*
Burn Dressing: *Arctostaphylos uva-ursi, Balsamorhiza sagittata, Pinus contorta, Symphoricarpos albus*
Cathartic: *Balsamorhiza sagittata, Frangula purshiana, Rhus glabra*
Ceremonial Medicine: *Juniperus scopulorum*
Cold Remedy: *Achillea millefolium, Artemisia ludoviciana, A. tridentata, Grindelia squarrosa, Hierochloe odorata, Juniperus scopulorum, Matricaria discoidea, Mentha arvensis, Monarda fistulosa, Populus balsamifera, P. deltoides*
Contraceptive: *Mahonia repens*

Cough Medicine: *Grindelia squarrosa, Mahonia repens, Mentha arvensis, Monarda fistulosa*
Dermatological Aid: *Abies lasiocarpa, Achillea millefolium, Artemisia dracunculus, A. ludoviciana, Mahonia repens, Nuphar lutea, Pinus contorta, P. ponderosa, Populus balsamifera, P. deltoides, Symphoricarpos albus*
Disinfectant: *Achillea millefolium*
Diuretic: *Equisetum hyemale*
Ear Medicine: *Arctostaphylos uva-ursi*
Eye Medicine: *Chimaphila umbellata, Monarda fistulosa, Prunus virginiana, Shepherdia canadensis, Symphoricarpos albus*
Febrifuge: *Achillea millefolium, Hierochloe odorata, Juniperus scopulorum, Mentha arvensis, Monarda fistulosa*
Gastrointestinal Aid: *Asclepias speciosa, Heuchera cylindrica, Matricaria discoidea*
Gynecological Aid: *Lewisia rediviva, Mahonia repens, Monarda fistulosa, Pinus ponderosa*
Heart Medicine: *Lewisia rediviva, Vaccinium membranaceum*
Misc. Disease Remedy: *Monarda fistulosa*
Nose Medicine: *Veratrum viride*
Oral Aid: *Abies lasiocarpa*
Other: *Populus tremuloides*
Pediatric Aid: *Abies lasiocarpa, Matricaria discoidea*
Poison: *Frangula purshiana*
Pulmonary Aid: *Artemisia tridentata, Balsamorhiza sagittata, Grindelia squarrosa, Juniperus scopulorum, Lewisia rediviva, Monarda fistulosa*
Respiratory Aid: *Grindelia squarrosa, Hierochloe odorata*
Tonic: *Mentha arvensis*
Toothache Remedy: *Mentha arvensis, Monarda fistulosa*
Tuberculosis Remedy: *Balsamorhiza sagittata, Grindelia squarrosa, Rhus glabra, Shepherdia canadensis*
Unspecified: *Ligusticum canbyi, Shepherdia canadensis*
Urinary Aid: *Balsamorhiza sagittata*
Venereal Aid: *Mahonia repens, Nuphar lutea, Populus balsamifera, P. deltoides*
Veterinary Aid: *Amelanchier alnifolia, Grindelia squarrosa, Juniperus scopulorum, Nuphar lutea*

Gabrielino

Hallucinogen: *Datura wrightii*
Unspecified: *Datura wrightii*

Gitksan

Analgesic: *Alnus rubra, Angelica genuflexa, Oplopanax horridus, Thalictrum occidentale, Viburnum edule*

Antihemorrhagic: *Alnus viridis, Calla palustris, Castilleja miniata, Lysichiton americanus, Nuphar lutea, Oplopanax horridus, Urtica dioica*

Antirheumatic (External): *Abies grandis, Heracleum maximum, Lysichiton americanus, Oplopanax horridus*

Antirheumatic (Internal): *Anemone multifida, Lysichiton americanus, Maianthemum racemosum, Malus fusca, Picea sitchensis, Shepherdia canadensis*

Blood Medicine: *Pinus contorta, Thalictrum occidentale*

Cancer Treatment: *Oplopanax horridus*

Cathartic: *Alnus rubra, A. viridis, Castilleja miniata, Maianthemum racemosum, Oplopanax horridus, Pinus contorta, Populus tremuloides, Sambucus racemosa, Sorbus sitchensis*

Cold Remedy: *Abies lasiocarpa, Oplopanax horridus, Picea glauca*

Cough Medicine: *Abies lasiocarpa, Alnus rubra, Castilleja miniata, Oplopanax horridus, Picea glauca, Shepherdia canadensis, Viburnum edule*

Dermatological Aid: *Abies grandis, Descurainia incana, Heracleum maximum, Lysichiton americanus, Maianthemum racemosum, Oplopanax horridus, Populus tremuloides*

Diaphoretic: *Anemone multifida*

Dietary Aid: *Malus fusca*

Diuretic: *Alnus incana, Castilleja miniata, Ledum groenlandicum, Malus fusca, Oplopanax horridus, Pinus contorta*

Emetic: *Alnus rubra, Sambucus racemosa*

Eye Medicine: *Angelica genuflexa, Calla palustris, Castilleja miniata, Lonicera involucrata, Malus fusca, Thalictrum occidentale, Viburnum edule*

Gastrointestinal Aid: *Oplopanax horridus, Tsuga heterophylla*

Gynecological Aid: *Nuphar lutea*

Hunting Medicine: *Veratrum viride*

Kidney Aid: *Castilleja miniata, Maianthemum racemosum*

Laxative: *Alnus incana, Malus fusca*

Liver Aid: *Tsuga heterophylla*

Misc. Disease Remedy: *Abies lasiocarpa, Calla palustris, Lysichiton americanus, Oplopanax horridus, Picea glauca*

Orthopedic Aid: *Castilleja miniata, Maianthemum racemosum, Oplopanax horridus, Thalictrum occidentale*

Other: *Oplopanax horridus, Tsuga heterophylla, Veratrum viride*

Poison: *Lysichiton americanus*

Pulmonary Aid: *Abies grandis, Castilleja miniata, Lysichiton americanus, Nuphar lutea, Oplopanax horridus, Thalictrum occidentale*

Respiratory Aid: *Calla palustris, Oplopanax horridus*

Sedative: *Lysichiton americanus*

Throat Aid: *Achillea millefolium*

Tonic: *Abies lasiocarpa, Alnus viridis, Calla palustris, Oplopanax horridus, Picea glauca, Pinus contorta*

Tuberculosis Remedy: *Malus fusca, Oplopanax horridus, Picea sitchensis, Pinus contorta, Viburnum edule*

Unspecified: *Alnus incana, A. rubra, Juniperus communis, Pinus contorta, Prunus pensylvanica, Ribes lacustre, Urtica dioica*

Urinary Aid: *Urtica dioica*

Venereal Aid: *Alnus incana, A. viridis, Oplopanax horridus, Pinus contorta, Shepherdia canadensis*

Witchcraft Medicine: *Heracleum maximum, Juniperus communis, Sambucus racemosa*

Gosiute

Analgesic: *Achillea millefolium, Aquilegia coerulea, Chaenactis douglasii, Mentha canadensis, Silene douglasii, S. scouleri*

Anthelmintic: *Pinus monophylla*

Antidiarrheal: *Geranium caespitosum*

Antirheumatic (External): *Achillea millefolium, Artemisia tridentata, Maianthemum stellatum, Valeriana edulis*

Antirheumatic (Internal): *Artemisia tridentata*

Blood Medicine: *Prunus virginiana, Rumex salicifolius*

Burn Dressing: *Cercocarpus ledifolius, Mentzelia albicaulis, Petrophyton caespitosum*

Cathartic: *Arenaria triflora, Rumex salicifolius*

Cold Remedy: *Artemisia tridentata, Juniperus californica, Lomatium graveolens, Mentha canadensis*

Cough Medicine: *Artemisia tridentata, Grindelia squarrosa, Juniperus californica, Mentha canadensis*

Dermatological Aid: *Achillea millefolium, Balsamorhiza sagittata, Cirsium eatonii, Collomia linearis, Geranium caespitosum, Heuchera rubescens, Linum lewisii, Lomatium dissectum, Mentzelia laevicaulis, Phlox gracilis, Potentilla*

glandulosa, Valeriana edulis, Wyethia amplexi-caulis
Disinfectant: *Lomatium dissectum*
Diuretic: *Lithospermum ruderale*
Emetic: *Silene douglasii, S. scouleri, Zigadenus nuttallii*
Eye Medicine: *Ambrosia psilostachya, Antennaria dioica, Cleome serrulata, Eriogonum ovalifolium*
Febrifuge: *Artemisia tridentata, Krascheninnikovia lanata*
Gastrointestinal Aid: *Achillea millefolium, Aquilegia coerulea, Arenaria congesta, A. triflora, Eriogonum ovalifolium, Heuchera rubescens, Lomatium graveolens, Mitella trifida, Petrophyton caespitosum, Prunus virginiana, Silene acaulis, S. douglasii, S. scouleri*
Heart Medicine: *Aquilegia coerulea*
Hemostat: *Balsamorhiza sagittata, Prunus virginiana*
Kidney Aid: *Lithospermum ruderale*
Narcotic: *Cornus sericea*
Orthopedic Aid: *Chaenactis douglasii, Lomatium dissectum, Wyethia amplexicaulis*
Panacea: *Aquilegia coerulea, Artemisia tridentata*
Pediatric Aid: *Arenaria triflora, Heuchera rubescens, Mitella trifida, Prunus virginiana, Silene acaulis*
Poison: *Aconitum fischeri, Brickellia grandiflora, Delphinium bicolor, Erigeron grandiflorus, Valeriana dioica*
Throat Aid: *Lomatium graveolens*
Unspecified: *Angelica pinnata, Brickellia grandiflora, Clematis ligusticifolia, Geum macrophyllum, Kalmia polifolia, Lomatium graveolens, Oenothera cespitosa, Potentilla glandulosa, Purshia mexicana*
Venereal Aid: *Chamaebatiaria millefolium, Eriogonum ovalifolium, Parnassia fimbriata, Spiranthes romanzoffiana, Zigadenus nuttallii*
Veterinary Aid: *Astragalus convallarius, Galium aparine, Lomatium dissectum, Lygodesmia grandiflora, Silene douglasii, S. scouleri*

Great Basin Indian
Analgesic: *Dugaldia hoopesii, Ipomopsis congesta*
Antidiarrheal: *Mahonia repens*
Antihemorrhagic: *Artemisia frigida*
Antirheumatic (External): *Pulsatilla patens*
Blood Medicine: *Ipomopsis aggregata, Mahonia repens*
Cold Remedy: *Lomatium dissectum*
Cough Medicine: *Lomatium dissectum*
Dermatological Aid: *Achillea millefolium, Clematis*

ligusticifolia, Lomatium dissectum, Thalictrum sparsiflorum
Eye Medicine: *Linum lewisii*
Gastrointestinal Aid: *Mentha canadensis*
Heart Medicine: *Chaenactis douglasii*
Laxative: *Achillea millefolium*
Misc. Disease Remedy: *Lomatium dissectum*
Other: *Ceanothus velutinus, Lomatium dissectum*
Pediatric Aid: *Chaenactis douglasii*
Respiratory Aid: *Dugaldia hoopesii, Lomatium dissectum*
Throat Aid: *Glycyrrhiza lepidota*
Tonic: *Lomatium dissectum*
Toothache Remedy: *Iris missouriensis*
Unspecified: *Lithospermum incisum, Lomatium dissectum*

Green River Group
Cathartic: *Cornus nuttallii*
Cold Remedy: *Abies grandis, Oplopanax horridus*
Cough Medicine: *Polypodium virginianum*
Dermatological Aid: *Oplopanax horridus, Stachys mexicana, Symphoricarpos albus*
Disinfectant: *Symphoricarpos albus*
Emetic: *Cornus nuttallii, Physocarpus capitatus*
Laxative: *Frangula purshiana*

Gros Ventre
Analgesic: *Mentha arvensis*
Antidiarrheal: *Prunus virginiana*
Ceremonial Medicine: *Helianthus annuus*
Febrifuge: *Artemisia ludoviciana*
Stimulant: *Helianthus annuus*

Haihais
Gastrointestinal Aid: *Taxus brevifolia*
Internal Medicine: *Taxus brevifolia*
Unspecified: *Aruncus dioicus*

Haisla
Analgesic: *Polypodium glycyrrhiza*
Antirheumatic (External): *Oplopanax horridus, Veratrum viride*
Cancer Treatment: *Oplopanax horridus*
Cold Remedy: *Oplopanax horridus, Veratrum viride*
Cough Medicine: *Oplopanax horridus*
Dermatological Aid: *Alnus rubra, Heracleum maximum, Oplopanax horridus, Ribes bracteosum, Thuja plicata*
Emetic: *Veratrum viride*
Gastrointestinal Aid: *Oplopanax horridus*
Hemostat: *Veratrum viride*

Laxative: *Populus tremuloides, Rumex aquaticus, Veratrum viride*

Misc. Disease Remedy: *Oplopanax horridus*

Reproductive Aid: *Ribes bracteosum*

Respiratory Aid: *Oplopanax horridus, Polypodium glycyrrhiza*

Sedative: *Veratrum viride*

Tonic: *Abies amabilis, Alnus rubra, Oplopanax horridus*

Tuberculosis Remedy: *Oplopanax horridus*

Unspecified: *Abies amabilis, Pseudotsuga menziesii*

Haisla & Hanaksiala

Abortifacient: *Sambucus racemosa*

Antirheumatic (External): *Nicotiana tabacum, Oplopanax horridus, Picea sitchensis, Pinus contorta, Urtica dioica*

Antirheumatic (Internal): *Malus fusca*

Burn Dressing: *Conocephalum conicum, Lysichiton americanus, Populus balsamifera*

Ceremonial Medicine: *Malus fusca, Veratrum viride*

Cold Remedy: *Ledum groenlandicum, Picea sitchensis, Polypodium glycyrrhiza*

Cough Medicine: *Picea sitchensis, Polypodium glycyrrhiza*

Dermatological Aid: *Clintonia uniflora, Oplopanax horridus, Picea sitchensis, Populus balsamifera*

Dietary Aid: *Ledum groenlandicum*

Emetic: *Oplopanax horridus*

Eye Medicine: *Clintonia uniflora, Oplopanax horridus*

Gastrointestinal Aid: *Oplopanax horridus, Sambucus racemosa*

Laxative: *Frangula purshiana, Oplopanax horridus*

Oral Aid: *Picea sitchensis, Populus tremuloides, Prunus virginiana*

Poison: *Bovista pila, B. plumbea, Bovistella sp., Calvatia sp., Cicuta douglasii, C. virosa, Lycoperdon sp., Oenanthe sarmentosa, Veratrum viride, Zigadenus venenosus*

Reproductive Aid: *Sambucus racemosa, Shepherdia canadensis*

Throat Aid: *Moneses uniflora, Polypodium glycyrrhiza*

Tuberculosis Remedy: *Fomitopsis officinalis, Ledum groenlandicum, Nuphar lutea, Picea sitchensis*

Unspecified: *Achillea millefolium, Nuphar lutea*

Urinary Aid: *Lysichiton americanus*

Hanaksiala

Analgesic: *Sambucus racemosa*

Antidiarrheal: *Thuja plicata*

Antirheumatic (External): *Rumex aquaticus, Sambucus racemosa, Veratrum viride*

Antirheumatic (Internal): *Veratrum viride*

Blood Medicine: *Veratrum viride*

Cold Remedy: *Oplopanax horridus*

Dermatological Aid: *Juniperus communis, Rumex aquaticus, Sambucus racemosa*

Gastrointestinal Aid: *Abies amabilis, Porphyra abbottae, Pseudotsuga menziesii*

Gynecological Aid: *Pseudotsuga menziesii*

Hemorrhoid Remedy: *Abies amabilis*

Hypotensive: *Veratrum viride*

Laxative: *Picea sitchensis*

Orthopedic Aid: *Porphyra abbottae*

Panacea: *Porphyra abbottae*

Respiratory Aid: *Veratrum viride*

Throat Aid: *Pseudotsuga menziesii*

Unspecified: *Ribes bracteosum, Veratrum viride*

Urinary Aid: *Taxus brevifolia*

Havasupai

Analgesic: *Aloysia wrightii, Eriogonum corymbosum, Mahonia repens, Porophyllum gracile*

Antirheumatic (External): *Mahonia repens, Phlox austromontana, P. longifolia, Porophyllum gracile*

Antirheumatic (Internal): *Aloysia wrightii, Porophyllum gracile*

Cold Remedy: *Artemisia tridentata, Frasera speciosa, Juniperus osteosperma, Mahonia repens, Phlox austromontana, P. longifolia, Purshia mexicana*

Cough Medicine: *Artemisia tridentata*

Dermatological Aid: *Artemisia tridentata, Atriplex canescens, Datura wrightii, Pinus edulis, P. monophylla, Porophyllum gracile*

Emetic: *Ephedra viridis, Thamnosma montana*

Gastrointestinal Aid: *Artemisia tridentata, Chaetopappa ericoides, Frasera speciosa, Mahonia repens, Phlox austromontana, P. longifolia, Porophyllum gracile, Ptelea trifoliata, Thamnosma montana*

Laxative: *Ephedra viridis, Erioneuron pulchellum, Mahonia repens, Purshia mexicana, Thamnosma montana*

Misc. Disease Remedy: *Atriplex canescens*

Narcotic: *Datura wrightii*

Nose Medicine: *Artemisia tridentata*

Pediatric Aid: *Chaetopappa ericoides, Mahonia repens, Phlox austromontana, P. longifolia, Ptelea trifoliata*

Poison: *Ptelea trifoliata, Shepherdia rotundifolia, Stanleya pinnata*

Psychological Aid: *Aloysia wrightii*
Throat Aid: *Artemisia tridentata, Pluchea sericea*
Unspecified: *Artemisia campestris, A. ludoviciana, Mahonia repens, Pseudotsuga menziesii*
Venereal Aid: *Frasera speciosa*
Veterinary Aid: *Pinus edulis, P. monophylla*

Hawaiian

Abortifacient: *Aleurites moluccana, Cocos nucifera*
Analgesic: *Alocasia macrorrhizos, Cibotium chamissoi, Eucalyptus* sp., *Freycinetia arborea, Ipomoea indica, Merremia dissecta, Metrosideros polymorpha, Pandanus tectorius, Piper methysticum, Ricinus communis, Zingiber zerumbet*
Antidiarrheal: *Psidium guajava*
Antiemetic: *Antidesma pulvinatum, Rubus hawaiensis, R. macraei*
Antihemorrhagic: *Digitaria setigera, Psidium guajava*
Antirheumatic (External): *Cibotium chamissoi, Conyza canadensis, Eucalyptus* sp., *Plumbago zeylanica*
Blood Medicine: *Asplenium horridum, Bobea* sp., *Caesalpinia bonduc, C. kavaiensis, Catharanthus roseus, Cibotium chamissoi, Curcuma longa, Ludwigia bonariensis, Murdannia nudiflora, Pelea* sp., *Polygonum densiflorum, Rumex giganteus*
Breast Treatment: *Carica papaya, Chamaesyce multiformis, Clermontia arborescens*
Burn Dressing: *Alocasia macrorrhizos*
Ceremonial Medicine: *Dodonaea viscosa, Pelea* sp.
Cold Remedy: *Cyperus laevigatus, Desmodium sandwicense, Piper methysticum*
Dermatological Aid: *Aleurites moluccana, Alyxia oliviformis, Antidesma pulvinatum, Artocarpus altilis, Asplenium nidus, A. pseudofalcatum, Bobea* sp., *Canavalia galeata, Carica papaya, Cenchrus calyculatus, Chenopodium oahuense, Clermontia arborescens, Cocos nucifera, Coprosma* sp., *Cucurbita maxima, Cyperus laevigatus, Diplazium meyenianum, Dodonaea viscosa, Eucalyptus* sp., *Ipomoea indica, Jacquemontia ovalifolia, Ludwigia bonariensis, Merremia dissecta, Morinda citrifolia, Nicotiana glauca, N. tabacum, Osteomeles anthyllidifolia, Pelea* sp., *Piper methysticum, Plumbago zeylanica, Psidium guajava, Rubus hawaiensis, R. macraei, Sadleria cyatheoides, Scaevola sericea, Senna occidentalis, Stenotaphrum secundatum, Styphelia tameiameiae, Syzygium malaccense, Tephrosia purpurea, Vigna luteola, Zingiber zerumbet*

Diaphoretic: *Acacia koa*
Dietary Aid: *Alocasia macrorrhizos, Chamaesyce multiformis, Chenopodium oahuense, Cibotium chamissoi, Phegopteris* sp., *Waltheria indica*
Emetic: *Syzygium malaccense*
Eye Medicine: *Digitaria setigera, Piper methysticum*
Febrifuge: *Artemisia australis, Cordyline fruticosa, Eucalyptus* sp., *Pleomele aurea, Ricinus communis*
Gastrointestinal Aid: *Abutilon incanum, Aleurites moluccana, Piper methysticum, Rubus hawaiensis, R. macraei, Syzygium malaccense*
Gynecological Aid: *Cassytha filiformis, Cucurbita maxima, Freycinetia arborea, Hibiscus tiliaceus, Peperomia* sp., *Phegopteris* sp., *Piper methysticum, Sida* sp., *Stenotaphrum secundatum*
Heart Medicine: *Rumex giganteus*
Herbal Steam: *Ochrosia compta*
Laxative: *Aleurites moluccana, Alocasia macrorrhizos, Caesalpinia bonduc, Chamaesyce multiformis, Colocasia esculenta, Cucurbita maxima, Digitaria setigera, Hibiscus tiliaceus, Ipomoea indica, I. tiliacea, Merremia dissecta, Mucuna gigantea, Odontoglossum chinensis, Opuntia tunicata, Osteomeles anthyllidifolia, Pandanus tectorius, Peperomia* sp., *Peucedanum sandwicense, Sida* sp., *Touchardia latifolia, Waltheria indica, Wikstroemia* sp.
Love Medicine: *Alocasia macrorrhizos*
Misc. Disease Remedy: *Dodonaea viscosa, Piper methysticum, Rumex giganteus*
Nose Medicine: *Cordyline fruticosa, Curcuma longa*
Oral Aid: *Artocarpus altilis, Asplenium horridum, A. nidus, A. pseudofalcatum, Curcuma longa, Piper methysticum, Stenotaphrum secundatum, Syzygium malaccense*
Orthopedic Aid: *Conyza canadensis, Eucalyptus* sp., *Ipomoea indica, Merremia dissecta, Morinda citrifolia, Psidium guajava, Zingiber zerumbet*
Other: *Cocos nucifera, Peperomia* sp.
Pediatric Aid: *Acacia koa, Aleurites moluccana, Asplenium nidus, Broussaisia arguta, Caesalpinia bonduc, Chamaesyce multiformis, Chenopodium oahuense, Cyrtandra* sp., *Digitaria setigera, Freycinetia arborea, Hibiscus tiliaceus, Ipomoea indica, Jacquemontia ovalifolia, Ludwigia bonariensis, Merremia dissecta, Ochrosia compta, Pandanus tectorius, Pelea* sp., *Peperomia* sp., *Peucedanum sandwicense, Piper methysticum, Pipturus* sp., *Psidium guajava, Ricinus communis, Sida* sp., *Stenotaphrum*

secundatum, *Syzygium malaccense, Touchardia latifolia, Vigna luteola, Waltheria indica*

Poison: *Tephrosia purpurea*

Psychological Aid: *Cucurbita maxima, Microlepia setosa*

Pulmonary Aid: *Artemisia australis, Caesalpinia bonduc, Cordyline fruticosa, Hibiscus tiliaceus, Hydrocotyle poltata, Peperomia* sp., *Piper methysticum, Pleomele aurea, Sadleria cyatheoides, Waltheria indica*

Reproductive Aid: *Artemisia australis, Broussaisia arguta, Chamaesyce multiformis, Cyrtandra* sp., *Ipomoea pes-caprae, Opuntia tunicata, Peucedanum sandwicense, Rumex giganteus*

Respiratory Aid: *Aleurites moluccana, Cassytha filiformis, Cheirodendron gaudicchaudii, Clermontia arborescens, Cordyline fruticosa, Desmodium sandwicense, Peperomia* sp., *Pleomele aurea, Sadleria cyatheoides, Sida* sp., *Vigna luteola, Waltheria indica, Wikstroemia* sp.

Sedative: *Cibotium chamissoi, Cordyline fruticosa, Piper methysticum*

Stimulant: *Asplenium horridum, Piper methysticum*

Strengthener: *Acacia koa, Aleurites moluccana, Asplenium nidus, Broussaisia arguta, Chamaesyce multiformis, Chenopodium oahuense, Cocos nucifera, Cyperus laevigatus, Cyrtandra* sp., *Desmodium sandwicense, Digitaria setigera, Freycinetia arborea, Hydrocotyle poltata, Ipomoea indica, Jacquemontia ovalifolia, Merremia dissecta, Musa ×paradisiaca, Ochrosia compta, Pandanus tectorius, Pelea* sp., *Peperomia* sp., *Piper methysticum, Pipturus* sp., *Portulaca oleracea, Rumex giganteus, Sida* sp., *Syzygium malaccense, Touchardia latifolia, Vigna luteola, Waltheria indica*

Throat Aid: *Hibiscus tiliaceus, Waltheria indica*

Toothache Remedy: *Zingiber zerumbet*

Tuberculosis Remedy: *Aleurites moluccana, Antidesma pulvinatum, Asplenium nidus, Cenchrus calyculatus, Chamaesyce multiformis, Coprosma* sp., *Desmodium sandwicense, Nicotiana glauca, N. tabacum, Pittosporum* sp., *Rumex giganteus, Styphelia tameiameiae*

Unspecified: *Chamaesyce multiformis, Cocos nucifera, Colocasia esculenta, Coprosma* sp., *Morinda citrifolia, Vitex trifolia*

Urinary Aid: *Piper methysticum*

Venereal Aid: *Cyperus laevigatus, Erythrina sandwicensis, Hydrocotyle poltata, Melicope cinerea*

Heiltzuk

Analgesic: *Salicornia virginica*

Antirheumatic (External): *Plagiomnium juniperinum, Salicornia virginica*

Dermatological Aid: *Sorbus sitchensis*

Hesquiat

Analgesic: *Achillea millefolium, Picea sitchensis, Ranunculus repens, Sambucus racemosa, Urtica dioica*

Anthelmintic: *Frangula purshiana*

Antidote: *Physocarpus capitatus*

Antirheumatic (External): *Physocarpus capitatus, Ranunculus repens, Sambucus racemosa, Urtica dioica*

Antirheumatic (Internal): *Physocarpus capitatus, Tsuga heterophylla*

Burn Dressing: *Lysichiton americanus*

Cancer Treatment: *Athyrium filix-femina, Blechnum spicant, Dryopteris campyloptera, Polystichum munitum, Pteridium aquilinum*

Carminative: *Polypodium glycyrrhiza*

Cough Medicine: *Achillea millefolium, Boschniakia hookeri, Polypodium glycyrrhiza*

Dermatological Aid: *Abies grandis, Blechnum spicant, Claytonia sibirica, Lysichiton americanus, Maianthemum dilatatum, Nicotiana tabacum, Picea sitchensis, Plantago major, Populus balsamifera, Ranunculus repens, Symphoricarpos albus, Tsuga heterophylla*

Emetic: *Physocarpus capitatus, Sambucus racemosa*

Eye Medicine: *Claytonia sibirica, Tsuga heterophylla*

Gastrointestinal Aid: *Achillea millefolium, Frangula purshiana, Geum macrophyllum, Rubus ursinus, Sambucus racemosa, Urtica dioica*

Gynecological Aid: *Geum macrophyllum, Ranunculus repens*

Internal Medicine: *Achillea millefolium*

Laxative: *Frangula purshiana, Physocarpus capitatus, Sambucus racemosa*

Misc. Disease Remedy: *Alnus rubra*

Oral Aid: *Menziesia ferruginea, Polypodium glycyrrhiza*

Other: *Ranunculus repens, Rubus ursinus, Tsuga heterophylla*

Poison: *Bromus carinatus, Kalmia polifolia, Sambucus racemosa*

Respiratory Aid: *Adiantum pedatum*

Strengthener: *Adiantum pedatum, Postelsia palmaeformis*

Throat Aid: *Polypodium glycyrrhiza*

Tuberculosis Remedy: *Alnus rubra, Maianthemum dilatatum, Tsuga heterophylla*

Unspecified: *Halosaccion glandiforme, Leathesia difformis, Lysichiton americanus, Nuphar lutea*

Hoh

Blood Medicine: *Mahonia nervosa, Prunus emarginata*
Ceremonial Medicine: *Equisetum hyemale, E. laevigatum*
Cold Remedy: *Sambucus racemosa*
Cough Medicine: *Pinus monticola, Sambucus racemosa*
Emetic: *Tsuga heterophylla, T. mertensiana*
Gynecological Aid: *Sambucus racemosa*
Pediatric Aid: *Nepeta cataria*
Tonic: *Cornus canadensis, C. nuttallii, C. sericea*
Unspecified: *Alnus rubra, Arctium minus, Arctostaphylos uva-ursi, Brassica nigra, Juncus ensifolius, Mentha canadensis, M. ×piperita, Moricandia arvensis, Oplopanax horridus, Populus balsamifera, Sinapis alba, Taraxacum officinale, Thuja plicata*
Venereal Aid: *Malus fusca*

Hopi

Adjuvant: *Psilostrophe sparsiflora*
Analgesic: *Conyza canadensis, Cryptantha cinerea, Cycloloma atriplicifolium, Epilobium ciliatum, Gaillardia pinnatifida, Heterotheca villosa, Ipomopsis longiflora, Petradoria pumila, Suaeda moquinii, Tetraneuris acaulis*
Anthelmintic: *Cirsium calcareum*
Anticonvulsive: *Atriplex confertifolia, A. obovata, Macromeria viridiflora, Salvia dorrii, Verbascum thapsus*
Antidiarrheal: *Opuntia whipplei, Sphaeralcea incana*
Antidote: *Physaria newberryi*
Antihemorrhagic: *Lithospermum incisum, Sphaeralcea grossulariifolia, S. parvifolia*
Antirheumatic (External): *Hymenoxys bigelovii, Juniperus monosperma, Poliomintha incana, Senecio flaccidus, S. spartioides, Tetraneuris acaulis*
Antirheumatic (Internal): *Cycloloma atriplicifolium*
Blood Medicine: *Lithospermum incisum*
Breast Treatment: *Petradoria pumila*
Burn Dressing: *Krascheninnikovia lanata*
Cancer Treatment: *Cryptantha flava*
Carminative: *Gutierrezia microcephala*
Cathartic: *Hymenoxys bigelovii*
Ceremonial Medicine: *Atriplex canescens, Calochortus aureus, Chrysothamnus parryi, Delphinium geraniifolium, D. scaposum, Equisetum*

laevigatum, Hymenopappus filifolius, Lesquerella intermedia, Lycium pallidum, Nicotiana attenuata, Oenothera albicaulis, Physaria newberryi, Poa fendleriana, Rhus trilobata, Sarcobatus vermiculatus, Suaeda moquinii, Yucca angustissima
Cold Remedy: *Rumex hymenosepalus*
Contraceptive: *Castilleja linariifolia*
Cough Medicine: *Machaeranthera grindelioides*
Dermatological Aid: *Artemisia filifolia, Chrysothamnus viscidiflorus, Cirsium calcareum, Cryptantha crassisepala, Dimorphocarpa wislizeni, Helianthus annuus, H. anomalus, H. petiolaris, Mirabilis coccineus, Pinus edulis, P. monophylla, Purshia stansburiana, Rhus trilobata, Rumex hymenosepalus, Senecio flaccidus, S. spartioides, Sphaeralcea parvifolia, Verbesina encelioides, Yucca angustissima*
Dietary Aid: *Chamaesyce fendleri*
Disinfectant: *Pinus edulis, P. monophylla, Yucca angustissima*
Diuretic: *Gaillardia pinnatifida, Sphaeralcea grossulariifolia, S. parvifolia, Stephanomeria exigua*
Ear Medicine: *Lupinus pusillus, Poliomintha incana*
Emetic: *Arenaria eastwoodiae, Croton texensis, Dalea candida, Delphinium scaposum, Hymenopappus filifolius, Lesquerella intermedia, Purshia stansburiana, Robinia neomexicana, Wyethia scabra*
Eye Medicine: *Croton texensis, Lupinus kingii, L. pusillus, Oenothera cespitosa*
Febrifuge: *Cycloloma atriplicifolium, Krascheninnikovia lanata, Verbesina encelioides*
Gastrointestinal Aid: *Artemisia filifolia, A. tridentata, Ipomopsis longiflora, Juniperus monosperma, Linum australe, Phoradendron juniperinum, Ribes cereum*
Gynecological Aid: *Asclepias subverticillata, A. verticillata, Castilleja linariifolia, Delphinium geraniifolium, D. scaposum, Hymenoxys bigelovii, Ipomopsis aggregata, Juniperus monosperma, J. osteosperma, Lesquerella intermedia, Linum australe, Lygodesmia grandiflora, Machaeranthera canescens, M. tanacetifolia, Mirabilis multiflora, Petradoria pumila, Reverchonia arenaria, Stephanomeria pauciflora, Tetradymia canescens, Tetraneuris acaulis*
Hallucinogen: *Datura wrightii, Mirabilis multiflora*
Laxative: *Cirsium calcareum, Juniperus monosperma, Yucca angustissima, Y. baileyi*
Narcotic: *Datura wrightii*
Nose Medicine: *Chaetopappa ericoides*

Oral Aid: *Chamaesyce fendleri, Mahonia fremontii*

Orthopedic Aid: *Artemisia tridentata, Krascheninnikovia lanata, Senecio flaccidus, Sphaeralcea grossulariifolia, S. parvifolia, Tetraneuris acaulis*

Other: *Datura wrightii, Helianthus petiolaris, Juniperus osteosperma, Salvia dorrii*

Panacea: *Chaetopappa ericoides*

Pediatric Aid: *Abronia elliptica, Chaetopappa ericoides, Chamaesyce fendleri, Juniperus monosperma, Sphaeralcea grossulariifolia, S. parvifolia, Tripterocalyx carnea*

Poison: *Datura wrightii, Oxytropis lambertii, Wyethia scabra*

Psychological Aid: *Datura wrightii, Macromeria viridiflora, Plantago patagonica, Verbascum thapsus*

Reproductive Aid: *Chaetopappa ericoides, Juniperus monosperma, Townsendia incana*

Sedative: *Abronia elliptica, Chaetopappa ericoides, Tripterocalyx carnea*

Snakebite Remedy: *Gaura parviflora, Lesquerella intermedia*

Stimulant: *Chaetopappa ericoides, Datura wrightii, Hymenoxys bigelovii, Machaeranthera canescens, M. tanacetifolia, Salvia dorrii, Tetraneuris acaulis*

Throat Aid: *Cirsium calcareum, Townsendia incana, T. strigosa*

Tonic: *Ephedra viridis, Tetradymia canescens*

Toothache Remedy: *Hymenopappus filifolius, Mentzelia albicaulis, M. pumila, Oenothera cespitosa, Parryella filifolia*

Tuberculosis Remedy: *Erysimum capitatum, E. inconspicuum, Pinus edulis, Rhus trilobata*

Unspecified: *Hymenoxys bigelovii, Lithospermum incisum, Marrubium vulgare, Phoradendron juniperinum, Rhus trilobata*

Venereal Aid: *Ephedra torreyana, E. viridis, Stephanomeria exigua*

Veterinary Aid: *Mirabilis multiflora, Phacelia crenulata*

Witchcraft Medicine: *Macromeria viridiflora, Phoradendron juniperinum, Pinus edulis, P. monophylla, Verbascum thapsus*

Houma

Abortifacient: *Rumex salicifolius, Sonchus oleraceus*

Analgesic: *Chenopodium ambrosioides, Desmodium paniculatum, Hypericum hypericoides, Lagenaria siceraria, Pleopeltis polypodioides, Polygonum punctatum, Sambucus canadensis, S. cerulea*

Anthelmintic: *Chenopodium ambrosioides, Myrica cerifera, Nyssa sylvatica, Solanum nigrum*

Antidiarrheal: *Quercus pagoda, Q. virginiana, Sonchus oleraceus, Ulmus americana*

Antiemetic: *Gonolobus* sp., *Panax quinquefolius*

Antirheumatic (External): *Quercus alba*

Antirheumatic (Internal): *Panax quinquefolius*

Blood Medicine: *Cocculus carolinus, Ipomoea sagittata, Magnolia virginiana, Passiflora incarnata, Salix caroliniana, S. nigra, Sequoia sempervirens*

Burn Dressing: *Plantago cordata*

Cold Remedy: *Gamochaeta purpurea, Magnolia virginiana*

Dermatological Aid: *Chamaesyce nutans, Cirsium horridulum, Ipomoea sagittata, Juglans nigra, Liquidambar styraciflua, Parthenocissus quinquefolia, Plantago cordata, Polymnia canadensis, Sambucus canadensis, S. cerulea, Solanum nigrum*

Diaphoretic: *Liquidambar styraciflua*

Expectorant: *Cirsium horridulum*

Eye Medicine: *Sabal minor*

Febrifuge: *Cornus florida, C. foemina, Eupatorium serotinum, Hypericum hypericoides, Laportea canadensis, Liquidambar styraciflua, Magnolia virginiana, Rumex salicifolius, Salix caroliniana, S. nigra, Tillandsia usneoides, Xanthium strumarium*

Gastrointestinal Aid: *Chamaesyce nutans, Rumex salicifolius*

Gynecological Aid: *Ambrosia artemisiifolia, Conyza canadensis, Erigeron philadelphicus, Hypericum hypericoides*

Heart Medicine: *Ipomoea sagittata, Sanicula canadensis*

Hypotensive: *Juglans nigra, Sabal minor*

Kidney Aid: *Arundinaria gigantea, Sabal minor, Verbena officinalis*

Liver Aid: *Rumex salicifolius, Sequoia sempervirens, Solidago nemoralis, Verbena officinalis*

Misc. Disease Remedy: *Bignonia capreolata, Cornus florida, C. foemina, Eupatorium serotinum, Gamochaeta purpurea, Modiola caroliniana, Parthenocissus quinquefolia, Sassafras albidum, Senna tora, Strophostyles helvula*

Oral Aid: *Pleopeltis polypodioides*

Orthopedic Aid: *Phoradendron leucarpum, Phyla nodiflora, Polygonum punctatum, Quercus pagoda, Zanthoxylum clava-herculis*

Panacea: *Forestiera acuminata, Phoradendron leucarpum*

Pediatric Aid: *Chamaesyce nutans, Chenopodium*

ambrosioides, Phyla nodiflora, Pleopeltis polypodioides, Solanum nigrum, Sonchus oleraceus
Pulmonary Aid: *Iresine diffusa, Typha latifolia*
Reproductive Aid: *Berchemia scandens*
Snakebite Remedy: *Ipomoea sagittata, Melothria pendula*
Stimulant: *Arundinaria gigantea, Desmodium paniculatum, Sabal minor*
Throat Aid: *Celtis laevigata, C. occidentalis, Cirsium horridulum, Modiola caroliniana, Quercus pagoda*
Tonic: *Quercus pagoda, Sambucus canadensis, S. cerulea, Toxicodendron radicans*
Toothache Remedy: *Hypericum hypericoides, Sonchus oleraceus, Zanthoxylum clava-herculis*
Tuberculosis Remedy: *Apium graveolens, Lepidium virginicum*
Urinary Aid: *Smilax bona-nox, S. laurifolia*
Venereal Aid: *Celtis laevigata, C. occidentalis*
Vertigo Medicine: *Pleopeltis polypodioides*

Hualapai

Antirheumatic (Internal): *Purshia mexicana*
Cold Remedy: *Larrea tridentata*
Dermatological Aid: *Acourtia wrightii, Agave* sp., *Eriodictyon angustifolium, Purshia mexicana*
Disinfectant: *Larrea tridentata*
Expectorant: *Pinus edulis*
Gastrointestinal Aid: *Eriodictyon angustifolium, Mahonia fremontii*
Laxative: *Eriodictyon angustifolium, Mahonia fremontii*
Liver Aid: *Mahonia fremontii*
Orthopedic Aid: *Eriodictyon angustifolium*
Other: *Pinus edulis*
Respiratory Aid: *Larrea tridentata*

Iroquois

Abortifacient: *Aralia racemosa, Ceanothus americanus, Celastrus scandens, Celtis occidentalis, Euonymus americana, Fagus grandifolia, Hypericum ellipticum, Malus coronaria, Taxus baccata, Triosteum perfoliatum, Vicia sativa, Zanthoxylum americanum*
Adjuvant: *Asarum canadense, Chimaphila umbellata, Lobelia cardinalis, Taxus baccata*
Alterative: *Rhus glabra*
Analgesic: *Achillea millefolium, Adiantum pedatum, Aesculus hippocastanum, Alnus incana, Angelica atropurpurea, Arisaema triphyllum, Asarum canadense, Cardamine concatenata, Chimaphila umbellata, Collinsonia canadensis, Cornus amomum, C. sericea, Cypripedium acaule, C. arietinum, C. pubescens, Dirca palus-*

tris, Epigaea repens, Epilobium angustifolium, Equisetum arvense, Eupatorium perfoliatum, Fraxinus nigra, Gentiana andrewsii, Hedeoma pulegioides, Hepatica nobilis, Heracleum maximum, Inula helenium, Ipomoea pandurata, Juglans cinerea, J. nigra, Lactuca canadensis, Larix laricina, Lobelia cardinalis, Lonicera oblongifolia, Mentha spicata, Mitchella repens, Nepeta cataria, Nuphar lutea, Osmunda cinnamomea, Panax trifolius, Platanthera psycodes, Polygonum hydropiper, Polystichum acrostichoides, Prunella vulgaris, Prunus serotina, Ranunculus acris, Rubus allegheniensis, R. idaeus, Salix interior, Sambucus canadensis, Sanguinaria canadensis, Sium suave, Smallanthus uvedalia, Solidago canadensis, Spiraea alba, Tanacetum vulgare, Taraxacum officinale, Triosteum perfoliatum, Veratrum viride, Viburnum acerifolium, Zanthoxylum americanum
Anthelmintic: *Achillea millefolium, Acorus calamus, Allium tricoccum, Anemone canadensis, Apocynum androsaemifolium, Aralia racemosa, Carya ovata, Chimaphila umbellata, Coptis trifolia, Elytrigia repens, Euonymus europaea, Gaultheria procumbens, Gentianella quinquefolia, Helianthus strumosus, Juglans cinerea, Magnolia acuminata, Maianthemum racemosum, Panax quinquefolius, Populus balsamifera, P. deltoides, P. tremuloides, Rudbeckia hirta, Sanguinaria canadensis, Sassafras albidum, Senna hebecarpa, S. marilandica, Symplocarpus foetidus, Verbena hastata, Viburnum lantanoides, Zanthoxylum americanum*
Anticonvulsive: *Achillea millefolium, Asarum canadense, Claytonia virginica, Conyza canadensis, Geum aleppicum, Lobelia cardinalis, Medeola virginiana, Mimulus ringens, Mitchella repens, Nuphar lutea, Osmunda regalis, Polystichum acrostichoides, Pyrola elliptica, Ranunculus abortivus, Sium suave, Verbascum thapsus*
Antidiarrheal: *Achillea millefolium, Agrimonia gryposepala, Ambrosia artemisiifolia, A. trifida, Anaphalis margaritacea, Anemone virginiana, Anthemis cotula, Apocynum cannabinum, Aralia racemosa, Argentina anserina, Arisaema triphyllum, Carpinus caroliniana, Ceanothus americanus, Chenopodium album, Collinsonia canadensis, Corylus americana, Epifagus virginiana, Eupatorium maculatum, Gentianella quinquefolia, Geranium maculatum, Geum aleppicum, G. rivale, Hamamelis virginiana, Hieracium pilosella, Hydrastis canadensis, Jeffersonia diphylla, Linaria vulgaris, Nepeta cataria, Polygonum aviculare, Polystichum*

acrostichoides, *Porteranthus trifoliatus, Potentilla canadensis, Prunella vulgaris, Prunus virginiana, Pteridium aquilinum, Quercus macrocarpa, Ranunculus acris, Rubus allegheniensis, R. occidentalis, R. odoratus, Rumex crispus, Sanguinaria canadensis, Ulmus americana, Verbascum thapsus, Veronicastrum virginicum*

Antidote: *Cardamine douglassii, Hydrophyllum canadense, Laportea canadensis, Maianthemum racemosum, Mentha arvensis, Mertensia virginica, Mimulus ringens, Nicotiana rustica, Parthenocissus quinquefolia, Portulaca oleracea, Quercus macrocarpa, Ranunculus abortivus, Rhamnus alnifolia, Ribes americanum, Sanicula marilandica*

Antiemetic: *Achillea millefolium, Agrimonia gryposepala, Anthemis cotula, Asarum canadense, Coptis trifolia, Corylus americana, Hamamelis virginiana, Mitchella repens, Nepeta cataria, Panax quinquefolius, Prunella vulgaris, Ribes americanum, Sanguinaria canadensis, Smallanthus uvedalia, Solidago juncea, Spiraea alba, Ulmus americana, Zanthoxylum americanum*

Antihemorrhagic: *Acer spicatum, Actaea rubra, Alnus incana, Corylus americana, Cynoglossum officinale, Prunus virginiana, Ranunculus acris, Sanguinaria canadensis, Scrophularia lanceolata, Tilia americana, Ulmus americana, Viburnum lentago*

Antirheumatic (External): *Abies balsamea, Actaea rubra, Adiantum pedatum, Angelica atropurpurea, Arctium minus, Asclepias syriaca, Asparagus officinalis, Carya ovata, Caulophyllum thalictroides, Cimicifuga racemosa, Collinsonia canadensis, Corylus cornuta, Eupatorium maculatum, Fraxinus nigra, Heracleum maximum, Inula helenium, Lathyrus japonicus, Lemna trisulca, Maianthemum racemosum, Osmunda cinnamomea, Phytolacca americana, Platanus occidentalis, Polygonum persicaria, Polystichum acrostichoides, Rumex crispus, Smilax herbacea, Stellaria media, Symplocarpus foetidus, Taxus baccata, Thuja occidentalis, Tsuga canadensis*

Antirheumatic (Internal): *Abies balsamea, Achillea millefolium, Adiantum pedatum, Aralia racemosa, Baptisia tinctoria, Carya ovata, Caulophyllum thalictroides, Chimaphila umbellata, Collinsonia canadensis, Epigaea repens, Equisetum arvense, Gaultheria procumbens, Hamamelis virginiana, Juniperus virginiana, Larix laricina, Maianthemum racemosum, Onoclea sensibilis, Pinus rigida, P. strobus, Populus balsamifera, Pteridium aquilinum, Pyrola ellip-*

tica, *Sagittaria latifolia, Sassafras albidum, Staphylea trifolia, Taxus baccata, Tsuga canadensis, Veronicastrum virginicum*

Basket Medicine: *Agrimonia gryposepala, Clintonia umbellulata, Corallorrhiza maculata, Desmodium glutinosum, Epilobium angustifolium, Lobelia cardinalis, Sarracenia purpurea*

Blood Medicine: *Acer rubrum, A. saccharum, Achillea millefolium, Acorus calamus, Ageratina altissima, Ambrosia trifida, Amelanchier arborea, A. canadensis, Angelica atropurpurea, Anthemis cotula, Apocynum cannabinum, Aralia nudicaulis, A. racemosa, Arctium minus, Arisaema triphyllum, Armoracia rusticana, Asarum canadense, Asparagus officinalis, Aster macrophyllus, Betula alleghaniensis, B. lenta, Ceanothus americanus, Celastrus scandens, Chimaphila umbellata, Cimicifuga racemosa, Collinsonia canadensis, Coptis trifolia, Cornus florida, Corylus americana, Cypripedium parviflorum, Dalibarda repens, Daucus carota, Diervilla lonicera, Dirca palustris, Fagus grandifolia, Fraxinus americana, Gaultheria procumbens, Gaylussacia baccata, Hamamelis virginiana, Hepatica nobilis, Huperzia lucidula, Ipomoea pandurata, Iris versicolor, Juglans cinerea, J. nigra, Larix laricina, Lobelia spicata, Lonicera canadensis, Lycopodium obscurum, Maianthemum racemosum, Mitchella repens, Myriophyllum sibiricum, Nuphar lutea, Onoclea sensibilis, Osmunda claytoniana, O. regalis, Oxalis stricta, Panax quinquefolius, Pinus strobus, Plantago major, Polystichum acrostichoides, Populus balsamifera, Prunella vulgaris, Prunus serotina, P. virginiana, Pteridium aquilinum, Pyrola elliptica, Ranunculus abortivus, R. acris, Rhamnus alnifolia, Rubus allegheniensis, R. idaeus, R. odoratus, Rumex crispus, R. obtusifolius, Sanguinaria canadensis, Sassafras albidum, Saxifraga pensylvanica, Scrophularia lanceolata, Senecio aureus, Senna marilandica, Taraxacum officinale, Thuja occidentalis, Toxicodendron rydbergii, Trifolium pratense, Tsuga canadensis, Ulmus rubra, Uvularia sessilifolia, Verbascum thapsus, Viburnum lantanoides, V. opulus, Vitis vulpina, Waldsteinia fragarioides*

Breast Treatment: *Cardamine diphylla*

Burn Dressing: *Chenopodium album, Fagus grandifolia, Physalis heterophylla, Pinus rigida, Portulaca oleracea, Prunus pensylvanica, P. serotina, Solidago squarrosa, Tilia americana*

Cancer Treatment: *Abies balsamea, Aralia nudicaulis, Chimaphila umbellata, Cirsium vulgare, Cynoglossum officinale, Ostrya virginiana*

purpurea, Asarum canadense, Heracleum maximum, Porteranthus trifoliatus, Senecio aureus, Taxus baccata, Triosteum perfoliatum, Tsuga canadensis

Dietary Aid: *Asarum canadense, Cardamine concatenata, Daucus carota, Euonymus europaea, Hamamelis virginiana, Panax quinquefolius, Pinus strobus, Rhus hirta, Rumex crispus, Sarracenia purpurea, Tiarella cordifolia, Triosteum perfoliatum*

Disinfectant: *Asarum canadense, Cicuta maculata, Smallanthus uvedalia*

Diuretic: *Adiantum pedatum, Argentina anserina, Asclepias incarnata, Celastrus scandens, Chimaphila umbellata, Cucurbita pepo, Daucus carota, Equisetum hyemale, Impatiens capensis, Inula helenium, Juniperus virginiana, Lithospermum officinale, Rubus odoratus, Tilia americana, Triosteum perfoliatum, Zanthoxylum americanum*

Ear Medicine: *Acorus calamus, Balsamita major, Coptis trifolia, Fraxinus americana, F. nigra, Hydrastis canadensis, Lobelia kalmii, Malus sylvestris, Panax quinquefolius, Sanguinaria canadensis, Verbascum thapsus, Verbena hastata*

Emetic: *Acer pensylvanicum, Achillea millefolium, Acorus calamus, Adiantum pedatum, Agrimonia gryposepala, Alnus incana, Anemone virginiana, Anthemis cotula, Apocynum cannabinum, Caltha palustris, Carex oligosperma, C. prasina, Caulophyllum thalictroides, Coptis trifolia, Cornus alternifolia, C. amomum, C. rugosa, C. sericea, Corylus cornuta, Dirca palustris, Elodea canadensis, Fraxinus americana, Galeopsis tetrahit, Geranium maculatum, Geum aleppicum, Hamamelis virginiana, Hydrastis canadensis, Ilex verticillata, Juglans cinerea, Juncus bufonius, J. tenuis, Laportea canadensis, Linaria vulgaris, Lobelia inflata, L. kalmii, L. spicata, Lonicera dioica, Lysimachia quadrifolia, Malva neglecta, Mentha canadensis, M. spicata, Mitella diphylla, Myriophyllum sibiricum, Onopordum acanthium, Pedicularis canadensis, Penstemon fruticosus, Physalis heterophylla, Phytolacca americana, Pinus strobus, Polystichum acrostichoides, Prunella vulgaris, Prunus serotina, Ranunculus abortivus, Rubus idaeus, R. occidentalis, Rumex crispus, Salix discolor, Sambucus canadensis, Sanguinaria canadensis, Sanicula marilandica, Silphium perfoliatum, Solidago canadensis, S. juncea, S. squarrosa, Taraxacum officinale, Tilia americana, Ulmus rubra, Veronica officinalis, Veronicastrum virginicum, Viburnum lentago, V. opulus, Zanthoxylum americanum*

Expectorant: *Phytolacca americana*

Eye Medicine: *Acer rubrum, A. saccharum, Anaphalis margaritacea, Apocynum cannabinum, Aralia nudicaulis, Arisaema triphyllum, Coptis trifolia, Cornus alternifolia, C. sericea, Dirca palustris, Equisetum hyemale, Gentiana andrewsii, Hydrastis canadensis, Impatiens capensis, Lactuca canadensis, Leucanthemum vulgare, Malus coronaria, M. sylvestris, Mitella diphylla, Panax quinquefolius, Polygonatum pubescens, Prenanthes trifoliolata, Pyrola elliptica, Ranunculus abortivus, Rosa acicularis, Sanguinaria canadensis, Sassafras albidum, Smilax tamnoides, Solanum tuberosum, Taraxacum officinale, Thalictrum dioicum, Tiarella cordifolia, Trifolium repens, Ulmus rubra, Uvularia perfoliata*

Febrifuge: *Achillea millefolium, Angelica atropurpurea, Anthemis cotula, Arisaema triphyllum, Asarum canadense, Aster lanceolatus, A. novae-angliae, A. prenanthoides, A. puniceus, Athyrium filix-femina, Betula lenta, Cardamine diphylla, Caulophyllum thalictroides, Celastrus scandens, Chimaphila umbellata, Clintonia umbellulata, Conyza canadensis, Cornus canadensis, Cypripedium parviflorum, Eupatorium maculatum, E. perfoliatum, Gentiana andrewsii, Geum aleppicum, G. rivale, Hydrastis canadensis, Hypericum perforatum, Impatiens capensis, I. pallida, Inula helenium, Larix laricina, Lindera benzoin, Linnaea borealis, Lobelia cardinalis, Lonicera dioica, Lythrum salicaria, Malva moschata, Melilotus officinalis, Mentha canadensis, M. ×piperita, M. spicata, Mitchella repens, Nepeta cataria, Nuphar lutea, Oxalis stricta, Panax quinquefolius, Polygonum hydropiper, Polystichum acrostichoides, Porteranthus trifoliatus, Prunella vulgaris, Prunus serotina, Rorippa sylvestris, Sambucus canadensis, Sanguinaria canadensis, Sarracenia purpurea, Sassafras albidum, Senecio aureus, Smallanthus uvedalia, Solidago juncea, Sparganium eurycarpum, Thuja occidentalis, Tsuga canadensis, Verbascum thapsus, Veronicastrum virginicum, Viburnum opulus*

Gastrointestinal Aid: *Acer spicatum, Achillea millefolium, Acorus calamus, Amphicarpaea bracteata, Anaphalis margaritacea, Anthemis cotula, Apocynum androsaemifolium, A. cannabinum, Aralia nudicaulis, Asclepias syriaca, Baptisia tinctoria, Bellis perennis, Cardamine concatenata, Carex prasina, Coptis trifolia, Cornus* amomum, C. racemosa, Corylus americana, Crataegus punctata, Cypripedium arietinum, Desmodium canadense, Epigaea repens, Eupatorium maculatum, E. perfoliatum, Euphorbia helioscopia, Fraxinus americana, Gentianella quinquefolia, Heracleum maximum, Hydrastis canadensis, Ilex verticillata, Inula helenium, Ipomoea pandurata, Leonurus cardiaca, Linnaea borealis, Lobelia cardinalis, Malva neglecta, Mentha spicata, Mitchella repens, Nepeta cataria, Nuphar lutea, Onoclea sensibilis, Oxalis stricta, Panax quinquefolius, Pedicularis canadensis, Physalis heterophylla, Picea glauca, P. mariana, Pinus strobus, Plantago major, Polygonum hydropiper, Populus tremuloides, Prunella vulgaris, Pyrola elliptica, Ranunculus abortivus, Rosa eglanteria, Rubus odoratus, Rumex crispus, Sambucus canadensis, Sanguinaria canadensis, Smilax herbacea, Solanum dulcamara, Solidago canadensis, S. flexicaulis, S. juncea, S. squarrosa, Sorbus americana, Triosteum perfoliatum, Ulmus americana, U. rubra, Verbena hastata, Veronicastrum virginicum, Viola pubescens, Vitis vulpina, Zanthoxylum americanum

Gland Medicine: *Chamaesyce glyptosperma*

Gynecological Aid: *Abies balsamea, Adiantum pedatum, Ageratina altissima, Alisma plantago-aquatica, Amelanchier arborea, A. canadensis, Angelica atropurpurea, Antennaria plantaginifolia, Apocynum androsaemifolium, Aralia racemosa, Arisaema triphyllum, Asclepias syriaca, Betula alleghaniensis, B. lenta, B. papyrifera, Campanula aparinoides, Carex brevior, Carpinus caroliniana, Celastrus scandens, Celtis occidentalis, Cerastium arvense, Chamaesyce glyptosperma, Chenopodium album, Chimaphila umbellata, Cimicifuga racemosa, Coeloglossum viride, Cornus alternifolia, Corylus americana, Crataegus punctata, Daucus carota, Diervilla lonicera, Dirca palustris, Echium vulgare, Epigaea repens, Euonymus americana, Eupatorium maculatum, Hamamelis virginiana, Hepatica nobilis, Impatiens pallida, Inula helenium, Iris versicolor, Juglans cinerea, Laportea canadensis, Lilium philadelphicum, Lobelia cardinalis, Lonicera dioica, L. oblongifolia, Lycopodium obscurum, Lysimachia thyrsiflora, Maianthemum racemosum, M. stellatum, Malus coronaria, Mitchella repens, Onoclea sensibilis, Osmunda cinnamomea, O. regalis, Panax quinquefolius, Penstemon fruticosus, Physocarpus opulifolius, Plantago major, Platanthera psycodes, Polygonum arenastrum,*

Polystichum acrostichoides, Prunella vulgaris, Prunus serotina, P. virginiana, Pteridium aquilinum, Quercus ilicifolia, Rhus hirta, Rosa acicularis, Rubus idaeus, R. odoratus, Rumex obtusifolius, Sanguinaria canadensis, Sassafras albidum, Scrophularia lanceolata, S. marilandica, Staphylea trifolia, Streptopus roseus, Symplocarpus foetidus, Thelypteris palustris, Thuja occidentalis, Tilia americana, Trifolium hybridum, T. pratense, Triosteum perfoliatum, Typha latifolia, Ulmus americana, U. rubra, Viburnum acerifolium, V. lantanoides, V. opulus, Vicia sativa, Zanthoxylum americanum

Hallucinogen: *Cardamine concatenata, Clematis virginiana*

Heart Medicine: *Ambrosia artemisiifolia, Cardamine concatenata, Clintonia borealis, Collinsonia canadensis, Festuca subverticillata, Geranium maculatum, Hamamelis virginiana, Hydrastis canadensis, Inula helenium, Nuphar lutea, Pedicularis canadensis, Polygonum persicaria, Rudbeckia hirta, Sambucus canadensis, Sanguinaria canadensis, Thalictrum dioicum, Veronicastrum virginicum, Viburnum opulus*

Hemorrhoid Remedy: *Betula populifolia, Cirsium discolor, C. vulgare, Corydalis sempervirens, Eupatorium perfoliatum, Lactuca tatarica, Mentha canadensis, Oenothera biennis, Prunella vulgaris, Rumex crispus, Salix discolor, Sanguinaria canadensis, Ulmus americana, Verbascum thapsus*

Hemostat: *Cirsium vulgare, Cornus sericea, Juglans cinerea, Lactuca canadensis, Mitchella repens, Rumex crispus, Sanguinaria canadensis, Sassafras albidum, Thalictrum pubescens, Typha latifolia*

Hunting Medicine: *Acer rubrum, Cardamine concatenata, Corallorrhiza maculata, Fraxinus americana, Heracleum maximum, Maianthemum racemosum, Panax trifolius, Polygonatum pubescens, Prenanthes trifoliolata, Thuja occidentalis, Tiarella cordifolia*

Hypotensive: *Rubus idaeus, Sassafras albidum*

Internal Medicine: *Dirca palustris, Epilobium angustifolium*

Kidney Aid: *Alisma plantago-aquatica, Aquilegia canadensis, Aralia racemosa, Asclepias incarnata, A. syriaca, Aster prenanthoides, Celastrus scandens, Chimaphila umbellata, Clematis virginiana, Collinsonia canadensis, Cornus rugosa, Cynoglossum officinale, Dirca palustris, Elymus canadensis, Epigaea repens, Epilobium angustifolium, Equisetum hyemale, Eupatorium maculatum, E. perfoliatum, Gaultheria pro-*

cumbens, Hamamelis virginiana, Impatiens capensis, Juniperus communis, Lactuca canadensis, Maianthemum canadense, Mitchella repens, Osmunda regalis, Ribes americanum, Rubus idaeus, R. odoratus, Rumex crispus, Sambucus canadensis, Sanguinaria canadensis, Sanicula marilandica, Saxifraga pensylvanica, Scrophularia lanceolata, Senecio aureus, Smallanthus uvedalia, Solidago nemoralis, Taraxacum officinale, Ulmus rubra, Viburnum opulus, Vitis vulpina, Zanthoxylum americanum

Laxative: Acer pensylvanicum, Apocynum cannabinum, Aster macrophyllus, Chimaphila umbellata, Cornus amomum, Dirca palustris, Eupatorium perfoliatum, Fraxinus americana, F. nigra, Geranium maculatum, Juglans cinerea, J. nigra, Lycopus asper, Nepeta cataria, Pinus rigida, Podophyllum peltatum, Populus balsamifera, Ranunculus recurvatus, Rubus odoratus, Sagittaria latifolia, Sambucus canadensis, Sanguinaria canadensis, Sanicula marilandica, Senna hebecarpa, Sisyrinchium angustifolium, Taraxacum officinale, Triosteum perfoliatum, Verbascum thapsus, Viburnum opulus

Liver Aid: Adiantum pedatum, Apocynum androsaemifolium, Aralia racemosa, Baptisia tinctoria, Caulophyllum thalictroides, Chelone glabra, Eupatorium maculatum, Fagus grandifolia, Gaylussacia baccata, Gentiana andrewsii, Hydrastis canadensis, Impatiens capensis, Ipomoea pandurata, Jeffersonia diphylla, Juglans cinerea, Panax quinquefolius, Phytolacca americana, Pinus strobus, Prunus serotina, Pteridium aquilinum, Rubus idaeus, R. occidentalis, Sambucus canadensis, Sanguinaria canadensis, Sarracenia purpurea, Sedum telephium, Solidago canadensis, S. juncea, S. rugosa, Tanacetum vulgare, Thalictrum pubescens, Viburnum opulus

Love Medicine: Anemone virginiana, Aster novaeangliae, Caltha palustris, Cardamine concatenata, C. diphylla, Corallorrhiza maculata, Dirca palustris, Eupatorium maculatum, Galium triflorum, Geranium maculatum, Geum aleppicum, G. canadense, Lilium philadelphicum, Linaria vulgaris, Lobelia cardinalis, L. inflata, L. kalmii, L. spicata, Lonicera dioica, Malva neglecta, Mitchella repens, Penstemon fruticosus, Phytolacca americana, Polygonum arenastrum, Populus alba, Prenanthes trifoliolata, Rumex crispus, Sarracenia purpurea, Solidago canadensis, Taraxacum officinale, Viburnum lantanoides, Vicia americana, V. sativa

Misc. Disease Remedy: Achillea millefolium,

Acorus calamus, Angelica atropurpurea, Aralia nudicaulis, Armoracia rusticana, Asarum canadense, Aster puniceus, Ceanothus americanus, Cinna arundinacea, Clintonia borealis, Dirca palustris, Eupatorium perfoliatum, Hamamelis virginiana, Heracleum maximum, Inula helenium, Ipomoea pandurata, Lindera benzoin, Mentha spicata, Mitchella repens, Nuphar lutea, Panax quinquefolius, Pinus strobus, Polypodium virginianum, Populus tremuloides, Porteranthus trifoliatus, Prunella vulgaris, Prunus virginiana, Quercus bicolor, Ranunculus abortivus, Rumex crispus, Sambucus canadensis, Scutellaria lateriflora, Sisyrinchium montanum, Tsuga canadensis, Typha latifolia, Verbascum thapsus

Nose Medicine: Arisaema triphyllum

Oral Aid: Ceanothus americanus, Cirsium arvense, Coptis trifolia, Cornus sericea, Geranium maculatum, Hydrophyllum virginianum, Juglans cinerea, Nepeta cataria, Oxalis stricta, Populus ×jackii, Salix sericea, Syringa vulgaris, Tiarella cordifolia, Toxicodendron pubescens

Orthopedic Aid: Abies balsamea, Acer pensylvanicum, Adiantum pedatum, Alisma plantago-aquatica, Ambrosia artemisiifolia, Angelica atropurpurea, A. venenosa, Aralia racemosa, Arisaema triphyllum, Asclepias incarnata, Baptisia tinctoria, Betula lenta, Cicuta maculata, Cimicifuga racemosa, Cornus racemosa, Cypripedium parviflorum, Dirca palustris, Epilobium angustifolium, Equisetum arvense, Eupatorium perfoliatum, Galium triflorum, Gentiana andrewsii, Gnaphalium uliginosum, Hamamelis virginiana, Hepatica nobilis, Iris versicolor, Lactuca canadensis, Malus sylvestris, Malva neglecta, Mitchella repens, Oenothera perennis, Osmunda cinnamomea, Parthenocissus quinquefolia, Pedicularis canadensis, Phytolacca americana, Pinus strobus, Polygala paucifolia, Polygonum arenastrum, P. aviculare, Polystichum acrostichoides, Prunella vulgaris, Pyrola elliptica, Quercus bicolor, Ranunculus abortivus, Rhamnus alnifolia, Ribes americanum, Rumex crispus, Sassafras albidum, Senecio aureus, Silphium perfoliatum, Sium suave, Smallanthus uvedalia, Tanacetum vulgare, Taraxacum officinale, Taxus baccata, Thuja occidentalis, Tiarella cordifolia, Tilia americana, Tsuga canadensis, Typha latifolia, Ulmus americana, Uvularia perfoliata, U. sessilifolia, Verbascum thapsus, Viburnum dentatum, Zanthoxylum americanum

Other: Agrimonia gryposepala, Alisma plantago-aquatica, *Angelica atropurpurea, Anthemis cotula, Asclepias incarnata, A. syriaca, A. tuberosa, Cardamine diphylla, Carex platyphylla, C. vulpinoidea, Carpinus caroliniana, Ceanothus americanus, Celastrus scandens, Circaea lutetiana, Elymus canadensis, Equisetum hyemale, Euonymus obovata, Eupatorium perfoliatum, E. purpureum, Festuca subverticillata, Fraxinus nigra, Hepatica nobilis, Ilex verticillata, Ipomoea pandurata, Lobelia cardinalis, L. inflata, Maianthemum racemosum, Mentha ×piperita, M. spicata, Myriophyllum verticillatum, Nepeta cataria, Nuphar lutea, Oxalis stricta, Parthenocissus quinquefolia, Phragmites australis, Pinus strobus, Polygala verticillata, Quercus ilicifolia, Ribes americanum, R. rotundifolium, Rubus alleghheniensis, Sanguinaria canadensis, Sedum telephium, Sisyrinchium angustifolium, Solanum nigrum, Solidago canadensis, S. rugosa, Thalictrum dioicum, Tiarella cordifolia, Tilia americana, Ulmus americana, Verbena hastata, Vitis vulpina*

Panacea: *Achillea millefolium, Ageratina altissima, Cardamine concatenata, Collinsonia canadensis, Cornus sericea, Epilobium angustifolium, Geum canadense, Hamamelis virginiana, Inula helenium, Lindera benzoin, Lobelia cardinalis, Medeola virginiana, Osmunda cinnamomea, Panax quinquefolius, Pinus strobus, Platanthera psycodes, Prunella vulgaris, Rumex crispus, Sanguinaria canadensis, Saxifraga pensylvanica, Tanacetum vulgare, Tilia americana, Veronicastrum virginicum*

Pediatric Aid: *Achillea millefolium, Acorus calamus, Adiantum pedatum, Agrimonia gryposepala, Allium tricoccum, Anthemis cotula, Apocynum cannabinum, Argentina anserina, Arisaema triphyllum, Asarum canadense, Asclepias incarnata, Aster prenanthoides, Carpinus caroliniana, Castanea dentata, Ceanothus americanus, Celastrus scandens, Chimaphila umbellata, Cimicifuga racemosa, Claytonia virginica, Collinsonia canadensis, Conyza canadensis, Coptis trifolia, Cornus alternifolia, C. amomum, Corylus americana, C. cornuta, Cucurbita pepo, Diervilla lonicera, Equisetum arvense, Euonymus europaea, Euphorbia helioscopia, Fagopyrum esculentum, Galium triflorum, Geranium maculatum, Helianthus strumosus, Hepatica nobilis, Inula helenium, Jeffersonia diphylla, Linaria vulgaris, Linnaea borealis, Lithospermum officinale, Lonicera canadensis, L. dioica, Lycopus asper, Malva neglecta, Medeola virginiana, Mentha canaden-*

sis, *M. spicata, Mitchella repens, Myriophyllum sibiricum, M. verticillatum, Nepeta cataria, Nuphar lutea, Onoclea sensibilis, Osmunda regalis, Panax quinquefolius, Pinus strobus, Platanthera psycodes, Polygala paucifolia, P. verticillata, Polygonum aviculare, P. hydropiper, Polystichum acrostichoides, Populus tremuloides, Prunella vulgaris, Prunus serotina, P. virginiana, Pyrola elliptica, Rhamnus alnifolia, Rorippa sylvestris, Rubus alleghheniensis, R. occidentalis, R. odoratus, Rudbeckia hirta, Rumex obtusifolius, Sagittaria latifolia, Sambucus canadensis, Sanguinaria canadensis, Sanicula marilandica, Sedum telephium, Senecio aureus, Silphium perfoliatum, Solidago canadensis, Sonchus asper, Staphylea trifolia, Symplocarpus foetidus, Syringa vulgaris, Tiarella cordifolia, Tilia americana, Toxicodendron pubescens, Triosteum perfoliatum, Uvularia perfoliata, Verbascum thapsus, Viburnum opulus, Vitis vulpina*

Poison: *Angelica atropurpurea, A. venenosa, Cardamine rhomboidea, Celastrus scandens, Cicuta maculata, Datura stramonium, Dipsacus fullonum, Eupatorium perfoliatum, Lycopus asper, L. virginicus, Onopordum acanthium, Parthenocissus quinquefolia, Podophyllum peltatum, Sisyrinchium montanum, Veronicastrum virginicum*

Poultice: *Cornus amomum, Verbena hastata*

Psychological Aid: *Actaea rubra, Asarum canadense, Cannabis sativa, Cardamine diphylla, Cornus sericea, Corylus cornuta, Eupatorium perfoliatum, Gentiana andrewsii, Ilex verticillata, Juglans cinerea, J. nigra, Laportea canadensis, Lobelia cardinalis, L. inflata, Lonicera canadensis, L. oblongifolia, Mitchella repens, Nicotiana rustica, Pinus strobus, Polygonum punctatum, Prunella vulgaris, Quercus alba, Ranunculus abortivus, Salix discolor, Smilax herbacea*

Pulmonary Aid: *Acer saccharum, Aesculus hippocastanum, Angelica atropurpurea, Anthemis cotula, Aralia racemosa, Asarum canadense, Aster puniceus, Campanulastrum americanum, Cardamine diphylla, Cornus amomum, C. sericea, Cypripedium pubescens, Erigeron philadelphicus, Eupatorium perfoliatum, Gentianella quinquefolia, Hamamelis virginiana, Hepatica nobilis, Hydrastis canadensis, Inula helenium, Nuphar lutea, Panax trifolius, Pinus strobus, Prunella vulgaris, Prunus serotina, Rubus occidentalis, Rumex obtusifolius, Sanguinaria canadensis, Sarracenia purpurea, Taraxacum officinale, Triosteum perfoliatum, Veronicas-trum virginicum, Viburnum lantanoides, V. opulus*

Reproductive Aid: *Athyrium filix-femina, Fraxinus americana, F. nigra, Hypericum perforatum, Lycopodium complanatum, Rhus hirta, Rumex crispus*

Respiratory Aid: *Acorus calamus, Anaphalis margaritacea, Arisaema triphyllum, Asarum canadense, Cornus alternifolia, Corylus americana, Gnaphalium uliginosum, Hamamelis virginiana, Ilex verticillata, Inula helenium, Iris versicolor, Mentha spicata, Panax quinquefolius, Pilea pumila, Plantago major, Prunella vulgaris, Prunus serotina, Quercus bicolor, Rubus allegheniensis, Sanguinaria canadensis, Taxus baccata, Trifolium repens, Ulmus rubra, Veratrum viride, Verbascum thapsus*

Sedative: *Anthemis cotula, Cornus amomum, Cypripedium parviflorum, Leonurus cardiaca, Linaria vulgaris, Linnaea borealis, Lonicera canadensis, L. oblongifolia, Nepeta cataria, Prunella vulgaris, Rhamnus alnifolia, Smallanthus uvedalia, Solidago canadensis, Sonchus asper, Staphylea trifolia, Toxicodendron pubescens*

Snakebite Remedy: *Adiantum pedatum, Calla palustris, Fraxinus americana, Maianthemum racemosum, Prenanthes alba, P. altissima, P. trifoliolata, Ranunculus abortivus, Scirpus tabernaemontani, Waldsteinia fragarioides*

Sports Medicine: *Asclepias tuberosa, Cornus sericea, Dicentra cucullaria, Juncus tenuis, Panax trifolius, Sarracenia purpurea*

Stimulant: *Achillea millefolium, Arisaema triphyllum, Asarum canadense, Betula lenta, Cannabis sativa, Chimaphila umbellata, Collinsonia canadensis, Cypripedium parviflorum, Hydrastis canadensis, Larix laricina, Malva moschata, Myriophyllum verticillatum, Oenothera biennis, Panax quinquefolius, Polystichum acrostichoides, Prenanthes alba, Prunus serotina, Rubus idaeus, Thuja occidentalis, Tilia americana, Tsuga canadensis, Ulmus rubra*

Strengthener: *Aralia racemosa, Asclepias incarnata, Collinsonia canadensis, Dirca palustris, Juncus bufonius, Oenothera biennis, Podophyllum peltatum, Rumex crispus, Viburnum opulus*

Throat Aid: *Acorus calamus, Aralia nudicaulis, Asarum canadense, Coptis trifolia, Geranium maculatum, Nepeta cataria, Pinus strobus, Polystichum acrostichoides, Porteranthus trifoliatus, Prunus serotina, Salix nigra, Sanguinaria canadensis, Scutellaria lateriflora, Thlaspi arvense, Triosteum perfoliatum, Ulmus rubra*

Tonic: *Allium tricoccum, Aralia racemosa, Asarum canadense, Caulophyllum thalictroides, Chimaphila umbellata, Dirca palustris, Juniperus communis, Leonurus cardiaca, Panax quinquefolius, Populus alba, Rhamnus alnifolia, Rubus idaeus, Rumex crispus, R. obtusifolius, Sassafras albidum, Tiarella cordifolia*

Toothache Remedy: *Acorus calamus, Antennaria plantaginifolia, Anthemis cotula, Asclepias incarnata, Celastrus scandens, Corylus americana, C. cornuta, Equisetum arvense, Hamamelis virginiana, Juglans cinerea, Magnolia acuminata, Polymnia canadensis, Ranunculus abortivus, R. bulbosus, R. hispidus, R. recurvatus, Taraxacum officinale, Verbascum thapsus, Zanthoxylum americanum*

Tuberculosis Remedy: *Abies balsamea, Alisma plantago-aquatica, Amphicarpaea bracteata, Anemone virginiana, Aralia nudicaulis, A. racemosa, Arisaema triphyllum, Asarum canadense, Aster puniceus, Botrychium virginianum, Cardamine diphylla, Carpinus caroliniana, Corallorrhiza maculata, Cornus alternifolia, C. canadensis, C. rugosa, C. sericea, Cynoglossum officinale, Cypripedium parviflorum, C. pubescens, Dirca palustris, Epilobium angustifolium, Erigeron pulchellus, Eupatorium maculatum, Fagus grandifolia, Hamamelis virginiana, Hydrastis canadensis, Inula helenium, Ipomoea pandurata, Juglans cinerea, Laportea canadensis, Lobelia cardinalis, Lonicera dioica, Malus coronaria, Nicotiana rustica, Onoclea sensibilis, Ostrya virginiana, Panax quinquefolius, Pedicularis canadensis, Pinus strobus, Platanthera orbiculata, Polystichum acrostichoides, Prunella vulgaris, Prunus serotina, P. virginiana, Pteridium aquilinum, Quercus alba, Q. bicolor, Rubus allegheniensis, Salix discolor, Sanguinaria canadensis, Scirpus tabernaemontani, Symplocarpus foetidus, Taxus baccata, Tilia americana, Tsuga canadensis, Tussilago farfara, Ulmus rubra, Veratrum viride, Verbascum thapsus, Viburnum lentago, Zanthoxylum americanum*

Unspecified: *Acer saccharinum, A. saccharum, Asclepias syriaca, Betula lenta, Coptis trifolia, Fragaria virginiana, Rubus canadensis, Sambucus canadensis*

Urinary Aid: *Abies balsamea, Actaea pachypoda, Alnus incana, Aralia racemosa, Asarum canadense, Asclepias incarnata, Ceanothus americanus, Celastrus scandens, Chimaphila umbellata, Citrullus lanatus, Clematis virginiana, Cornus amomum, Diervilla lonicera, Dirca*

Isleta

Febrifuge: *Gutierrezia sarothrae, Thymophylla acerosa*

Gastrointestinal Aid: *Artemisia frigida, Hymenopappus newberryi, Lactuca sativa, Plantago major, Rumex crispus*

Gynecological Aid: *Juniperus monosperma*

Laxative: *Croton texensis, Solanum elaeagnifolium*

Orthopedic Aid: *Populus tremuloides, Pseudotsuga menziesii*

Pediatric Aid: *Hymenopappus newberryi, Rosa woodsii*

Poison: *Atriplex canescens, Chrysothamnus nauseosus, Hackelia floribunda, Heterotheca villosa*

Psychological Aid: *Hymenoxys richardsonii*

Pulmonary Aid: *Anemopsis californica, Cucurbita foetidissima, Frasera speciosa, Nolina microcarpa*

Reproductive Aid: *Quercus gambelii*

Respiratory Aid: *Asclepias latifolia*

Throat Aid: *Allium cernuum, Frasera speciosa*

Venereal Aid: *Gutierrezia sarothrae*

Jemez

Analgesic: *Croton texensis*

Antirheumatic (Internal): *Croton texensis*

Cathartic: *Dalea formosa*

Dermatological Aid: *Atriplex canescens, Gutierrezia sarothrae, Helianthus annuus*

Gastrointestinal Aid: *Juniperus monosperma*

Gynecological Aid: *Erodium cicutarium, Gutierrezia sarothrae, Juniperus monosperma*

Misc. Disease Remedy: *Croton texensis*

Oral Aid: *Rhus trilobata*

Stimulant: *Atriplex canescens, Senecio flaccidus*

Veterinary Aid: *Macranthera* sp.

Karok

Analgesic: *Artemisia vulgaris, Osmorhiza berteroi, Pentagrama triangularis, Umbellularia californica*

Antidiarrheal: *Arctostaphylos nevadensis*

Antidote: *Arctostaphylos nevadensis*

Antirheumatic (External): *Aralia californica, Artemisia douglasiana*

Blood Medicine: *Taxus brevifolia*

Cathartic: *Frangula purshiana*

Ceremonial Medicine: *Arbutus menziesii, Equisetum hyemale, Pyrola asarifolia, Rhododendron macrophyllum, Salix sitchensis, Sambucus cerulea*

Cold Remedy: *Artemisia vulgaris, Eriodictyon californicum, Prunus virginiana, Pseudotsuga menziesii, Umbellularia californica*

Contraceptive: *Toxicodendron diversilobum*

Dermatological Aid: *Achillea millefolium, Ceanothus velutinus, Maianthemum racemosum, Marah oreganus, Trillium ovatum, Umbellularia californica*

Diaphoretic: *Monardella odoratissima*

Dietary Aid: *Ligusticum apiifolium, Lomatium californicum, Oxalis oregana, Rubus parviflorus*

Disinfectant: *Pseudotsuga menziesii, Umbellularia californica*

Eye Medicine: *Equisetum hyemale, Gnaphalium microcephalum*

Gastrointestinal Aid: *Eriogonum nudum, Lupinus albifrons, Taxus brevifolia*

Gynecological Aid: *Anthemis cotula, Artemisia vulgaris, Ceanothus integerrimus, Chimaphila menziesii, Darmera peltata, Hierochloe occidentalis, Lotus humistratus, Pentagrama triangularis, Quercus garryana, Umbellularia californica*

Herbal Steam: *Cornus nuttallii, Pseudotsuga menziesii, Rumex conglomeratus*

Kidney Aid: *Chimaphila menziesii, Satureja douglasii*

Love Medicine: *Acer circinatum, Calystegia occidentalis, Galium triflorum, Monardella odoratissima, Populus balsamifera, Satureja douglasii*

Misc. Disease Remedy: *Mahonia aquifolium*

Orthopedic Aid: *Chimaphila umbellata*

Other: *Elymus glaucus, Mahonia aquifolium*

Panacea: *Artemisia vulgaris, Mahonia aquifolium, Osmorhiza berteroi, Petasites frigidus, Pyrola picta, Sambucus cerulea, Umbellularia californica*

Pediatric Aid: *Maianthemum racemosum, Mimulus cardinalis, Mirabilis greenei, Petasites frigidus, Prunus virginiana, Pyrola asarifolia, P. picta, Sambucus cerulea, Silene campanulata*

Poison: *Heracleum maximum, Mahonia aquifolium, Marah oreganus, Solanum nigrum, Toxicodendron diversilobum*

Preventive Medicine: *Fraxinus latifolia, Osmorhiza berteroi*

Psychological Aid: *Osmorhiza berteroi, Penstemon laetus*

Pulmonary Aid: *Eriodictyon californicum*

Sedative: *Pyrola asarifolia*

Tonic: *Abies grandis, Mahonia pumila, Rubus parviflorus*

Tuberculosis Remedy: *Eriodictyon californicum*

Unspecified: *Juncus effusus, Nicotiana quadrivalvis, Silene campanulata*

Urinary Aid: *Chimaphila menziesii*

Veterinary Aid: *Hierochloe occidentalis*

Kawaiisu

Abortifacient: *Artemisia douglasiana, Phoradendron villosum*

Analgesic: *Acamptopappus sphaerocephalus, Arenaria macradenia, Artemisia tridentata, Aster subulatus, Astragalus pachypus, A. purshii, Chaenactis santolinoides, Cicuta douglasii, Croton setigerus, Cupressus nevadensis, Datura wrightii, Dicentra chrysantha, Encelia virginensis, Erigeron foliosus, Gnaphalium stramineum, Grindelia camporum, Larrea tridentata, Lessingia glandulifera, Lomatium dissectum, Mentha arvensis, Mimulus guttatus, Nicotiana quadrivalvis, Purshia glandulosa, Rhamnus crocea, Rumex salicifolius, Salvia dorrii, Sambucus cerulea, Tauschia parishii, Thamnosma montana, Urtica dioica*

Antidiarrheal: *Salix bonplandiana*

Antidote: *Frangula californica*

Antirheumatic (External): *Arenaria macradenia, Artemisia dracunculus, Datura wrightii, Encelia virginensis, Ericameria linearifolia, Phoradendron villosum, Turricula parryi*

Antirheumatic (Internal): *Quercus wislizeni, Rhamnus crocea*

Blood Medicine: *Ephedra viridis, Rhamnus crocea, Sambucus cerulea*

Burn Dressing: *Argemone munita, Frangula californica, Mentzelia albicaulis, Quercus douglasii, Q. lobata, Q. wislizeni*

Carminative: *Pinus lambertiana*

Cathartic: *Fremontodendron californicum*

Ceremonial Medicine: *Datura wrightii*

Cold Remedy: *Anemopsis californica, Artemisia tridentata, Balsamorhiza deltoidea, Corethrogyne filaginifolia, Cupressus nevadensis, Eriodictyon californicum, Eriogonum nudum, Garrya flavescens, Lomatium californicum, Marrubium vulgare, Osmorhiza brachypoda, Phacelia californica, Rhamnus crocea, Sambucus cerulea, Tauschia parishii, Thamnosma montana, Trichostema lanceolatum*

Contraceptive: *Pinus monophylla*

Cough Medicine: *Anemopsis californica, Artemisia tridentata, Balsamorhiza deltoidea, Cercocarpus montanus, Cupressus nevadensis, Eriogonum nudum, Marrubium vulgare, Osmorhiza brachypoda, Phacelia californica, Rhamnus crocea*

Dermatological Aid: *Anemopsis californica, Arenaria macradenia, Artemisia douglasiana, Asclepias californica, Castilleja stenantha, Chenopodium californicum, Datura wrightii, Distichlis spicata, Eriastrum densifolium, Ericameria linearifolia, Eriogonum umbellatum, Eschscholzia parishii, Frangula californica, Lomatium dissectum, L. utriculatum, Lythrum californicum, Marah horridus, Mentha arvensis, Nicotiana quadrivalvis, Osmorhiza brachypoda, Pinus monophylla, Quercus douglasii, Q. lobata, Ranunculus cymbalaria, Rhamnus crocea, Rumex salicifolius, Solanum xantii, Solidago californica, S. confinis, Tauschia parishii, Tetradymia stenolepis, Thamnosma montana, Turricula parryi, Urtica dioica*

Diaphoretic: *Corethrogyne filaginifolia, Sambucus cerulea, Thamnosma montana*

Disinfectant: *Frangula californica, Larrea tridentata*

Diuretic: *Rhamnus crocea*

Ear Medicine: *Cercocarpus ledifolius, Marah horridus, Nicotiana quadrivalvis, Plantago lanceolata, P. major*

Emetic: *Chenopodium californicum, Lomatium californicum, Nicotiana quadrivalvis, Phacelia ramosissima, Purshia glandulosa*

Eye Medicine: *Pinus lambertiana, Quercus douglasii, Q. lobata, Salvia columbariae, Stephanomeria virgata, Tauschia parishii*

Febrifuge: *Sambucus cerulea*

Gastrointestinal Aid: *Eriodictyon californicum, Garrya flavescens, Lomatium californicum, Nicotiana quadrivalvis, Phacelia californica, P. ramosissima, Rhamnus crocea, Rumex salicifolius, Salvia dorrii, Trichostema lanceolatum*

Gynecological Aid: *Astragalus pachypus, A. purshii, Cercocarpus ledifolius, Cupressus nevadensis, Nicotiana quadrivalvis, Pinus monophylla, Purshia glandulosa, Rhamnus crocea*

Hallucinogen: *Datura wrightii, Nicotiana quadrivalvis, Thamnosma montana*

Heart Medicine: *Croton setigerus, Dicentra chrysantha, Distichlis spicata*

Hemorrhoid Remedy: *Aesculus californica*

Hemostat: *Cuscuta californica, Frangula californica, Nicotiana quadrivalvis*

Herbal Steam: *Artemisia tridentata, Corethrogyne filaginifolia, Mimulus guttatus, Sambucus cerulea*

Hunting Medicine: *Thamnosma montana*

Internal Medicine: *Cercocarpus montanus*

Kidney Aid: *Cupressus nevadensis, Rhamnus crocea*

Laxative: *Distichlis spicata, Frangula californica, Garrya flavescens, Pinus lambertiana, Prunus virginiana, Purshia glandulosa, Rhamnus crocea, Senecio flaccidus*

Liver Aid: *Rhamnus crocea*

Misc. Disease Remedy: *Anemopsis californica, Artemisia tridentata, Rumex salicifolius, Sambucus cerulea*

Orthopedic Aid: *Chaenactis santolinoides, Cicuta douglasii, Cupressus nevadensis, Datura wrightii, Delphinium parryi, Ephedra viridis, Ericameria linearifolia, Grindelia camporum, Gutierrezia californica, Larrea tridentata, Lomatium dissectum, L. utriculatum, Mimulus guttatus, Penstemon rostriflorus, Populus fremontii, Rumex salicifolius, Solanum xantii, Tauschia parishii, Urtica dioica*

Other: *Artemisia douglasiana, Nicotiana quadrivalvis*

Pediatric Aid: *Artemisia douglasiana, Datura wrightii, Pinus lambertiana, P. monophylla, Urtica dioica*

Poison: *Aesculus californica, Chenopodium californicum, Cicuta douglasii, Datura wrightii, Nicotiana quadrivalvis, Thalictrum polycarpum*

Poultice: *Populus fremontii*

Psychological Aid: *Nicotiana quadrivalvis, Urtica dioica*

Respiratory Aid: *Arenaria macradenia, Marrubium vulgare, Nicotiana quadrivalvis*

Sedative: *Nicotiana quadrivalvis*

Snakebite Remedy: *Achillea millefolium, Chamaesyce albomarginata, Thamnosma montana*

Stimulant: *Nicotiana quadrivalvis, Phacelia californica, Rhamnus crocea*

Throat Aid: *Lomatium californicum*

Toothache Remedy: *Aster subulatus, Erigeron foliosus, Melica imperfecta, Nicotiana quadrivalvis, Tauschia parishii*

Unspecified: *Alnus rhombifolia, Frangula californica, Larrea tridentata, Lythrum californicum, Platanus racemosa, Rumex salicifolius, Senecio flaccidus*

Venereal Aid: *Calystegia longipes, Cercocarpus ledifolius, Coleogyne ramosissima, Distichlis spicata, Eriastrum densifolium, Eriodictyon californicum, Eriogonum umbellatum, Eschscholzia parishii, Garrya flavescens, Mahonia dictyota, Phacelia ramosissima, Purshia glandulosa, Rhamnus crocea*

Veterinary Aid: *Anemopsis californica, Chamaesyce albomarginata, Encelia virginensis, Ericameria linearifolia, Larrea tridentata, Thamnosma montana*

Witchcraft Medicine: *Salvia dorrii, Urtica dioica*

Keresan

Dermatological Aid: *Yucca baccata*

Febrifuge: *Glycyrrhiza lepidota, Mentha canadensis*

Gynecological Aid: *Solanum elaeagnifolium*

Veterinary Aid: *Ipomoea leptophylla*

Keres, Western

Analgesic: *Mentha canadensis, Plantago patagonica*

Antidiarrheal: *Juniperus monosperma, Phoradendron juniperinum, Plantago patagonica, Portulaca oleracea*

Antirheumatic (External): *Abies concolor, Artemisia ludoviciana, Brickellia ambigens, B. grandiflora, Chaetopappa ericoides, Epixiphium wislizeni, Erysimum capitatum, Gilia rigidula, Gutierrezia sarothrae, Lesquerella fendleri, Lygodesmia juncea, Oenothera albicaulis, Phacelia crenulata, Phoradendron juniperinum, Picea parryana, Zigadenus elegans, Zinnia acerosa*

Antirheumatic (Internal): *Abies concolor, Calochortus gunnisonii*

Blood Medicine: *Aquilegia elegantula, Plantago major, Portulaca oleracea*

Burn Dressing: *Anemopsis californica, Aristida divaricata, Conyza canadensis, Rumex salicifolius*

Carminative: *Brickellia ambigens, B. grandiflora*

Cathartic: *Aletes acaulis, Bahia dissecta, Croton texensis, Gutierrezia sarothrae, Solidago gigantea*

Cold Remedy: *Gnaphalium canescens, Picea parryana, Thalictrum fendleri*

Cough Medicine: *Ephedra torreyana, Glycyrrhiza lepidota, Prunus virginiana*

Dermatological Aid: *Alnus incana, Anemopsis californica, Baileya multiradiata, Buchloe dactyloides, Conyza canadensis, Croton texensis, Cucurbita foetidissima, Dalea candida, Datura wrightii, Geranium caespitosum, Gnaphalium canescens, Juniperus monosperma, Opuntia clavata, O. imbricata, Pinus edulis, Psorothamnus scoparius, Sarcobatus vermiculatus, Senecio flaccidus, Silene laciniata, Tragia ramosa, Vicia americana, Xanthium strumarium*

Diaphoretic: *Artemisia ludoviciana, Ephedra torreyana, Gutierrezia sarothrae, Juniperus monosperma, Zigadenus elegans*

Dietary Aid: *Abronia fragrans, Brickellia ambigens, B. grandiflora*

Diuretic: *Cirsium pallidum, Mentzelia multiflora*

Ear Medicine: *Geastrum sp., Juniperus monosperma, Opuntia imbricata*

Emetic: *Aletes acaulis, Bahia dissecta, Chenopo-*

dium graveolens, Dalea formosa, Eriogonum rotundifolium, Gutierrezia sarothrae, Ipomopsis laxiflora, I. longiflora, Juniperus monosperma, Lesquerella fendleri, Panicum capillare, Penstemon ambiguus, Psorothamnus scoparius, Pterospora andromedea, Quercus gambelii, Rhus trilobata, Sarcobatus vermiculatus

Eye Medicine: Chamaesyce albomarginata, Gutierrezia sarothrae, Houstonia rubra, Prosopis glandulosa, Stephanomeria runcinata

Febrifuge: Dyssodia papposa, Eriogonum tenellum, Gaura parviflora, Mentha canadensis

Gastrointestinal Aid: Amaranthus hybridus, A. retroflexus, Arabis fendleri, Asclepias involucrata, Cymopterus bulbosus, Grindelia decumbens, G. fastigiata, Houstonia rubra, Ipomoea leptophylla, Juniperus monosperma, Pectis angustifolia, Picea parryana, Pinus edulis, Polygonum lapathifolium, Psorothamnus scoparius, Rhus trilobata, Senecio flaccidus

Gynecological Aid: Ambrosia psilostachya, Apocynum cannabinum, Asclepias subverticillata, Chamaesyce albomarginata, Cheilanthes fendleri, Eriogonum tenellum, Euphorbia dentata, Gaillardia pinnatifida, G. pulchella, Ratibida columnifera, Rhus trilobata, Senecio spartioides, Sphaeralcea angustifolia, S. coccinea, Townsendia strigosa, Woodsia neomexicana

Heart Medicine: Eriogonum jamesii

Hemorrhoid Remedy: Croton texensis, Equisetum laevigatum

Hemostat: Helianthus niveus

Herbal Steam: Yucca glauca

Hunting Medicine: Ratibida tagetes

Kidney Aid: Ephedra torreyana, Zinnia grandiflora

Laxative: Juniperus monosperma

Liver Aid: Brickellia ambigens, B. grandiflora

Misc. Disease Remedy: Rosa nutkana

Nose Medicine: Dimorphocarpa wislizeni

Oral Aid: Ceanothus fendleri, Portulaca oleracea, Quercus gambelii, Rhus trilobata

Other: Artemisia ludoviciana, Draba helleriana, Dyssodia papposa, Mahonia aquifolium, Silene laciniata, Zinnia grandiflora

Panacea: Zea mays

Pediatric Aid: Dalea nana, Phoradendron juniperinum, Phragmites australis, Quercus gambelii, Rosa nutkana, Thelesperma filifolium, T. megapotamicum, Tragia ramosa

Poison: Cryptantha crassisepala, Datura wrightii, Hymenoxys richardsonii, Ranunculus sceleratus, Zigadenus elegans

Preventive Medicine: Mahonia aquifolium

Psychological Aid: Abronia fragrans, Berlandiera lyrata, Crepis runcinata, Datura ferox, Eriogonum jamesii, E. rotundifolium, Gaillardia pinnatifida, G. pulchella, Linum rigidum, Mentzelia multiflora, Pectis angustifolia, Senecio fendleri, Zinnia acerosa

Pulmonary Aid: Orobanche fasciculata

Sedative: Berlandiera lyrata, Eriogonum rotundifolium, Gaura parviflora, Ratibida tagetes

Snakebite Remedy: Epixiphium wislizeni, Glandularia bipinnatifida, Gutierrezia sarothrae

Stimulant: Nepeta cataria

Strengthener: Cercocarpus montanus, Dalea formosa, D. nana, Opuntia imbricata, Tragia ramosa, Yucca glauca, Zigadenus elegans

Throat Aid: Glandularia bipinnatifida, Phacelia crenulata

Tuberculosis Remedy: Commelina dianthifolia, Conopholis alpina, Mentzelia multiflora, Thelesperma filifolium, T. megapotamicum

Unspecified: Ratibida tagetes

Urinary Aid: Ephedra torreyana

Veterinary Aid: Cynodon dactylon, Gutierrezia sarothrae, Opuntia clavata

Kiowa

Analgesic: Lophophora williamsii

Anthelmintic: Artemisia vulgaris, Juglans nigra

Antihemorrhagic: Cephalanthus occidentalis

Antirheumatic (External): Lophophora williamsii

Burn Dressing: Cirsium ochrocentrum

Cold Remedy: Lophophora williamsii

Cough Medicine: Echinacea angustifolia

Dermatological Aid: Ambrosia psilostachya, Artemisia ludoviciana, Centaurea americana, Cirsium ochrocentrum, Hierochloe odorata, Lophophora williamsii, Monarda pectinata, Sapindus saponaria, Toxicodendron radicans, Vernonia missurica, Yucca glauca

Emetic: Aesculus glabra, Cucurbita foetidissima

Febrifuge: Lophophora williamsii

Gastrointestinal Aid: Artemisia ludoviciana, Lophophora williamsii, Penstemon grandiflorus, Rhus trilobata

Gynecological Aid: Taraxacum officinale

Herbal Steam: Artemisia ludoviciana

Misc. Disease Remedy: Lophophora williamsii, Quincula lobata, Rhus trilobata

Narcotic: Lophophora williamsii

Oral Aid: Bothriochloa saccharoides, Helianthus annuus, Juniperus virginiana, Oxalis stricta, Ulmus rubra

Orthopedic Aid: Lophophora williamsii

Other: Rhus glabra

Panacea: Lophophora williamsii

Poison: *Citrullus lanatus*
Pulmonary Aid: *Artemisia ludoviciana, Lophophora williamsii*
Snakebite Remedy: *Ribes aureum*
Throat Aid: *Artemisia ludoviciana, Echinacea angustifolia*
Tuberculosis Remedy: *Carya illinoinensis, Lophophora williamsii, Rhus glabra*
Venereal Aid: *Lophophora williamsii*
Veterinary Aid: *Ambrosia psilostachya*

Kitasoo

Antirheumatic (External): *Veratrum viride*
Cathartic: *Oenanthe sarmentosa*
Cold Remedy: *Ledum groenlandicum*
Cough Medicine: *Polypodium glycyrrhiza*
Dietary Aid: *Elliottia pyroliflorus*
Emetic: *Oenanthe sarmentosa*
Gastrointestinal Aid: *Taxus brevifolia*
Gynecological Aid: *Nuphar lutea*
Internal Medicine: *Taxus brevifolia*
Respiratory Aid: *Ledum groenlandicum*
Throat Aid: *Polypodium glycyrrhiza*
Unspecified: *Abies amabilis, Aruncus dioicus, Maianthemum racemosum*

Klallam

Analgesic: *Taxus brevifolia, Urtica dioica, Viola adunca*
Antidiarrheal: *Alnus rubra, Sambucus cerulea*
Antihemorrhagic: *Tsuga heterophylla*
Burn Dressing: *Gaultheria shallon*
Cold Remedy: *Achillea millefolium, Symphoricarpos albus*
Cough Medicine: *Polypodium virginianum*
Dermatological Aid: *Achillea millefolium, Aruncus dioicus, Dryopteris expansa, Galium triflorum, Lonicera ciliosa, Lysichiton americanus*
Dietary Aid: *Tsuga heterophylla*
Eye Medicine: *Malus fusca, Populus balsamifera, Ribes divaricatum*
Gynecological Aid: *Achillea millefolium, Geum macrophyllum*
Laxative: *Frangula purshiana*
Love Medicine: *Conium maculatum*
Orthopedic Aid: *Urtica dioica*
Panacea: *Urtica dioica*
Poison: *Conium maculatum, Disporum hookeri*
Tonic: *Salix sitchensis*
Tuberculosis Remedy: *Acer macrophyllum, Lysichiton americanus, Thuja plicata, Tsuga heterophylla*

Klamath

Antidiarrheal: *Artemisia tridentata*
Antirheumatic (External): *Artemisia tridentata, Wyethia mollis*
Burn Dressing: *Eriogonum umbellatum*
Cough Medicine: *Purshia tridentata*
Dermatological Aid: *Chrysothamnus nauseosus, Ericameria bloomeri, Wyethia mollis*
Emetic: *Frangula purshiana, Iris missouriensis, Purshia tridentata, Zigadenus venenosus*
Eye Medicine: *Artemisia tridentata, Pinus contorta*
Herbal Steam: *Calocedrus decurrens*
Orthopedic Aid: *Artemisia tridentata*
Poison: *Cicuta maculata*
Pulmonary Aid: *Purshia tridentata*
Respiratory Aid: *Purshia tridentata*
Unspecified: *Heracleum maximum*

Koasati

Analgesic: *Bignonia capreolata, Pteridium aquilinum, Pycnanthemum incanum, Salix nigra, Smilax rotundifolia*
Anthelmintic: *Chenopodium ambrosioides*
Antidiarrheal: *Parthenium hysterophorus*
Antirheumatic (Internal): *Baptisia alba, Bignonia capreolata, Cephalanthus occidentalis, Hypericum hypericoides, Liatris acidota*
Cough Medicine: *Berchemia scandens*
Dermatological Aid: *Acer rubrum, Chionanthus virginicus, Helenium amarum, Ilex opaca, Magnolia grandiflora, Nyssa sylvatica, Sassafras albidum, Ulmus americana*
Emetic: *Eryngium aquaticum, Eupatorium perfoliatum*
Eye Medicine: *Aralia spinosa*
Febrifuge: *Gnaphalium obtusifolium, Monarda fistulosa, Salix nigra*
Gastrointestinal Aid: *Callicarpa americana, Castanea pumila, Myrica cerifera, Salix nigra, Ulmus americana*
Gynecological Aid: *Gossypium herbaceum, Xanthium strumarium*
Heart Medicine: *Sassafras albidum*
Hemostat: *Pycnanthemum incanum*
Herbal Steam: *Helenium amarum*
Kidney Aid: *Helenium amarum*
Orthopedic Aid: *Cephalanthus occidentalis, Prunus persica, Rhus copallinum*
Other: *Liquidambar styraciflua*
Pediatric Aid: *Gnaphalium obtusifolium, Myrica cerifera, Rhus copallinum*
Snakebite Remedy: *Tephrosia florida*
Stimulant: *Pycnanthemum incanum*
Urinary Aid: *Eupatorium perfoliatum*

Koyukon

Ceremonial Medicine: *Picea glauca*
Dermatological Aid: *Picea glauca, P. mariana*
Hunting Medicine: *Picea glauca, P. mariana*
Kidney Aid: *Picea glauca, P. mariana*
Panacea: *Picea glauca, P. mariana*
Unspecified: *Betula papyrifera, Picea glauca, P. mariana*

Kuper Island Indian

Hemostat: *Sedum spathulifolium*

Kutenai

Abortifacient: *Alnus incana, Symphoricarpos albus*
Antidiarrheal: *Prunus virginiana*
Antirheumatic (External): *Heuchera cylindrica, Mentha arvensis*
Blood Medicine: *Mahonia repens*
Cathartic: *Frangula purshiana*
Cold Remedy: *Juniperus scopulorum, Mentha arvensis*
Cough Medicine: *Mentha arvensis*
Dermatological Aid: *Abies lasiocarpa, Achillea millefolium, Artemisia ludoviciana, Balsamorhiza sagittata, Cicuta douglasii, Larix occidentalis, Nuphar lutea, Populus balsamifera, P. deltoides*
Disinfectant: *Achillea millefolium*
Emetic: *Cicuta douglasii*
Eye Medicine: *Chimaphila umbellata, Shepherdia canadensis*
Febrifuge: *Juniperus scopulorum, Mentha arvensis*
Kidney Aid: *Chimaphila umbellata, Mahonia repens, Mentha arvensis, Monarda fistulosa*
Misc. Disease Remedy: *Juniperus scopulorum*
Nose Medicine: *Veratrum viride*
Pulmonary Aid: *Juniperus scopulorum*
Respiratory Aid: *Populus balsamifera, P. deltoides*
Throat Aid: *Rhus glabra*
Tonic: *Mentha arvensis*
Tuberculosis Remedy: *Heuchera cylindrica, Larix occidentalis, Pinus contorta, Populus deltoides*
Unspecified: *Ligusticum canbyi*
Veterinary Aid: *Apocynum cannabinum*

Kwakiutl

Abortifacient: *Veratrum viride*
Analgesic: *Alnus rubra, Angelica lucida, Argentina anserina, Galium triflorum, Lomatium nudicaule, Lonicera involucrata, Menziesia ferruginea, Moneses uniflora, Nuphar lutea, Oemleria cerasiformis, Oplopanax horridus, Picea sitchensis, Symphoricarpos albus, Urtica dioica, Veratrum viride*
Antidiarrheal: *Blechnum spicant, Cicuta douglasii,*
Juniperus communis, Picea sitchensis, Polypodium glycyrrhiza, Pseudotsuga menziesii, Ribes lobbii, Rubus ursinus, Tsuga heterophylla
Antiemetic: *Menyanthes trifoliata, Polypodium glycyrrhiza, Rubus parviflorus, R. ursinus*
Antihemorrhagic: *Alnus rubra, Aralia nudicaulis, Kalmia polifolia, Malus fusca, Menyanthes trifoliata, Polypodium glycyrrhiza, Rubus parviflorus, R. ursinus*
Antirheumatic (External): *Achillea millefolium, Chamaecyparis nootkatensis, Conioselinum gmelinii, Lomatium nudicaule, Lonicera involucrata*
Blood Medicine: *Juniperus communis*
Burn Dressing: *Rubus spectabilis, Tsuga heterophylla*
Cancer Treatment: *Epilobium angustifolium, Prunus emarginata*
Cathartic: *Cicuta douglasii, Physocarpus capitatus*
Ceremonial Medicine: *Abies grandis, Tsuga mertensiana*
Cold Remedy: *Achillea millefolium, Lomatium nudicaule, Picea sitchensis, Veratrum viride*
Cough Medicine: *Abies grandis, Aralia nudicaulis, Aruncus dioicus, Lomatium nudicaule, Picea sitchensis, Pinus contorta, P. monticola*
Dermatological Aid: *Abies grandis, Acer macrophyllum, Achillea millefolium, Allium cernuum, Alnus rubra, Anaphalis margaritacea, Argentina anserina, A. egedii, Chamaecyparis nootkatensis, Cicuta douglasii, Crataegus douglasii, Drosera rotundifolia, Epilobium angustifolium, Equisetum arvense, E. telmateia, Heracleum maximum, Kalmia polifolia, Lomatium nudicaule, Lonicera involucrata, Lysichiton americanus, Malus fusca, Menziesia ferruginea, Moneses uniflora, Oemleria cerasiformis, Oplopanax horridus, Picea sitchensis, Pinus monticola, Plantago major, Populus balsamifera, Prunus emarginata, Pseudotsuga menziesii, Ribes lobbii, Rubus parviflorus, R. spectabilis, Rumex aquaticus, Scirpus americanus, Thuja plicata, Tsuga heterophylla, T. mertensiana, Urtica dioica, Veratrum viride*
Dietary Aid: *Menyanthes trifoliata, Prunus emarginata*
Disinfectant: *Picea sitchensis*
Emetic: *Cicuta douglasii, Oenanthe sarmentosa, Osmorhiza berteroi, Physocarpus capitatus, Sambucus racemosa, Veratrum viride*
Eye Medicine: *Argentina egedii, Symphoricarpos albus, Thuja plicata, Tsuga heterophylla*
Gastrointestinal Aid: *Frangula purshiana, Lomatium nudicaule, Menyanthes trifoliata, Menziesia*

ferruginea, Oplopanax horridus, Pinus contorta, P. monticola, Rumex aquaticus

Gynecological Aid: *Achillea millefolium, Heracleum maximum, Lomatium nudicaule, Lonicera involucrata, Polystichum munitum, Prunus emarginata, Rubus parviflorus, Sambucus racemosa, Tsuga heterophylla, Urtica dioica*

Heart Medicine: *Menziesia ferruginea, Prunus emarginata*

Hemostat: *Prunus emarginata, Thuja plicata*

Herbal Steam: *Achillea millefolium, Angelica lucida, Chamaecyparis nootkatensis, Conioselinum gmelinii, Lomatium nudicaule, Lonicera involucrata, Lysichiton americanus, Oplopanax horridus, Sambucus racemosa*

Hunting Medicine: *Angelica lucida, Lomatium nudicaule, Tsuga heterophylla, Veratrum viride*

Internal Medicine: *Anaphalis margaritacea, Rubus parviflorus*

Kidney Aid: *Chamaecyparis nootkatensis, Picea sitchensis*

Laxative: *Abies grandis, Frangula purshiana, Lomatium nudicaule, Oplopanax horridus, Physocarpus capitatus, Veratrum viride*

Love Medicine: *Aruncus dioicus, Drosera rotundifolia, Monotropa hypopithys, Platanthera stricta*

Misc. Disease Remedy: *Cicuta douglasii, Menyanthes trifoliata*

Narcotic: *Arctostaphylos uva-ursi, Ledum groenlandicum*

Oral Aid: *Abies grandis, Cirsium remotifolium, Prunus emarginata, Ribes lobbii*

Orthopedic Aid: *Lomatium nudicaule, Lonicera involucrata, Nuphar lutea, Sambucus racemosa, Thuja plicata, Veratrum viride*

Other: *Lysichiton americanus, Picea sitchensis, Urtica dioica*

Panacea: *Achillea millefolium, Chamaecyparis nootkatensis, Lomatium nudicaule, Veratrum viride*

Pediatric Aid: *Cirsium remotifolium, Heracleum maximum, Lupinus littoralis, Lysichiton americanus, Phyllospadix torreyi, Prunus emarginata, Rubus spectabilis, Scirpus americanus, Tsuga mertensiana, Veratrum viride*

Poison: *Cicuta douglasii, Oplopanax horridus, Osmorhiza berteroi, Veratrum viride*

Preventive Medicine: *Prunus emarginata*

Reproductive Aid: *Pinus monticola*

Respiratory Aid: *Alnus rubra, Juniperus communis, Nuphar lutea*

Sedative: *Glaux maritima, Lupinus littoralis*

Stimulant: *Angelica lucida, Conioselinum gmelinii, Lysichiton americanus*

Strengthener: *Chamaecyparis nootkatensis, Phyllospadix torreyi*

Throat Aid: *Lomatium nudicaule*

Tonic: *Abies grandis*

Tuberculosis Remedy: *Abies grandis, Alnus rubra, Oplopanax horridus, Prunus emarginata*

Unspecified: *Angelica lucida, Pseudotsuga menziesii*

Venereal Aid: *Physocarpus capitatus, Urtica dioica*

Witchcraft Medicine: *Oplopanax horridus*

Kwakiutl, Southern

Analgesic: *Alnus rubra, Fucus gardneri, Lonicera involucrata, Urtica dioica*

Antirheumatic (External): *Chamaecyparis nootkatensis, Fucus gardneri, Urtica dioica*

Burn Dressing: *Nereocystis luetkeana*

Dermatological Aid: *Nereocystis luetkeana*

Orthopedic Aid: *Nereocystis luetkeana*

Pediatric Aid: *Nereocystis luetkeana*

Strengthener: *Chamaecyparis nootkatensis, Fucus gardneri*

Venereal Aid: *Fucus gardneri*

Kwakwaka'wakw

Antiemetic: *Kalmia microphylla*

Antihemorrhagic: *Kalmia microphylla*

Ceremonial Medicine: *Tsuga heterophylla*

Dermatological Aid: *Moneses uniflora*

Emetic: *Oenanthe sarmentosa*

Unspecified: *Pinus contorta*

Lakota

Abortifacient: *Yucca glauca*

Analgesic: *Astragalus canadensis, Clematis ligusticifolia, Dyssodia papposa, Psoralidium tenuiflorum, Ratibida columnifera*

Antidiarrheal: *Artemisia ludoviciana, Asclepias pumila, A. viridiflora, Heuchera richardsonii, Lygodesmia juncea, Rumex altissimus*

Antihemorrhagic: *Astragalus canadensis, Dyssodia papposa, Glycyrrhiza lepidota, Grindelia squarrosa, Rumex altissimus*

Antirheumatic (External): *Ambrosia artemisiifolia, Amphicarpaea bracteata, Antennaria parvifolia, Echinacea angustifolia, Euphorbia marginata, Onosmodium molle*

Cancer Treatment: *Fritillaria atropurpurea*

Cathartic: *Dalea villosa*

Ceremonial Medicine: *Xanthium strumarium*

Cold Remedy: *Artemisia ludoviciana, Gutierrezia sarothrae, Juniperus virginiana*

Cough Medicine: *Acorus calamus, Astragalus cana-*

densis, Gutierrezia sarothrae, Monarda fistulosa, Pycnanthemum virginianum

Dermatological Aid: *Achillea millefolium, Echinacea angustifolia, Heuchera richardsonii, Sphaeralcea coccinea, Thalictrum dasycarpum, Yucca glauca*

Dietary Aid: *Asclepias stenophylla, Physalis heterophylla*

Diuretic: *Artemisia campestris, Eriogonum annuum, Mirabilis linearis*

Eye Medicine: *Monarda fistulosa*

Gastrointestinal Aid: *Artemisia campestris, Croton texensis, Echinacea angustifolia, Ipomoea leptophylla, Ratibida columnifera, Rumex altissimus, Sium suave, Solanum triflorum, Urtica dioica, Yucca glauca*

Gynecological Aid: *Artemisia campestris, Asclepias verticillata, A. viridiflora, Astragalus gracilis, Euphorbia marginata, Rumex venosus, Yucca glauca*

Hemostat: *Monarda fistulosa*

Hypotensive: *Acorus calamus*

Kidney Aid: *Lepidium densiflorum*

Misc. Disease Remedy: *Acorus calamus, Glycyrrhiza lepidota*

Oral Aid: *Echinacea angustifolia, Eriogonum annuum*

Orthopedic Aid: *Acorus calamus*

Other: *Echinacea angustifolia*

Pediatric Aid: *Asclepias pumila, A. viridiflora, Eriogonum annuum, Lygodesmia juncea*

Poison: *Astragalus racemosus, Cicuta maculata, Conium maculatum, Delphinium carolinianum, Dichanthelium oligosanthes, Oxytropis lambertii, Toxicodendron rydbergii, Zigadenus venenosus*

Preventive Medicine: *Chamaesyce geyeri*

Pulmonary Aid: *Astragalus canadensis, Lithospermum caroliniense, Monarda fistulosa*

Reproductive Aid: *Dyssodia papposa*

Sedative: *Artemisia campestris*

Snakebite Remedy: *Opuntia humifusa*

Stimulant: *Monarda fistulosa*

Throat Aid: *Acorus calamus, Artemisia ludoviciana, Dalea villosa, Echinacea angustifolia*

Toothache Remedy: *Acorus calamus, Echinacea angustifolia, Glycyrrhiza lepidota*

Unspecified: *Ambrosia trifida, Artemisia cana, A. tridentata, Asclepias speciosa, Glycyrrhiza lepidota, Pediomelum argophyllum, P. cuspidatum, Sagittaria latifolia*

Vertigo Medicine: *Gutierrezia sarothrae*

Veterinary Aid: *Astragalus crassicarpus, Hymenopappus tenuifolius, Onosmodium molle, Pedi-*

omelum argophyllum, Ratibida columnifera, Thalictrum dasycarpum, Yucca glauca

Luiseño

Abortifacient: *Croton californicus*

Analgesic: *Woodwardia radicans*

Cathartic: *Marah macrocarpus, Mirabilis californica, Sisyrinchium bellum*

Ceremonial Medicine: *Datura wrightii*

Cold Remedy: *Satureja douglasii*

Dermatological Aid: *Baccharis douglasii, Hoita macrostachya, Quercus dumosa*

Emetic: *Ambrosia artemisiifolia*

Eye Medicine: *Solanum douglasii*

Febrifuge: *Centaurium venustum, Satureja douglasii*

Gynecological Aid: *Sambucus cerulea*

Hallucinogen: *Datura wrightii*

Narcotic: *Datura wrightii*

Snakebite Remedy: *Chamaesyce polycarpa*

Toothache Remedy: *Ribes indecorum, R. malvaceum*

Unspecified: *Artemisia dracunculus, A. furcata, Cneoridium dumosum, Datura wrightii, Ericameria parishii, Eriodictyon crassifolium, E. tomentosum, Monardella lanceolata, Pellaea mucronata, Satureja douglasii, Tauschia arguta, Turricula parryi*

Lummi

Analgesic: *Achillea millefolium, Ribes lacustre*

Antidiarrheal: *Holodiscus discolor, Spiraea douglasii*

Antiemetic: *Thuja plicata*

Dermatological Aid: *Achlys triphylla, Adiantum aleuticum, Aruncus dioicus*

Diaphoretic: *Achillea millefolium*

Emetic: *Achlys triphylla, Petasites frigidus*

Eye Medicine: *Holodiscus discolor, Trillium ovatum*

Gynecological Aid:, *Oplopanax horridus, Polystichum munitum, Prunus emarginata, Urtica dioica*

Laxative: *Cornus nuttallii, Frangula purshiana*

Misc. Disease Remedy: *Achillea millefolium, Aruncus dioicus*

Oral Aid: *Holodiscus discolor*

Orthopedic Aid: *Holodiscus discolor*

Pulmonary Aid: *Thuja plicata*

Tonic: *Ribes laxiflorum*

Tuberculosis Remedy: *Lonicera ciliosa, Pinus monticola*

Mahuna

Abortifacient: *Chenopodium ambrosioides, Iva axillaris*

Analgesic: *Malva neglecta, Phytolacca americana, Rosa californica, Saponaria officinalis*

Anthelmintic: *Sisyrinchium angustifolium*

Antidiarrheal: *Capsella bursa-pastoris, Diplacus aurantiacus, Hedeoma pulegioides, Rubus procumbens*

Antihemorrhagic: *Dennstaedtia punctilobula*

Antirheumatic (External): *Nicotiana glauca, Urtica dioica*

Antirheumatic (Internal): *Adiantum capillus-veneris, Eriodictyon californicum, Phlox subulata, Phyla lanceolata, Pinus monticola, Tanacetum parthenium, Xanthium strumarium*

Blood Medicine: *Eriogonum elongatum, Fouquieria splendens, Lotus scoparius, Pellaea atropurpurea, Salix washingtonia*

Burn Dressing: *Solidago nemoralis*

Cathartic: *Eriogonum elatum, Frangula californica*

Cold Remedy: *Spiraea salicifolia*

Contraceptive: *Iva axillaris*

Cough Medicine: *Eriodictyon californicum, Marrubium vulgare, Prunus ilicifolia, P. serotina, Rumex hymenosepalus, Salvia mellifera, Spiraea salicifolia*

Dermatological Aid: *Allium canadense, A. vineale, Ambrosia artemisiifolia, Anaphalis margaritacea, Anemopsis californica, Brodiaea sp., Clematis ligusticifolia, Datura wrightii, Grindelia humilis, G. squarrosa, Kalmia latifolia, Keckiella cordifolia, Larrea tridentata, Marah macrocarpus, Phytolacca americana, Piperia sp., Plantago major, Saponaria officinalis, Solidago nemoralis*

Dietary Aid: *Allium bisceptrum, Claytonia perfoliata, Lepidium densiflorum, Panicum capillare, Rhus trilobata*

Disinfectant: *Anemopsis californica, Grindelia squarrosa, Larrea tridentata, Solidago nemoralis*

Eye Medicine: *Piperia sp., Salvia columbariae*

Febrifuge: *Centaurium muehlenbergii, Juniperus californica, Mirabilis californica, Paeonia brownii, Rosa californica, R. gallica, Verbena hastata*

Gastrointestinal Aid: *Centaurium muehlenbergii, Chamaemelum nobile, Eriogonum umbellatum, Larrea tridentata, Malva neglecta, Monardella villosa, Platanus occidentalis, Rhus trilobata, Rosa californica, Sisyrinchium angustifolium, Verbena hastata*

Gynecological Aid: *Artemisia californica, Salvia apiana, Tephrosia virginiana*

Hemostat: *Quercus agrifolia, Typha latifolia*

Hypotensive: *Eriogonum elongatum*

Kidney Aid: *Centaurea melitensis, Croton pottsii, Pellaea atropurpurea, Xanthium spinosum, X. strumarium*

Laxative: *Centaurium muehlenbergii, Eupatorium purpureum*

Liver Aid: *Rorippa nasturtium-aquaticum*

Misc. Disease Remedy: *Juniperus californica, Sambucus racemosa*

Narcotic: *Datura wrightii*

Oral Aid: *Persea planifolia*

Orthopedic Aid: *Ulmus rubra, Xanthium strumarium*

Panacea: *Trichostema lanatum*

Pediatric Aid: *Chamaemelum nobile, Quercus agrifolia, Typha latifolia*

Poison: *Astragalus mollissimus, Datura wrightii, Eschscholzia californica, Kalmia latifolia, Phytolacca americana*

Preventive Medicine: *Pellaea atropurpurea, Toxicodendron diversilobum*

Pulmonary Aid: *Eriodictyon californicum, Paeonia brownii*

Respiratory Aid: *Andromeda polifolia, Eriodictyon californicum, Helenium autumnale, Platanus occidentalis, Salvia mellifera*

Sedative: *Mentha canadensis, M. spicata, Satureja douglasii*

Snakebite Remedy: *Allium canadense, A. vineale, Datura wrightii, Piperia sp.*

Throat Aid: *Marrubium vulgare, Nicotiana glauca, Rumex hymenosepalus*

Toothache Remedy: *Achillea millefolium, Persea planifolia, Quercus rubra*

Tuberculosis Remedy: *Nicotiana glauca, Xanthium strumarium*

Unspecified: *Quercus virginiana*

Urinary Aid: *Equisetum hyemale*

Venereal Aid: *Anagallis sp., Cercocarpus montanus, Xanthium strumarium*

Makah

Abortifacient: *Lysichiton americanus*

Adjuvant: *Frangula purshiana*

Analgesic: *Allium cernuum, Lysichiton americanus, Rubus spectabilis*

Antidiarrheal: *Equisetum hyemale, Malus fusca*

Antidote: *Salix hookeriana*

Antihemorrhagic: *Adiantum aleuticum*

Antirheumatic (External): *Aruncus dioicus, Lysich-*

Malecite

Gastrointestinal Aid: *Asarum canadense, Mentha canadensis*

Heart Medicine: *Inula helenium*

Hemorrhoid Remedy: *Sanguinaria canadensis*

Kidney Aid: *Aralia racemosa, Ledum groenlandicum, Nemopanthus mucronatus, Polygonum hydropiper, Sanicula odorata, Tanacetum vulgare, Tsuga canadensis, Typha angustifolia*

Laxative: *Abies balsamea*

Liver Aid: *Impatiens capensis*

Misc. Disease Remedy: *Heracleum maximum*

Oral Aid: *Alnus incana, Coptis trifolia*

Orthopedic Aid: *Achillea millefolium, Kalmia angustifolia*

Pediatric Aid: *Asarum canadense, Cardamine diphylla, Coptis trifolia, Geum aleppicum, G. rivale, Mentha canadensis, Prunus pensylvanica, Tiarella cordifolia, Tsuga canadensis*

Preventive Medicine: *Acorus calamus*

Pulmonary Aid: *Geum aleppicum, Mentha canadensis, Polypodium virginianum*

Respiratory Aid: *Comptonia peregrina, Cornus sericea, Verbascum thapsus*

Sedative: *Mentha canadensis*

Strengthener: *Aralia racemosa, Larix laricina*

Throat Aid: *Cardamine diphylla, Cornus sericea, Iris versicolor, Polystichum acrostichoides, Scirpus microcarpus*

Tonic: *Cardamine diphylla, Juniperus communis*

Toothache Remedy: *Thuja occidentalis*

Tuberculosis Remedy: *Aralia racemosa, Chimaphila umbellata, Juniperus communis, Larix laricina, Lilium philadelphicum, Nemopanthus mucronatus, Prunus serotina, Rhus hirta, Sanguinaria canadensis, Sarracenia purpurea, Thuja occidentalis*

Unspecified: *Abies balsamea, Acorus calamus, Coptis trifolia, Larix laricina, Picea glauca, P. mariana, Populus ×jackii, Symplocarpus foetidus, Taxus canadensis, Tsuga canadensis*

Venereal Aid: *Abies balsamea, Aralia racemosa, Arctium lappa, Larix laricina*

Veterinary Aid: *Tanacetum vulgare*

Mandan

Ceremonial Medicine: *Helianthus annuus*

Stimulant: *Helianthus annuus*

Maricopa

Antirheumatic (External): *Atriplex polycarpa*

Mendocino Indian

Abortifacient: *Phoradendron leucarpum*

Analgesic: *Achillea millefolium, Artemisia furcata,* *Eschscholzia californica, Heteromeles arbutifolia, Umbellularia californica, Wyethia longicaulis, Zigadenus venenosus*

Antidiarrheal: *Alnus rhombifolia, Artemisia furcata, Prunus virginiana, Rubus vitifolius, Salix lasiolepis*

Antidote: *Artemisia furcata*

Antihemorrhagic: *Alnus rhombifolia*

Antirheumatic (External): *Anthemis cotula, Artemisia furcata, Marah oreganus, Umbellularia californica, Wyethia longicaulis, Zigadenus venenosus*

Blood Medicine: *Alnus rhombifolia, Mahonia repens, Monardella villosa, Satureja douglasii*

Burn Dressing: *Alnus rhombifolia, Pinus sabiniana, Wyethia longicaulis*

Cathartic: *Frangula californica, Pinus lambertiana*

Cold Remedy: *Anthemis cotula, Aralia californica, Artemisia furcata, Clematis ligusticifolia, Eriodictyon californicum, Lithophragma affine*

Dermatological Aid: *Achillea millefolium, Asclepias eriocarpa, Chlorogalum pomeridianum, Eschscholzia californica, Marah oreganus, Mentzelia laevicaulis, Pinus sabiniana, Polygonum aviculare, Populus fremontii, Salix lasiolepis, Sambucus cerulea, Toxicodendron diversilobum, Umbellularia californica, Wyethia longicaulis, Zigadenus venenosus*

Diaphoretic: *Alnus rhombifolia, Salix lasiolepis*

Emetic: *Alnus rhombifolia, Eschscholzia californica, Wyethia longicaulis*

Eye Medicine: *Achillea millefolium, Anthemis cotula, Artemisia furcata, Clarkia purpurea, Lonicera interrupta, Polypodium californicum, Wyethia longicaulis*

Febrifuge: *Aralia californica, Artemisia furcata, Cercis canadensis, Salix lasiolepis, Sambucus cerulea, Scutellaria californica*

Gastrointestinal Aid: *Achillea millefolium, Alnus rhombifolia, Aralia californica, Arceuthobium occidentale, Artemisia furcata, Calocedrus decurrens, Chenopodium album, Eschscholzia californica, Heteromeles arbutifolia, Lithophragma affine, Mahonia repens, Mentzelia laevicaulis, Monardella villosa, Satureja douglasii, Thysanocarpus curvipes, Umbellularia californica, Wyethia longicaulis*

Gynecological Aid: *Alnus rhombifolia, Artemisia furcata, Eschscholzia californica*

Herbal Steam: *Artemisia furcata*

Kidney Aid: *Frangula californica*

Misc. Disease Remedy: *Frangula californica*

Narcotic: *Delphinium nudicaule, Eschscholzia californica*

Orthopedic Aid: *Achillea millefolium, Lathyrus jepsonii, Sambucus cerulea, Zigadenus venenosus*

Panacea: *Salix lasiolepis, Thalictrum polycarpum, Umbellularia californica*

Poison: *Aesculus californica, Allium unifolium, Arctostaphylos manzanita, Asclepias fascicularis, Chlorogalum pomeridianum, Crataegus rivularis, Delphinium hesperium, Marah oreganus, Phoradendron leucarpum, Quercus chrysolepis, Solanum nigrum, Taxus brevifolia, Thalictrum polycarpum, Zigadenus venenosus*

Psychological Aid: *Frangula californica*

Pulmonary Aid: *Aralia californica*

Respiratory Aid: *Artemisia furcata, Eriodictyon californicum*

Sedative: *Prunus virginiana*

Stimulant: *Umbellularia californica*

Throat Aid: *Clematis ligusticifolia*

Tonic: *Prunus virginiana*

Toothache Remedy: *Aesculus californica, Eschscholzia californica, Phoradendron leucarpum*

Tuberculosis Remedy: *Achillea millefolium, Alnus rhombifolia, Aralia californica, Eschscholzia californica*

Urinary Aid: *Marah oreganus*

Venereal Aid: *Helenium puberulum, Marah oreganus*

Veterinary Aid: *Aesculus californica, Populus fremontii, Pteridium aquilinum, Sambucus cerulea*

Menominee

Abortifacient: *Acorus calamus, Artemisia campestris, Quercus ellipsoidalis, Q. macrocarpa, Sanguinaria canadensis, Thuja occidentalis, Trillium grandiflorum*

Adjuvant: *Abies balsamea, Arctostaphylos uva-ursi, Chimaphila umbellata, Comptonia peregrina, Corylus americana, Fraxinus nigra, Ptelea trifoliata, Robinia pseudoacacia, Rubus idaeus, Sanguinaria canadensis, Symplocarpus foetidus, Taenidia integerrima, Thuja occidentalis, Zanthoxylum americanum*

Alterative: *Alnus incana, Helenium autumnale*

Analgesic: *Abies balsamea, Acorus calamus, Angelica atropurpurea, Aralia racemosa, Echinocystis lobata, Gnaphalium obtusifolium, Helenium autumnale, Heuchera americana, Hydrophyllum virginianum, Pinus strobus, Polygonatum biflorum, Solidago flexicaulis, Symplocarpus foetidus, Trillium grandiflorum, Tsuga canadensis, Valeriana edulis, V. uliginosa, Viburnum acerifolium, Zanthoxylum americanum*

Anthelmintic: *Apocynum cannabinum, Valeriana edulis*

Anticonvulsive: *Symplocarpus foetidus*

Antidiarrheal: *Adiantum pedatum, Betula papyrifera, Cornus alternifolia, C. amomum, Geranium maculatum, Hepatica nobilis, Heuchera americana, Hydrophyllum virginianum, Prunella vulgaris, Prunus virginiana, Rubus canadensis, Salix humilis*

Antidote: *Clintonia borealis, Sambucus racemosa, Sisyrinchium albidum*

Antihemorrhagic: *Polygonum pensylvanicum*

Antirheumatic (External): *Taxus canadensis, Zanthoxylum americanum*

Antirheumatic (Internal): *Gaultheria procumbens*

Blood Medicine: *Aralia racemosa, Chimaphila umbellata, Diervilla lonicera*

Burn Dressing: *Plantago rugelii*

Cancer Treatment: *Cornus alternifolia*

Cathartic: *Acorus calamus, Juglans cinerea, Sambucus racemosa, Ulmus rubra, Valeriana uliginosa, Veronicastrum virginicum*

Ceremonial Medicine: *Cornus amomum, Hamamelis virginiana, Veronicastrum virginicum*

Cold Remedy: *Abies balsamea, Acorus calamus, Alnus incana, Helenium autumnale, Populus balsamifera, Tsuga canadensis, Zanthoxylum americanum*

Cough Medicine: *Ceanothus americanus, Rhus hirta*

Dermatological Aid: *Abies balsamea, Achillea millefolium, Alnus incana, Anemone virginiana, Angelica atropurpurea, Aralia nudicaulis, A. racemosa, Arctium lappa, Asclepias tuberosa, Capsella bursa-pastoris, Castilleja sessiliflora, Epilobium angustifolium, Hierochloe odorata, Lactuca canadensis, Larix laricina, Lepidium virginicum, Lilium philadelphicum, Nuphar lutea, Petasites frigidus, Picea glauca, Pinus strobus, Plantago rugelii, Populus balsamifera, Prunus virginiana, Rhus hirta, Sanguinaria canadensis, Symplocarpus foetidus, Thuja occidentalis, Tsuga canadensis, Ulmus rubra, Uvularia grandiflora, Valeriana edulis, V. uliginosa, Zanthoxylum americanum*

Diaphoretic: *Nepeta cataria, Thuja occidentalis, Tsuga canadensis*

Dietary Aid: *Osmorhiza claytonii*

Disinfectant: *Gnaphalium obtusifolium, Trillium grandiflorum*

Diuretic: *Cucurbita pepo, Diervilla lonicera, Dirca palustris, Trillium grandiflorum*

Emetic: *Sambucus racemosa, Veronicastrum virginicum*

Eye Medicine: *Arisaema triphyllum, Osmorhiza claytonii, Quercus velutina, Rubus alleghenien-sis, Trillium grandiflorum, Vitis vulpina*

Febrifuge: *Achillea millefolium, Eupatorium perfo-liatum, Leucanthemum vulgare, Mentha cana-densis, Sambucus canadensis*

Gastrointestinal Aid: *Acorus calamus, Aralia race-mosa, Asarum canadense, Cardamine maxima, Ceanothus americanus, Heuchera americana, Rhus hirta, Rosa carolina, Salix humilis, Tsuga canadensis, Viburnum acerifolium*

Gynecological Aid: *Adiantum pedatum, Arisaema dracontium, Caulophyllum thalictroides, Chi-maphila umbellata, Comptonia peregrina, Cypripedium pubescens, Equisetum hyemale, Eupatorium purpureum, Hepatica nobilis, Mitchella repens, Osmunda cinnamomea, Physo-carpus opulifolius, Polygonum pensylvanicum, Pteridium aquilinum, Rhus hirta, Sisyrinchium atlanticum*

Hallucinogen: *Cypripedium pubescens*

Heart Medicine: *Liatris spicata, Symplocarpus foetidus*

Hemorrhoid Remedy: *Cornus alternifolia, Rhus hirta*

Hemostat: *Equisetum sylvaticum, Solidago flexi-caulis, Symplocarpus foetidus, Valeriana edulis*

Herbal Steam: *Maianthemum racemosum, Taxus canadensis, Tsuga canadensis*

Hunting Medicine: *Heracleum maximum, Panax quinquefolius, Valeriana uliginosa*

Internal Medicine: *Picea glauca*

Kidney Aid: *Dirca palustris, Equisetum hyemale, E. sylvaticum, Galium triflorum, Hypericum ascyron*

Laxative: *Veronicastrum virginicum*

Love Medicine: *Castilleja coccinea, Dicentra cucul-laria, Echinocystis lobata, Pedicularis cana-densis*

Oral Aid: *Coptis trifolia*

Orthopedic Aid: *Asclepias tuberosa, Hamamelis virginiana*

Other: *Hamamelis virginiana, Larix laricina, Zan-thoxylum americanum*

Panacea: *Echinocystis lobata, Ligusticum filici-num, Ptelea trifoliata*

Pediatric Aid: *Achillea millefolium, Coptis trifolia, Monarda fistulosa, Prunella vulgaris, Prunus virginiana, Symplocarpus foetidus*

Poison: *Comptonia peregrina*

Psychological Aid: *Diervilla lonicera, Gnaphalium obtusifolium, Panax quinquefolius, Valeriana uliginosa*

Pulmonary Aid: *Abies balsamea, Aralia nudicaulis,*

Asclepias syriaca, Hypericum ascyron, Mentha arvensis, M. ×piperita, Nepeta cataria, Prunus virginiana, Rhus hirta, Taenidia integerrima, Valeriana uliginosa, Verbascum thapsus, Zan-thoxylum americanum

Respiratory Aid: *Maianthemum racemosum, Monarda fistulosa, Taenidia integerrima*

Sedative: *Lithospermum canescens, Mitchella repens, Nepeta cataria, Valeriana uliginosa, Zanthoxylum americanum*

Snakebite Remedy: *Carex plantaginea*

Stimulant: *Gnaphalium obtusifolium, Polygona-tum biflorum, Thuja occidentalis*

Throat Aid: *Coptis trifolia, Valeriana uliginosa*

Tonic: *Asclepias tuberosa, Betula papyrifera, Comptonia peregrina, Echinocystis lobata, Panax quinquefolius, Salix humilis*

Toothache Remedy: *Coptis trifolia*

Tuberculosis Remedy: *Arctium lappa, Hypericum ascyron, Rhus hirta, Rubus occidentalis*

Unspecified: *Abies balsamea, Fagus grandifolia, Menyanthes trifoliata, Myriophyllum spicatum, Osmunda regalis, Pinus banksiana, Quercus alba, Rubus alleghaniensis, Salix bebbiana, Saxifraga pensylvanica, Silene noctiflora, Soli-dago gigantea*

Urinary Aid: *Cypripedium acaule, Eupatorium pur-pureum, Lonicera canadensis, Verbena hastata*

Venereal Aid: *Lonicera canadensis*

Veterinary Aid: *Alnus incana, Larix laricina, Lupi-nus perennis, Pedicularis canadensis, Prunus virginiana, Sisyrinchium albidum*

Witchcraft Medicine: *Arisaema triphyllum, Gnaphalium obtusifolium, Heracleum maxi-mum, Lupinus perennis, Sanicula marilandica, S. odorata, Sarracenia purpurea, Sisyrinchium albidum, Symplocarpus foetidus*

Meskwaki

Adjuvant: *Aralia racemosa, Asarum canadense, Cirsium vulgare, Desmodium illinoense, Juni-perus virginiana, Panax quinquefolius, Ptelea trifoliata, Rubus idaeus, Sanguinaria canaden-sis, Taenidia integerrima*

Alterative: *Pycnanthemum virginianum*

Analgesic: *Acorus calamus, Actaea pachypoda, Anemone cylindrica, Arctium minus, Asarum canadense, Athyrium filix-femina, Celastrus scandens, Cirsium discolor, Comandra umbel-lata, Coreopsis tripteris, Cornus racemosa, Cra-taegus calpodendron, Dioscorea villosa, Echina-cea angustifolia, Echinocystis lobata, Erigeron philadelphicus, Geranium maculatum, Heracle-um maximum, Lycopus americanus, Monarda*

maculatum, Napaea dioica, Polygonum pensyl-vanicum, Prunus virginiana, Rosa blanda

Hemostat: *Agrimonia gryposepala, Gentianella quinquefolia, Platanus occidentalis, Ranunculus abortivus, Salix humilis, Sanicula odorata, Valeriana edulis, Zanthoxylum americanum*

Herbal Steam: *Aster ericoides, A. laevis, A. lateriflorus, Silphium integrifolium*

Hunting Medicine: *Asarum canadense, Napaea dioica*

Internal Medicine: *Pedicularis canadensis*

Kidney Aid: *Apocynum androsaemifolium, A. cannabinum, Baptisia alba, Galium concinnum, Liatris scariosa, Silphium integrifolium, Veronicastrum virginicum, Zanthoxylum americanum*

Laxative: *Carya cordiformis, Fraxinus nigra, Maianthemum racemosum, Pediomelum argophyllum, Rhamnus alnifolia, Salix humilis, Veronicastrum virginicum*

Love Medicine: *Aquilegia canadensis, Cypripedium acaule, Eupatorium purpureum, Filipendula rubra, Iodanthus pinnatifidus, Lobelia cardinalis, L. siphilitica, Panax quinquefolius, Pedicularis canadensis, Phlox pilosa, Thalictrum dasycarpum*

Misc. Disease Remedy: *Achillea millefolium, Apocynum cannabinum, Dalea purpurea, Galium concinnum, Gleditsia triacanthos, Heracleum maximum, Maianthemum racemosum, Malus ioensis, Platanus occidentalis, Pycnanthemum virginianum, Veronicastrum virginicum*

Oral Aid: *Cornus racemosa, Geranium maculatum, Polygonum amphibium, Prunus americana*

Orthopedic Aid: *Coreopsis palmata, Silphium integrifolium*

Other: *Hepatica nobilis, Juniperus virginiana*

Panacea: *Apocynum cannabinum, Carya cordiformis, Clematis viorna, Echinocystis lobata, Fraxinus nigra, Heuchera americana, Morus rubra, Osmorhiza longistylis, Panax quinquefolius*

Pediatric Aid: *Adiantum pedatum, Alnus incana, Cornus racemosa, Maianthemum racemosum, Panax quinquefolius, Polygonum amphibium, Populus tremuloides, Triosteum perfoliatum*

Poison: *Arisaema triphyllum, Helenium autumnale*

Poultice: *Iodanthus pinnatifidus*

Psychological Aid: *Ambrosia trifida, Anemone cylindrica, Aster lateriflorus, Gnaphalium obtusifolium, Gymnocladus dioicus, Maianthemum racemosum, Solidago canadensis, Tradescantia occidentalis, Vitis vulpina*

Pulmonary Aid: *Asarum canadense, Comandra umbellata, Helianthus strumosus, Heliopsis helianthoides, Iris versicolor, Platanus occidentalis, Ptelea trifoliata, Quercus alba, Q. velutina, Sambucus canadensis, Taraxacum officinale, Tilia americana*

Respiratory Aid: *Anemone virginiana, Baptisia alba, Comandra umbellata, Erigeron philadelphicus, Helenium autumnale, Monarda punctata, Ranunculus flabellaris, Sisyrinchium campestre*

Sedative: *Arisaema triphyllum, Humulus lupulus, Maianthemum racemosum, Prunus virginiana*

Snakebite Remedy: *Arisaema triphyllum, Baptisia alba, Ceanothus americanus, Eryngium yuccifolium, Eupatorium perfoliatum, Fraxinus americana, Gentiana andrewsii, Hypericum ascyron, Juglans nigra, Triosteum perfoliatum*

Stimulant: *Actaea pachypoda, Ageratina altissima, Anemone cylindrica, A. virginiana, Aralia nudicaulis, Aster ericoides, A. laevis, A. novae-angliae, A. praealtus, Cornus racemosa, Crataegus calpodendron, Gnaphalium obtusifolium, Juniperus virginiana, Maianthemum racemosum, Monarda punctata, Physalis virginiana, Polygonatum biflorum, Pycnanthemum virginianum, Solidago ulmifolia, Verbena urticifolia, Veronicastrum virginicum*

Strengthener: *Zanthoxylum americanum*

Throat Aid: *Artemisia ludoviciana, Asarum canadense, Senna marilandica*

Tonic: *Gleditsia triacanthos*

Toothache Remedy: *Geranium maculatum, Symplocarpus foetidus, Zanthoxylum americanum*

Tuberculosis Remedy: *Acorus calamus, Artemisia ludoviciana, Campanulastrum americanum, Cornus racemosa, Hypericum ascyron, Zanthoxylum americanum*

Unspecified: *Agastache scrophulariifolia, Capsella bursa-pastoris, Hypericum punctatum, Physalis heterophylla, Salix candida, Scrophularia marilandica, Symplocarpus foetidus*

Urinary Aid: *Actaea pachypoda, Aquilegia canadensis, Caulophyllum thalictroides, Crataegus calpodendron, Diervilla lonicera, Eryngium yuccifolium, Galium concinnum, Laportea canadensis, Liatris punctata, L. scariosa, Mirabilis nyctaginea, Silphium integrifolium*

Venereal Aid: *Diervilla lonicera, Equisetum hyemale, Liatris punctata*

Veterinary Aid: *Artemisia ludoviciana, Celtis occidentalis, Liatris punctata, Maianthemum racemosum, Osmorhiza longistylis*

Mewuk

Antidote: *Angelica tomentosa*

Antiemetic: *Dryopteris arguta*
Antihemorrhagic: *Dryopteris arguta*
Antirheumatic (External): *Heracleum maximum*
Blood Medicine: *Grindelia camporum*
Cathartic: *Artemisia ludoviciana, Frangula californica*
Dermatological Aid: *Artemisia ludoviciana*
Disinfectant: *Artemisia ludoviciana*
Febrifuge: *Salix lasiolepis*
Gastrointestinal Aid: *Artemisia ludoviciana*
Misc. Disease Remedy: *Heracleum maximum, Salix lasiolepis*
Other: *Artemisia ludoviciana*
Panacea: *Artemisia ludoviciana*
Poison: *Chlorogalum pomeridianum*
Unspecified: *Artemisia ludoviciana, Sambucus cerulea*
Veterinary Aid: *Artemisia ludoviciana*

Micmac

Abortifacient: *Aletris farinosa, Fragaria virginiana, Lilium canadense, Rubus pubescens, Sanguinaria canadensis, Sanicula marilandica, Viburnum lentago*
Analgesic: *Aralia racemosa, Asarum canadense, Comptonia peregrina, Cornus sericea, Inula helenium, Kalmia angustifolia, Myrica cerifera, Ranunculus acris, Sanicula marilandica, Sorbus americana, Symplocarpus foetidus, Taxus canadensis, Thuja occidentalis*
Anthelmintic: *Apocynum cannabinum, Tilia americana*
Anticonvulsive: *Aristolochia serpentaria, Cornus canadensis*
Antidiarrheal: *Abies balsamea, Geum rivale, Prunus virginiana, Quercus rubra, Rubus fruticosus, Tiarella cordifolia, Tsuga canadensis*
Antiemetic: *Mentha canadensis, Solanum dulcamara*
Antihemorrhagic: *Acer pensylvanicum, Aralia racemosa, Baptisia tinctoria, Galium aparine, Pyrola asarifolia, Sarracenia purpurea, Streptopus amplexifolius*
Antirheumatic (External): *Achillea millefolium, Myrica cerifera*
Antirheumatic (Internal): *Chimaphila umbellata, Juniperus communis, Sanicula marilandica*
Blood Medicine: *Chimaphila umbellata, Panax quinquefolius, Taxus canadensis*
Burn Dressing: *Abies balsamea, Thuja occidentalis*
Cathartic: *Daucus carota, Juglans cinerea, Ribes uva-crispa, Rumex crispus, Sambucus canadensis*
Cold Remedy: *Abies balsamea, Acer pensylvani-*

cum, Achillea millefolium, Acorus calamus, Angelica sylvestris, Aralia racemosa, Brassica napus, Geum rivale, Inula helenium, Larix laricina, Ledum groenlandicum, Nymphaea odorata, Pinus strobus, Polygala senega, Populus tremuloides, Prunus serotina, Salix cordata, Sanguinaria canadensis, Tsuga canadensis
Contraceptive: *Chelone glabra, Pontederia cordata, Tanacetum vulgare*
Cough Medicine: *Acer alba, A. pensylvanicum, Acorus calamus, Angelica sylvestris, Aralia nudicaulis, A. racemosa, Brassica napus, Geum aleppicum, G. rivale, Ilex aquifolium, Lilium philadelphicum, Nymphaea odorata, Picea glauca, Pinus strobus, Prunus serotina, Rubus chamaemorus, R. hispidus, Thuja occidentalis, Tsuga canadensis*
Dermatological Aid: *Abies balsamea, Achillea millefolium, Aralia racemosa, Arctium lappa, A. minus, Arisaema triphyllum, Betula populifolia, Chimaphila umbellata, Comptonia peregrina, Hydrastis canadensis, Iris versicolor, Juniperus communis, Kalmia angustifolia, Larix americana, L. laricina, Lilium philadelphicum, Maianthemum racemosum, Myrica cerifera, Nuphar lutea, Nymphaea odorata, Picea glauca, Pinus strobus, Populus balsamifera, Prunus pensylvanica, Salix cordata, S. nigra, Sanguinaria canadensis, Scirpus microcarpus, Sedum telephium, Sorbus americana, Tilia americana, Tsuga canadensis, Typha latifolia, Ulmus rubra, Verbascum thapsus*
Diaphoretic: *Achillea millefolium*
Dietary Aid: *Populus tremuloides, Quercus alba, Rhus hirta, Salix cordata*
Diuretic: *Larix americana, Ledum groenlandicum, Polypodium virginianum*
Ear Medicine: *Nicotiana tabacum, Rhus glabra*
Emetic: *Betula populifolia, Euphorbia corollata, Sambucus canadensis, S. racemosa, Sorbus americana*
Eye Medicine: *Acer spicatum, Aralia racemosa, Cornus sericea*
Febrifuge: *Ilex aquifolium, Lilium philadelphicum, Rubus chamaemorus, R. hispidus, Taxus canadensis*
Gastrointestinal Aid: *Abies balsamea, Aletris farinosa, Asarum canadense, Chimaphila umbellata, Picea glauca, Sorbus americana, Taxus canadensis, Tsuga canadensis*
Gland Medicine: *Nymphaea odorata*
Gynecological Aid: *Aralia racemosa, Fraxinus americana, Heracleum sphondylium, Leonurus cardiaca, Sanicula marilandica, Sorbus ameri-*

cana, *Taxus canadensis, Viburnum pruni-folium*

Heart Medicine: *Inula helenium*

Hemorrhoid Remedy: *Quercus alba*

Hemostat: *Nicotiana tabacum, Phytolacca americana, Pinus strobus, Salix lucida, Sanguinaria canadensis*

Kidney Aid: *Acer pensylvanicum, Aralia racemosa, Baptisia tinctoria, Chimaphila umbellata, Cimicifuga racemosa, Eupatorium perfoliatum, Galium aparine, Ledum groenlandicum, Pinus strobus, Pyrola asarifolia, Sanicula marilandica, Sarracenia purpurea, Streptopus amplexifolius, Tanacetum vulgare, Tsuga canadensis*

Laxative: *Abies balsamea*

Liver Aid: *Impatiens capensis*

Love Medicine: *Sanguinaria canadensis*

Misc. Disease Remedy: *Acer pensylvanicum, Acorus calamus, Brassica napus, Chimaphila umbellata, Heracleum maximum, Iris versicolor, Ledum groenlandicum, Nymphaea odorata, Picea glauca, Pinus strobus, Prunus pensylvanica, P. serotina, Sarracenia purpurea, Taxus canadensis, Tsuga canadensis, Viburnum opulus*

Oral Aid: *Alnus incana, Berberis vulgaris, Coptis trifolia*

Orthopedic Aid: *Abies balsamea, Acer pensylvanicum, Achillea millefolium, Arisaema triphyllum, Comptonia peregrina, Juniperus communis, Kalmia angustifolia, Nuphar lutea, Nymphaea odorata, Salix nigra, Thuja occidentalis*

Other: *Adiantum pedatum, Betula alleghaniensis*

Panacea: *Acorus calamus, Iris versicolor, Kalmia angustifolia*

Pediatric Aid: *Geum rivale, Mentha canadensis, Pteridium aquilinum, Rubus fruticosus*

Poison: *Kalmia angustifolia*

Pulmonary Aid: *Acorus calamus, Geum aleppicum, Mentha canadensis, Polypodium virginianum, Sarracenia purpurea, Ulmus rubra*

Respiratory Aid: *Comptonia peregrina, Cornus sericea, Ledum groenlandicum, Salix lucida, Verbascum thapsus*

Sedative: *Cardamine diphylla, Cypripedium acaule, Sambucus canadensis*

Snakebite Remedy: *Sanicula marilandica*

Stimulant: *Aralia racemosa, Comptonia peregrina, Larix laricina, Myrica cerifera, Pteridium aquilinum*

Throat Aid: *Angelica sylvestris, Aralia racemosa, Berberis vulgaris, Cardamine diphylla, Cornus sericea, Iris versicolor, Polystichum acrostichoides, Rhexia virginica, Rhus hirta, Sangui-*

naria canadensis, Sarracenia purpurea, Scirpus microcarpus

Tonic: *Aletris farinosa, Asarum canadense, Cardamine diphylla, Juniperus communis, Ledum groenlandicum, Prunus serotina*

Toothache Remedy: *Thuja occidentalis*

Tuberculosis Remedy: *Aralia racemosa, Chimaphila umbellata, Ilex aquifolium, Juniperus communis, Larix laricina, Lilium philadelphicum, Limonium carolinianum, L. vulgare, Prunus serotina, Rubus chamaemorus, R. hispidus, Sanguinaria canadensis, Sarracenia purpurea, Sinapis alba, Thuja occidentalis*

Unspecified: *Acorus calamus, Coptis trifolia, Gaultheria hispidula, Heracleum sphondylium, Menyanthes trifoliata, Sorbus americana*

Urinary Aid: *Chimaphila umbellata, Clintonia uniflora, Conioselinum chinense, Heracleum sphondylium, Ilex aquifolium, Petroselinum crispum, Platanthera dilatata, Rumex crispus, Tsuga canadensis, Typha angustifolia*

Venereal Aid: *Abies balsamea, Acer pensylvanicum, Aralia racemosa, Arctium lappa, Baptisia tinctoria, Eupatorium perfoliatum, Fagus grandifolia, Galium aparine, Larix laricina, Populus balsamifera, Pyrola asarifolia, Streptopus amplexifolius*

Midoo

Throat Aid: *Quercus douglasii*

Miwok

Analgesic: *Achillea millefolium, Angelica breweri, Artemisia douglasiana, A. vulgaris, Balsamorhiza sagittata, Centaurium exaltatum, Lepechinia calycina, Monardella lanceolata, Polygala cornuta, Rosa californica, Trichostema lanceolatum, Umbellularia californica, Urtica dioica*

Antidiarrheal: *Mentha spicata*

Antihemorrhagic: *Epilobium canum, Pellaea mucronata*

Antirheumatic (External): *Chenopodium ambrosioides, Datisca glomerata, Ericameria arborescens, Eriodictyon californicum, Eriophyllum lanatum, Geranium oreganum, Gnaphalium viscosum, Malva parviflora, Navarretia cotulifolia, Solidago californica, Urtica dioica*

Antirheumatic (Internal): *Agastache urticifolia, Artemisia douglasiana, A. vulgaris, Balsamorhiza sagittata, Chamaebatia foliolosa, Eriodictyon californicum, Mahonia pinnata*

Blood Medicine: *Chamaesyce ocellata, Pellaea mucronata*

Burn Dressing: *Clematis lasiantha, Pinus sabiniana*

Cathartic: *Epilobium canum, Frangula rubra*

Ceremonial Medicine: *Artemisia douglasiana, A. vulgaris*

Cold Remedy: *Achillea millefolium, Angelica breweri, Aristolochia californica, Chamaebatia foliolosa, Ericameria cuneata, Eriodictyon californicum, Gnaphalium viscosum, Keckiella breviflora, Monardella lanceolata, M. odoratissima, Polygala cornuta, Pycnanthemum californicum, Symphoricarpos albus, Trichostema lanceolatum*

Cough Medicine: *Chamaebatia foliolosa, Eriodictyon californicum, Polygala cornuta, Quercus lobata, Q. wislizeni*

Dermatological Aid: *Asclepias speciosa, Chamaesyce serpyllifolia, Chenopodium ambrosioides, Clematis lasiantha, Datisca glomerata, Ericameria arborescens, Erigeron foliosus, Eriodictyon californicum, Grindelia robusta, Hypericum concinnum, Mahonia pinnata, Malva parviflora, Phacelia heterophylla, Pinus sabiniana, Polygonum bistortoides, Quercus lobata, Q. wislizeni, Rumex conglomeratus, Sanicula crassicaulis, Solidago californica, Trichostema lanceolatum*

Diaphoretic: *Balsamorhiza sagittata, Wyethia angustifolia*

Dietary Aid: *Arbutus menziesii, Arctostaphylos manzanita, A. tomentosa, A. viscida*

Emetic: *Polygala cornuta*

Eye Medicine: *Pinus lambertiana, Scutellaria angustifolia, Solanum nigrum*

Febrifuge: *Centaurium venustum, Erigeron foliosus, Holocarpha virgata, Lepechinia calycina, Monardella odoratissima, Wyethia angustifolia*

Gastrointestinal Aid: *Arbutus menziesii, Arctostaphylos manzanita, A. tomentosa, A. viscida, Centaurium exaltatum, Ericameria arborescens, Eriodictyon californicum, Gnaphalium viscosum, Mahonia pinnata, Mentha spicata, Rosa californica, Symphoricarpos albus*

Gynecological Aid: *Epilobium canum, Ericameria arborescens, Trichostema lanceolatum*

Hallucinogen: *Datura wrightii*

Kidney Aid: *Epilobium canum, Galium triflorum*

Misc. Disease Remedy: *Achillea millefolium, Agastache urticifolia, Centaurium venustum, Chamaebatia foliolosa, Erigeron foliosus, Holocarpha virgata, Lepechinia calycina, Mahonia pinnata, Sambucus cerulea, Trichostema lanceolatum*

Orthopedic Aid: *Ericameria arborescens, Eriodictyon californicum*

Other: *Pellaea mucronata*

Panacea: *Sanicula bipinnatifida*

Pediatric Aid: *Quercus lobata, Q. wislizeni*

Pulmonary Aid: *Centaurium venustum*

Snakebite Remedy: *Chamaesyce ocellata, C. serpyllifolia, Daucus pusillus, Sanicula bipinnata, S. bipinnatifida, S. crassicaulis*

Stimulant: *Trichostema lanceolatum*

Toothache Remedy: *Centaurium exaltatum, Chenopodium ambrosioides, Erigeron foliosus, Pentagrama triangularis, Solidago californica, Trichostema lanceolatum*

Tuberculosis Remedy: *Centaurium exaltatum, Epilobium canum, Mahonia pinnata*

Unspecified: *Asclepias cordifolia*

Urinary Aid: *Epilobium canum, Trichostema lanceolatum*

Venereal Aid: *Asclepias speciosa, Chamaebatia foliolosa, Chenopodium ambrosioides, Epilobium canum*

Witchcraft Medicine: *Artemisia douglasiana, A. vulgaris, Sitanion* sp.

Modesse

Antidote: *Rhododendron occidentale*

Antirheumatic (External): *Frangula californica*

Cathartic: *Frangula californica*

Cough Medicine: *Ceanothus velutinus*

Febrifuge: *Ceanothus velutinus*

Kidney Aid: *Croton setigerus*

Mohegan

Abortifacient: *Acorus calamus, Pedicularis canadensis*

Analgesic: *Acorus calamus, Alnus incana, Arctium minus, Arisaema triphyllum, Brassica nigra, Capsella bursa-pastoris, Humulus lupulus, Iris versicolor, Monotropa uniflora, Picea abies, Pinus strobus, Quercus alba, Vitis labrusca*

Anthelmintic: *Artemisia absinthium, Capsella bursa-pastoris, Mentha ×piperita, M. spicata, Rubus hispidus, Salvia officinalis*

Anticonvulsive: *Symplocarpus foetidus*

Antidiarrheal: *Prunus serotina, Rubus hispidus, Spiraea tomentosa*

Antirheumatic (External): *Aesculus glabra, A. hippocastanum, Arctium minus, Arisaema triphyllum, Quercus alba*

Antirheumatic (Internal): *Acorus calamus, Castanea dentata*

Blood Medicine: *Crotalaria sagittalis, Rumex crispus, Sanguinaria canadensis*

Burn Dressing: *Impatiens capensis, Plantago major*

Cathartic: *Euonymus atropurpurea, Sambucus canadensis, Taraxacum officinale*

Cold Remedy: *Acorus calamus, Allium cepa, Anaphalis margaritacea, Arctium minus, Castanea dentata, Eupatorium perfoliatum, Monotropa uniflora, Pinus strobus, Prunus serotina, Quercus alba, Trifolium repens, Ulmus americana, Verbascum thapsus*

Cough Medicine: *Acer saccharinum, A. saccharum, Barbarea vulgaris, Maianthemum racemosum, Pinus strobus, Trifolium repens, Ulmus americana, U. rubra, Verbascum thapsus*

Dermatological Aid: *Baptisia tinctoria, Chimaphila umbellata, Comptonia peregrina, Datura stramonium, Hamamelis virginiana, Impatiens capensis, Picea abies, Pinus strobus, Plantago major, Zea mays*

Dietary Aid: *Achillea millefolium, Tanacetum vulgare*

Ear Medicine: *Humulus lupulus, Nicotiana tabacum*

Emetic: *Sambucus canadensis, Sanguinaria canadensis*

Eye Medicine: *Sassafras albidum*

Febrifuge: *Anthemis cotula, Berberis vulgaris, Eupatorium perfoliatum, Monarda punctata, Monotropa uniflora, Prunella vulgaris, Vitis labrusca*

Gastrointestinal Aid: *Achillea millefolium, Aster umbellatus, Capsella bursa-pastoris, Eupatorium perfoliatum, Hedeoma pulegioides, Maianthemum racemosum, Mentha canadensis, Nepeta cataria, Prunus serotina, Rumex acetosella, Sambucus canadensis, Tanacetum vulgare*

Gynecological Aid: *Leonurus cardiaca, Phytolacca americana*

Heart Medicine: *Zanthoxylum americanum*

Kidney Aid: *Achillea millefolium, Caulophyllum thalictroides, Echium vulgare, Gaultheria procumbens*

Laxative: *Sambucus canadensis*

Liver Aid: *Achillea millefolium*

Misc. Disease Remedy: *Daucus carota*

Oral Aid: *Cirsium arvense, Coptis trifolia, Goodyera pubescens, Pyrola elliptica*

Orthopedic Aid: *Alnus incana, Arisaema triphyllum, Impatiens capensis, Quercus alba*

Panacea: *Acorus calamus, Anthemis cotula, Eupatorium perfoliatum, Panax quinquefolius, Salvia officinalis*

Pediatric Aid: *Cirsium arvense, Coptis trifolia,*

Goodyera pubescens, Mentha ×piperita, Nepeta cataria, Sambucus canadensis

Poison: *Arisaema triphyllum, Phytolacca americana*

Pulmonary Aid: *Asclepias tuberosa, Castanea dentata, Cirsium arvense, Inula helenium, Ulmus rubra*

Respiratory Aid: *Prunus americana, Verbascum thapsus*

Sedative: *Humulus lupulus*

Snakebite Remedy: *Aristolochia serpentaria, Plantago major*

Throat Aid: *Amaranthus retroflexus, Arisaema triphyllum, Berberis vulgaris, Pyrola elliptica, Rhus hirta, Ulmus rubra, Verbascum thapsus*

Tonic: *Acorus calamus, Aralia nudicaulis, Betula lenta, Eupatorium perfoliatum, Leonurus cardiaca, Leucanthemum vulgare, Maianthemum racemosum, Panax quinquefolius, Prunus serotina, Rumex crispus, Salvia officinalis, Sanguinaria canadensis, Sassafras albidum, Taraxacum officinale*

Toothache Remedy: *Armoracia rusticana, Brassica nigra, Humulus lupulus, Rorippa nasturtium-aquaticum*

Tuberculosis Remedy: *Cirsium arvense, Inula helenium*

Unspecified: *Vaccinium oxycoccos*

Veterinary Aid: *Inula helenium, Quercus alba*

Montagnais

Analgesic: *Iris versicolor, Kalmia angustifolia, Maianthemum canadense, Ranunculus acris, Salix lucida*

Anthelmintic: *Populus tremuloides*

Blood Medicine: *Hudsonia tomentosa, Ledum groenlandicum, Sorbus americana*

Cathartic: *Lycopodium dendroideum*

Cold Remedy: *Kalmia angustifolia, Pinus strobus*

Cough Medicine: *Anaphalis margaritacea, Gnaphalium obtusifolium, Hypericum perforatum, Picea mariana, Polygala polygama*

Dermatological Aid: *Platanthera orbiculata*

Diaphoretic: *Chimaphila umbellata, Streptopus roseus, Thuja occidentalis*

Dietary Aid: *Abies balsamea, Sorbus americana*

Diuretic: *Lonicera canadensis*

Expectorant: *Larix laricina*

Eye Medicine: *Viburnum opulus*

Febrifuge: *Achillea millefolium, Ledum groenlandicum, Lycopodium clavatum, Mitchella repens, Taxus canadensis*

Gastrointestinal Aid: *Kalmia angustifolia, Lycopodium dendroideum*

Liver Aid: *Ledum groenlandicum*

Misc. Disease Remedy: *Sarracenia purpurea*

Orthopedic Aid: *Cornus canadensis, Linnaea borealis, Moneses uniflora, Pteridium aquilinum*

Panacea: *Asarum canadense, Pontederia cordata, Pyrola asarifolia, Streptopus amplexifolius, Trientalis borealis*

Pediatric Aid: *Ledum groenlandicum, Pteridium aquilinum*

Poison: *Kalmia angustifolia*

Pulmonary Aid: *Picea rubens, Vaccinium macrocarpon*

Stimulant: *Aralia nudicaulis, Lycopodium clavatum, Pyrola elliptica, Taxus canadensis*

Throat Aid: *Picea rubens, Pinus strobus, Rhexia virginica*

Tonic: *Aralia nudicaulis, Picea glauca*

Tuberculosis Remedy: *Anaphalis margaritacea, Cirsium arvense, Gnaphalium obtusifolium, Pinus strobus, Trientalis borealis*

Montana Indian

Adjuvant: *Salix exigua, S. melanopsis*

Alterative: *Rubus parviflorus*

Analgesic: *Cicuta douglasii, Clematis hirsutissima, Zigadenus venenosus*

Antidiarrheal: *Artemisia tridentata, Geranium oreganum, Matricaria discoidea*

Antirheumatic (External): *Juniperus scopulorum, Pseudotsuga menziesii, Salix exigua, S. melanopsis, Sambucus cerulea, Zigadenus venenosus*

Burn Dressing: *Typha latifolia*

Cancer Treatment: *Orobanche fasciculata, Ulmus americana*

Cathartic: *Achillea millefolium, Apocynum androsaemifolium, Aralia nudicaulis*

Ceremonial Medicine: *Catabrosa aquatica, Glyceria fluitans, Juniperus scopulorum, Oplopanax horridus*

Cold Remedy: *Abies lasiocarpa, Clematis ligusticifolia, Salix exigua, S. melanopsis*

Dermatological Aid: *Abies lasiocarpa, Artemisia cana, Cornus sericea, Dalea purpurea, Erythronium grandiflorum, Geranium oreganum, Mentzelia laevicaulis, Pediomelum argophyllum, Sambucus cerulea, Yucca glauca, Zigadenus venenosus*

Dietary Aid: *Artemisia cana, Scirpus acutus*

Emetic: *Frangula purshiana, Iris missouriensis, Purshia tridentata, Sambucus cerulea*

Eye Medicine: *Artemisia tridentata*

Febrifuge: *Abies lasiocarpa, Apocynum androsaemifolium, Chimaphila umbellata, Mahonia*

repens, Salix exigua, S. melanopsis, Sambucus cerulea

Gastrointestinal Aid: *Mahonia repens, Mentzelia laevicaulis, Sambucus cerulea*

Gynecological Aid: *Matricaria discoidea, Monarda fistulosa*

Kidney Aid: *Juniperus chinense, Mahonia repens*

Misc. Disease Remedy: *Rhus trilobata, Rubus parviflorus*

Oral Aid: *Echinacea angustifolia*

Orthopedic Aid: *Artemisia tridentata*

Poison: *Apocynum androsaemifolium, Cicuta maculata, Lomatium dissectum, Orobanche fasciculata*

Pulmonary Aid: *Abies lasiocarpa, Artemisia frigida, Purshia tridentata, Sambucus cerulea*

Snakebite Remedy: *Cicuta douglasii, Echinacea angustifolia*

Throat Aid: *Clematis ligusticifolia, Glycyrrhiza lepidota*

Tonic: *Apocynum androsaemifolium, Aralia nudicaulis, Artemisia cana, Glycyrrhiza lepidota, Mahonia repens*

Tuberculosis Remedy: *Artemisia frigida*

Unspecified: *Artemisia cana, Frangula purshiana, Mentha canadensis*

Venereal Aid: *Grindelia squarrosa, Pseudotsuga menziesii*

Veterinary Aid: *Clematis hirsutissima*

Montauk

Toothache Remedy: *Nicotiana tabacum*

Nanticoke

Analgesic: *Pinus echinata*

Anthelmintic: *Aristolochia serpentaria*

Burn Dressing: *Impatiens capensis*

Cathartic: *Pinus echinata*

Cold Remedy: *Acorus calamus, Monarda punctata, Symplocarpus foetidus*

Dermatological Aid: *Arctium minus, Impatiens capensis, Opuntia humifusa*

Diaphoretic: *Hedeoma pulegioides, Tanacetum vulgare*

Febrifuge: *Eupatorium perfoliatum, Hepatica nobilis, Sassafras albidum, Verbascum thapsus*

Gastrointestinal Aid: *Acorus calamus*

Kidney Aid: *Hedeoma pulegioides*

Liver Aid: *Hedeoma pulegioides*

Misc. Disease Remedy: *Chimaphila maculata, C. umbellata, Sassafras albidum*

Orthopedic Aid: *Baptisia tinctoria, Impatiens capensis, Pinus echinata, Populus deltoides, Yucca filamentosa*

Pediatric Aid: *Acorus calamus, Peltandra virginica*
Tonic: *Leiophyllum buxifolium*
Unspecified: *Peltandra virginica*

Narraganset
Cold Remedy: *Prunus serotina*

Natchez
Anthelmintic: *Chenopodium ambrosioides*
Antidiarrheal: *Eryngium yuccifolium*
Cold Remedy: *Collinsia violacea*
Cough Medicine: *Collinsia violacea, Tephrosia virginiana*
Dermatological Aid: *Rhus aromatica, R. hirta*
Emetic: *Ilex vomitoria*
Febrifuge: *Aristolochia serpentaria, Chenopodium ambrosioides*
Hemostat: *Eryngium yuccifolium*
Pediatric Aid: *Chenopodium ambrosioides, Hypericum hypericoides*
Pulmonary Aid: *Collinsia violacea*
Tuberculosis Remedy: *Collinsia violacea*
Urinary Aid: *Hypericum hypericoides*
Witchcraft Medicine: *Potentilla canadensis*

Navajo
Abortifacient: *Tetradymia canescens*
Analgesic: *Artemisia tridentata, A. tripartita, Clematis ligusticifolia, Cryptantha fulvocanescens, Dalea candida, Eriogonum alatum, Gentiana affinis, Gutierrezia sarothrae, Hedeoma drummondii, Juniperus osteosperma, Machaeranthera pinnatifida, Monarda fistulosa, M. pectinata, Portulaca oleracea, Sagittaria cuneata*
Antidiarrheal: *Lactuca virosa*
Antidote: *Eupatorium purpureum*
Antiemetic: *Dugaldia hoopesii, Lactuca virosa, Yucca baccata*
Antihemorrhagic: *Krascheninnikovia lanata*
Antirheumatic (Internal): *Corydalis aurea, Mahonia repens, Mirabilis multiflora*
Blood Medicine: *Hymenopappus filifolius*
Burn Dressing: *Castilleja integra, Gaura parviflora, Phlox caespitosa*
Carminative: *Pectis angustifolia, Solanum fendleri*
Cathartic: *Chamaesyce lata, Euphorbia robusta, Machaeranthera parviflora, Phlox caespitosa, Prunus persica*
Ceremonial Medicine: *Artemisia tridentata, A. tripartita, Gutierrezia sarothrae, Hedeoma nana, Helianthus annuus, Ipomopsis longiflora, Juniperus scopulorum, Kochia scoparia, Lomatium dissectum, Oreoxis alpina, Parthenocissus vitacea, Pectis angustifolia, Phlox caespitosa, Pinus*

edulis, P. ponderosa, Sphaeralcea angustifolia, Townsendia exscapa, Tribulus terrestris, Vicia faba, Zea mays
Cold Remedy: *Artemisia tridentata, Cryptantha fulvocanescens, Lithospermum incisum, Sphaeralcea angustifolia, Tagetes micrantha*
Contraceptive: *Lithospermum incisum, L. ruderale, Ricinus communis*
Cough Medicine: *Cryptantha fulvocanescens, Ephedra viridis, Lithospermum incisum, Sphaeralcea angustifolia*
Dermatological Aid: *Abronia fragrans, Achillea millefolium, Artemisia tripartita, Atriplex canescens, Camissonia tanacetifolia, Chrysothamnus greenei, Comandra umbellata, Eupatorium purpureum, Euphorbia robusta, Gaura parviflora, Gutierrezia sarothrae, Juniperus osteosperma, J. scopulorum, Kochia scoparia, Krascheninnikovia lanata, Lesquerella fendleri, Lithospermum incisum, Lupinus brevicaulis, L. lyallii, Machaeranthera alta, Mirabilis multiflora, Orobanche fasciculata, Phoradendron juniperinum, Pinus edulis, Salsola australis, Sarcobatus vermiculatus, Senecio multicapitatus, Thelypodium wrightii, Xanthium strumarium, Yucca glauca*
Diaphoretic: *Sanvitalia abertii*
Dietary Aid: *Chenopodium album, Helianthus annuus*
Disinfectant: *Lepidium lasiocarpum*
Diuretic: *Draba rectifructa, Penstemon barbatus, Phlox caespitosa*
Emetic: *Chrysothamnus viscidiflorus, Cirsium vulgare, Cordylanthus ramosus, Eriogonum rotundifolium, Ipomopsis longiflora, Mentzelia multiflora, Pinus edulis*
Eye Medicine: *Solanum elaeagnifolium*
Febrifuge: *Artemisia tridentata, Cirsium neomexicanum, Shepherdia argentea, Tagetes micrantha*
Gastrointestinal Aid: *Abronia fragrans, Artemisia tridentata, Castilleja angustifolia, C. integra, C. lineata, Cercocarpus montanus, Chamaesyce fendleri, C. lata, Cucurbita pepo, Dalea candida, Ephedra trifurca, Fendlera rupicola, Helianthus nuttallii, Heuchera bracteata, Ipomopsis aggregata, I. longiflora, Lactuca virosa, Pectis angustifolia, Plantago patagonica, Portulaca oleracea, Solanum fendleri, Stenotus lanuginosus, Tagetes micrantha, Townsendia strigosa, Verbesina encelioides, Yucca baccata*
Gland Medicine: *Stanleya pinnata*
Gynecological Aid: *Ambrosia tenuifolia, Amelanchier utahensis, Artemisia tridentata, Asclepias hallii, Clematis ligusticifolia, Cordylanthus*

ramosus, Cryptantha fulvocanescens, Erigeron divergens, Euphorbia robusta, Lappula occidentalis, Phlox caespitosa, Purshia tridentata, Rorippa alpina, Townsendia incana, T. strigosa

Heart Medicine: *Echinocereus coccineus*

Hemostat: *Cordylanthus ramosus, Lappula occidentalis, Sphaeralcea coccinea*

Kidney Aid: *Ephedra nevadensis, E. trifurca*

Laxative: *Plantago patagonica, Yucca glauca*

Love Medicine: *Vitis arizonica*

Misc. Disease Remedy: *Astragalus kentrophyta, Chrysothamnus greenei, Gaillardia pinnatifida, Krascheninnikovia lanata, Sphaeralcea angustifolia*

Nose Medicine: *Asclepias verticillata, Machaeranthera canescens, Sisyrinchium mucronatum, Solanum elaeagnifolium, Stenotus lanuginosus, Townsendia strigosa, Zinnia grandiflora*

Oral Aid: *Heuchera bracteata, Mirabilis multiflora, Sanvitalia abertii, Stenotus lanuginosus*

Orthopedic Aid: *Cordylanthus ramosus*

Other: *Tagetes micrantha*

Panacea: *Argythamnia cyanophylla, Portulaca oleracea*

Pediatric Aid: *Lithospermum incisum, Plantago patagonica*

Poison: *Echinocereus coccineus, Opuntia polyacantha, Vicia faba*

Pulmonary Aid: *Dalea purpurea*

Reproductive Aid: *Lupinus brevicaulis*

Respiratory Aid: *Amorpha nana, Physaria newberryi*

Sedative: *Ceanothus fendleri, Frasera speciosa, Gutierrezia sarothrae, Shinnersoseris rostrata*

Snakebite Remedy: *Gutierrezia sarothrae*

Sports Medicine: *Artemisia tridentata*

Stimulant: *Achillea millefolium, Gentiana affinis, Rumex crispus, Thelesperma megapotamicum, Yucca glauca*

Throat Aid: *Asclepias verticillata, Eriogonum rotundifolium, Machaeranthera canescens, Marrubium vulgare, Sisyrinchium mucronatum, Solanum elaeagnifolium, Stenotus lanuginosus, Townsendia strigosa, Zea mays, Zinnia grandiflora*

Tonic: *Achillea millefolium, Clematis ligusticifolia*

Toothache Remedy: *Dalea candida, Heuchera bracteata, Phlox caespitosa, Stenotus lanuginosus, Thelesperma megapotamicum*

Unspecified: *Artemisia ludoviciana, Delphinium menziesii, D. scaposum, Eriogonum rotundifolium, Juniperus scopulorum, Prunus virginiana, Rumex hymenosepalus*

Venereal Aid: *Cordylanthus ramosus, C. wrightii,*

Ephedra nevadensis, E. trifurca, E. viridis, Ranunculus cymbalaria

Veterinary Aid: *Atriplex confertifolia, Datura wrightii, Gutierrezia microcephala, G. sarothrae, Ipomopsis longiflora, Muhlenbergia dubia, Verbascum thapsus*

Witchcraft Medicine: *Eriogonum fasciculatum, Gentiana affinis, Sphaeralcea coccinea*

Navajo, Kayenta

Analgesic: *Achillea millefolium, Androsace septentrionalis, Aquilegia triternata, Cymopterus purpurascens, Equisetum laevigatum, Erigeron concinnus, E. divergens, Eriogonum racemosum, Euphorbia robusta, Juniperus scopulorum, Linum lewisii, Pseudotsuga menziesii, Shepherdia rotundifolia*

Anticonvulsive: *Arabis perennans, Mimulus eastwoodiae*

Antidiarrheal: *Asclepias nyctaginifolia, Corydalis aurea, Dracocephalum parviflorum, Gutierrezia sarothrae, Psilostrophe sparsiflora, Pyrola chlorantha*

Antidote: *Senecio neomexicanus*

Antiemetic: *Cymopterus purpurascens, Malacothrix sonchoides*

Blood Medicine: *Antennaria parvifolia, Conioselinum scopulorum, Ipomopsis gunnisonii, I. longiflora, Psilostrophe sparsiflora*

Burn Dressing: *Chenopodium album, Potentilla hippiana, Senecio neomexicanus*

Cathartic: *Abronia fragrans, Fendlera rupicola, Ipomopsis aggregata*

Ceremonial Medicine: *Apocynum cannabinum, Aquilegia triternata, Arctostaphylos patula, Artemisia campestris, Asclepias speciosa, Astragalus sesquiflorus, Brickellia californica, Bromus tectorum, Ceanothus fendleri, Chrysothamnus nauseosus, Cleome lutea, Cordylanthus wrightii, Cornus sericea, Epipactis gigantea, Eriogonum divaricatum, Fendlera rupicola, Frangula betulifolia, Gutierrezia sarothrae, Helianthus annuus, Heterotheca villosa, Lesquerella intermedia, Maianthemum stellatum, Mentzelia multiflora, Oenothera cespitosa, O. elata, O. pallida, Petrophyton caespitosum, Psathyrotes pilifera, Pseudocymopterus montanus, Pseudostellaria jamesiana, Ribes cereum, Shepherdia rotundifolia, Sphaeralcea coccinea, Tetraneuris argentea*

Cold Remedy: *Oenothera elata*

Dermatological Aid: *Abronia fragrans, Adiantum capillus-veneris, Astragalus calycosus, A. sesquiflorus, Brickellia californica, B. oblongifolia,*

*Castilleja angustifolia, Chamaesaracha corono-
pus, Chamaesyce revoluta, Chenopodium capi-
tatum, Clematis ligusticifolia, Cleome lutea,
Conyza canadensis, Corallorrhiza maculata,
Corydalis aurea, Cryptantha crassisepala, Cy-
mopterus newberryi, Dalea candida, D. lanata,
Descurainia incana, Dimorphocarpa wislizeni,
Encelia frutescens, Erigeron neomexicanus,
Eriogonum alatum, E. cernuum, E. inflatum,
Erodium cicutarium, Frasera albomarginata,
Gayophytum ramosissimum, Gilia leptomeria,
Heuchera parvifolia, Hymenopappus filifolius,
Ipomopsis aggregata, I. gunnisonii, Isocoma
pluriflora, Iva xanthifolia, Lappula occidenta-
lis, Leptodactylon pungens, Lygodesmia grandi-
flora, Mentha arvensis, Mentzelia multiflora,
Mirabilis oxybaphoides, M. pumila, Nama hispidum, Oenothera brachycarpa, O. cespitosa, O.
elata, O. pallida, Orobanche ludoviciana,
Penstemon ambiguus, P. eatonii, Petradoria
pumila, Phyla cuneifolia, Poliomintha incana,
Potentilla hippiana, Psathyrotes pilifera, Pseudostellaria jamesiana, Psilostrophe sparsiflora,
Psoralidium lanceolatum, Rhus trilobata, Ribes
cereum, Senecio flaccidus, Shepherdia rotundifolia, Sphaeralcea coccinea, S. fendleri, Tetraneuris argentea, Vanclevea stylosa, Verbesina
encelioides*

Diaphoretic: *Abronia fragrans*

Dietary Aid: *Sphaeralcea coccinea*

Disinfectant: *Artemisia campestris, Conyza canadensis, Corydalis aurea, Cryptantha cinerea,
Eriogonum umbellatum, Erodium cicutarium,
Gaura parviflora, Gutierrezia sarothrae, Helianthus annuus, Linum lewisii, Lupinus pusillus, Mentha arvensis, Mentzelia multiflora, Penstemon ambiguus, P. eatonii, Pseudotsuga
menziesii, Sambucus cerulea, Senecio neomexicanus, Sphaeralcea coccinea*

Ear Medicine: *Astragalus pattersonii, Conyza canadensis, Lupinus pusillus*

Emetic: *Abronia fragrans, Apocynum cannabinum, Arctostaphylos patula, Asclepias speciosa,
Astragalus lonchocarpus, A. pattersonii, A.
sesquiflorus, Atriplex canescens, Brickellia californica, Ceanothus fendleri, Chrysothamnus
nauseosus, Cornus sericea, Eriogonum umbellatum, E. wrightii, Frangula betulifolia, Ipomopsis aggregata, Oenothera elata, O. pallida, Penstemon eatonii, P. jamesii, Psathyrotes pilifera,
Pseudocymopterus montanus, Ribes cereum,
Shepherdia rotundifolia, Wyethia scabra*

Eye Medicine: *Achillea millefolium, Astragalus pattersonii, Chenopodium capitatum, Comandra*

*umbellata, Cryptantha flava, Lesquerella inter-
media, Streptanthus cordatus, Thelypodium
wrightii*

Febrifuge: *Achillea millefolium, Baccharis salicifolia, Cirsium rothrockii*

Gastrointestinal Aid: *Abronia fragrans, Atriplex
canescens, Celtis laevigata, Conyza canadensis,
Cryptantha flava, Cymopterus purpurascens,
Epilobium angustifolium, Erigeron neomexicanus, Eriogonum umbellatum, Gutierrezia sarothrae, Ipomopsis aggregata, Lepidium densiflorum, L. montanum, Mentzelia multiflora,
Mirabilis linearis, Monarda pectinata, Penstemon eatonii, Pseudotsuga menziesii, Rhus trilobata, Rumex maritimus, Suaeda moquinii,
Tiquilia latior, Wyethia scabra*

Gynecological Aid: *Acourtia wrightii, Aquilegia
micrantha, Campanula parryi, Conioselinum
scopulorum, Cordylanthus wrightii, Corydalis
aurea, Cryptantha flava, Delphinium scaposum,
Erigeron concinnus, Euphorbia incisa, Gaura
parviflora, Gilia subnuda, Houstonia rubra,
Ipomopsis longiflora, Lathyrus eucosmus, Mirabilis linearis, Oenothera cespitosa, Potentilla
hippiana, Psilostrophe sparsiflora, Pyrola
chlorantha, Townsendia incana*

Heart Medicine: *Polypogon monspeliensis, Sonchus asper*

Hemorrhoid Remedy: *Dimorphocarpa wislizeni*

Hemostat: *Aquilegia micrantha, Lupinus pusillus,
Nicotiana attenuata, Penstemon eatonii, Pyrola
chlorantha*

Kidney Aid: *Chaetopappa ericoides, Eriogonum
cernuum, Leptodactylon pungens, Linum australe, Oenothera pallida*

Laxative: *Artemisia tridentata, Oxytropis lambertii*

Love Medicine: *Tradescantia occidentalis*

Misc. Disease Remedy: *Astragalus pattersonii,
Cirsium rothrockii, Oenothera elata, Portulaca
oleracea, Stephanomeria exigua*

Narcotic: *Comandra umbellata, Datura wrightii,
Nicotiana attenuata, Petrophyton caespitosum,
Stephanomeria pauciflora*

Nose Medicine: *Evolvulus nuttallianus*

Oral Aid: *Comandra umbellata, Sphaeralcea
fendleri*

Orthopedic Aid: *Cymopterus purpurascens, Datura
wrightii, Epilobium ciliatum, Equisetum laevigatum, Eriogonum divaricatum, E. racemosum,
Penstemon eatonii*

Other: *Apocynum cannabinum, Astragalus calyco-
sus, A. pattersonii, Camissonia multijuga,
Chamaesaracha coronopus, Epipactis gigantea,
Gaillardia pinnatifida, Geranium atropurpure-*

um, *Hymenopappus filifolius, Lepidium montanum, Sphaeralcea coccinea*

Panacea: *Abronia fragrans, Cirsium rothrockii, Dalea candida, Dracocephalum parviflorum, Eriogonum alatum, Frasera speciosa, Mahonia repens, Mirabilis linearis, Psilostrophe sparsiflora, Ranunculus cymbalaria, Rumex hymenosepalus*

Pediatric Aid: *Asclepias nyctaginifolia, Brickellia californica, B. oblongifolia, Conyza canadensis, Cryptantha cinerea, Dimorphocarpa wislizeni, Dracocephalum parviflorum, Epipactis gigantea, Helianthus annuus, Isocoma pluriflora, Lepidium densiflorum, Mentha arvensis, Penstemon jamesii, Pyrola chlorantha, Ribes cereum, Shepherdia rotundifolia, Solidago velutina, Thelypodium wrightii*

Poison: *Sonchus asper*

Poultice: *Astragalus calycosus, A. lonchocarpus*

Psychological Aid: *Adiantum capillus-veneris, Arabis perennans, Eriogonum jamesii, Gayophytum ramosissimum, Solidago velutina, Tetraneuris argentea, Thymophylla pentachaeta*

Respiratory Aid: *Asclepias asperula, A. auriculata, Conioselinum scopulorum*

Sedative: *Gilia leptomeria, Ipomopsis polycladon, Lepidium densiflorum, Quercus ×pauciloba, Thelypodium wrightii*

Snakebite Remedy: *Artemisia tridentata, Conioselinum scopulorum, Cryptantha cinerea, Eremocrinum albomarginatum, Eriogonum divaricatum, Penstemon eatonii, P. palmeri, Tragia nepetifolia*

Strengthener: *Sphaeralcea coccinea*

Throat Aid: *Astragalus pattersonii, Descurainia incana, Shepherdia rotundifolia, Symphoricarpos oreophilus*

Tonic: *Gilia leptomeria, Ipomopsis polycladon*

Toothache Remedy: *Asclepias involucrata, Dimorphocarpa wislizeni, Lycium pallidum, Phlox austromontana, Shepherdia rotundifolia*

Unspecified: *Townsendia incana*

Urinary Aid: *Chaetopappa ericoides*

Venereal Aid: *Kochia americana, Oenothera pallida*

Veterinary Aid: *Asclepias hallii, Collinsia parviflora, Corydalis aurea, Cryptantha cinerea, Dalea candida, Delphinium scaposum, Euphorbia incisa, Frasera speciosa, Iva xanthifolia, Oenothera pallida, Penstemon ambiguus, P. eatonii, Reverchonia arenaria, Sambucus cerulea, Thelypodiopsis elegans, Vicia americana, Zigadenus paniculatus*

Witchcraft Medicine: *Androsace septentrionalis,*

Euphorbia robusta, Fallugia paradoxa, Gaillardia pinnatifida

Navajo, Ramah

Adjuvant: *Oenothera coronopifolia*

Analgesic: *Ageratina herbacea, Androsace septentrionalis, Apocynum cannabinum, Arabis perennans, Arenaria lanuginosa, Artemisia tridentata, Atriplex argentea, A. canescens, Bahia dissecta, Brickellia grandiflora, Campanula rotundifolia, Castilleja linariifolia, Chamaesyce albomarginata, C. fendleri, C. serpyllifolia, Chrysothamnus nauseosus, Clematis hirsutissima, C. ligusticifolia, Cordylanthus wrightii, Corydalis aurea, Dalea candida, Datura wrightii, Dracocephalum parviflorum, Erigeron concinnus, E. speciosus, Eriogonum jamesii, E. leptophyllum, Erysimum capitatum, Galium fendleri, Gutierrezia sarothrae, Heuchera novomexicana, H. parviflora, Ipomopsis longiflora, Juniperus monosperma, J. scopulorum, Lotus wrightii, Marrubium vulgare, Menodora scabra, Monarda pectinata, M. punctata, Nicotiana attenuata, Oenothera coronopifolia, Oxalis drummondii, Penstemon barbatus, P. jamesii, Pericome caudata, Pinus edulis, Polygonum aviculare, P. ramosissimum, Potentilla norvegica, Prunus virginiana, Psilostrophe tagetina, Psoralidium lanceolatum, Quercus gambelii, Q. ×pauciloba, Ratibida tagetes, Rhus trilobata, Sanvitalia abertii, Senecio multilobatus, Tetradymia canescens, Thermopsis rhombifolia, Zinnia grandiflora*

Antidiarrheal: *Chamaesyce fendleri, C. serpyllifolia, Eriogonum alatum*

Antidote: *Amaranthus retroflexus, Bouteloua gracilis, Chenopodium album, C. incanum, Gutierrezia sarothrae, Krascheninnikovia lanata*

Antiemetic: *Gaillardia pinnatifida, Gaura coccinea*

Antihemorrhagic: *Sphaeralcea fendleri*

Antirheumatic (Internal): *Bahia dissecta, Ipomopsis longiflora*

Blood Medicine: *Castilleja integra, Cleome serrulata, Eriogonum racemosum*

Burn Dressing: *Castilleja integra, Mirabilis linearis, M. oblongifolia, Oenothera flava, Penstemon barbatus, Pinus edulis, Silene laciniata*

Cathartic: *Chrysothamnus nauseosus, Glycyrrhiza lepidota, Lotus wrightii, Orthocarpus purpureoalbus, Petradoria pumila, Psilostrophe tagetina, Quercus gambelii, Ratibida tagetes, Senecio multicapitatus, Zinnia grandiflora*

Ceremonial Medicine: *Achillea millefolium, Agastache pallidiflora, Agoseris aurantiaca,*

Amelanchier utahensis, Antennaria parvifolia, Apocynum cannabinum, A. ×floribundum, Arceuthobium campylopodum, A. vaginatum, Arctostaphylos pungens, A. uva-ursi, Asclepias asperula, A. tuberosa, Aster praealtus, Astragalus allochrous, A. bisulcatus, A. humistratus, A. kentrophyta, A. mollissimus, A. praelongus, Atriplex canescens, Baccharis wrightii, Besseya plantaginea, Brickellia grandiflora, Calochortus gunnisonii, Campanula rotundifolia, Carex microptera, Ceanothus fendleri, Chamaesyce fendleri, C. serpyllifolia, Chrysothamnus nauseosus, Cleome serrulata, Coreopsis tinctoria, Cornus sericea, Cosmos parviflorus, Cryptantha cinerea, Cuscuta megalocarpa, Cyperus esculentus, Datura wrightii, Dichanthelium oligosanthes, Draba helleriana, Echinochloa crus-pavonis, Eleocharis montevidensis, E. rostellata, Erigeron bellidiastrum, E. canus, E. divergens, E. eximius, E. flagellaris, Eriogonum alatum, E. annuum, Erysimum capitatum, Fallugia paradoxa, Forestiera pubescens, Galium fendleri, Gnaphalium stramineum, Gutierrezia sarothrae, Heterotheca villosa, Houstonia wrightii, Hymenoxys richardsonii, Ipomopsis longiflora, I. multiflora, Iris missouriensis, Juniperus communis, J. monosperma, J. scopulorum, Lactuca serriola, Lesquerella rectipes, Limosella aquatica, Lonicera arizonica, L. involucrata, Lupinus caudatus, Luzula multiflora, Lycium pallidum, L. torreyi, Mahonia repens, Maianthemum stellatum, Monarda pectinata, Monolepis nuttalliana, Nicotiana attenuata, Oenothera albicaulis, O. pallida, O. primiveris, Orthocarpus purpureoalbus, Parryella filifolia, Paxistima myrsinites, Penstemon jamesii, Pericome caudata, Peteria scoparia, Petradoria pumila, Picea engelmannii, Pinus edulis, P. flexilis, P. ponderosa, Polygonum lapathifolium, Potamogeton natans, Prunus virginiana, Pseudocymopterus montanus, Pseudotsuga menziesii, Psilostrophe tagetina, Psoralidium lanceolatum, Purshia stansburiana, P. tridentata, Pyrrhopappus pauciflorus, Quercus gambelii, Ranunculus cymbalaria, Ratibida tagetes, Ribes pinetorum, Rorippa palustris, Rosa woodsii, Rumex crispus, R. hymenosepalus, R. salicifolius, Salix exigua, S. lucida, Schoenocrambe linearifolia, Scirpus acutus, S. pallidus, Senecio fendleri, S. multilobatus, Sinapis arvensis, Stachys rothrockii, Symphoricarpos oreophilus, Tetraclea coulteri, Tetradymia canescens, Thalictrum fendleri, Thlaspi montanum, Tragopogon porrifolius, T. pratensis, Trifolium dubium, *Typha latifolia, Verbena bracteata, V. macdougalii, Veronica americana, V. peregrina, Viola nephrophylla, Yucca baccata, Zinnia grandiflora*

Cold Remedy: *Chrysothamnus nauseosus, Juniperus scopulorum, Melilotus officinalis, Pinus edulis, Sanvitalia abertii, Tetradymia canescens*

Contraceptive: *Bahia dissecta, Erigeron speciosus, Eriogonum jamesii, Phlox stansburyi, Rhus trilobata, Yucca glauca*

Cough Medicine: *Agastache pallidiflora, Artemisia carruthii, A. frigida, A. tridentata, Atriplex canescens, Brickellia californica, B. eupatorioides, Chrysothamnus nauseosus, Cryptantha fendleri, Draba helleriana, Ephedra torreyana, Erigeron eximius, Eriogonum alatum, Humulus lupulus, Hymenopappus filifolius, Iva xanthifolia, Juniperus communis, J. monosperma, Mirabilis linearis, Monarda pectinata, M. punctata, Nicotiana attenuata, Penstemon barbatus, Pericome caudata, Pinus edulis, P. flexilis, P. ponderosa, Purshia stansburiana, Ratibida tagetes, Tetradymia canescens, Thermopsis rhombifolia, Valeriana acutiloba, Verbascum thapsus*

Dermatological Aid: *Abronia fragrans, Agastache pallidiflora, Agoseris aurantiaca, Allionia incarnata, Arenaria lanuginosa, Artemisia carruthii, A. dracunculus, A. tridentata, Asclepias tuberosa, Astragalus humistratus, Atriplex argentea, A. canescens, Besseya plantaginea, Bouteloua gracilis, B. simplex, Calochortus gunnisonii, Campanula parryi, Chamaesyce fendleri, C. serpyllifolia, Cheilanthes wootonii, Cleome serrulata, Convolvulus arvensis, Conyza canadensis, Cryptantha cinerea, Cystopteris fragilis, Dimorphocarpa wislizeni, Draba reptans, Drymaria glandulosa, Dyssodia papposa, Erigeron flagellaris, Eriogonum abertianum, E. alatum, E. annuum, E. cernuum, Geranium lentum, Grindelia nuda, Gutierrezia sarothrae, Helianthella parryi, Helianthus annuus, Heterotheca villosa, Heuchera novomexicana, Houstonia wrightii, Hymenopappus filifolius, Hymenoxys richardsonii, Ipomopsis longiflora, Juniperus monosperma, Krascheninnikovia lanata, Lappula occidentalis, Limosella aquatica, Lupinus argenteus, L. caudatus, L. kingii, Machaeranthera gracilis, Mahonia repens, Malacothrix fendleri, Mirabilis multiflora, Monarda fistulosa, Monolepis nuttalliana, Myosurus cupulatus, M. minimus, Oenothera primiveris, Opuntia macrorhiza, Oxalis drummondii, Parthenocissus vitacea, Pennisetum glaucum, Penstemon barbatus, P. fendleri, Pericome caudata, Peteria scoparia, Petradoria pumila, Phlox gracilis, P.*

stansburyi, Picradeniopsis oppositifolia, Potentilla hippiana, Psilostrophe tagetina, Rhus trilobata, Rumex crispus, Salsola australis, Sanvitalia abertii, Senecio fendleri, Silene douglasii, S. laciniata, S. noctiflora, Sphaeralcea fendleri, Stachys rothrockii, Talinum parviflorum, Taraxacum officinale, Thlaspi montanum, Tragopogon porrifolius, T. pratensis, Verbena bracteata, Woodsia neomexicana, Zigadenus elegans

Diaphoretic: *Artemisia carruthii, A. tridentata, Juniperus monosperma, Pericome caudata*

Dietary Aid: *Hilaria jamesii, Plantago patagonica*

Disinfectant: *Agastache pallidiflora, Agoseris aurantiaca, Apocynum ×floribundum, Brickellia brachyphylla, Campanula rotundifolia, Carex inops, Coreopsis tinctoria, Dalea candida, Dichanthelium oligosanthes, Equisetum laevigatum, Erigeron canus, E. concinnus, E. divergens, E. flagellaris, Eriogonum annuum, Forestiera pubescens, Gutierrezia sarothrae, Heuchera novomexicana, Houstonia wrightii, Ipomopsis longiflora, Lathyrus eucosmus, Leptodactylon pungens, Lotus wrightii, Marrubium vulgare, Oenothera villosa, Phlox stansburyi, Plantago major, Purshia tridentata, Salix lucida, Sinapis arvensis, Stachys rothrockii, Tetradymia canescens, Tetraneuris argentea, Tradescantia occidentalis, Veronica peregrina*

Diuretic: *Besseya plantaginea, Hieracium fendleri*

Ear Medicine: *Pinus edulis*

Emetic: *Achillea millefolium, Agoseris aurantiaca, Amelanchier utahensis, Apocynum cannabinum, A. ×floribundum, Arctostaphylos pungens, A. uva-ursi, Asclepias asperula, Astragalus allochrous, A. bisulcatus, A. mollissimus, A. praelongus, Atriplex canescens, Baccharis wrightii, Besseya plantaginea, Brickellia grandiflora, Carex microptera, Ceanothus fendleri, Chrysothamnus nauseosus, Cornus sericea, Cuscuta megalocarpa, Cyperus esculentus, Draba helleriana, Echinochloa crus-pavonis, Eleocharis montevidensis, E. rostellata, Erysimum capitatum, Fallugia paradoxa, Forestiera pubescens, Galium fendleri, Gnaphalium stramineum, Grindelia nuda, Heterotheca villosa, Hymenoxys richardsonii, Iris missouriensis, Juniperus communis, J. monosperma, Lactuca serriola, Lonicera arizonica, L. involucrata, Lupinus caudatus, Luzula multiflora, Lycium pallidum, L. torreyi, Mahonia repens, Maianthemum stellatum, Monolepis nuttalliana, Oenothera pallida, Parryella filifolia, Paxistima myrsinites, Pericome caudata, Petradoria pumila, Picea engelmannii, Pinus edulis, P. flexilis, P. ponder-*

osa, Potamogeton natans, Prunus virginiana, Pseudocymopterus montanus, Pseudotsuga menziesii, Purshia stansburiana, P. tridentata, Pyrrhopappus pauciflorus, Quercus gambelii, Ranunculus cymbalaria, Ribes pinetorum, Rosa woodsii, Rumex crispus, R. salicifolius, Salix exigua, S. lucida, Scirpus acutus, S. pallidus, Sinapis arvensis, Sisymbrium altissimum, Symphoricarpos oreophilus, Tetradymia canescens, Tragopogon porrifolius, Trifolium dubium, Typha latifolia, Veronica americana, V. peregrina, Viola nephrophylla, Zinnia grandiflora

Eye Medicine: *Arenaria lanuginosa, Aster praealtus, Astragalus bisulcatus, Campanula rotundifolia, Cirsium calcareum, C. neomexicanum, C. undulatum, Draba helleriana, Dracocephalum parviflorum, Erigeron divergens, Ipomopsis longiflora, Lesquerella rectipes, Lithospermum incisum, Machaeranthera gracilis, Malacothrix fendleri, Mentzelia laciniata, M. multiflora, Psilostrophe tagetina, Rorippa palustris, Schoenocrambe linearifolia, Thermopsis rhombifolia, Vicia americana*

Febrifuge: *Agastache pallidiflora, Ageratina herbacea, Arenaria lanuginosa, Artemisia carruthii, Brickellia californica, Chrysothamnus nauseosus, Dalea candida, Dracocephalum parviflorum, Erigeron eximius, Gilia inconspicua, Gutierrezia sarothrae, Juniperus communis, J. monosperma, J. scopulorum, Mentha arvensis, Monarda pectinata, M. punctata, Pericome caudata, Pinus edulis, P. flexilis, P. ponderosa, Purshia tridentata, Ratibida columnifera, R. tagetes, Sanvitalia abertii, Tetraclea coulteri, Tetradymia canescens, Verbascum thapsus, Verbena macdougalii*

Gastrointestinal Aid: *Apocynum cannabinum, Aster praealtus, Atriplex canescens, Brassica juncea, Carex inops, Castilleja linariifolia, Cercocarpus montanus, Chamaesyce albomarginata, C. fendleri, C. serpyllifolia, Convolvulus arvensis, Corydalis aurea, Dalea candida, Dyssodia papposa, Ephedra torreyana, Eriogonum jamesii, Gaillardia pinnatifida, Gaura hexandra, Grindelia nuda, Gutierrezia sarothrae, Heterotheca villosa, Heuchera parvifolia, Ipomopsis longiflora, Juniperus monosperma, J. scopulorum, Linum lewisii, L. puberulum, Lotus wrightii, Machaeranthera tanacetifolia, Marrubium vulgare, Menodora scabra, Myosurus cupulatus, Oenothera coronopifolia, Orthocarpus purpureoalbus, Penstemon barbatus, Phoradendron juniperinum, Picradeniopsis oppositifolia, Polygonum aviculare, P. ramosis-*

simum, Prunus virginiana, Pseudocymopterus montanus, Psilostrophe tagetina, Psoralidium lanceolatum, Ratibida tagetes, Rhus trilobata, Sarcobatus vermiculatus, Senecio fendleri, Sphaeralcea digitata, Tetradymia canescens, Tetraneuris argentea, Veronica peregrina, Zinnia grandiflora

Gynecological Aid: *Androsace occidentalis, Artemisia tridentata, Bahia dissecta, Bouteloua gracilis, Calochortus gunnisonii, Capsicum annuum, Castilleja integra, C. linariifolia, Cercocarpus montanus, Chamaesyce fendleri, C. serpyllifolia, Chrysothamnus depressus, C. nauseosus, Cordylanthus wrightii, Corydalis aurea, Echeandia flavescens, Erigeron speciosus, Eriogonum jamesii, E. leptophyllum, Erysimum capitatum, Euphorbia lurida, Gutierrezia sarothrae, Heuchera parvifolia, Ipomopsis longiflora, Juniperus monosperma, Leptodactylon pungens, Marrubium vulgare, Menodora scabra, Opuntia macrorhiza, Pennellia micrantha, Penstemon barbatus, P. linarioides, Pericome caudata, Phlox stansburyi, Psoralidium lanceolatum, Purshia tridentata, Quercus gambelii, Rhus trilobata, Rumex hymenosepalus, Sanvitalia abertii, Senecio multicapitatus, S. multilobatus, Stephanomeria pauciflora, Taraxacum officinale, Townsendia exscapa, Yucca baccata, Y. glauca*

Hallucinogen: *Datura wrightii*

Heart Medicine: *Heterotheca villosa*

Hemostat: *Chamaesyce albomarginata, C. fendleri, C. serpyllifolia, Erigeron flagellaris, Gayophytum ramosissimum, Trifolium dubium*

Herbal Steam: *Picradeniopsis oppositifolia, Tetradymia canescens*

Hunting Medicine: *Antennaria rosulata, Aster praealtus, Besseya plantaginea, Campanula rotundifolia, Castilleja miniata, Cercocarpus montanus, Chamaebatiaria millefolium, Datura wrightii, Erigeron eximius, E. formosissimus, Helianthus petiolaris, Hieracium fendleri, Humulus lupulus, Ipomopsis aggregata, Limosella aquatica, Lonicera utahensis, Mirabilis linearis, Monolepis nuttalliana, Oenothera villosa, Pinus flexilis, Purshia tridentata, Ranunculus inamoenus, Senecio neomexicanus, Thermopsis rhombifolia, Valeriana acutiloba, Verbesina encelioides, Veronica peregrina*

Internal Medicine: *Aster praealtus, Machaeranthera gracilis, Sidalcea neomexicana, Tradescantia occidentalis*

Kidney Aid: *Draba helleriana, Juniperus scopulorum*

Laxative: *Mahonia repens*

Misc. Disease Remedy: *Artemisia carruthii, Asclepias tuberosa, Brickellia grandiflora, Erigeron eximius, Galium fendleri, Hedeoma drummondii, Holodiscus discolor, Humulus lupulus, Iva xanthifolia, Lycium pallidum, L. torreyi, Marrubium vulgare, Mentha arvensis, Monarda pectinata, Pericome caudata, Peteria scoparia, Pinus edulis, Psoralidium tenuiflorum, Salsola australis, Valeriana acutiloba*

Narcotic: *Datura wrightii*

Nose Medicine: *Atriplex canescens, Chaetopappa ericoides, Heterotheca villosa, Polygonum douglasii*

Oral Aid: *Abronia fragrans, Eriogonum alatum, Phlox gracilis, Rumex crispus, Sanvitalia abertii, Schkuhria multiflora, Schoenocrambe linearifolia*

Orthopedic Aid: *Agoseris aurantiaca, Clematis columbiana, C. ligusticifolia, Corydalis aurea, Hackelia floribunda, Heuchera novomexicana, Menodora scabra, Mirabilis oxybaphoides, Oenothera albicaulis, Tetradymia canescens*

Other: *Atriplex argentea, Brickellia eupatorioides, Corydalis aurea, Eriogonum annuum, Helianthus annuus, Malva neglecta, Pinus edulis, Tetraneuris argentea, Tripterocalyx carnea*

Panacea: *Acer glabrum, Agoseris aurantiaca, Amelanchier utahensis, Androsace septentrionalis, Arabis fendleri, Arenaria fendleri, Argythamnia cyanophylla, Artemisia carruthii, A. frigida, A. ludoviciana, Astragalus humistratus, A. kentrophyta, Besseya plantaginea, Bouteloua gracilis, Calliandra humilis, Calochortus aureus, C. gunnisonii, Calylophus hartwegii, Cercocarpus montanus, Cheilanthes wootonii, Cirsium neomexicanum, C. undulatum, Coreopsis tinctoria, Cryptantha cinerea, Cymopterus bulbosus, Dalea candida, Draba helleriana, Erigeron divergens, Eriogonum alatum, E. annuum, E. jamesii, E. leptophyllum, Fragaria vesca, Gaura coccinea, Geranium atropurpureum, G. lentum, G. richardsonii, Glandularia wrightii, Gnaphalium stramineum, Gutierrezia sarothrae, Helianthella parryi, Helianthus petiolaris, Heliomeris longifolia, Heterotheca villosa, Heuchera novomexicana, H. parvifolia, Houstonia wrightii, Hymenopappus filifolius, Ipomopsis longiflora, Krascheninnikovia lanata, Linanthus nuttallii, Linum puberulum, Lithospermum incisum, L. multiflorum, Lotus wrightii, Lupinus kingii, Lycium pallidum, L. torreyi, Menodora scabra, Myosurus aristatus, Oenothera albicaulis, O. cespitosa, O. coronopi-*

folia, O. elata, O. flava, Orobanche fasciculata, Penstemon barbatus, P. virgatus, Physalis pubescens, Picradeniopsis oppositifolia, Plantago major, Polygonum ramosissimum, Potentilla crinita, P. hippiana, P. pensylvanica, Prunus virginiana, Quercus gambelii, Ratibida tagetes, Rumex crispus, R. salicifolius, Sanvitalia abertii, Senecio fendleri, Silene drummondii, Sphaeralcea coccinea, S. digitata, Stephanomeria pauciflora, Tetraneuris argentea, Tragia nepetifolia, Vicia americana

Pediatric Aid: *Androsace occidentalis, Antennaria rosulata, Besseya plantaginea, Brickellia brachyphylla, Capsicum annuum, Cryptantha cinerea, Eriogonum alatum, Gaura coccinea, Grindelia nuda, Hilaria jamesii, Juniperus monosperma, Orobanche fasciculata, Ratibida tagetes, Salix lucida, Senecio fendleri*

Poison: *Hackelia floribunda, Hordeum jubatum, Hymenoxys richardsonii, Toxicodendron radicans, Urtica dioica, Yucca glauca*

Preventive Medicine: *Thlaspi montanum*

Psychological Aid: *Frasera speciosa, Verbascum thapsus*

Respiratory Aid: *Arenaria fendleri, A. lanuginosa, Clematis hirsutissima, Erysimum capitatum, Gaillardia pinnatifida, Lesquerella rectipes, Machaeranthera gracilis, M. tanacetifolia*

Snakebite Remedy: *Artemisia filifolia, Aster falcatus, A. praealtus, Chaetopappa ericoides, Conyza canadensis, Cryptantha fulvocanescens, Erigeron divergens, E. flagellaris, Eriogonum leptophyllum, Gutierrezia sarothrae, Mentzelia albicaulis, Oenothera pallida, Sanvitalia abertii*

Stimulant: *Juniperus monosperma, Mentha arvensis*

Strengthener: *Frasera speciosa, Verbascum thapsus*

Throat Aid: *Bouteloua simplex, Cleome serrulata, Corydalis aurea, Oenothera albicaulis, O. flava, O. pallida, Penstemon jamesii, Psilostrophe tagetina, Sanvitalia abertii, Tragopogon pratensis*

Toothache Remedy: *Artemisia frigida, Astragalus bisulcatus, Atriplex canescens, Chaetopappa ericoides, Chamaesyce fendleri, C. serpyllifolia, Cryptantha fulvocanescens, Descurainia pinnata, D. sophia, Erysimum capitatum, Heterotheca villosa, Lesquerella rectipes, Lycium pallidum, L. torreyi, Mentzelia albicaulis, Pennellia micrantha, Pericome caudata, Sanvitalia abertii*

Tuberculosis Remedy: *Valeriana acutiloba*

Urinary Aid: *Gutierrezia sarothrae*

Venereal Aid: *Androsace septentrionalis, Arenaria lanuginosa, Baccharis wrightii, Coreopsis tinctoria, Draba helleriana, Heterotheca villosa, Heuchera parvifolia, Potentilla norvegica, Psoralidium lanceolatum, Ratibida tagetes*

Veterinary Aid: *Artemisia carruthii, A. tridentata, Asclepias asperula, Atriplex canescens, Bouteloua gracilis, Cerastium beeringianum, Chamaesyce fendleri, C. serpyllifolia, Cirsium neomexicanum, C. undulatum, Commelina dianthifolia, Dalea candida, Datura wrightii, Echeandia flavescens, Elymus trachycaulus, Erigeron flagellaris, Eriogonum abertianum, Frasera speciosa, Grindelia nuda, Gutierrezia sarothrae, Ipomopsis longiflora, Juniperus monosperma, Lathyrus eucosmus, Mirabilis linearis, Nicotiana attenuata, Penstemon barbatus, Peteria scoparia, Psoralidium tenuiflorum, Ratibida columnifera, Rumex hymenosepalus, Silene douglasii, Solanum triflorum, Sporobolus cryptandrus, Talinum parviflorum, Tradescantia occidentalis, T. pinetorum, Tragopogon porrifolius, T. pratensis, Verbascum thapsus*

Witchcraft Medicine: *Agastache pallidiflora, Agoseris aurantiaca, Androsace septentrionalis, Antennaria parvifolia, A. rosulata, Aster oblongifolius, Besseya plantaginea, Campanula rotundifolia, Castilleja miniata, Clematis hirsutissima, C. ligusticifolia, Datura wrightii, Draba helleriana, Erigeron eximius, Eriogonum annuum, Heliomeris multiflora, Humulus lupulus, Iva xanthifolia, Juniperus scopulorum, Limosella aquatica, Myosurus aristatus, Pericome caudata, Peteria scoparia, Psoralidium lanceolatum, Solidago velutina, Tetradymia canescens, Tetraneuris argentea, Thermopsis rhombifolia, Thlaspi montanum, Tripterocalyx carnea, Valeriana acutiloba*

Neeshenam

Misc. Disease Remedy: *Croton setigerus*

Toothache Remedy: *Frangula californica*

Nevada Indian

Cold Remedy: *Corallorrhiza maculata, Eriogonum umbellatum*

Dermatological Aid: *Clematis ligusticifolia*

Heart Medicine: *Chaenactis stevioides, Peniocereus greggii*

Kidney Aid: *Iris missouriensis*

Pediatric Aid: *Chaenactis stevioides*

Urinary Aid: *Iris missouriensis*

Veterinary Aid: *Lomatium dissectum, Rumex crispus*

Nez Perce

Antidiarrheal: *Thuja plicata*

Antirheumatic (External): *Populus balsamifera, P. deltoides*

Blood Medicine: *Lewisia rediviva*

Cold Remedy: *Juniperus scopulorum, Larix occidentalis, Thuja plicata*

Cough Medicine: *Larix occidentalis, Thuja plicata*

Dermatological Aid: *Lomatium dissectum, Rhus glabra*

Dietary Aid: *Lomatium dissectum*

Eye Medicine: *Lomatium dissectum*

Febrifuge: *Juniperus scopulorum, Symphoricarpos albus*

Gynecological Aid: *Lewisia rediviva*

Pediatric Aid: *Symphoricarpos albus, Thuja plicata*

Pulmonary Aid: *Juniperus scopulorum*

Respiratory Aid: *Lomatium dissectum*

Throat Aid: *Larix occidentalis*

Tuberculosis Remedy: *Lomatium dissectum*

Veterinary Aid: *Clematis ligusticifolia, Populus balsamifera, P. deltoides*

Nitinaht

Anticonvulsive: *Postelsia palmaeformis*

Antirheumatic (External): *Urtica dioica*

Antirheumatic (Internal): *Oplopanax horridus*

Burn Dressing: *Lysichiton americanus, Maianthemum dilatatum*

Cathartic: *Huperzia selago, Sambucus racemosa*

Ceremonial Medicine: *Adiantum pedatum, Lomatium nudicaule*

Cold Remedy: *Achillea millefolium, Lomatium nudicaule*

Cough Medicine: *Malus fusca, Polypodium glycyrrhiza*

Dermatological Aid: *Alectoria sarmentosa, Alnus rubra, Galium aparine, Maianthemum dilatatum, Nereocystis luetkeana, Pinus contorta, P. monticola, Plantago major, Populus balsamifera, Tsuga heterophylla, Usnea longissima*

Dietary Aid: *Ledum groenlandicum, Malus fusca*

Disinfectant: *Frangula purshiana, Plantago major, Sphagnum* sp.

Diuretic: *Symphoricarpos albus*

Emetic: *Huperzia selago, Sambucus racemosa*

Eye Medicine: *Conocephalum conicum*

Febrifuge: *Aruncus dioicus*

Gastrointestinal Aid: *Frangula purshiana, Gaultheria shallon, Huperzia selago, Plantago major*

Gynecological Aid: *Oenanthe sarmentosa, Polytrichum commune*

Internal Medicine: *Abies amabilis, A. grandis, Alnus rubra, Tsuga heterophylla*

Kidney Aid: *Conocephalum conicum*

Laxative: *Frangula purshiana, Mahonia aquifolium, M. nervosa, Ribes bracteosum, Sambucus racemosa*

Misc. Disease Remedy: *Aruncus dioicus*

Orthopedic Aid: *Alnus rubra, Oplopanax horridus, Tsuga heterophylla*

Other: *Anaphalis margaritacea, Nuphar lutea*

Panacea: *Achillea millefolium, Malus fusca, Prunus emarginata*

Preventive Medicine: *Abies amabilis*

Psychological Aid: *Conocephalum conicum, Lonicera involucrata, Postelsia palmaeformis, Sambucus racemosa, Tellima grandiflora*

Pulmonary Aid: *Alnus rubra*

Reproductive Aid: *Gaultheria shallon, Halosaccion glandiforme*

Respiratory Aid: *Polypodium glycyrrhiza*

Strengthener: *Ledum groenlandicum, Lessoniopsis littoralis, Leymus mollis, Postelsia palmaeformis, Sambucus racemosa*

Throat Aid: *Achillea millefolium*

Tonic: *Malus fusca, Urtica dioica*

Tuberculosis Remedy: *Alnus rubra, Mahonia aquifolium, M. nervosa, Peltigera aphthosa*

Unspecified: *Abies grandis, Alnus rubra, Mahonia aquifolium, M. nervosa, Malus fusca, Nuphar lutea, Oplopanax horridus, Rosa nutkana, Tellima grandiflora, Urtica dioica*

Urinary Aid: *Peltigera aphthosa, P. canina*

Witchcraft Medicine: *Menziesia ferruginea*

Nootka

Alterative: *Polypodium glycyrrhiza*

Cancer Treatment: *Pyrola elliptica*

Gastrointestinal Aid: *Solanum dulcamara*

Strengthener: *Postelsia palmaeformis*

Unspecified: *Ledum groenlandicum*

Venereal Aid: *Polypodium glycyrrhiza*

Nootka, Manhousat

Love Medicine: *Lonicera involucrata*

Nuxalkmc

Cough Medicine: *Lonicera involucrata*

Dermatological Aid: *Lonicera involucrata*

Emetic: *Oenanthe sarmentosa*

Venereal Aid: *Lonicera involucrata*

Oglala

Poison: *Celastrus scandens*

Ojibwa

Adjuvant: *Betula papyrifera, Rubus idaeus, Tsuga canadensis*

Analgesic: *Acorus calamus, Apocynum androsaemifolium, Arctium minus, Aster macrophyllus, Betula papyrifera, Caulophyllum thalictroides, Cirsium vulgare, Comarum palustre, Comptonia peregrina, Cynoglossum virginianum, Erigeron strigosus, Euthamia graminifolia, Fragaria virginiana, Impatiens capensis, Maianthemum canadense, M. racemosum, Picea mariana, Polygonum amphibium, Pteridium aquilinum, Sanguinaria canadensis, Thuja occidentalis, Uvularia grandiflora, Viburnum opulus*

Anthelmintic: *Corylus cornuta*

Anticonvulsive: *Aralia nudicaulis, Monarda fistulosa, Picea mariana, Pinus banksiana, Sanguinaria canadensis*

Antidiarrheal: *Comptonia peregrina, Cornus racemosa, Geranium maculatum, Hydrophyllum virginianum, Ilex verticillata, Rubus allegheniensis, Rumex crispus*

Antidote: *Clintonia borealis*

Antiemetic: *Spiraea tomentosa, Vaccinium oxycoccos*

Antirheumatic (External): *Arctostaphylos alpina, A. uva-ursi, Populus alba, P. balsamifera, Sanguinaria canadensis, Saururus cernuus*

Antirheumatic (Internal): *Gaultheria procumbens, Silphium perfoliatum*

Blood Medicine: *Aralia nudicaulis, Arctium lappa, Arctostaphylos alpina, A. uva-ursi, Betula alleghaniensis, B. papyrifera, Mentha canadensis, Nepeta cataria, Populus alba, P. balsamifera, Quercus rubra, Sanguinaria canadensis, Taraxacum officinale, Thuja occidentalis, Vaccinium angustifolium*

Burn Dressing: *Plantago major*

Cathartic: *Acorus calamus, Euphorbia corollata, Iris versicolor, Polygonatum biflorum, Potentilla norvegica, Sambucus racemosa, Silene latifolia, Streptopus roseus, Viburnum opulus*

Ceremonial Medicine: *Abies balsamea, Achillea millefolium, Anemone canadensis, Apocynum androsaemifolium, Arctostaphylos alpina, A. uva-ursi, Cornus sericea, Mitchella repens, Rhus aromatica, R. copallinum, R. glabra, Sanguinaria canadensis, Solanum nigrum, Thuja occidentalis*

Cold Remedy: *Abies balsamea, Acorus calamus, Erigeron philadelphicus, Populus balsamifera, Prunus serotina*

Cough Medicine: *Abies balsamea, Nymphaea odorata, Polygonatum biflorum, Prunus pensylvanica, P. serotina, Streptopus roseus, Thuja occidentalis*

Dermatological Aid: *Abies balsamea, Achillea millefolium, Aralia nudicaulis, Athyrium filixfemina, Clintonia borealis, Corylus americana, C. cornuta, Epilobium angustifolium, Galium trifidum, Heracleum maximum, Impatiens pallida, Nuphar lutea, Oenothera biennis, Plantago major, Populus balsamifera, P. tremuloides, Quercus macrocarpa, Rhus glabra, Rosa virginiana, Rumex crispus, Salix fragilis, S. lucida, Sanguinaria canadensis, Tsuga canadensis, Typha latifolia, Ulmus rubra, Urtica dioica*

Diaphoretic: *Abies balsamea, Mentha canadensis, Thuja occidentalis*

Dietary Aid: *Asarum canadense*

Disinfectant: *Larix laricina, Picea glauca*

Diuretic: *Apocynum androsaemifolium, Cucurbita maxima, Dirca palustris, Galium aparine, Humulus lupulus, Laportea canadensis, Lycopodium obscurum, Malaxis unifolia, Prenanthes alba, Rubus allegheniensis, Viburnum lentago*

Emetic: *Acer negundo, Caulophyllum thalictroides, Cornus alternifolia, Iris versicolor, Sambucus racemosa*

Eye Medicine: *Abies balsamea, Acer rubrum, A. spicatum, Arisaema triphyllum, Melampyrum lineare, Rhus glabra, Rubus idaeus*

Febrifuge: *Achillea millefolium, Erigeron philadelphicus, Hedeoma pulegioides, Mentha canadensis, Monarda fistulosa, Sanicula marilandica, Tanacetum vulgare, Thalictrum dasycarpum*

Gastrointestinal Aid: *Acorus calamus, Actaea rubra, Alnus incana, Aquilegia canadensis, Arctium minus, Asarum canadense, Betula papyrifera, Cardamine maxima, Celastrus scandens, Chimaphila umbellata, Cirsium arvense, C. vulgare, Comarum palustre, Comptonia peregrina, Cornus canadensis, Dryopteris cristata, Echinocystis lobata, Equisetum palustre, Fragaria virginiana, Hedeoma pulegioides, Lathyrus ochroleucus, Mentha canadensis, Monarda punctata, Pedicularis canadensis, Picea mariana, Polygonum amphibium, Rosa blanda, Sagittaria cuneata, Salix candida, S. discolor, S. pedicellaris, S. pyrifolia, Sanguinaria canadensis, Saururus cernuus, Silphium perfoliatum, Taraxacum officinale, Ulmus rubra, Uvularia grandiflora, Viburnum opulus, Vitis vulpina*

Gynecological Aid: *Actaea rubra, Amelanchier laevis, Antennaria howellii, Apocynum androsaemifolium, Asclepias syriaca, Athyrium filixfemina, Betula pumila, Caulophyllum thalictroides, Clintonia borealis, Cypripedium pubescens, Geum macrophyllum, Glyceria canadensis, Lactuca biennis, Maianthemum canadense, M. racemosum, Onoclea sensibilis, Osmorhiza claytonii, O. longistylis, Pastinaca sativa, Prenanthes alba, Prunella vulgaris, Pteridium aquilinum, Ribes triste, Sarracenia purpurea, Spiraea tomentosa, Symphoricarpos albus, Vitis vulpina*

Heart Medicine: *Acorus calamus, Quercus rubra, Scutellaria galericulata, Verbascum thapsus, Viola conspersa*

Hemorrhoid Remedy: *Cornus racemosa*

Hemostat: *Eriophorum callitrix, Populus grandidentata, Rhus glabra, R. hirta, Rosa virginiana, Salix fragilis, S. lucida, Sanguinaria canadensis, Silphium perfoliatum, Tsuga canadensis, Ulmus rubra*

Herbal Steam: *Linaria vulgaris*

Hunting Medicine: *Acorus calamus, Aralia nudicaulis, Aster cordifolius, A. macrophyllus, Cicuta maculata, Conyza canadensis, Euthamia graminifolia, Heracleum maximum, Hieracium canadense, Polygonum amphibium, Prunella vulgaris, Pyrola americana, Ranunculus pensylvanicus, Rumex crispus, Sium suave, Spiraea salicifolia, Spiranthes lacera, Taenidia integerrima, Uvularia sessilifolia*

Kidney Aid: *Equisetum arvense, E. sylvaticum, Galium aparine, Maianthemum canadense, M. racemosum*

Laxative: *Equisetum palustre, Monarda punctata, Sanguinaria canadensis*

Love Medicine: *Coeloglossum viride, Pedicularis canadensis*

Narcotic: *Arctostaphylos alpina, A. uva-ursi*

Oral Aid: *Apocynum androsaemifolium, Coptis trifolia, Geranium maculatum, Rhus hirta*

Orthopedic Aid: *Mirabilis nyctaginea, Plantago major, Populus tremuloides, Quercus macrocarpa*

Other: *Nepeta cataria, Typha latifolia*

Panacea: *Arctostaphylos alpina, A. uva-ursi, Populus alba, P. balsamifera, Sanguinaria canadensis, Saururus cernuus*

Pediatric Aid: *Coptis trifolia, Cornus canadensis, Eupatorium purpureum, Fragaria virginiana, Hydrophyllum virginianum, Monarda fistulosa*

Poison: *Clintonia borealis, Pastinaca sativa*

Pulmonary Aid: *Anemone cylindrica, Botrychium virginianum, Campanula rotundifolia, Galium tinctorium, Prunus virginiana, Smilax herbacea, Uvularia grandiflora*

Respiratory Aid: *Betula pumila, Linaria vulgaris,*

Monarda fistulosa, Populus balsamifera, Quercus rubra, Zanthoxylum americanum

Sedative: *Salix candida, S. discolor, S. pyrifolia*

Snakebite Remedy: *Plantago major, Sanicula marilandica*

Stimulant: *Abies balsamea, Anaphalis margaritacea, Aralia nudicaulis, Corydalis aurea, Lycopodium complanatum, Maianthemum racemosum, Picea mariana, Pinus banksiana, P. resinosa, P. strobus, Salix candida, S. discolor, S. pyrifolia, Sanguinaria canadensis*

Throat Aid: *Acorus calamus, Anemone canadensis, Apocynum androsaemifolium, Maianthemum canadense, M. racemosum, Osmorhiza claytonii, O. longistylis, Pedicularis canadensis, Rhus hirta, Sanguinaria canadensis, Ulmus rubra, Zanthoxylum americanum*

Tonic: *Arctium minus, Echinocystis lobata, Fraxinus pennsylvanica*

Tuberculosis Remedy: *Anemone cylindrica, Botrychium virginianum, Galium trifidum, Nymphaea odorata*

Unspecified: *Aralia racemosa, Arctostaphylos alpina, A. uva-ursi, Arisaema triphyllum, Aster macrophyllus, Baptisia tinctoria, Brassica rapa, Celastrus scandens, Cicuta maculata, Cornus sericea, Equisetum hyemale, Fraxinus americana, Impatiens capensis, Larix laricina, Maianthemum canadense, Monarda punctata, Nemopanthus mucronatus, Picea mariana, Pinus resinosa, P. strobus, Plantago major, Polygala senega, Populus alba, Quercus rubra, Rhus aromatica, R. copallinum, R. glabra, Ribes americanum, R. hudsonianum, R. oxyacanthoides, R. rubrum, Rosa virginiana, Rumex altissimus, Sagittaria cuneata, Salix candida, S. discolor, S. pyrifolia, Sambucus racemosa, Sorbus americana*

Urinary Aid: *Agrimonia gryposepala, Diervilla lonicera, Dirca palustris, Galium aparine, Laportea canadensis*

Venereal Aid: *Acer saccharinum, Quercus rubra, Sanguinaria canadensis, Sorbus americana, Ulmus americana, U. rubra*

Veterinary Aid: *Artemisia ludoviciana, Lathyrus ochroleucus, L. palustris, Sagittaria cuneata*

Ojibwa, South

Analgesic: *Actaea rubra, Amorpha canescens, Anemone canadensis, Chamaecyparis thyoides, Geum aleppicum, Juniperus virginiana, Lappula squarrosa, Larix laricina, Maianthemum racemosum, Monarda fistulosa, Pinus resinosa,*

P. strobus, Prunus pensylvanica, P. serotina, Rubus idaeus, R. occidentalis, Viola canadensis

Antidiarrheal: Acer nigrum, A. saccharinum, Crataegus chrysocarpa, Picea glauca, Prunus americana, Quercus alba, Q. rubra, Rhus aromatica

Antirheumatic (Internal): Phryma leptostachya

Cathartic: Veronicastrum virginicum

Cold Remedy: Abies balsamea, Polygala senega

Cough Medicine: Geum aleppicum, Polygala senega, Salix candida

Dermatological Aid: Abies balsamea, Botrychium virginianum, Helianthus occidentalis, Populus deltoides, Prunus serotina, Rumex crispus, Sporobolus heterolepis, Typha latifolia

Diaphoretic: Abies balsamea

Diuretic: Acer saccharinum, Betula alleghaniensis

Emetic: Acer pensylvanicum, Sporobolus heterolepis

Eye Medicine: Fraxinus nigra, Rosa blanda, R. virginiana, Symphoricarpos orbiculatus

Gastrointestinal Aid: Actaea rubra, Amorpha canescens, Monarda fistulosa, Polygala senega, Prunus pensylvanica, Rubus idaeus, R. occidentalis

Gynecological Aid: Maianthemum racemosum, Prunus virginiana

Hemostat: Maianthemum racemosum, Panax trifolius

Herbal Steam: Larix laricina, Pinus strobus

Liver Aid: Sporobolus heterolepis

Orthopedic Aid: Anemone canadensis

Pulmonary Aid: Geum aleppicum, Prunus serotina

Throat Aid: Polygala senega, Viola pubescens

Unspecified: Picea mariana

Venereal Aid: Abies balsamea

Okanagan-Colville

Abortifacient: Pinus ponderosa

Analgesic: Achillea millefolium, Artemisia dracunculus, Erigeron philadelphicus, Gaillardia aristata, Mentha arvensis, Penstemon fruticosus, Potentilla gracilis, Ranunculus glaberrimus, Rorippa nasturtium-aquaticum, Spiraea betulifolia

Antidiarrheal: Achillea millefolium, Arabis sparsiflora, Crataegus douglasii, Epilobium minutum, Lactuca tatarica, Lesquerella douglasii, Potentilla gracilis, Prunus virginiana, Ribes lacustre, Rubus idaeus, Solidago canadensis

Antihemorrhagic: Arctostaphylos uva-ursi, Juniperus scopulorum, Leymus cinereus, Lithospermum ruderale, Pinus ponderosa

Antirheumatic (External): Achillea millefolium, Artemisia dracunculus, Asclepias speciosa, Cra-

taegus douglasii, Juniperus scopulorum, Larix occidentalis, Pseudoroegneria spicata, Ranunculus glaberrimus, Sambucus cerulea, Thuja plicata, Urtica dioica, Veratrum viride, Wyethia amplexicaulis

Antirheumatic (Internal): Equisetum arvense, E. hyemale, E. laevigatum, Frangula purshiana, Larix occidentalis, Lomatium dissectum, Mentha arvensis, Potentilla gracilis

Blood Medicine: Arctostaphylos uva-ursi, Chimaphila umbellata, Cornus sericea, Frangula purshiana, Heuchera cylindrica, Larix occidentalis, Lomatium dissectum, Lonicera utahensis, Mahonia aquifolium, Phlox longifolia, Potentilla gracilis, Pseudotsuga menziesii

Burn Dressing: Balsamorhiza sagittata, Ceanothus sanguineus, Holodiscus discolor, Taxus brevifolia

Cancer Treatment: Larix occidentalis

Carminative: Artemisia ludoviciana

Cathartic: Achillea millefolium, Philadelphus lewisii, Rubus idaeus, Symphoricarpos albus

Ceremonial Medicine: Antennaria rosea, Ceanothus velutinus, Ligusticum canbyi, Rosa acicularis, R. gymnocarpa, R. nutkana, R. woodsii, Vicia americana

Cold Remedy: Achillea millefolium, Agastache urticifolia, Amelanchier alnifolia, Artemisia absinthium, A. frigida, A. tridentata, A. tripartita, Asarum caudatum, Chimaphila umbellata, Cornus sericea, Equisetum laevigatum, Eriogonum compositum, E. heracleoides, E. niveum, Erythronium grandiflorum, Geum triflorum, Juniperus communis, Ligusticum canbyi, Lomatium ambiguum, L. macrocarpum, L. triternatum, Maianthemum racemosum, Mentha arvensis, Monardella odoratissima, Nepeta cataria, Paxistima myrsinites, Penstemon fruticosus, Polygonum amphibium, Prunus virginiana, Ribes lacustre, Salvia dorrii, Spiraea betulifolia, Veratrum viride

Contraceptive: Amelanchier alnifolia, Apocynum cannabinum, Arabis sparsiflora, Clematis ligusticifolia, Cornus sericea

Cough Medicine: Abies grandis, A. lasiocarpa, Oplopanax horridus, Prunus virginiana

Dermatological Aid: Abies grandis, A. lasiocarpa, Achillea millefolium, Agoseris glauca, Artemisia dracunculus, Asclepias speciosa, Aster conspicuus, Calochortus macrocarpus, Castilleja hispida, C. thompsonii, Ceanothus velutinus, Clematis columbiana, C. ligusticifolia, Cornus sericea, Disporum trachycarpum, Epilobium brachycarpum, Equisetum arvense, E. hyemale,

E. laevigatum, Eriogonum compositum, E. her-
acleoides, E. niveum, Erysimum asperum, Fra-
garia vesca, F. virginiana, Goodyera oblongifo-
lia, Heracleum maximum, Heuchera cylindrica,
Juniperus scopulorum, Larix occidentalis, Lew-
isia rediviva, Leymus cinereus, Lomatium dis-
sectum, Lonicera utahensis, Opuntia fragilis, O.
polyacantha, Penstemon fruticosus, Pinus pon-
derosa, Plantago major, P. patagonica, Populus
tremuloides, Potentilla gracilis, P. recta, Prunus
virginiana, Pseudotsuga menziesii, Pteryxia
terebinthina, Rhus glabra, Rosa acicularis, R.
gymnocarpa, R. nutkana, R. woodsii, Rubus
parviflorus, Salix bebbiana, S. scouleriana,
Shepherdia canadensis, Symphoricarpos albus,
Thuja plicata, Typha latifolia

Diaphoretic: *Artemisia tridentata, A. tripartita,*
Balsamorhiza sagittata

Dietary Aid: *Abies grandis, A. lasiocarpa, Alnus*
incana, A. viridis, Chimaphila umbellata, Geum
triflorum, Lomatium dissectum, Maianthemum
racemosum

Disinfectant: *Fragaria vesca, F. virginiana*

Diuretic: *Equisetum arvense, E. hyemale, E. laevi-*
gatum, Opuntia fragilis, O. polyacantha

Emetic: *Pseudotsuga menziesii*

Eye Medicine: *Arabis sparsiflora, Arctostaphylos*
uva-ursi, Chaenactis douglasii, Dodecatheon
pulchellum, Equisetum hyemale, Erigeron pum-
ilus, Lupinus sericeus, L. sulphureus, L. wyethii,
Mahonia aquifolium, Pinus ponderosa, Populus
tremuloides, Ribes cereum, Silene menziesii,
Symphoricarpos albus

Febrifuge: *Agastache urticifolia, Collomia grandi-*
flora, Geum triflorum, Ipomopsis aggregata,
Mentha arvensis, Osmorhiza occidentalis, Pinus
ponderosa, Pseudotsuga menziesii, Solidago
canadensis

Gastrointestinal Aid: *Abies grandis, A. lasiocarpa,*
Achillea millefolium, Anaphalis margaritacea,
Arabis sparsiflora, Artemisia absinthium, Cor-
nus sericea, Lesquerella douglasii, Mentha ar-
vensis, Penstemon fruticosus, Pinus contorta,
P. ponderosa, Prunus emarginata, P. virgin-
iana, Rubus idaeus, R. parviflorus, Salix sitch-
ensis, Spiraea betulifolia

Gland Medicine: *Abies grandis, A. lasiocarpa*

Gynecological Aid: *Alnus incana, A. viridis, Arte-*
misia absinthium, A. dracunculus, Chryso-
thamnus nauseosus, Cornus sericea, Geum
macrophyllum, G. triflorum, Lonicera involu-
crata, Potentilla arguta, Rhus glabra, Salix
bebbiana, S. scouleriana, Sedum lanceolatum,
Spiraea betulifolia

Heart Medicine: *Cornus sericea, Rhus glabra*

Hemorrhoid Remedy: *Aster conspicuus*

Hemostat: *Disporum trachycarpum, Salix bebbi-*
ana, S. scouleriana

Hunting Medicine: *Acer glabrum, Physocarpus*
malvaceus, Shepherdia canadensis, Veratrum
viride

Internal Medicine: *Ligusticum canbyi, Potentilla*
recta

Kidney Aid: *Arctostaphylos uva-ursi, Chimaphila*
umbellata, Gaillardia aristata, Ledum groen-
landicum, Mahonia aquifolium, Paxistima
myrsinites, Spiraea betulifolia

Laxative: *Achillea millefolium, Agoseris glauca,*
Asarum caudatum, Collomia grandiflora, Fran-
gula purshiana, Ipomopsis aggregata, Lonicera
utahensis, Rubus idaeus, Sedum lanceolatum

Love Medicine: *Apocynum androsaemifolium,*
Arnica cordifolia, A. latifolia, Geum triflorum,
Matricaria discoidea

Misc. Disease Remedy: *Artemisia absinthium, A.*
frigida, Geum triflorum, Juniperus scopulorum,
Lewisia rediviva, Lomatium macrocarpum,
Penstemon fruticosus, P. richardsonii, Solidago
canadensis

Oral Aid: *Artemisia tridentata, A. tripartita, Cra-*
taegus douglasii, Fragaria vesca, F. virginiana,
Lomatium macrocarpum

Orthopedic Aid: *Artemisia absinthium, Ceanothus*
velutinus, Crepis atribarba, Equisetum arvense,
E. hyemale, E. laevigatum, Gaillardia aristata,
Heracleum maximum, Lomatium dissectum,
Salix amygdaloides, S. bebbiana, S. lucida, S.
scouleriana, Veratrum viride

Other: *Abies grandis, A. lasiocarpa, Cornus seri-*
cea, Juniperus scopulorum, Ligusticum canbyi,
Lomatium dissectum, Rhus glabra, Spiraea
betulifolia

Panacea: *Cornus sericea, Salvia dorrii*

Pediatric Aid: *Agastache urticifolia, Alnus incana,*
A. viridis, Artemisia dracunculus, Ceanothus
velutinus, Cornus sericea, Crataegus douglasii,
Epilobium minutum, Equisetum hyemale, E.
laevigatum, Fragaria vesca, F. virginiana, Heu-
chera cylindrica, Lactuca tatarica, Ligusticum
canbyi, Lomatium macrocarpum, Mentha ar-
vensis, Monardella odoratissima, Phlox longi-
folia, Salix bebbiana, S. scouleriana, Solidago
canadensis, Sorbus scopulina, S. sitchensis,
Symphoricarpos albus

Poison: *Aconitum columbianum, Cicuta douglasii,*
Juniperus scopulorum, Lomatium dissectum,
Lonicera involucrata, Nuphar lutea, Nymphaea
odorata, Pteridium aquilinum, Ranunculus

Okanagon

Tonic: *Achillea millefolium, Aralia nudicaulis, Arctostaphylos uva-ursi, Clematis ligusticifolia, Heracleum maximum, Juniperus communis, Oplopanax horridus, Potentilla glandulosa, Rubus pubescens, Streptopus roseus*

Toothache Remedy: *Sambucus racemosa*

Urinary Aid: *Arabis drummondii, Arctostaphylos uva-ursi, Juniperus scopulorum, Pseudotsuga menziesii*

Omaha

Abortifacient: *Artemisia dracunculus, A. frigida*

Analgesic: *Amorpha canescens, Aquilegia canadensis, Cucurbita foetidissima, Dyssodia papposa, Echinacea angustifolia, Heracleum maximum, Lespedeza capitata, Physalis lanceolata, Pulsatilla patens, Rhus glabra, Silphium perfoliatum*

Anesthetic: *Echinacea angustifolia*

Antidiarrheal: *Chamaesyce serpyllifolia*

Antidote: *Echinacea angustifolia, Rhus glabra*

Antirheumatic (External): *Amorpha canescens, Lespedeza capitata, Pulsatilla patens*

Antirheumatic (Internal): *Silphium perfoliatum*

Blood Medicine: *Echinacea angustifolia*

Burn Dressing: *Echinacea angustifolia, Typha latifolia*

Carminative: *Acorus calamus, Mentha canadensis*

Cathartic: *Heracleum maximum*

Ceremonial Medicine: *Acorus calamus, Artemisia ludoviciana, Asclepias tuberosa, Fraxinus pennsylvanica, Hierochloe odorata, Juniperus virginiana, Lophophora williamsii, Populus deltoides, Prunus virginiana, Typha latifolia*

Cold Remedy: *Acorus calamus, Juniperus virginiana, Silphium perfoliatum*

Cough Medicine: *Acorus calamus, Juniperus virginiana*

Dermatological Aid: *Amorpha canescens, Asclepias tuberosa, Echinacea angustifolia, Eriogonum fasciculatum, Humulus lupulus, Impatiens capensis, I. pallida, Iris versicolor, Liatris scariosa, Osmorhiza longistylis, Oxalis stricta, Physalis lanceolata, P. viscosa, Prunus americana, Rhus glabra, Typha latifolia*

Diaphoretic: *Juniperus virginiana*

Dietary Aid: *Cucurbita foetidissima, Gymnocladus dioicus, Liatris scariosa*

Diuretic: *Rhus glabra*

Ear Medicine: *Iris versicolor*

Eye Medicine: *Echinacea angustifolia, Iris versicolor, Lygodesmia juncea, Rosa arkansana, Symphoricarpos occidentalis, S. orbiculatus*

Febrifuge: *Acorus calamus, Andropogon gerardii, Aquilegia canadensis, Artemisia ludoviciana, Caulophyllum thalictroides*

Gastrointestinal Aid: *Acorus calamus, Asclepias exaltata, Chamaesyce serpyllifolia, Heracleum maximum, Liatris scariosa, Physalis lanceolata, Rubus idaeus, R. occidentalis*

Gynecological Aid: *Cucurbita foetidissima, Gymnocladus dioicus, Lygodesmia juncea, Rhus glabra*

Hemostat: *Artemisia ludoviciana, Gymnocladus dioicus, Rhus glabra*

Herbal Steam: *Juniperus virginiana, Silphium perfoliatum*

Kidney Aid: *Gymnocladus dioicus, Ribes americanum*

Laxative: *Gymnocladus dioicus, Ulmus rubra*

Love Medicine: *Aquilegia canadensis, Artemisia dracunculus, Lomatium foeniculaceum*

Misc. Disease Remedy: *Echinacea angustifolia*

Other: *Echinacea angustifolia, Echinocactus williamsii*

Panacea: *Acorus calamus, Anemone canadensis, Cucurbita foetidissima*

Pediatric Aid: *Rubus idaeus, R. occidentalis, Typha latifolia*

Poison: *Toxicodendron pubescens*

Pulmonary Aid: *Asclepias tuberosa*

Respiratory Aid: *Asclepias tuberosa*

Snakebite Remedy: *Echinacea angustifolia*

Stimulant: *Andropogon gerardii, Gymnocladus dioicus*

Throat Aid: *Smilax herbacea*

Tonic: *Acorus calamus, Cucurbita foetidissima, Gymnocladus dioicus, Liatris scariosa*

Toothache Remedy: *Acorus calamus, Echinacea angustifolia*

Unspecified: *Artemisia dracunculus, Physalis lanceolata, Yucca glauca*

Urinary Aid: *Rhus glabra*

Veterinary Aid: *Acorus calamus, Echinacea angustifolia, Juniperus virginiana, Liatris scariosa, Silphium laciniatum*

Witchcraft Medicine: *Silphium laciniatum*

Oregon Indian

Antidiarrheal: *Prunus virginiana*

Dermatological Aid: *Clematis ligusticifolia*

Febrifuge: *Clematis ligusticifolia, Cleome serrulata*

Veterinary Aid: *Lomatium dissectum*

Oregon Indian, Warm Springs

Unspecified: *Ceanothus velutinus*

Oto

Antiemetic: *Ambrosia artemisiifolia*
Laxative: *Gymnocladus dioicus*
Pulmonary Aid: *Arctium minus*

Oweekeno

Analgesic: *Oplopanax horridus*
Antirheumatic (External): *Oplopanax horridus, Picea sitchensis, Plagiomnium insigne, Veratrum viride*
Ceremonial Medicine: *Thuja plicata, Tsuga heterophylla*
Cold Remedy: *Abies amabilis, Ledum groenlandicum, Oplopanax horridus*
Cough Medicine: *Polypodium glycyrrhiza*
Dermatological Aid: *Maianthemum dilatatum, Oplopanax horridus, Picea sitchensis, Plagiomnium insigne, Populus balsamifera*
Gastrointestinal Aid: *Picea sitchensis*
Internal Medicine: *Plagiomnium insigne*
Oral Aid: *Malus fusca*
Panacea: *Oplopanax horridus*
Poison: *Oplopanax horridus, Ribes lacustre, Veratrum viride*
Throat Aid: *Ledum groenlandicum, Polypodium glycyrrhiza*
Tonic: *Oplopanax horridus*
Unspecified: *Picea sitchensis*

Paiute

Abortifacient: *Porophyllum gracile*
Adjuvant: *Ephedra nevadensis*
Analgesic: *Achillea millefolium, Agastache urticifolia, Aquilegia formosa, Artemisia douglasiana, A. ludoviciana, A. spinescens, A. tridentata, Asclepias cryptoceras, Balsamorhiza sagittata, Cercocarpus ledifolius, Chaenactis douglasii, Cicuta maculata, Erigeron aphanactis, Eriogonum umbellatum, Hypericum scouleri, Iris missouriensis, Juniperus occidentalis, J. osteosperma, Larrea tridentata, Marrubium vulgare, Mentha canadensis, Mirabilis alipes, Monardella odoratissima, Osmorhiza occidentalis, Phragmites australis, Pinus monophylla, Prunus virginiana, Psathyrotes ramosissima, Psorothamnus polydenius, Purshia tridentata, Rumex crispus, R. venosus, Salvia dorrii, Stanleya pinnata, Symphoricarpos longiflorus, Zigadenus paniculatus, Z. venenosus*
Anthelmintic: *Nicotiana attenuata*
Antidiarrheal: *Artemisia ludoviciana, Cercocarpus ledifolius, Ephedra viridis, Eriastrum eremicum, Ericameria nana, Erigeron caespitosus, Eriodictyon angustifolium, Eriogonum sphaeroceph-*

alum, Eryngium alismifolium, Haplopappus sp., *Heliotropium curassavicum, Holodiscus dumosus, Ipomopsis congesta, Mahonia repens, Pinus monophylla, Pluchea sericea, Prunus andersonii, Psathyrotes ramosissima, Psorothamnus polydenius, Rosa woodsii, Rumex crispus, R. venosus, Sambucus cerulea, S. racemosa, Sarcobatus vermiculatus, Solanum physalifolium, Stephanomeria spinosa*
Antiemetic: *Eriodictyon angustifolium, Mirabilis alipes, Pinus monophylla*
Antihemorrhagic: *Juniperus occidentalis, J. osteosperma, Psorothamnus fremontii, Sarcobatus vermiculatus*
Antirheumatic (External): *Achillea millefolium, Aquilegia formosa, Artemisia dracunculus, A. ludoviciana, A. spinescens, Asclepias speciosa, Brachyactis frondosa, Cicuta douglasii, C. maculata, Eriogonum umbellatum, Gutierrezia sarothrae, Helianthus annuus, Heracleum maximum, Juniperus occidentalis, J. osteosperma, Larrea tridentata, Lomatium dissectum, Nicotiana attenuata, Psorothamnus polydenius, Rumex crispus, Sambucus cerulea, Urtica dioica, Veratrum californicum, Zigadenus paniculatus, Z. venenosus*
Antirheumatic (Internal): *Ephedra viridis, Pinus monophylla, Prunus andersonii, Rumex venosus*
Blood Medicine: *Achillea millefolium, Brachyactis frondosa, Cercocarpus ledifolius, Corallorrhiza maculata, Datura wrightii, Ephedra viridis, Juniperus communis, J. occidentalis, J. osteosperma, Mahonia nervosa, M. repens, Rumex crispus, R. venosus, Wyethia mollis*
Burn Dressing: *Argemone polyanthemos, Cercocarpus ledifolius, Ephedra nevadensis, Larrea tridentata, Mirabilis alipes, Rosa woodsii, Rumex crispus, R. hymenosepalus, R. venosus, Veratrum californicum, Zigadenus venenosus*
Carminative: *Linum lewisii, Mentha canadensis*
Cathartic: *Cucurbita foetidissima, Eriastrum filifolium, Erigeron aphanactis, Ipomopsis aggregata, I. congesta, Mirabilis alipes, Nicotiana attenuata, Osmorhiza occidentalis, Phlox longifolia, Psathyrotes ramosissima, Purshia mexicana, P. tridentata, Stephanomeria spinosa, Thymophylla pentachaeta, Wyethia mollis*
Ceremonial Medicine: *Artemisia tridentata*
Cold Remedy: *Abies procera, Achillea millefolium, Agastache urticifolia, Angelica breweri, Aquilegia formosa, Artemisia spinescens, A. tridentata, A. vulgaris, Calocedrus decurrens, Cercocarpus ledifolius, Chaenactis douglasii,*

Chrysothamnus viscidiflorus, Ephedra viridis, Ericameria nana, Eriodictyon angustifolium, Eriogonum ovalifolium, E. sphaerocephalum, E. umbellatum, Heracleum maximum, Holodiscus dumosus, Ipomopsis aggregata, I. congesta, Juniperus monosperma, J. occidentalis, J. osteosperma, Larrea tridentata, Lomatium dissectum, Mentha canadensis, Monardella odoratissima, Nicotiana attenuata, Orobanche californica, Osmorhiza occidentalis, Pinus monophylla, Plantago major, Prunus andersonii, P. virginiana, Psorothamnus polydenius, Purshia mexicana, P. tridentata, Rosa woodsii, Rumex venosus, Salvia dorrii, Sambucus racemosa, Tetradymia comosa, Urtica dioica, Wyethia mollis

Contraceptive: Veratrum californicum

Cough Medicine: Abies procera, Achillea millefolium, Angelica breweri, Aquilegia formosa, Artemisia spinescens, Asclepias speciosa, Cercocarpus ledifolius, Chaenactis douglasii, Chrysothamnus viscidiflorus, Ericameria nana, Eriodictyon angustifolium, Grindelia nana, G. squarrosa, Juniperus occidentalis, J. osteosperma, Ligusticum filicinum, Lomatium dissectum, Mahonia repens, Maianthemum stellatum, Paeonia brownii, Populus tremuloides, Prunus virginiana, Psorothamnus polydenius, Rumex venosus, Salvia dorrii, Sambucus racemosa, Tetradymia comosa

Dermatological Aid: Abies concolor, A. procera, Achillea millefolium, Agastache urticifolia, Angelica breweri, Antennaria anaphaloides, Aquilegia formosa, Argemone hispida, A. polyanthemos, Artemisia dracunculus, A. ludoviciana, A. spinescens, A. tridentata, A. vulgaris, Asclepias cryptoceras, A. speciosa, Balsamorhiza sagittata, Cercocarpus ledifolius, Chaenactis douglasii, Chamaesyce ocellata, Cicuta maculata, Crepis modocensis, Cucurbita foetidissima, Descurainia sophia, Ephedra viridis, Helianthella uniflora, Heracleum maximum, Hypericum scouleri, Iris missouriensis, Iva axillaris, Juniperus monosperma, J. occidentalis, J. osteosperma, Keckiella breviflora, Krameria grayi, Krascheninnikovia lanata, Larrea tridentata, Leucocrinum montanum, Linum lewisii, Lomatium dissectum, Maianthemum stellatum, Mentha canadensis, Mirabilis alipes, M. bigelovii, Nicotiana attenuata, Nothochelone nemorosa, Osmorhiza occidentalis, Paeonia brownii, Penstemon deustus, P. richardsonii, Pinus monophylla, P. ponderosa, Plantago major, Prunus virginiana, Psathyrotes ramosissima,

Psorothamnus polydenius, Purshia tridentata, Rhus trilobata, Ribes aureum, Rosa woodsii, Rumex crispus, R. hymenosepalus, R. venosus, Sambucus racemosa, Stephanomeria spinosa, Suaeda moquinii, Veratrum californicum, Wyethia mollis, Zigadenus paniculatus, Z. venenosus

Diaphoretic: Artemisia tridentata, Chrysothamnus viscidiflorus, Urtica dioica

Dietary Aid: Paeonia brownii

Disinfectant: Artemisia ludoviciana, A. tridentata, Balsamorhiza sagittata, Juniperus occidentalis, J. osteosperma, Krameria grayi, Lomatium dissectum, Osmorhiza occidentalis, Psorothamnus polydenius, Veratrum californicum

Diuretic: Abronia villosa, Artemisia spinescens, Heliotropium curassavicum, Juniperus occidentalis, J. osteosperma, Psorothamnus polydenius

Ear Medicine: Iris missouriensis, Maianthemum stellatum, Salvia dorrii

Emetic: Achillea millefolium, Artemisia tridentata, Chenopodium album, Cucurbita foetidissima, Eriastrum filifolium, Erigeron aphanactis, Heliotropium curassavicum, Ipomopsis aggregata, I. congesta, Nicotiana attenuata, Psathyrotes ramosissima, Purshia tridentata, Sambucus tridentata, Stephanomeria spinosa, Tanacetum vulgare, Wyethia amplexicaulis, Zigadenus paniculatus

Expectorant: Eriodictyon angustifolium, Grindelia nana, G. squarrosa, Phragmites australis

Eye Medicine: Achillea millefolium, Achlys triphylla, Artemisia ludoviciana, Chamaesyce ocellata, Cornus canadensis, Desmanthus illinoensis, Ericameria nana, Erigeron caespitosus, Heuchera rubescens, Krameria grayi, Krascheninnikovia lanata, Leymus condensatus, Linum lewisii, Maianthemum stellatum, Marah oreganus, Monardella odoratissima, Osmorhiza occidentalis, Paeonia brownii, Penstemon deustus, Phlox longifolia, Physaria chambersii, Prosopis pubescens, Prunus emarginata, P. virginiana, Psathyrotes annua, Salvia dorrii, Trientalis borealis, Trillium ovatum

Febrifuge: Achillea millefolium, Artemisia furcata, A. ludoviciana, A. tridentata, Ericameria nana, Juniperus occidentalis, J. osteosperma, Mentha canadensis, Osmorhiza occidentalis, Pinus monophylla, Populus tremuloides, Salvia dorrii, Veratrum californicum, Wyethia mollis

Gastrointestinal Aid: Achillea millefolium, Agastache urticifolia, Aquilegia formosa, Artemisia ludoviciana, A. spinescens, A. tridentata, Balsamorhiza hookeri, B. sagittata, Cercocarpus ledifolius, Ephedra viridis, Eriastrum eremicum, Ericameria nana, Erigeron aphanactis, Eriogonum umbellatum, Frangula purshiana, Haplopappus sp., Holodiscus dumosus, Ipomopsis congesta, Iris missouriensis, Juniperus occidentalis, J. osteosperma, Larrea tridentata, Linum lewisii, Mahonia repens, Maianthemum stellatum, Mentha canadensis, Monardella odoratissima, Osmorhiza occidentalis, Penstemon deustus, Phlox longifolia, Pinus monophylla, Pluchea sericea, Populus balsamifera, Psathyrotes ramosissima, Psorothamnus polydenius, Rumex crispus, R. venosus, Salvia dorrii, Sambucus cerulea, Symphoricarpos longiflorus, Tetradymia comosa

Gland Medicine: *Veratrum californicum*

Gynecological Aid: *Achillea millefolium, Artemisia dracunculus, A. ludoviciana, A. tridentata, Juniperus occidentalis, J. osteosperma, Maianthemum stellatum, Phoenicaulis cheiranthoides, Pinus monophylla, Sambucus racemosa, Thamnosma montana, Veratrum californicum*

Hallucinogen: *Datura wrightii*

Heart Medicine: *Cercocarpus ledifolius, Chaenactis douglasii, Helianthus cusickii, Paeonia brownii*

Hemostat: *Gutierrezia sarothrae, Mahonia nervosa, Sambucus racemosa*

Herbal Steam: *Artemisia ludoviciana, Lomatium dissectum, Prunus virginiana, Salvia dorrii, Urtica dioica*

Kidney Aid: *Achillea millefolium, Angelica breweri, Clematis ligusticifolia, Ephedra viridis, Juniperus occidentalis, J. osteosperma, Nicotiana attenuata, Paeonia brownii, Psorothamnus polydenius, Rumex venosus, Suaeda moquinii*

Laxative: *Anemopsis californica, Psathyrotes ramosissima, Sambucus tridentata*

Liver Aid: *Psathyrotes ramosissima, Purshia tridentata*

Misc. Disease Remedy: *Artemisia douglasiana, A. ludoviciana, A. tridentata, Asclepias speciosa, Ericameria nana, Juniperus monosperma, J. occidentalis, J. osteosperma, Larrea tridentata, Lomatium dissectum, Nicotiana attenuata, Osmorhiza occidentalis, Pinus monophylla, Prunus andersonii, Psorothamnus polydenius, Purshia tridentata, Rosa woodsii, Rumex venosus, Salvia dorrii, Stanleya pinnata, Suaeda moquinii, Tetradymia comosa, Thamnosma montana, Urtica dioica*

Narcotic: *Datura wrightii*

Orthopedic Aid: *Achillea millefolium, Anemopsis californica, Artemisia dracunculus, A. ludovici-*

ana, A. tridentata, A. vulgaris, Chaenactis douglasii, Chamaebatiaria millefolium, Cicuta maculata, Eriogonum umbellatum, Gutierrezia sarothrae, Helianthella uniflora, Hypericum scouleri, Juniperus communis, Lomatium dissectum, Maianthemum stellatum, Pinus monophylla, Psorothamnus polydenius, Ribes aureum, Wyethia mollis, Zigadenus paniculatus

Other: *Datura wrightii, Glycyrrhiza lepidota, Mentha arvensis*

Panacea: *Aquilegia formosa, Larrea tridentata, Lomatium dissectum, Veratrum californicum*

Pediatric Aid: *Artemisia furcata, A. ludoviciana, A. tridentata, Cercocarpus ledifolius, Ephedra viridis, Eriastrum eremicum, Mentha canadensis, Penstemon deustus, Phlox longifolia, Rosa woodsii, Salvia dorrii, Sambucus racemosa*

Poison: *Toxicodendron pubescens, Zigadenus venenosus*

Poultice: *Linum lewisii, Salvia dorrii*

Psychological Aid: *Mirabilis alipes*

Pulmonary Aid: *Abies concolor, Artemisia spinescens, A. tridentata, Cercocarpus ledifolius, Corallorrhiza maculata, Eriodictyon angustifolium, Grindelia nana, G. squarrosa, Juniperus occidentalis, J. osteosperma, Lomatium dissectum, Orobanche californica, Osmorhiza occidentalis, Phragmites australis, Pinus monophylla, Plantago major, Psorothamnus polydenius, Purshia tridentata, Rumex venosus, Salvia dorrii, Tetradymia comosa, Urtica dioica*

Respiratory Aid: *Achillea millefolium, Artemisia tridentata, Lomatium dissectum, Nicotiana attenuata*

Snakebite Remedy: *Asclepias speciosa, Chaenactis douglasii, Cicuta maculata, Nicotiana attenuata, Osmorhiza occidentalis, Psathyrotes ramosissima, Veratrum californicum, Zigadenus venenosus*

Stimulant: *Mirabilis alipes*

Throat Aid: *Angelica breweri, Aquilegia formosa, Eriastrum virgatum, Heliotropium curassavicum, Lomatium dissectum, Machaeranthera canescens, Mentha canadensis, Osmorhiza occidentalis, Pinus monophylla, Stanleya pinnata, Veratrum californicum*

Tonic: *Artemisia dracunculus, A. ludoviciana, A. tridentata, Brachyactis frondosa, Ephedra viridis, Juniperus communis, J. occidentalis, J. osteosperma, Phoenicaulis cheiranthoides, Pinus monophylla, Prunus andersonii, Purshia tridentata, Rosa woodsii, Rumex crispus, R. venosus, Sambucus racemosa, Stanleya pinnata, Wyethia mollis*

Toothache Remedy: *Achillea millefolium, Iris missouriensis, Psathyrotes annua, P. ramosissima, Psorothamnus polydenius, Stephanomeria spinosa, Veratrum californicum, Zigadenus paniculatus*

Tuberculosis Remedy: *Abies concolor, Achillea millefolium, Asclepias speciosa, Balsamorhiza sagittata, Cercocarpus ledifolius, Eriastrum eremicum, Eriodictyon angustifolium, Eriogonum microthecum, Helianthus cusickii, Lomatium dissectum, Nicotiana attenuata, Paeonia brownii, Pastinaca sativa, Pinus monophylla, Prunus andersonii, P. virginiana, Psorothamnus polydenius, Purshia tridentata, Wyethia mollis*

Unspecified: *Linum lewisii, Lophophora williamsii, Urtica dioica*

Urinary Aid: *Achillea millefolium, Artemisia spinescens, Balsamorhiza hookeri, Ephedra viridis, Eriogonum microthecum, Grindelia nana, G. squarrosa, Iris missouriensis, Mahonia repens, Suaeda moquinii*

Venereal Aid: *Abies concolor, Achillea millefolium, Anemopsis californica, Artemisia ludoviciana, A. vulgaris, Balsamorhiza sagittata, Cercocarpus ledifolius, Cucurbita foetidissima, Ephedra nevadensis, E. viridis, Heuchera rubescens, Ipomopsis congesta, Iris missouriensis, Juniperus communis, J. occidentalis, J. osteosperma, Krameria grayi, Larrea tridentata, Lomatium dissectum, Mahonia repens, Osmorhiza occidentalis, Phlox longifolia, Pinus monophylla, Psathyrotes ramosissima, Psorothamnus polydenius, Purshia mexicana, P. tridentata, Rumex crispus, R. venosus, Salvia dorrii, Sphenosciadium capitellatum, Veratrum californicum, Wyethia mollis*

Veterinary Aid: *Achillea millefolium, Descurainia sophia, Geum triflorum, Juniperus occidentalis, Lomatium dissectum, Paeonia brownii, Veratrum californicum*

Paiute, Northern

Analgesic: *Artemisia tridentata, Juniperus osteosperma, Lomatium dissectum, Osmorhiza occidentalis, Salvia dorrii*

Anthelmintic: *Purshia tridentata*

Antidiarrheal: *Artemisia tridentata*

Antihemorrhagic: *Angelica lineariloba, Cercocarpus ledifolius*

Antirheumatic (External): *Artemisia tridentata, Atriplex confertifolia, Heracleum maximum, Juniperus osteosperma, Lomatium dissectum, Osmorhiza occidentalis, Urtica dioica, Veratrum californicum, Zigadenus paniculatus, Z. venenosus*

Cathartic: *Psorothamnus polydenius*

Cold Remedy: *Achillea millefolium, Artemisia douglasiana, A. tridentata, Atriplex confertifolia, Juniperus osteosperma, Lomatium dissectum, Mentha canadensis, Osmorhiza occidentalis, Psorothamnus polydenius, Salvia dorrii, Veratrum californicum*

Cough Medicine: *Achillea millefolium*

Dermatological Aid: *Achillea millefolium, Asclepias cryptoceras, Ephedra viridis, Lomatium dissectum, Mirabilis alipes, Osmorhiza occidentalis, Penstemon deustus, Rumex crispus, Urtica dioica, Veratrum californicum*

Diaphoretic: *Achillea millefolium*

Diuretic: *Lomatium dissectum*

Emetic: *Artemisia tridentata*

Eye Medicine: *Osmorhiza occidentalis*

Febrifuge: *Artemisia douglasiana, A. tridentata, Mentha canadensis*

Gastrointestinal Aid: *Eriastrum sparsiflorum, Purshia tridentata*

Hallucinogen: *Datura wrightii*

Kidney Aid: *Achillea millefolium*

Laxative: *Purshia tridentata*

Misc. Disease Remedy: *Achillea millefolium, Psorothamnus polydenius*

Oral Aid: *Xanthium strumarium*

Orthopedic Aid: *Veratrum californicum*

Panacea: *Lomatium dissectum*

Pediatric Aid: *Artemisia tridentata*

Poison: *Datura wrightii*

Pulmonary Aid: *Angelica lineariloba, Psorothamnus polydenius*

Stimulant: *Artemisia tridentata*

Throat Aid: *Achillea millefolium, Lomatium dissectum, Psorothamnus polydenius*

Toothache Remedy: *Sarcobatus vermiculatus*

Tuberculosis Remedy: *Cercocarpus ledifolius*

Venereal Aid: *Salix exigua, Salvia dorrii*

Vertigo Medicine: *Lomatium dissectum*

Papago

Analgesic: *Larrea tridentata, Taraxacum officinale*

Antirheumatic (External): *Larrea tridentata*

Dermatological Aid: *Larrea tridentata, Peniocereus greggii, Prosopis velutina, Rumex hymenosepalus, Simmondsia chinensis*

Emetic: *Anemopsis californica, Larrea tridentata*

Gynecological Aid: *Larrea tridentata, Taraxacum officinale*

Orthopedic Aid: *Larrea tridentata*

Pediatric Aid: *Larrea tridentata*

Snakebite Remedy: *Larrea tridentata*
Throat Aid: *Rumex hymenosepalus*
Toothache Remedy: *Phaseolus acutifolius*

Pawnee

Abortifacient: *Artemisia frigida*
Analgesic: *Aquilegia canadensis, Arisaema triphyllum, Echinacea angustifolia, Gymnocladus dioicus, Ipomoea leptophylla*
Antidiarrheal: *Liatris scariosa, Rhus glabra, Rumex hymenosepalus*
Antidote: *Echinacea angustifolia*
Antirheumatic (External): *Arisaema triphyllum, Artemisia dracunculus*
Burn Dressing: *Echinacea angustifolia, Rosa arkansana, Typha latifolia*
Carminative: *Acorus calamus, Mentha canadensis*
Ceremonial Medicine: *Acorus calamus, Hierochloe odorata, Prunus virginiana*
Cold Remedy: *Acorus calamus, Juniperus virginiana*
Cough Medicine: *Acorus calamus, Juniperus virginiana*
Dermatological Aid: *Desmanthus illinoensis, Heracleum maximum, Opuntia humifusa, Typha latifolia*
Ear Medicine: *Glycyrrhiza lepidota*
Febrifuge: *Acorus calamus, Aquilegia canadensis, Glycyrrhiza lepidota, Penstemon grandiflorus*
Gastrointestinal Aid: *Acorus calamus, Baptisia bracteata*
Gynecological Aid: *Helianthus annuus, Mirabilis nyctaginea, Rhus glabra*
Herbal Steam: *Yucca glauca*
Laxative: *Ulmus rubra*
Love Medicine: *Aquilegia canadensis, Cuscuta compacta, Lobelia cardinalis, Lomatium foeniculaceum, Panax quinquefolius*
Misc. Disease Remedy: *Echinacea angustifolia*
Oral Aid: *Mirabilis nyctaginea*
Other: *Echinacea angustifolia*
Panacea: *Acorus calamus, Cucurbita foetidissima, Dalea candida, D. purpurea*
Pediatric Aid: *Croton texensis, Glycyrrhiza lepidota, Liatris scariosa, Mirabilis nyctaginea, Typha latifolia*
Poison: *Euphorbia marginata*
Sedative: *Ipomoea leptophylla, Juniperus virginiana*
Snakebite Remedy: *Echinacea angustifolia*
Stimulant: *Gymnocladus dioicus, Ipomoea leptophylla, Osmorhiza longistylis*
Tonic: *Silphium laciniatum*

Toothache Remedy: *Acorus calamus, Echinacea angustifolia, Glycyrrhiza lepidota*
Unspecified: *Artemisia dracunculus*
Veterinary Aid: *Echinacea angustifolia, Grindelia squarrosa, Juniperus virginiana, Oxalis violacea, Thalictrum dasycarpum, Zanthoxylum americanum*
Witchcraft Medicine: *Silphium laciniatum*

Penobscot

Analgesic: *Kalmia angustifolia, Thuja occidentalis*
Anthelmintic: *Apocynum cannabinum*
Anticonvulsive: *Aristolochia serpentaria*
Antidiarrheal: *Prunus virginiana*
Antihemorrhagic: *Acer pensylvanicum, Aralia racemosa, Baptisia tinctoria, Eupatorium perfoliatum, Galium aparine, Pyrola asarifolia, Sarracenia purpurea, Streptopus amplexifolius, Ulmus americana*
Burn Dressing: *Abies balsamea, Impatiens capensis*
Cold Remedy: *Populus tremuloides, Taxus canadensis*
Cough Medicine: *Aralia nudicaulis, Prunus serotina*
Dermatological Aid: *Abies balsamea, Acer pensylvanicum, Arctium minus, Chimaphila umbellata, Comptonia peregrina, Impatiens capensis, Nuphar lutea, Nymphaea odorata, Thuja occidentalis*
Diaphoretic: *Populus tremuloides*
Dietary Aid: *Quercus alba*
Emetic: *Sorbus americana*
Gynecological Aid: *Fraxinus americana*
Hemorrhoid Remedy: *Quercus alba*
Herbal Steam: *Iris versicolor*
Kidney Aid: *Acer pensylvanicum, Aralia racemosa, Baptisia tinctoria, Cimicifuga racemosa, Eupatorium perfoliatum, Galium aparine, Pyrola asarifolia, Sarracenia purpurea, Streptopus amplexifolius*
Misc. Disease Remedy: *Iris versicolor, Viburnum opulus*
Oral Aid: *Berberis vulgaris, Coptis trifolia*
Orthopedic Aid: *Arisaema triphyllum, Impatiens capensis*
Panacea: *Kalmia angustifolia, Thuja occidentalis*
Poison: *Arisaema triphyllum*
Preventive Medicine: *Iris versicolor, Sanguinaria canadensis*
Pulmonary Aid: *Ulmus americana*
Reproductive Aid: *Panax quinquefolius*
Respiratory Aid: *Salix lucida, Verbascum thapsus*
Sedative: *Cypripedium acaule*

Throat Aid: *Berberis vulgaris*

Tonic: *Acer pensylvanicum, Aralia racemosa, Baptisia tinctoria, Eupatorium perfoliatum, Galium aparine, Prunus serotina, Pyrola asarifolia, Streptopus amplexifolius*

Unspecified: *Lycopodium dendroideum, Mitchella repens*

Venereal Aid: *Acer pensylvanicum, Aralia racemosa, Baptisia tinctoria, Eupatorium perfoliatum, Galium aparine, Pyrola asarifolia, Streptopus amplexifolius*

Pima

Analgesic: *Ambrosia ambrosioides, Datura discolor, Encelia farinosa, Isocoma pluriflora, Krameria grayi, Larrea tridentata, Proboscidea althaeifolia, P. parviflora, Prosopis velutina, Ricinus communis, Ziziphus obtusifolia*

Anthelmintic: *Helianthus annuus*

Antidiarrheal: *Larrea tridentata, Plantago ovata, Pluchea sericea, Prosopis velutina, Sphaeralcea angustifolia, S. emoryi, Xanthium strumarium*

Antihemorrhagic: *Ambrosia ambrosioides*

Antirheumatic (External): *Atriplex polycarpa, Larrea tridentata, Proboscidea althaeifolia, P. parviflora, Ziziphus obtusifolia*

Antirheumatic (Internal): *Larrea tridentata*

Burn Dressing: *Prosopis velutina*

Carminative: *Larrea tridentata*

Cathartic: *Asclepias subulata, Phoradendron californicum, Prosopis velutina, Ricinus communis, Sonchus oleraceus, Yucca baccata*

Cold Remedy: *Anemopsis californica, Cyperus esculentus, Larrea tridentata, Rumex hymenosepalus, Sambucus cerulea, Solanum elaeagnifolium*

Cough Medicine: *Ambrosia ambrosioides, Anemopsis californica, Cyperus esculentus, Isocoma pluriflora, Krameria grayi, Rumex hymenosepalus*

Dermatological Aid: *Anemopsis californica, Atriplex lentiformis, Chamaesyce polycarpa, Cucurbita pepo, Datura discolor, Descurainia pinnata, Ephedra fasciculata, E. trifurca, Heliotropium curassavicum, Krameria erecta, K. grayi, Larrea tridentata, Malva parviflora, Orobanche ludoviciana, Phoradendron californicum, Pluchea sericea, Populus fremontii, Prosopis pubescens, P. velutina, Ricinus communis, Rumex hymenosepalus, Ziziphus obtusifolia*

Diaphoretic: *Anemopsis californica, Chamaesyce polycarpa*

Disinfectant: *Krameria grayi, Prosopis velutina*

Ear Medicine: *Datura discolor, Mammillaria grahamii*

Emetic: *Anemopsis californica, Asclepias subulata, Chamaesyce polycarpa, Larrea tridentata, Prosopis velutina*

Eye Medicine: *Asclepias subulata, Datura discolor, Krameria grayi, Pluchea sericea, Prosopis velutina, Sisymbrium irio, Xanthium strumarium, Ziziphus obtusifolia*

Febrifuge: *Helianthus annuus, Krameria grayi, Larrea tridentata, Salix gooddingii, Sambucus cerulea*

Gastrointestinal Aid: *Anemopsis californica, Asclepias subulata, Chamaesyce polycarpa, Datura discolor, Larrea tridentata, Opuntia acanthocarpa, Phoradendron californicum, Pluchea sericea, Prosopis velutina, Sambucus cerulea, Sphaeralcea angustifolia*

Gynecological Aid: *Ambrosia ambrosioides, Carnegia gigantea, Datura discolor, Opuntia engelmannii, O. phaeacantha, Prosopis pubescens*

Hemorrhoid Remedy: *Datura discolor*

Hemostat: *Acourtia wrightii*

Laxative: *Chamaesyce polycarpa, Pectis papposa, Ricinus communis, Xanthium strumarium*

Misc. Disease Remedy: *Peniocereus greggii*

Oral Aid: *Larrea tridentata, Prosopis velutina, Rumex hymenosepalus*

Orthopedic Aid: *Carnegia gigantea, Isocoma pluriflora*

Other: *Anemopsis californica, Datura discolor, Ephedra trifurca, Prosopis velutina, Sonchus oleraceus*

Panacea: *Asclepias subulata, Larrea tridentata*

Pediatric Aid: *Krameria grayi, Pluchea sericea, Prosopis velutina*

Poison: *Asclepias subulata, Chamaesyce polycarpa, Ricinus communis*

Sedative: *Pluchea sericea*

Snakebite Remedy: *Chamaesyce polycarpa, Cyperus esculentus*

Strengthener: *Larrea tridentata*

Throat Aid: *Anemopsis californica, Krameria grayi, Rumex hymenosepalus, Sambucus cerulea*

Toothache Remedy: *Larrea tridentata*

Tuberculosis Remedy: *Anemopsis californica, Larrea tridentata*

Unspecified: *Larrea tridentata, Rumex hymenosepalus*

Urinary Aid: *Larrea tridentata*

Venereal Aid: *Anemopsis californica, Ephedra antisyphilitica, E. fasciculata, E. trifurca, Thamnosma montana*

Veterinary Aid: *Cyperus esculentus, Helianthus an-nuus, Pluchea sericea, Xanthium strumarium*

Plains Indian
Dermatological Aid: *Typha latifolia*
Pediatric Aid: *Typha latifolia*
Veterinary Aid: *Hierochloe odorata*

Poliklah
Eye Medicine: *Artemisia ludoviciana*
Pediatric Aid: *Ceanothus thyrsiflorus*
Poison: *Lonicera involucrata*

Pomo
Abortifacient: *Phoradendron villosum*
Analgesic: *Umbellularia californica, Urtica dioica*
Antidiarrheal: *Arctostaphylos columbiana, Croton setigerus*
Antiemetic: *Perideridia kelloggii*
Antihemorrhagic: *Ligusticum apiifolium*
Antirheumatic (External): *Heracleum maximum, Oxalis oregana, Umbellularia californica, Urtica dioica*
Blood Medicine: *Satureja douglasii*
Cold Remedy: *Calycanthus occidentalis*
Dermatological Aid: *Alnus rhombifolia, Aralia californica, Arbutus menziesii, Artemisia vulgaris, Asarum caudatum, Chlorogalum pomeridianum, Gnaphalium stramineum, Heracleum maximum, Marah fabaceus, Sambucus racemosa, Scrophularia californica*
Dietary Aid: *Satureja douglasii*
Ear Medicine: *Sequoia sempervirens*
Expectorant: *Eriodictyon californicum*
Eye Medicine: *Thermopsis macrophylla*
Gastrointestinal Aid: *Satureja douglasii*
Gynecological Aid: *Amelanchier alnifolia, Artemisia vulgaris, Convolvulus arvensis, Iris macrosiphon, I. tenuissima*
Laxative: *Frangula californica*
Panacea: *Aralia californica*
Pediatric Aid: *Alnus rhombifolia, Artemisia vulgaris*
Poison: *Aesculus californica, Clintonia andrewsiana, Croton setigerus, Frangula californica*
Pulmonary Aid: *Ligusticum apiifolium*
Stimulant: *Sequoia sempervirens*
Tonic: *Sequoia sempervirens*
Tuberculosis Remedy: *Torreya californica*
Unspecified: *Arctostaphylos glandulosa, Pinus lambertiana*

Pomo, Calpella
Blood Medicine: *Linanthus ciliatus*

Cold Remedy: *Arctostaphylos manzanita, Linanthus ciliatus*
Cough Medicine: *Linanthus ciliatus*
Pediatric Aid: *Linanthus ciliatus*

Pomo, Kashaya
Abortifacient: *Garrya elliptica, Phoradendron villosum*
Analgesic: *Artemisia douglasiana, Umbellularia californica, Urtica dioica*
Antidiarrheal: *Arctostaphylos columbiana, A. glandulosa, Croton setigerus, Rubus leucodermis, R. ursinus*
Antiemetic: *Perideridia kelloggii*
Antirheumatic (External): *Heracleum maximum, Oxalis oregana, Umbellularia californica, Urtica dioica*
Blood Medicine: *Eriodictyon californicum, Horkelia californica, Ligusticum apiifolium, Satureja douglasii*
Cold Remedy: *Angelica tomentosa, Calycanthus occidentalis, Salix lucida, Satureja douglasii, Umbellularia californica*
Cough Medicine: *Eriodictyon californicum, Lithocarpus densiflorus*
Dermatological Aid: *Achillea millefolium, Alnus rhombifolia, A. rubra, Angelica tomentosa, Aralia californica, Arbutus menziesii, Artemisia douglasiana, Asarum caudatum, Chlorogalum pomeridianum, Equisetum arvense, Eriodictyon californicum, Marah fabaceus, Phacelia californica, Pteridium aquilinum, Scrophularia californica, Stachys bullata, Umbellularia californica, Xerophyllum tenax*
Ear Medicine: *Sequoia sempervirens*
Expectorant: *Calycanthus occidentalis, Nereocystis luetkeana*
Eye Medicine: *Diplacus aurantiacus, Foeniculum vulgare, Thermopsis macrophylla*
Febrifuge: *Eriodictyon californicum, Sambucus cerulea*
Gastrointestinal Aid: *Angelica tomentosa, Artemisia douglasiana, Calycanthus occidentalis, Foeniculum vulgare, Rubus leucodermis, Satureja douglasii, Sisyrinchium bellum*
Gynecological Aid: *Amelanchier pallida, Angelica tomentosa, Artemisia douglasiana, Convolvulus arvensis, Equisetum telmateia, Eschscholzia californica, Rubus ursinus, Thermopsis macrophylla, Umbellularia californica*
Kidney Aid: *Equisetum laevigatum*
Laxative: *Frangula californica, Melilotus indicus*
Love Medicine: *Arbutus menziesii*
Misc. Disease Remedy: *Vaccinium ovatum*

Oral Aid: *Angelica tomentosa*
Other: *Angelica tomentosa, Rubus leucodermis*
Poison: *Amanita muscaria, Clintonia andrewsiana, Lycoperdon* sp., *Zigadenus venenosus*
Pulmonary Aid: *Ligusticum apiifolium*
Respiratory Aid: *Sisyrinchium bellum, Umbellularia californica*
Sedative: *Dodecatheon hendersonii, Satureja douglasii*
Stimulant: *Sequoia sempervirens*
Throat Aid: *Angelica tomentosa, Arbutus menziesii, Calycanthus occidentalis, Nereocystis luetkeana, Salix hindsiana, S. lucida, Umbellularia californica*
Toothache Remedy: *Asarum caudatum*
Tuberculosis Remedy: *Ligusticum apiifolium, Torreya californica*

Pomo, Little Lakes

Analgesic: *Arctostaphylos manzanita*
Antidiarrheal: *Arctostaphylos manzanita*
Antihemorrhagic: *Sambucus cerulea*
Antirheumatic (External): *Pseudotsuga menziesii*
Cold Remedy: *Arbutus menziesii*
Herbal Steam: *Pseudotsuga menziesii*
Tuberculosis Remedy: *Sambucus cerulea*
Venereal Aid: *Pseudotsuga menziesii*

Pomo, Potter Valley

Disinfectant: *Sambucus cerulea*
Emetic: *Sambucus cerulea*
Gastrointestinal Aid: *Cynoglossum grande, Sambucus cerulea*
Venereal Aid: *Cynoglossum grande*

Ponca

Abortifacient: *Artemisia frigida*
Analgesic: *Aquilegia canadensis, Echinacea angustifolia, Lespedeza capitata, Physalis lanceolata, Silphium perfoliatum*
Antidiarrheal: *Lygodesmia juncea, Prunus virginiana*
Antidote: *Echinacea angustifolia*
Antirheumatic (External): *Lespedeza capitata*
Antirheumatic (Internal): *Silphium perfoliatum*
Burn Dressing: *Artemisia dracunculus, Echinacea angustifolia, Typha latifolia*
Carminative: *Acorus calamus, Mentha canadensis*
Ceremonial Medicine: *Acorus calamus, Hierochloe odorata, Prunus virginiana*
Cold Remedy: *Acorus calamus, Juniperus virginiana, Silphium perfoliatum*
Cough Medicine: *Acorus calamus, Juniperus virginiana*

Dermatological Aid: *Iris versicolor, Mirabilis nyctaginea, Physalis lanceolata, Plantago major, Typha latifolia*
Ear Medicine: *Iris versicolor*
Eye Medicine: *Iris versicolor, Lygodesmia juncea, Symphoricarpos occidentalis, S. orbiculatus*
Febrifuge: *Acorus calamus, Aquilegia canadensis, Caulophyllum thalictroides*
Gastrointestinal Aid: *Acorus calamus, Asclepias exaltata, Physalis lanceolata*
Gynecological Aid: *Chamaesyce serpyllifolia, Lygodesmia juncea*
Hallucinogen: *Lophophora williamsii*
Herbal Steam: *Juniperus virginiana, Silphium perfoliatum*
Laxative: *Gymnocladus dioicus, Ulmus rubra*
Love Medicine: *Aquilegia canadensis, Lomatium foeniculaceum, Sanguinaria canadensis, Thalictrum dasycarpum*
Misc. Disease Remedy: *Echinacea angustifolia*
Other: *Echinacea angustifolia*
Panacea: *Acorus calamus, Anemone canadensis, Cucurbita foetidissima*
Pediatric Aid: *Typha latifolia*
Poison: *Toxicodendron pubescens*
Pulmonary Aid: *Asclepias tuberosa*
Respiratory Aid: *Asclepias tuberosa*
Snakebite Remedy: *Echinacea angustifolia*
Stimulant: *Gymnocladus dioicus*
Toothache Remedy: *Acorus calamus, Echinacea angustifolia*
Tuberculosis Remedy: *Grindelia squarrosa*
Unspecified: *Artemisia dracunculus, Lophophora williamsii, Physalis lanceolata*
Veterinary Aid: *Echinacea angustifolia, Juniperus virginiana, Silphium laciniatum*
Witchcraft Medicine: *Silphium laciniatum*

Potawatomi

Adjuvant: *Betula alleghaniensis, B. papyrifera, Cirsium vulgare, Panax quinquefolius, Prunus serotina, Thuja occidentalis*
Alterative: *Aralia hispida, Gentiana alba*
Analgesic: *Aster furcatus, Coptis trifolia, Equisetum arvense, Gaultheria procumbens, Impatiens capensis, Prunus pensylvanica, Rosa blanda, Ulmus americana, Uvularia grandiflora*
Anthelmintic: *Rhus hirta*
Antidiarrheal: *Alnus incana, Cornus sericea, Epilobium ciliatum, Ostrya virginiana, Quercus rubra, Tsuga canadensis, Ulmus americana*
Antiemetic: *Asarum canadense*
Antihemorrhagic: *Acorus calamus, Ostrya virginiana*

Veterinary Aid: *Alnus incana, Conyza canadensis, Larix laricina, Populus tremuloides*

Witchcraft Medicine: *Achillea millefolium, Anaphalis margaritacea, Aster umbellatus, Thuja occidentalis*

Puyallup

Dermatological Aid: *Stachys mexicana*

Quileute

Abortifacient: *Castilleja angustifolia*

Analgesic: *Lysichiton americanus*

Antidiarrheal: *Alnus rubra*

Antidote: *Lonicera involucrata*

Antirheumatic (External): *Achillea millefolium, Urtica dioica*

Antirheumatic (Internal): *Anaphalis margaritacea, Urtica dioica*

Blood Medicine: *Mahonia nervosa, Prunus emarginata*

Burn Dressing: *Fragaria chiloensis, Rubus spectabilis*

Ceremonial Medicine: *Equisetum hyemale, E. laevigatum*

Cold Remedy: *Sambucus racemosa*

Cough Medicine: *Petasites frigidus, Pinus monticola, Sambucus racemosa, Tiarella trifoliata*

Dermatological Aid: *Actaea rubra, Aquilegia formosa, Aruncus dioicus, Claytonia sibirica, Gaultheria shallon, Geum macrophyllum, Leucanthemum vulgare, Lysichiton americanus, Oxalis oregana, Polystichum munitum, Prunella vulgaris, Rosa nutkana, Trillium ovatum, Tsuga heterophylla*

Emetic: *Lonicera involucrata, Tsuga heterophylla, T. mertensiana*

Eye Medicine: *Claytonia sibirica*

Febrifuge: *Achillea millefolium, Lysichiton americanus*

Gynecological Aid: *Lysichiton americanus, Sambucus racemosa*

Laxative: *Frangula purshiana*

Love Medicine: *Galium triflorum*

Orthopedic Aid: *Blechnum spicant*

Panacea: *Achillea millefolium, Blechnum spicant, Frangula purshiana*

Pediatric Aid: *Achillea millefolium, Nepeta cataria*

Pulmonary Aid: *Malus fusca*

Sports Medicine: *Equisetum hyemale, Salix hookeriana*

Tonic: *Aruncus dioicus, Cornus canadensis, C. nuttallii, C. sericea*

Tuberculosis Remedy: *Boykinia occidentalis*

Unspecified: *Alnus rubra, Arctium minus, Arctostaphylos uva-ursi, Brassica nigra, Juncus ensifolius, Leymus mollis, Mentha canadensis, M. ×piperita, Moricandia arvensis, Oplopanax horridus, Populus balsamifera, Sinapis alba, Taraxacum officinale, Thuja plicata*

Urinary Aid: *Claytonia sibirica*

Venereal Aid: *Frangula purshiana, Malus fusca*

Quinault

Abortifacient: *Equisetum hyemale*

Analgesic: *Allium cernuum, Heracleum maximum, Malus fusca, Nuphar lutea, Rubus spectabilis, Urtica dioica*

Antidiarrheal: *Gaultheria shallon*

Antirheumatic (External): *Nuphar lutea*

Antirheumatic (Internal): *Ledum groenlandicum, Veratrum viride*

Blood Medicine: *Malus fusca, Pinus monticola*

Burn Dressing: *Polystichum munitum, Rubus spectabilis*

Cold Remedy: *Tsuga heterophylla*

Cough Medicine: *Polypodium virginianum*

Dermatological Aid: *Actaea rubra, Aruncus dioicus, Galium triflorum, Geum macrophyllum, Lonicera involucrata, Petasites frigidus, Picea sitchensis, Pinus contorta, Polystichum munitum, Populus balsamifera, Prunella vulgaris, Pseudotsuga menziesii, Rosa nutkana, Rubus spectabilis, Taxus brevifolia, Thuja plicata*

Disinfectant: *Populus balsamifera, Rubus spectabilis*

Emetic: *Sambucus cerulea*

Eye Medicine: *Achillea millefolium, Equisetum hyemale, Maianthemum dilatatum, Malus fusca, Oxalis oregana, Petasites frigidus*

Febrifuge: *Thuja plicata*

Gastrointestinal Aid: *Blechnum spicant, Gaultheria shallon, Pinus monticola*

Gynecological Aid: *Claytonia sibirica, Geum macrophyllum, Lonicera involucrata, Prunus emarginata, Rubus spectabilis, Sambucus racemosa, Urtica dioica*

Hemostat: *Urtica dioica*

Kidney Aid: *Thuja plicata*

Laxative: *Frangula purshiana, Prunus emarginata, Tsuga heterophylla*

Love Medicine: *Menziesia ferruginea, Vicia nigricans*

Oral Aid: *Lonicera involucrata*

Orthopedic Aid: *Heracleum maximum, Urtica dioica*

Panacea: *Geum macrophyllum, Lysichiton americanus*

Pediatric Aid: *Tsuga heterophylla*

Poison: *Veratrum viride*
Pulmonary Aid: *Allium cernuum, Taxus brevifolia*
Throat Aid: *Picea sitchensis, Pinus contorta*
Tonic: *Achillea millefolium*
Tuberculosis Remedy: *Achillea millefolium, Populus balsamifera*
Urinary Aid: *Lysichiton americanus*
Venereal Aid: *Rosa nutkana, Thuja plicata*

Rappahannock
Abortifacient: *Lindera benzoin*
Analgesic: *Brassica oleracea, Liriodendron tulipifera, Nepeta cataria*
Anthelmintic: *Chenopodium ambrosioides*
Antidiarrheal: *Cornus florida, Hieracium scabrum, Juglans nigra, Liquidambar styraciflua, Phytolacca americana, Rubus hispidus*
Antirheumatic (Internal): *Nepeta cataria, Phytolacca americana, Sambucus canadensis*
Blood Medicine: *Chimaphila umbellata, Cornus florida, Eupatorium purpureum, Gentianopsis crinita, Perilla frutescens, Rumex crispus, Taraxacum officinale, Trifolium pratense*
Burn Dressing: *Sassafras albidum*
Cold Remedy: *Gleditsia triacanthos, Marrubium vulgare, Prunus serotina*
Cough Medicine: *Gleditsia triacanthos, Marrubium vulgare, Prunus serotina*
Dermatological Aid: *Andropogon glomeratus, Aralia spinosa, Arisaema triphyllum, Aristolochia serpentaria, Asclepias syriaca, Datura stramonium, Fagus grandifolia, Morus rubra, Nuphar lutea, Phytolacca americana, Pinus echinata, Polygonatum biflorum, Portulaca oleracea, Rubus hispidus, Sambucus canadensis, Sassafras albidum, Solanum tuberosum, Verbascum thapsus, Vicia villosa, Xanthium strumarium*
Dietary Aid: *Chimaphila umbellata, Prunus serotina, Quercus rubra*
Ear Medicine: *Nicotiana tabacum*
Emetic: *Pinus echinata*
Eye Medicine: *Sassafras albidum*
Febrifuge: *Aralia spinosa, Aristolochia serpentaria, Datura stramonium, Gnaphalium obtusifolium, Hexastylis arifolia, Juglans nigra, Nuphar lutea, Plantago major, Sassafras albidum*
Gastrointestinal Aid: *Acorus calamus, Chimaphila umbellata, Juglans nigra, Taraxacum officinale, Vicia villosa*
Gynecological Aid: *Aletris farinosa, Hedeoma pulegioides, Lindera benzoin*
Hallucinogen: *Magnolia virginiana*
Hemorrhoid Remedy: *Andropogon glomeratus, Phytolacca americana*

Hypotensive: *Allium vineale*
Kidney Aid: *Citrullus lanatus, Pinus virginiana, Prunus persica*
Love Medicine: *Liriodendron tulipifera*
Misc. Disease Remedy: *Sassafras albidum*
Oral Aid: *Diospyros virginiana*
Orthopedic Aid: *Polygonatum biflorum, Verbascum thapsus*
Other: *Juniperus virginiana*
Panacea: *Alnus glutinosa, Cypripedium acaule, Iris versicolor, Rhus hirta, Xanthium strumarium*
Pediatric Aid: *Acorus calamus, Nepeta cataria*
Poison: *Datura stramonium, Prunus serotina, Solanum nigrum*
Pulmonary Aid: *Allium vineale, Datura stramonium, Hexastylis arifolia, Juniperus virginiana*
Respiratory Aid: *Gnaphalium obtusifolium, Hexastylis arifolia, Juniperus virginiana*
Sedative: *Acorus calamus, Sassafras albidum, Solanum nigrum*
Snakebite Remedy: *Aristolochia serpentaria, Asclepias tuberosa*
Stimulant: *Liriodendron tulipifera, Sassafras albidum*
Throat Aid: *Datura stramonium, Diospyros virginiana*
Tonic: *Acorus calamus, Chenopodium ambrosioides, Chimaphila umbellata, Cornus florida, Eupatorium perfoliatum, Nepeta cataria, Prunus serotina, Quercus rubra, Rubus hispidus, Sassafras albidum*
Toothache Remedy: *Nicotiana tabacum*
Unspecified: *Prunus americana*
Veterinary Aid: *Chimaphila umbellata, Citrullus lanatus, Liquidambar styraciflua, Pinus echinata, Verbascum thapsus*

Ree
Ceremonial Medicine: *Helianthus annuus*
Stimulant: *Helianthus annuus*

Round Valley Indian
Analgesic: *Eriogonum latifolium*
Antidiarrheal: *Marrubium vulgare*
Antirheumatic (Internal): *Eriodictyon californicum*
Blood Medicine: *Eriodictyon californicum*
Cold Remedy: *Marrubium vulgare*
Dermatological Aid: *Humulus lupulus, Rhus trilobata*
Eye Medicine: *Eriogonum latifolium*
Febrifuge: *Eriodictyon californicum*
Gastrointestinal Aid: *Eriogonum latifolium*

Gynecological Aid: *Eriogonum latifolium*

Misc. Disease Remedy: *Eriodictyon californicum, Rhus trilobata*

Respiratory Aid: *Eriodictyon californicum*

Tuberculosis Remedy: *Eriodictyon californicum*

Saanich

Antidiarrheal: *Rubus parviflorus*

Antirheumatic (External): *Chimaphila umbellata, Goodyera oblongifolia*

Blood Medicine: *Equisetum arvense, E. telmateia, Satureja douglasii*

Burn Dressing: *Symphoricarpos albus*

Cold Remedy: *Achillea millefolium, Arbutus menziesii, Lomatium nudicaule, Polypodium virginianum, Prunus emarginata*

Dermatological Aid: *Abies grandis, Symphoricarpos albus, Vicia nigricans*

Gastrointestinal Aid: *Cornus sericea, Polypodium virginianum, Rubus parviflorus*

Laxative: *Physocarpus capitatus*

Misc. Disease Remedy: *Juniperus scopulorum*

Panacea: *Malus fusca, Prunus emarginata*

Psychological Aid: *Prunus emarginata, Ribes divaricatum, R. lacustre, R. lobbii*

Respiratory Aid: *Cornus sericea*

Throat Aid: *Achillea millefolium, Lomatium nudicaule, Polypodium virginianum*

Tonic: *Alnus rubra, Stachys ciliata*

Toothache Remedy: *Achillea millefolium*

Salish

Cathartic: *Shepherdia canadensis*

Cold Remedy: *Artemisia tridentata, Veratrum viride*

Dermatological Aid: *Ipomopsis aggregata, Nicotiana attenuata*

Disinfectant: *Juniperus virginiana*

Eye Medicine: *Achillea millefolium, Ipomopsis aggregata*

Gastrointestinal Aid: *Shepherdia canadensis*

Oral Aid: *Geranium oreganum*

Pediatric Aid: *Ipomopsis aggregata*

Poison: *Veratrum viride*

Tonic: *Ledum groenlandicum, Lupinus polyphyllus, Shepherdia canadensis*

Tuberculosis Remedy: *Verbascum thapsus*

Unspecified: *Aconitum delphiniifolium, Apocynum androsaemifolium, Mentha canadensis, Penstemon fruticosus*

Venereal Aid: *Arabis drummondii, Populus tremuloides*

Salish, Coast

Analgesic: *Lomatium utriculatum, Oplopanax horridus, Veratrum viride*

Antirheumatic (External): *Oplopanax horridus, Veratrum viride*

Cathartic: *Cicuta douglasii*

Dermatological Aid: *Abies grandis, Heracleum maximum, Moneses uniflora, Pinus contorta, Prunella vulgaris*

Diaphoretic: *Veratrum viride*

Emetic: *Cicuta douglasii*

Gastrointestinal Aid: *Lomatium utriculatum*

Internal Medicine: *Lomatium nudicaule*

Misc. Disease Remedy: *Pinus contorta*

Other: *Ribes divaricatum, R. lacustre, R. lobbii*

Tonic: *Frangula purshiana*

Salish, Cowichan

Throat Aid: *Arbutus menziesii*

Samish

Cough Medicine: *Gaultheria shallon*

Dermatological Aid: *Malus fusca*

Gastrointestinal Aid: *Malus fusca*

Other: *Lysichiton americanus*

Tonic: *Mahonia aquifolium, Urtica dioica*

Tuberculosis Remedy: *Gaultheria shallon*

Sanpoil

Abortifacient: *Achillea millefolium*

Adjuvant: *Equisetum hyemale*

Analgesic: *Artemisia ludoviciana, Balsamorhiza sagittata, Heracleum maximum*

Antidiarrheal: *Eriogonum compositum, E. heracleoides, Prunus virginiana, Salix scouleriana*

Antiemetic: *Mahonia aquifolium*

Antihemorrhagic: *Purshia tridentata*

Cathartic: *Chaenactis douglasii, Frangula purshiana*

Cold Remedy: *Achillea millefolium, Artemisia dracunculus, A. ludoviciana, A. tridentata, Mentha canadensis, Monardella odoratissima, Oplopanax horridus, Ribes bracteosum*

Dermatological Aid: *Alnus incana, Arctostaphylos uva-ursi, Artemisia ludoviciana, Balsamorhiza sagittata, Ceanothus sanguineus, Clematis ligusticifolia, Geranium viscosissimum, Heracleum maximum, Holodiscus discolor, Juniperus scopulorum, Rhus glabra, Symphoricarpos albus*

Diaphoretic: *Artemisia tridentata*

Diuretic: *Symphoricarpos albus*

Eye Medicine: *Geranium viscosissimum, Heracle-*

um maximum, Mahonia aquifolium, Symphori-carpos albus

Gastrointestinal Aid: *Artemisia tridentata, Mahonia aquifolium*

Gynecological Aid: *Apocynum androsaemifolium*

Laxative: *Artemisia tridentata, Purshia tridentata*

Misc. Disease Remedy: *Artemisia tridentata*

Oral Aid: *Rhus glabra*

Panacea: *Mentha canadensis*

Pediatric Aid: *Arctostaphylos uva-ursi, Equisetum hyemale, Mentha canadensis, Monardella odoratissima, Ribes bracteosum*

Tuberculosis Remedy: *Artemisia tridentata, Chaenactis douglasii, Grindelia nana, Juniperus scopulorum, Mahonia aquifolium*

Unspecified: *Juniperus scopulorum, Symphoricarpos albus*

Veterinary Aid: *Chrysothamnus nauseosus, Clematis ligusticifolia, Symphoricarpos albus*

Sanpoil & Nespelem

Unspecified: *Prunus virginiana*

Seminole

Abortifacient: *Persea borbonia, Pterocaulon virgatum*

Analgesic: *Andropogon floridanus, Bidens coronata, Cephalanthus occidentalis, Desmodium incanum, Dichanthelium laxiflorum, D. strigosum, Eleocharis geniculata, Eryngium yuccifolium, Galactia volubilis, Juniperus virginiana, Lagenaria siceraria, Lechea minor, Liatris laxa, Licania michauxii, Myrica cerifera, Pediomelum canescens, Persea borbonia, Phytolacca americana, Pinguicula lutea, P. pumila, Pinus elliottii, Quercus phellos, Q. virginiana, Rudbeckia hirta, Sabal palmetto, Sabatia campanulata, Salix caroliniana, S. humilis, Sassafras albidum, Sisyrinchium nashii, Solanum donianum, Vaccinium myrsinites, Verbesina virginica, Vitis aestivalis*

Antidiarrheal: *Andropogon floridanus, Bidens coronata, Cephalanthus occidentalis, Eleocharis geniculata, Eryngium yuccifolium, Galactia volubilis, Juniperus virginiana, Lechea minor, Liatris laxa, Licania michauxii, Persea borbonia, Pterocaulon virgatum, Sabatia campanulata, Salix caroliniana, S. humilis, Sassafras albidum, Stillingia sylvatica, Vaccinium myrsinites*

Antiemetic: *Andropogon floridanus, Cephalanthus occidentalis, Chamaecrista fasciculata, Erythrina herbacea, Galactia volubilis, Lechea minor, Liatris laxa, Licania michauxii, Persea borbonia, Sassafras albidum, Stillingia sylvatica*

Antihemorrhagic: *Eryngium yuccifolium, Pterocaulon virgatum*

Antirheumatic (External): *Barbula unguiculata, Bidens coronata, Bryum capillare, Chaptalia tomentosa, Dichanthelium laxiflorum, D. strigosum, Eleocharis geniculata, Eryngium yuccifolium, Erythrina herbacea, Juniperus virginiana, Liatris laxa, Octoblepharum albidum, Panax quinquefolius, Pediomelum canescens, Persea borbonia, Phoradendron leucarpum, Pinus elliottii, Polygala lutea, P. rugelii, Quercus phellos, Q. virginiana, Salix caroliniana, Saururus cernuus, Verbesina virginica, Ximenia americana*

Antirheumatic (Internal): *Eryngium yuccifolium, Phytolacca americana, Salix caroliniana*

Blood Medicine: *Cephalanthus occidentalis, Chenopodium ambrosioides, Polygala lutea, P. rugelii, Salix caroliniana, Stillingia sylvatica*

Cathartic: *Arundinaria gigantea, Cephalanthus occidentalis, Hypericum brachyphyllum, H. fasciculatum, Ricinus communis, Sassafras albidum*

Ceremonial Medicine: *Eryngium yuccifolium, Persea borbonia, Piloblephis rigida, Salix caroliniana, Sambucus canadensis, Sassafras albidum, Vaccinium myrsinites, Verbesina virginica, Vitis aestivalis, V. munsoniana*

Cold Remedy: *Conyza canadensis, Juniperus virginiana, Pediomelum canescens, Piloblephis rigida, Pityopsis graminifolia, Pterocaulon virgatum, Sassafras albidum, Vaccinium myrsinites, Xyris ambigua*

Cough Medicine: *Andropogon floridanus, Bacopa caroliniana, Conyza canadensis, Dichanthelium laxiflorum, D. strigosum, Hydrocotyle umbellata, Juniperus virginiana, Nymphoides cordata, Pediomelum canescens, Sassafras albidum*

Dermatological Aid: *Acer rubrum, Angadenia berteroi, Aster carolinianus, Callicarpa americana, Drosera capillaris, Eryngium yuccifolium, Ficus aurea, Hyptis pectinata, Ludwigia virgata, Mikania batatifolia, Panax quinquefolius, Paspalidium geminatum, Phragmites australis, Piloblephis rigida, Pinus elliottii, Quercus phellos, Q. virginiana, Rhus copallinum, Sagittaria lancifolia, Salix caroliniana, Sassafras albidum, Saururus cernuus*

Dietary Aid: *Eryngium yuccifolium, Galactia volubilis, Lechea minor, Liatris laxa, Persea borbonia, Sabal palmetto, Sassafras albidum, Stillingia sylvatica*

Emetic: *Eleocharis geniculata, Eryngium yucci-*

folium, Eupatorium perfoliatum, Juniperus virginiana, Persea borbonia, Phoradendron leucarpum, Piloblephis rigida, Salix caroliniana, Sambucus canadensis, Sassafras albidum, Saururus cernuus, Vaccinium myrsinites, Verbesina virginica, Vitis aestivalis, V. munsoniana

Eye Medicine: *Bidens coronata, Juniperus virginiana, Persea borbonia, Sabatia campanulata, Salix caroliniana, S. humilis, Sassafras albidum, Vaccinium myrsinites, Verbesina virginica*

Febrifuge: *Acrostichum danaeifolium, Barbula unguiculata, Bidens coronata, Bryum capillare, Cephalanthus occidentalis, Cicuta maculata, Desmodium incanum, Eleocharis geniculata, Eryngium yuccifolium, Eupatorium perfoliatum, Galactia volubilis, Juniperus virginiana, Lechea minor, Myrica cerifera, Octoblephorum albidum, Persea borbonia, Piloblephis rigida, Pityopsis graminifolia, Pterocaulon virgatum, Rudbeckia hirta, Sabal palmetto, Sabatia campanulata, Salix caroliniana, S. humilis, Sassafras albidum, Saururus cernuus, Vaccinium myrsinites, Verbesina virginica, Vitis aestivalis*

Gastrointestinal Aid: *Andropogon floridanus, Cephalanthus occidentalis, Chenopodium ambrosioides, Desmodium incanum, Eryngium yuccifolium, Lechea minor, Liatris laxa, Licania michauxii, Myrica cerifera, Persea borbonia, Pinguicula lutea, P. pumila, Pterocaulon virgatum, Rubus trivialis, Salix caroliniana, Sambucus canadensis, Sassafras albidum, Verbesina virginica, Vitis aestivalis*

Gynecological Aid: *Pterocaulon virgatum, Zeuxine strateumatica*

Heart Medicine: *Eryngium yuccifolium, Polygala lutea, P. rugelii*

Hemorrhoid Remedy: *Acer rubrum, Pinus elliottii, Quercus phellos, Q. virginiana*

Hemostat: *Tephrosia purpurea*

Hunting Medicine: *Salix caroliniana, S. humilis*

Kidney Aid: *Annona reticulata, Mitchella repens*

Laxative: *Cephalanthus occidentalis, Erythrina herbacea, Persea borbonia, Sassafras albidum, Verbesina virginica*

Love Medicine: *Chrysobalanus icaco, Chrysophyllum oliviforme, Conyza canadensis, Myrica cerifera, Panax quinquefolius, Persea borbonia, Quercus phellos, Q. virginiana, Salix caroliniana, Sideroxylon foetidissimum*

Oral Aid: *Persea borbonia, Salix caroliniana, Sassafras albidum, Verbesina virginica, Ximenia americana*

Orthopedic Aid: *Acer rubrum, Eryngium yuccifolium, Juniperus virginiana, Persea borbonia,*

Pinus elliottii, Pteridium caudatum, Pterocaulon virgatum, Quercus phellos, Q. virginiana, Salix caroliniana, Thelypteris kunthii, Ximenia americana

Other: *Angadenia berteroi, Aster simmondsii, Bacopa caroliniana, Berchemia scandens, Cephalanthus occidentalis, Clematis baldwinii, Commelina erecta, Coreopsis leavenworthii, Juniperus virginiana, Licania michauxii, Nymphoides cordata, Osmunda regalis, Persea borbonia, Phlebodium aureum, Polygala lutea, Polypodium incanum, Pterocaulon virgatum, Rubus cuneifolius, Salix caroliniana, S. humilis, Sassafras albidum, Saururus cernuus, Smilax auriculata, Stillingia sylvatica, Vittaria lineata*

Panacea: *Eryngium yuccifolium, Persea borbonia*

Pediatric Aid: *Galactia volubilis, Juniperus virginiana, Lechea minor, Liatris laxa, Osmunda regalis, Panax quinquefolius, Persea borbonia, Phlebodium aureum, Phoradendron leucarpum, Piloblephis rigida, Sassafras albidum, Stenandrium dulce, Stillingia sylvatica, Vaccinium myrsinites, Vitis aestivalis, V. munsoniana, Vittaria lineata*

Preventive Medicine: *Salix caroliniana*

Psychological Aid: *Hyptis pectinata, Ilex vomitoria, Juniperus virginiana, Lagenaria siceraria, Licania michauxii, Osmunda regalis, Persea borbonia, Phlebodium aureum, Polypodium incanum, Thelypteris kunthii, Vittaria lineata*

Pulmonary Aid: *Andropogon floridanus, Chenopodium ambrosioides, Dichanthelium laxiflorum, D. strigosum, Persea borbonia, Pterocaulon virgatum, Xyris ambigua*

Reproductive Aid: *Galactia volubilis, Justicia crassifolia, Licania michauxii, Persea borbonia, Trema micranthum, Zeuxine strateumatica*

Respiratory Aid: *Bacopa caroliniana, Conyza canadensis, Eryngium yuccifolium, Hydrocotyle umbellata, Nymphoides cordata, Panax quinquefolius, Persea borbonia, Polygala lutea, P. rugelii, Salix caroliniana*

Sedative: *Bacopa caroliniana, Chenopodium ambrosioides, Hydrocotyle umbellata, Juniperus virginiana, Nymphoides cordata, Panax quinquefolius, Persea borbonia, Stenandrium dulce*

Snakebite Remedy: *Eryngium yuccifolium, Manfreda virginica, Platanthera ciliaris, Polygala rugelii, Vitis munsoniana*

Stimulant: *Chenopodium ambrosioides, Eryngium yuccifolium, Galactia volubilis, Juniperus virginiana, Persea borbonia, Piloblephis rigida,*

Salix caroliniana, Stenandrium dulce, Vaccinium myrsinites

Strengthener: *Cephalanthus occidentalis, Habenaria odontopetala, Salix caroliniana, Stillingia sylvatica*

Throat Aid: *Andropogon floridanus, Crotalaria rotundifolia, Dichanthelium laxiflorum, D. strigosum, Sassafras albidum*

Tonic: *Panax quinquefolius*

Toothache Remedy: *Zephyranthes* sp.

Unspecified: *Cephalanthus occidentalis, Eleocharis geniculata, Eryngium yuccifolium, Galactia volubilis, Juniperus virginiana, Licania michauxii, Osmunda regalis, Panax quinquefolius, Pediomelum canescens, Persea borbonia, Phlebodium aureum, Pterocaulon virgatum, Salix caroliniana, Sassafras albidum, Saururus cernuus, Vaccinium myrsinites, Verbesina virginica, Vittaria lineata, Ximenia americana*

Urinary Aid: *Andropogon floridanus, Callicarpa americana, Cephalanthus occidentalis, Chaptalia tomentosa, Eleocharis geniculata, Erythrina herbacea, Hypericum fasciculatum, Licania michauxii, Persea borbonia, Rhus copallinum, Sassafras albidum, Verbesina virginica*

Venereal Aid: *Rhus copallinum*

Vertigo Medicine: *Eleocharis geniculata, Juniperus virginiana, Persea borbonia, Salix caroliniana*

Witchcraft Medicine: *Juniperus virginiana, Panax quinquefolius*

Seri

Poison: *Sapium biloculare*

Unspecified: *Guajacum coulteri*

Shasta

Analgesic: *Helianthus cusickii*

Carminative: *Helianthus cusickii*

Cold Remedy: *Clematis lasiantha*

Dermatological Aid: *Helianthus cusickii*

Disinfectant: *Helianthus cusickii*

Febrifuge: *Helianthus cusickii*

Herbal Steam: *Clematis lasiantha, Helianthus cusickii*

Preventive Medicine: *Helianthus cusickii*

Shinnecock

Analgesic: *Brassica nigra, Hedeoma pulegioides, Quercus alba, Tanacetum vulgare*

Antidiarrheal: *Rubus hispidus*

Antirheumatic (External): *Aesculus hippocastanum*

Antirheumatic (Internal): *Nepeta cataria*

Blood Medicine: *Acorus calamus*

Cancer Treatment: *Trifolium pratense*

Cold Remedy: *Allium cepa, Eupatorium perfoliatum, Prunus serotina, Verbascum thapsus*

Cough Medicine: *Barbarea vulgaris, Pinus strobus*

Dermatological Aid: *Alcea rosea, Comptonia peregrina, Impatiens capensis, Pinus rigida, Plantago major*

Diaphoretic: *Eupatorium perfoliatum*

Disinfectant: *Allium cepa*

Ear Medicine: *Allium cepa, Nicotiana tabacum*

Emetic: *Brassica nigra*

Eye Medicine: *Plantago major*

Febrifuge: *Allium cepa, Eupatorium perfoliatum*

Gastrointestinal Aid: *Prunus serotina*

Gynecological Aid: *Leonurus cardiaca*

Kidney Aid: *Gaultheria procumbens*

Liver Aid: *Berberis vulgaris*

Misc. Disease Remedy: *Allium cepa*

Oral Aid: *Acorus calamus*

Orthopedic Aid: *Quercus alba*

Pulmonary Aid: *Humulus lupulus*

Sedative: *Humulus lupulus*

Tonic: *Leucanthemum vulgare, Taraxacum officinale*

Toothache Remedy: *Brassica nigra, Nicotiana tabacum*

Urinary Aid: *Hibiscus moscheutos*

Shoshoni

Abortifacient: *Porophyllum gracile*

Adjuvant: *Angelica breweri*

Analgesic: *Achillea millefolium, Angelica breweri, Aquilegia formosa, Artemisia ludoviciana, A. tridentata, Chamaebatiaria millefolium, Claytonia perfoliata, Clematis ligusticifolia, Crepis acuminata, Eriastrum filifolium, Ericameria nana, Erigeron aphanactis, Eriodictyon angustifolium, Grindelia nana, G. squarrosa, Helianthella uniflora, Hypericum scouleri, Ipomopsis aggregata, Iris missouriensis, Iva axillaris, Machaeranthera canescens, Mahonia repens, Monardella odoratissima, Opuntia basilaris, Osmorhiza occidentalis, Penstemon deustus, P. eatonii, Pinus monophylla, Populus balsamifera, Psathyrotes ramosissima, Psorothamnus polydenius, Rumex crispus, Salvia dorrii, Stanleya pinnata, Zigadenus paniculatus*

Anesthetic: *Achillea millefolium*

Anthelmintic: *Juniperus occidentalis, J. osteosperma, Nicotiana attenuata*

Anticonvulsive: *Anemopsis californica*

Antidiarrheal: *Achillea millefolium, Aquilegia formosa, Artemisia ludoviciana, Asclepias speciosa, Cercocarpus ledifolius, Chrysothamnus nauseosus, Enceliopsis nudicaulis, Ephedra viridis, Eriogonum sphaerocephalum, Heuchera rubescens, Ipomopsis congesta, Iva axillaris, Lithospermum ruderale, Mahonia repens, Osmorhiza occidentalis, Paeonia brownii, Phlox longifolia, Psathyrotes ramosissima, Psorothamnus polydenius, Rosa woodsii, Sambucus racemosa, Tanacetum vulgare, Tetradymia comosa*

Antidote: *Artemisia tridentata*

Antiemetic: *Achillea millefolium, Pinus monophylla, Prunus virginiana, Sphaeralcea ambigua, Stephanomeria spinosa*

Antihemorrhagic: *Purshia tridentata*

Antirheumatic (External): *Achillea millefolium, Angelica breweri, Arabis puberula, Arenaria congesta, Artemisia tridentata, Chrysothamnus viscidiflorus, Claytonia perfoliata, Clematis ligusticifolia, Eriastrum filifolium, Eriodictyon angustifolium, Eriogonum microthecum, E. umbellatum, Helianthella uniflora, Ipomopsis aggregata, Iris missouriensis, Lomatium dissectum, Lonicera interrupta, Nicotiana attenuata, Plantago major, Rumex crispus, Sphaeralcea ambigua, Stanleya pinnata, Urtica dioica, Veratrum californicum, Zigadenus paniculatus*

Antirheumatic (Internal): *Mahonia repens, Penstemon deustus*

Blood Medicine: *Arenaria congesta, Castilleja linariifolia, Caulanthus crassicaulis, Cercocarpus ledifolius, Corallorrhiza maculata, Ephedra viridis, Ipomopsis aggregata, Juniperus communis, Machaeranthera canescens, Mahonia repens, Monardella odoratissima, Populus balsamifera, Rosa woodsii, Rumex crispus, R. venosus, Sambucus racemosa, Urtica dioica*

Burn Dressing: *Abronia villosa, Argemone polyanthemos, Cercocarpus ledifolius, Clematis ligusticifolia, Ephedra viridis, Iris missouriensis, Juniperus occidentalis, J. osteosperma, Paeonia brownii, Penstemon eatonii, Rosa woodsii, Rumex crispus, R. venosus*

Carminative: *Achillea millefolium, Mentha canadensis*

Cathartic: *Agastache urticifolia, Argemone hispida, A. polyanthemos, Artemisia dracunculus, A. ludoviciana, Atriplex canescens, Castilleja linariifolia, Cucurbita foetidissima, Ephedra viridis, Eriastrum filifolium, Hedeoma nana, Ipomopsis aggregata, I. congesta, Machaeranthera canescens, Monardella odoratissima, Nicotiana attenuata, Osmorhiza occidentalis, Psathyrotes ramosissima, Purshia mexicana, P. tridentata, Rumex crispus, R. venosus, Sphaer-*

alcea ambigua, Tetradymia canescens, Wyethia mollis

Cold Remedy: *Abies lasiocarpa, Achillea millefolium, Anemopsis californica, Angelica breweri, Artemisia dracunculus, A. ludoviciana, A. nova, A. tridentata, Cercocarpus ledifolius, Chrysothamnus nauseosus, Ephedra viridis, Ericameria nana, Eriodictyon angustifolium, Eriogonum ovalifolium, E. umbellatum, Gutierrezia sarothrae, Heracleum maximum, Ipomopsis congesta, Iva axillaris, Juniperus monosperma, J. occidentalis, J. osteosperma, Larrea tridentata, Lomatium dissectum, Mentha canadensis, Monardella odoratissima, Osmorhiza occidentalis, Penstemon deustus, Pinus monophylla, Psorothamnus polydenius, Rosa woodsii, Salvia dorrii, Sambucus racemosa, Sphaeralcea ambigua, Tetradymia comosa, Thamnosma montana, Urtica dioica, Veratrum californicum*

Contraceptive: *Lithospermum ruderale, Sphaeralcea ambigua, Veratrum californicum*

Cough Medicine: *Artemisia ludoviciana, A. nova, A. tridentata, Cercocarpus ledifolius, Chrysothamnus nauseosus, Enceliopsis nudicaulis, Ericameria nana, Eriodictyon angustifolium, Eriogonum microthecum, Grindelia nana, G. squarrosa, Heracleum maximum, Juniperus occidentalis, J. osteosperma, Lomatium dissectum, Mahonia repens, Osmorhiza occidentalis, Paeonia brownii, Pinus monophylla, Psathyrotes ramosissima, Psorothamnus polydenius, Sambucus racemosa, Tetradymia comosa*

Dermatological Aid: *Abies concolor, Abronia turbinata, Achillea millefolium, Anemopsis californica, Aquilegia formosa, Arenaria congesta, Argemone polyanthemos, Artemisia dracunculus, A. ludoviciana, A. spinescens, A. tridentata, Asclepias speciosa, Balsamorhiza sagittata, Cercocarpus ledifolius, Chaenactis douglasii, Clematis ligusticifolia, Ephedra nevadensis, E. viridis, Grindelia nana, G. squarrosa, Gutierrezia sarothrae, Hypericum scouleri, Ipomopsis aggregata, I. congesta, Iris missouriensis, Juniperus monosperma, J. occidentalis, J. osteosperma, Krameria grayi, Krascheninnikovia lanata, Leucocrinum montanum, Linum lewisii, Lomatium dissectum, Mimulus guttatus, Nicotiana attenuata, Opuntia basilaris, Osmorhiza occidentalis, Paeonia brownii, Penstemon deustus, Phlox longifolia, Pinus aristata, P. monophylla, Plantago major, Psathyrotes ramosissima, Purshia mexicana, P. tridentata, Rosa woodsii, Rubus leucodermis, Rumex crispus, R. venosus, Sphaeralcea ambigua, Tanacetum vulgare,*

Tetradymia comosa, Veratrum californicum, Wyethia amplexicaulis, Zigadenus paniculatus

Diaphoretic: *Artemisia tridentata*

Disinfectant: *Anemopsis californica, Artemisia ludoviciana, A. tridentata, Grindelia nana, G. squarrosa, Gutierrezia sarothrae, Holodiscus dumosus, Ipomopsis aggregata, I. congesta, Juniperus occidentalis, J. osteosperma, Lomatium dissectum, Osmorhiza occidentalis, Penstemon deustus, Pinus monophylla, Plantago major, Psorothamnus polydenius, Purshia mexicana, Tanacetum vulgare, Veratrum californicum*

Diuretic: *Ephedra nevadensis, Heliotropium curassavicum, Juniperus occidentalis, J. osteosperma, Larrea tridentata, Rosa woodsii*

Ear Medicine: *Iris missouriensis, Penstemon deustus, Stanleya pinnata*

Emetic: *Aquilegia formosa, Argemone polyanthemos, Artemisia tridentata, Castilleja linariifolia, Chaenactis douglasii, Cucurbita foetidissima, Eriastrum filifolium, Grindelia nana, G. squarrosa, Heliotropium curassavicum, Holodiscus dumosus, Ipomopsis aggregata, I. congesta, Nicotiana attenuata, Psathyrotes ramosissima, Purshia tridentata, Ribes cereum, Sphaeralcea ambigua, Wyethia amplexicaulis, Zigadenus paniculatus*

Expectorant: *Eriodictyon angustifolium, Grindelia nana, G. squarrosa*

Eye Medicine: *Arenaria aculeata, Argemone polyanthemos, Artemisia dracunculus, A. ludoviciana, A. tridentata, Balsamorhiza sagittata, Cercocarpus ledifolius, Chamaesyce polycarpa, Cicuta maculata, Crepis acuminata, C. modocensis, Ericameria nana, Erigeron aphanactis, Frasera albomarginata, Ipomopsis congesta, Krascheninnikovia lanata, Leptodactylon pungens, Leymus condensatus, Linum lewisii, Lomatium dissectum, Machaeranthera canescens, Maianthemum stellatum, Osmorhiza occidentalis, Paeonia brownii, Penstemon deustus, Phlox longifolia, Physaria chambersii, Prunus virginiana, Sphaeralcea ambigua, Stephanomeria spinosa*

Febrifuge: *Artemisia ludoviciana, A. tridentata, Heuchera rubescens, Mentha canadensis, Osmorhiza occidentalis, Pinus monophylla*

Gastrointestinal Aid: *Achillea millefolium, Anemopsis californica, Aquilegia formosa, Artemisia ludoviciana, A. tridentata, Brickellia oblongifolia, Chaenactis douglasii, Chamaebatiaria millefolium, Chrysothamnus nauseosus, Clematis ligusticifolia, Ephedra viridis, Ericameria nana, Erigeron aphanactis, Eriodictyon angusti-*

folium, Grindelia nana, G. squarrosa, Hedeoma nana, Holodiscus dumosus, Ipomopsis congesta, Iris missouriensis, Iva axillaris, Maianthemum stellatum, Mentha canadensis, Monardella odoratissima, Osmorhiza occidentalis, Pedicularis centranthera, Penstemon deustus, Phlox longifolia, Pinus monophylla, Plantago major, Prunus virginiana, Psathyrotes annua, P. ramosissima, Psorothamnus fremontii, P. polydenius, Salvia dorrii, Tetradymia comosa

Gland Medicine: *Veratrum californicum*

Gynecological Aid: *Artemisia ludoviciana, A. tridentata, Crepis acuminata, C. modocensis, Maianthemum stellatum, Osmorhiza occidentalis, Veratrum californicum*

Hallucinogen: *Datura wrightii*

Heart Medicine: *Cercocarpus ledifolius, Heuchera rubescens, Juniperus occidentalis, J. osteosperma*

Hemostat: *Artemisia spinescens*

Herbal Steam: *Artemisia dracunculus, Lomatium dissectum, Prunus virginiana*

Kidney Aid: *Chaenactis douglasii, Clematis ligusticifolia, Ephedra viridis, Grindelia squarrosa, Ipomopsis congesta, Juniperus occidentalis, J. osteosperma, Mahonia repens, Paeonia brownii, Pinus monophylla, Plantago major, Psorothamnus polydenius, Purshia mexicana, Suaeda moquinii*

Laxative: *Psathyrotes ramosissima*

Liver Aid: *Heuchera rubescens, Ipomopsis congesta, Linum lewisii, Psathyrotes ramosissima, Pyrola asarifolia, Rumex crispus*

Misc. Disease Remedy: *Artemisia ludoviciana, A. spinescens, Cercocarpus ledifolius, Chrysothamnus viscidiflorus, Grindelia nana, G. squarrosa, Gutierrezia sarothrae, Heliotropium curassavicum, Ipomopsis congesta, Juniperus monosperma, J. occidentalis, J. osteosperma, Lomatium dissectum, Osmorhiza occidentalis, Pinus monophylla, Psorothamnus polydenius, Purshia mexicana, P. tridentata, Wyethia amplexicaulis*

Narcotic: *Datura wrightii*

Oral Aid: *Juniperus occidentalis, J. osteosperma*

Orthopedic Aid: *Achillea millefolium, Artemisia tridentata, Cicuta maculata, Clematis ligusticifolia, Eriogonum microthecum, E. umbellatum, Grindelia nana, G. squarrosa, Hypericum scouleri, Lomatium dissectum, Penstemon deustus, Pinus monophylla, Ribes aureum, Zigadenus paniculatus*

Other: *Purshia tridentata, Salvia dorrii*

Panacea: *Frasera speciosa, Lomatium dissectum*

Pediatric Aid: *Angelica breweri, Artemisia ludovi-*

ciana, A. tridentata, Cercocarpus ledifolius, Ephedra viridis, Iva axillaris, Mentha canadensis, Pedicularis centranthera, Penstemon deustus, Phlox longifolia, Psathyrotes annua, Salvia dorrii

Poison: *Cicuta maculata*

Poultice: *Pinus monophylla*

Pulmonary Aid: *Abies concolor, Angelica breweri, Artemisia spinescens, A. tridentata, Corallorrhiza maculata, Eriodictyon angustifolium, Lomatium dissectum, Osmorhiza occidentalis, Pinus monophylla, Psorothamnus polydenius*

Respiratory Aid: *Lomatium dissectum*

Snakebite Remedy: *Chamaesyce albomarginata, Osmorhiza occidentalis, Psathyrotes ramosissima, Veratrum californicum*

Stimulant: *Aquilegia formosa, Catabrosa aquatica*

Throat Aid: *Artemisia dracunculus, A. tridentata, Heliotropium curassavicum, Heracleum maximum, Juniperus occidentalis, J. osteosperma, Lomatium dissectum, Osmorhiza occidentalis, Paeonia brownii, Salvia dorrii, Veratrum californicum*

Tonic: *Anemopsis californica, Angelica breweri, Artemisia tridentata, Catabrosa aquatica, Chamaesyce albomarginata, C. polycarpa, Chrysothamnus nauseosus, Ephedra viridis, Frasera speciosa, Heuchera rubescens, Ipomopsis aggregata, Juniperus communis, J. occidentalis, J. osteosperma, Machaeranthera canescens, Monardella odoratissima, Osmorhiza occidentalis, Populus balsamifera, Purshia tridentata, Rosa woodsii, Rumex crispus, R. venosus, Stephanomeria spinosa, Thamnosma montana, Urtica dioica*

Toothache Remedy: *Achillea millefolium, Argemone polyanthemos, Artemisia tridentata, Chrysothamnus viscidiflorus, Heracleum maximum, Hypericum scouleri, Iris missouriensis, Juniperus occidentalis, J. osteosperma, Nicotiana attenuata, Osmorhiza occidentalis, Stanleya pinnata, Zigadenus paniculatus*

Tuberculosis Remedy: *Angelica breweri, Cercocarpus ledifolius, Eriodictyon angustifolium, Eriogonum microthecum, Glossopetalon spinescens, Heracleum maximum, Lomatium dissectum, Nicotiana attenuata, Paeonia brownii, Populus balsamifera, Psathyrotes ramosissima, Psorothamnus polydenius, Sambucus racemosa*

Unspecified: *Cercocarpus ledifolius, Holodiscus dumosus, Ribes aureum, Sphaeralcea ambigua*

Urinary Aid: *Ephedra viridis, Grindelia nana, G. squarrosa, Psathyrotes annua, Psorothamnus polydenius, Suaeda moquinii*

Venereal Aid: *Anemopsis californica, Angelica breweri, Aquilegia formosa, Arctostaphylos patula, Arenaria congesta, Artemisia dracunculus, Asclepias speciosa, Astragalus calycosus, Balsamorhiza sagittata, Castilleja linariifolia, Cercocarpus ledifolius, Clematis ligusticifolia, Cordylanthus ramosus, Cucurbita foetidissima, Enceliopsis nudicaulis, Ephedra nevadensis, E. viridis, Eriastrum filifolium, Erigeron concinnus, Eriodictyon angustifolium, Grindelia nana, G. squarrosa, Heliotropium curassavicum, Heuchera rubescens, Holodiscus dumosus, Hypericum scouleri, Ipomopsis aggregata, I. congesta, Iris missouriensis, Juniperus occidentalis, J. osteosperma, J. scopulorum, Larrea tridentata, Lomatium dissectum, Mahonia repens, Maianthemum stellatum, Osmorhiza occidentalis, Paeonia brownii, Penstemon deustus, Pinus monophylla, Populus balsamifera, P. tremuloides, Psathyrotes ramosissima, Psorothamnus polydenius, Purshia mexicana, P. tridentata, Rumex crispus, R. venosus, Sphaeralcea ambigua, Stephanomeria tenuifolia, Tetradymia canescens, Thalictrum fendleri, Wyethia amplexicaulis*

Veterinary Aid: *Angelica breweri, Asclepias cryptoceras, Cucurbita foetidissima, Heuchera rubescens, Ipomopsis congesta, Lomatium dissectum, Pinus monophylla, Sphaeralcea ambigua*

Shuswap

Analgesic: *Betula papyrifera, Lysichiton americanus, Nuphar lutea, Urtica dioica, U. urens*

Antidiarrheal: *Heuchera cylindrica, Rubus arcticus, Spiraea betulifolia*

Antirheumatic (External): *Nuphar lutea, Urtica dioica, U. urens*

Blood Medicine: *Achillea millefolium, Mahonia repens, Maianthemum racemosum*

Cathartic: *Shepherdia canadensis*

Cold Remedy: *Artemisia campestris, A. tridentata, Matricaria discoidea, Phacelia linearis*

Cough Medicine: *Artemisia campestris, Pinus contorta*

Dermatological Aid: *Abies grandis, Achillea millefolium, Alnus incana, Artemisia campestris, Balsamorhiza sagittata, Heracleum maximum, Heuchera cylindrica, Ledum groenlandicum, Lesquerella douglasii, Lithospermum ruderale, Lomatium dissectum, Lysichiton americanus, Nuphar lutea, Opuntia fragilis, Picea glauca, Pinus ponderosa, Plantago major, Populus balsamifera, Urtica dioica, U. urens, Veratrum viride*

Diaphoretic: *Alnus incana, Juniperus communis, J. scopulorum, Lesquerella douglasii, Plantago major*

Disinfectant: *Artemisia tridentata, Lithospermum ruderale*

Eye Medicine: *Arnica cordifolia, Castilleja angustifolia, Ledum groenlandicum, Rudbeckia hirta, Symphoricarpos mollis*

Gastrointestinal Aid: *Cirsium undulatum, Shepherdia canadensis, Spiraea betulifolia*

Gynecological Aid: *Artemisia dracunculus, Solidago canadensis*

Heart Medicine: *Matricaria discoidea*

Herbal Steam: *Urtica dioica, U. urens*

Internal Medicine: *Heracleum maximum*

Kidney Aid: *Cornus sericea*

Laxative: *Frangula purshiana*

Misc. Disease Remedy: *Ceanothus velutinus, Juniperus scopulorum*

Orthopedic Aid: *Lysichiton americanus, Nuphar lutea, Zigadenus venenosus*

Panacea: *Abies grandis, Artemisia campestris, Juniperus communis, J. scopulorum, Lysichiton americanus, Picea glauca, Pinus ponderosa, Ribes lacustre*

Pediatric Aid: *Cornus sericea, Pinus ponderosa*

Poison: *Cicuta douglasii, Galium boreale, Platanthera dilatata, Sium suave, Veratrum viride, Zigadenus venenosus*

Stimulant: *Artemisia dracunculus, Pinus ponderosa*

Throat Aid: *Opuntia fragilis*

Toothache Remedy: *Abies grandis, Picea glauca*

Tuberculosis Remedy: *Abies grandis, Artemisia campestris, Picea glauca, Pinus contorta, P. monticola, Shepherdia canadensis, Tsuga heterophylla*

Unspecified: *Alnus incana, Shepherdia canadensis*

Urinary Aid: *Cornus sericea, Heracleum maximum, Nicotiana attenuata, Penstemon fruticosus*

Witchcraft Medicine: *Artemisia dracunculus, A. tridentata*

Sia

Febrifuge: *Mentha canadensis*

Veterinary Aid: *Ipomoea leptophylla*

Sikani

Analgesic: *Heracleum maximum*

Anthelmintic: *Populus tremuloides*

Antirheumatic (External): *Heracleum maximum*

Cathartic: *Sambucus racemosa*

Cough Medicine: *Picea sitchensis, Pinus contorta*

Dermatological Aid: *Heracleum maximum, Populus tremuloides*

Sioux

Abortifacient: *Artemisia frigida*

Adjuvant: *Prunus virginiana*

Analgesic: *Echinacea pallida*

Antidiarrheal: *Prunus virginiana, Shepherdia canadensis*

Antidote: *Echinacea pallida*

Antihemorrhagic: *Rhus glabra*

Burn Dressing: *Echinacea pallida, Typha latifolia*

Cathartic: *Shepherdia canadensis*

Ceremonial Medicine: *Prunus virginiana*

Cold Remedy: *Juniperus scopulorum*

Dermatological Aid: *Opuntia polyacantha, Rhus glabra, Typha latifolia*

Diuretic: *Symphoricarpos albus, Urtica dioica*

Ear Medicine: *Glycyrrhiza lepidota, Polygala alba*

Eye Medicine: *Lygodesmia juncea, Symphoricarpos albus*

Febrifuge: *Glycyrrhiza lepidota, Juniperus scopulorum*

Gastrointestinal Aid: *Grindelia squarrosa, Monarda fistulosa*

Gynecological Aid: *Lygodesmia juncea, Monarda fistulosa*

Hemostat: *Nuphar lutea, Prunus virginiana*

Kidney Aid: *Grindelia squarrosa*

Misc. Disease Remedy: *Juniperus scopulorum, Typha latifolia*

Pediatric Aid: *Glycyrrhiza lepidota*

Poison: *Shepherdia canadensis*

Pulmonary Aid: *Juniperus scopulorum*

Toothache Remedy: *Echinacea pallida, Glycyrrhiza lepidota*

Urinary Aid: *Rhus glabra*

Veterinary Aid: *Echinacea pallida, Glycyrrhiza lepidota*

Sioux, Fort Peck

Abortifacient: *Acorus calamus*

Panacea: *Acorus calamus*

Sioux, Teton

Analgesic: *Echinacea angustifolia, Erysimum asperum*

Antidiarrheal: *Heuchera americana*

Cold Remedy: *Monarda fistulosa*

Dermatological Aid: *Mirabilis nyctaginea*

Febrifuge: *Monarda fistulosa*

Gastrointestinal Aid: *Echinacea angustifolia, Erysimum asperum*

Orthopedic Aid: *Mirabilis nyctaginea*

Pulmonary Aid: *Lithospermum incisum*
Throat Aid: *Echinacea angustifolia*
Toothache Remedy: *Echinacea angustifolia*

Skagit

Anthelmintic: *Dicentra formosa*
Antidiarrheal: *Achillea millefolium, Frangula purshiana*
Antidote: *Symphoricarpos albus*
Antirheumatic (External): *Petasites frigidus, Pinus monticola*
Cold Remedy: *Aruncus dioicus, Prunus emarginata, Ribes laxiflorum, Urtica dioica, Vaccinium parvifolium*
Cough Medicine: *Thuja plicata*
Dermatological Aid: *Achlys triphylla, Aruncus dioicus, Dicentra formosa, Eriophyllum lanatum, Frangula purshiana, Heuchera micrantha, Pinus monticola, Pseudotsuga menziesii, Rubus parviflorus, Tsuga heterophylla*
Dietary Aid: *Asarum caudatum, Tellima grandiflora*
Disinfectant: *Pseudotsuga menziesii*
Eye Medicine: *Ribes lacustre, Rosa nutkana, Trillium ovatum, Tsuga heterophylla*
Gastrointestinal Aid: *Rubus ursinus*
Gynecological Aid: *Oplopanax horridus, Prunus emarginata, Ribes lacustre*
Laxative: *Frangula purshiana*
Oral Aid: *Symphoricarpos albus*
Panacea: *Tellima grandiflora*
Pediatric Aid: *Symphoricarpos albus*
Poison: *Trillium ovatum*
Throat Aid: *Aruncus dioicus, Claytonia sibirica, Rosa nutkana, Tsuga heterophylla*
Tonic: *Asarum caudatum, Claytonia sibirica, Gaultheria shallon, Lonicera ciliosa, Salix sitchensis*
Toothache Remedy: *Dicentra formosa*
Tuberculosis Remedy: *Achlys triphylla, Asarum caudatum, Oplopanax horridus, Petasites frigidus, Pinus monticola, Symphoricarpos albus*
Venereal Aid: *Mahonia nervosa*

Skagit, Upper

Cold Remedy: *Ribes laxiflorum, Vaccinium parvifolium*
Dermatological Aid: *Polypodium virginianum*
Expectorant: *Polypodium virginianum*
Gastrointestinal Aid: *Rubus ursinus*
Gynecological Aid: *Ribes lacustre*
Laxative: *Frangula purshiana, Polypodium virginianum*
Other: *Gaultheria shallon*

Throat Aid: *Claytonia sibirica, Ribes divaricatum, Rosa nutkana*

Skokomish

Analgesic: *Lysichiton americanus*
Cathartic: *Lysichiton americanus*
Cold Remedy: *Arbutus menziesii, Prunus emarginata, Rhododendron albiflorum*
Dermatological Aid: *Adiantum aleuticum, Claytonia sibirica, Lysichiton americanus, Rhododendron albiflorum, Urtica dioica*
Febrifuge: *Lysichiton americanus*
Gastrointestinal Aid: *Arbutus menziesii, Rhododendron albiflorum*
Gynecological Aid: *Prunus emarginata*
Oral Aid: *Thuja plicata*
Throat Aid: *Arbutus menziesii, Rhododendron albiflorum*
Tuberculosis Remedy: *Epilobium angustifolium, Ribes laxiflorum*

Snake

Poison: *Valeriana edulis*

Snohomish

Analgesic: *Vicia sativa*
Antidiarrheal: *Achillea millefolium*
Cold Remedy: *Linnaea borealis, Urtica dioica*
Dermatological Aid: *Claytonia sibirica, Dryopteris expansa, Geum macrophyllum, Philadelphus lewisii*
Eye Medicine: *Cornus sericea*
Poison: *Conium maculatum*
Throat Aid: *Epilobium angustifolium, Rosa pisocarpa*

Songish

Cold Remedy: *Lomatium nudicaule*
Gynecological Aid: *Sedum spathulifolium*
Love Medicine: *Osmorhiza purpurea*
Throat Aid: *Lomatium nudicaule*

Squaxin

Analgesic: *Marah oreganus, Vicia americana*
Blood Medicine: *Holodiscus discolor, Mahonia aquifolium, Sambucus racemosa*
Cold Remedy: *Pseudotsuga menziesii*
Dermatological Aid: *Achillea millefolium, Adenocaulon bicolor, Frangula purshiana, Populus balsamifera*
Disinfectant: *Populus balsamifera, Sambucus racemosa*
Emetic: *Zigadenus venenosus*
Gastrointestinal Aid: *Achillea millefolium*

Gynecological Aid: *Lonicera ciliosa, Rosa piso-carpa, Urtica dioica*

Laxative: *Frangula purshiana*

Orthopedic Aid: *Marah oreganus*

Poison: *Marah oreganus*

Throat Aid: *Mahonia aquifolium, Populus balsamifera*

Tuberculosis Remedy: *Adenocaulon bicolor, Rumex acetosella*

Stony Indian

Antihemorrhagic: *Juniperus scopulorum*

Swinomish

Analgesic: *Pseudotsuga menziesii*

Antirheumatic (External): *Juniperus scopulorum*

Cold Remedy: *Alnus rubra, Lonicera ciliosa, Pseudotsuga menziesii*

Cough Medicine: *Gaultheria shallon*

Dermatological Aid: *Alnus rubra, Malus fusca*

Disinfectant: *Juniperus scopulorum*

Gastrointestinal Aid: *Alnus rubra, Malus fusca*

Gynecological Aid: *Lonicera ciliosa*

Laxative: *Frangula purshiana*

Love Medicine: *Osmorhiza berteroi*

Oral Aid: *Pseudotsuga menziesii*

Other: *Achillea millefolium, Epilobium angustifolium, Lysichiton americanus*

Panacea: *Juniperus scopulorum*

Poison: *Epilobium angustifolium, Ribes lacustre*

Strengthener: *Taxus brevifolia*

Throat Aid: *Lonicera ciliosa, Polystichum munitum, Pseudotsuga menziesii, Ribes divaricatum*

Tonic: *Juniperus scopulorum, Mahonia aquifolium, Pseudotsuga menziesii, Urtica dioica*

Tuberculosis Remedy: *Alnus rubra, Gaultheria shallon, Ribes divaricatum*

Venereal Aid: *Ribes divaricatum*

Tanaina

Antirheumatic (Internal): *Artemisia tilesii, Petasites frigidus, Urtica dioica*

Misc. Disease Remedy: *Artemisia tilesii, Petasites frigidus, Urtica dioica*

Tuberculosis Remedy: *Artemisia tilesii, Petasites frigidus, Urtica dioica*

Unspecified: *Heracleum maximum*

Tanana, Upper

Analgesic: *Huperzia selago, Linnaea borealis, Nuphar lutea*

Antidiarrheal: *Empetrum nigrum*

Antirheumatic (External): *Artemisia tilesii, Juniperus communis, Ledum palustre, Shepherdia canadensis*

Antirheumatic (Internal): *Ledum palustre, Picea glauca*

Blood Medicine: *Artemisia tilesii, Ledum palustre, Rosa acicularis*

Cancer Treatment: *Artemisia alaskana, A. arctica, A. frigida*

Carminative: *Alnus viridis*

Cold Remedy: *Artemisia alaskana, A. arctica, A. frigida, Empetrum nigrum, Gentianella propinqua, Juniperus communis, Ledum palustre, Picea glauca, Polygonum alpinum, Populus balsamifera, P. tremuloides, Ribes hudsonianum, Rosa acicularis, Vaccinium vitis-idaea, Viburnum edule*

Cough Medicine: *Artemisia alaskana, A. arctica, A. frigida, A. tilesii, Gentianella propinqua, Juniperus communis, Ledum palustre, Picea glauca, Polygonum alpinum, Populus balsamifera, P. tremuloides, Vaccinium vitis-idaea*

Dermatological Aid: *Artemisia tilesii, Ledum palustre, Picea glauca, Populus balsamifera, Shepherdia canadensis*

Disinfectant: *Artemisia tilesii, Ledum palustre, Picea glauca*

Emetic: *Rosa acicularis*

Eye Medicine: *Artemisia alaskana, A. arctica, A. frigida, A. tilesii, Empetrum nigrum, Ribes triste*

Febrifuge: *Alnus viridis, Rosa acicularis*

Gastrointestinal Aid: *Ledum palustre, Rosa acicularis, Viburnum edule*

Gynecological Aid: *Pentaphylloides floribunda*

Hemorrhoid Remedy: *Picea glauca*

Kidney Aid: *Empetrum nigrum, Juniperus communis*

Laxative: *Arctostaphylos uva-ursi*

Misc. Disease Remedy: *Artemisia alaskana, A. arctica, A. frigida, Ledum palustre*

Oral Aid: *Artemisia tilesii, Picea glauca*

Orthopedic Aid: *Betula papyrifera*

Panacea: *Juniperus communis, Ledum palustre, Populus balsamifera, Ribes hudsonianum, Shepherdia canadensis*

Pediatric Aid: *Linnaea borealis*

Poison: *Hedysarum boreale*

Psychological Aid: *Linnaea borealis*

Pulmonary Aid: *Picea glauca*

Respiratory Aid: *Ledum palustre, Picea glauca*

Stimulant: *Alnus viridis*

Throat Aid: *Juniperus communis, Ledum palustre, Picea glauca, Vaccinium vitis-idaea, Viburnum edule*

Tuberculosis Remedy: *Juniperus communis, Picea glauca, Shepherdia canadensis*
Unspecified: *Ribes triste*
Vertigo Medicine: *Ledum palustre*

Tarahumara

Ceremonial Medicine: *Dasylirion durangensis*

Tewa

Analgesic: *Gutierrezia sarothrae, Ipomopsis longiflora, Juniperus monosperma, Monarda fistulosa, Zea mays*
Antidiarrheal: *Ephedra antisyphilitica, Kallstroemia californica, Xanthium strumarium*
Antiemetic: *Artemisia campestris, Xanthium strumarium*
Antirheumatic (External): *Juniperus monosperma, Poliomintha incana*
Burn Dressing: *Krascheninnikovia lanata*
Carminative: *Artemisia filifolia, A. frigida, A. tridentata, Gutierrezia microcephala*
Ceremonial Medicine: *Nicotiana attenuata, Yucca baccata*
Contraceptive: *Castilleja linariifolia*
Cough Medicine: *Artemisia tridentata, Nicotiana attenuata*
Dermatological Aid: *Abies concolor, Argyrochosma fendleri, Artemisia filifolia, Fallugia paradoxa, Ipomopsis longiflora, Juniperus monosperma, Kallstroemia californica, Penstemon barbatus, Pinus edulis, Sphaeralcea angustifolia, Taraxacum officinale, Zea mays*
Disinfectant: *Gutierrezia sarothrae, Juniperus monosperma, Sphaeralcea angustifolia*
Diuretic: *Juniperus monosperma*
Ear Medicine: *Gutierrezia sarothrae, Poliomintha incana, Prosopis pubescens*
Emetic: *Yucca baccata*
Expectorant: *Artemisia tridentata*
Eye Medicine: *Monarda fistulosa*
Febrifuge: *Artemisia campestris, Krascheninnikovia lanata, Monarda fistulosa*
Gastrointestinal Aid: *Artemisia filifolia, A. frigida, A. tridentata, Cleome serrulata, Gutierrezia sarothrae, Juniperus monosperma, Phoradendron juniperinum*
Gynecological Aid: *Castilleja linariifolia, Gutierrezia sarothrae, Juniperus monosperma, Nicotiana attenuata, Yucca baccata, Zea mays*
Heart Medicine: *Zea mays*
Herbal Steam: *Juniperus monosperma*
Internal Medicine: *Juniperus monosperma*
Kidney Aid: *Mirabilis multiflora*

Laxative: *Cercocarpus montanus, Cucurbita foetidissima, Juniperus monosperma*
Misc. Disease Remedy: *Gutierrezia sarothrae*
Nose Medicine: *Nicotiana attenuata*
Oral Aid: *Chrysothamnus nauseosus*
Orthopedic Aid: *Juniperus monosperma, Taraxacum officinale*
Pediatric Aid: *Chrysothamnus nauseosus, Gutierrezia sarothrae, Juniperus monosperma, Xanthium strumarium, Zea mays*
Reproductive Aid: *Juniperus monosperma*
Snakebite Remedy: *Sphaeralcea angustifolia*
Throat Aid: *Monarda fistulosa*
Tonic: *Ephedra viridis*
Toothache Remedy: *Juniperus monosperma, Nicotiana attenuata, Parryella filifolia*
Urinary Aid: *Populus tremuloides, Xanthium strumarium*
Venereal Aid: *Ephedra viridis*

Thompson

Adjuvant: *Triteleia grandiflora, Valeriana dioica, V. sitchensis*
Analgesic: *Arabis drummondii, Artemisia dracunculus, Asclepias speciosa, Ceanothus velutinus, Cicuta douglasii, Eriogonum androsaceum, E. heracleoides, Frangula purshiana, Gaillardia aristata, Geum triflorum, Luetkea pectinata, Maianthemum racemosum, M. stellatum, Malus fusca, Mentha canadensis, Nuphar lutea, Paxistima myrsinites, Pinus contorta, Platanthera leucostachys, Streptopus amplexifolius, Valeriana dioica, V. sitchensis, Zigadenus elegans*
Anthelmintic: *Cornus sericea*
Anticonvulsive: *Calypso bulbosa, Lonicera ciliosa*
Antidiarrheal: *Acer circinatum, Achillea millefolium, Artemisia campestris, Balsamorhiza sagittata, Ceanothus velutinus, Chrysothamnus nauseosus, Cornus sericea, Crataegus douglasii, Fragaria vesca, F. virginiana, Picea sitchensis, Polygonum aviculare, Prunus virginiana, Ribes cereum, Rosa acicularis, R. nutkana, R. pisocarpa, R. woodsii, Solidago canadensis, Symphoricarpos albus, Valeriana dioica, V. sitchensis*
Antiemetic: *Acer glabrum, Cornus sericea, Rosa acicularis, R. nutkana, R. pisocarpa, R. woodsii, Rubus pubescens*
Antihemorrhagic: *Arctostaphylos uva-ursi, Athyrium filix-femina, Pteridium aquilinum, Rubus idaeus, R. pubescens*
Antirheumatic (External): *Achillea millefolium, Arnica cordifolia, Artemisia dracunculus, A. ludoviciana, A. tridentata, Ceanothus veluti-*

nus, *Eriogonum androsaceum, E. heracleoides, Geum triflorum, Juniperus scopulorum, Mahonia aquifolium, M. nervosa, Mentha canadensis, Nuphar lutea, Penstemon fruticosus, Philadelphus lewisii, Pinus contorta, P. ponderosa, Platanthera leucostachys, Populus tremuloides, Pseudotsuga menziesii, Pteridium aquilinum, Pulsatilla occidentalis, Ranunculus uncinatus, Urtica dioica, Veratrum viride, Zigadenus venenosus*

Antirheumatic (Internal): *Actaea rubra, Ceanothus velutinus, Juniperus communis, Mahonia aquifolium, M. nervosa, Maianthemum racemosum, M. stellatum, Populus tremuloides, Sambucus cerulea, S. racemosa*

Blood Medicine: *Aralia nudicaulis, Cornus nuttallii, Mahonia aquifolium, M. nervosa, Oplopanax horridus, Veratrum californicum, V. viride*

Breast Treatment: *Philadelphus lewisii*

Burn Dressing: *Equisetum laevigatum, Larix occidentalis, Lomatium dissectum*

Cancer Treatment: *Ceanothus velutinus, Gaillardia aristata, Larix occidentalis, Maianthemum racemosum, Picea engelmannii, Shepherdia canadensis, Trifolium pratense*

Cathartic: *Abies grandis, Frangula purshiana, Heracleum maximum, Juniperus communis, Penstemon confertus, Shepherdia canadensis*

Ceremonial Medicine: *Eriogonum heracleoides, Heracleum maximum, Populus balsamifera, Valeriana dioica, V. sitchensis*

Cold Remedy: *Abies amabilis, A. grandis, A. lasiocarpa, Achillea millefolium, Artemisia dracunculus, A. ludoviciana, A. tridentata, Aruncus dioicus, Betula papyrifera, Chrysothamnus nauseosus, Cornus sericea, Juniperus communis, J. scopulorum, Lomatium dissectum, L. nudicaule, Maianthemum stellatum, Mentha arvensis, M. canadensis, Osmorhiza occidentalis, Pinus contorta, Polypodium glycyrrhiza, P. hesperium, Prunus virginiana, Pseudotsuga menziesii, Pteridium aquilinum, Ribes hudsonianum, Spiraea betulifolia, Tsuga heterophylla, T. mertensiana, Valeriana dioica, V. sitchensis, Verbascum thapsus*

Contraceptive: *Amelanchier alnifolia, Betula papyrifera*

Cough Medicine: *Abies lasiocarpa, Betula papyrifera, Larix occidentalis, Picea engelmannii, Pinus contorta, Prunus virginiana, Rosa woodsii, Rumex crispus, Verbascum thapsus*

Dermatological Aid: *Abies lasiocarpa, Achillea millefolium, Agoseris glauca, Alnus rubra, Aquilegia formosa, Arabis drummondii, Aralia nudicaulis, Arnica cordifolia, Artemisia dracunculus, Aruncus dioicus, Asarum caudatum, Asclepias speciosa, Astragalus purshii, Caltha leptosepala, Chaenactis douglasii, Chimaphila umbellata, Clematis columbiana, C. ligusticifolia, Comandra umbellata, Cornus canadensis, Crataegus douglasii, Epilobium angustifolium, Equisetum arvense, Erigeron compositus, E. filifolius, Eriogonum androsaceum, E. heracleoides, Fragaria virginiana, Helianthus annuus, H. petiolaris, Heuchera cylindrica, H. micrantha, Hierochloe odorata, Juniperus scopulorum, Larix occidentalis, Leptarrhena pyrolifolia, Linum lewisii, Lomatium dissectum, Lonicera involucrata, Luetkea pectinata, Lysichiton americanus, Mentha canadensis, Monotropa uniflora, Nicotiana attenuata, N. tabacum, Nuphar lutea, Oplopanax horridus, Oxytropis monticola, Paxistima myrsinites, Penstemon confertus, Philadelphus lewisii, Picea engelmannii, Pinus contorta, P. ponderosa, Plantago major, Polemonium elegans, P. pulcherrimum, Populus balsamifera, P. tremuloides, Potentilla gracilis, Pseudotsuga menziesii, Pteridium aquilinum, Ranunculus glaberrimus, Rhododendron albiflorum, Rosa acicularis, R. nutkana, R. pisocarpa, R. woodsii, Rubus parviflorus, Salix cordata, Sambucus racemosa, Shepherdia canadensis, Symphoricarpos albus, Thalictrum occidentale, Urtica dioica, Valeriana dioica, V. sitchensis, Verbascum thapsus*

Diaphoretic: *Artemisia dracunculus, Lomatium nudicaule*

Dietary Aid: *Actaea rubra, Arctostaphylos uva-ursi, Asclepias speciosa, Aster foliaceus, Balsamorhiza sagittata, Ceanothus velutinus, Larix occidentalis, Lonicera involucrata, Oplopanax horridus, Pteridium aquilinum, Solidago simplex, Streptopus amplexifolius*

Disinfectant: *Artemisia ludoviciana, Astragalus purshii, Eriogonum heracleoides, Geum triflorum, Heracleum maximum, Juniperus scopulorum, Oxytropis campestris, Pinus contorta, Platanthera leucostachys, Populus tremuloides, Pseudotsuga menziesii, Ranunculus uncinatus, Shepherdia canadensis, Tsuga heterophylla, T. mertensiana*

Diuretic: *Arabis drummondii, Arctostaphylos uva-ursi, Juniperus scopulorum, Pseudotsuga menziesii*

Ear Medicine: *Pinus ponderosa, Sorbus sitchensis*

Eye Medicine: *Abies grandis, Achillea millefolium, Arctostaphylos uva-ursi, Calochortus macrocarpus, Campanula rotundifolia, Claytonia* perfoliata, Comandra umbellata, Cryptogramma sitchensis, Equisetum hyemale, E. laevigatum, Eriogonum heracleoides, Juniperus communis, Mahonia aquifolium, M. nervosa, Penstemon fruticosus, Picea sitchensis, Pinus ponderosa, Pulsatilla occidentalis, Ribes lacustre, Rosa gymnocarpa, Symphoricarpos albus, Trillium ovatum

Febrifuge: Lomatium nudicaule

Gastrointestinal Aid: Achillea millefolium, Amelanchier alnifolia, Artemisia ludoviciana, Aruncus dioicus, Asarum caudatum, Aster foliaceus, Chaenactis douglasii, Chrysothamnus nauseosus, Cornus nuttallii, Crataegus douglasii, Eriogonum androsaceum, E. heracleoides, Frangula purshiana, Juniperus communis, J. scopulorum, Larix occidentalis, Luetkea pectinata, Maianthemum racemosum, Mentha canadensis, Nuphar lutea, Oplopanax horridus, Penstemon confertus, P. fruticosus, Populus tremuloides, Pulsatilla occidentalis, Rhododendron albiflorum, Rhus glabra, Ribes hudsonianum, R. lacustre, R. oxyacanthoides, Rubus idaeus, R. pubescens, Shepherdia canadensis, Spiraea betulifolia, Streptopus amplexifolius, Symphoricarpos albus, Valeriana dioica, V. sitchensis

Gynecological Aid: Acer glabrum, Amelanchier alnifolia, Artemisia campestris, A. dracunculus, Calamagrostis rubescens, Chimaphila umbellata, Cornus sericea, Equisetum hyemale, E. laevigatum, Geranium viscosissimum, Goodyera oblongifolia, Juniperus scopulorum, Larix occidentalis, Luetkea pectinata, Maianthemum racemosum, Phacelia hastata, Populus balsamifera, Prunus virginiana, Ribes lacustre, Rosa acicularis, R. nutkana, R. pisocarpa, R. woodsii, Symphoricarpos albus, Thuja plicata

Heart Medicine: Juniperus communis, J. scopulorum, Maianthemum racemosum, Shepherdia canadensis

Hemorrhoid Remedy: Philadelphus lewisii, Plantago major, Sedum divergens, S. spathulifolium, Urtica dioica

Hemostat: Anemone multifida, Scirpus acutus

Herbal Steam: Eriogonum androsaceum, E. heracleoides, Geum triflorum, Mentha canadensis, Platanthera leucostachys, Ranunculus uncinatus

Hunting Medicine: Astragalus purshii, Platanthera leucostachys, Polystichum munitum, Rosa gymnocarpa, Valeriana dioica, V. sitchensis

Hypotensive: Juniperus communis, Shepherdia canadensis

Internal Medicine: Paxistima myrsinites, Rhus glabra

Kidney Aid: Arabis drummondii, Arctostaphylos uva-ursi, Juniperus communis, J. scopulorum, Penstemon fruticosus, Pseudotsuga menziesii, Sorbus sitchensis

Laxative: Frangula purshiana, Mahonia aquifolium, M. nervosa, Oplopanax horridus, Prunus virginiana, Sedum divergens, S. spathulifolium, Shepherdia canadensis, Symphoricarpos albus

Liver Aid: Cryptogramma sitchensis, Frangula purshiana, Heuchera cylindrica, H. micrantha, Sambucus racemosa, Shepherdia canadensis

Love Medicine: Aquilegia formosa, Delphinium menziesii, Dodecatheon jeffreyi, Geranium viscosissimum, Platanthera leucostachys, Sagittaria latifolia

Misc. Disease Remedy: Acer circinatum, Achillea millefolium, Anaphalis margaritacea, Artemisia ludoviciana, Aruncus dioicus, Gaillardia aristata, Juniperus scopulorum, Mentha arvensis, Oplopanax horridus, Pinus contorta, Prunus virginiana, Rubus leucodermis, Solidago spathulata, Thuja plicata, Tsuga heterophylla, T. mertensiana, Valeriana dioica, V. sitchensis, Veratrum viride

Oral Aid: Arctostaphylos uva-ursi, Heuchera cylindrica, H. micrantha, Polypodium glycyrrhiza, P. hesperium, Pseudotsuga menziesii, Rhus glabra, Sedum spathulifolium

Orthopedic Aid: Abies lasiocarpa, Achillea millefolium, Arabis drummondii, Arctostaphylos uva-ursi, Artemisia dracunculus, A. ludoviciana, Aruncus dioicus, Ceanothus velutinus, Chimaphila umbellata, Cicuta douglasii, Erigeron compositus, Eriogonum androsaceum, E. heracleoides, Geum triflorum, Larix occidentalis, Lomatium dissectum, Lonicera involucrata, Paxistima myrsinites, Penstemon fruticosus, Pinus contorta, Platanthera leucostachys, Populus balsamifera, Prunus emarginata, Pseudotsuga menziesii, Pteridium aquilinum, Ranunculus uncinatus, Solidago canadensis, Urtica dioica, Veratrum viride, Zigadenus venenosus

Other: Chrysothamnus nauseosus, Clematis ligusticifolia, Eriogonum androsaceum, E. heracleoides, Juniperus scopulorum, Ribes lacustre

Panacea: Abies amabilis, A. grandis, A. lasiocarpa, Achillea millefolium, Artemisia tridentata, Ceanothus velutinus, Chrysothamnus nauseosus, Cicuta douglasii, Cornus sericea, Crataegus douglasii, Larix occidentalis, Oplopanax horridus, Picea sitchensis, Pinus monticola, Ribes hudsonianum, Taxus brevifolia

Pediatric Aid: *Abies grandis, Achillea millefolium, Artemisia dracunculus, Asarum caudatum, Clematis ligusticifolia, Cornus sericea, Fragaria vesca, F. virginiana, Larix occidentalis, Linum lewisii, Lomatium macrocarpum, Mentha canadensis, Pinus contorta, P. ponderosa, Polygonum aviculare, Populus tremuloides, Ribes cereum, R. hudsonianum, Rosa woodsii, Rubus parviflorus, Scirpus acutus, Sedum divergens, S. spathulifolium, Solidago canadensis, Symphoricarpos albus, Veratrum viride*

Poison: *Actaea rubra, Anemone multifida, Artemisia dracunculus, Asclepias speciosa, Cicuta douglasii, Cornus sericea, Lonicera involucrata, Lupinus polyphyllus, L. sericeus, Ranunculus glaberrimus, R. repens, R. sceleratus, R. uncinatus, Rhus glabra, Rosa gymnocarpa, Symphoricarpos albus, Toxicodendron radicans, Veratrum californicum, Zigadenus elegans*

Psychological Aid: *Cornus nuttallii, Lewisia pygmaea, Lysichiton americanus, Mahonia nervosa, Picea engelmannii, Populus tremuloides, Thuja plicata*

Pulmonary Aid: *Actaea rubra, Cornus nuttallii, Eriogonum heracleoides, Philadelphus lewisii, Pinus contorta*

Reproductive Aid: *Lomatium macrocarpum, Lonicera ciliosa*

Respiratory Aid: *Larix occidentalis, Veratrum californicum*

Sedative: *Asarum caudatum, Balsamorhiza sagittata, Lomatium macrocarpum, Lonicera ciliosa, Pinus ponderosa, Ribes hudsonianum, Sedum spathulifolium, Shepherdia canadensis, Solidago canadensis*

Snakebite Remedy: *Acer glabrum, Achillea millefolium, Chaenactis douglasii, Chamaesyce glyptosperma*

Stimulant: *Aralia nudicaulis, Artemisia tridentata, Chaenactis douglasii, Potentilla glandulosa*

Strengthener: *Aquilegia formosa, Cornus sericea, Larix occidentalis, Ribes cereum*

Throat Aid: *Artemisia tridentata, Corylus cornuta, Heuchera cylindrica, H. micrantha, Lonicera involucrata, Maianthemum racemosum, Pinus contorta, Polypodium glycyrrhiza, P. hesperium, Ribes hudsonianum, Rosa woodsii, Veratrum viride*

Tonic: *Acer macrophyllum, Achillea millefolium, Amelanchier alnifolia, Aralia nudicaulis, Arctostaphylos uva-ursi, Asarum caudatum, Asclepias speciosa, Chaenactis douglasii, Chimaphila umbellata, Clematis ligusticifolia, Geum triflorum, Heracleum maximum, Juniperus communis, Lonicera ciliosa, Mahonia aquifolium, Oplopanax horridus, Potentilla glandulosa, Prunella vulgaris, Prunus virginiana, Pseudotsuga menziesii, Ribes lacustre, R. oxyacanthoides, Rosa gymnocarpa, Rubus idaeus, R. pubescens, Shepherdia canadensis, Solidago simplex, Spiraea ×pyramidata, Streptopus roseus*

Toothache Remedy: *Achillea millefolium, Alnus rubra, A. viridis, Arabis holboellii, Clematis ligusticifolia, Sambucus canadensis, S. cerulea, S. racemosa*

Tuberculosis Remedy: *Abies amabilis, A. grandis, A. lasiocarpa, Arnica cordifolia, Artemisia tridentata, Cassiope mertensiana, Chrysothamnus nauseosus, Eriogonum heracleoides, Gaillardia aristata, Juniperus communis, J. scopulorum, Larix occidentalis, Paxistima myrsinites, Phyllodoce empetriformis, Ribes hudsonianum, Shepherdia canadensis, Valeriana dioica, V. sitchensis*

Unspecified: *Abies amabilis, A. grandis, A. lasiocarpa, Achillea millefolium, Apocynum cannabinum, Arnica latifolia, Artemisia campestris, A. frigida, Asarum caudatum, Calypso bulbosa, Castilleja miniata, Ceanothus velutinus, Chaenactis douglasii, Dicentra formosa, Erigeron filifolius, Eriogonum heracleoides, Geranium richardsonii, G. viscosissimum, Hackelia hispida, Heracleum maximum, Heuchera cylindrica, H. micrantha, Kalmia polifolia, Ligusticum canbyi, Linnaea borealis, Lupinus polyphyllus, L. rivularis, Mentha canadensis, Mentzelia laevicaulis, Pedicularis bracteosa, P. racemosa, Phacelia linearis, Picea sitchensis, Pinus monticola, Populus balsamifera, Prunus emarginata, P. virginiana, Pulsatilla occidentalis, Salix interior, Stenanthium occidentale, Stephanomeria tenuifolia, Streptopus roseus, Triteleia grandiflora, Urtica dioica*

Urinary Aid: *Achillea millefolium, Arabis drummondii, Arctostaphylos uva-ursi, Chrysothamnus nauseosus, Clematis ligusticifolia, Equisetum arvense, E. hyemale, E. laevigatum, E. telmateia, Juniperus scopulorum, Lonicera involucrata, Pseudotsuga menziesii*

Venereal Aid: *Abies grandis, Achillea millefolium, Actaea rubra, Apocynum cannabinum, Arabis drummondii, Artemisia frigida, Aster foliaceus, Ceanothus velutinus, Chrysothamnus nauseosus, Elaeagnus commutata, Eriogonum androsaceum, E. heracleoides, Heracleum maximum, Mahonia aquifolium, M. nervosa, Populus tremuloides, Rhus glabra, Rosa acicularis, R. nutkana, R. pisocarpa, R. woodsii, Sambucus* cerulea, Solidago simplex, Spiraea betulifolia, Veratrum californicum

Veterinary Aid: Achlys triphylla, Aquilegia formosa, Artemisia dracunculus, Cicuta douglasii, Juniperus scopulorum, Leymus cinereus, Lomatium dissectum, Lupinus polyphyllus, L. sericeus, Penstemon fruticosus, Pinus ponderosa, Solidago canadensis, Valeriana dioica, V. sitchensis, Zigadenus elegans

Witchcraft Medicine: Abies grandis, Geranium viscosissimum, Lithospermum ruderale

Tlingit

Antidiarrheal: Picea glauca
Blood Medicine: Aruncus dioicus
Cough Medicine: Osmorhiza claytonii
Dermatological Aid: Boschniakia glabra, Kalmia polifolia, Oplopanax horridus, Petasites frigidus
Herbal Steam: Artemisia vulgaris
Pulmonary Aid: Artemisia vulgaris, Coptis macrosepala, Sorbus americana
Toothache Remedy: Picea sitchensis, Tsuga mertensiana
Unspecified: Menyanthes trifoliata
Venereal Aid: Claytonia sibirica, Heuchera glabra, Ledum palustre, Picea sitchensis, Pinus contorta, Sequoia sempervirens, Thuja excelsa, Tsuga mertensiana

Tolowa

Anthelmintic: Artemisia douglasiana
Anticonvulsive: Pteridium aquilinum
Antidote: Toxicodendron diversilobum
Antirheumatic (External): Artemisia douglasiana, Lysichiton americanus, Oxalis oregana, Petasites frigidus
Blood Medicine: Mahonia pumila
Cough Medicine: Mahonia pumila
Dermatological Aid: Oxalis oregana, Plantago australis, Urtica dioica
Disinfectant: Asarum caudatum, Oxalis oregana
Eye Medicine: Viola adunca
Laxative: Frangula purshiana
Oral Aid: Equisetum telmateia
Orthopedic Aid: Artemisia douglasiana
Other: Lysichiton americanus
Pediatric Aid: Artemisia douglasiana, Equisetum telmateia
Poison: Lonicera involucrata, Toxicodendron diversilobum
Unspecified: Vancouveria chrysantha

Tsimshian

Antirheumatic (External): Veratrum viride
Cancer Treatment: Taxus brevifolia
Ceremonial Medicine: Oenanthe sarmentosa
Dermatological Aid: Veratrum viride
Hunting Medicine: Picea sitchensis
Internal Medicine: Taxus brevifolia
Psychological Aid: Veratrum viride
Respiratory Aid: Veratrum viride
Unspecified: Argentina egedii

Tubatulabal

Analgesic: Trichostema lanceolatum
Antidiarrheal: Eriogonum fasciculatum, Heliotropium curassavicum
Antirheumatic (External): Encelia virginensis, Ericameria cooperi, E. linearifolia
Antirheumatic (Internal): Datura wrightii
Blood Medicine: Ephedra viridis
Cold Remedy: Anemopsis californica, Loeseliastrum matthewsii
Dermatological Aid: Argemone polyanthemos, Chorizanthe staticoides, Datura wrightii, Echinocystis brandegei, Eriogonum baileyi, E. gracillimum, E. roseum, Marah horridus
Gastrointestinal Aid: Datura wrightii, Diplacus aurantiacus, D. longiflorus, Eriogonum fasciculatum
Hemorrhoid Remedy: Argemone polyanthemos
Hemostat: Trichostema lanceolatum
Laxative: Datura wrightii
Pediatric Aid: Echinocystis brandegei, Eriogonum fasciculatum, Marah horridus
Sedative: Datura wrightii
Venereal Aid: Ephedra viridis

Umatilla

Gynecological Aid: Shepherdia canadensis

Ute

Analgesic: Comandra umbellata
Cold Remedy: Grindelia squarrosa
Dermatological Aid: Achillea millefolium, Collinsia parviflora, Lomatium dissectum, Phlox gracilis
Diuretic: Lithospermum ruderale
Gastrointestinal Aid: Abronia fragrans, Castilleja parviflora, Cryptantha sericea
Narcotic: Datura wrightii
Panacea: Achillea millefolium
Poison: Fritillaria atropurpurea, Zigadenus nuttallii
Unspecified: Artemisia tridentata, Descurainia pinnata, Eriogonum ovalifolium, Fritillaria

atropurpurea, Hedysarum boreale, Iva axillaris, Matricaria discoidea, Viola cucullata
Veterinary Aid: *Lomatium dissectum*

Wailaki

Analgesic: *Chlorogalum pomeridianum, Thalictrum polycarpum*
Antirheumatic (External): *Chlorogalum pomeridianum, Polypodium californicum*
Antirheumatic (Internal): *Pinus sabiniana*
Carminative: *Chlorogalum pomeridianum*
Dermatological Aid: *Chlorogalum pomeridianum, Erythronium oregonum, Evernia vulpina, Polypodium californicum, Trillium sessile*
Disinfectant: *Chlorogalum pomeridianum*
Diuretic: *Chlorogalum pomeridianum*
Gastrointestinal Aid: *Chlorogalum pomeridianum*
Laxative: *Chlorogalum pomeridianum*
Other: *Trillium sessile*
Panacea: *Trillium sessile*
Snakebite Remedy: *Toxicodendron diversilobum*

Walapai

Venereal Aid: *Aloysia wrightii*

Washo

Adjuvant: *Angelica breweri*
Analgesic: *Artemisia douglasiana, A. ludoviciana, Juniperus occidentalis, J. osteosperma, Monardella odoratissima, Osmorhiza occidentalis, Paeonia brownii, Zigadenus paniculatus*
Antidiarrheal: *Heracleum maximum, Ipomopsis congesta, Mentha canadensis, Typha latifolia*
Antirheumatic (External): *Arenaria congesta, Artemisia douglasiana, Veratrum californicum, Zigadenus paniculatus*
Blood Medicine: *Maianthemum stellatum*
Burn Dressing: *Argemone polyanthemos*
Cathartic: *Ipomopsis congesta, Osmorhiza occidentalis, Purshia tridentata, Wyethia mollis*
Cold Remedy: *Artemisia ludoviciana, A. tridentata, Ipomopsis congesta, Juniperus occidentalis, J. osteosperma, Lomatium dissectum, Mentha canadensis, Monardella odoratissima, Osmorhiza occidentalis, Pinus monophylla, Rosa woodsii, Salvia dorrii, Thalictrum fendleri*
Contraceptive: *Veratrum californicum*
Cough Medicine: *Angelica breweri, Artemisia ludoviciana, Lomatium dissectum*
Dermatological Aid: *Achillea millefolium, Argemone polyanthemos, Lomatium dissectum, Maianthemum stellatum, Pedicularis attollens, Veratrum californicum, Zigadenus paniculatus*

Disinfectant: *Artemisia tridentata, Balsamorhiza sagittata, Juniperus occidentalis, J. osteosperma*
Emetic: *Ipomopsis congesta, Veratrum californicum, Wyethia mollis*
Eye Medicine: *Phlox longifolia*
Febrifuge: *Mentha canadensis*
Gastrointestinal Aid: *Ipomopsis congesta, Mentha canadensis, Monardella odoratissima, Osmorhiza occidentalis*
Gynecological Aid: *Balsamorhiza hookeri, Ephedra viridis*
Hemostat: *Maianthemum stellatum*
Herbal Steam: *Lomatium dissectum*
Kidney Aid: *Ipomopsis congesta*
Misc. Disease Remedy: *Angelica breweri, Lomatium dissectum, Osmorhiza occidentalis*
Orthopedic Aid: *Zigadenus paniculatus*
Panacea: *Lomatium dissectum*
Pediatric Aid: *Lomatium dissectum, Mentha canadensis*
Pulmonary Aid: *Lomatium dissectum, Osmorhiza occidentalis*
Respiratory Aid: *Angelica breweri, Lomatium dissectum, Salvia dorrii*
Throat Aid: *Angelica breweri, Lomatium dissectum*
Tonic: *Artemisia tridentata, Maianthemum stellatum, Pedicularis attollens*
Toothache Remedy: *Heracleum maximum, Zigadenus paniculatus*
Tuberculosis Remedy: *Abies concolor, Lomatium dissectum, Paeonia brownii*
Venereal Aid: *Pinus monophylla*

West Coast Indian

Cathartic: *Frangula purshiana*
Panacea: *Frangula purshiana*
Poison: *Frangula purshiana*
Venereal Aid: *Frangula purshiana*

Wet'suwet'en

Antirheumatic (External): *Oplopanax horridus*
Burn Dressing: *Lonicera involucrata*
Cancer Treatment: *Oplopanax horridus*
Cold Remedy: *Abies lasiocarpa, Oplopanax horridus, Picea glauca*
Cough Medicine: *Abies lasiocarpa, Oplopanax horridus, Picea glauca, Prunus pensylvanica*
Dermatological Aid: *Cornus sericea, Lonicera involucrata, Oplopanax horridus*
Disinfectant: *Lonicera involucrata*
Eye Medicine: *Symphoricarpos albus*
Febrifuge: *Cornus sericea, Sorbus scopulina*
Gastrointestinal Aid: *Oplopanax horridus*
Hemorrhoid Remedy: *Cornus sericea*

Cold Remedy: *Distichlis spicata*
Diaphoretic: *Eriodictyon californicum*
Dietary Aid: *Distichlis spicata*
Emetic: *Sambucus cerulea*
Gastrointestinal Aid: *Datura wrightii*
Other: *Datura wrightii*
Unspecified: *Artemisia ludoviciana*

Yuki

Analgesic: *Artemisia douglasiana, Lomatium californicum, Umbellularia californica*
Antidiarrheal: *Artemisia douglasiana, Quercus lobata, Rumex crispus*
Antirheumatic (External): *Artemisia douglasiana, Lomatium californicum, Umbellularia californica*
Cold Remedy: *Achillea millefolium, Lomatium californicum, Populus fremontii*
Cough Medicine: *Eriodictyon californicum, Marrubium vulgare*
Dermatological Aid: *Arbutus menziesii, Artemisia douglasiana, Eriodictyon californicum, Evernia vulpina, Lonicera interrupta, Populus fremontii, Rumex crispus, Symphoricarpos albus, Toxicodendron diversilobum, Trillium sessile*
Diuretic: *Equisetum telmateia*
Emetic: *Arbutus menziesii, Wyethia angustifolia*
Eye Medicine: *Equisetum variegatum*
Febrifuge: *Sambucus cerulea*
Gastrointestinal Aid: *Arbutus menziesii*
Gynecological Aid: *Artemisia douglasiana*
Orthopedic Aid: *Artemisia douglasiana, Thalictrum polycarpum*
Other: *Lomatium californicum, Trillium sessile*
Panacea: *Trillium sessile*
Pediatric Aid: *Rumex crispus*
Poison: *Anthemis cotula, Zigadenus venenosus*
Respiratory Aid: *Achillea millefolium, Umbellularia californica*
Throat Aid: *Populus fremontii*
Unspecified: *Boykinia occidentalis, Rhamnus crocea*
Veterinary Aid: *Arbutus menziesii, Artemisia douglasiana*

Yuma

Narcotic: *Datura wrightii*

Yurok

Anthelmintic: *Artemisia douglasiana*
Antirheumatic (External): *Artemisia douglasiana, Chimaphila umbellata, Lysichiton americanus*
Blood Medicine: *Satureja douglasii, Taxus brevifolia*

Burn Dressing: *Trillium chloropetalum*
Cold Remedy: *Eriodictyon californicum*
Cough Medicine: *Eriodictyon californicum, Vancouveria hexandra*
Dermatological Aid: *Asarum caudatum, Plantago australis, P. major*
Disinfectant: *Polypodium californicum*
Eye Medicine: *Achillea millefolium*
Kidney Aid: *Chimaphila umbellata*
Laxative: *Frangula purshiana*
Misc. Disease Remedy: *Lysichiton americanus*
Orthopedic Aid: *Artemisia douglasiana*
Pediatric Aid: *Artemisia douglasiana, Asarum caudatum*
Poison: *Toxicodendron diversilobum*
Strengthener: *Lithocarpus densiflorus*
Unspecified: *Populus balsamifera, Rosa pisocarpa, Umbellularia californica*

Yurok, South Coast (Nererner)

Cathartic: *Frangula purshiana*
Dermatological Aid: *Artemisia ludoviciana*
Eye Medicine: *Artemisia ludoviciana*

Zuni

Abortifacient: *Ambrosia acanthicarpa*
Analgesic: *Artemisia carruthii, Bahia dissecta, Chaetopappa ericoides, Chenopodium graveolens, Ipomopsis multiflora, Senecio multicapitatus, Solidago canadensis, Verbesina encelioides*
Anesthetic: *Datura wrightii*
Antidiarrheal: *Plantago patagonica*
Antiemetic: *Croton texensis*
Antirheumatic (External): *Ageratina occidentalis, Artemisia tridentata, Bahia dissecta, Berula erecta, Chaetopappa ericoides, Cucurbita foetidissima, C. pepo, Erysimum capitatum, Gutierrezia sarothrae, Juniperus monosperma, Ligusticum porteri, Lobelia cardinalis, Oenothera coronopifolia, O. elata, O. triloba*
Burn Dressing: *Achillea millefolium, Krascheninnikovia lanata*
Carminative: *Pectis papposa*
Cathartic: *Chamaesyce serpyllifolia, Croton texensis, Polygonum lapathifolium*
Ceremonial Medicine: *Ligusticum porteri, Lithospermum incisum, Senecio multicapitatus, Xanthium strumarium*
Cold Remedy: *Artemisia frigida, A. tridentata, Chaetopappa ericoides*
Contraceptive: *Cirsium ochrocentrum, Juniperus monosperma*
Cough Medicine: *Salix exigua*
Dermatological Aid: *Ageratina occidentalis, Arte-*

*misia tridentata, Aster falcatus, A. lanceolatus,
Atriplex argentea, A. canescens, Berula erecta,
Calliandra humilis, Campanula parryi, Chaetopappa ericoides, Cryptantha cinerea, Cucurbita
pepo, Dalea compacta, Datura wrightii, Dimorphocarpa wislizeni, Eriogonum fasciculatum,
Erodium cicutarium, Hymenopappus filifolius,
Hymenoxys richardsonii, Ipomopsis longiflora,
I. multiflora, Lithospermum incisum, Lobelia
cardinalis, Oenothera triloba, Phacelia neomexicana, Picradeniopsis woodhousei, Pinus
edulis, Rumex crispus, Stanleya pinnata, Verbascum thapsus, Xanthium strumarium, Zinnia
grandiflora*

Diaphoretic: *Cirsium ochrocentrum, Gutierrezia
sarothrae, Pinus edulis, Tripterocalyx carnea,
Zinnia grandiflora*

Dietary Aid: *Mirabilis multiflora*

Disinfectant: *Pinus edulis, Psoralidium tenuiflorum*

Diuretic: *Cirsium ochrocentrum, Croton texensis,
Gutierrezia sarothrae, Mirabilis linearis, Pinus
edulis*

Emetic: *Chamaesyce serpyllifolia, Cirsium ochrocentrum, Dimorphocarpa wislizeni, Eriogonum
alatum, Erysimum capitatum, Hymenopappus
filifolius, Machaeranthera canescens, Mirabilis
linearis, Phoradendron juniperinum, Picradeniopsis woodhousei, Polygonum lapathifolium,
Ratibida columnifera, Verbesina encelioides*

Eye Medicine: *Eriogonum jamesii, Linum puberulum, Pectis papposa, Rorippa sinuata, Senecio
multicapitatus, Tetraneuris scaposa, Zinnia
grandiflora*

Febrifuge: *Zinnia grandiflora*

Gastrointestinal Aid: *Abronia fragrans, Atriplex
argentea, Croton texensis, Dalea compacta,
Eriogonum jamesii, Erodium cicutarium,
Hymenoxys richardsonii, Lithospermum incisum, Mirabilis linearis, M. multiflora, Picradeniopsis woodhousei, Psoralidium lanceolatum, Solanum rostratum, Verbesina encelioides*

Gynecological Aid: *Chaetopappa ericoides,
Chamaesyce albomarginata, C. polycarpa, C.
serpyllifolia, Eriogonum fasciculatum, Juniperus monosperma, Phoradendron juniperinum*

Hemorrhoid Remedy: *Orobanche fasciculata*

Hemostat: *Aster lanceolatus, Juniperus monosperma, Phoradendron juniperinum*

Herbal Steam: *Chenopodium graveolens*

Hunting Medicine: *Atriplex canescens, Penstemon
barbatus*

Kidney Aid: *Lithospermum incisum*

Laxative: *Mentzelia pumila*

Misc. Disease Remedy: *Cirsium ochrocentrum*

Narcotic: *Datura wrightii*

Oral Aid: *Eriogonum jamesii, Glycyrrhiza lepidota*

Orthopedic Aid: *Senecio multicapitatus*

Other: *Eriogonum alatum*

Pediatric Aid: *Aster falcatus, Ipomopsis longiflora,
Iris missouriensis, Mentzelia pumila, Mirabilis
multiflora, Phaseolus angustissimus*

Poultice: *Grindelia nuda*

Psychological Aid: *Dimorphocarpa wislizeni*

Pulmonary Aid: *Ipomopsis multiflora*

Reproductive Aid: *Coreopsis tinctoria, Rumex
salicifolius*

Respiratory Aid: *Conyza canadensis*

Snakebite Remedy: *Amsonia tomentosa, Astragalus
amphioxys, Croton texensis, Gaura parviflora,
Grindelia nuda, Helianthus annuus, Nicotiana
attenuata, Psilostrophe tagetina, Solanum
elaeagnifolium, Stephanomeria tenuifolia,
Tripterocalyx carnea, Verbesina encelioides*

Stimulant: *Cryptantha crassisepala*

Strengthener: *Aster falcatus, Gutierrezia sarothrae,
Iris missouriensis, Mentzelia pumila, Phaseolus
angustissimus*

Throat Aid: *Eriogonum fasciculatum, Ligusticum
porteri, Lithospermum incisum, Rumex salicifolius, Salix exigua, Tripterocalyx carnea*

Toothache Remedy: *Ambrosia acanthicarpa, Solanum elaeagnifolium*

Unspecified: *Asclepias involucrata, Machaeranthera tanacetifolia*

Urinary Aid: *Gutierrezia sarothrae*

Venereal Aid: *Cirsium ochrocentrum, Croton texensis, Ephedra nevadensis, Pinus edulis, Stanleya pinnata*

Veterinary Aid: *Caesalpinia jamesii*

Witchcraft Medicine: *Lotus wrightii, Tripterocalyx
carnea*

Index of Plant Usages

Plants are listed alphabetically under each category of usage. For all usages given below, check all entries under that genus in the Catalog of Plants. For example, one may find Cold Remedy below and see that *Rhus* was used by the Cahuilla, Cheyenne, Chippewa, Comanche, and Iroquois. The specific ethnobotanical information and the sources from which the information was obtained may be found by turning to *Rhus* in the Catalog of Plants and examining Cold Remedy under the entries for that genus.

Abortifacient

Abies: Cree, Woodlands
Achillea: Sanpoil
Acorus: Delaware; Delaware, Oklahoma; Menominee; Mohegan; Sioux, Fort Peck
Aletris: Micmac
Aleurites: Hawaiian
Alnus: Cree, Woodlands; Kutenai
Ambrosia: Zuni
Anemone: Blackfoot
Angelica: Cherokee
Apocynum: Cherokee
Aralia: Chippewa; Iroquois
Arctostaphylos: Cree, Woodlands
Aristolochia: Cherokee
Armoracia: Cherokee
Artemisia: Blackfoot; Chippewa; Dakota; Kawaiisu; Menominee; Omaha; Pawnee; Ponca; Sioux
Asarum: Cherokee
Asplenium: Cherokee
Aster: Cree, Woodlands
Betula: Blackfoot
Carya: Cherokee
Castilleja: Quileute
Ceanothus: Iroquois
Celastrus: Iroquois
Celtis: Iroquois
Chamaemelum: Cherokee
Chenopodium: Mahuna
Cimicifuga: Cherokee
Cocos: Hawaiian
Croton: Luiseño
Draba: Blackfoot

Echinocystis: Cherokee
Equisetum: Costanoan; Cree; Quinault
Erigeron: Cherokee
Euonymus: Iroquois
Eupatorium: Chippewa
Fagus: Iroquois
Fragaria: Malecite; Micmac
Fraxinus: Abnaki
Galium: Choctaw
Garrya: Pomo, Kashaya
Grindelia: Cree
Hedeoma: Cherokee
Hepatica: Chippewa
Heteromeles: Costanoan (Olhonean)
Hydrangea: Cherokee
Hypericum: Cherokee; Iroquois
Hyssopus: Cherokee
Iva: Mahuna
Juniperus: Cherokee
Lilium: Malecite; Micmac
Lindera: Cherokee; Rappahannock
Lysichiton: Makah
Malus: Iroquois
Mitchella: Delaware; Delaware, Oklahoma
Monarda: Cherokee
Nepeta: Cherokee
Orbexilum: Cherokee
Pedicularis: Mohegan
Persea: Seminole
Petroselinum: Cherokee
Phoradendron: Kawaiisu; Mendocino Indian; Pomo; Pomo, Kashaya
Physaria: Blackfoot
Pinus: Okanagan-Colville
Platanus: Cherokee
Polygala: Cherokee
Populus: Cree
Porophyllum: Paiute; Shoshoni
Pterocaulon: Seminole
Pycnanthemum: Chippewa
Quercus: Menominee
Ribes: Chippewa
Rubus: Chippewa; Malecite; Micmac
Rumex: Houma
Sambucus: Haisla & Hanaksiala

Sanguinaria: Abnaki; Menominee; Micmac
Sanicula: Chippewa; Malecite; Micmac
Sarracenia: Cree, Woodlands
Scutellaria: Cherokee
Silphium: Chippewa
Solidago: Cherokee
Sonchus: Houma
Stylosanthes: Cherokee
Symphoricarpos: Kutenai
Tanacetum: Chippewa
Taxus: Algonquin, Tête-de-Boule; Iroquois
Tephrosia: Creek
Tetradymia: Navajo
Thuja: Chehalis; Menominee
Trillium: Menominee
Triosteum: Iroquois
Vaccinium: Cree, Woodlands
Veratrum: Kwakiutl
Verbena: Cherokee
Verbesina: Chickasaw
Viburnum: Malecite; Micmac
Vicia: Iroquois
Yucca: Lakota
Zanthoxylum: Iroquois

Adjuvant

Abies: Menominee
Acorus: Cree, Woodlands
Angelica: Shoshoni; Washo
Aralia: Meskwaki
Arctostaphylos: Menominee
Asarum: Chippewa; Iroquois; Meskwaki
Betula: Ojibwa; Potawatomi
Chamaecyparis: Bella Coola
Chimaphila: Iroquois; Menominee
Cirsium: Meskwaki; Potawatomi
Comptonia: Menominee
Corylus: Menominee
Desmodium: Meskwaki
Ephedra: Paiute
Equisetum: Sanpoil
Eupatorium: Cherokee
Frangula: Makah
Fraxinus: Menominee
Gleditsia: Cherokee
Gnaphalium: Creek
Juniperus: Meskwaki
Lilium: Malecite
Lobelia: Iroquois
Matricaria: Eskimo, Kuskokwagmiut; Eskimo, Western
Mentha: Cherokee
Oenothera: Navajo, Ramah
Osmorhiza: Cheyenne

Panax: Meskwaki; Potawatomi
Poliomintha: Comanche
Prunella: Cherokee
Prunus: Potawatomi; Sioux
Psilostrophe: Hopi
Ptelea: Menominee; Meskwaki
Robinia: Menominee
Rubus: Menominee; Meskwaki; Ojibwa
Salix: Montana Indian
Sanguinaria: Menominee; Meskwaki
Sphaeralcea: Cheyenne
Symplocarpus: Menominee
Taenidia: Menominee; Meskwaki
Taxus: Iroquois
Thuja: Menominee; Potawatomi
Triteleia: Thompson
Tsuga: Ojibwa
Valeriana: Thompson
Zanthoxylum: Menominee

Alternative

Alnus: Menominee
Aralia: Potawatomi
Gentiana: Potawatomi
Helenium: Menominee
Persea: Creek
Polypodium: Nootka
Pycnanthemum: Meskwaki
Rhus: Iroquois
Rubus: Montana Indian

Analgesic

Abies: Blackfoot; Chippewa; Menominee
Acamptopappus: Kawaiisu
Acer: Cherokee
Achillea: Aleut; Algonquin, Quebec; Algonquin, Tête-de-Boule; Blackfoot; Cheyenne; Chippewa; Cree, Woodlands; Gosiute; Hesquiat; Iroquois; Lummi; Mendocino Indian; Miwok; Navajo, Kayenta; Okanagan-Colville; Paiute; Shoshoni
Acorus: Blackfoot; Cherokee; Cheyenne; Cree, Woodlands; Delaware, Oklahoma; Menominee; Meskwaki; Mohegan; Ojibwa
Actaea: Algonquin; Meskwaki; Ojibwa, South
Adenostoma: Coahuilla
Adiantum: Costanoan; Iroquois
Aesculus: Iroquois
Agastache: Cheyenne; Chippewa; Paiute
Ageratina: Navajo, Ramah
Allium: Makah; Quinault
Alnus: Bella Coola; Cherokee; Cowlitz; Gitksan; Iroquois; Kwakiutl; Kwakiutl, Southern
Alocasia: Hawaiian
Aloysia: Havasupai

Ambrosia: Cheyenne; Pima
Amorpha: Ojibwa, South; Omaha
Anaphalis: Cherokee
Andropogon: Catawba; Chippewa; Seminole
Androsace: Navajo, Kayenta; Navajo, Ramah
Anemone: Blackfoot; Meskwaki; Ojibwa, South
Anemopsis: Costanoan
Angelica: Aleut; Gitksan; Iroquois; Kwakiutl;
    Menominee; Miwok; Shoshoni; Yana
Antennaria: Bella Coola
Anthemis: Cherokee
Aplectrum: Catawba
Apocynum: Chippewa; Navajo, Ramah; Ojibwa
Aquilegia: Gosiute; Navajo, Kayenta; Omaha; Paiute;
    Pawnee; Ponca; Shoshoni
Arabis: Navajo, Ramah; Okanagon; Thompson
Aralia: Bella Coola; Choctaw; Malecite; Menomi-
    nee; Micmac
Arctium: Abnaki; Delaware, Ontario; Meskwaki;
    Mohegan; Ojibwa
Arctostaphylos: Cheyenne; Chippewa; Pomo, Little
    Lakes
Arenaria: Kawaiisu; Navajo, Ramah
Argentina: Kwakiutl
Arisaema: Cherokee; Iroquois; Mohegan; Pawnee
Aristolochia: Cherokee; Choctaw
Armoracia: Delaware, Ontario
Arnica: Catawba
Artemisia: Carrier, Northern; Cherokee; Cheyenne;
    Costanoan; Cree, Woodlands; Karok; Kawaiisu;
    Mendocino Indian; Miwok; Navajo; Navajo,
    Ramah; Okanagan-Colville; Okanagon; Paiute;
    Paiute, Northern; Pomo, Kashaya; Sanpoil;
    Shoshoni; Thompson; Washo; Yuki; Zuni
Aruncus: Bella Coola
Arundinaria: Choctaw
Asarum: Bella Coola; Cherokee; Iroquois;
    Meskwaki; Micmac
Asclepias: Cherokee; Okanagon; Paiute; Thompson
Aster: Cherokee; Kawaiisu; Ojibwa; Potawatomi
Astragalus: Kawaiisu; Lakota
Athyrium: Cowlitz; Meskwaki
Atriplex: Navajo, Ramah
Bahia: Navajo, Ramah; Zuni
Balsamorhiza: Cheyenne; Miwok; Paiute; Sanpoil
Betula: Chippewa; Eskimo, Western; Ojibwa;
    Shuswap
Bidens: Seminole
Bignonia: Koasati
Blephilia: Cherokee
Brassica: Mohegan; Rappahannock; Shinnecock
Brickellia: Navajo, Ramah
Callirhoe: Dakota
Campanula: Navajo, Ramah

Capsella: Cheyenne; Chippewa; Mohegan
Cardamine: Cherokee; Iroquois
Carum: Abnaki
Carya: Cherokee; Chippewa
Castanea: Cherokee
Castilleja: Navajo, Ramah
Caulophyllum: Chippewa; Ojibwa
Ceanothus: Okanagon; Thompson
Celastrus: Cherokee; Creek; Meskwaki
Centaurium: Miwok
Cephalanthus: Seminole
Cercocarpus: Paiute
Chaenactis: Gosiute; Kawaiisu; Paiute
Chaetopappa: Zuni
Chamaebatiaria: Shoshoni
Chamaecyparis: Ojibwa, South
Chamaesyce: Navajo, Ramah
Chenopodium: Cherokee; Houma; Zuni
Chimaphila: Catawba; Cherokee; Iroquois
Chlorogalum: Wailaki
Chrysothamnus: Coahuilla; Navajo, Ramah
Cibotium: Hawaiian
Cicuta: Kawaiisu; Montana Indian; Paiute;
    Thompson
Cimicifuga: Cherokee
Cirsium: Cherokee; Chippewa; Meskwaki; Ojibwa
Claytonia: Shoshoni
Clematis: Cherokee; Costanoan; Lakota; Montana
    Indian; Navajo; Navajo, Ramah; Shoshoni
Collinsonia: Iroquois
Comandra: Meskwaki; Ute
Comarum: Ojibwa
Comptonia: Algonquin, Quebec; Micmac; Ojibwa
Conyza: Chippewa; Hopi
Coptis: Potawatomi
Cordylanthus: Navajo, Ramah
Coreopsis: Meskwaki
Cornus: Abnaki; Carrier; Cherokee; Delaware;
    Delaware, Oklahoma; Iroquois; Malecite;
    Meskwaki; Micmac
Corydalis: Navajo, Ramah
Corylus: Chippewa
Crataegus: Meskwaki
Crepis: Shoshoni
Croton: Concow; Jemez; Kawaiisu
Cryptantha: Hopi; Navajo
Cucurbita: Omaha
Cunila: Cherokee
Cupressus: Kawaiisu
Cycloloma: Hopi
Cymopterus: Navajo, Kayenta
Cynoglossum: Ojibwa
Cypripedium: Cherokee; Iroquois
Dalea: Navajo; Navajo, Ramah

Liatris: Blackfoot; Cherokee; Seminole
Licania: Seminole
Ligusticum: Atsugewi
Lindera: Creek
Linnaea: Tanana, Upper
Linum: Navajo, Kayenta
Liriodendron: Rappahannock
Lithospermum: Cheyenne
Lobelia: Cherokee; Iroquois
Lomatium: Cheyenne; Kawaiisu; Kwakiutl; Paiute,
    Northern; Salish, Coast; Yuki
Lonicera: Iroquois; Kwakiutl; Kwakiutl, Southern
Lophophora: Kiowa
Lotus: Navajo, Ramah
Luetkea: Okanagon; Thompson
Lycopodium: Aleut; Carrier, Southern
Lycopus: Meskwaki
Lysichiton: Makah; Quileute; Shuswap; Skokomish
Machaeranthera: Navajo; Shoshoni
Magnolia: Cherokee
Mahonia: Havasupai; Shoshoni
Maianthemum: Chippewa; Montagnais; Ojibwa;
    Ojibwa, South; Thompson
Malus: Quinault; Thompson
Malva: Costanoan; Mahuna
Marah: Squaxin
Marrubium: Navajo, Ramah; Paiute
Matricaria: Aleut; Costanoan
Menodora: Navajo, Ramah
Mentha: Bella Coola; Blackfoot; Cherokee; Cree,
    Woodlands; Gosiute; Gros Ventre; Iroquois;
    Kawaiisu; Keres, Western; Okanagan-Colville;
    Okanagon; Paiute; Thompson
Menyanthes: Aleut
Menziesia: Kwakiutl
Merremia: Hawaiian
Metrosideros: Hawaiian
Mimulus: Kawaiisu
Mirabilis: Paiute
Mitchella: Cherokee; Iroquois
Monarda: Cherokee; Chippewa; Choctaw; Dakota;
    Meskwaki; Navajo; Navajo, Ramah; Ojibwa,
    South; Tewa
Monardella: Miwok; Paiute; Shoshoni; Washo
Moneses: Kwakiutl
Monotropa: Mohegan
Myrica: Micmac; Seminole
Nepeta: Iroquois; Rappahannock
Nicotiana: Cherokee; Kawaiisu; Navajo, Ramah
Nuphar: Bella Coola; Cree, Woodlands; Iroquois;
    Kwakiutl; Quinault; Shuswap; Tanana, Upper;
    Thompson
Oemleria: Kwakiutl
Oenothera: Navajo, Ramah

Oplopanax: Carrier; Carrier, Northern; Cheyenne;
    Crow; Gitksan; Kwakiutl; Oweekeno; Salish,
    Coast
Opuntia: Flathead; Shoshoni
Osmorhiza: Karok; Paiute; Paiute, Northern;
    Shoshoni; Washo
Osmunda: Iroquois
Oxalis: Navajo, Ramah
Paeonia: Washo
Panax: Cherokee; Iroquois
Pandanus: Hawaiian
Papaver: Cherokee
Pastinaca: Cherokee
Paxistima: Thompson
Pedicularis: Catawba
Pediomelum: Seminole
Penstemon: Blackfoot; Dakota; Navajo, Ramah;
    Okanagan-Colville; Shoshoni
Pentagrama: Karok
Pericome: Navajo, Ramah
Persea: Seminole
Petradoria: Hopi
Phoradendron: Cherokee
Phragmites: Paiute
Physalis: Omaha; Ponca; Winnebago
Physaria: Blackfoot
Physocarpus: Bella Coola
Phytolacca: Mahuna; Seminole
Picea: Bella Coola; Carrier, Southern; Hesquiat;
    Kwakiutl; Mohegan; Ojibwa
Pinguicula: Seminole
Pinus: Carrier, Southern; Delaware, Ontario; Flat-
    head; Menominee; Mohegan; Nanticoke; Navajo,
    Ramah; Ojibwa, South; Paiute; Seminole;
    Shoshoni; Thompson; Yokia
Piper: Hawaiian
Plantago: Abnaki; Cherokee; Iroquois; Keres,
    Western
Platanthera: Cherokee; Thompson
Platanus: Meskwaki
Pleopeltis: Houma
Pogogyne: Concow
Polygala: Miwok
Polygonatum: Chippewa; Menominee
Polygonum: Cherokee; Chippewa; Houma;
    Iroquois; Navajo, Ramah; Ojibwa
Polypodium: Bella Coola; Haisla
Polystichum: Iroquois
Populus: Bella Coola; Cahuilla; Carrier, Southern;
    Chippewa; Shoshoni
Porophyllum: Havasupai
Portulaca: Navajo
Potentilla: Chippewa; Navajo, Ramah; Okanagan-
    Colville

Prenanthes: Bella Coola; Cherokee; Choctaw
Proboscidea: Pima
Prosopis: Pima
Prunella: Iroquois
Prunus: Chippewa; Iroquois; Navajo, Ramah; Ojibwa, South; Paiute; Potawatomi
Psathyrotes: Paiute; Shoshoni
Pseudotsuga: Bella Coola; Navajo, Kayenta; Swinomish
Psilostrophe: Navajo, Ramah
Psoralidium: Arapaho; Lakota; Navajo, Ramah
Psorothamnus: Paiute; Shoshoni
Pteridium: Koasati; Ojibwa
Pulsatilla: Chippewa; Omaha
Purshia: Kawaiisu; Paiute
Pycnanthemum: Cherokee; Choctaw; Koasati
Quercus: Chippewa; Choctaw; Delaware, Oklahoma; Mohegan; Navajo, Ramah; Seminole; Shinnecock
Ranunculus: Abnaki; Hesquiat; Iroquois; Micmac; Montagnais; Okanagan-Colville
Ratibida: Cheyenne; Dakota; Lakota; Navajo, Ramah
Rhamnus: Kawaiisu
Rhododendron: Cherokee
Rhus: Chippewa; Coahuilla; Navajo, Ramah; Omaha
Ribes: Chippewa; Lummi
Ricinus: Hawaiian; Pima
Rorippa: Okanagan-Colville
Rosa: Cahuilla; Chehalis; Mahuna; Miwok; Potawatomi
Rubus: Cherokee; Chippewa; Iroquois; Makah; Ojibwa, South; Quinault
Rudbeckia: Seminole
Rumex: Bella Coola; Kawaiisu; Paiute; Shoshoni
Sabal: Seminole
Sabatia: Cherokee; Seminole
Sagittaria: Navajo
Salicornia: Heiltzuk
Salix: Blackfoot; Eskimo, Nunivak; Iroquois; Koasati; Montagnais; Seminole
Salvia: Costanoan; Kawaiisu; Paiute; Paiute, Northern; Shoshoni
Sambucus: Bella Coola; Chickasaw; Hanaksiala; Hesquiat; Houma; Iroquois; Kawaiisu
Sanguinaria: Chippewa; Iroquois; Meskwaki; Ojibwa
Sanicula: Cherokee; Malecite; Micmac
Sanvitalia: Navajo, Ramah
Saponaria: Mahuna
Sassafras: Seminole
Satureja: Cherokee
Sedum: Eskimo, Western
Senecio: Cheyenne; Navajo, Ramah; Zuni

Senna: Cherokee
Shepherdia: Navajo, Kayenta
Silene: Gosiute
Silphium: Chippewa; Meskwaki; Omaha; Ponca; Winnebago
Sisyrinchium: Meskwaki; Seminole
Sium: Iroquois
Smallanthus: Iroquois
Smilax: Cherokee; Chippewa; Koasati
Solanum: Seminole
Solidago: Iroquois; Menominee; Zuni
Sorbus: Malecite; Micmac
Sphaeralcea: Dakota
Spiraea: Iroquois; Okanagan-Colville
Stanleya: Paiute; Shoshoni
Streptopus: Thompson
Suaeda: Hopi
Symphoricarpos: Kwakiutl; Paiute
Symplocarpus: Delaware; Delaware, Oklahoma; Menominee; Micmac
Tanacetum: Cherokee; Iroquois; Shinnecock
Taraxacum: Bella Coola; Iroquois; Papago
Tauschia: Kawaiisu
Taxus: Klallam; Micmac
Tephrosia: Catawba
Tetradymia: Navajo, Ramah
Tetraneuris: Hopi
Thalictrum: Gitksan; Wailaki
Thamnosma: Kawaiisu
Thermopsis: Cheyenne; Navajo, Ramah
Thuja: Bella Coola; Chippewa; Micmac; Ojibwa; Penobscot
Torreya: Costanoan
Tradescantia: Cherokee
Trichostema: Concow; Costanoan; Miwok; Tubatulabal
Trillium: Iroquois; Menominee
Triosteum: Iroquois; Meskwaki
Tsuga: Menominee
Ulmus: Choctaw; Potawatomi
Umbellularia: Cahuilla; Karok; Mendocino Indian; Miwok; Pomo; Pomo, Kashaya; Yuki
Urtica: Bella Coola; Cahuilla; Carrier; Costanoan; Hesquiat; Kawaiisu; Klallam; Kwakiutl; Kwakiutl, Southern; Miwok; Pomo; Pomo, Kashaya; Quinault; Shuswap
Uvularia: Ojibwa; Potawatomi
Vaccinium: Seminole
Valeriana: Cree, Woodlands; Menominee; Okanagon; Thompson
Veratrum: Bella Coola; Blackfoot; Cherokee; Cowlitz; Iroquois; Kwakiutl; Salish, Coast
Verbascum: Catawba; Cherokee; Delaware, Oklahoma; Delaware, Ontario

Verbena: Cherokee; Dakota
Verbesina: Seminole; Zuni
Vernonia: Cherokee
Veronicastrum: Cherokee
Viburnum: Algonquin, Tête-de-Boule; Chippewa; Gitksan; Iroquois; Menominee; Meskwaki; Ojibwa
Vicia: Cherokee; Snohomish; Squaxin
Viola: Carrier, Southern; Cherokee; Klallam; Ojibwa, South
Vitis: Meskwaki; Mohegan; Seminole
Woodwardia: Luiseño
Wyethia: Mendocino Indian
Xanthorhiza: Cherokee
Zanthoxylum: Iroquois; Menominee
Zea: Tewa
Zigadenus: Mendocino Indian; Montana Indian; Paiute; Shoshoni; Thompson; Washo
Zingiber: Hawaiian
Zinnia: Navajo, Ramah
Zizia: Meskwaki
Ziziphus: Pima

Anesthetic

Achillea: Shoshoni
Datura: Zuni
Echinacea: Omaha
Salix: Eskimo, Alaska

Anthelmintic

Achillea: Iroquois
Acorus: Cherokee; Iroquois
Allium: Iroquois
Amelanchier: Cherokee
Amorpha: Meskwaki
Anemone: Iroquois
Apocynum: Iroquois; Menominee; Micmac; Penobscot
Aralia: Iroquois
Aristolochia: Nanticoke
Artemisia: Cherokee; Kiowa; Mohegan; Tolowa; Yurok
Asarum: Cherokee
Asclepias: Meskwaki
Bidens: Cherokee
Capsella: Mohegan
Carya: Iroquois
Cerastium: Cherokee
Chelone: Cherokee
Chenopodium: Cherokee; Houma; Koasati; Natchez; Rappahannock
Chimaphila: Iroquois
Cirsium: Abnaki; Hopi
Comptonia: Cherokee

Coptis: Iroquois
Cornus: Cherokee; Thompson
Corylus: Ojibwa
Cucurbita: Cherokee
Cypripedium: Cherokee
Dicentra: Skagit
Dryopteris: Cherokee
Echinacea: Dakota
Elytrigia: Iroquois
Eryngium: Delaware; Delaware, Oklahoma
Euonymus: Iroquois
Eupatorium: Meskwaki
Euphorbia: Meskwaki
Fagus: Cherokee
Frangula: Hesquiat
Fraxinus: Cowlitz
Gaultheria: Iroquois
Gentianella: Iroquois
Gleditsia: Cherokee
Helianthus: Iroquois; Pima
Juglans: Delaware; Iroquois; Kiowa
Juniperus: Cherokee; Shoshoni
Liriodendron: Cherokee
Lobelia: Cherokee
Lonicera: Meskwaki
Magnolia: Iroquois
Maianthemum: Iroquois
Manfreda: Cherokee
Melia: Cherokee
Mentha: Mohegan
Mirabilis: Dakota
Monarda: Chippewa
Morus: Cherokee
Myrica: Houma
Nepeta: Cherokee
Nicotiana: Cherokee; Paiute; Shoshoni
Nyssa: Cherokee; Houma
Oxalis: Cherokee
Panax: Iroquois
Pinus: Cherokee; Choctaw; Gosiute
Podophyllum: Cherokee
Populus: Abnaki; Iroquois; Montagnais; Sikani
Portulaca: Cherokee
Prunus: Cherokee; Chippewa; Delaware; Flathead
Purshia: Paiute, Northern
Quercus: Meskwaki
Rhus: Meskwaki; Potawatomi
Ribes: Meskwaki
Rosa: Cherokee
Rubus: Mohegan
Rudbeckia: Cherokee; Iroquois
Ruta: Cherokee
Salvia: Mohegan
Sanguinaria: Iroquois

Sassafras: Cherokee; Iroquois
Satureja: Costanoan
Senna: Iroquois
Sisyrinchium: Mahuna
Solanum: Cherokee; Houma
Spigelia: Cherokee; Creek
Symplocarpus: Iroquois
Tanacetum: Cherokee
Tephrosia: Cherokee
Tilia: Malecite; Micmac
Valeriana: Menominee
Verbena: Iroquois
Viburnum: Iroquois
Zanthoxylum: Iroquois

Anticonvulsive

Achillea: Iroquois
Acorus: Cherokee
Actaea: Chippewa
Anemopsis: Shoshoni
Anthemis: Cherokee
Apocynum: Chippewa
Arabis: Navajo, Kayenta
Aralia: Ojibwa
Aristolochia: Micmac; Penobscot
Artemisia: Chippewa
Asarum: Algonquin, Quebec; Iroquois
Astragalus: Chippewa
Atriplex: Hopi
Calypso: Thompson
Caulophyllum: Cherokee
Claytonia: Iroquois
Conyza: Iroquois
Cornus: Malecite; Micmac
Cypripedium: Cherokee
Echinacea: Meskwaki
Erigeron: Cherokee
Geum: Iroquois
Hepatica: Chippewa
Heracleum: Winnebago
Juniperus: Apache, White Mountain
Lathyrus: Chippewa
Ligusticum: Flathead
Lobelia: Iroquois
Lonicera: Thompson
Macromeria: Hopi
Maianthemum: Meskwaki
Matricaria: Costanoan
Medeola: Iroquois
Mimulus: Iroquois; Navajo, Kayenta
Mitchella: Iroquois
Monarda: Ojibwa
Monotropa: Cherokee
Nepeta: Cherokee

Nicotiana: Cherokee
Nuphar: Iroquois
Osmunda: Iroquois
Panax: Cherokee
Papaver: Cherokee
Phoradendron: Cherokee
Picea: Ojibwa
Pinus: Ojibwa
Polygala: Chippewa
Polygonum: Chippewa
Polystichum: Iroquois
Postelsia: Nitinaht
Pteridium: Tolowa
Pyrola: Iroquois
Ranunculus: Iroquois
Rosa: Chippewa
Salvia: Hopi
Sanguinaria: Ojibwa
Sium: Iroquois
Solidago: Chippewa
Symplocarpus: Delaware, Oklahoma; Menominee;
   Mohegan
Valeriana: Cree, Woodlands
Verbascum: Hopi; Iroquois
Veronicastrum: Meskwaki
Viburnum: Cherokee

Antidiarrheal

Abies: Micmac
Acer: Cherokee; Ojibwa, South; Thompson
Achillea: Chehalis; Iroquois; Okanagan-Colville;
   Shoshoni; Skagit; Snohomish; Thompson
Acorus: Cherokee
Adiantum: Menominee
Agalinis: Meskwaki
Ageratina: Cherokee
Agrimonia: Cherokee; Iroquois
Aletris: Catawba
Alnus: Klallam; Mendocino Indian; Potawatomi;
   Quileute
Ambrosia: Cheyenne; Dakota; Iroquois
Amelanchier: Cherokee; Chippewa
Amphicarpaea: Cherokee
Anaphalis: Iroquois
Andropogon: Cherokee; Seminole
Anemone: Iroquois
Angelica: Yana
Anthemis: Iroquois
Apocynum: Iroquois
Aquilegia: Meskwaki; Shoshoni
Arabis: Okanagan-Colville
Aralia: Iroquois
Arctostaphylos: Cahuilla; Cree, Woodlands; Karok;
   Pomo; Pomo, Kashaya; Pomo, Little Lakes

Argentina: Blackfoot; Iroquois
Arisaema: Iroquois
Artemisia: Chippewa; Costanoan; Klamath; Lakota;
  Mendocino Indian; Montana Indian; Okanagon;
  Paiute; Paiute, Northern; Shoshoni; Thompson;
  Yuki
Aruncus: Bella Coola
Asarum: Cherokee
Asclepias: Cherokee; Lakota; Navajo, Kayenta;
  Shoshoni
Aster: Cherokee
Aureolaria: Cherokee
Balsamorhiza: Thompson
Berberis: Cherokee
Betula: Cherokee; Chippewa; Menominee
Bidens: Seminole
Blechnum: Kwakiutl
Callicarpa: Choctaw
Campanula: Cherokee
Capsella: Chippewa; Costanoan; Mahuna
Carpinus: Cherokee; Iroquois
Ceanothus: Iroquois; Meskwaki; Thompson
Cephalanthus: Choctaw; Seminole
Cercocarpus: Paiute; Shoshoni
Chamaesyce: Navajo, Ramah; Omaha
Chenopodium: Iroquois
Chrysothamnus: Shoshoni; Thompson
Cicuta: Kwakiutl
Collinsonia: Iroquois
Comarum: Chippewa
Comptonia: Ojibwa
Conyza: Blackfoot; Cahuilla; Cree, Hudson Bay
Coptis: Algonquin, Quebec
Coreopsis: Cherokee
Cornus: Cherokee; Chippewa; Menominee;
  Meskwaki; Ojibwa; Potawatomi; Rappahannock;
  Thompson
Corydalis: Navajo, Kayenta
Corylus: Iroquois
Crataegus: Ojibwa, South; Okanagan-Colville;
  Thompson
Croton: Costanoan; Pomo; Pomo, Kashaya
Dalea: Dakota; Meskwaki
Delphinium: Blackfoot
Diospyros: Cherokee
Diplacus: Mahuna
Dracocephalum: Navajo, Kayenta
Eleocharis: Seminole
Empetrum: Tanana, Upper
Enceliopsis: Shoshoni
Ephedra: Paiute; Shoshoni; Tewa
Epifagus: Iroquois
Epigaea: Cherokee
Epilobium: Okanagan-Colville; Potawatomi

Equisetum: Makah
Eriastrum: Paiute
Ericameria: Paiute
Erigeron: Blackfoot; Paiute
Eriodictyon: Paiute
Eriogonum: Diegueño; Navajo, Ramah; Paiute;
  Sanpoil; Shoshoni; Tubatulabal
Eryngium: Natchez; Paiute; Seminole
Escobaria: Blackfoot
Eupatorium: Iroquois
Fragaria: Blackfoot; Cherokee; Diegueño; Skokom-
  ish; Thompson
Frangula: Skagit
Frasera: Cherokee; Cheyenne
Galactia: Seminole
Gaultheria: Cherokee; Quinault
Gaylussacia: Cherokee
Gentianella: Iroquois
Geranium: Chippewa; Gosiute; Iroquois; Menomi-
  nee; Meskwaki; Montana Indian; Ojibwa
Geum: Iroquois; Malecite; Micmac
Glycyrrhiza: Cheyenne
Gutierrezia: Diegueño; Navajo, Kayenta
Hamamelis: Iroquois
Hedeoma: Cherokee; Mahuna
Heliotropium: Paiute; Tubatulabal
Hepatica: Menominee
Heracleum: Blackfoot; Washo
Heuchera: Blackfoot; Cherokee; Cree, Woodlands;
  Flathead; Lakota; Menominee; Shoshoni; Shus-
  wap; Sioux, Teton
Hieracium: Iroquois; Rappahannock
Holodiscus: Lummi; Paiute
Hydrastis: Iroquois
Hydrophyllum: Menominee; Ojibwa
Hypericum: Alabama; Cherokee
Ilex: Ojibwa
Ipomopsis: Paiute; Shoshoni; Washo
Iva: Shoshoni
Jeffersonia: Iroquois
Juglans: Cherokee; Rappahannock
Juniperus: Cree, Woodlands; Crow; Keres, Western;
  Kwakiutl; Seminole
Kallstroemia: Tewa
Kalmia: Cree, Hudson Bay
Lactuca: Bella Coola; Navajo; Okanagan-Colville
Larrea: Pima
Lechea: Seminole
Lesquerella: Okanagan-Colville
Liatris: Pawnee; Seminole
Licania: Seminole
Lilium: Cherokee
Linaria: Iroquois
Liquidambar: Cherokee; Rappahannock

Liriodendron: Cherokee
Lithospermum: Shoshoni
Lomatium: Cheyenne
Lygodesmia: Lakota; Ponca
Magnolia: Cherokee
Mahonia: Great Basin Indian; Paiute; Shoshoni
Malus: Makah
Malvella: Choctaw
Manfreda: Cherokee
Marrubium: Round Valley Indian
Matricaria: Blackfoot; Cahuilla; Flathead; Montana Indian; Yokia
Menispermum: Cherokee
Mentha: Miwok; Washo
Mitchella: Cherokee
Morus: Cherokee
Nepeta: Iroquois
Nyssa: Cherokee
Opuntia: Flathead; Hopi
Osmorhiza: Shoshoni
Ostrya: Potawatomi
Oxydendrum: Cherokee
Paeonia: Shoshoni
Parthenium: Koasati
Parthenocissus: Meskwaki
Pedicularis: Cherokee
Pediomelum: Cheyenne
Perideridia: Blackfoot
Persea: Seminole
Phlox: Shoshoni
Phoradendron: Keres, Western
Phragmites: Apache, White Mountain
Phytolacca: Rappahannock
Picea: Cree, Woodlands; Kwakiutl; Ojibwa, South; Thompson; Tlingit
Pinus: Cherokee; Paiute
Plantago: Cherokee; Keres, Western; Pima; Zuni
Platanthera: Cherokee
Platanus: Cherokee
Pluchea: Paiute; Pima
Polygonatum: Cherokee
Polygonum: Cherokee; Iroquois; Meskwaki; Thompson
Polypodium: Kwakiutl
Polystichum: Iroquois
Polytaenia: Meskwaki
Porteranthus: Iroquois
Portulaca: Keres, Western
Potentilla: Cherokee; Chippewa; Iroquois; Okanagan-Colville
Prosopis: Pima
Prunella: Iroquois; Menominee
Prunus: Blackfoot; Cheyenne; Cree, Hudson Bay; Cree, Woodlands; Crow; Delaware; Delaware,

Oklahoma; Flathead; Gros Ventre; Iroquois; Kutenai; Mendocino Indian; Menominee; Micmac; Mohegan; Ojibwa, South; Okanagan-Colville; Oregon Indian; Paiute; Penobscot; Ponca; Sanpoil; Sioux; Thompson
Psathyrotes: Paiute; Shoshoni
Pseudotsuga: Bella Coola; Kwakiutl
Psidium: Hawaiian
Psilostrophe: Navajo, Kayenta
Psorothamnus: Paiute; Shoshoni
Pteridium: Iroquois
Pterocaulon: Seminole
Pycnanthemum: Cherokee
Pyrola: Navajo, Kayenta
Quercus: Cherokee; Creek; Houma; Iroquois; Malecite; Meskwaki; Micmac; Ojibwa, South; Potawatomi; Yuki
Ranunculus: Iroquois
Rheum: Cherokee
Rhus: Chippewa; Creek; Delaware, Ontario; Ojibwa, South; Pawnee
Ribes: Cherokee; Kwakiutl; Okanagan-Colville; Thompson
Rosa: Blackfoot; Cherokee; Paiute; Shoshoni; Thompson
Rubus: Algonquin, Quebec; Cherokee; Chippewa; Costanoan; Delaware; Delaware, Oklahoma; Diegueño; Iroquois; Kwakiutl; Mahuna; Mendocino Indian; Menominee; Micmac; Mohegan; Ojibwa; Okanagan-Colville; Pomo, Kashaya; Rappahannock; Saanich; Shinnecock; Shuswap
Rumex: Cherokee; Eskimo, Inuktitut; Eskimo, Kuskokwagmiut; Iroquois; Lakota; Ojibwa; Paiute; Pawnee; Yuki
Sabatia: Seminole
Salix: Bella Coola; Cherokee; Cheyenne; Cree, Woodlands; Kawaiisu; Mendocino Indian; Menominee; Meskwaki; Sanpoil; Seminole
Salvia: Cherokee
Sambucus: Clallam; Klallam; Paiute; Shoshoni
Sanguinaria: Iroquois
Sarcobatus: Paiute
Sassafras: Cherokee; Seminole
Scutellaria: Cherokee; Meskwaki
Sesamum: Cherokee
Shepherdia: Sioux
Sisyrinchium: Cherokee
Solanum: Blackfoot; Paiute
Solidago: Cherokee; Delaware; Delaware, Oklahoma; Okanagan-Colville; Thompson
Sonchus: Houma
Sphaeralcea: Hopi; Pima
Spiraea: Lummi; Meskwaki; Mohegan; Shuswap
Stephanomeria: Paiute

Stillingia: Seminole
Symphoricarpos: Thompson
Symphytum: Cherokee
Tanacetum: Shoshoni
Tetradymia: Shoshoni
Thalictrum: Cherokee
Thuja: Hanaksiala; Nez Perce
Tiarella: Malecite; Micmac
Tilia: Cherokee
Tsuga: Cherokee; Chippewa; Kwakiutl; Malecite; Micmac; Potawatomi
Typha: Washo
Ulmus: Cherokee; Houma; Iroquois; Potawatomi
Urtica: Chippewa
Uvularia: Cherokee
Vaccinium: Seminole
Valeriana: Thompson
Verbascum: Iroquois
Verbena: Cherokee
Veronicastrum: Iroquois
Viburnum: Carrier, Northern
Viola: Cherokee
Vitis: Cherokee
Xanthium: Pima; Tewa
Xyris: Cherokee

Antidote

Amaranthus: Navajo, Ramah
Angelica: Mewuk
Arctostaphylos: Karok
Artemisia: Chippewa; Mendocino Indian; Shoshoni
Asarum: Meskwaki
Bouteloua: Navajo, Ramah
Cardamine: Iroquois
Chenopodium: Navajo, Ramah
Clintonia: Menominee; Ojibwa
Cornus: Cherokee
Cuscuta: Diegueño
Datura: Cahuilla
Dryopteris: Bella Coola
Echinacea: Dakota; Omaha; Pawnee; Ponca; Sioux; Winnebago
Eryngium: Choctaw; Meskwaki
Eupatorium: Navajo
Frangula: Kawaiisu
Gutierrezia: Navajo, Ramah
Hydrophyllum: Iroquois
Krascheninnikovia: Navajo, Ramah
Laportea: Iroquois
Lespedeza: Meskwaki
Lonicera: Quileute
Maianthemum: Iroquois
Mentha: Iroquois
Mertensia: Iroquois

Mimulus: Iroquois
Nicotiana: Iroquois
Parthenocissus: Iroquois
Physaria: Hopi
Physocarpus: Hesquiat
Plantago: Cherokee
Portulaca: Iroquois
Quercus: Iroquois
Ranunculus: Iroquois
Rhamnus: Iroquois
Rhododendron: Modesse
Rhus: Omaha
Ribes: Iroquois
Rubus: Meskwaki
Rumex: Meskwaki
Salix: Makah
Sambucus: Menominee
Sanicula: Iroquois
Senecio: Navajo, Kayenta
Sisyrinchium: Menominee
Symphoricarpos: Skagit
Toxicodendron: Tolowa
Vitis: Meskwaki

Antiemetic

Acer: Thompson
Achillea: Cheyenne; Iroquois; Shoshoni
Agrimonia: Iroquois
Ambrosia: Dakota; Oto
Andropogon: Seminole
Anthemis: Iroquois
Antidesma: Hawaiian
Artemisia: Tewa
Asarum: Iroquois; Potawatomi
Baptisia: Cherokee
Cephalanthus: Seminole
Cercis: Delaware; Delaware, Oklahoma
Chamaecrista: Seminole
Chamaemelum: Cherokee
Clethra: Cherokee
Coptis: Iroquois
Cornus: Thompson
Corylus: Iroquois
Croton: Zuni
Cymopterus: Navajo, Kayenta
Dryopteris: Mewuk
Dugaldia: Navajo
Eriodictyon: Paiute
Erythrina: Seminole
Frasera: Cherokee
Gaillardia: Navajo, Ramah
Galactia: Seminole
Gaura: Navajo, Ramah
Gnaphalium: Creek

Hamamelis: Iroquois
Hydrangea: Cherokee
Juniperus: Blackfoot
Kalmia: Kwakwaka'wakw
Lactuca: Bella Coola; Navajo
Larix: Cree, Woodlands
Lechea: Seminole
Liatris: Seminole
Licania: Seminole
Lupinus: Cherokee
Mahonia: Sanpoil
Malacothrix: Navajo, Kayenta
Mentha: Cherokee; Cheyenne; Micmac
Menyanthes: Kwakiutl
Mirabilis: Paiute
Mitchella: Iroquois
Nepeta: Iroquois
Oxalis: Cherokee
Panax: Houma; Iroquois
Penstemon: Blackfoot
Perideridia: Blackfoot; Pomo; Pomo, Kashaya
Persea: Seminole
Pinus: Paiute; Shoshoni
Polypodium: Kwakiutl
Prunella: Iroquois
Prunus: Cherokee; Delaware; Meskwaki; Shoshoni
Pteridium: Cherokee
Quercus: Delaware, Ontario
Rhus: Cherokee
Ribes: Iroquois
Rosa: Thompson
Rubus: Hawaiian; Kwakiutl; Okanagon; Thompson
Sanguinaria: Delaware, Ontario; Iroquois
Sassafras: Seminole
Silphium: Meskwaki
Smallanthus: Iroquois
Solanum: Malecite; Micmac
Solidago: Iroquois
Sphaeralcea: Shoshoni
Spiraea: Iroquois; Ojibwa
Stephanomeria: Shoshoni
Stillingia: Seminole
Thalictrum: Cherokee
Thuja: Lummi
Ulmus: Iroquois
Vaccinium: Cheyenne; Ojibwa
Xanthium: Tewa
Yucca: Navajo
Zanthoxylum: Iroquois

Antihemorrhagic

Acer: Iroquois; Micmac; Penobscot
Achillea: Cherokee; Cree, Woodlands
Acorus: Cree, Woodlands; Potawatomi

Actaea: Iroquois
Adiantum: Makah
Agastache: Cree, Woodlands
Allium: Cherokee
Alnus: Gitksan; Iroquois; Kwakiutl; Mendocino Indian; Meskwaki
Ambrosia: Cheyenne; Pima
Anemone: Aleut
Angelica: Blackfoot; Paiute, Northern
Aralia: Kwakiutl; Micmac; Penobscot
Arceuthobium: Bella Coola; Carrier, Southern
Arctostaphylos: Costanoan (Olhonean); Okanagan-Colville; Okanagon; Thompson
Artemisia: Great Basin Indian
Astragalus: Blackfoot; Lakota
Athyrium: Thompson
Baptisia: Micmac; Penobscot
Boykinia: Cheyenne
Calla: Gitksan
Castilleja: Gitksan
Caulophyllum: Chippewa
Cephalanthus: Kiowa
Cercocarpus: Paiute, Northern
Chimaphila: Cree, Woodlands
Conyza: Blackfoot
Coreopsis: Meskwaki
Corylus: Iroquois
Cynoglossum: Iroquois
Dennstaedtia: Mahuna
Digitaria: Hawaiian
Dryopteris: Mewuk
Dyssodia: Lakota
Epilobium: Cheyenne; Miwok
Equisetum: Eskimo, Alaska
Erigeron: Blackfoot; Cherokee
Eryngium: Seminole
Euonymus: Cherokee
Eupatorium: Penobscot
Galium: Micmac; Penobscot
Geum: Algonquin, Tête-de-Boule
Glycyrrhiza: Lakota
Grindelia: Lakota
Hosta: Cherokee
Hyptis: Cahuilla
Juniperus: Crow; Okanagan-Colville; Paiute; Stony Indian
Kalmia: Kwakiutl; Kwakwaka'wakw
Krascheninnikovia: Navajo
Lachnanthes: Cherokee
Lactuca: Bella Coola
Ledum: Eskimo, Alaska
Leymus: Okanagan-Colville
Ligusticum: Pomo
Lithospermum: Hopi; Okanagan-Colville

Lupinus: Cherokee
Lysichiton: Gitksan
Mahonia: Blackfoot
Maianthemum: Abnaki
Malus: Kwakiutl
Matricaria: Eskimo, Alaska
Mentha: Cree, Woodlands
Menyanthes: Kwakiutl
Nuphar: Gitksan
Oplopanax: Gitksan
Ostrya: Chippewa; Potawatomi
Pellaea: Costanoan; Diegueño; Miwok
Pinus: Okanagan-Colville
Polygonatum: Abnaki
Polygonum: Menominee
Polypodium: Kwakiutl
Prunus: Chippewa; Iroquois
Psidium: Hawaiian
Psorothamnus: Paiute
Pteridium: Thompson
Pterocaulon: Seminole
Pterospora: Cheyenne
Purshia: Sanpoil; Shoshoni
Pyrola: Cree, Woodlands; Micmac; Penobscot
Ranunculus: Iroquois
Rhus: Sioux
Rubus: Kwakiutl; Okanagon; Thompson
Rumex: Cheyenne; Lakota
Sambucus: Pomo, Little Lakes
Sanguinaria: Iroquois; Malecite
Sarcobatus: Paiute
Sarracenia: Micmac; Penobscot
Scrophularia: Iroquois
Selaginella: Blackfoot
Shepherdia: Cree, Woodlands
Silphium: Chippewa
Solidago: Chippewa
Sphaeralcea: Hopi; Navajo, Ramah
Streptopus: Micmac; Penobscot
Tilia: Iroquois
Tradescantia: Cherokee
Tsuga: Clallam; Cowlitz; Klallam
Ulmus: Iroquois; Penobscot
Urtica: Gitksan
Viburnum: Iroquois

Antirheumatic (External)

Abies: Chippewa; Gitksan; Iroquois; Keres, Western
Achillea: Blackfoot; Carrier; Flathead; Gosiute; Kwakiutl; Micmac; Okanagan-Colville; Paiute; Quileute; Shoshoni; Thompson
Acorus: Cree, Woodlands
Actaea: Iroquois
Adenostoma: Cahuilla

Adiantum: Cherokee; Iroquois
Aesculus: Cherokee; Delaware; Mohegan; Shinnecock
Ageratina: Zuni
Alnus: Bella Coola
Ambrosia: Lakota
Amorpha: Omaha
Amphicarpaea: Lakota
Anaphalis: Chippewa
Angelica: Blackfoot; Iroquois; Shoshoni
Antennaria: Lakota
Anthemis: Mendocino Indian
Aquilegia: Paiute
Arabis: Shoshoni
Aralia: Karok
Arctium: Abnaki; Iroquois; Mohegan
Arctostaphylos: Ojibwa
Arenaria: Kawaiisu; Shoshoni; Washo
Arisaema: Mohegan; Pawnee
Arnica: Thompson
Artemisia: Aleut; Blackfoot; Costanoan; Eskimo, Alaska; Flathead; Gosiute; Karok; Kawaiisu; Keres, Western; Klamath; Mendocino Indian; Okanagan-Colville; Okanagon; Paiute; Paiute, Northern; Pawnee; Shoshoni; Tanana, Upper; Thompson; Tolowa; Washo; Yuki; Yurok; Zuni
Aruncus: Makah
Asarum: Bella Coola
Asclepias: Blackfoot; Delaware; Iroquois; Okanagan-Colville; Paiute
Asparagus: Iroquois
Atriplex: Maricopa; Paiute, Northern; Pima
Baccharis: Western; Yavapai
Bahia: Zuni
Barbula: Seminole
Berula: Zuni
Bidens: Seminole
Brachyactis: Paiute
Brickellia: Keres, Western
Bryum: Seminole
Callicarpa: Alabama
Carya: Iroquois
Caulophyllum: Iroquois
Ceanothus: Thompson
Celastrus: Cherokee
Chaetopappa: Keres, Western; Zuni
Chamaecyparis: Kwakiutl; Kwakiutl, Southern
Chaptalia: Seminole
Chenopodium: Cree, Woodlands; Miwok
Chimaphila: Saanich; Yurok
Chlorogalum: Wailaki
Chrysothamnus: Shoshoni
Cibotium: Hawaiian
Cicuta: Cree, Woodlands; Paiute

Cimicifuga: Iroquois
Cirsium: Delaware; Delaware, Oklahoma
Claytonia: Shoshoni
Clematis: Shoshoni
Collinsonia: Iroquois
Conioselinum: Kwakiutl
Conyza: Hawaiian
Coronilla: Cherokee
Corylus: Iroquois
Crataegus: Okanagan-Colville
Cucurbita: Zuni
Datisca: Miwok
Datura: Cahuilla; Kawaiisu
Dichanthelium: Seminole
Echinacea: Lakota
Eleocharis: Seminole
Encelia: Kawaiisu; Tubatulabal
Epixiphium: Keres, Western
Eriastrum: Shoshoni
Ericameria: Kawaiisu; Miwok; Tubatulabal
Eriodictyon: Atsugewi; Cahuilla; Costanoan; Miwok; Shoshoni
Eriogonum: Paiute; Shoshoni; Thompson
Eriophyllum: Miwok
Eryngium: Seminole
Erysimum: Keres, Western; Zuni
Erythrina: Seminole
Eupatorium: Chippewa; Iroquois
Euphorbia: Lakota
Frangula: Modesse
Fraxinus: Iroquois
Fucus: Kwakiutl, Southern
Gaultheria: Delaware
Geranium: Miwok
Geum: Thompson
Gilia: Keres, Western
Glycyrrhiza: Blackfoot
Gnaphalium: Miwok
Goodyera: Delaware; Saanich
Gutierrezia: Keres, Western; Paiute; Zuni
Hazardia: Diegueño
Helianthella: Shoshoni
Helianthus: Paiute
Heracleum: Bella Coola; Carrier; Cree, Woodlands; Gitksan; Iroquois; Mewuk; Paiute; Paiute, Northern; Pomo; Pomo, Kashaya; Sikani
Heuchera: Blackfoot; Cheyenne; Kutenai
Hymenoxys: Hopi
Inula: Iroquois
Ipomoea: Cherokee
Ipomopsis: Shoshoni
Iris: Delaware; Shoshoni
Juniperus: Blackfoot; Chippewa; Delaware, Oklahoma; Hopi; Isleta; Montana Indian; Okanagan-Colville; Paiute; Paiute, Northern; Seminole; Swinomish; Tanana, Upper; Tewa; Thompson; Zuni
Kalmia: Cherokee
Larix: Okanagan-Colville
Larrea: Cahuilla; Diegueño; Isleta; Paiute; Papago; Pima; Yavapai
Lathyrus: Iroquois
Ledum: Cree, Hudson Bay; Tanana, Upper
Lemna: Iroquois
Lespedeza: Omaha; Ponca
Lesquerella: Keres, Western
Leucothoe: Cherokee
Liatris: Seminole
Ligusticum: Zuni
Lithospermum: Cheyenne
Lobelia: Zuni
Lomatium: Crow; Kwakiutl; Paiute; Paiute, Northern; Shoshoni; Yuki
Lonicera: Kwakiutl; Shoshoni
Lophophora: Kiowa
Lycopodium: Chippewa
Lygodesmia: Keres, Western
Lysichiton: Cowlitz; Gitksan; Makah; Tolowa; Yurok
Mahonia: Flathead; Havasupai; Thompson
Maianthemum: Gosiute; Iroquois
Malva: Miwok
Marah: Mendocino Indian
Marrubium: Isleta
Mentha: Kutenai; Thompson
Mitchella: Abnaki; Delaware; Delaware, Oklahoma
Mnium: Carrier, Southern; Makah
Myrica: Micmac
Navarretia: Miwok
Nicotiana: Haisla & Hanaksiala; Mahuna; Paiute; Shoshoni
Nuphar: Cree, Woodlands; Flathead; Quinault; Shuswap; Thompson
Octoblephorum: Seminole
Oenothera: Keres, Western; Zuni
Onosmodium: Cheyenne; Lakota
Oplopanax: Cowlitz; Gitksan; Haisla; Haisla & Hanaksiala; Makah; Oweekeno; Salish, Coast; Wet'suwet'en
Osmorhiza: Paiute, Northern
Osmunda: Cherokee; Iroquois
Ostrya: Chippewa
Oxalis: Pomo; Pomo, Kashaya; Tolowa
Panax: Seminole
Pediomelum: Blackfoot; Seminole
Penstemon: Thompson
Persea: Seminole
Petasites: Skagit; Tolowa
Phacelia: Cherokee; Keres, Western

Philadelphus: Thompson
Phlox: Havasupai
Phoradendron: Kawaiisu; Keres, Western; Seminole
Physaria: Blackfoot
Physocarpus: Hesquiat
Phytolacca: Delaware; Delaware, Oklahoma;
   Iroquois
Picea: Bella Coola; Chippewa; Haisla & Hanaksiala;
   Oweekeno
Pinus: Bella Coola; Cherokee; Flathead; Haisla &
   Hanaksiala; Keres, Western; Seminole; Skagit;
   Thompson; Yokia
Plagiomnium: Bella Coola; Heiltzuk; Oweekeno
Plantago: Abnaki; Chippewa; Shoshoni
Platanthera: Thompson
Platanus: Iroquois
Plumbago: Hawaiian
Poliomintha: Hopi; Tewa
Polygala: Seminole
Polygonum: Iroquois
Polypodium: Wailaki
Polystichum: Cherokee; Iroquois
Populus: Algonquin, Tête-de-Boule; Bella Coola;
   Cahuilla; Nez Perce; Ojibwa; Okanagon;
   Thompson
Porophyllum: Havasupai
Porteranthus: Cherokee
Proboscidea: Pima
Pseudoroegneria: Okanagan-Colville
Pseudotsuga: Isleta; Montana Indian; Okanagon;
   Pomo, Little Lakes; Thompson
Psorothamnus: Paiute
Pteridium: Thompson
Pulsatilla: Great Basin Indian; Omaha; Thompson
Quercus: Houma; Mohegan; Seminole
Ranunculus: Hesquiat; Okanagan-Colville;
   Thompson
Rhizomnium: Bella Coola
Rhododendron: Cherokee
Rosa: Arapaho
Rubus: Cherokee
Rumex: Bella Coola; Blackfoot; Cree, Woodlands;
   Hanaksiala; Iroquois; Paiute; Shoshoni
Salicornia: Heiltzuk
Salix: Kiowa; Montana Indian; Seminole
Sambucus: Hanaksiala; Hesquiat; Montana Indian;
   Okanagan-Colville; Paiute
Sanguinaria: Ojibwa
Saururus: Ojibwa; Seminole
Senecio: Hopi
Shepherdia: Cree, Woodlands; Tanana, Upper
Smilax: Iroquois
Solidago: Miwok
Sorbus: Cree, Woodlands

Sphaeralcea: Shoshoni
Stanleya: Shoshoni
Stellaria: Iroquois
Symplocarpus: Abnaki; Iroquois
Taxus: Abnaki; Chippewa; Iroquois; Menominee
Tephrosia: Catawba
Tetraneuris: Hopi
Thuja: Abnaki; Bella Coola; Iroquois; Okanagan-
   Colville
Trillium: Chippewa
Tsuga: Abnaki; Algonquin, Quebec; Bella Coola;
   Delaware; Delaware, Oklahoma; Iroquois
Turricula: Kawaiisu
Umbellularia: Mendocino Indian; Pomo; Pomo,
   Kashaya; Yuki
Urtica: Bella Coola; Cahuilla; Chehalis; Diegueño;
   Haisla & Hanaksiala; Hesquiat; Kwakiutl, South-
   ern; Mahuna; Miwok; Nitinaht; Okanagan-
   Colville; Paiute; Paiute, Northern; Pomo; Pomo,
   Kashaya; Quileute; Shoshoni; Shuswap; Thompson
Valeriana: Gosiute
Veratrum: Bella Coola; Cherokee; Haisla;
   Hanaksiala; Kitasoo; Okanagan-Colville;
   Oweekeno; Paiute; Paiute, Northern; Salish,
   Coast; Shoshoni; Thompson; Tsimshian; Washo
Verbascum: Delaware; Delaware, Oklahoma
Verbesina: Seminole
Viola: Blackfoot
Wyethia: Klamath; Mendocino Indian; Okanagan-
   Colville
Ximenia: Seminole
Yucca: Blackfoot
Zanthoxylum: Cherokee; Menominee
Zigadenus: Keres, Western; Mendocino Indian;
   Montana Indian; Okanagon; Paiute; Paiute,
   Northern; Shoshoni; Thompson; Washo
Zinnia: Keres, Western
Ziziphus: Pima

Antirheumatic (Internal)

Abies: Iroquois; Keres, Western
Achillea: Iroquois
Acorus: Mohegan
Actaea: Okanagon; Thompson
Adiantum: Cherokee; Iroquois; Mahuna
Agastache: Miwok
Aletris: Cherokee
Alnus: Eskimo, Inuktitut
Aloysia: Havasupai
Anaphalis: Quileute
Anemone: Gitksan
Anthemis: Cherokee
Apocynum: Cherokee
Aralia: Cherokee; Iroquois

Arctium: Abnaki; Cherokee; Delaware; Delaware, Oklahoma
Aristolochia: Cherokee
Armoracia: Cherokee
Artemisia: Gosiute; Miwok; Tanaina
Asclepias: Delaware, Oklahoma
Bahia: Navajo, Ramah
Balsamorhiza: Blackfoot; Miwok
Baptisia: Iroquois; Koasati
Bignonia: Koasati
Calochortus: Keres, Western
Carya: Iroquois
Castanea: Mohegan
Caulophyllum: Cherokee; Iroquois
Ceanothus: Thompson
Cephalanthus: Koasati
Chamaebatia: Miwok
Chenopodium: Cree, Woodlands
Chimaphila: Cherokee; Iroquois; Micmac
Cimicifuga: Cherokee
Collinsonia: Iroquois
Corydalis: Navajo
Croton: Jemez
Cupressus: Costanoan; *Cycloloma*: Hopi
Datura: Tubatulabal
Dryopteris: Cherokee
Echinacea: Cheyenne
Echinocystis: Cherokee
Ephedra: Paiute
Epigaea: Iroquois
Equisetum: Iroquois; Okanagan-Colville
Eriodictyon: Cahuilla; Mahuna; Miwok; Round Valley Indian
Eryngium: Creek; Seminole
Eupatorium: Cherokee
Euphorbia: Meskwaki
Frangula: Okanagan-Colville
Gaultheria: Delaware, Oklahoma; Iroquois; Menominee; Ojibwa; Potawatomi
Gnaphalium: Cherokee
Goodyera: Delaware, Oklahoma
Hamamelis: Iroquois
Heracleum: California Indian
Heuchera: Cheyenne
Humulus: Cherokee
Hypericum: Koasati
Ipomopsis: Navajo, Ramah
Iris: Delaware, Oklahoma
Juniperus: Cherokee; Chippewa; Iroquois; Micmac; Thompson
Larix: Iroquois; Okanagan-Colville
Larrea: Pima
Ledum: Quinault; Tanana, Upper
Leucothoe: Cherokee

Liatris: Koasati
Lilium: Cherokee
Lindera: Creek
Liriodendron: Cherokee
Lobelia: Cherokee
Lomatium: Okanagan-Colville
Lysichiton: Gitksan
Mahonia: Miwok; Navajo; Shoshoni; Thompson
Maianthemum: Algonquin, Quebec; Gitksan; Iroquois; Thompson
Malus: Gitksan; Haisla & Hanaksiala
Mentha: Okanagan-Colville
Mentzelia: Cheyenne
Menyanthes: Aleut
Mirabilis: Navajo
Nepeta: Rappahannock; Shinnecock
Nolina: Isleta
Nuphar: Bella Coola
Onoclea: Iroquois
Oplopanax: Bella Coola; Nitinaht
Panax: Cherokee; Houma
Penstemon: Shoshoni
Petasites: Tanaina
Phlox: Mahuna
Phryma: Ojibwa, South
Phyla: Mahuna
Physocarpus: Hesquiat
Phytolacca: Cherokee; Delaware, Oklahoma; Rappahannock; Seminole
Picea: Cree, Woodlands; Gitksan; Tanana, Upper
Pinus: Cherokee; Costanoan; Iroquois; Mahuna; Paiute; Wailaki
Podophyllum: Cherokee; Meskwaki
Polygala: Cherokee
Polystichum: Cherokee
Populus: Cherokee; Iroquois; Okanagon; Thompson
Porophyllum: Havasupai
Potentilla: Okanagan-Colville
Prunus: Paiute
Pseudotsuga: Bella Coola
Pteridium: Iroquois
Purshia: Hualapai
Pyrola: Iroquois
Quercus: Kawaiisu
Rhamnus: Kawaiisu
Rhododendron: Cherokee
Rhus: Algonquin, Quebec
Rosa: Costanoan
Rubus: Cherokee
Rumex: Paiute
Sagittaria: Iroquois
Salix: Seminole
Sambucus: Cherokee; Okanagon; Rappahannock; Thompson

Sanicula: Micmac
Sassafras: Cherokee; Iroquois
Shepherdia: Gitksan
Silphium: Ojibwa; Omaha; Ponca; Winnebago
Smilax: Cherokee
Sorbus: Bella Coola
Staphylea: Iroquois
Tanacetum: Mahuna
Taxus: Abnaki; Algonquin, Quebec; Chippewa;
   Iroquois
Tephrosia: Catawba
Thuja: Algonquin, Quebec
Tsuga: Abnaki; Hesquiat; Iroquois
Urtica: Quileute; Tanaina
Vaccinium: Flathead
Veratrum: Hanaksiala; Quinault
Verbascum: Atsugewi
Veronicastrum: Iroquois
Vicia: Cherokee
Vitis: Chippewa
Xanthium: Mahuna

Basket Medicine

Agrimonia: Iroquois
Clintonia: Iroquois
Corallorrhiza: Iroquois
Desmodium: Iroquois
Epilobium: Iroquois
Lobelia: Iroquois
Sarracenia: Iroquois

Blood Medicine

Acer: Iroquois
Achillea: Iroquois; Makah; Paiute; Shuswap
Acorus: Iroquois; Shinnecock
Actaea: Cheyenne
Adiantum: Costanoan
Ageratina: Iroquois
Agrimonia: Cherokee
Alnus: Cherokee; Chippewa; Mendocino Indian
Ambrosia: Delaware; Delaware, Oklahoma;
   Iroquois
Amelanchier: Iroquois
Anemopsis: Isleta
Angelica: Iroquois
Antennaria: Navajo, Kayenta
Anthemis: Iroquois
Apocynum: Iroquois
Aquilegia: Keres, Western
Aralia: Abnaki; Cherokee; Chippewa; Iroquois;
   Menominee; Ojibwa; Okanagon; Thompson
Arctium: Cherokee; Delaware; Delaware, Okla-
   homa; Delaware, Ontario; Iroquois; Ojibwa;
   Potawatomi

Arctostaphylos: Ojibwa; Okanagan-Colville
Arenaria: Shoshoni
Arisaema: Choctaw; Iroquois
Armoracia: Iroquois
Artemisia: Tanana, Upper
Aruncus: Tlingit
Asarum: Cherokee; Iroquois
Asparagus: Iroquois
Asplenium: Hawaiian
Aster: Iroquois
Barbarea: Cherokee
Berchemia: Choctaw
Betula: Iroquois; Ojibwa
Bignonia: Cherokee
Brachyactis: Paiute
Caesalpinia: Hawaiian
Castilleja: Navajo, Ramah; Shoshoni
Catharanthus: Hawaiian
Caulanthus: Shoshoni
Ceanothus: Iroquois
Celastrus: Iroquois
Cephalanthus: Seminole
Cercocarpus: Paiute; Shoshoni
Chamaesyce: Costanoan; Miwok
Chenopodium: Carrier; Seminole
Chimaphila: Delaware; Delaware, Oklahoma;
   Iroquois; Malecite; Menominee; Micmac;
   Okanagan-Colville; Rappahannock
Cibotium: Hawaiian
Cimicifuga: Iroquois
Cleome: Navajo, Ramah
Cocculus: Houma
Collinsonia: Iroquois
Comptonia: Delaware; Delaware, Oklahoma
Conioselinum: Navajo, Kayenta
Coptis: Iroquois
Corallorrhiza: Paiute; Shoshoni
Cornus: Cherokee; Iroquois; Okanagan-Colville;
   Rappahannock; Thompson
Corylus: Iroquois
Crotalaria: Mohegan
Curcuma: Hawaiian
Cypripedium: Iroquois
Dalibarda: Iroquois
Datura: Paiute
Daucus: Costanoan; Iroquois
Diervilla: Iroquois; Menominee
Dirca: Iroquois
Echinacea: Omaha
Ephedra: Cahuilla; Diegueño; Kawaiisu; Paiute;
   Shoshoni; Tubatulabal
Equisetum: Saanich
Eriodictyon: Cahuilla; Costanoan; Pomo, Kashaya;
   Round Valley Indian

Sambucus: Delaware; Delaware, Oklahoma; Kawaiisu; Shoshoni; Squaxin
Sanguinaria: Delaware, Ontario; Iroquois; Mohegan; Ojibwa
Sarcobatus: Cheyenne
Sassafras: Cherokee; Chippewa; Choctaw; Delaware; Delaware, Oklahoma; Iroquois
Satureja: Mendocino Indian; Pomo; Pomo, Kashaya; Saanich; Yurok
Saxifraga: Iroquois
Scrophularia: Iroquois
Senecio: Iroquois
Senna: Iroquois
Sequoia: Houma
Sorbus: Montagnais
Stillingia: Seminole
Taraxacum: Algonquin, Quebec; Cherokee; Iroquois; Ojibwa; Rappahannock
Taxus: Karok; Micmac; Yurok
Thalictrum: Gitksan
Thuja: Iroquois; Ojibwa
Toxicodendron: Iroquois
Trifolium: Iroquois; Rappahannock
Tsuga: Iroquois
Ulmus: Iroquois
Urtica: Shoshoni
Uvularia: Iroquois
Vaccinium: Ojibwa
Veratrum: Hanaksiala; Okanagon; Thompson
Verbascum: Iroquois
Vernonia: Cherokee
Veronicastrum: Chippewa
Viburnum: Iroquois
Viola: Cherokee
Vitis: Cherokee; Iroquois
Waldsteinia: Iroquois
Wyethia: Paiute
Xanthium: Apache, White Mountain
Xanthorhiza: Cherokee

Breast Treatment

Achillea: Bella Coola
Asarum: Cherokee
Asplenium: Cherokee
Cardamine: Iroquois
Carica: Hawaiian
Chamaesyce: Hawaiian
Clermontia: Hawaiian
Collinsonia: Cherokee
Eupatorium: Cherokee
Gaillardia: Blackfoot
Hepatica: Cherokee
Humulus: Cherokee
Ledum: Cree, Woodlands

Lewisia: Flathead
Lygodesmia: Cheyenne
Marrubium: Cherokee
Mertensia: Cheyenne
Osmorhiza: Blackfoot
Panax: Cherokee
Perideridia: Blackfoot
Petradoria: Hopi
Philadelphus: Thompson
Plagiomnium: Bella Coola
Polygonatum: Cherokee
Rhizomnium: Bella Coola
Sambucus: Creek
Scutellaria: Cherokee
Verbena: Cherokee

Burn Dressing

Abies: Carrier, Northern; Micmac; Penobscot
Abronia: Shoshoni
Achillea: Bella Coola; Crow; Zuni
Acorus: Meskwaki
Agastache: Chippewa
Alnus: Mendocino Indian
Alocasia: Hawaiian
Anaphalis: Algonquin, Tête-de-Boule
Anemone: Meskwaki
Anemopsis: Keres, Western
Aralia: Cherokee; Meskwaki
Arbutus: Cowichan
Arctostaphylos: Atsugewi; Flathead
Argemone: Kawaiisu; Paiute; Shoshoni; Washo
Aristida: Keres, Western
Artemisia: Meskwaki; Ponca
Balsamorhiza: Flathead; Okanagan-Colville
Betula: Cree, Woodlands
Castilleja: Navajo; Navajo, Ramah
Ceanothus: Okanagan-Colville
Cercocarpus: Apache, White Mountain; Gosiute; Paiute; Shoshoni
Chenopodium: Iroquois; Navajo, Kayenta
Cirsium: Kiowa
Clematis: Miwok; Shoshoni
Clintonia: Chippewa
Conocephalum: Haisla & Hanaksiala
Conyza: Keres, Western
Cynoglossum: Concow
Echinacea: Cheyenne; Dakota; Omaha; Pawnee; Ponca; Sioux; Winnebago
Ephedra: Paiute; Shoshoni
Equisetum: Okanagon; Thompson
Eriogonum: Klamath
Eupatorium: Potawatomi
Fagus: Iroquois; Potawatomi
Fragaria: Quileute

Frangula: Kawaiisu
Gaultheria: Klallam
Gaura: Navajo
Geranium: Meskwaki
Goodyera: Cherokee
Helianthus: Meskwaki
Holodiscus: Okanagan-Colville
Hydrangea: Cherokee
Impatiens: Mohegan; Nanticoke; Penobscot
Iris: Algonquin, Tête-de-Boule; Meskwaki; Shoshoni
Juniperus: Shoshoni
Krascheninnikovia: Hopi; Tewa; Zuni
Larix: Chippewa; Thompson
Larrea: Paiute
Ledum: Chippewa; Cree; Cree, Woodlands
Lomatium: Thompson
Lonicera: Wet'suwet'en
Lysichiton: Haisla & Hanaksiala; Hesquiat; Nitinaht
Maianthemum: Nitinaht
Malvella: Choctaw
Mentzelia: Gosiute; Kawaiisu
Mirabilis: Meskwaki; Navajo, Ramah; Paiute
Monarda: Chippewa
Navarretia: Costanoan
Nereocystis: Kwakiutl, Southern
Oenothera: Navajo, Ramah
Opuntia: Cahuilla;
Paeonia: Shoshoni
Parthenium: Catawba
Pediomelum: Cheyenne
Penstemon: Navajo, Ramah; Shoshoni
Petrophyton: Gosiute
Phlox: Navajo
Physalis: Iroquois
Picea: Bella Coola; Cree, Woodlands
Pinus: Flathead; Iroquois; Mendocino Indian; Miwok; Navajo, Ramah
Plantago: Algonquin, Tête-de-Boule; Cherokee; Houma; Menominee; Meskwaki; Mohegan; Ojibwa
Polystichum: Quinault
Populus: Haisla & Hanaksiala
Portulaca: Iroquois
Potentilla: Navajo, Kayenta
Prenanthes: Bella Coola
Prosopis: Pima
Prunella: Cherokee
Prunus: Chippewa; Crow; Iroquois
Pteridium: Yana
Quercus: Kawaiisu;
Rhus: Cherokee; Cheyenne
Rosa: Paiute; Pawnee; Shoshoni
Rubus: Cowlitz; Kwakiutl; Quileute; Quinault

Rudbeckia: Chippewa
Rumex: Keres, Western; Paiute; Shoshoni
Sambucus: Cherokee; Yokut
Sanguinaria: Meskwaki
Sassafras: Rappahannock
Senecio: Navajo, Kayenta
Silene: Navajo, Ramah
Smallanthus: Cherokee
Smilax: Cherokee
Solidago: Chippewa; Costanoan; Iroquois; Mahuna; Meskwaki
Sphaeralcea: Dakota
Symphoricarpos: Cowichan; Flathead; Saanich
Taxus: Okanagan-Colville
Thuja: Malecite; Micmac
Tilia: Iroquois
Trillium: Yurok
Tsuga: Bella Coola; Kwakiutl
Typha: Dakota; Montana Indian; Omaha; Pawnee; Ponca; Sioux; Winnebago
Ulmus: Cherokee
Veratrum: Paiute
Wyethia: Mendocino Indian
Zanthoxylum: Comanche
Zigadenus: Paiute

Cancer Treatment

Abies: Iroquois
Aesculus: Cherokee
Aralia: Iroquois
Arnoglossum: Cherokee
Artemisia: Eskimo; Tanana, Upper
Athyrium: Hesquiat
Blechnum: Hesquiat
Ceanothus: Thompson
Celastrus: Chippewa
Chamaesyce: Cherokee
Chimaphila: Cherokee; Iroquois
Cirsium: Iroquois
Cornus: Menominee
Crepis: Meskwaki
Cryptantha: Hopi
Cynoglossum: Cherokee; Iroquois
Dryopteris: Hesquiat
Epilobium: Kwakiutl
Euphorbia: Cherokee
Fritillaria: Lakota
Gaillardia: Thompson
Hackelia: Cherokee
Hydrangea: Cherokee
Hydrastis: Cherokee
Lachnanthes: Cherokee
Larix: Okanagan-Colville; Thompson
Larrea: Cahuilla

Maianthemum: Thompson
Oplopanax: Gitksan; Haisla; Wet'suwet'en
Orobanche: Montana Indian
Ostrya: Iroquois
Oxalis: Cherokee
Pedicularis: Meskwaki
Picea: Thompson
Polystichum: Hesquiat
Prunus: Kwakiutl
Pteridium: Hesquiat
Pyrola: Nootka
Shepherdia: Thompson
Taxus: Tsimshian
Tradescantia: Cherokee
Trifolium: Shinnecock; Thompson
Trillium: Cherokee
Ulmus: Montana Indian
Xanthorhiza: Cherokee

Carminative

Achillea: Shoshoni
Acorus: Abnaki; Cherokee; Dakota; Omaha;
  Pawnee; Ponca; Winnebago
Aletris: Cherokee
Allium: Cherokee
Alnus: Tanana, Upper
Angelica: Cherokee
Aralia: Cherokee
Arisaema: Cherokee
Artemisia: Okanagan-Colville; Tewa
Asclepias: Meskwaki
Brickellia: Keres, Western
Cardamine: Iroquois
Chenopodium: Eskimo, Inupiat
Chlorogalum: Wailaki
Eupatorium: Iroquois
Foeniculum: Cherokee
Gutierrezia: Hopi; Tewa
Helianthus: Shasta
Hydrastis: Iroquois
Inula: Iroquois
Larrea: Pima
Liatris: Cherokee
Linum: Paiute
Matricaria: Aleut
Mentha: Cherokee; Chippewa; Dakota; Omaha;
  Paiute; Pawnee; Ponca; Shoshoni; Winnebago
Menyanthes: Aleut
Mitchella: Iroquois
Monarda: Cherokee
Pectis: Navajo; Zuni
Pinus: Kawaiisu
Polygonatum: Iroquois
Polypodium: Hesquiat

Salix: Iroquois
Salvia: Costanoan
Sanguinaria: Iroquois
Solanum: Navajo

Cathartic

Abies: Okanagon; Thompson
Abronia: Navajo, Kayenta
Acer: Blackfoot
Achillea: Makah; Montana Indian; Okanagan-
  Colville
Acorus: Chippewa; Menominee; Meskwaki; Ojibwa
Acourtia: Coahuilla
Actaea: Cree, Hudson Bay
Adenostoma: Coahuilla
Agastache: Shoshoni
Ageratina: Iroquois
Aletes: Keres, Western
Allium: Cherokee
Alnus: Bella Coola; Cherokee; Iroquois
Amelanchier: Blackfoot
Amphicarpaea: Chippewa
Angelica: Bella Coola
Apocynum: Cree, Hudson Bay; Montana Indian
Aralia: Montana Indian
Arenaria: Gosiute
Argemone: Shoshoni
Artemisia: Mewuk; Shoshoni
Arundinaria: Seminole
Asarum: Iroquois
Asclepias: Meskwaki; Pima
Atriplex: Shoshoni
Bahia: Keres, Western
Balsamorhiza: Flathead
Baptisia: Cherokee
Betula: Chippewa; Delaware, Oklahoma
Castilleja: Gitksan; Shoshoni
Celastrus: Chippewa
Cephalanthus: Seminole
Chaenactis: Sanpoil
Chamaesyce: Cherokee; Navajo; Zuni
Chrysothamnus: Navajo, Ramah
Cicuta: Bella Coola; Kwakiutl; Salish, Coast
Cornus: Algonquin, Quebec; Green River Group;
  Iroquois
Croton: Apache, White Mountain; Keres, Western;
  Zuni
Cucurbita: Cahuilla; Paiute; Shoshoni
Dalea: Jemez; Lakota
Datura: Costanoan
Daucus: Micmac
Dirca: Chippewa; Iroquois
Empetrum: Bella Coola
Ephedra: Shoshoni

Sonchus: Pima
Sorbus: Gitksan
Sphaeralcea: Shoshoni
Stephanomeria: Paiute
Streptopus: Ojibwa
Symphoricarpos: Okanagan-Colville
Taraxacum: Mohegan
Tetradymia: Shoshoni
Thymophylla: Paiute
Triosteum: Meskwaki
Ulmus: Menominee
Valeriana: Menominee
Veronicastrum: Cherokee; Chippewa; Iroquois;
    Menominee; Ojibwa, South
Viburnum: Carrier, Northern; Ojibwa
Wyethia: Paiute; Shoshoni; Washo
Yucca: Pima
Zinnia: Navajo, Ramah

Ceremonial Medicine

Abies: Blackfoot; Cheyenne; Crow; Kwakiutl; Ojibwa
Acer: Cheyenne
Achillea: Navajo, Ramah; Ojibwa
Acorus: Cheyenne; Dakota; Omaha; Pawnee; Ponca;
    Winnebago
Actaea: Cheyenne
Adiantum: Nitinaht
Agastache: Cree; Navajo, Ramah
Agoseris: Navajo, Ramah
Amaranthus: Cherokee
Ambrosia: Cherokee
Amelanchier: Navajo, Ramah
Anaphalis: Cheyenne
Andropogon: Cherokee
Anemone: Ojibwa
Angelica: Blackfoot
Antennaria: Navajo, Ramah; Okanagan-Colville
Apocynum: Navajo, Kayenta; Navajo, Ramah; Ojibwa
Aquilegia: Meskwaki; Navajo, Kayenta
Arbutus: Karok
Arceuthobium: Navajo, Ramah
Arctostaphylos: Navajo, Kayenta; Navajo, Ramah;
    Ojibwa
Arisaema: Meskwaki
Artemisia: Cheyenne; Delaware, Oklahoma; Miwok;
    Navajo; Navajo, Kayenta; Omaha; Paiute
Asclepias: Navajo, Kayenta; Navajo, Ramah; Omaha
Aster: Navajo, Ramah
Astragalus: Navajo, Kayenta; Navajo, Ramah
Atriplex: Hopi; Navajo, Ramah
Baccharis: Navajo, Ramah
Besseya: Navajo, Ramah
Brickellia: Navajo, Kayenta; Navajo, Ramah
Bromus: Navajo, Kayenta

Calochortus: Hopi; Navajo, Ramah
Campanula: Navajo, Ramah
Carex: Cheyenne; Navajo, Ramah
Catabrosa: Crow; Montana Indian
Ceanothus: Navajo, Kayenta; Navajo, Ramah;
    Okanagan-Colville
Chamaesyce: Navajo, Ramah
Chrysothamnus: Hopi; Navajo, Kayenta; Navajo,
    Ramah
Cicuta: Cherokee
Clematis: Cherokee
Cleome: Navajo, Kayenta; Navajo, Ramah
Comptonia: Chippewa
Cordylanthus: Navajo, Kayenta
Coreopsis: Navajo, Ramah
Cornus: Apache, White Mountain; Menominee;
    Navajo, Kayenta; Navajo, Ramah; Ojibwa
Cosmos: Navajo, Ramah
Cryptantha: Navajo, Ramah
Cucurbita: Cherokee
Cuscuta: Navajo, Ramah
Cynoglossum: Cherokee
Cyperus: Navajo, Ramah
Dasylirion: Tarahumara
Datura: Apache, White Mountain; Kawaiisu;
    Luiseño; Navajo, Ramah; Yokut
Delphinium: Hopi
Dichanthelium: Navajo, Ramah
Dimorphocarpa: Apache, White Mountain
Dodonaea: Hawaiian
Draba: Navajo, Ramah
Echinochloa: Navajo, Ramah
Eleocharis: Navajo, Ramah
Elymus: Iroquois
Epipactis: Navajo, Kayenta
Equisetum: Hoh; Hopi; Karok; Quileute
Erigeron: Navajo, Ramah
Eriogonum: Apache, White Mountain; Navajo,
    Kayenta; Navajo, Ramah; Thompson
Eryngium: Meskwaki; Seminole
Erysimum: Navajo, Ramah
Fallugia: Navajo, Ramah
Fendlera: Navajo, Kayenta
Forestiera: Navajo, Ramah
Frangula: Navajo, Kayenta
Fraxinus: Omaha
Galium: Navajo, Ramah
Gaylussacia: Iroquois
Glyceria: Crow; Montana Indian
Glycyrrhiza: Cheyenne
Gnaphalium: Navajo, Ramah
Gutierrezia: Navajo; Navajo, Kayenta; Navajo,
    Ramah
Hamamelis: Menominee

Sphaeralcea: Cheyenne; Navajo; Navajo, Kayenta
Stachys: Navajo, Ramah
Staphylea: Meskwaki
Suaeda: Hopi
Symphoricarpos: Navajo, Ramah
Tetraclea: Navajo, Ramah
Tetradymia: Navajo, Ramah
Tetraneuris: Navajo, Kayenta
Thalictrum: Navajo, Ramah
Thlaspi: Navajo, Ramah
Thuja: Chippewa; Ojibwa; Oweekeno
Townsendia: Navajo
Tragopogon: Navajo, Ramah
Tribulus: Navajo
Trifolium: Navajo, Ramah
Tsuga: Kwakiutl; Kwakwaka'wakw; Oweekeno
Typha: Cheyenne; Navajo, Ramah; Omaha
Vaccinium: Iroquois; Seminole
Valeriana: Thompson
Veratrum: Haisla & Hanaksiala
Verbena: Navajo, Ramah
Verbesina: Seminole
Veronica: Navajo, Ramah
Veronicastrum: Menominee
Vicia: Navajo; Okanagan-Colville
Viola: Navajo, Ramah
Vitis: Seminole
Xanthium: Lakota; Zuni
Yucca: Apache, Western; Cherokee; Hopi; Navajo, Ramah; Tewa
Zea: Navajo
Zinnia: Navajo, Ramah

Cold Remedy

Abies: Algonquin, Tête-de-Boule; Blackfoot; Chehalis; Cree, Woodlands; Crow; Gitksan; Green River Group; Iroquois; Menominee; Micmac; Montana Indian; Ojibwa; Ojibwa, South; Oweekeno; Paiute; Potawatomi; Shoshoni; Thompson; Wet'suwet'en
Acer: Micmac
Achillea: Abnaki; Aleut; Algonquin, Quebec; Carrier, Southern; Cheyenne; Clallam; Flathead; Klallam; Kwakiutl; Micmac; Miwok; Nitinaht; Okanagan-Colville; Paiute; Paiute, Northern; Saanich; Sanpoil; Shoshoni; Thompson; Yuki
Acorus: Algonquin, Quebec; Cherokee; Cheyenne; Chippewa; Cree, Woodlands; Dakota; Delaware; Delaware, Oklahoma; Delaware, Ontario; Iroquois; Malecite; Menominee; Micmac; Mohegan; Nanticoke; Ojibwa; Omaha; Pawnee; Ponca; Winnebago
Actaea: Blackfoot
Adenostoma: Cahuilla

Agastache: Cheyenne; Okanagan-Colville; Paiute
Allium: Cherokee; Chippewa; Mohegan; Shinnecock
Alnus: Menominee; Swinomish
Ambrosia: Cheyenne
Amelanchier: Cree, Woodlands; Okanagan-Colville
Anaphalis: Cherokee; Mohegan
Anemone: Carrier, Southern
Anemopsis: Cahuilla; Kawaiisu; Pima; Shoshoni; Tubatulabal
Angelica: Aleut; Cherokee; Iroquois; Micmac; Miwok; Paiute; Pomo, Kashaya; Shoshoni; Yana
Anthemis: Mendocino Indian
Apocynum: Chippewa
Aquilegia: Paiute
Arabis: Cheyenne
Aralia: Iroquois; Malecite; Mendocino Indian; Micmac
Arbutus: Pomo, Little Lakes; Saanich; Skokomish
Arctium: Mohegan
Arctostaphylos: Cheyenne; Pomo, Calpella
Arisaema: Cherokee
Aristolochia: Cherokee; Miwok
Armoracia: Cherokee
Aronia: Potawatomi
Artemisia: Blackfoot; Cahuilla; Costanoan; Diegueño; Flathead; Gosiute; Havasupai; Karok; Kawaiisu; Lakota; Mendocino Indian; Navajo; Okanagan-Colville; Paiute; Paiute, Northern; Salish; Sanpoil; Shoshoni; Shuswap; Tanana, Upper; Thompson; Washo; Zuni
Aruncus: Skagit; Thompson
Asarum: Abnaki; Cherokee; Iroquois; Okanagan-Colville
Asclepias: Costanoan
Aster: Iroquois
Atriplex: Cahuilla; Paiute, Northern
Balsamorhiza: Cheyenne; Kawaiisu
Betula: Cherokee; Iroquois; Thompson
Brassica: Meskwaki; Micmac
Callirhoe: Dakota
Calocedrus: Paiute
Caltha: Chippewa
Calycanthus: Pomo; Pomo, Kashaya
Capsicum: Cherokee
Cardamine: Cherokee; Iroquois
Carya: Cherokee
Castanea: Mohegan
Castilleja: Chippewa
Ceanothus: Iroquois
Celastrus: Iroquois
Celtis: Iroquois
Cercocarpus: Paiute; Shoshoni
Chaenactis: Paiute
Chaetopappa: Zuni

Okanagan-Colville; Okanogon; Paiute; Paiute, Northern; Sanpoil; Shoshoni; Thompson; Washo

Monarda: Cherokee; Chippewa; Flathead; Meskwaki; Nanticoke; Sioux, Teton

Monardella: Miwok; Okanagan-Colville; Paiute; Sanpoil; Shoshoni; Washo

Moneses: Eskimo, Alaska

Monotropa: Mohegan

Nepeta: Cherokee; Iroquois; Okanagan-Colville

Nicotiana: Paiute

Nymphaea: Micmac

Obolaria: Cherokee

Oenothera: Navajo, Kayenta

Oplopanax: Cowlitz; Gitksan; Green River Group; Haisla; Hanaksiala; Oweekeno; Sanpoil; Wet'suwet'en

Orobanche: Paiute

Osmorhiza: Blackfoot; Cheyenne; Kawaiisu; Paiute; Paiute, Northern; Shoshoni; Thompson; Washo

Osmunda: Iroquois

Paxistima: Okanagan-Colville

Pediomelum: Seminole

Penstemon: Okanagan-Colville; Shoshoni

Petasites: Eskimo, Inupiat

Phacelia: Kawaiisu; Shuswap

Phlox: Havasupai

Physostegia: Meskwaki

Phytolacca: Iroquois

Picea: Cherokee; Gitksan; Haisla & Hanaksiala; Kwakiutl; Tanana, Upper; Wet'suwet'en

Piloblephis: Seminole

Pinus: Algonquin, Tête-de-Boule; Apache, Mescalero; Cherokee; Eskimo, Alaska; Iroquois; Keres, Western; Micmac; Mohegan; Montagnais; Navajo, Ramah; Okanogon; Paiute; Shoshoni; Thompson; Washo

Piper: Hawaiian

Pityopsis: Seminole

Plantago: Paiute

Platanus: Delaware; Delaware, Oklahoma; Meskwaki

Polygala: Cherokee; Malecite; Micmac; Miwok; Ojibwa, South

Polygonum: Okanagan-Colville; Potawatomi; Tanana, Upper

Polypodium: Cowichan; Haisla & Hanaksiala; Saanich; Thompson

Populus: Delaware, Ontario; Flathead; Iroquois; Menominee; Meskwaki; Micmac; Ojibwa; Penobscot; Tanana, Upper; Yuki

Porteranthus: Cherokee; Iroquois

Prenanthes: Bella Coola

Prunella: Iroquois

Prunus: Cherokee; Cowichan; Iroquois; Karok;

Malecite; Micmac; Mohegan; Narraganset; Ojibwa; Okanagan-Colville; Paiute; Rappahannock; Saanich; Shinnecock; Skagit; Skokomish; Thompson

Pseudotsuga: Bella Coola; Cowlitz; Karok; Squaxin; Swinomish; Thompson

Psorothamnus: Paiute; Paiute, Northern; Shoshoni

Pteridium: Thompson

Pterocaulon: Seminole

Purshia: Havasupai; Paiute

Pycnanthemum: Cherokee; Choctaw; Miwok

Quercus: Delaware; Delaware, Oklahoma; Mohegan

Ranunculus: Meskwaki

Rhamnus: Kawaiisu

Rhododendron: Skokomish

Rhus: Cahuilla; Cheyenne; Chippewa; Comanche

Ribes: Bella Coola; Okanagan-Colville; Sanpoil; Skagit; Skagit, Upper; Tanana, Upper; Thompson

Rosa: Costanoan; Paiute; Shoshoni; Tanana, Upper; Washo

Rubus: Iroquois

Rudbeckia: Potawatomi

Rumex: Hopi; Paiute; Pima

Salix: Costanoan; Micmac; Montana Indian; Pomo, Kashaya

Salvia: Cahuilla; Cherokee; Diegueño; Okanagan-Colville; Paiute; Paiute, Northern; Shoshoni; Washo

Sambucus: Cahuilla; Costanoan; Hoh; Kawaiisu; Paiute; Pima; Quileute; Shoshoni

Sanguinaria: Iroquois; Micmac

Sanvitalia: Navajo, Ramah

Sassafras: Cherokee; Iroquois; Seminole

Satureja: Cahuilla; Luiseño; Pomo, Kashaya

Scrophularia: Iroquois

Senecio: Yavapai

Silphium: Omaha; Ponca; Winnebago

Solanum: Pima

Solidago: Cherokee

Sorbus: Algonquin, Quebec; Carrier, Southern; Potawatomi

Sphaeralcea: Navajo; Shoshoni

Spiraea: Mahuna; Okanagan-Colville; Thompson

Stachys: Meskwaki

Stephanomeria: Cheyenne

Symphoricarpos: Klallam; Miwok

Symplocarpus: Nanticoke

Tagetes: Navajo

Tanacetum: Iroquois

Tauschia: Kawaiisu

Taxus: Iroquois; Penobscot

Tetradymia: Navajo, Ramah; Paiute; Shoshoni

Thalictrum: Keres, Western; Washo

Thamnosma: Kawaiisu; Shoshoni
Thermopsis: Cheyenne
Thuja: Algonquin, Quebec; Cowlitz; Iroquois; Nez Perce
Trichostema: Costanoan; Kawaiisu; Miwok
Trifolium: Mohegan
Triosteum: Iroquois
Tsuga: Algonquin, Quebec; Iroquois; Malecite; Menominee; Micmac; Potawatomi; Quinault; Thompson
Ulmus: Cherokee; Delaware; Delaware, Oklahoma; Mohegan
Umbellularia: Karok; Pomo, Kashaya
Urtica: Paiute; Shoshoni; Skagit; Snohomish
Vaccinium: Seminole; Skagit; Skagit, Upper; Tanana, Upper
Valeriana: Cree, Woodlands; Okanagon; Thompson
Veratrum: Haisla; Iroquois; Kwakiutl; Okanagan-Colville; Paiute, Northern; Salish; Shoshoni
Verbascum: Atsugewi; Delaware, Oklahoma; Mohegan; Shinnecock; Thompson
Verbena: Cherokee
Viburnum: Bella Coola; Iroquois; Tanana, Upper
Viola: Cherokee
Wyethia: Paiute
Xanthorhiza: Catawba
Xyris: Seminole
Zanthoxylum: Chippewa; Menominee

Contraceptive

Amelanchier: Okanagan-Colville; Thompson
Apocynum: Okanagan-Colville
Arabis: Okanagan-Colville
Arisaema: Iroquois
Asclepias: Iroquois
Bahia: Navajo, Ramah
Betula: Thompson
Castilleja: Hopi; Tewa
Chelone: Malecite; Micmac
Cicuta: Cherokee
Cirsium: Zuni
Claytonia: Iroquois
Clematis: Okanagan-Colville
Cornus: Okanagan-Colville
Equisetum: Costanoan
Erigeron: Navajo, Ramah
Eriogonum: Navajo, Ramah
Erythronium: Iroquois
Galium: Choctaw
Geum: Chehalis
Hepatica: Iroquois
Iva: Mahuna
Juniperus: Zuni
Lithospermum: Navajo; Shoshoni

Lonicera: Chehalis
Mahonia: Flathead
Maianthemum: Costanoan
Phlox: Navajo, Ramah
Pinus: Kawaiisu
Pontederia: Malecite; Micmac
Rhus: Navajo, Ramah
Ricinus: Navajo
Rumex: Iroquois
Sphaeralcea: Shoshoni
Tanacetum: Malecite; Micmac
Toxicodendron: Karok
Vaccinium: Cree, Woodlands
Veratrum: Paiute; Shoshoni; Washo
Viburnum: Iroquois
Yucca: Navajo, Ramah

Cough Medicine

Abies: Cree, Woodlands; Crow; Gitksan; Iroquois; Kwakiutl; Ojibwa; Okanagan-Colville; Paiute; Thompson; Wet'suwet'en
Acer: Micmac; Mohegan; Potawatomi
Achillea: Cheyenne; Hesquiat; Paiute; Paiute, Northern
Acorus: Algonquin, Quebec; Chippewa; Cree, Woodlands; Dakota; Delaware; Delaware, Oklahoma; Lakota; Meskwaki; Micmac; Omaha; Pawnee; Ponca; Winnebago
Actaea: Blackfoot
Agastache: Chippewa; Navajo, Ramah
Aletris: Cherokee
Alnus: Cherokee; Gitksan
Ambrosia: Pima
Amelanchier: Cree, Woodlands
Anaphalis: Cherokee; Montagnais
Andropogon: Seminole
Anemopsis: Kawaiisu; Pima
Angelica: Micmac; Paiute; Washo
Apocynum: Cherokee
Aquilegia: Paiute
Aralia: Cherokee; Chippewa; Iroquois; Kwakiutl; Micmac; Penobscot
Arctium: Chippewa
Arctostaphylos: Cheyenne
Arisaema: Cherokee
Aristolochia: Cherokee
Artemisia: Arapaho; Blackfoot; Costanoan; Diegueño; Gosiute; Havasupai; Kawaiisu; Navajo, Ramah; Paiute; Shoshoni; Shuswap; Tanana, Upper; Tewa; Washo
Aruncus: Kwakiutl
Asarum: Abnaki; Cherokee; Iroquois
Asclepias: Paiute
Asplenium: Cherokee

Astragalus: Lakota
Atriplex: Navajo, Ramah
Baccharis: Diegueño
Bacopa: Seminole
Balsamorhiza: Kawaiisu
Barbarea: Mohegan; Shinnecock
Berchemia: Koasati
Betula: Thompson
Boschniakia: Hesquiat
Botrychium: Iroquois
Brassica: Micmac
Brickellia: Navajo, Ramah
Campanulastrum: Meskwaki
Castanea: Cherokee
Castilleja: Gitksan
Ceanothus: Chippewa; Menominee; Modesse
Celastrus: Cherokee
Cercocarpus: Kawaiisu; Paiute; Shoshoni
Chaenactis: Paiute
Chamaebatia: Miwok
Chrysothamnus: Cheyenne; Coahuilla; Navajo, Ramah; Paiute; Shoshoni
Cimicifuga: Cherokee
Collinsia: Natchez
Conyza: Seminole
Coptis: Abnaki
Cornus: Chippewa; Cree, Hudson Bay; Iroquois
Croton: Diegueño
Cryptantha: Navajo; Navajo, Ramah
Cupressus: Kawaiisu
Cyperus: Pima
Dichanthelium: Seminole
Draba: Navajo, Ramah
Echinacea: Choctaw; Kiowa
Enceliopsis: Shoshoni
Ephedra: Keres, Western; Navajo; Navajo, Ramah
Epilobium: Abnaki
Ericameria: Paiute; Shoshoni
Erigeron: Cherokee; Iroquois; Navajo, Ramah
Eriodictyon: Cahuilla; Diegueño; Mahuna; Miwok; Paiute; Pomo, Kashaya; Shoshoni; Yuki; Yurok
Eriogonum: Costanoan; Kawaiisu; Navajo, Ramah; Shoshoni
Galium: Cherokee
Gaultheria: Samish; Swinomish
Gentianella: Tanana, Upper
Geum: Blackfoot; Malecite; Micmac; Ojibwa, South
Gleditsia: Delaware; Delaware, Oklahoma; Rappahannock
Glycyrrhiza: Blackfoot; Cherokee; Keres, Western
Gnaphalium: Cherokee; Montagnais
Grindelia: Crow; Flathead; Gosiute; Paiute; Shoshoni
Gutierrezia: Lakota

Hamamelis: Iroquois
Hedeoma: Cherokee
Heracleum: Shoshoni
Hierochloe: Blackfoot
Hosta: Cherokee
Humulus: Navajo, Ramah
Hydrocotyle: Seminole
Hymenopappus: Navajo, Ramah
Hypericum: Montagnais
Hyssopus: Cherokee
Ilex: Micmac
Inula: Cherokee; Iroquois
Ipomoea: Cherokee; Iroquois
Isocoma: Pima
Iva: Navajo, Ramah
Juniperus: Apache, White Mountain; Bella Coola; Carrier, Northern; Cheyenne; Cree, Woodlands; Dakota; Eskimo, Inupiat; Gosiute; Iroquois; Navajo, Ramah; Omaha; Paiute; Pawnee; Ponca; Seminole; Shoshoni; Tanana, Upper
Krameria: Pima
Larix: Abnaki; Algonquin, Quebec; Iroquois; Nez Perce; Thompson
Ledum: Tanana, Upper
Ligusticum: Atsugewi; Crow; Paiute
Lilium: Malecite; Micmac
Linanthus: Pomo, Calpella
Lindera: Cherokee
Linum: Cherokee
Liriodendron: Cherokee
Lithocarpus: Pomo, Kashaya
Lithospermum: Navajo
Lobelia: Iroquois
Lomatium: Great Basin Indian; Kwakiutl; Paiute; Shoshoni; Washo
Lonicera: Bella Coola; Nuxalkmc
Lotus: Costanoan
Lygodesmia: Blackfoot
Machaeranthera: Hopi
Mahonia: Flathead; Paiute; Shoshoni; Tolowa
Maianthemum: Mohegan; Paiute
Malus: Nitinaht
Marrubium: Cherokee; Costanoan; Kawaiisu; Mahuna; Rappahannock; Yuki
Mentha: Flathead; Gosiute; Kutenai
Mirabilis: Navajo, Ramah
Monarda: Blackfoot; Flathead; Lakota; Navajo, Ramah
Moneses: Eskimo, Alaska
Nemopanthus: Malecite
Nepeta: Cherokee; Iroquois
Nicotiana: Navajo, Ramah; Tewa
Nymphaea: Micmac; Ojibwa
Nymphoides: Seminole

Obolaria: Cherokee

Oplopanax: Gitksan; Haisla; Okanagan-Colville; Wet'suwet'en

Osmorhiza: Blackfoot; Kawaiisu; Shoshoni; Tlingit

Ostrya: Chippewa; Iroquois

Paeonia: Paiute; Shoshoni

Pedicularis: Cherokee; Cheyenne

Pediomelum: Seminole

Penstemon: Navajo, Ramah

Penthorum: Meskwaki

Pericome: Navajo, Ramah

Perideridia: Blackfoot

Petasites: Delaware; Delaware, Oklahoma; Quileute

Phacelia: Kawaiisu

Picea: Algonquin, Quebec; Eskimo, Kuskokwagmiut; Eskimo, Western; Gitksan; Haisla & Hanaksiala; Kwakiutl; Micmac; Montagnais; Sikani; Tanana, Upper; Thompson; Wet'suwet'en

Pinus: Abnaki; Cherokee; Eskimo, Alaska; Hoh; Iroquois; Kwakiutl; Micmac; Mohegan; Navajo, Ramah; Okanagon; Quileute; Shinnecock; Shoshoni; Shuswap; Sikani; Thompson

Plantago: Carrier

Platanus: Cherokee

Polygala: Miwok; Montagnais; Ojibwa, South

Polygonatum: Ojibwa

Polygonum: Tanana, Upper

Polypodium: Green River Group; Haisla & Hanaksiala; Hesquiat; Kitasoo; Klallam; Makah; Nitinaht; Oweekeno; Quinault

Populus: Carrier, Southern; Meskwaki; Paiute; Tanana, Upper

Prunella: Iroquois

Prunus: Algonquin, Quebec; Cherokee; Delaware; Delaware, Oklahoma; Diegueño; Iroquois; Keres, Western; Mahuna; Malecite; Micmac; Ojibwa; Okanagan-Colville; Paiute; Penobscot; Potawatomi; Rappahannock; Thompson; Wet'suwet'en

Psathyrotes: Shoshoni

Pseudotsuga: Apache, White Mountain

Psorothamnus: Paiute; Shoshoni

Purshia: Klamath; Navajo, Ramah

Pycnanthemum: Lakota

Quercus: Delaware; Delaware, Oklahoma; Miwok

Ratibida: Navajo, Ramah

Rhamnus: Kawaiisu

Rhus: Cahuilla; Coahuilla; Malecite; Menominee

Rosa: Cree, Woodlands; Thompson

Rubus: Cherokee; Iroquois; Micmac

Rumex: Mahuna; Paiute; Pima; Thompson; Yavapai

Ruta: Costanoan

Salix: Iroquois; Ojibwa, South; Zuni

Salvia: Cherokee; Costanoan; Diegueño; Mahuna; Paiute

Sambucus: Hoh; Paiute; Quileute; Shoshoni

Sanguinaria: Cherokee; Iroquois

Sassafras: Seminole

Shepherdia: Gitksan

Solidago: Cherokee

Sphaeralcea: Navajo

Spiraea: Mahuna

Streptopus: Ojibwa; Potawatomi

Symplocarpus: Chippewa; Delaware, Oklahoma

Taxus: Iroquois

Tephrosia: Choctaw; Natchez

Tetradymia: Navajo, Ramah; Paiute; Shoshoni

Thermopsis: Navajo, Ramah

Thuja: Bella Coola; Chippewa; Makah; Malecite; Micmac; Nez Perce; Ojibwa; Skagit

Tiarella: Quileute

Tilia: Cherokee

Trifolium: Mohegan

Trillium: Cherokee

Tsuga: Iroquois; Micmac

Tussilago: Iroquois

Ulmus: Cherokee; Delaware; Delaware, Oklahoma; Mohegan

Uvularia: Iroquois

Vaccinium: Tanana, Upper

Valeriana: Navajo, Ramah

Vancouveria: Yurok

Veratrum: Bella Coola

Verbascum: Cherokee; Creek; Delaware; Delaware, Oklahoma; Mohegan; Navajo, Ramah; Thompson

Verbena: Cherokee

Veronica: Cherokee

Veronicastrum: Iroquois

Viburnum: Carrier; Gitksan

Viola: Cherokee

Zanthoxylum: Chippewa; Meskwaki

Dermatological Aid

Abies: Abnaki; Algonquin, Quebec; Blackfoot; Cherokee; Chippewa; Cree, Woodlands; Flathead; Gitksan; Hesquiat; Iroquois; Kutenai; Kwakiutl; Menominee; Micmac; Montana Indian; Ojibwa; Ojibwa, South; Okanagan-Colville; Paiute; Penobscot; Potawatomi; Saanich; Salish, Coast; Shoshoni; Shuswap; Tewa; Thompson

Abronia: Navajo; Navajo, Kayenta; Navajo, Ramah; Shoshoni

Acer: Algonquin, Tête-de-Boule; Cherokee; Chippewa; Iroquois; Koasati; Kwakiutl; Penobscot; Seminole

Achillea: Bella Coola; Blackfoot; Carrier, Southern; Cherokee; Chippewa; Costanoan; Cowlitz; Crow; Flathead; Gosiute; Great Basin Indian; Karok; Klallam; Kutenai; Kwakiutl; Lakota; Malecite;

Mendocino Indian; Menominee; Meskwaki; Micmac; Navajo; Ojibwa; Okanagan-Colville; Okanagon; Paiute; Paiute, Northern; Pomo, Kashaya; Shoshoni; Shuswap; Squaxin; Thompson; Ute; Washo; Winnebago

Achlys: Lummi; Skagit

Acorus: Cherokee; Cree, Woodlands; Iroquois

Acourtia: Hualapai

Actaea: Cherokee; Cheyenne; Quileute; Quinault

Adenocaulon: Cowlitz; Squaxin

Adenostoma: Coahuilla

Adiantum: Lummi; Makah; Navajo, Kayenta; Skokomish

Aesculus: Cherokee

Agastache: Iroquois; Navajo, Ramah; Paiute

Ageratina: Zuni

Agoseris: Navajo, Ramah; Okanagan-Colville; Thompson

Agrimonia: Cherokee

Alcea: Shinnecock

Alectoria: Nitinaht

Aleurites: Hawaiian

Alisma: Cherokee

Allionia: Navajo, Ramah

Allium: Cherokee; Cheyenne; Isleta; Kwakiutl; Mahuna

Alnus: Abnaki; Carrier, Southern; Cherokee; Clallam; Cree, Hudson Bay; Eskimo, Alaska; Haisla; Keres, Western; Kwakiutl; Menominee; Nitinaht; Pomo; Pomo, Kashaya; Potawatomi; Sanpoil; Shuswap; Swinomish; Thompson

Alyxia: Hawaiian

Amaranthus: Cherokee

Ambrosia: Cherokee; Delaware, Oklahoma; Diegueño; Kiowa; Mahuna

Amianthium: Cherokee

Amorpha: Meskwaki; Omaha

Amphiachyris: Comanche

Anaphalis: Kwakiutl; Mahuna

Andropogon: Cherokee; Rappahannock

Anemone: Chippewa; Menominee

Anemopsis: Cahuilla; Costanoan; Isleta; Kawaiisu; Keres, Western; Mahuna; Pima; Shoshoni

Angadenia: Seminole

Angelica: Blackfoot; Menominee; Paiute; Pomo, Kashaya

Antennaria: Paiute

Anthemis: Cherokee

Antidesma: Hawaiian

Aplectrum: Catawba

Apocynum: Blackfoot; Cherokee; Cree, Hudson Bay; Iroquois

Aquilegia: Iroquois; Paiute; Quileute; Shoshoni; Thompson

Arabis: Thompson

Aralia: Cherokee; Chippewa; Choctaw; Cree, Woodlands; Iroquois; Menominee; Meskwaki; Micmac; Ojibwa; Okanagon; Pomo; Pomo, Kashaya; Potawatomi; Rappahannock; Thompson

Arbutus: Cowichan; Pomo; Pomo, Kashaya; Yuki

Arctium: Cherokee; Iroquois; Malecite; Menominee; Micmac; Nanticoke; Penobscot

Arctostaphylos: Atsugewi; Blackfoot; Cahuilla; Carrier; Concow; Sanpoil

Arenaria: Kawaiisu; Navajo, Ramah; Shoshoni

Argemone: Paiute; Shoshoni; Tubatulabal; Washo

Argentina: Blackfoot; Kwakiutl

Argyrochosma: Tewa

Arisaema: Cherokee; Iroquois; Malecite; Micmac; Rappahannock

Aristolochia: Cherokee; Rappahannock

Arnica: Thompson

Arnoglossum: Cherokee

Artemisia: Aleut; Blackfoot; Carrier, Southern; Cherokee; Chippewa; Comanche; Costanoan; Crow; Eskimo, Inuktitut; Eskimo, Kuskokwagmiut; Flathead; Havasupai; Hopi; Kawaiisu; Kiowa; Kutenai; Meskwaki; Mewuk; Montana Indian; Navajo; Navajo, Ramah; Okanagan-Colville; Paiute; Pomo; Pomo, Kashaya; Sanpoil; Shoshoni; Shuswap; Tanana, Upper; Tewa; Thompson; Yuki; Yurok, South Coast (Nererner); Zuni

Artocarpus: Hawaiian

Aruncus: Cherokee; Klallam; Lummi; Makah; Quileute; Quinault; Skagit; Thompson

Asarum: Cherokee; Chippewa; Iroquois; Pomo; Pomo, Kashaya; Thompson; Yurok

Asclepias: Blackfoot; Cherokee; Costanoan; Iroquois; Kawaiisu; Mendocino Indian; Menominee; Miwok; Navajo, Ramah; Okanagan-Colville; Omaha; Paiute; Paiute, Northern; Rappahannock; Shoshoni; Thompson

Asplenium: Hawaiian

Aster: Iroquois; Okanagan-Colville; Seminole; Zuni

Astragalus: Blackfoot; Cheyenne; Navajo, Kayenta; Navajo, Ramah; Thompson

Athyrium: Ojibwa

Atriplex: Havasupai; Jemez; Navajo, Ramah; Pima; Zuni

Baccharis: Cahuilla; Costanoan; Diegueño; Luiseño

Baileya: Keres, Western

Balsamorhiza: Blackfoot; Gosiute; Kutenai; Paiute; Sanpoil; Shoshoni; Shuswap

Baptisia: Choctaw; Delaware; Delaware, Oklahoma; Meskwaki; Mohegan

Berula: Zuni

Besseya: Navajo, Ramah

Betula: Algonquin, Quebec; Cree, Hudson Bay; Cree, Woodlands; Iroquois; Malecite; Micmac

Blechnum: Hesquiat

Bobea: Hawaiian

Boschniakia: Tlingit

Botrychium: Ojibwa, South

Bouteloua: Navajo, Ramah

Brassica: Cherokee; Iroquois

Brickellia: Navajo, Kayenta

Buchloe: Keres, Western

Bursera: Cahuilla

Calla: Potawatomi

Calliandra: Zuni

Callicarpa: Seminole

Calochortus: Navajo, Ramah; Okanagan-Colville

Caltha: Chippewa; Okanagon; Thompson

Calycanthus: Cherokee

Camissonia: Navajo

Campanula: Navajo, Ramah; Zuni

Canavalia: Hawaiian

Capsella: Menominee

Cardamine: Iroquois

Carica: Hawaiian

Carpinus: Cherokee; Iroquois

Carya: Cherokee; Comanche; Iroquois

Castanea: Cherokee; Iroquois

Castela: Yavapai

Castilleja: Costanoan; Kawaiisu; Menominee; Navajo, Kayenta; Okanagan-Colville

Caulophyllum: Cherokee

Ceanothus: Diegueño; Iroquois; Karok; Meskwaki; Okanagan-Colville; Sanpoil

Celastrus: Cherokee; Chippewa; Delaware

Cenchrus: Hawaiian

Centaurea: Kiowa

Cerastium: Iroquois

Cercocarpus: Paiute; Shoshoni

Chaenactis: Okanagon; Paiute; Shoshoni; Thompson

Chaetopappa: Zuni

Chamaecyparis: Kwakiutl

Chamaedaphne: Potawatomi

Chamaemelum: Cherokee

Chamaesaracha: Navajo, Kayenta

Chamaesyce: Cahuilla; Cherokee; Costanoan; Diegueño; Houma; Miwok; Navajo, Kayenta; Navajo, Ramah; Paiute; Pima

Cheilanthes: Navajo, Ramah

Chelone: Cherokee

Chenopodium: Hawaiian; Kawaiisu; Meskwaki; Miwok; Navajo, Kayenta

Chimaphila: Cherokee; Delaware; Delaware, Oklahoma; Iroquois; Micmac; Mohegan; Okanagon; Penobscot; Thompson

Chionanthus: Choctaw; Koasati

Chlorogalum: Cahuilla; Costanoan; Mendocino Indian; Pomo; Pomo, Kashaya; Wailaki

Chorizanthe: Tubatulabal

Chrysothamnus: Cheyenne; Hopi; Klamath; Navajo

Cichorium: Iroquois

Cicuta: Iroquois; Kutenai; Kwakiutl; Paiute

Cimicifuga: Cherokee

Circaea: Iroquois

Cirsium: Cree; Gosiute; Hopi; Houma; Iroquois; Kiowa

Claytonia: Cowlitz; Hesquiat; Quileute; Skokomish; Snohomish

Clematis: Great Basin Indian; Iroquois; Mahuna; Miwok; Navajo, Kayenta; Nevada Indian; Okanagan-Colville; Oregon Indian; Sanpoil; Shoshoni; Thompson

Cleome: Navajo, Kayenta; Navajo, Ramah

Clermontia: Hawaiian

Clintonia: Algonquin, Quebec; Algonquin, Tête-de-Boule; Bella Coola; Chippewa; Cowlitz; Haisla & Hanaksiala; Ojibwa

Cocos: Hawaiian

Collinsia: Ute

Collinsonia: Cherokee; Iroquois

Collomia: Gosiute

Comandra: Cherokee; Navajo; Thompson

Comptonia: Delaware; Delaware, Oklahoma; Malecite; Micmac; Mohegan; Penobscot; Potawatomi; Shinnecock

Convolvulus: Navajo, Ramah

Conyza: Keres, Western; Navajo, Kayenta; Navajo, Ramah

Corallorrhiza: Navajo, Kayenta

Cornus: Carrier, Northern; Cherokee; Chippewa; Iroquois; Montana Indian; Okanagan-Colville; Thompson; Wet'suwet'en

Corydalis: Navajo, Kayenta

Corylus: Cherokee; Iroquois; Ojibwa; Potawatomi

Crataegus: Kwakiutl; Okanagon; Thompson

Crepis: Meskwaki; Paiute

Croton: Keres, Western

Cryptantha: Hopi; Navajo, Kayenta; Navajo, Ramah; Zuni

Cucurbita: Cahuilla; Hawaiian; Keres, Western; Paiute; Pima; Zuni

Cuscuta: Cherokee

Cymopterus: Navajo, Kayenta

Cynoglossum: Cherokee; Iroquois

Cyperus: Hawaiian

Cypripedium: Chippewa; Iroquois

Cystopteris: Navajo, Ramah

Dalea: Keres, Western; Montana Indian; Navajo, Kayenta; Zuni

Datisca: Miwok
Datura: Cherokee; Costanoan; Delaware; Delaware, Oklahoma; Havasupai; Kawaiisu; Keres, Western; Mahuna; Mohegan; Pima; Rappahannock; Tubatulabal; Zuni
Daucus: Cherokee; Costanoan; Iroquois
Delphinium: Blackfoot; Chehalis
Descurainia: Gitksan; Navajo, Kayenta; Paiute; Pima
Desmanthus: Pawnee
Dicentra: Skagit
Dimorphocarpa: Apache, White Mountain; Hopi; Navajo, Kayenta; Navajo, Ramah; Zuni
Diospyros: Cherokee
Diplazium: Hawaiian
Dipsacus: Iroquois
Dirca: Chippewa; Iroquois
Disporum: Okanagan-Colville
Distichlis: Kawaiisu
Dodonaea: Hawaiian
Draba: Navajo, Ramah
Drosera: Kwakiutl; Seminole
Drymaria: Navajo, Ramah
Dryopteris: Costanoan; Klallam; Snohomish
Dudleya: Diegueño
Dyssodia: Navajo, Ramah
Echinacea: Cheyenne; Dakota; Lakota; Omaha
Echinocystis: Tubatulabal
Elaeagnus: Blackfoot
Encelia: Navajo, Kayenta
Ephedra: Cocopa; Isleta; Paiute; Paiute, Northern; Pima; Shoshoni
Epilobium: Algonquin, Tête-de-Boule; Bella Coola; Blackfoot; Chippewa; Costanoan; Cree, Woodlands; Eskimo, Inupiat; Kwakiutl; Menominee; Ojibwa; Okanagan-Colville; Thompson
Equisetum: Blackfoot; Costanoan; Kwakiutl; Okanagan-Colville; Pomo, Kashaya; Thompson
Eriastrum: Kawaiisu
Ericameria: Cahuilla; Diegueño; Kawaiisu; Klamath; Miwok
Erigeron: Cherokee; Iroquois; Miwok; Navajo, Kayenta; Navajo, Ramah; Thompson
Eriodictyon: Coahuilla; Costanoan; Hualapai; Miwok; Pomo, Kashaya; Yuki
Eriogonum: Kawaiisu; Navajo, Kayenta; Navajo, Ramah; Okanagan-Colville; Omaha; Thompson; Tubatulabal; Zuni
Eriophorum: Eskimo, Western
Eriophyllum: Skagit
Erodium: Navajo, Kayenta; Zuni
Eryngium: Seminole
Erysimum: Chippewa; Okanagan-Colville
Erythronium: Cherokee; Iroquois; Montana Indian; Wailaki

Eschscholzia: Kawaiisu; Mendocino Indian
Euonymus: Cherokee; Meskwaki
Eupatorium: Iroquois; Navajo
Euphorbia: Cherokee; Navajo
Evernia: Blackfoot; Wailaki; Yuki
Fagus: Iroquois; Malecite; Potawatomi; Rappahannock
Fallugia: Tewa
Ficus: Seminole
Fragaria: Okanagan-Colville; Thompson
Frangula: Clallam; Costanoan; Diegueño; Kawaiisu; Skagit; Squaxin
Frasera: Navajo, Kayenta
Fraxinus: Iroquois; Meskwaki; Yokia
Gaillardia: Blackfoot
Galium: Chippewa; Choctaw; Iroquois; Klallam; Makah; Nitinaht; Ojibwa; Quinault
Gaultheria: Bella Coola; Quileute
Gaura: Isleta; Navajo
Gayophytum: Navajo, Kayenta
Gelsemium: Delaware, Oklahoma
Geocaulon: Cree, Hudson Bay
Geranium: Cherokee; Choctaw; Gosiute; Iroquois; Keres, Western; Montana Indian; Navajo, Ramah; Sanpoil
Geum: Aleut; Bella Coola; Blackfoot; Carrier, Southern; Clallam; Quileute; Quinault; Snohomish
Gilia: Navajo, Kayenta
Glechoma: Cherokee
Glycyrrhiza: Isleta
Gnaphalium: Keres, Western; Pomo
Goodyera: Okanagan-Colville
Grindelia: Cheyenne; Costanoan; Mahuna; Miwok; Navajo, Ramah; Shoshoni
Gutierrezia: Isleta; Jemez; Navajo; Navajo, Ramah; Shoshoni
Hackelia: Cherokee
Hamamelis: Cherokee; Chippewa; Iroquois; Mohegan
Helenium: Costanoan; Koasati
Helianthella: Navajo, Ramah; Paiute
Helianthus: Hopi; Jemez; Meskwaki; Navajo, Ramah; Ojibwa, South; Shasta; Thompson
Heliotropium: Pima
Hepatica: Chippewa
Heracleum: Aleut; Bella Coola; Blackfoot; Carrier, Northern; Chippewa; Cree; Cree, Woodlands; Gitksan; Haisla; Iroquois; Kwakiutl; Meskwaki; Ojibwa; Okanagan-Colville; Paiute; Pawnee; Pomo; Salish, Coast; Sanpoil; Shuswap; Sikani
Heteranthera: Cherokee
Heteromeles: Diegueño
Heterotheca: Navajo, Ramah

Heuchera: Blackfoot; Cherokee; Cheyenne; Chickasaw; Choctaw; Creek; Gosiute; Lakota; Meskwaki; Navajo, Kayenta; Navajo, Ramah; Okanagan-Colville; Shuswap; Skagit; Thompson

Hierochloe: Blackfoot; Kiowa; Menominee; Thompson

Hoita: Luiseño

Holodiscus: Sanpoil

Hosta: Cherokee

Houstonia: Navajo, Ramah

Humulus: Dakota; Omaha; Round Valley Indian

Huperzia: Iroquois

Hydrangea: Cherokee

Hydrastis: Cherokee; Micmac

Hymenopappus: Navajo, Kayenta; Navajo, Ramah; Zuni

Hymenoxys: Navajo, Ramah; Zuni

Hypericum: Cherokee; Miwok; Paiute; Shoshoni

Hyptis: Seminole

Ilex: Catawba; Koasati

Impatiens: Cherokee; Chippewa; Iroquois; Meskwaki; Mohegan; Nanticoke; Ojibwa; Omaha; Penobscot; Potawatomi; Shinnecock

Inula: Iroquois

Ipomoea: Hawaiian; Houma

Ipomopsis: Navajo, Kayenta; Navajo, Ramah; Salish; Shoshoni; Tewa; Zuni

Iris: Algonquin, Tête-de-Boule; Cherokee; Chippewa; Meskwaki; Micmac; Omaha; Paiute; Ponca; Potawatomi; Shoshoni

Isocoma: Cahuilla; Navajo, Kayenta

Iva: Navajo, Kayenta; Paiute

Jacquemontia: Hawaiian

Jeffersonia: Cherokee

Juglans: Cherokee; Comanche; Delaware; Delaware, Oklahoma; Houma; Iroquois

Juncus: Iroquois

Juniperus: Cherokee; Cree, Hudson Bay; Hanaksiala; Keres, Western; Malecite; Micmac; Navajo; Navajo, Ramah; Okanagan-Colville; Paiute; Sanpoil; Shoshoni; Tewa; Thompson

Kallstroemia: Tewa

Kalmia: Cherokee; Kwakiutl; Mahuna; Malecite; Micmac; Tlingit

Keckiella: Mahuna; Paiute

Kochia: Navajo

Koeleria: Cheyenne

Krameria: Paiute; Pima; Shoshoni

Krascheninnikovia: Navajo; Navajo, Ramah; Paiute; Shoshoni

Lachnanthes: Cherokee

Lactuca: Chippewa; Menominee

Lagenaria: Cherokee

Lappula: Navajo, Kayenta; Navajo, Ramah

Larix: Cree, Woodlands; Kutenai; Menominee; Micmac; Okanagan-Colville; Potawatomi; Thompson

Larrea: Cahuilla; Isleta; Mahuna; Paiute; Papago; Pima; Yavapai

Ledum: Chippewa; Cree, Hudson Bay; Cree, Woodlands; Shuswap; Tanana, Upper

Lepidium: Cahuilla; Cherokee; Menominee

Leptarrhena: Thompson

Leptodactylon: Navajo, Kayenta

Lesquerella: Navajo; Shuswap

Leucanthemum: Quileute

Leucocrinum: Paiute; Shoshoni

Leucothoe: Cherokee

Lewisia: Okanagan-Colville

Leymus: Okanagan-Colville

Liatris: Blackfoot; Meskwaki; Omaha

Lilium: Chippewa; Dakota; Malecite; Menominee; Micmac

Limosella: Navajo, Ramah

Lindera: Cherokee

Linum: Gosiute; Okanagon; Paiute; Shoshoni; Thompson

Liquidambar: Cherokee; Choctaw; Houma

Liriodendron: Cherokee

Lithocarpus: Costanoan

Lithospermum: Navajo; Shuswap; Zuni

Lobelia: Cherokee; Iroquois; Zuni

Lomatium: Gosiute; Great Basin Indian; Kawaiisu; Kwakiutl; Nez Perce; Okanagan-Colville; Paiute; Paiute, Northern; Shoshoni; Shuswap; Thompson; Ute; Washo

Lonicera: Bella Coola; Carrier; Carrier, Northern; Chehalis; Iroquois; Klallam; Kwakiutl; Makah; Nuxalkmc; Okanagan-Colville; Quinault; Thompson; Wet'suwet'en; Yuki

Lophophora: Kiowa

Ludwigia: Hawaiian; Seminole

Luetkea: Okanagon; Thompson

Lupinus: Navajo; Navajo, Ramah

Lycopodium: Blackfoot

Lygodesmia: Blackfoot; Navajo, Kayenta

Lyonia: Cherokee

Lysichiton: Clallam; Gitksan; Hesquiat; Klallam; Kwakiutl; Quileute; Shuswap; Skokomish; Thompson

Lythrum: Kawaiisu

Machaeranthera: Navajo; Navajo, Ramah

Magnolia: Choctaw; Koasati

Mahonia: Blackfoot; Flathead; Miwok; Navajo, Ramah

Maianthemum: Gitksan; Hesquiat; Iroquois; Karok; Malecite; Micmac; Nitinaht; Oweekeno; Paiute; Washo

Malacothrix: Navajo, Ramah

Malus: Iroquois; Kwakiutl; Makah; Samish; Swinomish

Malva: Cherokee; Costanoan; Diegueño; Iroquois; Miwok; Pima

Marah: Chehalis; Costanoan; Karok; Kawaiisu; Mahuna; Mendocino Indian; Pomo; Pomo, Kashaya; Tubatulabal

Marrubium: Costanoan

Matelea: Comanche

Matricaria: Cheyenne; Costanoan

Melia: Cherokee

Melilotus: Iroquois

Menispermum: Cherokee; Delaware, Oklahoma

Mentha: Cheyenne; Kawaiisu; Navajo, Kayenta; Okanagan; Paiute; Thompson

Mentzelia: Gosiute; Mendocino Indian; Montana Indian; Navajo, Kayenta

Menziesia: Kwakiutl

Merremia: Hawaiian

Mertensia: Cheyenne

Mikania: Seminole

Mimulus: Shoshoni

Mirabilis: Cherokee; Dakota; Hopi; Navajo; Navajo, Kayenta; Navajo, Ramah; Paiute; Paiute, Northern; Ponca; Sioux, Teton

Mitchella: Cherokee; Iroquois

Monarda: Blackfoot; Cheyenne; Chippewa; Delaware; Kiowa; Navajo, Ramah; Winnebago

Moneses: Cowichan; Kwakiutl; Kwakwaka'wakw; Salish, Coast

Monolepis: Navajo, Ramah

Monotropa: Cherokee; Thompson

Morinda: Hawaiian

Morus: Rappahannock

Myosotis: Makah

Myosurus: Navajo, Ramah

Myrica: Micmac

Nama: Navajo, Kayenta

Napaea: Meskwaki

Nepeta: Cherokee

Nereocystis: Kwakiutl, Southern; Nitinaht

Nicotiana: Cahuilla; Cherokee; Hawaiian; Hesquiat; Iroquois; Kawaiisu; Paiute; Salish; Shoshoni; Thompson

Nothochelone: Paiute

Nuphar: Algonquin, Quebec; Cree, Woodlands; Flathead; Kutenai; Menominee; Micmac; Ojibwa; Penobscot; Potawatomi; Rappahannock; Shuswap; Thompson

Nymphaea: Micmac; Penobscot

Nyssa: Koasati

Obolaria: Choctaw

Oemleria: Kwakiutl

Oenothera: Blackfoot; Iroquois; Isleta; Navajo, Kayenta; Navajo, Ramah; Ojibwa; Zuni

Onoclea: Iroquois

Onosmodium: Cheyenne

Oplopanax: Gitksan; Green River Group; Haisla; Haisla & Hanaksiala; Kwakiutl; Okanagon; Oweekeno; Thompson; Tlingit; Wet'suwet'en

Opuntia: Cahuilla; Dakota; Keres, Western; Nanticoke; Navajo, Ramah; Okanagan-Colville; Pawnee; Shoshoni; Shuswap; Sioux

Orbexilum: Catawba

Orobanche: Blackfoot; Navajo; Navajo, Kayenta; Pima

Osmorhiza: Blackfoot; Chippewa; Kawaiisu; Omaha; Paiute; Paiute, Northern; Shoshoni; Winnebago

Osteomeles: Hawaiian

Ostrya: Iroquois

Oxalis: Cherokee; Navajo, Ramah; Omaha; Quileute; Tolowa

Oxydendrum: Cherokee

Oxytropis: Blackfoot; Thompson

Paeonia: Paiute; Shoshoni

Panax: Cherokee; Creek; Iroquois; Seminole

Panicum: Isleta

Parthenocissus: Houma; Navajo, Ramah

Paspalidium: Seminole

Passiflora: Cherokee

Pastinaca: Iroquois; Potawatomi

Paxistima: Thompson

Pedicularis: Cherokee; Meskwaki; Washo

Pediomelum: Montana Indian

Pellaea: Costanoan; Yavapai

Peniocereus: Papago

Pennisetum: Navajo, Ramah

Penstemon: Costanoan; Navajo, Kayenta; Navajo, Ramah; Okanagan-Colville; Paiute; Paiute, Northern; Shoshoni; Tewa; Thompson

Pericome: Navajo, Ramah

Perideridia: Blackfoot

Petasites: Concow; Cree, Woodlands; Menominee; Quinault; Tlingit

Peteria: Navajo, Ramah

Petradoria: Navajo, Kayenta; Navajo, Ramah

Phacelia: Miwok; Pomo, Kashaya; Zuni

Philadelphus: Snohomish; Thompson

Phlox: Gosiute; Meskwaki; Navajo, Ramah; Shoshoni; Ute

Phoradendron: Diegueño; Navajo; Pima

Phragmites: Seminole

Phyla: Navajo, Kayenta

Physalis: Omaha; Ponca; Winnebago

Physaria: Blackfoot

Phytolacca: Cherokee; Delaware; Iroquois; Mahuna; Rappahannock

Picea: Algonquin, Quebec; Bella Coola; Cree, Woodlands; Eskimo, Alaska; Eskimo, Inuktitut; Eskimo, Nunivak; Haisla & Hanaksiala; Hesquiat; Koyukon; Kwakiutl; Makah; Menominee; Micmac; Mohegan; Oweekeno; Potawatomi; Quinault; Shuswap; Tanana, Upper; Thompson

Picradeniopsis: Navajo, Ramah; Zuni

Pilea: Cherokee

Piloblephis: Seminole

Pinus: Apache, Western; Bella Coola; Cahuilla; Carrier, Northern; Cherokee; Cheyenne; Chippewa; Cree, Woodlands; Delaware, Ontario; Flathead; Havasupai; Hopi; Iroquois; Isleta; Kawaiisu; Keres, Western; Kwakiutl; Mendocino Indian; Menominee; Micmac; Miwok; Mohegan; Navajo; Nitinaht; Okanagan-Colville; Paiute; Potawatomi; Quinault; Rappahannock; Salish, Coast; Sanpoil; Seminole; Shinnecock; Shoshoni; Shuswap; Skagit; Tewa; Thompson; Yokia; Zuni

Piper: Cherokee; Hawaiian

Plagiomnium: Bella Coola; Oweekeno

Plantago: Algonquin, Tête-de-Boule; Cherokee; Chippewa; Delaware, Ontario; Hesquiat; Houma; Iroquois; Kwakiutl; Mahuna; Menominee; Meskwaki; Mohegan; Nitinaht; Ojibwa; Okanagan-Colville; Paiute; Ponca; Potawatomi; Shinnecock; Shoshoni; Shuswap; Thompson; Tolowa; Yurok

Platanthera: Iroquois; Montagnais

Platanus: Cherokee; Iroquois; Meskwaki

Pluchea: Pima

Plumbago: Hawaiian

Podophyllum: Cherokee; Iroquois

Polemonium: Thompson

Poliomintha: Navajo, Kayenta

Polygala: Choctaw; Iroquois

Polygonatum: Cherokee; Rappahannock

Polygonum: Cherokee; Iroquois; Mendocino Indian; Miwok

Polymnia: Houma

Polypodium: Cherokee; Skagit, Upper; Wailaki

Polystichum: Cowlitz; Iroquois; Quileute; Quinault

Populus: Algonquin, Quebec; Anticosti; Bella Coola; Cahuilla; Carrier, Northern; Cherokee; Chippewa; Choctaw; Cree, Woodlands; Diegueño; Flathead; Gitksan; Haisla & Hanaksiala; Hesquiat; Iroquois; Kutenai; Kwakiutl; Malecite; Mendocino Indian; Menominee; Micmac; Nitinaht; Ojibwa; Ojibwa, South; Okanagan-Colville; Oweekeno; Pima; Potawatomi; Quinault; Shuswap; Sikani; Squaxin; Tanana, Upper; Thompson; Yuki

Porophyllum: Havasupai

Porteranthus: Cherokee

Portulaca: Iroquois; Rappahannock

Potentilla: Cherokee; Chippewa; Gosiute; Navajo, Kayenta; Navajo, Ramah; Okanagan-Colville; Thompson

Prenanthes: Iroquois

Prosopis: Cahuilla; Papago; Pima

Prunella: Blackfoot; Cherokee; Quileute; Quinault; Salish, Coast

Prunus: Atsugewi; Cherokee; Chippewa; Crow; Iroquois; Kwakiutl; Malecite; Menominee; Meskwaki; Micmac; Ojibwa, South; Okanagan-Colville; Omaha; Paiute

Psathyrotes: Navajo, Kayenta; Paiute; Shoshoni

Pseudostellaria: Navajo, Kayenta

Pseudotsuga: Cowlitz; Kwakiutl; Okanagan-Colville; Quinault; Skagit; Thompson

Psidium: Hawaiian

Psilostrophe: Navajo, Kayenta; Navajo, Ramah

Psoralidium: Arapaho; Navajo, Kayenta

Psorothamnus: Keres, Western; Paiute

Pteridium: Costanoan; Pomo, Kashaya; Thompson

Pterospora: Cheyenne

Pteryxia: Okanagan-Colville

Pulsatilla: Blackfoot

Purshia: Hopi; Hualapai; Paiute; Shoshoni

Pycnanthemum: Cherokee

Pyrola: Cherokee; Iroquois

Pyrularia: Cherokee

Quercus: Cherokee; Delaware, Oklahoma; Diegueño; Iroquois; Kawaiisu; Luiseño; Miwok; Ojibwa; Seminole

Ranunculus: Bella Coola; Cherokee; Hesquiat; Kawaiisu; Potawatomi; Thompson

Ratibida: Cheyenne; Dakota

Rhamnus: Cherokee; Iroquois; Kawaiisu

Rheum: Cherokee

Rhizomnium: Bella Coola

Rhododendron: Okanagon; Skokomish; Thompson

Rhus: Cherokee; Delaware; Delaware, Oklahoma; Hopi; Menominee; Meskwaki; Natchez; Navajo, Kayenta; Navajo, Ramah; Nez Perce; Ojibwa; Okanagan-Colville; Omaha; Paiute; Round Valley Indian; Sanpoil; Seminole; Sioux; Yokia

Ribes: Bella Coola; Cowlitz; Haisla; Iroquois; Kwakiutl; Navajo, Kayenta; Paiute

Ricinus: Cahuilla; Cherokee; Diegueño; Pima

Rosa: Costanoan; Meskwaki; Ojibwa; Okanagan-Colville; Quileute; Quinault; Shoshoni; Thompson

Rubus: Cherokee; Costanoan; Hawaiian; Iroquois; Kwakiutl; Makah; Okanagan-Colville; Quinault; Rappahannock; Shoshoni; Skagit; Thompson

Rudbeckia: Cherokee

Typha: Algonquin, Quebec; Cahuilla; Dakota; Malecite; Meskwaki; Micmac; Ojibwa; Ojibwa, South; Okanagan-Colville; Omaha; Pawnee; Plains Indian; Ponca; Potawatomi; Sioux; Winnebago

Ulmus: Cherokee; Koasati; Menominee; Meskwaki; Micmac; Ojibwa; Potawatomi

Umbellularia: Karok; Mendocino Indian; Pomo, Kashaya

Urtica: Carrier; Chehalis; Kawaiisu; Kwakiutl; Ojibwa; Paiute, Northern; Shuswap; Skokomish; Thompson; Tolowa

Usnea: Nitinaht

Uvularia: Cherokee; Menominee

Valeriana: Carrier, Northern; Gosiute; Menominee; Okanagon; Thompson

Vanclevea: Navajo, Kayenta

Veratrum: Bella Coola; Iroquois; Kwakiutl; Paiute; Paiute, Northern; Shoshoni; Shuswap; Tsimshian; Washo

Verbascum: Atsugewi; Catawba; Cherokee; Delaware, Ontario; Iroquois; Malecite; Micmac; Rappahannock; Thompson; Zuni

Verbena: Cherokee; Navajo, Ramah

Verbesina: Hopi; Navajo, Kayenta

Vernonia: Kiowa

Veronica: Cherokee

Viburnum: Cree, Woodlands

Vicia: Keres, Western; Makah; Rappahannock; Saanich

Vigna: Hawaiian

Viola: Cherokee

Vitis: Delaware, Oklahoma; Diegueño

Woodsia: Navajo, Ramah

Wyethia: Costanoan; Gosiute; Klamath; Mendocino Indian; Paiute; Shoshoni

Xanthium: Keres, Western; Navajo; Rappahannock; Zuni

Xanthorhiza: Cherokee

Xerophyllum: Blackfoot; Pomo, Kashaya

Yucca: Blackfoot; Catawba; Cherokee; Cheyenne; Choctaw; Dakota; Hopi; Isleta; Keresan; Kiowa; Lakota; Montana Indian; Navajo

Zanthoxylum: Alabama; Menominee

Zea: Cherokee; Mohegan; Tewa

Zigadenus: Mendocino Indian; Montana Indian; Navajo, Ramah; Paiute; Shoshoni; Washo

Zingiber: Hawaiian

Zinnia: Zuni

Ziziphus: Pima

Diaphoretic

Abies: Ojibwa; Ojibwa, South

Abronia: Navajo, Kayenta

Acacia: Hawaiian

Achillea: Cheyenne; Lummi; Makah; Micmac; Paiute, Northern

Acorus: Cherokee

Agastache: Cheyenne

Ageratina: Iroquois; Meskwaki

Alnus: Mendocino Indian; Shuswap

Amelanchier: Cree, Woodlands

Anemone: Gitksan

Anemopsis: Pima

Angelica: Iroquois

Anthemis: Cherokee

Aralia: Cherokee

Arisaema: Cherokee

Artemisia: Keres, Western; Navajo, Ramah; Okanagan-Colville; Okanagon; Paiute; Sanpoil; Shoshoni; Thompson

Asarum: Iroquois

Asclepias: Choctaw

Aster: Cree, Woodlands

Balsamorhiza: Miwok; Okanagan-Colville

Betula: Cree, Woodlands

Botrychium: Chickasaw

Callicarpa: Alabama

Caltha: Chippewa

Carya: Cherokee

Chamaesyce: Pima

Chimaphila: Montagnais

Chrysothamnus: Paiute

Cirsium: Zuni

Conyza: Meskwaki

Corethrogyne: Kawaiisu

Cornus: Cherokee

Cunila: Cherokee

Daphne: Cherokee

Diphylleia: Cherokee

Ephedra: Keres, Western

Erigeron: Cherokee

Eriodictyon: Yokut

Eupatorium: Cherokee; Shinnecock

Euphorbia: Cherokee

Galium: Choctaw

Geum: Cree, Woodlands

Gutierrezia: Keres, Western; Zuni

Hedeoma: Cherokee; Nanticoke

Heracleum: Iroquois

Ilex: Cherokee

Juniperus: Cherokee; Costanoan; Keres, Western; Navajo, Ramah; Omaha; Shuswap

Lesquerella: Shuswap

Liatris: Cherokee

Lindera: Cherokee; Creek

Liquidambar: Houma

Lomatium: Thompson

Mentha: Ojibwa
Mitchella: Cherokee
Monarda: Cherokee
Monardella: Karok
Nepeta: Menominee
Nicotiana: Cherokee
Obolaria: Cherokee
Orbexilum: Cherokee
Panax: Creek
Pericome: Navajo, Ramah
Persea: Creek
Pinus: Yokia; Zuni
Plantago: Shuswap
Polygala: Cherokee
Populus: Bella Coola; Penobscot
Porteranthus: Iroquois
Pycnanthemum: Choctaw
Rosa: Bella Coola
Salix: Mendocino Indian
Salvia: Cherokee
Sambucus: Cherokee; Kawaiisu
Sanvitalia: Navajo
Senecio: Iroquois
Solidago: Cherokee
Stephanomeria: Cheyenne
Streptopus: Montagnais
Tanacetum: Chippewa; Nanticoke
Taxus: Chehalis; Iroquois
Thamnosma: Kawaiisu
Thuja: Menominee; Montagnais; Ojibwa
Torreya: Costanoan
Triosteum: Iroquois
Tripterocalyx: Zuni
Tsuga: Iroquois; Menominee; Potawatomi
Urtica: Paiute
Vaccinium: Cree, Woodlands
Veratrum: Salish, Coast
Verbascum: Atsugewi
Verbena: Cherokee
Veronicastrum: Cherokee
Viburnum: Cherokee
Wyethia: Miwok
Zigadenus: Keres, Western
Zinnia: Zuni

Dietary Aid

Abies: Montagnais; Okanagan-Colville
Abronia: Keres, Western
Achillea: Mohegan
Actaea: Cheyenne; Okanogan; Thompson
Agrimonia: Cherokee
Allium: Mahuna
Alnus: Okanagan-Colville
Alocasia: Hawaiian

Amelanchier: Cheyenne
Angelica: Blackfoot
Aplectrum: Cherokee
Arbutus: Miwok
Arceuthobium: Carrier, Southern
Arctium: Cherokee
Arctostaphylos: Miwok; Thompson
Armoracia: Cherokee
Artemisia: Montana Indian
Asarum: Iroquois; Ojibwa; Skagit
Asclepias: Lakota; Thompson
Asparagus: Cherokee
Aster: Okanagon; Thompson
Balsamorhiza: Thompson
Brassica: Cherokee
Brickellia: Keres, Western
Cardamine: Iroquois
Ceanothus: Thompson
Chamaesyce: Hawaiian; Hopi
Chelone: Cherokee
Chenopodium: Cherokee; Hawaiian; Navajo
Chimaphila: Okanagan-Colville; Rappahannock
Cibotium: Hawaiian
Claytonia: Mahuna
Crataegus: Cherokee
Cucurbita: Omaha
Daucus: Iroquois
Distichlis: Yokut
Echinacea: Cheyenne
Elliottia: Kitasoo
Ephedra: Diegueño
Eryngium: Seminole
Euonymus: Iroquois
Frasera: Cherokee
Galactia: Seminole
Geum: Okanagan-Colville
Goodyera: Cherokee
Gymnocladus: Omaha
Hamamelis: Iroquois
Hedeoma: Dakota
Helianthus: Navajo
Hilaria: Navajo, Ramah
Hydrastis: Cherokee
Juniperus: Crow
Larix: Thompson
Lechea: Seminole
Ledum: Haisla & Hanaksiala; Nitinaht
Lepidium: Mahuna
Liatris: Omaha; Seminole
Ligusticum: Karok
Lilium: Cherokee
Lomatium: Blackfoot; Karok; Nez Perce; Okanagan-Colville
Lonicera: Thompson

Maianthemum: Okanagan-Colville
Malus: Gitksan; Nitinaht
Mentzelia: Cheyenne
Menyanthes: Kwakiutl
Mirabilis: Zuni
Mitchella: Cherokee
Oenothera: Cherokee
Oplopanax: Thompson
Osmorhiza: Menominee; Meskwaki
Oxalis: Karok
Paeonia: Paiute
Panax: Iroquois
Panicum: Mahuna
Passiflora: Cherokee
Persea: Seminole
Phlox: Cherokee
Physalis: Lakota
Physaria: Blackfoot
Pilea: Cherokee
Pinus: Iroquois
Plantago: Navajo, Ramah
Platanus: Meskwaki
Populus: Malecite; Micmac
Prunus: Cheyenne; Kwakiutl; Rappahannock
Pteridium: Thompson
Quercus: Micmac; Penobscot; Rappahannock
Ranunculus: Eskimo, Kuskokwagmiut
Rhus: Algonquin, Quebec; Mahuna; Meskwaki; Micmac
Rubus: Karok
Rudbeckia: Cherokee
Rumex: Iroquois
Sabal: Seminole
Salix: Malecite; Micmac
Sarracenia: Iroquois
Sassafras: Cherokee; Seminole
Satureja: Pomo
Scirpus: Montana Indian
Sinapis: Cherokee
Solidago: Thompson
Sorbus: Montagnais
Sphaeralcea: Navajo, Kayenta
Stillingia: Seminole
Streptopus: Thompson
Tanacetum: Mohegan
Tellima: Skagit
Tiarella: Iroquois
Triosteum: Iroquois
Tsuga: Klallam
Vaccinium: Cheyenne
Waltheria: Hawaiian

Disinfectant

Abies: Abnaki

Achillea: Flathead; Kutenai
Adenostoma: Cahuilla
Agastache: Navajo, Ramah
Agoseris: Navajo, Ramah
Allium: Shinnecock
Ambrosia: Cherokee
Amelanchier: Chippewa
Anaphalis: Cheyenne
Anemopsis: Costanoan; Isleta; Mahuna; Shoshoni
Angelica: Eskimo, Kuskokwagmiut
Apocynum: Navajo, Ramah
Aralia: Cherokee; Potawatomi
Aristolochia: Cherokee
Artemisia: Cahuilla; Chippewa; Eskimo; Mewuk; Navajo, Kayenta; Paiute; Pawnee; Shoshoni; Shuswap; Tanana, Upper; Thompson; Washo
Asarum: Iroquois; Tolowa
Astragalus: Thompson
Baccharis: Costanoan
Balsamorhiza: Paiute; Washo
Brickellia: Navajo, Ramah
Campanula: Navajo, Ramah
Carex: Navajo, Ramah
Castilleja: Costanoan
Chionanthus: Choctaw
Chlorogalum: Wailaki
Cicuta: Iroquois
Clintonia: Algonquin, Quebec
Conyza: Navajo, Kayenta
Coreopsis: Navajo, Ramah
Cornus: Cherokee
Corydalis: Navajo, Kayenta
Cryptantha: Navajo, Kayenta
Dalea: Navajo, Ramah
Datura: Apache, White Mountain
Dichanthelium: Navajo, Ramah
Diphylleia: Cherokee
Epilobium: Costanoan
Equisetum: Chippewa; Navajo, Ramah
Erigeron: Navajo, Ramah
Eriodictyon: Costanoan
Eriogonum: Navajo, Kayenta; Navajo, Ramah; Thompson
Erodium: Navajo, Kayenta
Euonymus: Cherokee
Eupatorium: Cherokee
Forestiera: Navajo, Ramah
Fragaria: Okanagan-Colville
Frangula: Kawaiisu; Nitinaht
Frasera: Cherokee
Gaura: Navajo, Kayenta
Geum: Thompson
Gnaphalium: Menominee
Grindelia: Cheyenne, Northern; Mahuna; Shoshoni

Gutierrezia: Navajo, Kayenta; Navajo, Ramah; Shoshoni; Tewa
Helianthus: Navajo, Kayenta; Shasta
Heracleum: Thompson
Heterotheca: Cheyenne
Heuchera: Navajo, Ramah
Holodiscus: Shoshoni
Houstonia: Navajo, Ramah
Hydrangea: Cherokee
Ipomopsis: Navajo, Ramah; Shoshoni
Juniperus: Arapaho; Comanche; Cree, Hudson Bay; Paiute; Salish; Shoshoni; Swinomish; Tewa; Thompson; Washo
Kalmia: Cherokee
Krameria: Paiute; Pima
Larix: Algonquin, Quebec; Ojibwa
Larrea: Cahuilla; Hualapai; Isleta; Kawaiisu; Mahuna
Lathyrus: Navajo, Ramah
Ledum: Tanana, Upper
Lepidium: Navajo
Leptodactylon: Navajo, Ramah
Linum: Navajo, Kayenta
Lithospermum: Shuswap
Lomatium: Gosiute; Paiute; Shoshoni
Lonicera: Wet'suwet'en
Lotus: Navajo, Ramah
Lupinus: Navajo, Kayenta
Mahonia: Blackfoot
Marrubium: Navajo, Ramah
Matricaria: Costanoan
Mentha: Navajo, Kayenta
Mentzelia: Navajo, Kayenta
Nuphar: Algonquin, Quebec
Oenothera: Navajo, Ramah
Osmorhiza: Paiute; Shoshoni
Oxalis: Tolowa
Oxytropis: Thompson
Penstemon: Costanoan; Navajo, Kayenta; Shoshoni
Phlox: Navajo, Ramah
Picea: Bella Coola; Kwakiutl; Ojibwa; Potawatomi; Tanana, Upper
Pinus: Hopi; Shoshoni; Thompson; Zuni
Plantago: Navajo, Ramah; Nitinaht; Shoshoni
Platanthera: Thompson
Polypodium: Yurok
Populus: Algonquin, Quebec; Cree, Woodlands; Quinault; Squaxin; Thompson
Prosopis: Pima
Prunus: Algonquin, Quebec; Chippewa
Pseudotsuga: Karok; Navajo, Kayenta; Skagit; Thompson
Psoralidium: Zuni
Psorothamnus: Paiute; Shoshoni

Pteridium: Cherokee
Pterospora: Cheyenne
Purshia: Navajo, Ramah; Shoshoni
Quercus: Cherokee; Delaware; Delaware, Oklahoma
Ranunculus: Thompson
Rubus: Costanoan; Quinault
Salix: Navajo, Ramah
Salvia: Cahuilla
Sambucus: Cherokee; Navajo, Kayenta; Pomo, Potter Valley; Squaxin; Yokia
Scrophularia: Costanoan
Sedum: Delaware, Ontario
Senecio: Costanoan; Navajo, Kayenta
Shepherdia: Thompson
Sinapis: Navajo, Ramah
Smallanthus: Iroquois
Solidago: Mahuna
Sphaeralcea: Navajo, Kayenta; Tewa
Stachys: Costanoan; Navajo, Ramah
Symphoricarpos: Green River Group
Tanacetum: Shoshoni
Tetradymia: Navajo, Ramah
Tetraneuris: Navajo, Ramah
Thuja: Chippewa
Tradescantia: Navajo, Ramah
Trichostema: Costanoan
Trillium: Menominee
Tsuga: Algonquin, Quebec; Thompson
Typha: Algonquin, Quebec
Umbellularia: Karok
Veratrum: Paiute; Shoshoni
Veronica: Navajo, Ramah
Veronicastrum: Cherokee
Yucca: Hopi

Diuretic

Abronia: Paiute
Achillea: Blackfoot
Acorus: Cherokee; Cheyenne
Adiantum: Iroquois
Agastache: Meskwaki
Ageratina: Cherokee
Allium: Cherokee
Alnus: Gitksan
Andropogon: Chippewa
Apocynum: Ojibwa; Potawatomi
Arabis: Thompson
Arctostaphylos: Thompson
Argentina: Iroquois
Aristolochia: Cherokee
Armoracia: Cherokee
Artemisia: Lakota; Paiute
Aruncus: Bella Coola

Asclepias: Iroquois; Meskwaki
Athyrium: Chippewa
Besseya: Navajo, Ramah
Betula: Ojibwa, South
Caltha: Chippewa
Carya: Meskwaki
Castilleja: Gitksan
Celastrus: Chippewa; Iroquois
Chimaphila: Iroquois
Chlorogalum: Wailaki
Cimicifuga: Cherokee
Cirsium: Keres, Western; Zuni
Citrullus: Cheyenne
Croton: Zuni
Cucurbita: Cherokee; Iroquois; Menominee;
    Ojibwa
Daucus: Iroquois
Diervilla: Algonquin, Tête-de-Boule; Menominee;
    Potawatomi
Diphylleia: Cherokee
Dirca: Menominee; Ojibwa; Potawatomi
Draba: Navajo
Empetrum: Cree, Woodlands
Ephedra: Shoshoni
Equisetum: Blackfoot; Crow; Flathead; Iroquois;
    Okanagan-Colville; Yuki
Erigeron: Cherokee
Eriogonum: Lakota
Eryngium: Choctaw
Eupatorium: Cherokee
Gaillardia: Hopi
Galium: Choctaw; Cree, Hudson Bay; Ojibwa
Gutierrezia: Zuni
Heliotropium: Paiute; Shoshoni
Hieracium: Navajo, Ramah
Humulus: Ojibwa
Impatiens: Iroquois
Inula: Iroquois
Ipomoea: Cherokee; Creek
Juniperus: Cree, Hudson Bay; Iroquois; Paiute;
    Shoshoni; Tewa; Thompson
Laportea: Meskwaki; Ojibwa
Larix: Micmac
Larrea: Shoshoni
Ledum: Cree; Cree, Woodlands; Gitksan; Micmac
Liatris: Cherokee
Lithospermum: Gosiute; Iroquois; Ute
Lomatium: Paiute, Northern
Lonicera: Chippewa; Cree, Woodlands; Montagnais;
    Potawatomi
Lycopodium: Ojibwa
Lygodesmia: Blackfoot
Malaxis: Ojibwa
Malus: Gitksan

Mentzelia: Keres, Western
Mirabilis: Lakota; Zuni
Mitchella: Cherokee
Monarda: Cherokee
Myrica: Bella Coola
Nicotiana: Cherokee
Oplopanax: Gitksan
Opuntia: Okanagan-Colville
Penstemon: Navajo
Perideridia: Blackfoot
Phlox: Navajo
Picea: Bella Coola
Pinus: Gitksan; Zuni
Plantago: Meskwaki
Polemonium: Meskwaki
Polygala: Cherokee
Polypodium: Micmac
Prenanthes: Choctaw; Ojibwa
Pseudotsuga: Bella Coola; Thompson
Psorothamnus: Paiute
Rhamnus: Kawaiisu
Rhus: Cheyenne; Omaha
Rosa: Shoshoni
Rubus: Iroquois; Ojibwa
Sambucus: Cherokee; Meskwaki
Sarracenia: Algonquin, Tête-de-Boule
Solidago: Chippewa
Sphaeralcea: Hopi
Stephanomeria: Hopi
Symphoricarpos: Bella Coola; Chippewa; Nitinaht;
    Sanpoil; Sioux
Taxus: Potawatomi
Tilia: Iroquois
Tradescantia: Meskwaki
Trillium: Menominee
Triosteum: Iroquois
Urtica: Chippewa; Sioux
Verbesina: Chickasaw
Viburnum: Ojibwa
Zanthoxylum: Iroquois

Ear Medicine

Achillea: Winnebago
Acorus: Cree, Woodlands; Iroquois
Aesculus: Delaware; Delaware, Oklahoma
Allium: Cherokee; Shinnecock
Amelanchier: Blackfoot
Apocynum: Chippewa
Aralia: Algonquin, Tête-de-Boule
Arctostaphylos: Flathead
Artemisia: Costanoan
Asarum: Meskwaki
Aster: Cheyenne; Chippewa
Astragalus: Navajo, Kayenta

Balsamita: Iroquois
Campanula: Chippewa
Cercocarpus: Kawaiisu
Chamaesyce: Cahuilla
Conyza: Navajo, Kayenta
Coptis: Iroquois
Croton: Cahuilla; Isleta
Datura: Pima
Fraxinus: Iroquois
Glycyrrhiza: Dakota; Pawnee; Sioux
Gutierrezia: Tewa
Humulus: Delaware; Delaware, Oklahoma;
    Mohegan
Hydrastis: Iroquois
Iris: Omaha; Paiute; Ponca; Shoshoni
Juniperus: Keres, Western
Ligusticum: Crow
Lobelia: Iroquois
Lupinus: Hopi; Navajo, Kayenta
Maianthemum: Paiute
Malus: Iroquois
Mammillaria: Pima
Marah: Kawaiisu
Medicago: Costanoan
Mentzelia: Cheyenne
Mitella: Cree, Woodlands
Nicotiana: Cahuilla; Costanoan; Kawaiisu; Micmac;
    Mohegan; Rappahannock; Shinnecock
Opuntia: Keres, Western
Oxytropis: Blackfoot
Panax: Iroquois; Potawatomi
Passiflora: Cherokee
Pediomelum: Blackfoot
Penstemon: Shoshoni
Physaria: Blackfoot
Pinus: Navajo, Ramah; Thompson
Plantago: Kawaiisu
Podophyllum: Cherokee
Poliomintha: Hopi; Tewa
Polygala: Sioux
Portulaca: Cherokee
Prosopis: Apache, Mescalero; Apache, Western;
    Tewa
Rhus: Micmac
Rudbeckia: Cherokee
Ruta: Costanoan; Diegueño
Salvia: Costanoan; Paiute
Sanguinaria: Iroquois
Sempervivum: Cherokee
Sequoia: Pomo; Pomo, Kashaya
Sophora: Comanche
Sorbus: Thompson
Stachys: Costanoan
Stanleya: Shoshoni

Tanacetum: Chippewa
Trillium: Chippewa
Valeriana: Cree, Woodlands
Verbascum: Iroquois
Verbena: Iroquois
Veronica: Cherokee

Emetic

Abies: Blackfoot
Abronia: Navajo, Kayenta
Acer: Iroquois; Meskwaki; Ojibwa; Ojibwa, South
Achillea: Iroquois; Navajo, Ramah; Paiute
Achlys: Lummi
Acorus: Iroquois
Adenostoma: Cahuilla; Coahuilla
Adiantum: Cherokee; Iroquois
Aesculus: Kiowa
Agoseris: Navajo, Ramah
Agrimonia: Iroquois
Aletes: Keres, Western
Allium: Chippewa
Alnus: Algonquin, Quebec; Cherokee; Chippewa;
    Gitksan; Iroquois; Mendocino Indian
Ambrosia: Luiseño
Amelanchier: Navajo, Ramah
Anemone: Iroquois
Anemopsis: Papago; Pima
Anthemis: Cherokee; Iroquois
Apocynum: Cree, Hudson Bay; Iroquois; Navajo,
    Kayenta; Navajo, Ramah
Aquilegia: Shoshoni
Aralia: Cherokee
Arbutus: Concow; Yuki
Arctostaphylos: Navajo, Kayenta; Navajo, Ramah
Arenaria: Hopi
Argemone: Shoshoni
Argentina: Blackfoot
Artemisia: Paiute; Paiute, Northern; Shoshoni
Asarum: Cherokee
Asclepias: Meskwaki; Navajo, Kayenta; Navajo,
    Ramah; Pima
Asplenium: Cherokee
Astragalus: Navajo, Kayenta; Navajo, Ramah
Atriplex: Navajo, Kayenta; Navajo, Ramah
Aureolaria: Chickasaw
Baccharis: Navajo, Ramah
Bahia: Keres, Western
Baptisia: Cherokee
Besseya: Navajo, Ramah
Betula: Delaware, Oklahoma; Micmac
Botrychium: Cherokee; Chickasaw
Brassica: Shinnecock
Brickellia: Navajo, Kayenta; Navajo, Ramah
Caltha: Chippewa; Iroquois

Calycanthus: Cherokee
Carex: Iroquois; Navajo, Ramah
Carya: Cherokee
Castilleja: Shoshoni
Caulophyllum: Chippewa; Iroquois; Ojibwa
Ceanothus: Navajo, Kayenta; Navajo, Ramah
Cephalanthus: Meskwaki
Chaenactis: Shoshoni
Chaerophyllum: Chickasaw
Chamaesyce: Pima; Zuni
Chenopodium: Kawaiisu; Keres, Western; Paiute
Chimaphila: Cherokee
Chrysothamnus: Navajo; Navajo, Kayenta; Navajo,
    Ramah
Cicuta: Bella Coola; Kutenai; Kwakiutl; Salish, Coast
Cirsium: Navajo; Zuni
Clethra: Cherokee
Collinsonia: Cherokee
Coptis: Iroquois
Cordylanthus: Navajo
Cornus: Cree, Hudson Bay; Green River Group; Iro-
    quois; Navajo, Kayenta; Navajo, Ramah; Ojibwa
Coronilla: Cherokee
Corylus: Cherokee; Iroquois
Croton: Hopi
Cucurbita: Cahuilla; Kiowa; Paiute; Shoshoni
Cuscuta: Navajo, Ramah
Cyperus: Navajo, Ramah
Dalea: Hopi; Keres, Western
Delphinium: Hopi
Dimorphocarpa: Zuni
Dirca: Iroquois
Draba: Navajo, Ramah
Dryopteris: Cherokee
Echinochloa: Navajo, Ramah
Eleocharis: Navajo, Ramah; Seminole
Elodea: Iroquois
Ephedra: Havasupai
Epigaea: Cherokee
Eriastrum: Paiute; Shoshoni
Erigeron: Paiute
Eriogonum: Diegueño; Keres, Western; Navajo;
    Navajo, Kayenta; Zuni
Eryngium: Alabama; Cherokee; Koasati; Seminole
Erysimum: Navajo, Ramah; Zuni
Eschscholzia: Mendocino Indian
Eupatorium: Cherokee; Koasati; Seminole
Euphorbia: Cherokee; Micmac
Fallugia: Navajo, Ramah
Forestiera: Navajo, Ramah
Frangula: Delaware, Oklahoma; Klamath; Montana
    Indian; Navajo, Kayenta
Fraxinus: Delaware, Oklahoma; Iroquois
Galeopsis: Iroquois

Galium: Meskwaki; Navajo, Ramah
Geocaulon: Cree, Hudson Bay
Geranium: Iroquois
Geum: Iroquois
Gnaphalium: Navajo, Ramah
Goodyera: Cherokee
Grindelia: Navajo, Ramah; Shoshoni
Gutierrezia: Keres, Western
Hamamelis: Chippewa; Iroquois
Heliotropium: Paiute; Shoshoni
Hepatica: Cherokee
Heterotheca: Navajo, Ramah
Holodiscus: Shoshoni
Huperzia: Nitinaht
Hydrangea: Cherokee
Hydrastis: Iroquois
Hymenopappus: Hopi; Zuni
Hymenoxys: Navajo, Ramah
Ilex: Alabama; Cherokee; Creek; Iroquois; Natchez
Ipomopsis: Keres, Western; Navajo; Navajo, Kayenta;
    Paiute; Shoshoni; Washo
Iris: Klamath; Montana Indian; Navajo, Ramah;
    Ojibwa
Juglans: Delaware, Oklahoma; Iroquois
Juncus: Cherokee; Iroquois
Juniperus: Isleta; Keres, Western; Navajo, Ramah;
    Seminole
Lactuca: Navajo, Ramah
Laportea: Iroquois
Larrea: Cahuilla; Papago; Pima
Lathyrus: Chippewa; Costanoan
Ledum: Cree
Lesquerella: Hopi; Keres, Western
Linaria: Iroquois
Lindera: Creek
Lobelia: Cherokee; Cree, Hudson Bay; Iroquois
Lomatium: Kawaiisu
Lonicera: Blackfoot; Iroquois; Makah; Navajo,
    Ramah; Quileute
Lupinus: Navajo, Ramah
Luzula: Navajo, Ramah
Lycium: Navajo, Ramah
Lysimachia: Iroquois
Machaeranthera: Zuni
Mahonia: Navajo, Ramah
Maianthemum: Navajo, Ramah
Malva: Costanoan; Iroquois
Mentha: Iroquois
Mentzelia: Navajo
Mirabilis: Zuni
Mitella: Iroquois
Monarda: Blackfoot
Monolepis: Navajo, Ramah
Morus: Creek; Delaware, Oklahoma

Myriophyllum: Iroquois
Nicotiana: Cahuilla; Cherokee; Costanoan; Kawaiisu; Paiute; Shoshoni
Nyssa: Cherokee
Oenanthe: Kitasoo; Kwakiutl; Kwakwaka'wakw; Nuxalkmc
Oenothera: Navajo, Kayenta; Navajo, Ramah
Onopordum: Iroquois
Oplopanax: Bella Coola; Haisla & Hanaksiala
Osmorhiza: Bella Coola; Kwakiutl
Panicum: Keres, Western
Parryella: Navajo, Ramah
Paxistima: Navajo, Ramah
Pedicularis: Iroquois
Pellaea: Costanoan
Penstemon: Iroquois; Keres, Western; Navajo, Kayenta
Pericome: Navajo, Ramah
Persea: Seminole
Petasites: Lummi
Petradoria: Navajo, Ramah
Phacelia: Kawaiisu
Phoradendron: Seminole; Zuni
Phragmites: Blackfoot
Physalis: Iroquois
Physocarpus: Bella Coola; Carrier, Southern; Chippewa; Green River Group; Hesquiat; Kwakiutl
Phytolacca: Iroquois
Picea: Navajo, Ramah
Picradeniopsis: Zuni
Piloblephis: Seminole
Pinus: Iroquois; Navajo; Navajo, Ramah; Rappahannock
Platanus: Cherokee
Podophyllum: Meskwaki
Polygala: Miwok
Polygonum: Zuni
Polystichum: Cherokee; Iroquois
Porteranthus: Cherokee
Potamogeton: Navajo, Ramah
Prosopis: Pima
Prunella: Iroquois
Prunus: Iroquois; Navajo, Ramah
Psathyrotes: Navajo, Kayenta; Paiute; Shoshoni
Pseudocymopterus: Navajo, Kayenta; Navajo, Ramah
Pseudotsuga: Bella Coola; Navajo, Ramah; Okanagan-Colville
Psorothamnus: Keres, Western
Pterospora: Keres, Western
Purshia: Hopi; Kawaiisu; Klamath; Montana Indian; Navajo, Ramah; Paiute; Shoshoni
Pyrrhopappus: Navajo, Ramah
Pyrularia: Cherokee

Quercus: Cherokee; Keres, Western; Navajo, Ramah
Ranunculus: Iroquois; Navajo, Ramah
Ratibida: Zuni
Rhus: Chippewa; Keres, Western
Ribes: Navajo, Kayenta; Navajo, Ramah; Shoshoni
Robinia: Cherokee; Hopi
Rosa: Navajo, Ramah; Tanana, Upper
Rubus: Cherokee; Iroquois
Rumex: Iroquois; Navajo, Ramah
Salix:; Iroquois; Navajo, Ramah; Seminole
Sambucus: Algonquin, Quebec; Bella Coola; Cherokee; Chippewa; Gitksan; Hesquiat; Iroquois; Kwakiutl; Malecite; Menominee; Micmac; Mohegan; Montana Indian; Nitinaht; Ojibwa; Paiute; Pomo, Potter Valley; Potawatomi; Quinault; Seminole; Yokia; Yokut
Sanguinaria: Iroquois; Mohegan
Sanicula: Iroquois
Sarcobatus: Keres, Western
Sassafras: Seminole
Saururus: Seminole
Scirpus: Cherokee; Navajo, Ramah
Scutellaria: Cherokee
Shepherdia: Navajo, Kayenta
Silene: Gosiute
Silphium: Iroquois; Meskwaki; Winnebago
Sinapis: Navajo, Ramah
Sisymbrium: Navajo, Ramah
Smallanthus: Cherokee
Solanum: Cherokee
Solidago: Iroquois
Sorbus: Micmac; Penobscot; Potawatomi
Sphaeralcea: Shoshoni
Sporobolus: Ojibwa, South
Stachys: Meskwaki
Stephanomeria: Paiute
Symphoricarpos: Navajo, Ramah
Syzygium: Hawaiian
Tanacetum: Paiute
Taraxacum: Iroquois
Tetradymia: Navajo, Ramah
Thamnosma: Havasupai
Tilia: Iroquois
Toxicodendron: Cherokee
Tragopogon: Navajo, Ramah
Trifolium: Navajo, Ramah
Triodanis: Meskwaki
Triosteum: Cherokee
Tsuga: Hoh; Quileute
Typha: Navajo, Ramah
Ulmus: Iroquois
Vaccinium: Seminole
Veratrum: Bella Coola; Carrier, Southern; Haisla; Kwakiutl; Washo

Verbena: Cherokee
Verbesina: Seminole; Zuni
Veronica: Iroquois; Navajo, Ramah
Veronicastrum: Iroquois; Menominee
Viburnum: Chippewa; Iroquois
Vicia: Cherokee
Viola: Navajo, Ramah
Vitis: Seminole
Wyethia: Hopi; Mendocino Indian; Navajo, Kayenta; Paiute; Shoshoni; Washo; Yuki
Xanthium: Cherokee
Yucca: Tewa
Zanthoxylum: Iroquois
Zigadenus: Chehalis; Gosiute; Klamath; Paiute; Shoshoni; Squaxin
Zinnia: Navajo, Ramah

Expectorant

Acer: Potawatomi
Allium: Cherokee
Aralia: Cherokee; Choctaw
Arisaema: Cherokee
Artemisia: Tewa
Asclepias: Cherokee
Botrychium: Chickasaw
Calycanthus: Pomo, Kashaya
Chimaphila: Delaware, Oklahoma
Cirsium: Houma
Comptonia: Delaware, Oklahoma
Eriodictyon: Paiute; Pomo; Shoshoni
Eryngium: Choctaw
Euonymus: Cherokee
Euphorbia: Cherokee
Galium: Cherokee
Glycyrrhiza: Cherokee
Grindelia: Paiute; Shoshoni
Hedeoma: Cherokee
Ipomoea: Cherokee
Larix: Montagnais
Liatris: Cherokee
Nereocystis: Pomo, Kashaya
Nicotiana: Cherokee
Panax: Cherokee
Phragmites: Paiute
Phytolacca: Iroquois
Pinus: Hualapai
Polygala: Cherokee
Polypodium: Skagit, Upper
Zanthoxylum: Meskwaki

Eye Medicine

Abies: Bella Coola; Ojibwa; Okanagon; Thompson
Acer: Cherokee; Iroquois; Malecite; Micmac; Ojibwa; Potawatomi

Achillea: Mendocino Indian; Navajo, Kayenta; Okanagon; Paiute; Quinault; Salish; Thompson; Yurok
Achlys: Paiute
Alnus: Cherokee; Chippewa; Cree, Woodlands
Ambrosia: Gosiute
Amelanchier: Blackfoot
Anaphalis: Cherokee; Iroquois
Anemone: Meskwaki
Angelica: Gitksan
Antennaria: Gosiute
Anthemis: Mendocino Indian
Apocynum: Cree, Woodlands; Iroquois
Arabis: Okanagan-Colville
Aralia: Choctaw; Iroquois; Koasati; Micmac
Arctostaphylos: Okanagan-Colville; Okanagon; Thompson
Arenaria: Navajo, Ramah; Shoshoni
Argemone: Comanche; Shoshoni
Argentina: Kwakiutl
Arisaema: Chippewa; Iroquois; Menominee; Ojibwa
Arnica: Shuswap
Artemisia: Blackfoot; Crow; Klamath; Mendocino Indian; Montana Indian; Paiute; Poliklah; Shoshoni; Tanana, Upper; Yurok, South Coast (Nererner)
Aruncus: Cherokee
Asarum: Cherokee
Asclepias: Blackfoot; Cheyenne; Pima
Aster: Navajo, Ramah
Astragalus: Navajo, Kayenta; Navajo, Ramah
Athyrium: Bella Coola
Baccharis: Coahuilla
Balsamorhiza: Shoshoni
Bidens: Seminole
Calla: Gitksan
Calochortus: Thompson
Calycanthus: Cherokee
Campanula: Navajo, Ramah; Thompson
Castilleja: Gitksan; Shuswap
Cephalanthus: Chickasaw; Choctaw
Cercocarpus: Shoshoni
Chaenactis: Okanagan-Colville
Chamaesyce: Costanoan; Keres, Western; Paiute; Shoshoni
Chenopodium: Navajo, Kayenta
Chimaphila: Chippewa; Flathead; Kutenai
Cicuta: Shoshoni
Cirsium: Navajo, Ramah
Clarkia: Mendocino Indian
Claytonia: Hesquiat; Quileute; Thompson
Cleome: Gosiute
Clintonia: Bella Coola; Cowlitz; Haisla & Hanaksiala

Comandra: Navajo, Kayenta; Thompson
Conocephalum: Nitinaht
Coptis: Algonquin, Quebec; Iroquois
Cornus: Abnaki; Bella Coola; Carrier, Southern; Chippewa; Cree, Woodlands; Iroquois; Malecite; Micmac; Paiute; Potawatomi; Snohomish
Corylus: Abnaki
Crepis: Shoshoni
Croton: Hopi
Cryptantha: Navajo, Kayenta
Cryptogramma: Thompson
Datura: Costanoan; Pima
Desmanthus: Paiute
Diervilla: Chippewa; Cree, Woodlands
Digitaria: Hawaiian
Diplacus: Pomo, Kashaya
Dirca: Iroquois
Disporum: Blackfoot
Dodecatheon: Blackfoot; Okanagan-Colville
Draba: Navajo, Ramah
Dracocephalum: Navajo, Ramah
Echinacea: Dakota; Omaha
Empetrum: Tanana, Upper
Epilobium: Eskimo, Inupiat
Equisetum: Iroquois; Karok; Okanagan-Colville; Quinault; Thompson; Yuki
Ericameria: Paiute; Shoshoni
Erigeron: Cherokee; Navajo, Ramah; Okanagan-Colville; Paiute; Shoshoni
Eriodictyon: Costanoan
Eriogonum: Coahuilla; Gosiute; Round Valley Indian; Thompson; Zuni
Eriophorum: Eskimo, Western
Escobaria: Blackfoot
Euonymus: Meskwaki
Foeniculum: Pomo, Kashaya
Frasera: Shoshoni
Fraxinus: Ojibwa, South
Gaillardia: Blackfoot
Gentiana: Iroquois
Geranium: Blackfoot; Sanpoil
Geum: Blackfoot
Gnaphalium: Karok
Goodyera: Cherokee
Grindelia: Cheyenne; Cheyenne, Northern
Gutierrezia: Keres, Western
Hamamelis: Chippewa
Hedeoma: Chickasaw
Hepatica: Meskwaki
Heracleum: Makah; Sanpoil
Heuchera: Blackfoot; Chippewa; Cree, Woodlands; Paiute
Hierochloe: Blackfoot
Holodiscus: Lummi

Hordeum: Chippewa
Houstonia: Keres, Western
Hydrastis: Iroquois
Hypericum: Alabama; Choctaw
Ilex: Alabama; Choctaw
Impatiens: Iroquois
Ipomopsis: Navajo, Ramah; Salish; Shoshoni
Iris: Omaha; Ponca
Juniperus: Okanagon; Seminole; Thompson
Krameria: Paiute; Pima
Krascheninnikovia: Paiute; Shoshoni
Lactuca: Iroquois
Ledum: Shuswap
Leptodactylon: Shoshoni
Lesquerella: Navajo, Kayenta; Navajo, Ramah
Leucanthemum: Iroquois
Leymus: Paiute; Shoshoni
Linum: Apache, White Mountain; Great Basin Indian; Paiute; Shoshoni; Zuni
Lithospermum: Navajo, Ramah
Lomatium: Nez Perce; Shoshoni
Lonicera: Carrier; Carrier, Southern; Gitksan; Mendocino Indian
Lupinus: Hopi; Okanagan-Colville
Lygodesmia: Omaha; Ponca; Sioux
Machaeranthera: Navajo, Ramah; Shoshoni
Maclura: Comanche
Mahonia: Apache, Mescalero; Okanagan-Colville; Sanpoil; Thompson
Maianthemum: Cherokee; Paiute; Quinault; Shoshoni
Malacothrix: Navajo, Ramah
Malus: Bella Coola; Gitksan; Iroquois; Klallam; Quinault
Marah: Paiute
Melampyrum: Ojibwa
Mentha: Isleta
Mentzelia: Navajo, Ramah
Mitella: Iroquois
Monarda: Blackfoot; Flathead; Lakota; Tewa
Monardella: Paiute
Monotropa: Cherokee
Nyssa: Cherokee
Oenothera: Hopi
Oplopanax: Haisla & Hanaksiala
Orthilia: Carrier, Southern
Osmorhiza: Blackfoot; Menominee; Meskwaki; Paiute; Paiute, Northern; Potawatomi; Shoshoni
Oxalis: Cowlitz; Quinault
Paeonia: Paiute; Shoshoni
Panax: Iroquois; Potawatomi
Pectis: Zuni
Pediomelum: Blackfoot

Penstemon: Okanagon; Paiute; Shoshoni;
   Thompson
Persea: Seminole
Petasites: Quinault
Phlox: Paiute; Shoshoni; Washo
Physalis: Diegueño
Physaria: Blackfoot; Paiute; Shoshoni
Picea: Carrier, Southern; Thompson
Pinus: Carrier, Northern; Kawaiisu; Klamath;
   Miwok; Okanagan-Colville; Okanagon;
   Thompson
Piper: Hawaiian
Plantago: Cherokee; Shinnecock
Pluchea: Pima
Polygonatum: Iroquois
Polypodium: Mendocino Indian
Populus: Carrier, Northern; Klallam; Okanagan-
   Colville
Prenanthes: Iroquois
Prosopis: Apache, Mescalero; Cahuilla; Diegueño;
   Isleta; Keres, Western; Paiute; Pima
Prunella: Blackfoot
Prunus: Cree, Woodlands; Flathead; Paiute;
   Potawatomi; Shoshoni
Psathyrotes: Paiute
Psilostrophe: Navajo, Ramah
Pulsatilla: Thompson
Pyrola: Carrier, Southern; Cree, Woodlands;
   Iroquois
Quercus: Diegueño; Kawaiisu; Menominee
Ranunculus: Iroquois
Rhamnus: Cherokee
Rhus: Diegueño; Ojibwa
Ribes: Bella Coola; Klallam; Makah; Okanagan-
   Colville; Potawatomi; Skagit; Tanana, Upper;
   Thompson
Rorippa: Navajo, Ramah; Zuni
Rosa: Bella Coola; Carrier; Cree, Woodlands; Iro-
   quois; Ojibwa, South; Omaha; Skagit; Thompson
Rubus: Chippewa; Menominee; Meskwaki; Ojibwa;
   Potawatomi
Rudbeckia: Shuswap
Sabal: Houma
Sabatia: Seminole
Salix: Eskimo, Alaska; Eskimo, Kuskokwagmiut;
   Eskimo, Western; Seminole
Salvia: Cahuilla; Costanoan; Kawaiisu; Mahuna;
   Paiute
Sanguinaria: Iroquois
Sassafras: Cherokee; Iroquois; Mohegan; Rappa-
   hannock; Seminole
Schoenocrambe: Navajo, Ramah
Scrophularia: Costanoan
Scutellaria: Miwok

Senecio: Zuni
Shepherdia: Flathead; Kutenai
Silene: Okanagan-Colville
Sisymbrium: Pima
Smilax: Iroquois
Solanum: Cahuilla; Iroquois; Luiseño; Miwok;
   Navajo
Sorbus: Bella Coola
Sphaeralcea: Shoshoni
Stellaria: Chippewa
Stephanomeria: Kawaiisu; Keres, Western;
   Shoshoni
Streptanthus: Navajo, Kayenta
Streptopus: Chippewa
Symphoricarpos: Carrier, Southern; Cree, Wood-
   lands; Dakota; Flathead; Kwakiutl; Ojibwa,
   South; Okanagan-Colville; Omaha; Ponca; San-
   poil; Shuswap; Sioux; Thompson; Wet'suwet'en
Taraxacum: Iroquois
Tauschia: Kawaiisu
Tetraneuris: Zuni
Thalictrum: Gitksan; Iroquois
Thelypodium: Navajo, Kayenta
Thermopsis: Navajo, Ramah; Pomo; Pomo, Kashaya
Thuja: Kwakiutl
Tiarella: Iroquois
Tilia: Algonquin, Quebec
Toxicodendron: Diegueño
Trientalis: Cowlitz; Paiute
Trifolium: Iroquois
Trillium: Lummi; Menominee; Paiute; Skagit;
   Thompson
Tsuga: Cowlitz; Hesquiat; Kwakiutl; Skagit
Ulmus: Cherokee; Iroquois; Meskwaki; Potawatomi
Uvularia: Iroquois
Vaccinium: Seminole
Verbesina: Seminole
Viburnum: Gitksan; Montagnais
Vicia: Navajo, Ramah
Viola: Tolowa
Vitis: Menominee
Wyethia: Mendocino Indian
Xanthium: Pima
Xanthorhiza: Cherokee
Zinnia: Zuni
Ziziphus: Pima

Febrifuge

Abies: Blackfoot; Montana Indian
Achillea: Abnaki; Cherokee; Cheyenne; Cree,
   Woodlands; Flathead; Iroquois; Menominee;
   Meskwaki; Montagnais; Navajo, Kayenta; Ojibwa;
   Paiute; Quileute

Acorus: Cree, Woodlands; Dakota; Omaha; Pawnee; Ponca; Winnebago
Acrostichum: Seminole
Adiantum: Cherokee
Agastache: Cheyenne; Navajo, Ramah; Okanagan-Colville
Ageratina: Cherokee; Navajo, Ramah
Agrimonia: Cherokee
Aletris: Cherokee
Allium: Cherokee; Shinnecock
Alnus: Cherokee; Tanana, Upper
Ambrosia: Cherokee
Amelanchier: Cree, Woodlands
Andropogon: Omaha
Angelica: Cherokee; Iroquois
Anthemis: Cherokee; Iroquois; Mohegan
Apocynum: Montana Indian
Aquilegia: Omaha; Pawnee; Ponca
Aralia: Mendocino Indian; Rappahannock
Arctium: Abnaki
Arenaria: Navajo, Ramah
Arisaema: Iroquois
Aristolochia: Cherokee; Natchez; Rappahannock
Artemisia: Blackfoot; Cree, Woodlands; Eskimo; Gosiute; Gros Ventre; Hawaiian; Mendocino Indian; Navajo; Navajo, Ramah; Omaha; Paiute; Paiute, Northern; Shoshoni; Tewa; Winnebago
Aruncus: Nitinaht
Asarum: Algonquin, Quebec; Cherokee; Iroquois
Aster: Cherokee; Cree, Woodlands; Iroquois
Astragalus: Dakota
Athyrium: Iroquois
Baccharis: Navajo, Kayenta
Balsamorhiza: Cheyenne
Barbula: Seminole
Berberis: Mohegan
Betula: Iroquois
Bidens: Seminole
Boebera: Keres, Western
Brassica: Cherokee
Brickellia: Diegueño; Navajo, Ramah
Bryum: Seminole
Callicarpa: Alabama
Calycadenia: Yana
Capsicum: Cherokee
Cardamine: Algonquin, Quebec; Iroquois
Castanea: Cherokee
Caulophyllum: Iroquois; Omaha; Ponca
Ceanothus: Modesse
Celastrus: Iroquois
Centaurium: Luiseño; Mahuna; Miwok
Cephalanthus: Choctaw; Seminole
Cercis: Alabama; Delaware; Delaware, Oklahoma; Mendocino Indian

Chamaedaphne: Potawatomi
Chelone: Cherokee
Chenopodium: Creek; Natchez
Chimaphila: Cherokee; Iroquois; Montana Indian
Chrysothamnus: Navajo, Ramah
Cicuta: Seminole
Cirsium: Navajo; Navajo, Kayenta
Clematis: Oregon Indian
Cleome: Oregon Indian
Clethra: Cherokee
Clintonia: Iroquois
Collomia: Okanagan-Colville
Comptonia: Chippewa
Conyza: Iroquois
Cordyline: Hawaiian
Cornus: Cherokee; Costanoan; Cree, Hudson Bay; Houma; Iroquois; Wet'suwet'en
Croton: Concow
Cunila: Cherokee
Cycloloma: Hopi
Cypripedium: Iroquois
Cystopteris: Cherokee
Dalea: Navajo, Ramah
Datura: Rappahannock
Daucus: Costanoan
Dennstaedtia: Cherokee
Desmodium: Seminole
Dracocephalum: Navajo, Ramah
Echinacea: Cheyenne
Echinocystis: Cherokee
Eleocharis: Seminole
Epilobium: Costanoan
Ericameria: Paiute
Erigeron: Miwok; Navajo, Ramah; Ojibwa
Eriodictyon: Cahuilla; Pomo, Kashaya; Round Valley Indian
Eriogonum: Keres, Western
Eryngium: Seminole
Erythronium: Cherokee
Eupatorium: Cherokee; Delaware; Delaware, Oklahoma; Houma; Iroquois; Menominee; Mohegan; Nanticoke; Seminole; Shinnecock
Euthamia: Potawatomi
Fraxinus: Costanoan
Galactia: Seminole
Gaultheria: Potawatomi
Gaura: Keres, Western
Gentiana: Iroquois
Geum: Iroquois; Okanagan-Colville
Gilia: Navajo, Ramah
Gleditsia: Meskwaki
Glycyrrhiza: Dakota; Keresan; Pawnee; Sioux
Gnaphalium: Koasati; Rappahannock
Gutierrezia: Isleta; Navajo, Ramah

Hamamelis: Cherokee
Hedeoma: Cherokee; Ojibwa
Helenium: Comanche
Helianthus: Pima; Shasta
Hepatica: Nanticoke
Heuchera: Shoshoni
Hexastylis: Rappahannock
Hierochloe: Flathead
Hoita: Costanoan
Holocarpha: Miwok
Humulus: Dakota
Hydrastis: Iroquois
Hypericum: Cherokee; Houma; Iroquois
Hyssopus: Cherokee
Ilex: Micmac
Impatiens: Iroquois
Inula: Iroquois
Ipomopsis: Okanagan-Colville
Juglans: Rappahannock
Juniperus: Cheyenne; Cree, Woodlands; Flathead;
    Kutenai; Mahuna; Navajo, Ramah; Nez Perce;
    Paiute; Seminole; Sioux
Krameria: Pima
Krascheninnikovia: Gosiute; Hopi; Tewa
Laportea: Houma
Larix: Iroquois
Larrea: Pima
Lechea: Seminole
Ledum: Montagnais
Lepechinia: Miwok
Leucanthemum: Menominee
Lilium: Malecite; Micmac
Lindera: Iroquois
Linnaea: Iroquois
Linum: Cherokee
Liquidambar: Houma
Liriodendron: Cherokee
Lobelia: Cherokee; Iroquois
Lomatium: Thompson
Lonicera: Iroquois
Lophophora: Kiowa
Lycopodium: Montagnais
Lysichiton: Quileute; Skokomish
Lythrum: Iroquois
Magnolia: Houma
Mahonia: Montana Indian
Malva: Costanoan; Diegueño; Iroquois
Matricaria: Costanoan; Diegueño
Melilotus: Iroquois
Melissa: Cherokee
Mentha: Algonquin, Tête-de-Boule; Cherokee; Cree,
    Woodlands; Flathead; Iroquois; Keres, Western;
    Keresan; Kutenai; Menominee; Navajo, Ramah;

Ojibwa; Okanagan-Colville; Paiute; Paiute,
    Northern; Potawatomi; Shoshoni; Sia; Washo
Mentzelia: Cheyenne; Dakota
Mirabilis: Dakota; Mahuna
Mitchella: Iroquois; Montagnais
Monarda: Cherokee; Delaware; Delaware, Okla-
    homa; Flathead; Koasati; Mohegan; Navajo,
    Ramah; Ojibwa; Sioux, Teton; Tewa
Monardella: Miwok
Monotropa: Mohegan
Myrica: Choctaw; Seminole
Nemopanthus: Malecite
Nepeta: Cherokee; Chippewa; Iroquois
Nuphar: Iroquois; Rappahannock
Octoblephorum: Seminole
Osmorhiza: Okanagan-Colville; Paiute; Shoshoni
Osmunda: Cherokee
Oxalis: Iroquois
Paeonia: Mahuna
Panax: Creek; Iroquois
Pediomelum: Cheyenne
Pellaea: Costanoan
Penstemon: Pawnee
Pericome: Navajo, Ramah
Persea: Creek; Seminole
Phacelia: Costanoan
Phytolacca: Cherokee
Piloblephis: Seminole
Pinus: Cherokee; Navajo, Ramah; Okanagan-
    Colville; Paiute; Shoshoni
Pityopsis: Seminole
Plantago: Costanoan; Rappahannock
Pleomele: Hawaiian
Pluchea: Choctaw
Polygonum: Iroquois; Potawatomi
Polystichum: Cherokee; Iroquois
Populus: Paiute
Porteranthus: Iroquois
Potentilla: Cherokee
Prosopis: Diegueño
Prunella: Algonquin, Quebec; Delaware; Delaware,
    Oklahoma; Iroquois; Mohegan
Prunus: Cherokee; Iroquois
Pseudotsuga: Okanagan-Colville
Pterocaulon: Seminole
Purshia: Navajo, Ramah
Pycnanthemum: Cherokee; Chippewa; Meskwaki
Quercus: Cherokee
Ratibida: Navajo, Ramah
Rhus: Malecite
Ricinus: Hawaiian
Rorippa: Costanoan; Iroquois
Rosa: Costanoan; Diegueño; Mahuna; Tanana,
    Upper

Rubus: Micmac
Rudbeckia: Seminole
Rumex: Houma
Sabal: Seminole
Sabatia: Seminole
Sagittaria: Cherokee
Salix: Blackfoot; Cherokee; Costanoan; Houma; Koasati; Mendocino Indian; Mewuk; Montana Indian; Pima; Seminole
Salvia: Costanoan; Paiute
Sambucus: Cahuilla; Diegueño; Iroquois; Kawaiisu; Mendocino Indian; Menominee; Montana Indian; Pima; Pomo, Kashaya; Yuki
Sanguinaria: Iroquois
Sanicula: Ojibwa
Sanvitalia: Navajo, Ramah
Sarracenia: Iroquois
Sassafras: Iroquois; Nanticoke; Rappahannock; Seminole
Satureja: Cahuilla; Luiseño
Saururus: Seminole
Scrophularia: Diegueño
Scutellaria: Mendocino Indian
Senecio: Iroquois
Senna: Cherokee
Shepherdia: Navajo
Sinapis: Cherokee
Sisyrinchium: Costanoan
Smallanthus: Iroquois
Solanum: Delaware, Oklahoma
Solidago: Cherokee; Delaware; Delaware, Oklahoma; Iroquois; Okanagan-Colville; Potawatomi
Sorbus: Wet'suwet'en
Sparganium: Iroquois
Symphoricarpos: Cree, Woodlands; Nez Perce
Symplocos: Choctaw
Tagetes: Navajo
Tanacetum: Chippewa; Ojibwa
Taxus: Micmac; Montagnais
Tephrosia: Catawba
Tetraclea: Navajo, Ramah
Tetradymia: Navajo, Ramah
Thalictrum: Ojibwa
Thuja: Algonquin, Quebec; Iroquois; Quinault
Thymophylla: Isleta
Thymus: Delaware, Ontario
Tillandsia: Houma
Torreya: Costanoan
Toxicodendron: Cherokee
Triadenum: Potawatomi
Trichostema: Concow
Trifolium: Cherokee
Triosteum: Cherokee
Tsuga: Iroquois

Urtica: Potawatomi
Vaccinium: Seminole
Veratrum: Paiute
Verbascum: Iroquois; Nanticoke; Navajo, Ramah
Verbena: Cherokee; Costanoan; Delaware, Oklahoma; Mahuna; Navajo, Ramah
Verbesina: Choctaw; Hopi; Seminole
Veronica: Cherokee
Veronicastrum: Cherokee; Iroquois
Viburnum: Cherokee; Iroquois
Vitis: Choctaw; Mohegan; Seminole
Wyethia: Miwok; Paiute
Xanthium: Houma
Zanthoxylum: Comanche
Zinnia: Zuni
Zizia: Meskwaki

Gastrointestinal Aid

Abies: Bella Coola; Cherokee; Hanaksiala; Micmac; Okanagan-Colville
Abronia: Navajo; Navajo, Kayenta; Ute; Zuni
Abutilon: Hawaiian
Acer: Iroquois
Achillea: Aleut; Cherokee; Costanoan; Cowlitz; Gosiute; Hesquiat; Iroquois; Mendocino Indian; Mohegan; Okanagan-Colville; Paiute; Shoshoni; Squaxin; Thompson
Acorus: Blackfoot; Cherokee; Cheyenne; Cree; Cree, Woodlands; Dakota; Delaware; Iroquois; Menominee; Meskwaki; Nanticoke; Ojibwa; Omaha; Pawnee; Ponca; Rappahannock; Winnebago
Actaea: Ojibwa; Ojibwa, South
Adenostoma: Cahuilla; Coahuilla; Diegueño
Adiantum: Costanoan; Makah
Aesculus: Cherokee
Agastache: Paiute
Agrimonia: Cherokee
Aletris: Catawba; Micmac
Aleurites: Hawaiian
Alisma: Cherokee; Cree, Woodlands
Allium: Cherokee
Alnus: Carrier, Northern; Cherokee; Clallam; Mendocino Indian; Ojibwa; Swinomish
Amaranthus: Keres, Western
Ambrosia: Cheyenne; Diegueño
Amelanchier: Blackfoot; Thompson
Amorpha: Ojibwa, South
Amphicarpaea: Iroquois
Anaphalis: Iroquois; Okanagan-Colville
Andropogon: Chippewa; Seminole
Anemopsis: Cahuilla; Pima; Shoshoni
Angelica: Blackfoot; Delaware; Delaware, Oklahoma; Pomo, Kashaya

Antennaria: Cherokee
Anthemis: Iroquois
Apocynum: Iroquois; Navajo, Ramah
Aquilegia: Gosiute; Meskwaki; Ojibwa; Paiute; Shoshoni
Arabis: Keres, Western; Okanagan-Colville
Aralia: Bella Coola; Choctaw; Iroquois; Mendocino Indian; Menominee
Arbutus: Cahuilla; Miwok; Skokomish; Yuki
Arceuthobium: Mendocino Indian
Arctium: Ojibwa
Arctostaphylos: Miwok
Arenaria: Gosiute
Aristolochia: Cherokee; Choctaw
Armoracia: Cherokee
Artemisia: Blackfoot; Cherokee; Chippewa; Coahuilla; Costanoan; Eskimo, Western; Havasupai; Hopi; Isleta; Kiowa; Lakota; Mendocino Indian; Mewuk; Navajo; Okanagan-Colville; Paiute; Pomo, Kashaya; Sanpoil; Shoshoni; Tewa; Thompson
Aruncus: Bella Coola; Thompson
Asarum: Bella Coola; Cherokee; Chippewa; Malecite; Menominee; Meskwaki; Micmac; Ojibwa; Okanagon; Thompson
Asclepias: Flathead; Iroquois; Keres, Western; Omaha; Pima; Ponca
Aster: Mohegan; Navajo, Ramah; Okanagon; Thompson
Astragalus: Cree, Woodlands
Atriplex: Navajo, Kayenta; Navajo, Ramah; Zuni
Baccharis: Diegueño
Balsamorhiza: Cheyenne; Paiute
Baptisia: Iroquois; Pawnee
Bellis: Iroquois
Betula: Cherokee; Chippewa; Delaware, Oklahoma; Eskimo, Western; Ojibwa
Blechnum: Makah; Quinault
Brassica: Navajo, Ramah
Brickellia: Shoshoni
Callicarpa: Choctaw; Koasati
Calocedrus: Mendocino Indian
Calycanthus: Pomo, Kashaya
Capsella: Chippewa; Mohegan
Capsicum: Cherokee
Cardamine: Delaware; Delaware, Oklahoma; Iroquois; Menominee; Ojibwa
Carex: Iroquois; Navajo, Ramah
Carya: Cherokee
Castanea: Cherokee; Koasati
Castilleja: Navajo; Navajo, Ramah; Ute
Caulophyllum: Cherokee; Chippewa
Ceanothus: Cherokee; Chippewa; Menominee; Meskwaki

Celastrus: Cherokee; Ojibwa
Celtis: Navajo, Kayenta
Centaurium: Mahuna; Miwok
Cephalanthus: Seminole
Cercocarpus: Navajo; Navajo, Ramah; Paiute
Chaenactis: Shoshoni; Thompson
Chaetopappa: Havasupai
Chamaebatiaria: Shoshoni
Chamaemelum: Cherokee; Mahuna
Chamaesyce: Houma; Navajo; Navajo, Ramah; Omaha; Pima
Chenopodium: Cahuilla; Mendocino Indian; Seminole
Chimaphila: Micmac; Ojibwa; Rappahannock
Chlorogalum: Wailaki
Chrysothamnus: Shoshoni; Thompson
Cirsium: Cherokee; Meskwaki; Ojibwa; Shuswap
Clematis: Cherokee; Shoshoni; Yavapai
Cleome: Tewa
Clethra: Cherokee
Comarum: Ojibwa
Comptonia: Ojibwa
Convolvulus: Navajo, Ramah
Conyza: Chippewa; Navajo, Kayenta
Coptis: Iroquois
Cornus: Cherokee; Iroquois; Ojibwa; Okanagan-Colville; Saanich; Thompson
Corydalis: Navajo, Ramah
Corylus: Algonquin, Quebec; Iroquois
Crataegus: Iroquois; Okanagon; Potawatomi; Thompson
Croton: Apache, White Mountain; Lakota; Zuni
Cryptantha: Navajo, Kayenta; Ute
Cucurbita: Navajo
Cymopterus: Keres, Western; Navajo, Kayenta
Cynoglossum: Pomo, Potter Valley
Cypripedium: Algonquin, Tête-de-Boule; Cherokee; Chippewa; Iroquois
Dalea: Dakota; Navajo; Navajo, Ramah; Zuni
Datura: Pima; Tubatulabal; Yokut
Descurainia: Cahuilla
Desmodium: Iroquois; Seminole
Diervilla: Chippewa
Diospyros: Cherokee
Diplacus: Tubatulabal
Dryopteris: Eskimo, Western; Ojibwa
Dyssodia: Navajo, Ramah
Echinacea: Choctaw; Crow; Lakota; Meskwaki; Sioux, Teton
Echinocystis: Ojibwa
Ephedra: Diegueño; Navajo; Navajo, Ramah; Paiute; Shoshoni
Epigaea: Cherokee; Iroquois

Epilobium: Cheyenne; Eskimo, Western; Navajo, Kayenta
Equisetum: Ojibwa
Eriastrum: Paiute; Paiute, Northern
Ericameria: Miwok; Paiute; Shoshoni
Erigeron: Navajo, Kayenta; Paiute; Shoshoni
Eriodictyon: Hualapai; Kawaiisu; Miwok; Shoshoni
Eriogonum: Coahuilla; Comanche; Gosiute; Karok; Mahuna; Navajo, Kayenta; Navajo, Ramah; Paiute; Round Valley Indian; Thompson; Tubatulabal; Zuni
Erodium: Zuni
Eryngium: Cherokee; Creek; Seminole
Erysimum: Sioux, Teton
Erythrina: Alabama
Eschscholzia: Mendocino Indian
Eupatorium: Cherokee; Delaware, Ontario; Iroquois; Mohegan
Euphorbia: Iroquois
Evernia: Blackfoot
Fendlera: Navajo
Foeniculum: Cherokee; Pomo, Kashaya
Fragaria: Cherokee; Ojibwa; Potawatomi
Frangula: Delaware, Oklahoma; Hesquiat; Kwakiutl; Nitinaht; Paiute; Thompson
Frasera: Cherokee; Havasupai
Fraxinus: Cherokee; Delaware, Oklahoma; Iroquois
Gaillardia: Blackfoot; Navajo, Ramah
Galium: Cherokee
Garrya: Kawaiisu
Gaultheria: Algonquin, Quebec; Algonquin, Tête-de-Boule; Cherokee; Nitinaht; Quinault
Gaura: Navajo, Ramah
Gentianella: Cherokee; Iroquois
Gentianopsis: Delaware; Delaware, Oklahoma
Geum: Bella Coola; Chippewa; Hesquiat
Gleditsia: Cherokee
Glycyrrhiza: Cheyenne
Gnaphalium: Costanoan; Miwok
Goodyera: Potawatomi
Grindelia: Dakota; Keres, Western; Navajo, Ramah; Shoshoni; Sioux
Gutierrezia: Navajo, Kayenta; Navajo, Ramah; Tewa
Hedeoma: Delaware; Delaware, Oklahoma; Mohegan; Ojibwa; Shoshoni
Helenium: Meskwaki
Helianthus: Navajo
Hepatica: Cherokee
Heracleum: Iroquois; Meskwaki; Omaha
Heteromeles: Mendocino Indian
Heterotheca: Navajo, Ramah
Heuchera: Blackfoot; Cherokee; Chippewa; Flathead; Gosiute; Menominee; Navajo; Navajo, Ramah
Hexastylis: Catawba; Cherokee

Hieracium: Cherokee
Holodiscus: Paiute; Shoshoni
Houstonia: Keres, Western
Humulus: Dakota
Huperzia: Nitinaht
Hydrangea: Cherokee
Hydrastis: Cherokee; Iroquois
Hymenopappus: Isleta
Hymenoxys: Zuni
Hypericum: Cherokee; Choctaw
Ilex: Cherokee; Iroquois
Impatiens: Cherokee; Potawatomi
Inula: Delaware; Delaware, Oklahoma; Iroquois
Ipomoea: Iroquois; Keres, Western; Lakota
Ipomopsis: Hopi; Navajo; Navajo, Kayenta; Navajo, Ramah; Paiute; Shoshoni; Washo
Iris: Paiute; Shoshoni
Iva: Shoshoni
Juglans: Delaware; Delaware, Oklahoma; Rappahannock
Juniperus: Arapaho; Bella Coola; Crow; Hopi; Jemez; Keres, Western; Navajo, Ramah; Paiute; Tewa; Thompson
Kalmia: Cree, Hudson Bay; Montagnais
Lachnanthes: Cherokee
Lactuca: Isleta; Navajo
Larix: Thompson
Larrea: Cahuilla; Coahuilla; Mahuna; Paiute; Pima
Lathyrus: Ojibwa
Lechea: Seminole
Ledum: Bella Coola; Eskimo, Alaska; Eskimo, Western; Tanana, Upper
Leonurus: Cherokee; Iroquois
Lepidium: Diegueño; Navajo, Kayenta
Lesquerella: Okanagan-Colville
Liatris: Blackfoot; Cherokee; Omaha; Seminole
Licania: Seminole
Ligusticum: Atsugewi; Cherokee; Creek
Lilium: Algonquin, Quebec
Linnaea: Iroquois
Linum: Hopi; Navajo, Ramah; Paiute
Liriodendron: Cherokee
Lithophragma: Mendocino Indian
Lithospermum: Zuni
Lobelia: Cherokee; Iroquois
Lomatium: Cheyenne; Gosiute; Kawaiisu; Kwakiutl; Salish, Coast
Lonicera: Blackfoot
Lophophora: Kiowa
Lotus: Navajo, Ramah
Luetkea: Okanagon; Thompson
Lupinus: Karok
Lycopodium: Montagnais
Lycopus: Meskwaki

Pseudocymopterus: Navajo, Ramah
Pseudotsuga: Bella Coola; Hanaksiala; Navajo, Kayenta
Psilostrophe: Navajo, Ramah
Psoralidium: Navajo, Ramah; Zuni
Psorothamnus: Keres, Western; Paiute; Shoshoni
Ptelea: Havasupai
Pterocaulon: Seminole
Pulsatilla: Okanagon; Thompson
Purshia: Paiute, Northern
Pycnanthemum: Cherokee
Pyrola: Iroquois
Quercus: Cherokee; Chippewa; Choctaw; Delaware; Delaware, Oklahoma
Ranunculus: Iroquois
Ratibida: Lakota; Navajo, Ramah
Rhamnus: Kawaiisu
Rhododendron: Okanagon; Skokomish; Thompson
Rhus: Chippewa; Keres, Western; Kiowa; Mahuna; Menominee; Navajo, Kayenta; Navajo, Ramah; Thompson
Ribes: Hopi; Thompson
Rosa: Costanoan; Iroquois; Mahuna; Menominee; Meskwaki; Miwok; Ojibwa; Tanana, Upper
Rubus: Bella Coola; Cherokee; Hawaiian; Hesquiat; Iroquois; Meskwaki; Ojibwa, South; Okanagan-Colville; Okanagon; Omaha; Pomo, Kashaya; Saanich; Seminole; Skagit; Skagit, Upper; Thompson
Rudbeckia: Chippewa
Rumex: Houma; Iroquois; Isleta; Kawaiisu; Kwakiutl; Lakota; Mohegan; Navajo, Kayenta; Paiute; Yavapai
Ruta: Costanoan; Diegueño
Sagittaria: Chippewa; Ojibwa
Salix: Cheyenne; Koasati; Menominee; Ojibwa; Okanagan-Colville; Seminole
Salvia: Kawaiisu; Paiute; Shoshoni
Sambucus: Bella Coola; Cahuilla; Choctaw; Delaware, Oklahoma; Haisla & Hanaksiala; Hesquiat; Iroquois; Mohegan; Montana Indian; Paiute; Pima; Pomo, Potter Valley; Seminole; Yokia
Sanguinaria: Chippewa; Delaware; Delaware, Oklahoma; Iroquois; Ojibwa
Sanicula: Cherokee
Sarcobatus: Navajo, Ramah
Sassafras: Seminole
Satureja: Mendocino Indian; Pomo; Pomo, Kashaya
Saururus: Ojibwa
Scutellaria: Delaware
Sedum: Eskimo, Western
Senecio: Keres, Western; Navajo, Ramah; Yavapai
Shepherdia: Blackfoot; Salish; Shuswap; Thompson
Silene: Gosiute

Silphium: Ojibwa
Sisyrinchium: Cherokee; Costanoan; Mahuna; Pomo, Kashaya
Sium: Lakota
Smilax: Cherokee; Iroquois
Solanum: Iroquois; Lakota; Navajo; Nootka; Zuni
Solidago: Iroquois
Sorbus: Bella Coola; Iroquois; Micmac
Sphaeralcea: Navajo, Ramah; Pima
Spiraea: Okanagan-Colville; Shuswap; Thompson
Stachys: Chippewa; Costanoan
Stenotus: Navajo
Streptopus: Thompson
Suaeda: Navajo, Kayenta
Symphoricarpos: Miwok; Paiute; Thompson
Symphytum: Cherokee
Syzygium: Hawaiian
Tagetes: Navajo
Tanacetum: Delaware, Ontario; Mohegan
Taraxacum: Aleut; Bella Coola; Ojibwa; Rappahannock
Taxus: Haihais; Karok; Kitasoo; Micmac
Tetradymia: Navajo, Ramah; Paiute; Shoshoni
Tetraneuris: Navajo, Ramah
Thalictrum: Potawatomi
Thamnosma: Havasupai
Thaspium: Chippewa
Thuja: Algonquin, Quebec; Bella Coola
Thysanocarpus: Mendocino Indian
Tilia: Cherokee
Tiquilia: Navajo, Kayenta
Torreya: Costanoan
Townsendia: Navajo
Tradescantia: Cherokee
Trichostema: Cahuilla; Costanoan; Kawaiisu
Trillium: Cherokee
Triodanis: Cherokee
Triosteum: Iroquois
Tsuga: Gitksan; Menominee; Micmac
Typha: Cheyenne
Ulmus: Cherokee; Iroquois; Koasati; Ojibwa
Umbellularia: Mendocino Indian
Urtica: Cherokee; Hesquiat; Lakota
Uvularia: Ojibwa
Vaccinium: Algonquin, Quebec
Valeriana: Blackfoot; Eskimo; Eskimo, Inuktitut; Thompson
Veratrum: Bella Coola; Blackfoot
Verbena: Cherokee; Costanoan; Dakota; Iroquois; Mahuna
Verbesina: Navajo; Seminole; Zuni
Vernonia: Cherokee
Veronica: Navajo, Ramah
Veronicastrum: Cherokee; Iroquois

Viburnum: Chippewa; Menominee; Ojibwa; Tanana, Upper
Vicia: Cherokee; Rappahannock
Viola: Carrier, Southern; Iroquois
Vitis: Cherokee; Iroquois; Ojibwa; Seminole
Wyethia: Mendocino Indian; Navajo, Kayenta
Xanthium: Cherokee
Xanthorhiza: Catawba
Yucca: Lakota; Navajo
Zanthoxylum: Iroquois
Zinnia: Navajo, Ramah

Gland Medicine

Abies: Okanagan-Colville
Chamaesyce: Iroquois
Nymphaea: Micmac
Phytolacca: Delaware
Stanleya: Navajo
Veratrum: Paiute; Shoshoni
Verbascum: Cherokee

Gynecological Aid

Abies: Algonquin, Quebec; Cherokee; Iroquois
Acer: Cherokee; Thompson
Achillea: Blackfoot; Cherokee; Clallam; Klallam; Kwakiutl; Makah; Paiute
Acorus: Algonquin, Quebec
Acourtia: Navajo, Kayenta
Actaea: Cheyenne; Chippewa; Cree, Woodlands; Meskwaki; Ojibwa; Potawatomi
Adiantum: Costanoan; Iroquois; Menominee; Potawatomi
Aesculus: Cherokee
Ageratina: Iroquois
Agrimonia: Cherokee
Aletris: Cherokee; Rappahannock
Alisma: Iroquois
Alnus: Cherokee; Chippewa; Mendocino Indian; Okanagan-Colville; Potawatomi
Amaranthus: Cherokee
Ambrosia: Houma; Keres, Western; Navajo; Pima
Amelanchier: Chippewa; Iroquois; Navajo; Ojibwa; Pomo; Pomo, Kashaya; Thompson
Androsace: Navajo, Ramah
Anemopsis: Costanoan
Angelica: Iroquois; Pomo, Kashaya;
Antennaria: Cherokee; Iroquois; Meskwaki; Ojibwa
Anthemis: Karok
Apocynum: Cree, Woodlands; Iroquois; Keres, Western; Meskwaki; Ojibwa; Sanpoil
Aquilegia: Cherokee; Navajo, Kayenta
Aralia: Cherokee; Cree, Woodlands; Iroquois; Meskwaki; Micmac
Arctium: Cherokee; Meskwaki

Arctostaphylos: Cree, Woodlands
Arisaema: Iroquois; Menominee
Artemisia: Blackfoot; Cahuilla; Cherokee; Cheyenne; Chippewa; Comanche; Karok; Lakota; Mahuna; Mendocino Indian; Navajo; Navajo, Ramah; Okanagan-Colville; Okanagon; Paiute; Pomo; Pomo, Kashaya; Shoshoni; Shuswap; Thompson; Yuki
Aruncus: Cherokee
Asarum: Cherokee
Asclepias: Cherokee; Chippewa; Delaware; Delaware, Oklahoma; Hopi; Iroquois; Keres, Western; Lakota; Navajo; Ojibwa
Aster: Cree, Woodlands
Astragalus: Kawaiisu; Lakota
Athyrium: Makah; Meskwaki; Ojibwa; Potawatomi
Baccharis: Cahuilla
Bahia: Navajo, Ramah
Balsamorhiza: Cheyenne; Washo
Baptisia: Cherokee; Delaware; Delaware, Oklahoma
Betula: Cree, Woodlands; Iroquois; Ojibwa
Bouteloua: Navajo, Ramah
Calamagrostis: Thompson
Calliandra: Yavapai
Calochortus: Navajo, Ramah
Caltha: Chippewa
Camassia: Blackfoot
Campanula: Iroquois; Navajo, Kayenta
Capsicum: Navajo, Ramah
Carex: Iroquois
Carnegia: Pima
Carpinus: Delaware, Ontario; Iroquois
Carya: Delaware, Ontario
Cassytha: Hawaiian
Castanea: Cherokee
Castilleja: Hopi; Navajo, Ramah; Tewa
Caulophyllum: Cherokee; Menominee; Meskwaki; Ojibwa; Potawatomi
Ceanothus: Karok
Celastrus: Cherokee; Creek; Iroquois; Meskwaki
Celtis: Iroquois
Cerastium: Iroquois
Cercocarpus: Kawaiisu; Navajo, Ramah
Chaetopappa: Zuni
Chamaesyce: Cherokee; Iroquois; Keres, Western; Navajo, Ramah; Ponca; Zuni
Cheilanthes: Keres, Western
Chenopodium: Iroquois
Chimaphila: Iroquois; Karok; Menominee; Okanagon; Thompson
Chrysothamnus: Navajo, Ramah; Okanagan-Colville
Cimicifuga: Iroquois
Claytonia: Quinault

Clematis: Navajo
Clintonia: Ojibwa
Coeloglossum: Iroquois
Comptonia: Menominee
Conioselinum: Navajo, Kayenta
Convolvulus: Pomo; Pomo, Kashaya
Conyza: Chippewa; Houma
Cordylanthus: Navajo; Navajo, Kayenta; Navajo, Ramah
Cornus: Algonquin, Tête-de-Boule; Cherokee; Iroquois; Okanagan-Colville; Okanagon; Thompson
Corydalis: Navajo, Kayenta; Navajo, Ramah
Corylus: Iroquois
Crataegus: Iroquois
Crepis: Shoshoni
Cryptantha: Navajo; Navajo, Kayenta
Cucurbita: Hawaiian; Meskwaki; Omaha
Cunila: Cherokee
Cupressus: Kawaiisu
Cypripedium: Algonquin, Quebec; Cherokee; Menominee; Ojibwa
Darmera: Karok
Datura: Pima
Daucus: Iroquois
Delphinium: Hopi; Navajo, Kayenta
Diervilla: Cree, Woodlands; Iroquois
Dioscorea: Meskwaki
Dirca: Iroquois
Echeandia: Navajo, Ramah
Echium: Iroquois
Ephedra: Washo
Epigaea: Iroquois
Epilobium: Miwok
Equisetum: Menominee; Pomo, Kashaya; Thompson
Ericameria: Miwok
Erigeron: Houma; Navajo; Navajo, Kayenta; Navajo, Ramah
Eriogonum: Cheyenne; Keres, Western; Navajo, Ramah; Round Valley Indian; Zuni
Erodium: Jemez
Erysimum: Navajo, Ramah
Eschscholzia: Mendocino Indian; Pomo, Kashaya
Euonymus: Cherokee; Iroquois; Winnebago
Eupatorium: Algonquin, Quebec; Cherokee; Chippewa; Iroquois; Menominee; Potawatomi
Euphorbia: Cherokee; Keres, Western; Lakota; Navajo; Navajo, Kayenta; Navajo, Ramah
Foeniculum: Cherokee
Fraxinus: Cherokee; Micmac; Penobscot
Freycinetia: Hawaiian
Gaillardia: Keres, Western
Gaura: Navajo, Kayenta
Gentiana: Meskwaki
Geranium: Thompson

Geum: Chippewa; Hesquiat; Klallam; Ojibwa; Okanagan-Colville; Quinault
Gilia: Navajo, Kayenta
Glyceria: Ojibwa
Glycyrrhiza: Meskwaki
Goodyera: Delaware; Delaware, Oklahoma; Okanagon; Potawatomi; Thompson
Gossypium: Koasati
Grindelia: Cree
Gutierrezia: Jemez; Navajo, Ramah; Tewa
Gymnocladus: Omaha
Hamamelis: Cherokee; Iroquois
Hedeoma: Rappahannock
Helenium: Cherokee; Comanche
Helianthus: Pawnee
Hepatica: Iroquois; Menominee
Heracleum: Kwakiutl; Micmac
Heuchera: Cherokee; Navajo, Ramah
Hibiscus: Hawaiian
Hierochloe: Karok
Houstonia: Navajo, Kayenta
Humulus: Cherokee
Hydrangea: Cherokee
Hymenoxys: Hopi
Hypericum: Houma
Impatiens: Cherokee; Iroquois
Inula: Cherokee; Iroquois
Ipomopsis: Hopi; Navajo, Kayenta; Navajo, Ramah
Iris: Iroquois; Pomo
Juglans: Iroquois
Juniperus: Apache, White Mountain; Cheyenne; Comanche; Cree, Woodlands; Crow; Delaware, Ontario; Hopi; Isleta; Jemez; Navajo, Ramah; Paiute; Tewa; Thompson; Zuni
Lachnanthes: Cherokee
Lactuca: Meskwaki; Ojibwa
Laportea: Iroquois
Lappula: Navajo
Larix: Thompson
Larrea: Cahuilla; Papago
Lathyrus: Navajo, Kayenta
Ledum: Makah
Leonurus: Delaware; Delaware, Oklahoma; Micmac; Mohegan; Shinnecock
Leptodactylon: Navajo, Ramah
Lesquerella: Hopi
Lewisia: Flathead; Nez Perce
Lilium: Iroquois
Lindera: Rappahannock
Linnaea: Algonquin, Quebec; Potawatomi
Linum: Hopi
Liquidambar: Cherokee
Lobelia: Iroquois
Lomatium: Kwakiutl

Lonicera: Algonquin, Quebec; Cree, Woodlands; Iroquois; Kwakiutl; Makah; Okanagan-Colville; Quinault; Squaxin; Swinomish

Lotus: Karok

Luetkea: Okanagon; Thompson

Lycopodium: Aleut; Iroquois

Lygodesmia: Blackfoot; Cheyenne; Hopi; Omaha; Ponca; Sioux

Lysichiton: Quileute

Lysimachia: Cherokee; Iroquois

Machaeranthera: Hopi

Mahonia: Flathead

Maianthemum: Chippewa; Delaware; Delaware, Oklahoma; Iroquois; Ojibwa; Ojibwa, South; Paiute; Shoshoni; Thompson

Malus: Iroquois

Marrubium: Navajo, Ramah

Matelea: Comanche

Matricaria: Diegueño; Montana Indian

Matteuccia: Cree, Woodlands

Menispermum: Cherokee

Menodora: Navajo, Ramah

Mertensia: Cheyenne

Mirabilis: Hopi; Navajo, Kayenta; Pawnee

Mitchella: Cherokee; Delaware, Oklahoma; Iroquois; Menominee

Monarda: Flathead; Montana Indian; Sioux

Monotropa: Potawatomi

Napaea: Meskwaki

Nicotiana: Kawaiisu; Tewa

Nuphar: Gitksan; Kitasoo

Nyssa: Cherokee

Oenanthe: Nitinaht

Oenothera: Navajo, Kayenta

Onoclea: Iroquois; Ojibwa

Oplopanax: Carrier, Southern; Lummi; Skagit

Opuntia: Navajo, Ramah; Pima

Orbexilum: Cherokee

Osmorhiza: Blackfoot; Chippewa; Ojibwa; Shoshoni

Osmunda: Iroquois; Menominee

Ostrya: Delaware, Ontario

Oxydendrum: Catawba

Panax: Cherokee; Iroquois

Pastinaca: Ojibwa

Pellaea: Yavapai

Pennellia: Navajo, Ramah

Penstemon: Iroquois; Navajo, Ramah

Pentagrama: Karok

Pentaphylloides: Tanana, Upper

Peperomia: Hawaiian

Pericome: Navajo, Ramah

Petradoria: Hopi

Petroselinum: Cherokee

Phacelia: Thompson

Phegopteris: Hawaiian

Phlox: Navajo; Navajo, Ramah

Phoenicaulis: Paiute

Phoradendron: Cherokee; Zuni

Physocarpus: Iroquois; Menominee

Phytolacca: Mohegan

Picea: Algonquin, Quebec

Pinus: Cherokee; Flathead; Kawaiisu; Paiute

Piper: Hawaiian

Plantago: Cherokee; Delaware; Delaware, Oklahoma; Iroquois

Platanthera: Iroquois

Platanus: Cherokee

Polygonatum: Cherokee

Polygonum: Choctaw; Iroquois; Menominee; Meskwaki

Polystichum: Iroquois; Kwakiutl; Lummi

Polytaenia: Meskwaki

Polytrichum: Nitinaht

Populus: Blackfoot; Chippewa; Cree; Delaware, Oklahoma; Thompson

Potentilla: Navajo, Kayenta; Okanagan-Colville

Prenanthes: Chippewa; Ojibwa

Prosopis: Pima

Prunella: Iroquois; Ojibwa

Prunus: Cherokee; Delaware, Ontario; Iroquois; Kwakiutl; Lummi; Ojibwa, South; Quinault; Skagit; Skokomish; Thompson

Pseudotsuga: Hanaksiala

Psilostrophe: Navajo, Kayenta

Psoralidium: Navajo, Ramah

Pteridium: Iroquois; Menominee; Ojibwa

Pterocaulon: Seminole

Pulsatilla: Blackfoot

Purshia: Kawaiisu; Navajo; Navajo, Ramah

Pyrola: Navajo, Kayenta

Quercus: Cherokee; Choctaw; Delaware; Delaware, Oklahoma; Delaware, Ontario; Iroquois; Karok; Navajo, Ramah

Ranunculus: Hesquiat

Ratibida: Keres, Western

Reverchonia: Hopi

Rhamnus: Kawaiisu

Rhododendron: Cherokee

Rhus: Cherokee; Diegueño; Iroquois; Keres, Western; Menominee; Navajo, Ramah; Okanagan-Colville; Omaha; Pawnee

Ribes: Blackfoot; Chippewa; Cree, Woodlands; Meskwaki; Ojibwa; Potawatomi; Skagit; Skagit, Upper; Thompson; Winnebago

Rorippa: Navajo

Rosa: Chehalis; Iroquois; Squaxin; Thompson

Rubus: Cherokee; Chippewa; Cree, Woodlands; Iroquois; Kwakiutl; Pomo, Kashaya; Quinault

Rudbeckia: Cherokee
Rumex: Apache, White Mountain; Iroquois; Lakota; Navajo, Ramah
Sabatia: Cherokee
Salix: Algonquin, Tête-de-Boule; Catawba; Okanagan-Colville
Salvia: Cherokee; Mahuna
Sambucus: Creek; Hoh; Kwakiutl; Luiseño; Meskwaki; Paiute; Quileute; Quinault
Sanguinaria: Iroquois
Sanicula: Chippewa; Micmac
Sanvitalia: Navajo, Ramah
Sarracenia: Algonquin, Quebec; Cree, Woodlands; Ojibwa; Potawatomi
Sassafras: Iroquois
Scrophularia: Iroquois
Scutellaria: Cherokee
Sedum: Bella Coola; Okanagan-Colville; Songish
Selaginella: Blackfoot
Senecio: Cherokee; Costanoan; Keres, Western; Navajo, Ramah
Sesamum: Cherokee
Shepherdia: Carrier; Umatilla
Sida: Hawaiian
Silphium: Cherokee; Meskwaki
Sisyrinchium: Menominee; Meskwaki
Smallanthus: Cherokee
Smilax: Cherokee
Solanum: Keresan
Solidago: Cahuilla; Chippewa; Shuswap
Sonchus: Potawatomi
Sorbus: Micmac
Sphaeralcea: Keres, Western
Spiraea: Ojibwa; Okanagan-Colville
Staphylea: Iroquois
Stenotaphrum: Hawaiian
Stephanomeria: Hopi; Navajo, Ramah
Streptopus: Iroquois; Makah
Stylosanthes: Cherokee
Symphoricarpos: Meskwaki; Ojibwa; Thompson
Symphytum: Cherokee
Symplocarpus: Iroquois
Tanacetum: Cherokee
Taraxacum: Chippewa; Kiowa; Navajo, Ramah; Papago
Taxus: Algonquin, Quebec; Micmac
Tephrosia: Mahuna
Tetradymia: Hopi
Tetraneuris: Hopi
Thamnosma: Paiute
Thelypteris: Iroquois
Thermopsis: Pomo, Kashaya
Thuja: Algonquin, Quebec; Iroquois; Thompson
Tilia: Iroquois

Townsendia: Keres, Western; Navajo; Navajo, Kayenta; Navajo, Ramah
Tradescantia: Cherokee
Trichostema: Miwok
Trifolium: Cherokee; Iroquois
Trillium: Algonquin, Tête-de-Boule; Cherokee; Potawatomi
Triosteum: Iroquois
Tsuga: Algonquin, Quebec; Cherokee; Kwakiutl
Typha: Iroquois
Ulmus: Alabama; Cherokee; Cheyenne; Choctaw; Iroquois; Meskwaki
Umbellularia: Karok; Pomo, Kashaya
Urtica: Cowlitz; Cree, Woodlands; Kwakiutl; Lummi; Quinault; Squaxin
Vaccinium: Algonquin, Quebec; Cree, Woodlands; Makah
Valeriana: Cree, Woodlands
Veratrum: Paiute; Shoshoni
Verbascum: Cherokee
Verbena: Meskwaki
Verbesina: Chickasaw
Vernonia: Cherokee
Veronica: Cherokee
Veronicastrum: Meskwaki
Viburnum: Chippewa; Delaware, Oklahoma; Iroquois; Micmac
Vicia: Iroquois
Viola: Makah
Vitis: Cherokee; Choctaw; Delaware, Oklahoma; Ojibwa
Woodsia: Keres, Western
Xanthium: Koasati
Yucca: Lakota; Navajo, Ramah; Tewa
Zanthoxylum: Iroquois
Zea: Tewa
Zeuxine: Seminole

Hallucinogen

Acorus: Cree, Alberta
Cardamine: Iroquois
Clematis: Iroquois
Cypripedium: Menominee
Datura: Cahuilla; Chumash; Coahuilla; Costanoan; Diegueño; Gabrielino; Hopi; Kawaiisu; Luiseño; Miwok; Navajo, Ramah; Paiute; Paiute, Northern; Shoshoni
Ilex: Cherokee
Lophophora: Ponca
Magnolia: Rappahannock
Mirabilis: Hopi
Nicotiana: Kawaiisu
Thamnosma: Kawaiisu

Heart Medicine

Abies: Algonquin, Quebec
Achillea: Cheyenne
Acorus: Algonquin, Quebec; Ojibwa
Adiantum: Cherokee
Agastache: Cheyenne
Alisma: Cree, Woodlands
Alnus: Cherokee
Ambrosia: Iroquois
Apocynum: Chippewa; Potawatomi
Aquilegia: Cherokee; Gosiute
Aralia: Algonquin, Quebec
Artemisia: Chippewa
Asarum: Cherokee
Asclepias: Cherokee
Campanula: Cree, Woodlands
Cardamine: Algonquin, Quebec; Iroquois
Castanea: Cherokee
Cercocarpus: Paiute; Shoshoni
Chaenactis: Great Basin Indian; Nevada Indian; Paiute
Chimaphila: Cree, Woodlands
Clintonia: Iroquois
Collinsonia: Iroquois
Consolida: Cherokee
Coptis: Algonquin, Quebec
Cornus: Okanagan-Colville
Corylus: Algonquin, Quebec; Algonquin, Tête-de-Boule
Crataegus: Cherokee
Croton: Kawaiisu
Dalea: Chippewa
Delphinium: Cherokee
Dicentra: Kawaiisu
Distichlis: Kawaiisu
Echinocereus: Navajo
Erigeron: Catawba
Eriogonum: Diegueño; Keres, Western
Eryngium: Seminole
Festuca: Iroquois
Filipendula: Meskwaki
Geranium: Iroquois
Hamamelis: Iroquois
Helenium: Comanche
Helianthus: Paiute
Heterotheca: Navajo, Ramah
Heuchera: Shoshoni
Hexastylis: Catawba
Hydrastis: Iroquois
Hypoxis: Cherokee
Inula: Iroquois; Malecite; Micmac
Ipomoea: Houma
Juniperus: Shoshoni; Thompson
Lactuca: Bella Coola

Lewisia: Flathead
Liatris: Menominee
Ligusticum: Cree
Maianthemum: Thompson
Malus: Makah
Matricaria: Shuswap
Mentha: Blackfoot; Cheyenne
Menziesia: Kwakiutl
Monarda: Cherokee
Nuphar: Bella Coola; Iroquois
Paeonia: Paiute
Pedicularis: Iroquois
Peniocereus: Nevada Indian
Picea: Bella Coola
Pinus: Bella Coola
Polygala: Chippewa; Meskwaki; Seminole
Polygonum: Iroquois
Polypodium: Algonquin, Quebec
Polypogon: Navajo, Kayenta
Populus: Chippewa
Prunella: Bella Coola
Prunus: Bella Coola; Kwakiutl
Pycnanthemum: Cherokee
Quercus: Chippewa; Ojibwa
Rhododendron: Cherokee
Rhus: Okanagan-Colville
Rubus: Cree, Woodlands
Rudbeckia: Iroquois
Rumex: Hawaiian
Salvia: Costanoan
Sambucus: Iroquois
Sanguinaria: Algonquin, Quebec; Iroquois
Sanicula: Houma
Sassafras: Koasati
Scutellaria: Ojibwa
Senecio: Cherokee
Senna: Cherokee
Shepherdia: Thompson
Sonchus: Navajo, Kayenta
Symplocarpus: Menominee
Thalictrum: Iroquois
Thuja: Bella Coola
Tsuga: Bella Coola
Vaccinium: Flathead
Veratrum: Bella Coola
Verbascum: Ojibwa
Veronicastrum: Iroquois
Viburnum: Iroquois
Viola: Ojibwa; Potawatomi
Zanthoxylum: Delaware; Delaware, Oklahoma; Mohegan
Zea: Tewa

Hemorrhoid Remedy

Abies: Hanaksiala
Acer: Seminole
Achillea: Cherokee
Aesculus: Cherokee; Costanoan; Kawaiisu
Alnus: Cherokee; Potawatomi
Andropogon: Rappahannock
Argemone: Tubatulabal
Aster: Okanagan-Colville
Baptisia: Meskwaki
Betula: Iroquois
Cirsium: Iroquois
Cornus: Algonquin, Quebec; Menominee; Ojibwa; Wet'suwet'en
Corydalis: Iroquois
Croton: Keres, Western
Datura: Delaware; Delaware, Oklahoma; Pima
Dimorphocarpa: Navajo, Kayenta
Diospyros: Cherokee
Equisetum: Keres, Western
Eupatorium: Iroquois
Geranium: Meskwaki
Heuchera: Cherokee
Lachnanthes: Cherokee
Lactuca: Iroquois
Malus: Cherokee
Mentha: Cherokee; Iroquois
Mitchella: Cherokee
Napaea: Meskwaki
Oenothera: Cherokee; Iroquois
Orobanche: Zuni
Philadelphus: Thompson
Phytolacca: Rappahannock
Picea: Tanana, Upper
Pinus: Cherokee; Seminole
Plantago: Thompson
Polygonum: Meskwaki
Prunella: Iroquois
Prunus: Meskwaki
Quercus: Micmac; Penobscot; Seminole
Rhus: Menominee
Rosa: Meskwaki
Rubus: Cherokee
Rumex: Iroquois
Salix: Iroquois
Sanguinaria: Iroquois; Malecite
Sedum: Okanagon; Thompson
Ulmus: Iroquois
Urtica: Thompson
Verbascum: Iroquois
Xanthorhiza: Cherokee

Hemostat

Achillea: Aleut; Cheyenne

Acorus: Cree, Woodlands
Acourtia: Pima
Agrimonia: Meskwaki; Potawatomi
Anemone: Chippewa; Okanagon; Thompson
Apocynum: Chippewa
Aquilegia: Navajo, Kayenta
Aralia: Chippewa
Artemisia: Blackfoot; Cheyenne; Chippewa; Eskimo, Alaska; Omaha; Shoshoni
Aster: Zuni
Astragalus: Chippewa
Balsamorhiza: Gosiute
Camellia: Makah
Chamaesyce: Navajo, Ramah
Cirsium: Iroquois
Cordylanthus: Navajo
Cornus: Iroquois
Cuscuta: Kawaiisu
Disporum: Okanagan-Colville
Equisetum: Menominee
Erigeron: Navajo, Ramah
Eriophorum: Ojibwa
Eryngium: Natchez
Frangula: Kawaiisu
Gayophytum: Navajo, Ramah
Gentianella: Meskwaki
Geranium: Cherokee; Cheyenne
Gutierrezia: Paiute
Gymnocladus: Omaha
Helianthus: Keres, Western
Heuchera: Blackfoot
Hypericum: Cherokee
Juglans: Iroquois
Juniperus: Zuni
Lactuca: Iroquois
Lappula: Navajo
Lathyrus: Chippewa
Lobelia: Cherokee
Lupinus: Navajo, Kayenta
Lycopodium: Blackfoot; Potawatomi
Mahonia: Paiute
Maianthemum: Ojibwa, South; Washo
Mentha: Cree, Woodlands
Mitchella: Iroquois
Monarda: Cherokee; Lakota
Nicotiana: Kawaiisu; Micmac; Navajo, Kayenta
Nuphar: Sioux
Panax: Creek; Ojibwa, South
Penstemon: Navajo, Kayenta
Phoradendron: Zuni
Phytolacca: Micmac
Pinus: Micmac
Platanus: Meskwaki
Polygala: Chippewa

Populus: Cree, Woodlands; Ojibwa
Prunus: Algonquin, Tête-de-Boule; Gosiute; Kwakiutl; Sioux
Pterospora: Cheyenne
Pycnanthemum: Koasati
Pyrola: Navajo, Kayenta
Quercus: Mahuna
Ranunculus: Meskwaki
Rhus: Cheyenne; Ojibwa; Omaha; Potawatomi
Rosa: Chippewa; Ojibwa
Rumex: Iroquois
Salix: Cheyenne; Meskwaki; Micmac; Ojibwa; Okanagan-Colville; Potawatomi
Sambucus: Paiute
Sanguinaria: Iroquois; Micmac; Ojibwa
Sanicula: Meskwaki
Sassafras: Iroquois
Scirpus: Cree, Woodlands; Thompson
Sedum: Kuper Island Indian
Silphium: Chippewa; Ojibwa
Solidago: Menominee
Sphaeralcea: Navajo
Symplocarpus: Menominee
Tephrosia: Seminole
Thalictrum: Iroquois
Thuja: Kwakiutl
Trichostema: Tubatulabal
Trifolium: Navajo, Ramah
Tsuga: Chippewa; Makah; Ojibwa
Typha: Iroquois; Mahuna
Ulmus: Ojibwa
Urtica: Abnaki; Bella Coola; Quinault
Valeriana: Menominee; Meskwaki
Veratrum: Haisla
Verbena: Chippewa
Xerophyllum: Blackfoot
Yucca: Blackfoot
Zanthoxylum: Meskwaki

Herbal Steam

Abies: Chippewa
Achillea: Chippewa; Kwakiutl
Agastache: Cheyenne
Anaphalis: Chippewa
Angelica: Kwakiutl
Artemisia: Chippewa; Kawaiisu; Kiowa; Mendocino Indian; Paiute; Shoshoni; Tlingit
Aster: Meskwaki
Callicarpa: Alabama
Calocedrus: Klamath
Carya: Chippewa
Chamaecyparis: Kwakiutl
Chenopodium: Zuni
Cirsium: Delaware, Oklahoma

Clematis: Shasta
Conioselinum: Kwakiutl
Corethrogyne: Kawaiisu
Cornus: Karok
Eriodictyon: Atsugewi
Eriogonum: Thompson
Geum: Thompson
Gutierrezia: Blackfoot
Helenium: Koasati
Helianthus: Shasta
Iris: Penobscot
Juniperus: Cheyenne; Chippewa; Delaware, Oklahoma; Omaha; Ponca; Tewa
Larix: Ojibwa, South
Linaria: Ojibwa
Lindera: Creek
Lomatium: Kwakiutl; Paiute; Shoshoni; Washo
Lonicera: Kwakiutl
Lysichiton: Kwakiutl
Madia: Cheyenne
Maianthemum: Menominee
Mentha: Thompson
Mimulus: Kawaiisu
Mitchella: Delaware, Oklahoma
Ochrosia: Hawaiian
Oplopanax: Kwakiutl
Phytolacca: Delaware, Oklahoma
Picradeniopsis: Navajo, Ramah
Pinus: Ojibwa, South
Platanthera: Thompson
Polygonatum: Chippewa
Populus: Choctaw
Prunus: Paiute; Shoshoni
Pseudotsuga: Karok; Pomo, Little Lakes
Ranunculus: Thompson
Rumex: Bella Coola; Karok
Salvia: Paiute
Sambucus: Kawaiisu; Kwakiutl
Silphium: Meskwaki; Omaha; Ponca; Winnebago
Stephanomeria: Cheyenne
Taxus: Chippewa; Menominee
Tetradymia: Navajo, Ramah
Tsuga: Delaware, Oklahoma; Menominee
Urtica: Bella Coola; Paiute; Shuswap
Yucca: Blackfoot; Keres, Western; Pawnee

Hunting Medicine

Acer: Iroquois; Okanagan-Colville
Acorus: Chippewa; Ojibwa
Angelica: Kwakiutl
Antennaria: Navajo, Ramah
Aralia: Ojibwa
Arctostaphylos: Chippewa
Asarum: Meskwaki

Aster: Chippewa; Navajo, Ramah; Ojibwa
Astragalus: Thompson
Atriplex: Zuni
Besseya: Navajo, Ramah
Campanula: Navajo, Ramah
Cardamine: Iroquois
Castilleja: Navajo, Ramah
Cercocarpus: Navajo, Ramah
Chamaebatiaria: Navajo, Ramah
Cicuta: Ojibwa
Conyza: Ojibwa
Corallorrhiza: Iroquois
Cornus: Chippewa
Datura: Cahuilla; Navajo, Ramah; Yavapai
Erigeron: Navajo, Ramah
Erythronium: Cherokee
Eupatorium: Chippewa
Euthamia: Ojibwa
Fraxinus: Iroquois
Helianthus: Navajo, Ramah
Hepatica: Chippewa
Heracleum: Iroquois; Menominee; Ojibwa
Hieracium: Navajo, Ramah; Ojibwa
Humulus: Navajo, Ramah
Ipomopsis: Navajo, Ramah
Limosella: Navajo, Ramah
Lomatium: Kwakiutl
Lonicera: Navajo, Ramah
Maianthemum: Iroquois
Mirabilis: Navajo, Ramah
Monolepis: Navajo, Ramah
Napaea: Meskwaki
Nicotiana: Cahuilla
Oenothera: Navajo, Ramah
Panax: Iroquois; Menominee
Penstemon: Zuni
Physocarpus: Okanagan-Colville
Picea: Koyukon; Tsimshian
Pinus: Navajo, Ramah
Platanthera: Thompson
Polygonatum: Iroquois
Polygonum: Ojibwa
Polystichum: Thompson
Prenanthes: Iroquois
Prunella: Ojibwa
Purshia: Navajo, Ramah
Pyrola: Ojibwa
Ranunculus: Navajo, Ramah; Ojibwa
Ratibida: Keres, Western
Rosa: Thompson
Rumex: Ojibwa
Salix: Seminole
Salvia: Cahuilla
Senecio: Navajo, Ramah

Shepherdia: Okanagan-Colville
Sium: Ojibwa
Spiraea: Ojibwa
Spiranthes: Ojibwa
Taenidia: Ojibwa
Thalictrum: Potawatomi
Thamnosma: Kawaiisu
Thermopsis: Navajo, Ramah
Thuja: Iroquois
Tiarella: Iroquois
Tsuga: Kwakiutl
Urtica: Makah
Uvularia: Ojibwa
Valeriana: Menominee; Navajo, Ramah; Thompson
Veratrum: Gitksan; Kwakiutl; Okanagan-Colville
Verbesina: Navajo, Ramah
Veronica: Navajo, Ramah

Hypotensive

Acorus: Lakota
Allium: Rappahannock
Alnus: Cherokee
Equisetum: Diegueño
Eriogonum: Mahuna
Helenium: Comanche
Hydrangea: Cherokee
Juglans: Houma
Juniperus: Diegueño; Thompson
Phoradendron: Cherokee
Rubus: Iroquois
Sabal: Houma
Sassafras: Iroquois
Shepherdia: Thompson
Veratrum: Hanaksiala

Internal Medicine

Abies: Nitinaht
Achillea: Hesquiat
Alnus: Nitinaht
Anaphalis: Kwakiutl
Aruncus: Makah
Aster: Navajo, Ramah
Cercocarpus: Kawaiisu
Dirca: Iroquois
Epilobium: Iroquois
Heracleum: Shuswap
Juniperus: Tewa
Ligusticum: Okanagan-Colville
Lomatium: Salish, Coast
Machaeranthera: Navajo, Ramah
Malus: Makah
Paxistima: Thompson
Pedicularis: Meskwaki; Potawatomi
Picea: Algonquin, Quebec; Menominee

Plagiomnium: Oweekeno
Potentilla: Okanagan-Colville
Rhus: Thompson
Rubus: Kwakiutl
Sidalcea: Navajo, Ramah
Taxus: Haihais; Kitasoo; Tsimshian
Tradescantia: Navajo, Ramah
Tsuga: Bella Coola; Makah; Nitinaht

Kidney Aid

Abies: Anticosti; Cherokee
Acalypha: Cherokee
Acer: Micmac; Penobscot
Achillea: Delaware; Delaware, Oklahoma;
   Mohegan; Paiute; Paiute, Northern
Acorus: Cherokee
Alisma: Iroquois
Allium: Cherokee
Alnus: Cherokee; Cree, Hudson Bay
Angelica: Paiute
Annona: Seminole
Anthemis: Cherokee
Apocynum: Cherokee; Meskwaki; Potawatomi
Aquilegia: Iroquois
Arabis: Okanagon; Thompson
Aralia: Algonquin, Quebec; Iroquois; Malecite;
   Micmac; Penobscot
Arctostaphylos: Cherokee; Okanagan-Colville;
   Okanagon; Thompson
Aruncus: Makah
Arundinaria: Houma
Asclepias: Cherokee; Iroquois
Aster: Iroquois
Baccharis: Costanoan
Baptisia: Meskwaki; Micmac; Penobscot
Bignonia: Choctaw
Brassica: Cherokee
Castilleja: Gitksan
Caulophyllum: Mohegan
Celastrus: Iroquois
Centaurea: Mahuna
Chaenactis: Shoshoni
Chaetopappa: Navajo, Kayenta
Chamaecyparis: Kwakiutl
Chimaphila: Iroquois; Karok; Kutenai; Micmac;
   Okanagan-Colville; Yurok
Cimicifuga: Micmac; Penobscot
Citrullus: Cherokee; Rappahannock
Clematis: Cherokee; Iroquois; Paiute; Shoshoni
Collinsonia: Iroquois
Comandra: Cherokee
Conocephalum: Nitinaht
Cornus: Iroquois; Shuswap
Croton: Mahuna; Modesse

Cucurbita: Cherokee
Cupressus: Kawaiisu
Cynoglossum: Iroquois
Cypripedium: Algonquin, Tête-de-Boule; Cherokee
Diplacus: Costanoan
Dirca: Iroquois; Menominee
Disporum: Costanoan
Draba: Navajo, Ramah
Echinocystis: Cherokee
Echium: Mohegan
Elymus: Iroquois
Empetrum: Tanana, Upper
Ephedra: Diegueño; Keres, Western; Navajo; Paiute;
   Shoshoni
Epigaea: Algonquin, Quebec; Cherokee; Iroquois
Epilobium: Iroquois; Miwok
Equisetum: Carrier; Cherokee; Iroquois; Menomi-
   nee; Ojibwa; Pomo, Kashaya; Potawatomi
Erigeron: Cherokee
Eriogonum: Navajo, Kayenta
Eryngium: Creek
Eupatorium: Cherokee; Iroquois; Micmac; Penob-
   scot
Fragaria: Cherokee
Frangula: Mendocino Indian
Gaillardia: Okanagan-Colville
Galax: Cherokee
Galium: Menominee; Meskwaki; Micmac; Miwok;
   Ojibwa; Penobscot
Gaultheria: Delaware; Iroquois; Mohegan;
   Shinnecock
Gaylussacia: Cherokee
Goodyera: Cherokee
Grindelia: Cree; Shoshoni; Sioux
Gymnocladus: Omaha
Hackelia: Cherokee
Hamamelis: Iroquois
Hedeoma: Nanticoke
Helenium: Koasati
Helianthemum: Cherokee
Humulus: Cherokee
Hydrangea: Delaware
Hypericum: Menominee
Ilex: Cherokee
Impatiens: Iroquois
Ipomoea: Cherokee; Creek
Ipomopsis: Shoshoni; Washo
Iris: Delaware; Delaware, Oklahoma; Nevada
   Indian
Jeffersonia: Cherokee
Juniperus: Blackfoot; Cree, Woodlands; Iroquois;
   Montana Indian; Navajo, Ramah; Okanagon;
   Paiute; Shoshoni; Tanana, Upper; Thompson
Lactuca: Iroquois

Larix: Anticosti
Ledum: Makah; Malecite; Micmac; Okanagan-Colville
Lepidium: Lakota
Leptodactylon: Navajo, Kayenta
Liatris: Cherokee; Meskwaki
Linum: Navajo, Kayenta
Lithospermum: Gosiute; Zuni
Lonicera: Algonquin, Quebec
Lygodesmia: Blackfoot
Lysimachia: Cherokee
Lythrum: Cherokee
Magnolia: Choctaw
Mahonia: Blackfoot; Kutenai; Montana Indian; Okanagan-Colville; Shoshoni
Maianthemum: Gitksan; Iroquois; Ojibwa
Manfreda: Catawba
Marrubium: Cahuilla
Mentha: California Indian; Kutenai
Mirabilis: Tewa
Mitchella: Iroquois; Seminole
Monarda: Blackfoot; Kutenai
Nemopanthus: Malecite
Nicotiana: Cherokee; Paiute
Oenothera: Navajo, Kayenta
Osmorhiza: Cheyenne
Osmunda: Iroquois
Ostrya: Chippewa
Paeonia: Paiute; Shoshoni
Panax: Cherokee
Paxistima: Okanagan-Colville
Pellaea: Mahuna
Penstemon: Okanagon; Thompson
Persea: Creek
Petroselinum: Cherokee
Phytolacca: Cherokee
Picea: Koyukon; Kwakiutl
Pinus: Cherokee; Delaware, Ontario; Micmac; Rappahannock; Shoshoni
Plantago: Shoshoni
Polygala: Cherokee
Polygonum: Malecite
Porteranthus: Cherokee
Prunus: Cherokee; Rappahannock
Pseudotsuga: Okanagon; Thompson
Psorothamnus: Paiute; Shoshoni
Purshia: Shoshoni
Pyrola: Micmac; Penobscot
Rhamnus: Kawaiisu
Ribes: Blackfoot; Iroquois; Omaha
Rorippa: Costanoan
Rosa: Costanoan
Rubus: Iroquois
Rudbeckia: Cherokee

Rumex: Cherokee; Iroquois; Paiute
Sabal: Houma
Sambucus: Cherokee; Iroquois
Sanguinaria: Iroquois
Sanicula: Iroquois; Malecite; Micmac
Sarracenia: Micmac; Penobscot
Satureja: Karok
Saxifraga: Iroquois
Scrophularia: Iroquois
Scutellaria: Cherokee
Senecio: Costanoan; Iroquois
Silphium: Meskwaki
Sinapis: Cherokee
Smallanthus: Iroquois
Smilax: Chippewa
Solidago: Iroquois
Sorbus: Thompson
Spiraea: Okanagan-Colville
Streptopus: Micmac; Penobscot
Suaeda: Paiute; Shoshoni
Tanacetum: Malecite; Micmac
Taraxacum: Iroquois
Tephrosia: Cherokee
Thuja: Quinault
Tradescantia: Cherokee
Trifolium: Cherokee
Tsuga: Cherokee; Malecite; Micmac
Typha: Delaware; Delaware, Oklahoma; Malecite
Ulmus: Iroquois
Verbascum: Cherokee
Verbena: Cherokee; Houma
Veronicastrum: Meskwaki
Viburnum: Iroquois
Vitis: Iroquois
Xanthium: Mahuna
Zanthoxylum: Iroquois; Meskwaki
Zea: Cherokee
Zinnia: Keres, Western

Laxative

Abies: Algonquin, Quebec; Cherokee; Crow; Kwakiutl; Malecite; Micmac
Acer: Iroquois
Achillea: Great Basin Indian; Okanagan-Colville
Acorus: Cheyenne
Adenostoma: Cahuilla
Agoseris: Okanagan-Colville
Aleurites: Hawaiian
Alisma: Cree, Woodlands
Alnus: Algonquin, Quebec; Cree, Woodlands; Gitksan
Alocasia: Hawaiian
Ambrosia: Cheyenne
Amelanchier: Blackfoot

Anemopsis: Paiute
Apocynum: Blackfoot; Iroquois
Arctostaphylos: Tanana, Upper
Artemisia: Eskimo, Alaska; Navajo, Kayenta;
  Sanpoil
Asarum: Okanagan-Colville
Asclepias: Cherokee
Aster: Iroquois
Caesalpinia: Hawaiian
Caltha: Eskimo, Western
Carya: Meskwaki
Ceanothus: Chippewa
Centaurium: Mahuna
Cephalanthus: Seminole
Cercocarpus: Tewa
Chamaesyce: Hawaiian; Pima
Chelone: Cherokee
Chimaphila: Iroquois
Chlorogalum: Wailaki
Cimicifuga: Cherokee
Cirsium: Hopi
Collomia: Okanagan-Colville
Colocasia: Hawaiian
Cornus: Iroquois; Lummi
Crataegus: Blackfoot
Croton: Isleta
Cucurbita: Hawaiian; Tewa
Datura: Tubatulabal
Diervilla: Chippewa
Digitaria: Hawaiian
Dirca: Algonquin, Quebec; Iroquois
Distichlis: Kawaiisu
Ephedra: Havasupai
Epilobium: Blackfoot; Eskimo, Alaska
Equisetum: Cherokee; Ojibwa
Eriodictyon: Hualapai
Erioneuron: Havasupai
Erythrina: Seminole
Eupatorium: Cherokee; Iroquois; Mahuna
Fomes: Eskimo, Inuktitut
Frangula: Bella Coola; Cahuilla; Costanoan;
  Cowlitz; Green River Group; Haisla & Hanaksiala;
  Hesquiat; Kawaiisu; Klallam; Kwakiutl; Lummi;
  Makah; Nitinaht; Okanagan-Colville; Pomo;
  Pomo, Kashaya; Quileute; Quinault; Shuswap;
  Skagit; Skagit, Upper; Squaxin; Swinomish;
  Thompson; Tolowa; Yurok
Fraxinus: Iroquois; Meskwaki
Galium: Cherokee
Garrya: Kawaiisu
Gentianella: Cherokee
Geranium: Iroquois
Gymnocladus: Dakota; Omaha; Oto; Ponca;
  Winnebago

Hepatica: Cherokee
Hibiscus: Hawaiian
Inula: Delaware, Oklahoma
Ipomoea: Cherokee
Ipomopsis: Okanagan-Colville
Iris: Aleut
Juglans: Iroquois
Juniperus: Hopi; Keres, Western; Tewa
Larix: Algonquin, Tête-de-Boule
Lomatium: Kwakiutl
Lonicera: Okanagan-Colville
Lycopus: Iroquois
Mahonia: Havasupai; Hualapai; Navajo, Ramah;
  Nitinaht; Thompson
Maianthemum: Meskwaki
Malus: Gitksan; Makah
Matricaria: Aleut
Melilotus: Pomo, Kashaya
Menispermum: Cherokee
Mentzelia: Apache, White Mountain; Zuni
Menyanthes: Aleut
Merremia: Hawaiian
Monarda: Ojibwa
Morus: Cherokee
Mucuna: Hawaiian
Nepeta: Iroquois
Odontoglossum: Hawaiian
Oemleria: Makah
Oenanthe: Makah
Oplopanax: Haisla & Hanaksiala; Kwakiutl;
  Thompson
Opuntia: Cahuilla; Hawaiian
Osteomeles: Hawaiian
Oxytropis: Navajo, Kayenta
Paeonia: Costanoan
Pandanus: Hawaiian
Pectis: Pima
Pediomelum: Meskwaki
Perideridia: Blackfoot
Persea: Seminole
Peucedanum: Hawaiian
Phlox: Blackfoot
Physocarpus: Bella Coola; Hesquiat; Kwakiutl;
  Saanich
Phytolacca: Cherokee
Picea: Algonquin, Quebec; Bella Coola; Hanaksiala
Pinus: Cherokee; Iroquois; Kawaiisu
Plantago: Carrier; Costanoan; Navajo
Podophyllum: Cherokee; Delaware; Delaware,
  Oklahoma; Iroquois
Polypodium: Skagit, Upper
Populus: Haisla; Iroquois
Prunus: Kawaiisu; Makah; Quinault; Thompson
Psathyrotes: Paiute; Shoshoni

Pseudotsuga: Bella Coola
Purshia: Havasupai; Kawaiisu; Paiute, Northern;
    Sanpoil
Ranunculus: Iroquois
Rhamnus: Kawaiisu; Meskwaki
Rheum: Cherokee
Ribes: Bella Coola; Nitinaht
Ricinus: Pima
Rubus: Iroquois; Okanagan-Colville
Rumex: Cherokee; Haisla
Sagittaria: Iroquois
Salix: Meskwaki
Salvia: Cherokee
Sambucus: Algonquin, Quebec; Cahuilla;
    Diegueño; Hesquiat; Iroquois; Mohegan;
    Nitinaht; Paiute
Sanguinaria: Iroquois; Ojibwa
Sanicula: Iroquois
Sassafras: Seminole
Scutellaria: Delaware; Delaware, Oklahoma
Sebastiania: Alabama
Sedum: Okanagan-Colville; Okanagon; Thompson
Senecio: Kawaiisu
Senna: Iroquois
Shepherdia: Blackfoot; Carrier; Cree, Woodlands;
    Thompson
Sisyrinchium: Iroquois
Solanum: Isleta
Spiraea: Blackfoot
Symphoricarpos: Thompson
Symphytum: Cherokee
Taraxacum: Delaware; Delaware, Oklahoma;
    Iroquois
Thamnosma: Havasupai
Touchardia: Hawaiian
Tradescantia: Cherokee
Triosteum: Iroquois
Tsuga: Quinault
Ulmus: Cherokee; Dakota; Omaha; Pawnee; Ponca;
    Winnebago
Veratrum: Bella Coola; Haisla; Kwakiutl
Verbascum: Iroquois
Verbesina: Seminole
Veronicastrum: Menominee; Meskwaki
Viburnum: Iroquois
Vicia: Costanoan
Waltheria: Hawaiian
Xanthium: Pima
Yucca: Hopi; Navajo

Liver Aid

Achillea: Blackfoot; Delaware; Delaware, Okla-
    homa; Mohegan
Adiantum: Iroquois

Aletris: Cherokee
Allium: Cherokee
Apocynum: Iroquois
Aralia: Iroquois
Asplenium: Cherokee
Baptisia: Iroquois
Berberis: Shinnecock
Betula: Delaware, Oklahoma
Brickellia: Keres, Western
Carya: Cherokee
Caulophyllum: Iroquois
Celastrus: Delaware
Chelone: Iroquois
Clethra: Cherokee
Cornus: Blackfoot
Cryptogramma: Thompson
Diospyros: Cherokee
Eupatorium: Iroquois
Fagus: Iroquois
Fragaria: Cherokee
Frangula: Creek; Delaware, Oklahoma; Thompson
Fraxinus: Delaware, Oklahoma
Gaylussacia: Iroquois
Gentiana: Iroquois
Grindelia: Blackfoot
Hedeoma: Nanticoke
Hepatica: Cherokee; Chippewa
Heuchera: Shoshoni; Thompson
Hydrangea: Cherokee; Delaware, Oklahoma
Hydrastis: Iroquois
Impatiens: Iroquois; Malecite; Micmac
Ipomoea: Iroquois
Ipomopsis: Shoshoni
Iris: Cherokee; Cree, Hudson Bay; Delaware; Dela-
    ware, Oklahoma
Jeffersonia: Iroquois
Juglans: Delaware, Oklahoma; Iroquois
Ledum: Montagnais
Linum: Shoshoni
Mahonia: Hualapai
Manfreda: Cherokee
Morus: Delaware, Oklahoma
Panax: Cherokee; Iroquois
Parthenocissus: Cherokee
Passiflora: Cherokee
Phytolacca: Iroquois
Pinus: Iroquois
Porteranthus: Cherokee
Prunus: Iroquois
Psathyrotes: Paiute; Shoshoni
Pteridium: Iroquois
Purshia: Paiute
Pyrola: Shoshoni
Rhamnus: Kawaiisu

Rorippa: Costanoan; Mahuna
Rubus: Iroquois
Rumex: Delaware; Delaware, Oklahoma; Houma; Shoshoni
Sambucus: Choctaw; Delaware; Delaware, Oklahoma; Iroquois; Thompson
Sanguinaria: Iroquois
Sarracenia: Iroquois
Sedum: Iroquois
Sequoia: Houma
Shepherdia: Thompson
Solidago: Houma; Iroquois
Sporobolus: Ojibwa, South
Tanacetum: Iroquois
Thalictrum: Iroquois
Tsuga: Gitksan
Verbena: Houma
Veronicastrum: Cherokee
Viburnum: Iroquois
Vitis: Cherokee
Xanthorhiza: Catawba

Love Medicine

Acer: Karok
Alocasia: Hawaiian
Anemone: Iroquois
Apocynum: Okanagan-Colville
Aquilegia: Meskwaki; Omaha; Pawnee; Ponca; Thompson
Arbutus: Pomo, Kashaya
Arnica: Okanagan-Colville
Artemisia: Omaha; Winnebago
Aruncus: Kwakiutl
Aster: Iroquois
Caltha: Iroquois
Calystegia: Karok
Cardamine: Iroquois
Castilleja: Menominee
Chrysobalanus: Seminole
Chrysophyllum: Seminole
Coeloglossum: Ojibwa
Conium: Klallam
Conyza: Seminole
Corallorhiza: Iroquois
Cuscuta: Pawnee
Cypripedium: Meskwaki
Datura: Costanoan
Delphinium: Thompson
Dicentra: Menominee
Dirca: Iroquois
Disporum: Makah
Dodecatheon: Thompson
Drosera: Kwakiutl
Echinocystis: Menominee

Eriophyllum: Chehalis
Eupatorium: Iroquois; Meskwaki
Filipendula: Meskwaki
Galium: Cowlitz; Iroquois; Karok; Quileute
Geranium: Iroquois; Thompson
Geum: Iroquois; Okanagan-Colville
Hackelia: Cherokee
Iodanthus: Meskwaki
Juniperus: Cheyenne
Lilium: Iroquois
Linaria: Iroquois
Liriodendron: Rappahannock
Lobelia: Iroquois; Meskwaki; Pawnee
Lomatium: Dakota; Omaha; Pawnee; Ponca; Winnebago
Lonicera: Iroquois; Nootka, Manhousat
Madia: Cheyenne
Malva: Iroquois
Matricaria: Okanagan-Colville
Mentha: Cheyenne
Menziesia: Quinault
Mitchella: Iroquois
Monardella: Karok
Monotropa: Kwakiutl
Myrica: Seminole
Osmorhiza: Songish; Swinomish
Panax: Meskwaki; Pawnee; Seminole
Pedicularis: Menominee; Meskwaki; Ojibwa
Penstemon: Iroquois
Persea: Seminole
Phlox: Meskwaki
Phoradendron: Cherokee
Phytolacca: Iroquois
Platanthera: Kwakiutl; Potawatomi; Thompson
Podophyllum: Delaware, Oklahoma
Polygonum: Iroquois
Populus: Iroquois; Karok
Prenanthes: Iroquois
Quercus: Seminole
Rumex: Iroquois
Sagittaria: Thompson
Salix: Seminole
Sanguinaria: Algonquin; Micmac; Ponca
Sarracenia: Iroquois
Satureja: Karok
Scirpus: Potawatomi
Sideroxylon: Seminole
Solidago: Iroquois
Taraxacum: Iroquois
Thalictrum: Meskwaki; Ponca; Potawatomi
Tradescantia: Navajo, Kayenta
Trillium: Makah
Valeriana: Cree, Woodlands
Viburnum: Iroquois

Vicia: Iroquois; Makah; Quinault
Vitis: Navajo

Miscellaneous Disease Remedy

Abies: Gitksan; Wet'suwet'en
Acalypha: Cherokee
Acer: Cherokee; Micmac; Thompson
Achillea: Abnaki; Iroquois; Lummi; Meskwaki; Miwok; Paiute, Northern; Thompson
Acorus: Iroquois; Lakota; Micmac
Adiantum: Cherokee
Agastache: Miwok
Ageratina: Cherokee
Alisma: Cree, Woodlands
Allium: Cherokee; Shinnecock
Alnus: Hesquiat
Amelanchier: Cree, Woodlands
Anaphalis: Thompson
Anemopsis: Kawaiisu
Angelica: Blackfoot; Cherokee; Iroquois; Washo
Apocynum: Meskwaki
Aralia: Algonquin, Quebec; Iroquois
Arbutus: Cowichan
Arctium: Abnaki
Aristolochia: Cherokee
Armoracia: Iroquois
Artemisia: Blackfoot; Kawaiisu; Navajo, Ramah; Okanagan-Colville; Paiute; Sanpoil; Shoshoni; Tanaina; Tanana, Upper; Thompson
Aruncus: Bella Coola; Lummi; Nitinaht; Thompson
Asarum: Cherokee; Iroquois
Asclepias: Navajo, Ramah; Paiute
Aster: Iroquois
Astragalus: Cree, Woodlands; Navajo; Navajo, Kayenta
Atriplex: Havasupai
Aureolaria: Chickasaw
Bignonia: Houma
Brassica: Cherokee; Micmac
Brickellia: Navajo, Ramah
Calla: Gitksan
Carya: Cherokee
Castanea: Cherokee
Ceanothus: Iroquois; Shuswap
Centaurium: Miwok
Cercocarpus: Shoshoni
Chamaebatia: Miwok
Chenopodium: Cherokee; Potawatomi
Chimaphila: Micmac; Nanticoke
Chrysothamnus: Cheyenne; Navajo; Shoshoni
Cicuta: Kwakiutl
Cinna: Iroquois
Cirsium: Navajo, Kayenta; Zuni
Clintonia: Iroquois

Cornus: Cherokee; Houma
Croton: Concow; Jemez; Neeshenam
Cypripedium: Cherokee
Dalea: Meskwaki
Daucus: Delaware; Delaware, Oklahoma; Mohegan
Diphylleia: Cherokee
Dirca: Iroquois
Dodonaea: Hawaiian
Echinacea: Cheyenne; Dakota; Omaha; Pawnee; Ponca; Winnebago
Ericameria: Diegueño; Paiute
Erigeron: Miwok; Navajo, Ramah
Eriodictyon: Round Valley Indian
Erodium: Costanoan
Eupatorium: Cherokee; Houma; Iroquois
Fragaria: Cherokee; Chippewa
Frangula: Mendocino Indian; Yokia
Gaillardia: Navajo; Thompson
Galium: Choctaw; Meskwaki; Navajo, Ramah
Gamochaeta: Houma
Gaultheria: Algonquin, Tête-de-Boule
Geum: Okanagan-Colville
Glechoma: Cherokee
Gleditsia: Cherokee; Creek; Meskwaki
Glycyrrhiza: Lakota
Gnaphalium: Cherokee; Creek
Grindelia: Shoshoni
Gutierrezia: Shoshoni; Tewa
Hamamelis: Iroquois
Hedeoma: Navajo, Ramah
Heliotropium: Shoshoni
Heracleum: Iroquois; Malecite; Meskwaki; Mewuk; Micmac
Holocarpha: Miwok
Holodiscus: Chehalis; Navajo, Ramah
Humulus: Navajo, Ramah
Ilex: Catawba
Impatiens: Cherokee
Inula: Iroquois
Ipomoea: Cherokee; Iroquois
Ipomopsis: Shoshoni
Iris: Micmac; Penobscot
Iva: Navajo, Ramah
Juglans: Cherokee
Juniperus: Arapaho; Cherokee; Dakota; Eskimo, Inupiat; Kutenai; Mahuna; Okanagan-Colville; Paiute; Saanich; Shoshoni; Shuswap; Sioux; Thompson
Krascheninnikovia: Navajo
Larrea: Paiute
Ledum: Micmac; Tanana, Upper
Lepechinia: Miwok
Leptarrhena: Aleut
Lewisia: Okanagan-Colville

Lindera: Cherokee; Iroquois
Liriodendron: Cherokee
Lobelia: Delaware; Delaware, Oklahoma
Lomatium: Great Basin Indian; Okanagan-Colville; Paiute; Shoshoni; Washo
Lonicera: Cree, Woodlands
Lophophora: Kiowa
Lycium: Navajo, Ramah
Lygodesmia: Cheyenne
Lysichiton: Gitksan; Yurok
Mahonia: Karok; Miwok
Maianthemum: Meskwaki
Malus: Meskwaki
Marrubium: Navajo, Ramah
Marshallia: Catawba
Matelea: Comanche
Melissa: Cherokee
Mentha: Cherokee; Iroquois; Navajo, Ramah; Thompson
Mentzelia: Cheyenne
Menyanthes: Kwakiutl
Mertensia: Cheyenne
Mitchella: Iroquois
Modiola: Houma
Monarda: Cherokee; Flathead; Navajo, Ramah
Nicotiana: Cherokee; Paiute
Nuphar: Iroquois
Nymphaea: Micmac
Oenothera: Navajo, Kayenta
Oplopanax: Gitksan; Haisla; Thompson; Wet'suwet'en
Osmorhiza: Paiute; Shoshoni; Washo
Panax: Cherokee; Iroquois
Parthenocissus: Houma
Peniocereus: Pima
Penstemon: Okanagan-Colville
Pericome: Navajo, Ramah
Petasites: Concow; Tanaina
Peteria: Navajo, Ramah
Picea: Cherokee; Gitksan; Micmac; Wet'suwet'en
Pinus: Cherokee; Iroquois; Micmac; Navajo, Ramah; Paiute; Salish, Coast; Shoshoni; Thompson
Piper: Hawaiian
Platanus: Cherokee; Meskwaki
Polygonatum: Chippewa
Polypodium: Cowlitz; Iroquois
Populus: Iroquois
Porteranthus: Iroquois
Portulaca: Navajo, Kayenta
Prunella: Catawba; Iroquois
Prunus: Cherokee; Chippewa; Iroquois; Micmac; Paiute; Thompson
Psoralidium: Navajo, Ramah

Psorothamnus: Paiute; Paiute, Northern; Shoshoni
Pteridium: Cherokee
Purshia: Paiute; Shoshoni
Pycnanthemum: Meskwaki
Quercus: Iroquois
Quincula: Kiowa
Ranunculus: Iroquois
Rhus: Blackfoot; Kiowa; Montana Indian; Potawatomi; Round Valley Indian; Yokia
Ribes: Cherokee
Rosa: Keres, Western; Paiute
Rubus: Chippewa; Montana Indian; Thompson
Rumex: Choctaw; Hawaiian; Iroquois; Kawaiisu; Paiute
Salix: Mewuk
Salsola: Navajo, Ramah
Salvia: Diegueño; Paiute
Sambucus: Cahuilla; Iroquois; Kawaiisu; Mahuna; Miwok
Sanguinaria: Potawatomi
Sarracenia: Micmac; Montagnais
Sassafras: Cherokee; Choctaw; Houma; Nanticoke; Rappahannock
Scutellaria: Iroquois
Senna: Cherokee; Houma
Sesamum: Cherokee
Sinapis: Cherokee
Sisyrinchium: Iroquois
Solanum: Costanoan
Solidago: Cherokee; Okanagan-Colville; Thompson
Sorbus: Potawatomi
Sphaeralcea: Navajo
Stanleya: Paiute
Stephanomeria: Cheyenne; Navajo, Kayenta
Strophostyles: Houma
Suaeda: Paiute
Symplocarpus: Delaware
Taxus: Micmac
Tetradymia: Paiute
Thamnosma: Paiute
Thuja: Chippewa; Thompson
Toxicodendron: Cherokee
Trichostema: Concow; Miwok
Tsuga: Iroquois; Micmac; Thompson
Typha: Iroquois; Sioux
Urtica: Cherokee; Paiute; Tanaina
Vaccinium: Pomo, Kashaya
Valeriana: Navajo, Ramah; Thompson
Veratrum: Thompson
Verbascum: Cherokee; Iroquois
Verbena: Costanoan
Veronicastrum: Cherokee; Meskwaki
Viburnum: Cherokee; Delaware, Ontario; Micmac; Penobscot

Vicia: Cherokee
Vitis: Chippewa
Wyethia: Shoshoni
Yucca: Cherokee

Narcotic

Arctostaphylos: Kwakiutl; Ojibwa
Broussonetia: Apache, Chiricahua & Mescalero
Comandra: Navajo, Kayenta
Cornus: Gosiute
Crotalaria: Delaware; Delaware, Oklahoma
Datura: Apache, White Mountain; Havasupai; Hopi;
  Luiseño; Mahuna; Navajo, Kayenta; Navajo,
  Ramah; Paiute; Shoshoni; Ute; Yuma; Zuni
Delphinium: Mendocino Indian
Eschscholzia: Mendocino Indian
Ledum: Kwakiutl
Lophophora: Comanche; Kiowa
Nicotiana: Navajo, Kayenta
Opuntia: Apache, Chiricahua & Mescalero
Petrophyton: Navajo, Kayenta
Selaginella: Blackfoot
Stephanomeria: Navajo, Kayenta

Nose Medicine

Arisaema: Iroquois
Aristolochia: Cherokee
Artemisia: Cheyenne; Havasupai
Asclepias: Navajo
Atriplex: Cahuilla; Navajo, Ramah
Chaetopappa: Hopi; Navajo, Ramah
Chimaphila: Abnaki
Cordyline: Hawaiian
Curcuma: Hawaiian
Dimorphocarpa: Keres, Western
Draba: Blackfoot
Evolvulus: Navajo, Kayenta
Gaillardia: Blackfoot
Geranium: Cheyenne
Helenium: Cherokee
Helianthus: Cherokee
Heterotheca: Navajo, Ramah
Kalmia: Abnaki
Ledum: Abnaki
Machaeranthera: Navajo
Nicotiana: Tewa
Osmorhiza: Blackfoot
Polygonum: Navajo, Ramah
Pterospora: Cheyenne
Sanguinaria: Cherokee
Senecio: Yavapai
Sisyrinchium: Navajo
Solanum: Navajo
Stenotus: Navajo

Townsendia: Navajo
Veratrum: Blackfoot; Flathead; Kutenai
Zinnia: Navajo

Oral Aid

Abies: Blackfoot; Flathead; Kwakiutl
Abronia: Navajo, Ramah
Achillea: Cree, Woodlands
Acorus: Shinnecock
Alnus: Cherokee; Malecite; Micmac
Angelica: Cherokee; Pomo, Kashaya
Apocynum: Ojibwa
Aralia: Cree, Woodlands
Arctostaphylos: Blackfoot; Crow; Thompson
Armoracia: Cherokee
Artemisia: Blackfoot; Okanagan-Colville; Tanana,
  Upper
Artocarpus: Hawaiian
Asclepias: Blackfoot
Asplenium: Hawaiian
Balsamorhiza: Cheyenne
Berberis: Micmac; Penobscot
Bothriochloa: Kiowa
Carya: Cherokee
Ceanothus: Iroquois; Keres, Western
Chamaesyce: Apache, White Mountain; Hopi
Chrysothamnus: Jemez; Tewa
Cirsium: Iroquois; Kwakiutl; Mohegan
Clitoria: Cherokee
Comandra: Navajo, Kayenta
Coptis: Iroquois; Malecite; Menominee; Micmac;
  Mohegan; Ojibwa; Penobscot; Potawatomi
Cornus: Iroquois; Meskwaki
Crataegus: Okanagan-Colville
Curcuma: Hawaiian
Delphinium: Blackfoot
Desmodium: Cherokee
Diospyros: Cherokee; Rappahannock
Dodecatheon: Blackfoot
Echinacea: Cheyenne; Lakota; Montana Indian
Equisetum: Tolowa
Eriodictyon: Cahuilla
Eriogonum: Apache, White Mountain; Lakota;
  Navajo, Ramah; Zuni
Fragaria: Okanagan-Colville
Gaultheria: Cherokee; Makah
Geranium: Cherokee; Chippewa; Iroquois;
  Meskwaki; Ojibwa; Salish
Geum: Blackfoot
Glycyrrhiza: Blackfoot; Zuni
Gnaphalium: Cherokee
Goodyera: Mohegan
Helianthus: Kiowa
Heuchera: Blackfoot; Cherokee; Navajo; Thompson

Holodiscus: Lummi
Hydrophyllum: Iroquois
Iris: Yokia
Juglans: Iroquois
Juncus: Cherokee
Juniperus: Kiowa; Shoshoni
Lachnanthes: Cherokee
Larrea: Pima
Lomatium: Okanagan-Colville
Lonicera: Quinault
Mahonia: Hopi
Malus: Cherokee; Oweekeno
Mentha: Cree, Woodlands
Menziesia: Hesquiat
Mirabilis: Navajo; Pawnee
Nepeta: Iroquois
Nymphaea: Chippewa
Oxalis: Cherokee; Iroquois; Kiowa
Oxydendrum: Cherokee
Panax: Cherokee
Persea: Mahuna; Seminole
Phlox: Navajo, Ramah
Picea: Cree, Woodlands; Haisla & Hanaksiala; Tanana, Upper
Piper: Hawaiian
Pityopsis: Choctaw
Pleopeltis: Houma
Polygala: Cree, Woodlands
Polygonum: Cree, Woodlands; Meskwaki
Polypodium: Bella Coola; Hesquiat; Thompson
Populus: Haisla & Hanaksiala; Iroquois
Portulaca: Keres, Western
Potentilla: Cherokee
Prosopis: Pima
Prunus: Cherokee; Cheyenne; Haisla & Hanaksiala; Kwakiutl; Meskwaki
Pseudotsuga: Swinomish; Thompson
Pyrola: Mohegan
Quercus: Cherokee; Keres, Western
Ranunculus: Cherokee
Rhus: Chippewa; Delaware; Delaware, Oklahoma; Jemez; Keres, Western; Ojibwa; Okanagon; Sanpoil; Thompson
Ribes: Kwakiutl
Rubus: Cherokee
Rumex: Navajo, Ramah; Pima
Salix: Catawba; Eskimo, Alaska; Eskimo, Inupiat; Eskimo, Kuskokwagmiut; Eskimo, Nunivak; Eskimo, Western; Iroquois; Seminole
Sanvitalia: Navajo; Navajo, Ramah
Sassafras: Cherokee; Seminole
Schkuhria: Navajo, Ramah
Schoenocrambe: Navajo, Ramah
Scirpus: Cherokee

Sedum: Eskimo, Alaska; Thompson
Solanum: Cherokee
Solidago: Cherokee
Sphaeralcea: Navajo, Kayenta
Stenotaphrum: Hawaiian
Stenotus: Navajo
Symphoricarpos: Skagit
Syringa: Iroquois
Syzygium: Hawaiian
Thuja: Skokomish
Tiarella: Cherokee; Iroquois
Toxicodendron: Iroquois
Trollius: Cherokee
Ulmus: Kiowa
Urtica: Makah
Veratrum: Blackfoot
Verbesina: Seminole
Viburnum: Cherokee
Vitis: Cherokee
Xanthium: Paiute, Northern
Xanthorhiza: Cherokee
Ximenia: Seminole

Orthopedic Aid

Abies: Iroquois; Micmac; Thompson
Acer: Iroquois; Micmac; Seminole
Achillea: Carrier, Southern; Malecite; Mendocino Indian; Micmac; Paiute; Shoshoni; Thompson
Acorus: Cree, Woodlands; Lakota
Adiantum: Iroquois
Aesculus: Cherokee
Agoseris: Navajo, Ramah
Alisma: Iroquois
Alnus: Cherokee; Cowlitz; Mohegan; Nitinaht
Ambrosia: Costanoan; Iroquois
Anaphalis: Chippewa
Andropogon: Catawba
Anemone: Ojibwa, South
Anemopsis: Paiute
Arabis: Okanagon; Thompson
Aralia: Cherokee; Chippewa; Iroquois
Arctium: Iroquois
Arctostaphylos: Cheyenne; Thompson
Arisaema: Cherokee; Iroquois; Micmac; Mohegan; Penobscot
Arnica: Catawba
Artemisia: Aleut; Carrier, Southern; Chippewa; Eskimo, Kuskokwagmiut; Eskimo, Western; Hopi; Klamath; Montana Indian; Okanagan-Colville; Okanagon; Paiute; Shoshoni; Thompson; Tolowa; Yuki; Yurok
Aruncus: Cherokee; Thompson
Arundo: Cahuilla
Asarum: Chippewa

Asclepias: Iroquois; Menominee
Aster: Cree, Woodlands
Baptisia: Iroquois; Nanticoke
Betula: Cree, Woodlands; Iroquois; Tanana, Upper
Blechnum: Quileute
Brassica: Cherokee
Calla: Cree, Woodlands
Carnegia: Pima
Carya: Cherokee
Castilleja: Chippewa; Gitksan
Ceanothus: Alabama; Okanagan-Colville; Thompson
Celastrus: Creek
Cephalanthus: Koasati
Chaenactis: Gosiute; Kawaiisu; Paiute
Chamaebatiaria: Paiute
Chenopodium: Costanoan
Chimaphila: Catawba; Cree, Woodlands; Karok; Thompson
Cicuta: Iroquois; Kawaiisu; Paiute; Shoshoni; Thompson
Cimicifuga: Iroquois
Clematis: Cherokee; Navajo, Ramah; Shoshoni
Comptonia: Micmac
Conyza: Hawaiian
Cordylanthus: Navajo
Coreopsis: Meskwaki
Cornus: Carrier, Northern; Iroquois; Montagnais
Coronilla: Cherokee
Corydalis: Navajo, Ramah
Crepis: Okanagan-Colville
Cupressus: Kawaiisu
Cymopterus: Navajo, Kayenta
Cypripedium: Iroquois
Datura: Kawaiisu; Navajo, Kayenta
Delphinium: Kawaiisu
Dirca: Iroquois
Echinacea: Cheyenne
Elytrigia: Cherokee
Ephedra: Kawaiisu
Epilobium: Iroquois; Navajo, Kayenta
Equisetum: Blackfoot; Iroquois; Navajo, Kayenta; Okanagan-Colville; Potawatomi
Ericameria: Coahuilla; Kawaiisu; Miwok
Erigeron: Cheyenne; Thompson
Eriodictyon: Coahuilla; Hualapai; Miwok
Eriogonum: Navajo, Kayenta; Paiute; Shoshoni; Thompson
Eryngium: Seminole
Euonymus: Cherokee
Eupatorium: Abnaki; Iroquois
Gaillardia: Blackfoot; Okanagan-Colville
Galium: Iroquois
Gentiana: Iroquois

Geum: Thompson
Glyceria: Catawba
Gnaphalium: Cherokee; Iroquois
Grindelia: Kawaiisu; Shoshoni
Gutierrezia: Kawaiisu; Paiute
Hackelia: Navajo, Ramah
Hamamelis: Iroquois; Menominee; Potawatomi
Helianthella: Paiute
Hepatica: Iroquois
Heracleum: Aleut; Bella Coola; Okanagan-Colville; Quinault
Heuchera: Cheyenne; Navajo, Ramah
Hexastylis: Catawba
Holodiscus: Lummi
Hydrangea: Cherokee
Hypericum: Alabama; Paiute; Shoshoni
Ilex: Cherokee
Impatiens: Mohegan; Nanticoke; Penobscot; Potawatomi
Ipomoea: Hawaiian
Iris: Iroquois
Isocoma: Pima
Juncus: Cherokee
Juniperus: Micmac; Paiute; Seminole; Tewa
Kalmia: Cherokee; Malecite; Micmac
Krascheninnikovia: Hopi
Lactuca: Iroquois
Larix: Thompson
Larrea: Diegueño; Kawaiisu; Papago
Lathyrus: Mendocino Indian
Ledum: Cree, Hudson Bay
Linnaea: Montagnais
Liriodendron: Cherokee
Lithospermum: Cheyenne
Lobelia: Cherokee
Lomatium: Gosiute; Kawaiisu; Kwakiutl; Okanagan-Colville; Paiute; Shoshoni; Thompson
Lonicera: Carrier, Northern; Kwakiutl; Thompson
Lophophora: Kiowa
Lygodesmia: Blackfoot
Lysichiton: Shuswap
Maianthemum: Gitksan; Paiute
Malus: Iroquois; Makah
Malva: Iroquois
Marah: Squaxin
Matelea: Comanche
Matteuccia: Cree, Woodlands
Menodora: Navajo, Ramah
Merremia: Hawaiian
Mimulus: Kawaiisu
Mirabilis: Chippewa; Navajo, Ramah; Ojibwa; Sioux, Teton
Mitchella: Iroquois
Moneses: Montagnais

Other

Agrimonia: Iroquois
Alisma: Iroquois
Ambrosia: Makah
Anaphalis: Nitinaht
Anemopsis: Pima
Angadenia: Seminole
Angelica: Blackfoot; Iroquois; Pomo, Kashaya
Anthemis: Iroquois
Apocynum: Navajo, Kayenta
Artemisia: Kawaiisu; Keres, Western; Mewuk
Asclepias: Costanoan; Iroquois
Aster: Seminole
Astragalus: Navajo, Kayenta
Atriplex: Navajo, Ramah
Aureolaria: Cherokee
Bacopa: Seminole
Berchemia: Seminole
Betula: Micmac
Botrychium: Abnaki
Brickellia: Navajo, Ramah
Callicarpa: Choctaw
Camissonia: Navajo, Kayenta
Cardamine: Iroquois
Carex: Iroquois
Carpinus: Iroquois
Ceanothus: Great Basin Indian; Iroquois
Celastrus: Iroquois
Cephalanthus: Seminole
Chamaesaracha: Navajo, Kayenta
Chrysothamnus: Thompson
Circaea: Iroquois
Clematis: Seminole; Thompson
Cocos: Hawaiian
Commelina: Seminole
Coreopsis: Seminole
Cornus: Okanagan-Colville
Corydalis: Navajo, Ramah
Cucurbita: Cahuilla
Datura: Cahuilla; Hopi; Paiute; Pima; Yokut
Diervilla: Potawatomi
Draba: Keres, Western
Dyssodia: Keres, Western
Echinacea: Dakota; Lakota; Omaha; Pawnee; Ponca; Winnebago
Echinocactus: Omaha
Elymus: Iroquois; Karok
Ephedra: Cahuilla; Pima
Epilobium: Swinomish
Epipactis: Navajo, Kayenta
Equisetum: Iroquois
Erigeron: Cheyenne
Eriogonum: Navajo, Ramah; Thompson; Zuni
Euonymus: Cherokee; Iroquois
Eupatorium: Cherokee; Iroquois

Festuca: Iroquois
Fraxinus: Iroquois
Gaillardia: Navajo, Kayenta
Gaultheria: Skagit, Upper
Geranium: Blackfoot; Navajo, Kayenta
Glycyrrhiza: Paiute
Gymnocarpium: Abnaki
Hamamelis: Menominee
Helianthus: Hopi; Navajo, Ramah
Hepatica: Iroquois; Meskwaki; Potawatomi
Hymenopappus: Navajo, Kayenta
Ilex: Iroquois
Ipomoea: Iroquois
Juniperus: Algonquin; Comanche; Hopi; Meskwaki; Okanagan-Colville; Rappahannock; Seminole; Thompson
Larix: Menominee; Potawatomi
Lepidium: Navajo, Kayenta
Leucothoe: Cherokee
Licania: Seminole
Ligusticum: Okanagan-Colville
Liquidambar: Cherokee; Koasati
Lobelia: Cherokee; Iroquois
Lomatium: Great Basin Indian; Okanagan-Colville; Yuki
Lycopus: Cherokee
Lysichiton: Kwakiutl; Samish; Swinomish; Tolowa
Mahonia: Karok; Keres, Western
Maianthemum: Iroquois
Malva: Costanoan; Navajo, Ramah
Mentha: Iroquois; Paiute
Myriophyllum: Iroquois
Nepeta: Iroquois; Ojibwa
Nicotiana: Cherokee; Kawaiisu
Nuphar: Iroquois; Nitinaht
Nymphoides: Seminole
Nyssa: Cherokee
Oplopanax: Gitksan
Osmunda: Seminole
Oxalis: Iroquois; Makah
Panax: Cherokee
Parthenocissus: Iroquois
Pellaea: Miwok
Pentaphylloides: Cheyenne
Persea: Seminole
Phlebodium: Seminole
Phragmites: Iroquois
Phytolacca: Cherokee
Picea: Kwakiutl
Pinus: Cherokee; Hualapai; Iroquois; Navajo, Ramah
Platanus: Cherokee
Polygala: Cherokee; Iroquois; Seminole
Polypodium: Seminole

Populus: Flathead
Prenanthes: Choctaw
Prosopis: Pima
Pterocaulon: Seminole
Purshia: Shoshoni
Quercus: Iroquois
Ranunculus: Hesquiat
Rhododendron: Cherokee
Rhus: Creek; Kiowa; Okanagan-Colville
Ribes: Iroquois; Salish, Coast; Thompson
Rubus: Hesquiat; Iroquois; Pomo, Kashaya;
   Seminole
Salix: Seminole
Salvia: Diegueño; Hopi; Shoshoni
Sambucus: Cherokee
Sanguinaria: Iroquois
Sassafras: Seminole
Saururus: Seminole
Scirpus: Clallam
Sedum: Iroquois
Senecio: Costanoan
Silene: Keres, Western
Sisyrinchium: Iroquois
Smallanthus: Cherokee
Smilax: Cherokee; Creek; Seminole
Solanum: Iroquois
Solidago: Iroquois
Sonchus: Pima
Sphaeralcea: Navajo, Kayenta
Spiraea: Okanagan-Colville
Stillingia: Seminole
Tagetes: Navajo
Tanacetum: Cheyenne
Taxus: Chippewa
Tetraneuris: Navajo, Ramah
Thalictrum: Iroquois
Thuja: Bella Coola
Tiarella: Iroquois
Tilia: Iroquois
Trillium: Wailaki; Yuki
Tripterocalyx: Navajo, Ramah
Tsuga: Gitksan; Hesquiat
Typha: Ojibwa
Ulmus: Iroquois
Urtica: Kwakiutl
Veratrum: Gitksan
Verbena: Iroquois
Vitis: Cherokee; Iroquois
Vittaria: Seminole
Zanthoxylum: Menominee
Zinnia: Keres, Western

Panacea

Abies: Abnaki; Shuswap; Thompson

Abronia: Navajo, Kayenta
Acer: Navajo, Ramah
Achillea: Blackfoot; Iroquois; Kwakiutl; Nitinaht;
   Quileute; Thompson; Ute
Acorus: Cheyenne; Cree, Woodlands; Dakota; Mic-
   mac; Mohegan; Omaha; Pawnee; Ponca; Sioux,
   Fort Peck; Winnebago
Ageratina: Iroquois
Agoseris: Navajo, Ramah
Alisma: Cree, Woodlands
Alnus: Rappahannock
Amelanchier: Navajo, Ramah
Androsace: Navajo, Ramah
Anemone: Carrier, Southern; Omaha; Ponca
Angelica: Eskimo; Yana
Anthemis: Mohegan
Apocynum: Meskwaki
Aquilegia: Gosiute; Paiute
Arabis: Cheyenne; Navajo, Ramah
Aralia: Cree, Woodlands; Pomo
Arctostaphylos: Ojibwa
Arenaria: Navajo, Ramah
Argythamnia: Navajo; Navajo, Ramah
Artemisia: Gosiute; Karok; Mewuk; Navajo, Ramah;
   Shuswap; Thompson
Asarum: Montagnais
Asclepias: Pima
Astragalus: Navajo, Ramah
Baccharis: Costanoan
Balsamorhiza: Cheyenne
Besseya: Navajo, Ramah
Blechnum: Quileute
Bouteloua: Navajo, Ramah
Bursera: Cahuilla
Calliandra: Navajo, Ramah
Calochortus: Navajo, Ramah
Calylophus: Navajo, Ramah
Cardamine: Iroquois
Carya: Meskwaki
Ceanothus: Thompson
Cercocarpus: Navajo, Ramah
Chaetopappa: Hopi
Chamaecyparis: Kwakiutl
Cheilanthes: Navajo, Ramah
Chenopodium: Creek
Chrysothamnus: Thompson
Cicuta: Thompson
Cirsium: Navajo, Kayenta; Navajo, Ramah
Clematis: Meskwaki
Collinsonia: Iroquois
Coreopsis: Navajo, Ramah
Cornus: Iroquois; Okanagan-Colville; Thompson
Crataegus: Thompson
Cryptantha: Navajo, Ramah

Rumex: Blackfoot; Iroquois; Navajo, Kayenta; Navajo, Ramah

Salix: Cheyenne; Mendocino Indian; Potawatomi

Salvia: Mohegan; Okanagan-Colville

Sambucus: Karok

Sanguinaria: Delaware, Oklahoma; Iroquois; Ojibwa

Sanicula: Miwok

Sanvitalia: Navajo, Ramah

Saururus: Ojibwa

Saxifraga: Iroquois

Senecio: Navajo, Ramah

Shepherdia: Tanana, Upper

Silene: Navajo, Ramah

Sphaeralcea: Navajo, Ramah

Stephanomeria: Cheyenne; Navajo, Ramah

Streptopus: Montagnais

Tanacetum: Iroquois

Taxus: Chehalis; Thompson

Tellima: Skagit

Tetraneuris: Navajo, Ramah

Thalictrum: Mendocino Indian

Thuja: Abnaki; Cree, Woodlands; Penobscot

Tilia: Iroquois

Tragia: Navajo, Ramah

Trichostema: Mahuna

Trientalis: Montagnais

Trillium: Abnaki; Wailaki; Yuki

Umbellularia: Karok; Mendocino Indian

Urtica: Klallam

Valeriana: Cree, Woodlands

Veratrum: Cherokee; Kwakiutl; Paiute

Veronicastrum: Iroquois

Vicia: Navajo, Ramah

Xanthium: Rappahannock

Zea: Keres, Western

Pediatric Aid

Abies: Flathead; Thompson

Abronia: Hopi

Acacia: Hawaiian

Achillea: Abnaki; Bella Coola; Cree, Woodlands; Iroquois; Menominee; Quileute; Thompson

Acorus: Cheyenne; Chippewa; Cree, Woodlands; Iroquois; Nanticoke; Rappahannock

Actaea: Chippewa

Adiantum: Iroquois; Meskwaki

Agastache: Okanagan-Colville

Agrimonia: Cherokee; Iroquois

Aleurites: Hawaiian

Allium: Cherokee; Chippewa; Iroquois

Alnus: Cherokee; Meskwaki; Okanagan-Colville; Pomo

Amelanchier: Blackfoot; Cherokee; Cheyenne; Cree, Woodlands

Androsace: Navajo, Ramah

Angelica: Blackfoot; Shoshoni

Antennaria: Cherokee; Navajo, Ramah

Anthemis: Iroquois

Aplectrum: Cherokee

Apocynum: Chippewa; Iroquois

Arabis: Cheyenne

Aralia: Algonquin, Quebec; Choctaw; Cree, Woodlands

Arctostaphylos: Blackfoot; Cree, Woodlands; Sanpoil

Arenaria: Gosiute

Argentina: Iroquois

Arisaema: Iroquois

Artemisia: Blackfoot; Cahuilla; Chippewa; Costanoan; Kawaiisu; Okanagan-Colville; Paiute; Paiute, Northern; Pomo; Shoshoni; Thompson; Tolowa; Yurok

Asarum: Algonquin, Quebec; Iroquois; Malecite; Thompson; Yurok

Asclepias: Blackfoot; Chippewa; Iroquois; Lakota; Navajo, Kayenta

Asplenium: Hawaiian

Aster: Cree, Woodlands; Iroquois; Zuni

Astragalus: Blackfoot; Dakota

Besseya: Navajo, Ramah

Betula: Algonquin, Quebec; Cree, Woodlands

Botrychium: Abnaki

Brickellia: Navajo, Kayenta; Navajo, Ramah

Broussaisia: Hawaiian

Caesalpinia: Hawaiian

Calycanthus: Cherokee

Capsicum: Navajo, Ramah

Cardamine: Algonquin, Quebec; Malecite

Carpinus: Iroquois

Carum: Cree, Woodlands

Castanea: Cherokee; Iroquois

Ceanothus: Iroquois; Okanagan-Colville; Poliklah

Celastrus: Chippewa; Iroquois

Cerastium: Cherokee

Cercocarpus: Paiute; Shoshoni

Chaenactis: Great Basin Indian; Nevada Indian

Chaetopappa: Havasupai; Hopi

Chamaemelum: Mahuna

Chamaesyce: Cherokee; Hawaiian; Hopi; Houma

Chenopodium: Hawaiian; Houma; Natchez

Chimaphila: Cherokee; Iroquois

Chrysopsis: Delaware

Chrysothamnus: Tewa

Cimicifuga: Cherokee; Iroquois

Cirsium: Abnaki; Kwakiutl; Mohegan

Citrullus: Cherokee

Claytonia: Iroquois
Clematis: Thompson
Coix: Cherokee
Collinsonia: Iroquois
Conyza: Iroquois; Navajo, Kayenta
Coptis: Iroquois; Malecite; Menominee; Mohegan; Ojibwa; Potawatomi
Cornus: Cherokee; Iroquois; Meskwaki; Ojibwa; Okanagan-Colville; Shuswap; Thompson
Corylus: Iroquois
Crataegus: Okanagan-Colville
Croton: Cahuilla; Pawnee
Cryptantha: Navajo, Kayenta; Navajo, Ramah
Cucurbita: Iroquois
Cypripedium: Algonquin, Tête-de-Boule
Dalea: Keres, Western
Datura: Kawaiisu
Delphinium: Blackfoot
Diervilla: Iroquois
Digitaria: Hawaiian
Dimorphocarpa: Navajo, Kayenta
Dodecatheon: Blackfoot
Dracocephalum: Navajo, Kayenta
Echinocystis: Tubatulabal
Elaeagnus: Blackfoot
Empetrum: Cree, Woodlands
Ephedra: Paiute; Shoshoni
Epigaea: Cherokee
Epilobium: Blackfoot; Costanoan; Okanagan-Colville
Epipactis: Navajo, Kayenta
Equisetum: Iroquois; Okanagan-Colville; Sanpoil; Tolowa
Eriastrum: Paiute
Eriogonum: Diegueño; Lakota; Navajo, Ramah; Tubatulabal
Eschscholzia: Costanoan
Euonymus: Iroquois
Eupatorium: Chippewa; Ojibwa
Euphorbia: Cherokee; Iroquois
Fagopyrum: Iroquois
Foeniculum: Cherokee
Fragaria: Chippewa; Ojibwa; Okanagan-Colville; Thompson
Freycinetia: Hawaiian
Galactia: Seminole
Galium: Iroquois
Gaura: Navajo, Ramah
Geranium: Cherokee; Chippewa; Iroquois
Geum: Cree, Woodlands; Malecite; Micmac
Glechoma: Cherokee
Gleditsia: Creek
Glycyrrhiza: Dakota; Pawnee; Sioux
Gnaphalium: Koasati

Goodyera: Mohegan
Gossypium: Tewa
Grindelia: Dakota; Navajo, Ramah
Helianthus: Iroquois; Navajo, Kayenta
Hepatica: Chippewa; Iroquois
Heracleum: Kwakiutl
Heuchera: Blackfoot; Gosiute; Okanagan-Colville
Hibiscus: Hawaiian
Hilaria: Navajo, Ramah
Hydrangea: Cherokee
Hydrophyllum: Ojibwa
Hymenopappus: Isleta
Hypericum: Alabama; Natchez
Impatiens: Cherokee
Inula: Iroquois
Ipomoea: Hawaiian
Ipomopsis: Salish; Zuni
Iris: Yokia; Zuni
Isocoma: Navajo, Kayenta
Iva: Shoshoni
Jacquemontia: Hawaiian
Jeffersonia: Iroquois
Juncus: Cherokee
Juniperus: Cree, Woodlands; Hopi; Navajo, Ramah; Seminole; Tewa
Krameria: Pima
Lactuca: Okanagan-Colville
Larix: Thompson
Larrea: Papago
Lechea: Seminole
Ledum: Cree, Woodlands; Eskimo, Kuskokwagmiut; Montagnais
Lepidium: Navajo, Kayenta
Liatris: Pawnee; Seminole
Ligusticum: Atsugewi; Okanagan-Colville
Lilium: Cherokee
Linanthus: Pomo, Calpella
Linaria: Iroquois
Linnaea: Iroquois; Tanana, Upper
Linum: Okanagon; Thompson
Liriodendron: Cherokee
Lithospermum: Iroquois; Navajo
Lomatium: Cheyenne; Okanagan-Colville; Thompson; Washo
Lonicera: Iroquois
Ludwigia: Hawaiian
Lupinus: Kwakiutl
Lycopus: Cherokee; Iroquois
Lygodesmia: Blackfoot; Cheyenne; Lakota
Lysichiton: Kwakiutl
Mahonia: Havasupai
Maianthemum: Karok; Meskwaki
Malva: Costanoan; Iroquois
Marah: Tubatulabal

Marrubium: Cherokee; Diegueño
Matelea: Comanche
Matricaria: Costanoan; Diegueño; Flathead
Medeola: Iroquois
Melissa: Costanoan
Mentha: Abnaki; Cherokee; Iroquois; Malecite; Micmac; Mohegan; Navajo, Kayenta; Okanagan-Colville; Okanagon; Paiute; Sanpoil; Shoshoni; Thompson; Washo
Mentzelia: Zuni
Merremia: Hawaiian
Mimulus: Karok
Mirabilis: Karok; Pawnee; Zuni
Mitchella: Cherokee; Iroquois
Mitella: Gosiute
Monarda: Choctaw; Menominee; Ojibwa
Monardella: Okanagan-Colville; Sanpoil
Monotropa: Cherokee
Myrica: Koasati
Myriophyllum: Iroquois
Nepeta: Cherokee; Delaware; Delaware, Oklahoma; Delaware, Ontario; Hoh; Iroquois; Mohegan; Quileute; Rappahannock
Nereocystis: Kwakiutl, Southern
Nuphar: Iroquois
Nyssa: Cherokee
Ochrosia: Hawaiian
Onoclea: Iroquois
Orobanche: Navajo, Ramah
Osmunda: Iroquois; Seminole
Oxalis: Cherokee
Panax: Cherokee;; Iroquois; Meskwaki; Seminole
Pandanus: Hawaiian
Parnassia: Cheyenne
Passiflora: Cherokee
Pedicularis: Shoshoni
Pediomelum: Blackfoot
Peltandra: Nanticoke
Penstemon: Navajo, Kayenta; Paiute; Shoshoni
Persea: Seminole
Petasites: Karok
Peucedanum: Hawaiian
Phaseolus: Zuni
Phlebodium: Seminole
Phlox: Blackfoot; Cherokee; Havasupai; Okanagan-Colville; Paiute; Shoshoni
Phoradendron: Keres, Western; Seminole
Phragmites: Keres, Western
Phyla: Houma
Phyllospadix: Kwakiutl
Physaria: Blackfoot
Picea: Cree, Woodlands; Makah
Pilea: Cherokee
Piloblephis: Seminole

Pinus: Delaware, Ontario; Iroquois; Kawaiisu; Shuswap; Thompson
Piper: Hawaiian
Plantago: Cherokee; Navajo
Platanthera: Iroquois
Platanus: Cherokee
Pleopeltis: Houma
Pluchea: Pima
Polygala: Iroquois
Polygonum: Cherokee; Iroquois; Meskwaki; Thompson
Polystichum: Iroquois
Populus: Iroquois; Meskwaki; Thompson
Prenanthes: Bella Coola
Prosopis: Apache, Mescalero; Pima
Prunella: Iroquois; Menominee
Prunus: Algonquin, Tête-de-Boule; Blackfoot; Cheyenne; Chippewa; Delaware; Gosiute; Iroquois; Karok; Kwakiutl; Malecite; Menominee
Psathyrotes: Shoshoni
Psidium: Hawaiian
Ptelea: Havasupai
Pteridium: Micmac; Montagnais
Pyrola: Iroquois; Karok; Navajo, Kayenta
Quercus: Alabama; Keres, Western; Mahuna; Miwok;
Ratibida: Navajo, Ramah
Rhamnus: Iroquois
Rhus: Chippewa; Diegueño; Koasati
Ribes: Navajo, Kayenta; Sanpoil; Thompson
Ricinus: Hawaiian
Rorippa: Iroquois
Rosa: Blackfoot; Cahuilla; Cherokee; Cowlitz; Diegueño; Isleta; Keres, Western; Paiute; Thompson
Rubus: Cree, Woodlands; Iroquois; Kwakiutl; Micmac; Omaha; Thompson
Rudbeckia: Chippewa; Iroquois
Rumex: Chippewa; Iroquois; Yavapai; Yuki
Sagittaria: Cherokee; Iroquois
Salix: Catawba; Navajo, Ramah; Okanagan-Colville
Salvia: Paiute; Shoshoni
Sambucus: Cahuilla; Cherokee; Delaware; Delaware, Oklahoma; Diegueño; Iroquois; Karok; Mohegan; Paiute
Sanguinaria: Iroquois
Sanicula: Iroquois
Sassafras: Cherokee; Seminole
Scirpus: Kwakiutl; Thompson
Sedum: Iroquois; Okanagon; Thompson
Senecio: Iroquois; Navajo, Ramah
Senna: Cherokee
Sesamum: Cherokee
Shepherdia: Navajo, Kayenta

Silene: Gosiute; Karok
Silphium: Iroquois
Sisyrinchium: Cherokee
Solanum: Blackfoot; Cherokee; Houma
Solidago: Iroquois; Navajo, Kayenta; Okanagan-Colville; Thompson
Sonchus: Houma; Iroquois
Sorbus: Okanagan-Colville
Sphaeralcea: Hopi
Spigelia: Creek
Spiranthes: Cherokee
Staphylea: Iroquois
Stenandrium: Seminole
Stenotaphrum: Hawaiian
Stillingia: Seminole
Symphoricarpos: Cree, Woodlands; Nez Perce; Okanagan-Colville; Skagit; Thompson
Symplocarpus: Iroquois; Menominee
Syringa: Iroquois
Syzygium: Hawaiian
Tanacetum: Cherokee
Tephrosia: Cherokee
Thaspium: Chippewa
Thelesperma: Keres, Western
Thelypodium: Navajo, Kayenta
Thuja: Algonquin, Quebec; Nez Perce
Tiarella: Iroquois; Malecite
Tilia: Iroquois
Touchardia: Hawaiian
Toxicodendron: Iroquois
Tragia: Keres, Western
Trillium: Abnaki
Triosteum: Iroquois; Meskwaki
Tripterocalyx: Hopi
Tsuga: Algonquin, Quebec; Kwakiutl; Malecite; Quinault
Typha: Dakota; Mahuna; Omaha; Pawnee; Plains Indian; Ponca; Winnebago
Ulmus: Cheyenne
Urtica: Kawaiisu
Uvularia: Iroquois
Vaccinium: Algonquin, Quebec; Cheyenne; Seminole
Valeriana: Cree, Woodlands
Veratrum: Kwakiutl; Thompson
Verbascum: Abnaki; Catawba; Iroquois
Viburnum: Cree, Woodlands; Iroquois
Vigna: Hawaiian
Viola: Blackfoot
Vitis: Cherokee; Iroquois; Seminole
Vittaria: Seminole
Waltheria: Hawaiian
Xanthium: Tewa
Xyris: Cherokee

Zanthoxylum: Chippewa
Zea: Tewa

Poison

Aconitum: Aleut; Cree, Hudson Bay; Eskimo, Inupiat; Gosiute; Okanagan-Colville
Actaea: Alaska Native; Eskimo, Arctic; Thompson
Aesculus: Costanoan; Delaware; Delaware, Oklahoma; Kawaiisu; Mendocino Indian; Pomo
Allium: Mendocino Indian
Amanita: Pomo, Kashaya
Amianthium: Cherokee
Anemone: Thompson
Angelica: Iroquois
Anthemis: Yuki
Apocynum: Montana Indian
Aralia: Cherokee
Arctostaphylos: Mendocino Indian
Arisaema: Meskwaki; Mohegan; Penobscot
Artemisia: Thompson
Asclepias: Mendocino Indian; Pima; Thompson
Astragalus: Lakota; Mahuna
Atriplex: Isleta
Bovista: Haisla & Hanaksiala
Brickellia: Gosiute
Bromus: Hesquiat
Calla: Cree, Woodlands
Caltha: Abnaki; Alaska Native; Eskimo, Inupiat
Calycanthus: Cherokee
Cardamine: Iroquois
Castilleja: Cherokee
Celastrus: Iroquois; Oglala
Chaerophyllum: Chickasaw
Chamaesyce: Pima
Chenopodium: Kawaiisu
Chimaphila: Cherokee
Chlorogalum: Costanoan; Mendocino Indian; Mewuk
Chrysothamnus: Isleta
Cicuta: Alaska Native; Eskimo, Inupiat; Eskimo, Kuskokwagmiut; Eskimo, Western; Haisla & Hanaksiala; Iroquois; Kawaiisu; Klamath; Kwakiutl; Lakota; Montana Indian; Okanagan-Colville; Shoshoni; Shuswap; Thompson
Citrullus: Kiowa
Clintonia: Ojibwa; Pomo; Pomo, Kashaya
Comptonia: Menominee
Conium: Klallam; Lakota; Snohomish
Consolida: Cherokee
Cornus: Blackfoot; Thompson
Crataegus: Mendocino Indian
Croton: Cahuilla; Pomo
Cryptantha: Keres, Western
Dalea: Dakota

Datura: Cahuilla; Coahuilla; Diegueño; Hopi; Iroquois; Kawaiisu; Keres, Western; Mahuna; Paiute, Northern; Rappahannock

Delphinium: Chehalis; Cherokee; Gosiute; Lakota; Mendocino Indian

Dichanthelium: Lakota

Dipsacus: Iroquois

Disporum: Klallam

Echinocereus: Navajo

Epilobium: Swinomish

Erigeron: Gosiute

Eschscholzia: Costanoan; Mahuna

Eupatorium: Iroquois

Euphorbia: Pawnee

Frangula: Flathead; Pomo; West Coast Indian

Fritillaria: Ute

Galium: Cowlitz; Shuswap

Hackelia: Isleta; Navajo, Ramah

Hedysarum: Alaska Native; Eskimo, Inupiat; Tanana, Upper

Helenium: Meskwaki

Heracleum: Cree; Karok

Heterotheca: Isleta

Hordeum: Navajo, Ramah

Hymenoxys: Keres, Western; Navajo, Ramah

Iris: Abnaki; Eskimo, Inupiat

Juglans: Cherokee

Juniperus: Okanagan-Colville

Kalmia: Algonquin, Quebec; Algonquin, Tête-de-Boule; Cree, Hudson Bay; Hesquiat; Mahuna; Micmac; Montagnais

Lathyrus: Eskimo, Inupiat

Ledum: Eskimo, Inupiat

Ligusticum: Eskimo, Western

Lomatium: Creek; Montana Indian; Okanagan-Colville

Lonicera: Makah; Okanagan-Colville; Poliklah; Thompson; Tolowa

Lupinus: Alaska Native; Eskimo, Inupiat; Thompson

Lycoperdon: Kashaya

Lycopus: Iroquois

Lysichiton: Gitksan

Mahonia: Karok

Marah: Karok; Mendocino Indian; Squaxin

Nicotiana: Kawaiisu

Nuphar: Okanagan-Colville

Nymphaea: Okanagan-Colville

Oenanthe: Haisla & Hanaksiala

Onopordum: Iroquois

Oplopanax: Cowlitz; Kwakiutl; Oweekeno

Opuntia: Navajo

Orobanche: Montana Indian

Osmorhiza: Kwakiutl

Oxytropis: Hopi; Lakota

Parthenocissus: Iroquois

Pastinaca: Ojibwa; Potawatomi

Pentaphylloides: Cheyenne

Phoradendron: Mendocino Indian

Phytolacca: Cherokee; Mahuna; Mohegan

Platanthera: Shuswap

Podophyllum: Cherokee; Iroquois

Polygonum: Cherokee

Prunus: Rappahannock

Ptelea: Havasupai

Pteridium: Alaska Native; Okanagan-Colville

Pulsatilla: Cheyenne

Quercus: Mendocino Indian

Ranunculus: Aleut; Eskimo, Inupiat; Keres, Western; Okanagan-Colville; Thompson

Rheum: Cherokee

Rhus: Thompson

Ribes: Oweekeno; Swinomish

Ricinus: Cahuilla; Pima

Rosa: Thompson

Sambucus: Hesquiat

Sapium: Seri

Senecio: Eskimo, Inuktitut; Eskimo, Western

Shepherdia: Eskimo, Inupiat; Havasupai; Sioux

Sisyrinchium: Iroquois

Sium: Shuswap

Solanum: Cahuilla; Karok; Mendocino Indian; Rappahannock

Sonchus: Navajo, Kayenta

Stanleya: Havasupai

Symphoricarpos: Okanagan-Colville; Thompson

Taxus: Mendocino Indian

Tephrosia: Hawaiian

Thalictrum: Kawaiisu; Mendocino Indian

Thuja: Okanagan-Colville

Toxicodendron: Cherokee; Chippewa; Karok; Lakota; Navajo, Ramah; Omaha; Paiute; Ponca; Potawatomi; Thompson; Tolowa; Yurok

Triglochin: Blackfoot

Trillium: Concow; Pomo, Kashaya; Skagit

Triteleia: Okanagan-Colville

Urtica: Navajo, Ramah

Valeriana: Blackfoot; Gosiute; Snake

Veratrum: Alaska Native; Bella Coola; Blackfoot; Carrier, Southern; Cowlitz; Haisla & Hanaksiala; Kwakiutl; Okanagan-Colville; Oweekeno; Quinault; Salish; Shuswap; Thompson

Veronicastrum: Iroquois

Vicia: Navajo

Wyethia: Hopi

Yucca: Navajo, Ramah

Zigadenus: Alaska Native; Eskimo, Inupiat; Haisla & Hanaksiala; Keres, Western; Lakota; Mendocino Indian; Okanagan-Colville; Paiute; Pomo, Kashaya; Shuswap; Thompson; Ute; Yuki

Poultice

Abies: Algonquin, Quebec
Achillea: Algonquin, Quebec
Aralia: Choctaw
Astragalus: Navajo, Kayenta
Capsicum: Cherokee
Cirsium: Cherokee
Cornus: Cherokee; Iroquois
Grindelia: Zuni
Iodanthus: Meskwaki
Linum: Paiute
Liriodendron: Cherokee
Pinus: Shoshoni
Plantago: Algonquin, Quebec
Polygonum: Cherokee
Populus: Kawaiisu
Ruta: Cherokee
Salvia: Paiute
Saururus: Cherokee
Taraxacum: Algonquin, Quebec
Taxus: Algonquin, Quebec
Verbena: Iroquois

Preventive Medicine

Abies: Nitinaht
Acorus: Algonquin, Quebec; Malecite
Angelica: Eskimo
Chamaesyce: Lakota
Crataegus: Cherokee
Fraxinus: Karok
Helianthus: Shasta
Iris: Penobscot
Mahonia: Keres, Western
Osmorhiza: Karok
Pellaea: Mahuna
Prunus: Kwakiutl
Salix: Seminole
Sanguinaria: Penobscot
Thlaspi: Navajo, Ramah
Toxicodendron: Mahuna

Psychological Aid

Abronia: Keres, Western
Acorus: Dakota
Actaea: Iroquois
Adiantum: Navajo, Kayenta
Aloysia: Havasupai
Ambrosia: Meskwaki
Anemone: Meskwaki
Angelica: Eskimo
Apocynum: Chippewa

Arabis: Navajo, Kayenta
Arctostaphylos: Cheyenne
Artemisia: Cheyenne
Asarum: Iroquois
Aster: Meskwaki
Berlandiera: Keres, Western
Cannabis: Iroquois
Cardamine: Iroquois
Chrysothamnus: Cheyenne
Conocephalum: Nitinaht
Cornus: Iroquois; Thompson
Corylus: Iroquois
Crepis: Keres, Western
Cucurbita: Hawaiian
Cynoglossum: Cherokee
Datura: Hopi; Keres, Western
Diervilla: Menominee
Dimorphocarpa: Zuni
Eriogonum: Keres, Western; Navajo, Kayenta
Eupatorium: Iroquois
Fragaria: Cherokee
Frangula: Mendocino Indian
Frasera: Navajo, Ramah
Fraxinus: Algonquin, Tête-de-Boule
Gaillardia: Keres, Western
Gayophytum: Navajo, Kayenta
Gentiana: Iroquois
Gnaphalium: Creek; Menominee; Meskwaki
Gymnocladus: Meskwaki
Hackelia: Cherokee
Hymenoxys: Isleta
Hyptis: Seminole
Ilex: Iroquois; Seminole
Juglans: Iroquois
Juniperus: Seminole
Lagenaria: Seminole
Laportea: Iroquois
Lewisia: Thompson
Licania: Seminole
Linnaea: Tanana, Upper
Linum: Keres, Western
Lithospermum: Cheyenne
Lobelia: Iroquois
Lonicera: Iroquois; Nitinaht
Lygodesmia: Cheyenne
Lysichiton: Thompson
Macromeria: Hopi
Madia: Cheyenne
Mahonia: Thompson
Maianthemum: Meskwaki
Mentzelia: Keres, Western
Microlepia: Hawaiian
Mirabilis: Paiute
Mitchella: Iroquois

Nicotiana: Iroquois; Kawaiisu
Osmorhiza: Karok
Osmunda: Seminole
Panax: Menominee
Pectis: Keres, Western
Penstemon: Karok
Persea: Seminole
Phlebodium: Seminole
Picea: Thompson
Pinus: Iroquois
Plantago: Hopi
Polygonum: Iroquois
Polypodium: Seminole
Populus: Thompson
Postelsia: Nitinaht
Prunella: Iroquois
Prunus: Saanich
Quercus: Iroquois
Ranunculus: Iroquois
Ribes: Saanich
Salix: Iroquois
Sambucus: Nitinaht
Senecio: Keres, Western
Smilax: Iroquois
Solanum: Cherokee
Solidago: Meskwaki; Navajo, Kayenta
Sorbus: Algonquin, Tête-de-Boule
Tellima: Nitinaht
Tetraneuris: Navajo, Kayenta
Thelypteris: Seminole
Thuja: Thompson
Thymophylla: Navajo, Kayenta
Tradescantia: Meskwaki
Urtica: Kawaiisu
Vaccinium: Chippewa
Valeriana: Menominee
Veratrum: Tsimshian
Verbascum: Hopi; Navajo, Ramah
Vitis: Meskwaki
Vittaria: Seminole
Zinnia: Keres, Western

Pulmonary Aid

Abies: Blackfoot; Cherokee; Gitksan; Menominee; Montana Indian; Paiute; Shoshoni
Acer: Iroquois
Acorus: Blackfoot; Cree, Woodlands; Micmac
Actaea: Thompson
Adenostoma: Cahuilla
Aesculus: Iroquois
Agastache: Cheyenne
Aletris: Cherokee
Allium: Cherokee; Makah; Quinault; Rappahannock
Alnus: Bella Coola; Clallam; Nitinaht

Ambrosia: Cherokee
Amelanchier: Cree, Woodlands
Andropogon: Seminole
Anemone: Cherokee; Ojibwa
Anemopsis: Cahuilla; Isleta
Angelica: Iroquois; Paiute, Northern; Shoshoni
Anthemis: Iroquois
Apocynum: Cherokee
Aralia: Cherokee; Cree, Woodlands; Iroquois; Mendocino Indian; Menominee
Arceuthobium: Bella Coola
Arctium: Cowlitz; Oto
Aristolochia: Cherokee
Artemisia: Blackfoot; Flathead; Hawaiian; Kiowa; Montana Indian; Paiute; Shoshoni; Tlingit
Asarum: Iroquois; Meskwaki
Asclepias: Cherokee; Delaware; Delaware, Oklahoma; Menominee; Mohegan; Omaha; Ponca
Aster: Iroquois
Astragalus: Blackfoot; Lakota
Balsamorhiza: Flathead
Betula: Chippewa
Blechnum: Makah
Botrychium: Ojibwa
Boykinia: Cheyenne
Brassica: Cherokee
Caesalpinia: Hawaiian
Campanula: Ojibwa
Campanulastrum: Iroquois
Cardamine: Iroquois
Castanea: Mohegan
Castilleja: Gitksan
Caulophyllum: Chippewa
Ceanothus: Chippewa
Centaurium: Miwok
Cercis: Alabama; Cherokee
Cercocarpus: Paiute
Chenopodium: Potawatomi; Seminole
Chimaphila: Cree, Woodlands; Delaware
Cirsium: Mohegan
Collinsia: Natchez
Comandra: Meskwaki
Comptonia: Delaware
Coptis: Tlingit
Corallorrhiza: Paiute; Shoshoni
Cordyline: Hawaiian
Cornus: Carrier; Iroquois; Thompson
Cucurbita: Isleta
Cypripedium: Iroquois
Dalea: Navajo
Datura: Rappahannock
Dichanthelium: Seminole
Dirca: Chippewa
Epigaea: Cherokee

Sanguinaria: Cherokee; Iroquois
Sarracenia: Iroquois; Micmac
Senna: Cherokee
Silphium: Chippewa
Sinapis: Cherokee
Sisymbrium: Cherokee
Smilax: Ojibwa
Solidago: Chippewa
Sorbus: Potawatomi; Tlingit
Symplocarpus: Delaware
Taenidia: Menominee
Taraxacum: Iroquois; Meskwaki
Taxus: Bella Coola; Quinault
Tetradymia: Paiute
Thalictrum: Blackfoot; Gitksan
Thuja: Cree, Woodlands; Lummi
Tilia: Meskwaki
Trifolium: Algonquin, Quebec
Triosteum: Iroquois
Typha: Houma
Ulmus: Micmac; Mohegan; Penobscot
Urtica: Paiute
Uvularia: Ojibwa
Vaccinium: Montagnais
Valeriana: Cree, Woodlands; Menominee
Verbascum: Catawba; Delaware; Delaware, Oklahoma; Menominee
Veronicastrum: Iroquois
Viburnum: Bella Coola; Iroquois
Waltheria: Hawaiian
Wyethia: Costanoan
Xanthium: Cherokee
Xyris: Seminole
Zanthoxylum: Chippewa; Menominee
Zea: Cherokee

Reproductive Aid

Antennaria: Okanagan-Colville
Artemisia: Hawaiian
Athyrium: Iroquois
Berchemia: Houma
Broussaisia: Hawaiian
Chaetopappa: Hopi
Chamaesyce: Hawaiian
Cinchona: Cherokee
Coreopsis: Zuni
Cypripedium: Okanagan-Colville
Dyssodia: Lakota
Fraxinus: Iroquois
Galactia: Seminole
Gaultheria: Nitinaht
Goodyera: Okanagan-Colville
Halosaccion: Nitinaht
Hypericum: Iroquois

Ipomoea: Hawaiian
Juniperus: Hopi; Tewa
Justicia: Seminole
Licania: Seminole
Lomatium: Thompson
Lonicera: Thompson
Lupinus: Navajo
Lycopodium: Iroquois
Maianthemum: Makah
Opuntia: Hawaiian
Panax: Penobscot
Persea: Seminole
Peucedanum: Hawaiian
Pinus: Kwakiutl
Quercus: Isleta
Rhus: Cheyenne; Iroquois
Ribes: Haisla
Rubus: Cree, Woodlands
Rumex: Hawaiian; Iroquois; Zuni
Salix: Delaware
Sambucus: Haisla & Hanaksiala
Shepherdia: Haisla & Hanaksiala
Tephrosia: Creek
Townsendia: Hopi
Trema: Seminole
Urtica: Makah
Vaccinium: Cree, Woodlands
Viburnum: Delaware
Vitis: Delaware; Delaware, Oklahoma
Zeuxine: Seminole

Respiratory Aid

Acer: Abnaki
Achillea: Algonquin, Quebec; Bella Coola; Cherokee; Cheyenne; Paiute; Yuki
Acorus: Chippewa; Iroquois; Potawatomi
Adiantum: Cherokee; Hesquiat
Aleurites: Hawaiian
Allium: Cherokee
Alnus: Kwakiutl
Amorpha: Navajo
Anaphalis: Cherokee; Iroquois
Andromeda: Mahuna
Anemone: Meskwaki
Anemopsis: Cahuilla
Angelica: Washo
Anthemis: Cherokee
Apocynum: Cherokee
Aralia: Cherokee
Arenaria: Kawaiisu; Navajo, Ramah
Arisaema: Iroquois
Armoracia: Cherokee
Artemisia: Blackfoot; Cahuilla; Cheyenne;

Costanoan; Diegueño; Eskimo, Alaska;
  Mendocino Indian; Paiute
Asarum: Iroquois
Asclepias: Costanoan; Isleta; Navajo, Kayenta;
  Omaha; Ponca
Aster: Cherokee
Bacopa: Seminole
Baptisia: Meskwaki
Betula: Ojibwa
Brassica: Cherokee
Calla: Gitksan
Cassytha: Hawaiian
Ceanothus: Chippewa
Cercis: Alabama
Cheirodendron: Hawaiian
Clematis: Navajo, Ramah
Clermontia: Hawaiian
Comandra: Meskwaki
Comptonia: Malecite; Micmac
Conioselinum: Navajo, Kayenta
Conyza: Seminole; Zuni
Coptis: Algonquin, Tête-de-Boule
Cordyline: Hawaiian
Cornus: Iroquois; Malecite; Micmac; Saanich
Corylus: Iroquois
Croton: Cahuilla
Datura: Cahuilla; Cherokee; Costanoan
Desmodium: Hawaiian
Dudleya: Diegueño
Dugaldia: Great Basin Indian
Erigeron: Meskwaki
Eriodictyon: Cahuilla; Costanoan; Mahuna;
  Mendocino Indian; Round Valley Indian
Eryngium: Seminole
Erysimum: Navajo, Ramah
Euonymus: Cherokee
Eupatorium: Cherokee
Gaillardia: Navajo, Ramah
Galium: Cherokee
Geum: Blackfoot
Glycyrrhiza: Cherokee
Gnaphalium: Cherokee; Iroquois; Rappahannock
Grindelia: Crow; Flathead
Gutierrezia: Blackfoot
Hamamelis: Iroquois
Helenium: Comanche; Mahuna; Meskwaki
Hexastylis: Rappahannock
Hierochloe: Flathead
Hydrocotyle: Seminole
Hyssopus: Cherokee
Ilex: Iroquois
Inula: Cherokee; Iroquois
Ipomoea: Cherokee
Iris: Iroquois

Juniperus: Chippewa; Cree, Woodlands; Eskimo,
  Inupiat; Kwakiutl; Rappahannock
Larix: Thompson
Larrea: Cahuilla; Hualapai
Ledum: Kitasoo; Micmac; Tanana, Upper
Lesquerella: Navajo, Ramah
Ligusticum: Crow
Limonium: Costanoan
Linaria: Ojibwa
Lindera: Cherokee
Lobelia: Cherokee
Lomatium: Great Basin Indian; Nez Perce;
  Okanagan-Colville; Paiute; Shoshoni; Washo
Machaeranthera: Navajo, Ramah
Magnolia: Cherokee
Maianthemum: Menominee
Marrubium: Kawaiisu
Mentha: Iroquois
Monarda: Crow; Menominee; Meskwaki; Ojibwa
Monardella: Costanoan
Nicotiana: Kawaiisu; Paiute
Nuphar: Kwakiutl
Nymphoides: Seminole
Oplopanax: Gitksan; Haisla; Wet'suwet'en
Oxydendrum: Cherokee
Panax: Iroquois; Seminole
Perideridia: Blackfoot
Persea: Seminole
Petasites: Delaware; Delaware, Oklahoma; Eskimo,
  Inupiat
Physaria: Navajo
Picea: Eskimo, Inuktitut; Okanagan-Colville;
  Tanana, Upper
Pilea: Iroquois
Pimpinella: Cherokee
Pinus: Cherokee
Plantago: Iroquois
Platanus: Diegueño; Mahuna
Pleomele: Hawaiian
Polygala: Blackfoot; Seminole
Polypodium: Haisla; Nitinaht
Populus: Kutenai; Ojibwa
Porteranthus: Cherokee
Prunella: Iroquois
Prunus: Iroquois; Mohegan
Purshia: Klamath
Quercus: Cherokee; Iroquois; Ojibwa
Ranunculus: Meskwaki
Rhus: Chippewa
Rubus: Iroquois
Sadleria: Hawaiian
Salix: Cherokee; Micmac; Penobscot; Seminole
Salvia: Cherokee; Mahuna; Washo
Sanguinaria: Cherokee; Iroquois

Sinapis: Cherokee
Sisyrinchium: Meskwaki; Pomo, Kashaya
Taenidia: Menominee
Taxus: Iroquois
Thuja: Bella Coola
Toxicodendron: Cherokee
Trifolium: Iroquois
Trillium: Cherokee
Ulmus: Cherokee; Iroquois
Umbellularia: Pomo, Kashaya; Yuki
Veratrum: Hanaksiala; Iroquois; Thompson; Tsimshian
Verbascum: Delaware; Delaware, Oklahoma; Iroquois; Malecite; Micmac; Mohegan; Penobscot; Potawatomi
Vicia: Cherokee
Vigna: Hawaiian
Viola: Blackfoot; Cherokee
Waltheria: Hawaiian
Zanthoxylum: Ojibwa

Sedative

Abronia: Hopi
Achillea: Cherokee
Acorus: Rappahannock
Angelica: Cherokee*Anthemis*: Cherokee; Iroquois
Arisaema: Meskwaki
Artemisia: Lakota
Asarum: Cherokee; Thompson
Bacopa: Seminole
Balsamorhiza: Thompson
Berlandiera: Keres, Western
Cardamine: Micmac
Carum: Cree, Woodlands
Caulophyllum: Cherokee
Ceanothus: Navajo
Chaetopappa: Hopi
Chamaemelum: Cherokee
Chenopodium: Seminole
Chrysopsis: Delaware; Delaware, Oklahoma
Cibotium: Hawaiian
Cimicifuga: Cherokee
Cordyline: Hawaiian
Cornus: Iroquois
Cypripedium: Cherokee; Iroquois; Micmac; Penobscot
Datura: Tubatulabal
Dodecatheon: Pomo, Kashaya
Eriogonum: Keres, Western
Eryngium: Creek
Eschscholzia: Costanoan
Eupatorium: Chippewa
Fragaria: Cherokee
Frasera: Navajo

Galax: Cherokee
Gaultheria: Anticosti
Gaura: Keres, Western
Gentianella: Cherokee
Gilia: Navajo, Kayenta
Glaux: Kwakiutl
Gnaphalium: Alabama; Creek
Gutierrezia: Navajo
Heterotheca: Cheyenne
Humulus: Cherokee; Delaware; Delaware, Oklahoma; Meskwaki; Mohegan; Shinnecock
Hydrocotyle: Seminole
Ipomoea: Pawnee
Ipomopsis: Navajo, Kayenta
Juniperus: Cheyenne; Pawnee; Seminole
Lactuca: Cherokee
Leonurus: Cherokee; Iroquois
Lepidium: Navajo, Kayenta
Linaria: Iroquois
Linnaea: Iroquois
Liquidambar: Cherokee
Liriodendron: Cherokee
Lithospermum: Cheyenne; Menominee
Lomatium: Thompson
Lonicera: Iroquois; Thompson
Lupinus: Kwakiutl
Lysichiton: Gitksan
Maianthemum: Meskwaki
Mentha: Abnaki; Cherokee; Mahuna; Malecite
Mitchella: Menominee
Monarda: Cherokee
Nepeta: Cherokee; Delaware, Ontario; Iroquois; Menominee
Nicotiana: Kawaiisu
Nymphoides: Seminole
Oxydendrum: Cherokee
Panax: Seminole
Papaver: Cherokee
Persea: Seminole
Pinus: Cherokee; Thompson
Piper: Hawaiian
Pluchea: Pima
Polygonatum: Chippewa
Prunella: Iroquois
Prunus: Mendocino Indian; Meskwaki
Pyrola: Karok
Quercus: Navajo, Kayenta
Ranunculus: Cherokee
Ratibida: Keres, Western
Rhamnus: Iroquois
Ribes: Cherokee; Thompson
Ruta: Cherokee
Salix: Ojibwa
Salvia: Cherokee

Sambucus: Micmac
Sassafras: Rappahannock
Satureja: Mahuna; Pomo, Kashaya
Sedum: Okanagon; Thompson
Senecio: Cheyenne
Shepherdia: Thompson
Shinnersoseris: Navajo
Smallanthus: Iroquois
Solanum: Rappahannock
Solidago: Cherokee; Iroquois; Thompson
Sonchus: Cherokee; Iroquois
Staphylea: Iroquois
Stenandrium: Seminole
Taraxacum: Cherokee
Thelypodium: Navajo, Kayenta
Toxicodendron: Iroquois
Tripterocalyx: Hopi
Valeriana: Menominee
Veratrum: Haisla
Xanthorhiza: Cherokee
Yucca: Cherokee
Zanthoxylum: Menominee

Snakebite Remedy

Acer: Thompson
Achillea: Kawaiisu; Okanagon; Thompson
Adiantum: Iroquois
Allium: Mahuna
Amphicarpaea: Cherokee
Amsonia: Zuni
Arisaema: Meskwaki
Aristolochia: Cherokee; Mohegan; Rappahannock
Artemisia: Navajo, Kayenta; Navajo, Ramah
Asclepias: California Indian; Choctaw; Paiute; Rappahannock
Aster: Navajo, Ramah
Astragalus: Zuni
Baptisia: Meskwaki
Botrychium: Cherokee; Chippewa
Calla: Iroquois
Carex: Menominee
Ceanothus: Meskwaki
Chaenactis: Okanagon; Paiute; Thompson
Chaetopappa: Navajo, Ramah
Chamaesyce: Kawaiisu; Luiseño; Miwok; Pima; Shoshoni; Thompson
Cicuta: Montana Indian; Paiute
Conioselinum: Navajo, Kayenta
Conyza: Navajo, Ramah
Croton: Zuni
Cryptantha: Navajo, Kayenta; Navajo, Ramah
Cunila: Cherokee
Cyperus: Pima
Datura: Cahuilla; Mahuna

Daucus: Costanoan; Miwok
Echinacea: Dakota; Montana Indian; Omaha; Pawnee; Ponca; Winnebago
Epixiphium: Keres, Western
Eremocrinum: Navajo, Kayenta
Erigeron: Navajo, Ramah
Eriogonum: Navajo, Kayenta; Navajo, Ramah
Eryngium: Cherokee; Choctaw; Creek; Meskwaki; Seminole
Eupatorium: Chippewa; Meskwaki
Fraxinus: Costanoan; Iroquois; Meskwaki
Gaura: Hopi; Zuni
Gentiana: Meskwaki
Glandularia: Keres, Western
Goodyera: Potawatomi
Grindelia: Zuni
Gutierrezia: Keres, Western; Navajo; Navajo, Ramah
Helianthus: Apache, White Mountain; Zuni
Heuchera: Blackfoot
Hypericum: Cherokee; Meskwaki
Ipomoea: Houma
Juglans: Meskwaki
Larrea: Papago
Lesquerella: Hopi
Lilium: Chippewa
Liriodendron: Cherokee
Lycopus: Cherokee
Maianthemum: Iroquois
Manfreda: Catawba; Creek; Seminole
Melothria: Houma
Mentzelia: Navajo, Ramah
Nicotiana: Cherokee; Paiute; Zuni
Oenothera: Navajo, Ramah
Opuntia: Lakota
Osmorhiza: Paiute; Shoshoni
Osmunda: Cherokee
Penstemon: Navajo, Kayenta
Plantago: Cherokee; Chippewa; Mohegan; Ojibwa
Platanthera: Seminole
Polygala: Cherokee; Seminole
Populus: Choctaw
Prenanthes: Iroquois
Psathyrotes: Paiute; Shoshoni
Psilostrophe: Zuni
Ranunculus: Iroquois
Ratibida: Cheyenne
Ribes: Kiowa
Rudbeckia: Cherokee
Sanicula: Micmac; Miwok; Ojibwa
Sanvitalia: Navajo, Ramah
Scirpus: Iroquois
Solanum: Zuni
Sphaeralcea: Tewa
Stephanomeria: Apache, White Mountain; Zuni

Tephrosia: Koasati
Thamnosma: Kawaiisu
Tilia: Cherokee
Toxicodendron: Wailaki
Tragia: Navajo, Kayenta
Triosteum: Meskwaki
Tripterocalyx: Zuni
Veratrum: Paiute; Shoshoni
Verbesina: Zuni
Vitis: Seminole
Waldsteinia: Iroquois
Xanthium: Cherokee
Yucca: Apache
Zigadenus: Paiute

Sports Medicine

Artemisia: Navajo
Asclepias: Iroquois
Chamaecrista: Cherokee
Cornus: Iroquois
Datura: Cahuilla
Dicentra: Iroquois
Equisetum: Quileute
Juncus: Iroquois
Panax: Iroquois
Salix: Quileute
Sarracenia: Iroquois

Stimulant

Abies: Blackfoot; Cheyenne; Ojibwa
Achillea: Chippewa; Iroquois; Navajo; Potawatomi
Acorus: Cherokee; Cree, Alberta
Actaea: Cherokee; Meskwaki
Aesculus: Cherokee
Ageratina: Cherokee; Choctaw; Meskwaki
Alisma: Cree, Woodlands
Allium: Cherokee
Alnus: Tanana, Upper
Anaphalis: Ojibwa
Andropogon: Omaha
Anemone: Meskwaki
Angelica: Kwakiutl
Aquilegia: Shoshoni
Aralia: Choctaw; Meskwaki; Micmac; Montagnais; Ojibwa; Thompson
Arctium: Delaware; Delaware, Oklahoma
Arisaema: Cherokee; Iroquois
Aristolochia: Cherokee
Artemisia: Blackfoot; Chippewa; Paiute, Northern; Potawatomi; Shuswap; Thompson
Arundinaria: Houma
Asarum: Cherokee; Iroquois
Asclepias: Choctaw
Asplenium: Hawaiian

Aster: Meskwaki; Potawatomi
Astragalus: Chippewa
Atriplex: Jemez
Betula: Iroquois
Brassica: Cherokee
Cannabis: Iroquois
Capsicum: Cherokee
Catabrosa: Shoshoni
Chaenactis: Thompson
Chaetopappa: Hopi
Chamaecrista: Cherokee
Chenopodium: Seminole
Chimaphila: Iroquois
Cimicifuga: Cherokee
Collinsonia: Iroquois
Comptonia: Micmac
Conioselinum: Kwakiutl
Cornus: Carrier, Northern; Cherokee; Meskwaki
Corydalis: Ojibwa
Crataegus: Meskwaki
Cryptantha: Zuni
Cunila: Cherokee
Cypripedium: Iroquois
Daphne: Cherokee
Datura: Hopi
Delphinium: Blackfoot
Desmodium: Houma
Equisetum: Okanagan-Colville
Erigeron: Cheyenne
Eryngium: Choctaw; Seminole
Erythronium: Cherokee
Eupatorium: Cherokee
Fraxinus: Algonquin, Tête-de-Boule
Galactia: Seminole
Gentiana: Navajo
Gentianella: Cherokee
Geum: Chippewa
Gnaphalium: Menominee; Meskwaki
Gymnocladus: Dakota; Omaha; Pawnee; Ponca; Winnebago
Hedeoma: Cherokee
Helianthus: Gros Ventre; Mandan; Ree
Heliopsis: Chippewa
Heracleum: Winnebago
Humulus: Delaware; Delaware, Oklahoma
Hydrangea: Cherokee
Hydrastis: Cherokee; Iroquois
Hymenoxys: Hopi
Ipomoea: Pawnee
Juniperus: Meskwaki; Navajo, Ramah; Seminole
Koeleria: Cheyenne
Lactuca: Cherokee
Larix: Iroquois; Micmac
Lathyrus: Chippewa

Leonurus: Cherokee
Leucothoe: Cherokee
Liatris: Cherokee
Liriodendron: Cherokee; Rappahannock
Lithospermum: Cheyenne
Lomatium: Blackfoot
Lonicera: Carrier, Northern
Lycopodium: Montagnais; Ojibwa
Lysichiton: Kwakiutl
Machaeranthera: Hopi
Maianthemum: Delaware, Oklahoma; Meskwaki;
    Ojibwa; Potawatomi
Malva: Iroquois
Melissa: Cherokee
Menispermum: Cherokee
Mentha: Cherokee; Cheyenne; Navajo, Ramah
Mirabilis: Paiute
Monarda: Lakota; Meskwaki
Morus: Creek
Myrica: Micmac
Myriophyllum: Iroquois
Nepeta: Cherokee; Keres, Western
Nicotiana: Kawaiisu
Oenothera: Iroquois
Osmorhiza: Cheyenne; Pawnee
Panax: Cherokee; Iroquois
Papaver: Cherokee
Parnassia: Cheyenne
Persea: Seminole
Phacelia: Kawaiisu
Phlox: Cheyenne
Physalis: Meskwaki
Phytolacca: Delaware; Delaware, Oklahoma
Picea: Ojibwa
Piloblephis: Seminole
Pinus: Carrier, Northern; Cherokee; Ojibwa;
    Potawatomi; Shuswap
Piper: Cherokee; Hawaiian
Polygala: Chippewa
Polygonatum: Menominee; Meskwaki
Polystichum: Iroquois
Populus: Cherokee
Potentilla: Okanagon; Thompson
Prenanthes: Choctaw; Iroquois
Prunus: Iroquois
Pteridium: Micmac
Pulsatilla: Cheyenne
Pycnanthemum: Koasati; Meskwaki
Pyrola: Montagnais
Rhamnus: Kawaiisu
Rosa: Chippewa
Rubus: Cherokee; Iroquois
Rumex: Navajo
Sabal: Houma

Salix: Ojibwa; Seminole
Salvia: Cherokee; Hopi
Sanguinaria: Ojibwa
Sassafras: Rappahannock
Senecio: Jemez
Senna: Cherokee
Sequoia: Pomo; Pomo, Kashaya
Silphium: Cherokee
Sinapis: Cherokee
Solidago: Cherokee; Chippewa; Meskwaki
Stenandrium: Seminole
Taxus: Montagnais
Tephrosia: Cherokee
Tetraneuris: Hopi
Thelesperma: Navajo
Thuja: Iroquois; Menominee
Tilia: Iroquois
Trichostema: Miwok
Tsuga: Iroquois
Ulmus: Iroquois
Umbellularia: Mendocino Indian
Urtica: Makah
Vaccinium: Seminole
Veratrum: Cherokee
Verbascum: Potawatomi
Verbena: Meskwaki
Verbesina: Chickasaw
Veronicastrum: Meskwaki
Yucca: Navajo

Strengthener
Abies: Okanagan-Colville
Acacia: Hawaiian
Adiantum: Hesquiat
Aleurites: Hawaiian
Ambrosia: Makah
Aquilegia: Thompson
Aralia: Iroquois; Malecite
Artemisia: Chippewa; Okanagan-Colville
Asclepias: Chippewa; Iroquois
Asplenium: Hawaiian
Aster: Zuni
Broussaisia: Hawaiian
Cephalanthus: Seminole
Cercocarpus: Keres, Western
Chamaecyparis: Kwakiutl; Kwakiutl, Southern
Chamaesyce: Hawaiian
Chenopodium: Hawaiian
Cocos: Hawaiian
Collinsonia: Iroquois
Cornus: Thompson
Cyperus: Hawaiian
Dalea: Keres, Western
Desmodium: Hawaiian

Digitaria: Hawaiian
Dirca: Iroquois
Frasera: Navajo, Ramah
Freycinetia: Hawaiian
Fucus: Kwakiutl, Southern
Gutierrezia: Zuni
Habenaria: Seminole
Hierochloe: Blackfoot
Hydrocotyle: Hawaiian
Hypericum: Cherokee
Ipomoea: Hawaiian
Iris: Zuni
Jacquemontia: Hawaiian
Juncus: Cherokee; Iroquois
Larix: Malecite; Thompson
Larrea: Pima
Ledum: Nitinaht
Lessoniopsis: Nitinaht
Leymus: Nitinaht
Lithocarpus: Yurok
Lomatium: Blackfoot
Mentzelia: Zuni
Merremia: Hawaiian
Musa: Hawaiian
Nephroma: Eskimo, Inuktitut
Ochrosia: Hawaiian
Oenothera: Iroquois
Opuntia: Keres, Western
Pandanus: Hawaiian
Perideridia: Blackfoot
Phaseolus: Zuni
Phyllospadix: Kwakiutl
Picea: Makah
Piper: Hawaiian
Podophyllum: Iroquois
Populus: Delaware
Portulaca: Hawaiian
Postelsia: Hesquiat; Nitinaht; Nootka
Rheum: Cherokee
Ribes: Thompson
Rosa: Cowlitz
Rumex: Hawaiian; Iroquois
Salix: Seminole
Salvia: Diegueño
Sambucus: Nitinaht
Sanguinaria: Delaware
Sorbus: Algonquin, Tête-de-Boule
Sphaeralcea: Navajo, Kayenta
Stillingia: Seminole
Syzygium: Hawaiian
Tanacetum: Cheyenne
Taxus: Swinomish
Touchardia: Hawaiian
Tragia: Keres, Western

Verbascum: Navajo, Ramah
Viburnum: Iroquois
Vigna: Hawaiian
Vitis: Delaware
Waltheria: Hawaiian
Yucca: Keres, Western
Zanthoxylum: Meskwaki
Zigadenus: Keres, Western

Throat Aid

Abies: Anticosti; Bella Coola
Achillea: Aleut; Blackfoot; Cheyenne; Gitksan; Makah; Nitinaht; Paiute, Northern; Saanich
Acorus: Blackfoot; Cherokee; Chippewa; Cree; Cree, Woodlands; Iroquois; Lakota; Ojibwa
Actaea: Cherokee
Allium: Cherokee; Isleta
Amaranthus: Mohegan
Anaphalis: Cherokee
Andropogon: Seminole
Anemone: Ojibwa
Anemopsis: Pima
Angelica: Aleut; Cherokee; Micmac; Paiute; Pomo, Kashaya; Washo
Apocynum: Ojibwa
Aquilegia: Paiute
Aralia: Iroquois; Micmac
Arbutus: Pomo, Kashaya; Salish, Cowichan; Skokomish
Arisaema: Cherokee; Mohegan
Aristolochia: Cherokee
Armoracia: Cherokee
Artemisia: Blackfoot; Havasupai; Kiowa; Lakota; Meskwaki; Okanagan-Colville; Shoshoni; Thompson
Aruncus: Skagit
Asarum: Iroquois; Meskwaki
Asclepias: Blackfoot; Navajo
Astragalus: Navajo, Kayenta
Balsamorhiza: Cheyenne
Berberis: Micmac; Mohegan; Penobscot
Bidens: Cherokee
Bouteloua: Navajo, Ramah
Calycanthus: Pomo, Kashaya
Cardamine: Cherokee; Malecite; Micmac
Celtis: Houma
Cirsium: Hopi; Houma
Claytonia: Skagit; Skagit, Upper
Clematis: Mendocino Indian; Montana Indian
Cleome: Navajo, Ramah
Conioselinum: Aleut
Coptis: Iroquois; Menominee
Cornus: Cherokee; Malecite; Micmac
Corydalis: Navajo, Ramah

Rubus: Cherokee

Rumex: Apache, White Mountain; Cherokee; Mahuna; Papago; Pima; Yavapai; Zuni

Salix: Algonquin, Tête-de-Boule; Cherokee; Iroquois; Pomo, Kashaya; Zuni

Salvia: Costanoan; Shoshoni

Sambucus: Pima

Sanguinaria: Iroquois; Micmac; Ojibwa; Potawatomi

Sanvitalia: Navajo, Ramah

Sarracenia: Micmac

Sassafras: Seminole

Scirpus: Malecite; Micmac

Scutellaria: Iroquois

Senna: Meskwaki

Shepherdia: Navajo, Kayenta

Sisyrinchium: Navajo

Smilax: Omaha

Solanum: Cherokee; Navajo

Solidago: Chippewa

Stachys: Costanoan

Stanleya: Paiute

Stenotus: Navajo

Symphoricarpos: Navajo, Kayenta

Tanacetum: Chippewa

Taraxacum: Aleut

Thlaspi: Iroquois

Townsendia: Hopi; Navajo

Tragopogon: Navajo, Ramah

Triosteum: Iroquois

Tripterocalyx: Zuni

Tsuga: Skagit

Ulmus: Cherokee; Chippewa; Iroquois; Mohegan; Ojibwa; Potawatomi

Umbellularia: Pomo, Kashaya

Vaccinium: Tanana, Upper

Valeriana: Menominee

Veratrum: Paiute; Shoshoni; Thompson

Verbascum: Mohegan

Viburnum: Cree, Woodlands; Eskimo, Chugach; Tanana, Upper

Viola: Ojibwa, South

Waltheria: Hawaiian

Xanthium: Cherokee

Xanthorhiza: Cherokee

Zanthoxylum: Chippewa; Comanche; Ojibwa

Zea: Navajo

Zinnia: Navajo

Tonic

Abies: Gitksan; Haisla; Karok; Kwakiutl; Wet'suwet'en

Acer: Penobscot; Thompson

Achillea: Navajo; Okanagon; Quinault; Thompson

Acorus: Mohegan; Omaha; Rappahannock; Winnebago

Ageratina: Cherokee; Choctaw

Aletris: Cherokee; Micmac

Allium: Iroquois

Alnus: Gitksan; Haisla; Saanich

Amelanchier: Cherokee; Okanagan-Colville; Potawatomi; Thompson

Anaphalis: Delaware, Oklahoma

Anemopsis: Shoshoni

Angelica: Aleut; Shoshoni

Anthemis: Cherokee

Apocynum: Montana Indian

Aralia: Cherokee; Delaware, Oklahoma; Iroquois; Mohegan; Montagnais; Montana Indian; Okanagon; Penobscot; Potawatomi; Thompson

Arctium: Ojibwa; Potawatomi

Arctostaphylos: Okanagon; Thompson

Aristolochia: Cherokee; Delaware; Delaware, Oklahoma

Armoracia: Cherokee

Artemisia: Aleut; Chippewa; Eskimo, Alaska; Montana Indian; Okanagan-Colville; Paiute; Shoshoni; Washo

Aruncus: Quileute

Asarum: Iroquois; Micmac; Skagit; Thompson

Asclepias: Menominee; Thompson

Astragalus: Chippewa

Baptisia: Penobscot

Betula: Menominee; Mohegan

Brachyactis: Paiute

Brassica: Cherokee

Calla: Gitksan

Cardamine: Malecite; Micmac

Carpinus: Delaware, Ontario

Carya: Delaware, Ontario

Catabrosa: Shoshoni

Caulophyllum: Iroquois

Cephalanthus: Choctaw

Chaenactis: Thompson

Chamaesyce: Shoshoni

Chenopodium: Creek; Rappahannock

Chimaphila: Iroquois; Rappahannock; Thompson

Chrysopsis: Delaware; Delaware, Oklahoma

Chrysothamnus: Shoshoni

Cichorium: Cherokee

Cimicifuga: Cherokee; Delaware; Delaware, Oklahoma

Cinchona: Cherokee

Claytonia: Skagit

Clematis: Navajo; Okanagon; Thompson

Comptonia: Menominee

Cornus: Cherokee; Delaware; Delaware, Oklahoma; Hoh; Quileute; Rappahannock

Cucurbita: Omaha
Cunila: Cherokee
Dirca: Iroquois
Echinocystis: Menominee; Ojibwa
Ephedra: Hopi; Paiute; Shoshoni; Tewa
Erythrina: Choctaw
Euonymus: Cherokee
Eupatorium: Cherokee; Mohegan; Penobscot; Rappahannock
Foeniculum: Cherokee
Frangula: Cahuilla; Salish, Coast
Frasera: Cherokee; Shoshoni
Fraxinus: Ojibwa
Galium: Penobscot
Gaultheria: Chippewa; Delaware; Delaware, Oklahoma; Skagit
Gentiana: Dakota; Winnebago
Gentianella: Cherokee
Geum: Aleut; Blackfoot; Thompson
Gilia: Navajo, Kayenta
Gleditsia: Delaware, Oklahoma; Meskwaki
Glycyrrhiza: Montana Indian
Goodyera: Cowlitz
Gymnocladus: Omaha
Helianthemum: Delaware, Oklahoma
Heracleum: Makah; Okanagon; Thompson
Heuchera: Chickasaw; Choctaw; Creek; Shoshoni
Hieracium: Okanagan-Colville
Holodiscus: Makah
Humulus: Delaware, Oklahoma
Hydrastis: Cherokee
Inula: Delaware; Delaware, Oklahoma
Ipomopsis: Navajo, Kayenta; Shoshoni
Ivesia: Arapaho
Juglans: Potawatomi
Juniperus: Delaware, Ontario; Iroquois; Malecite; Micmac; Okanagan-Colville; Okanagon; Paiute; Shoshoni; Swinomish; Thompson
Kalmia: Cree, Hudson Bay
Larrea: Cahuilla
Lathyrus: Chippewa
Ledum: Algonquin, Quebec; Micmac; Salish
Leiophyllum: Nanticoke
Leonurus: Iroquois; Mohegan
Leucanthemum: Mohegan; Shinnecock
Liatris: Omaha
Lindera: Cherokee
Lomatium: Blackfoot; Cheyenne; Great Basin Indian
Lonicera: Skagit; Thompson
Lupinus: Salish
Lygodesmia: Blackfoot
Machaeranthera: Shoshoni

Mahonia: Karok; Montana Indian; Samish; Swinomish; Thompson
Maianthemum: Delaware, Oklahoma; Mohegan; Washo
Malus: Makah; Nitinaht
Matricaria: Aleut
Melissa: Cherokee
Mentha: Delaware, Oklahoma; Flathead; Kutenai
Menyanthes: Aleut
Monardella: Shoshoni
Nemopanthus: Potawatomi
Nepeta: Cherokee; Delaware, Oklahoma; Rappahannock
Oplopanax: Gitksan; Haisla; Okanagon; Oweekeno; Thompson; Wet'suwet'en
Orbexilum: Cherokee
Osmorhiza: Shoshoni
Osmunda: Cherokee
Ostrya: Delaware, Ontario
Panax: Cherokee; Delaware; Delaware, Oklahoma; Iroquois; Menominee; Mohegan; Seminole
Pedicularis: Washo
Phoenicaulis: Paiute
Picea: Gitksan; Montagnais; Wet'suwet'en
Pimpinella: Delaware, Oklahoma
Pinus: Gitksan; Paiute
Plantago: Aleut
Podophyllum: Delaware; Delaware, Oklahoma
Polygala: Chippewa
Polygonatum: Cherokee
Polygonum: Aleut
Populus: Iroquois; Shoshoni
Potentilla: Okanagon; Thompson
Prunella: Thompson
Prunus: Delaware; Delaware, Oklahoma; Delaware, Ontario; Makah; Mendocino Indian; Micmac; Mohegan; Okanagan-Colville; Paiute; Penobscot; Potawatomi; Rappahannock; Thompson
Pseudotsuga: Swinomish; Thompson
Pteridium: Cherokee
Pteryxia: Okanagan-Colville
Purshia: Paiute; Shoshoni
Pyrola: Penobscot
Quercus: Cherokee; Delaware, Ontario; Houma; Rappahannock
Rhamnus: Iroquois
Ribes: Lummi; Thompson
Rosa: Chippewa; Paiute; Shoshoni; Thompson
Rubus: Cherokee; Iroquois; Karok; Okanagon; Rappahannock; Thompson
Rumex: Iroquois; Mohegan; Paiute; Shoshoni
Salix: Cherokee; Klallam; Menominee; Skagit
Salvia: Mohegan
Sambucus: Houma; Paiute

Sanguinaria: Algonquin, Quebec; Delaware, Oklahoma; Mohegan

Sassafras: Delaware, Oklahoma; Iroquois; Mohegan; Rappahannock

Sequoia: Pomo

Shepherdia: Salish; Thompson

Silphium: Pawnee

Sinapis: Cherokee

Smilax: Cherokee; Choctaw

Solidago: Cherokee; Chippewa; Cree, Hudson Bay; Thompson

Sorbus: Algonquin, Quebec; Wet'suwet'en

Spiraea: Thompson

Stachys: Saanich

Stanleya: Paiute

Stephanomeria: Shoshoni

Streptopus: Okanagon; Penobscot; Thompson

Tanacetum: Cherokee

Taraxacum: Delaware, Oklahoma; Mohegan; Potawatomi; Shinnecock

Tetradymia: Hopi

Thamnosma: Shoshoni

Thuja: Okanagan-Colville

Tiarella: Iroquois

Toxicodendron: Houma

Urtica: Nitinaht; Samish; Shoshoni; Swinomish

Verbena: Cherokee

Veronicastrum: Cherokee

Viburnum: Cherokee

Viola: Cherokee

Vitis: Cherokee; Choctaw; Delaware, Oklahoma

Wyethia: Paiute

Xanthorhiza: Cherokee

Zanthoxylum: Delaware, Oklahoma

Toothache Remedy

Abies: Shuswap

Achillea: Carrier; Costanoan; Cree, Woodlands; Creek; Mahuna; Okanagan-Colville; Paiute; Saanich; Shoshoni; Thompson

Acorus: Blackfoot; Chippewa; Cree, Woodlands; Dakota; Iroquois; Lakota; Omaha; Pawnee; Ponca; Winnebago

Actaea: Cherokee

Adenostoma: Diegueño

Aesculus: Costanoan; Mendocino Indian

Ageratina: Chickasaw; Choctaw

Alnus: Algonquin, Quebec; Cherokee; Okanagan-Colville; Thompson

Ambrosia: Zuni

Amelanchier: Cree, Woodlands

Antennaria: Iroquois

Anthemis: Iroquois

Arabis: Thompson

Aralia: Cherokee; Cree, Woodlands

Argemone: Shoshoni

Aristolochia: Cherokee

Armoracia: Mohegan

Artemisia: Costanoan; Navajo, Ramah; Shoshoni

Asarum: Pomo, Kashaya

Asclepias: Iroquois; Navajo, Kayenta

Aster: Cree, Woodlands; Kawaiisu; Okanagan-Colville

Astragalus: Navajo, Ramah

Atriplex: Navajo, Ramah

Balsamorhiza: Cheyenne

Baptisia: Cherokee

Betula: Cree, Woodlands

Brassica: Mohegan; Shinnecock

Caulophyllum: Cherokee

Ceanothus: Cherokee

Celastrus: Iroquois

Centaurium: Miwok

Cephalanthus: Choctaw

Chaetopappa: Navajo, Ramah

Chamaesyce: Cherokee; Navajo, Ramah

Chenopodium: Miwok

Chrysothamnus: Cahuilla; Shoshoni

Clematis: Thompson

Coix: Cherokee

Coptis: Algonquin, Quebec; Menominee

Corylus: Iroquois

Cryptantha: Navajo, Ramah

Cypripedium: Chippewa

Dalea: Navajo

Datura: Cahuilla

Descurainia: Navajo, Ramah

Dicentra: Skagit

Dimorphocarpa: Navajo, Kayenta

Diospyros: Cherokee

Dryopteris: Cherokee

Echinacea: Blackfoot; Cheyenne; Crow; Dakota; Lakota; Omaha; Pawnee; Ponca; Sioux; Sioux, Teton; Winnebago

Encelia: Cahuilla

Equisetum: Iroquois

Erigenia: Cherokee

Erigeron: Kawaiisu; Miwok

Eryngium: Cherokee

Erysimum: Navajo, Ramah

Eschscholzia: California Indian; Mendocino Indian

Euphorbia: Cherokee

Fragaria: Cherokee

Frangula: Neeshenam

Geranium: Meskwaki

Geum: Cree, Woodlands

Glycyrrhiza: Dakota; Lakota; Pawnee; Sioux

Goodyera: Cherokee

Gutierrezia: Cahuilla
Hamamelis: Iroquois
Hedeoma: Cherokee
Heracleum: Cree; Shoshoni; Washo
Heterotheca: Navajo, Ramah
Heuchera: Navajo
Humulus: Delaware; Delaware, Oklahoma; Mohegan
Hymenopappus: Hopi
Hypericum: Houma; Shoshoni
Iris: Great Basin Indian; Paiute; Shoshoni
Juglans: Cherokee; Iroquois
Juniperus: Cree, Woodlands; Shoshoni; Tewa
Larrea: Pima
Lesquerella: Navajo, Ramah
Lithocarpus: Costanoan
Lycium: Navajo, Kayenta; Navajo, Ramah
Magnolia: Cherokee; Iroquois
Melica: Kawaiisu
Mentha: Cree, Woodlands; Flathead
Mentzelia: Hopi; Navajo, Ramah
Monarda: Flathead
Monotropa: Cree, Woodlands
Nicotiana: Cherokee; Kawaiisu; Montauk; Rappa-
    hannock; Shinnecock; Shoshoni; Tewa
Nuphar: Okanagan-Colville
Nymphaea: Okanagan-Colville
Oenothera: Hopi
Osmorhiza: Okanagan-Colville; Shoshoni
Ostrya: Cherokee
Parryella: Hopi; Tewa
Pediomelum: Blackfoot
Pennellia: Navajo, Ramah
Penstemon: Okanagan-Colville
Pentagrama: Miwok
Pericome: Navajo, Ramah
Persea: Mahuna
Phaseolus: Papago
Phlox: Navajo; Navajo, Kayenta
Phoradendron: Mendocino Indian
Physaria: Blackfoot
Picea: Cree, Woodlands; Shuswap; Tlingit
Polygala: Cree, Woodlands
Polymnia: Iroquois
Polystichum: Cherokee
Populus: Cherokee
Porteranthus: Cherokee
Psathyrotes: Paiute
Psorothamnus: Paiute
Pteridium: Makah
Quercus: Mahuna
Ranunculus: Iroquois
Rhus: Cheyenne
Ribes: Luiseño
Robinia: Cherokee

Rorippa: Mohegan
Rubus: Cherokee; Cree, Woodlands; Makah
Rumex: Yavapai
Sambucus: Cahuilla; Okanagon; Thompson
Sanvitalia: Navajo, Ramah
Sarcobatus: Paiute, Northern
Satureja: Costanoan
Shepherdia: Navajo, Kayenta
Solanum: Costanoan; Zuni
Solidago: Miwok
Sonchus: Houma
Stanleya: Shoshoni
Stenotus: Navajo
Stephanomeria: Paiute
Symplocarpus: Meskwaki
Taraxacum: Cherokee; Iroquois
Tauschia: Kawaiisu
Thelesperma: Navajo
Thuja: Algonquin, Quebec; Cowlitz; Malecite;
    Micmac
Trichostema: Miwok
Tsuga: Tlingit
Veratrum: Paiute
Verbascum: Abnaki; Iroquois
Vernonia: Cherokee
Viburnum: Cree, Woodlands
Zanthoxylum: Alabama; Comanche; Houma;
    Iroquois; Meskwaki
Zigadenus: Paiute; Shoshoni; Washo
Zingiber: Hawaiian

Tuberculosis Remedy

Abies: Bella Coola; Blackfoot; Cree, Woodlands;
    Iroquois; Kwakiutl; Okanagan-Colville; Paiute;
    Potawatomi; Shuswap; Thompson; Washo
Acer: Klallam
Achillea: Aleut; Cheyenne; Mendocino Indian;
    Paiute; Quinault
Achlys: Cowlitz; Skagit
Acorus: Meskwaki
Adenocaulon: Squaxin
Aletris: Cherokee
Aleurites: Hawaiian
Alisma: Iroquois
Alnus: Blackfoot; Hesquiat; Kwakiutl; Mendocino
    Indian; Nitinaht; Swinomish
Amphicarpaea: Iroquois
Anaphalis: Bella Coola; Montagnais
Anemone: Iroquois; Ojibwa
Anemopsis: Pima
Angelica: Shoshoni
Antidesma: Hawaiian
Apium: Houma

Aralia: Algonquin, Quebec; Iroquois; Malecite; Mendocino Indian; Micmac
Arceuthobium: Carrier, Southern
Arctium: Menominee
Arisaema: Cherokee; Iroquois
Arnica: Thompson
Artemisia: Meskwaki; Montana Indian; Okanagan-Colville; Sanpoil; Shuswap; Tanaina; Thompson
Asarum: Iroquois; Skagit
Asclepias: Paiute
Asplenium: Hawaiian
Aster: Iroquois
Balsamorhiza: Flathead; Paiute
Botrychium: Iroquois; Ojibwa
Boykinia: Quileute
Caltha: Chippewa
Campanulastrum: Meskwaki
Cardamine: Delaware, Oklahoma; Iroquois
Carpinus: Iroquois
Carya: Kiowa
Cassiope: Thompson
Celastrus: Delaware, Ontario
Cenchrus: Hawaiian
Centaurium: Miwok
Cercocarpus: Paiute; Paiute, Northern; Shoshoni
Chaenactis: Sanpoil
Chamaesyce: Hawaiian
Chimaphila: Cherokee; Delaware, Oklahoma; Malecite; Micmac; Okanagan-Colville
Chrysothamnus: Cheyenne; Thompson
Cimicifuga: Cherokee
Cirsium: Mohegan; Montagnais
Collinsia: Creek; Natchez
Commelina: Keres, Western
Comptonia: Delaware, Oklahoma
Conopholis: Keres, Western
Corallorrhiza: Iroquois
Cornus: Iroquois; Meskwaki
Cynoglossum: Iroquois
Cypripedium: Iroquois
Desmodium: Hawaiian
Dirca: Iroquois
Epilobium: Iroquois; Miwok; Skokomish
Eriastrum: Paiute
Erigeron: Iroquois; Okanagan-Colville
Eriodictyon: Cahuilla; Costanoan; Karok; Paiute; Round Valley Indian; Shoshoni
Eriogonum: Paiute; Shoshoni; Thompson
Erysimum: Hopi
Eschscholzia: Mendocino Indian
Eupatorium: Iroquois
Fagus: Iroquois
Fomitopsis: Haisla & Hanaksiala
Frasera: Okanagan-Colville

Gaillardia: Thompson
Galium: Ojibwa
Gaultheria: Samish; Swinomish
Glossopetalon: Shoshoni
Gnaphalium: Montagnais
Grindelia: Flathead; Ponca; Sanpoil
Hamamelis: Cherokee; Iroquois
Helianthus: Paiute
Heracleum: Shoshoni
Heuchera: Kutenai
Hydrastis: Iroquois
Hypericum: Menominee; Meskwaki
Ilex: Micmac
Inula: Cherokee; Iroquois; Mohegan
Ipomoea: Cherokee; Iroquois
Iris: Chippewa; Delaware, Oklahoma
Juglans: Iroquois
Juniperus: Carrier; Malecite; Micmac; Okanagan-Colville; Sanpoil; Tanana, Upper; Thompson
Laportea: Iroquois
Larix: Kutenai; Malecite; Micmac; Thompson
Larrea: Coahuilla; Pima
Ledum: Haisla & Hanaksiala
Lepidium: Houma
Ligusticum: Pomo, Kashaya
Lilium: Malecite; Micmac
Limonium: Micmac
Lobelia: Iroquois
Lomatium: Nez Perce; Okanagan-Colville; Paiute; Shoshoni; Washo
Lonicera: Iroquois; Lummi
Lophophora: Delaware; Kiowa
Lysichiton: Klallam
Mahonia: Miwok; Nitinaht; Sanpoil
Maianthemum: Delaware, Oklahoma; Hesquiat
Malus: Gitksan; Iroquois; Makah
Marah: Chehalis
Mentzelia: Keres, Western
Mertensia: Cherokee
Nemopanthus: Malecite
Nicotiana: Hawaiian; Iroquois; Mahuna; Paiute; Shoshoni
Nuphar: Bella Coola; Haisla & Hanaksiala
Nymphaea: Ojibwa
Nyssa: Creek
Oemleria: Makah
Onoclea: Iroquois
Oplopanax: Gitksan; Haisla; Kwakiutl; Okanagan-Colville; Skagit; Wet'suwet'en
Ostrya: Iroquois
Paeonia: Paiute; Shoshoni; Washo
Panax: Cherokee; Iroquois
Pastinaca: Paiute
Paxistima: Okanagan-Colville; Thompson

Pedicularis: Iroquois
Peltigera: Nitinaht
Petasites: Concow; Skagit; Tanaina
Phoradendron: Creek
Phyllodoce: Thompson
Physocarpus: Bella Coola
Picea: Gitksan; Haisla & Hanaksiala; Okanagan-
    Colville; Shuswap; Tanana, Upper
Pinus: Bella Coola; Blackfoot; Cherokee; Gitksan;
    Hopi; Iroquois; Kutenai; Lummi; Montagnais;
    Paiute; Shuswap; Skagit; Yokia
Platanthera: Iroquois
Platanus: Creek
Polypodium: Cree, Woodlands
Polystichum: Iroquois
Populus: Bella Coola; Kutenai; Quinault; Shoshoni
Prunella: Iroquois
Prunus: Bella Coola; Chippewa; Iroquois; Kwakiutl;
    Malecite; Micmac; Paiute
Psathyrotes: Shoshoni
Psoralidium: Dakota
Psorothamnus: Paiute; Shoshoni
Pteridium: Iroquois
Purshia: Paiute
Quercus: Cowlitz; Iroquois
Rhus: Flathead; Hopi; Kiowa; Malecite; Menominee
Ribes: Skokomish; Swinomish; Thompson
Rubus: Iroquois; Menominee; Micmac
Rumex: Hawaiian; Squaxin
Salix: Delaware, Oklahoma; Iroquois
Sambucus: Pomo, Little Lakes; Shoshoni
Sanguinaria: Iroquois; Malecite; Micmac
Sarracenia: Malecite; Micmac
Scirpus: Iroquois
Sedum: Eskimo, Western
Senecio: Catawba
Shepherdia: Carrier; Flathead; Shuswap; Tanana,
    Upper; Thompson
Sinapis: Micmac
Solidago: Cherokee
Stephanomeria: Cheyenne
Styphelia: Hawaiian
Symphoricarpos: Skagit
Symplocarpus: Iroquois
Taxus: Iroquois
Tephrosia: Creek
Thelesperma: Keres, Western
Thuja: Clallam; Klallam; Malecite; Micmac
Tilia: Cherokee; Iroquois
Torreya: Pomo; Pomo, Kashaya
Trientalis: Montagnais
Tsuga: Chehalis; Hesquiat; Iroquois; Klallam;
    Shuswap
Tussilago: Iroquois

Ulmus: Catawba; Cherokee; Iroquois
Urtica: Tanaina
Valeriana: Navajo, Ramah; Thompson
Veratrum: Iroquois
Verbascum: Iroquois; Salish
Veronicastrum: Chippewa
Viburnum: Gitksan; Iroquois
Wyethia: Paiute
Xanthium: Mahuna
Zanthoxylum: Iroquois; Meskwaki

Unspecified

Abies: Abnaki; Algonquin, Quebec; Carrier, South-
    ern; Haisla; Kitasoo; Malecite; Menominee;
    Nitinaht; Thompson
Acer: Algonquin, Quebec; Iroquois
Achillea: Eskimo, Alaska; Eskimo, Nunivak; Haisla
    & Hanaksiala; Thompson
Aconitum: Salish
Acorus: Cree, Alberta; Malecite; Micmac
Agastache: Cheyenne; Meskwaki
Alnus: Bella Coola; Gitksan; Hoh; Kawaiisu;
    Nitinaht; Quileute; Shuswap
Ambrosia: Lakota
Amelanchier: Cheyenne
Amsinckia: Costanoan
Anaphalis: Cheyenne
Anemopsis: Diegueño
Angelica: Blackfoot; Eskimo, Inuktitut; Gosiute;
    Kwakiutl
Apocynum: Cahuilla; Cree, Hudson Bay; Salish;
    Thompson
Aralia: Algonquin, Quebec; Ojibwa
Arctium: Hoh; Quileute
Arctostaphylos: Cheyenne; Hoh; Ojibwa; Pomo;
    Quileute
Argentina: Tsimshian
Arisaema: Ojibwa
Arnica: Thompson
Artemisia: Bella Coola; Cahuilla; Cheyenne;
    Havasupai; Lakota; Luiseño; Mewuk; Montana
    Indian; Navajo; Omaha; Pawnee; Ponca; Thomp-
    son; Ute; Winnebago; Yokut
Aruncus: Haihais; Kitasoo; Makah
Asarum: Thompson
Asclepias: Iroquois; Lakota; Miwok; Potawatomi;
    Zuni
Aster: Ojibwa; Okanagan-Colville; Potawatomi
Baptisia: Ojibwa
Berula: Apache, White Mountain
Betula: Algonquin, Quebec; Iroquois; Koyukon
Bignonia: Creek
Botrychium: Abnaki; Potawatomi
Boykinia: Yuki

Veratrum: Hanaksiala
Verbascum: Atsugewi
Verbesina: Seminole
Viola: Ute
Vitex: Hawaiian
Vittaria: Seminole
Ximenia: Seminole
Yucca: Choctaw; Omaha

Urinary Aid

Abies: Cherokee; Iroquois
Acalypha: Cherokee
Achillea: Cherokee; Paiute; Thompson
Acorus: Cherokee
Actaea: Iroquois; Meskwaki
Ageratina: Cherokee
Agrimonia: Ojibwa
Aletris: Cherokee
Allium: Cherokee
Alnus: Cherokee; Iroquois
Ampelopsis: Cherokee
Andropogon: Seminole
Apocynum: Potawatomi
Aquilegia: Meskwaki
Arabis: Okanagon; Thompson
Aralia: Iroquois
Arctium: Cherokee
Arctostaphylos: Cherokee; Okanagan-Colville;
    Okanagon; Thompson
Aristolochia: Cherokee
Armoracia: Cherokee
Artemisia: Costanoan; Paiute
Aruncus: Cherokee
Asarum: Iroquois
Asclepias: Cherokee; Iroquois
Balsamorhiza: Flathead; Paiute
Betula: Cherokee
Callicarpa: Seminole
Calycanthus: Cherokee
Carpinus: Cherokee
Caulophyllum: Meskwaki
Ceanothus: Iroquois
Celastrus: Creek; Iroquois
Cephalanthus: Seminole
Chaetopappa: Navajo, Kayenta
Chamaesyce: Cherokee
Chaptalia: Seminole
Chimaphila: Cherokee; Delaware; Delaware,
    Oklahoma; Iroquois; Karok; Micmac
Chrysothamnus: Thompson
Citrullus: Cherokee; Chickasaw; Iroquois
Claytonia: Quileute
Clematis: Iroquois; Thompson
Clintonia: Micmac

Comptonia: Delaware; Delaware, Oklahoma
Conioselinum: Micmac
Cornus: Iroquois; Shuswap
Crataegus: Meskwaki
Cucurbita: Cherokee
Cynoglossum: Cherokee
Cypripedium: Algonquin, Tête-de-Boule;
    Menominee
Diervilla: Iroquois; Meskwaki; Ojibwa
Diplacus: Costanoan
Dirca: Iroquois; Ojibwa
Echium: Cherokee
Eleocharis: Seminole
Elytrigia: Cherokee; Iroquois
Ephedra: Keres, Western; Paiute; Shoshoni
Epilobium: Costanoan; Iroquois; Miwok
Equisetum: Carrier; Chippewa; Costanoan;
    Iroquois; Mahuna; Potawatomi; Thompson
Eriogonum: Costanoan; Paiute
Eryngium: Meskwaki
Erythrina: Seminole
Euonymus: Cherokee; Iroquois
Eupatorium: Cherokee; Koasati; Menominee
Euphorbia: Cherokee
Fragaria: Cherokee
Fraxinus: Iroquois
Galium: Iroquois; Meskwaki; Ojibwa
Goodyera: Potawatomi
Grindelia: Paiute; Shoshoni
Gutierrezia: Navajo, Ramah; Zuni
Heracleum: Micmac; Shuswap
Hibiscus: Shinnecock
Hordeum: Costanoan
Houstonia: Cherokee
Humulus: Cherokee
Hypericum: Natchez; Seminole
Ilex: Cherokee; Micmac
Impatiens: Iroquois
Ipomoea: Cherokee
Iris: Cherokee; Nevada Indian; Paiute
Jeffersonia: Cherokee
Juglans: Iroquois
Juniperus: Okanagon; Potawatomi; Thompson
Laportea: Meskwaki; Ojibwa
Larrea: Pima
Liatris: Comanche; Meskwaki
Licania: Seminole
Limonium: Costanoan
Linum: Cherokee
Liparis: Cherokee
Lonicera: Chippewa; Iroquois; Menominee;
    Thompson
Lysichiton: Haisla & Hanaksiala; Quinault
Lysimachia: Cherokee

Mahonia: Paiute
Marah: Mendocino Indian
Mentha: Cherokee
Mirabilis: Meskwaki
Mitchella: Iroquois
Morus: Alabama; Creek
Nicotiana: Shuswap
Nyssa: Cherokee
Parthenocissus: Iroquois
Peltigera: Nitinaht
Penstemon: Shuswap
Persea: Seminole
Petroselinum: Cherokee; Micmac
Picea: Abnaki
Pinus: Cherokee
Piper: Hawaiian
Plantago: Cherokee
Platanthera: Micmac
Platanus: Cherokee
Polygonum: Cherokee
Populus: Iroquois; Tewa
Prosopis: Apache, Mescalero
Prunus: Cherokee
Psathyrotes: Shoshoni
Pseudotsuga: Okanagon; Thompson
Psorothamnus: Shoshoni
Pteridium: Iroquois
Quercus: Cherokee
Rhus: Cherokee; Omaha; Seminole; Sioux
Ribes: Chippewa
Rosa: Iroquois
Rubus: Algonquin, Tête-de-Boule; Cherokee;
    Iroquois
Rumex: Costanoan; Micmac
Sambucus: Choctaw
Sarracenia: Algonquin, Quebec; Algonquin, Tête-
    de-Boule
Sassafras: Seminole
Saxifraga: Bella Coola
Silphium: Meskwaki
Smilax: Houma
Sorbus: Okanagan-Colville
Spiranthes: Cherokee
Suaeda: Paiute; Shoshoni
Taraxacum: Iroquois
Taxus: Hanaksiala
Tephrosia: Creek
Thuja: Cree, Woodlands
Toxicodendron: Cherokee
Trichostema: Miwok
Triosteum: Iroquois
Tsuga: Micmac
Typha: Micmac
Urtica: Gitksan

Verbena: Menominee
Verbesina: Seminole
Viburnum: Chippewa; Iroquois
Vitis: Cherokee; Iroquois
Xanthium: Costanoan; Tewa

Venereal Aid

Abies: Blackfoot; Cherokee; Iroquois; Malecite;
    Micmac; Ojibwa, South; Paiute; Thompson
Acer: Micmac; Ojibwa; Penobscot
Achillea: Iroquois; Paiute; Thompson
Acorus: Cree, Woodlands
Actaea: Thompson
Adiantum: Iroquois
Ageratina: Iroquois
Alnus: Gitksan; Iroquois
Aloysia: Walapai
Amelanchier: Bella Coola; Iroquois
Androsace: Navajo, Ramah
Anemopsis: Pima; Shoshoni
Angelica: Paiute; Shoshoni
Anthemis: Iroquois
Apocynum: Thompson
Aquilegia: Shoshoni
Arabis: Salish; Thompson
Aralia: Cherokee; Iroquois; Malecite; Micmac;
    Penobscot
Arctium: Cherokee; Malecite; Micmac
Arctostaphylos: Shoshoni
Arenaria: Navajo, Ramah; Shoshoni
Artemisia: Okanagan-Colville; Paiute; Shoshoni;
    Thompson
Aruncus: Bella Coola; Makah
Asarum: Iroquois
Asclepias: Cherokee; Miwok; Shoshoni
Aster: Iroquois; Okanagan-Colville; Thompson
Astragalus: Shoshoni
Athyrium: Iroquois
Baccharis: Navajo, Ramah; Yavapai
Balsamorhiza: Paiute; Shoshoni
Baptisia: Micmac; Penobscot
Betula: Cree, Woodlands
Calystegia: Kawaiisu
Cardamine: Delaware; Delaware, Oklahoma
Castilleja: Shoshoni
Ceanothus: Iroquois; Thompson
Celtis: Houma
Cercocarpus: Kawaiisu; Mahuna; Paiute; Shoshoni
Chamaebatia: Miwok
Chamaebatiaria: Gosiute
Chamaesyce: Cherokee
Chenopodium: Miwok
Chimaphila: Chippewa; Delaware; Iroquois
Chrysothamnus: Thompson

Cirsium: Comanche; Zuni
Claytonia: Tlingit
Clematis: Iroquois; Shoshoni
Coleogyne: Kawaiisu
Comptonia: Delaware
Coptis: Iroquois
Cordylanthus: Navajo; Shoshoni
Coreopsis: Navajo, Ramah
Cornus: Iroquois
Crotalaria: Delaware; Delaware, Oklahoma
Croton: Zuni
Cucurbita: Paiute; Shoshoni
Cynoglossum: Iroquois; Pomo, Potter Valley
Cyperus: Hawaiian
Cypripedium: Algonquin, Quebec
Dalibarda: Iroquois
Daphne: Cherokee
Diervilla: Iroquois; Meskwaki; Potawatomi
Diospyros: Cherokee
Dirca: Iroquois
Distichlis: Kawaiisu
Draba: Navajo, Ramah
Echinacea: Delaware; Delaware, Oklahoma
Elaeagnus: Thompson
Enceliopsis: Shoshoni
Ephedra: Apache, White Mountain; Hopi; Navajo;
   Paiute; Pima; Shoshoni; Tewa; Tubatulabal; Zuni
Epilobium: Miwok
Equisetum: Iroquois; Meskwaki; Okanagan-Colville
Eriastrum: Kawaiisu; Shoshoni
Erigeron: Shoshoni
Eriodictyon: Kawaiisu; Shoshoni
Eriogonum: Gosiute; Kawaiisu; Thompson
Eryngium: Choctaw; Creek; Delaware, Oklahoma
Erythrina: Hawaiian
Eschscholzia: Kawaiisu
Euonymus: Cherokee
Eupatorium: Algonquin, Quebec; Iroquois; Mic-
   mac; Penobscot
Euphorbia: Cherokee
Fagus: Micmac
Frangula: Quileute; West Coast Indian
Frasera: Havasupai
Fraxinus: Iroquois
Fucus: Kwakiutl, Southern
Gaillardia: Okanagan-Colville
Galium: Micmac; Penobscot
Garrya: Kawaiisu
Gaultheria: Iroquois
Geranium: Choctaw; Iroquois
Grindelia: Cree; Montana Indian; Shoshoni
Gutierrezia: Isleta
Hamamelis: Iroquois
Helenium: Mendocino Indian

Heliotropium: Shoshoni
Heracleum: Cree; Thompson
Heterotheca: Navajo, Ramah
Heuchera: Navajo, Ramah; Paiute; Shoshoni; Tlingit
Hierochloe: Blackfoot
Holodiscus: Shoshoni
Hydrocotyle: Hawaiian
Hypericum: Cherokee; Shoshoni
Ipomopsis: Paiute; Shoshoni
Iris: Delaware; Paiute; Shoshoni
Juglans: Iroquois
Juniperus: Blackfoot; Paiute; Shoshoni
Kochia: Navajo, Kayenta
Krameria: Paiute
Lachnanthes: Cherokee
Larix: Iroquois; Malecite; Micmac
Larrea: Paiute; Shoshoni; Yavapai
Ledum: Tlingit
Leymus: Okanagan-Colville
Liatris: Meskwaki
Limonium: Costanoan
Lindera: Iroquois
Lobelia: Cherokee; Iroquois
Lomatium: Paiute; Shoshoni
Lonicera: Bella Coola; Cree, Woodlands; Iroquois;
   Menominee; Nuxalkmc
Lophophora: Kiowa
Lycopodium: Blackfoot; Iroquois
Madia: Cheyenne
Magnolia: Iroquois
Mahonia: Flathead; Kawaiisu; Paiute; Shoshoni;
   Skagit; Thompson
Maianthemum: Delaware, Oklahoma; Shoshoni
Malus: Hoh; Quileute
Marah: Mendocino Indian
Melicope: Hawaiian
Menispermum: Cherokee
Mertensia: Iroquois
Mirabilis: Yavapai
Mitchella: Iroquois
Myrica: Bella Coola
Nuphar: Bella Coola; Flathead
Oenothera: Navajo, Kayenta
Onoclea: Iroquois
Oplopanax: Gitksan
Osmorhiza: Paiute; Shoshoni
Osmunda: Iroquois
Paeonia: Shoshoni
Panax: Cherokee; Iroquois
Parnassia: Gosiute
Penstemon: Shoshoni
Phacelia: Kawaiisu
Phlox: Paiute
Physalis: Iroquois

Physocarpus: Bella Coola; Kwakiutl
Picea: Bella Coola; Cree, Woodlands; Tlingit
Pinus: Apache, White Mountain; Cherokee; Gitksan; Iroquois; Paiute; Shoshoni; Tlingit; Washo; Zuni
Polygala: Iroquois
Polypodium: Nootka
Polystichum: Iroquois
Populus: Bella Coola; Cherokee; Cree, Woodlands; Flathead; Iroquois; Micmac; Okanagan-Colville; Salish; Shoshoni; Thompson
Potentilla: Navajo, Ramah; Okanagan-Colville
Prunella: Iroquois
Prunus: Iroquois
Psathyrotes: Paiute; Shoshoni
Pseudotsuga: Bella Coola; Montana Indian; Pomo, Little Lakes
Psoralidium: Navajo, Ramah
Psorothamnus: Paiute; Shoshoni
Pteridium: Iroquois
Pterospora: Okanagan-Colville
Purshia: Kawaiisu; Paiute; Shoshoni
Pyrola: Micmac; Penobscot
Quercus: Ojibwa
Ranunculus: Iroquois; Navajo
Ratibida: Navajo, Ramah
Rhamnus: Iroquois; Kawaiisu
Rhus: Delaware; Delaware, Oklahoma; Okanagan-Colville; Seminole; Thompson
Ribes: Bella Coola; Swinomish
Rosa: Quinault; Thompson
Rubus: Cherokee; Iroquois
Rudbeckia: Cherokee
Rumex: Iroquois; Paiute; Shoshoni; Yavapai
Salix: Delaware; Delaware, Oklahoma; Iroquois; Paiute, Northern
Salvia: Paiute; Paiute, Northern
Sambucus: Iroquois; Thompson
Sanguinaria: Iroquois; Ojibwa
Sanicula: Iroquois
Sarracenia: Cree, Woodlands
Sassafras: Cherokee
Schizachyrium: Comanche
Sedum: Okanagan-Colville
Senecio: Yavapai
Sequoia: Tlingit
Shepherdia: Cree, Woodlands; Gitksan
Sicyos: Iroquois
Solanum: Delaware, Oklahoma
Solidago: Iroquois; Thompson
Sorbus: Ojibwa
Sphaeralcea: Shoshoni
Sphenosciadium: Paiute
Spiraea: Blackfoot; Thompson
Spiranthes: Gosiute

Stachys: Delaware; Delaware, Oklahoma
Stanleya: Zuni
Stephanomeria: Hopi; Shoshoni
Stillingia: Cherokee
Streptopus: Micmac; Penobscot
Symphoricarpos: Bella Coola; Chehalis; Cree, Woodlands
Symphytum: Cherokee
Taxus: Potawatomi
Tetradymia: Shoshoni
Thalictrum: Shoshoni
Thamnosma: Pima
Thuja: Quinault; Tlingit
Toxicodendron: Cherokee
Triosteum: Iroquois
Tsuga: Chehalis; Iroquois; Tlingit
Typha: Iroquois
Ulmus: Ojibwa
Urtica: Kwakiutl
Veratrum: Bella Coola; Paiute; Thompson
Verbesina: Chickasaw
Viburnum: Iroquois
Wyethia: Paiute; Shoshoni
Xanthium: Mahuna
Zanthoxylum: Iroquois; Potawatomi
Zigadenus: Gosiute

Vertigo Medicine
Apocynum: Chippewa
Eleocharis: Seminole
Gutierrezia: Lakota
Juniperus: Seminole
Ledum: Tanana, Upper
Lomatium: Paiute, Northern
Nicotiana: Cherokee
Persea: Seminole
Pleopeltis: Houma
Rorippa: Okanagan-Colville
Salix: Seminole
Tanacetum: Cheyenne

Veterinary Aid
Abies: Blackfoot
Acer: Algonquin, Quebec
Achillea: Blackfoot; Chippewa; Paiute
Achlys: Thompson
Acorus: Omaha
Actaea: Blackfoot; Iroquois
Adenostoma: Cahuilla; Coahuilla
Aesculus: Mendocino Indian
Ageratina: Iroquois
Alnus: Menominee; Potawatomi
Ambrosia: Kiowa
Amelanchier: Flathead

Anaphalis: Cheyenne
Anemopsis: Cahuilla; Kawaiisu
Angelica: Blackfoot; Shoshoni
Apocynum: Cherokee; Iroquois; Kutenai
Aquilegia: Thompson
Aralia: Chippewa
Arbutus: Yuki
Arctostaphylos: Concow
Arisaema: Iroquois
Artemisia: Blackfoot; Meskwaki; Mewuk; Navajo,
　Ramah; Ojibwa; Thompson; Yuki
Asarum: Iroquois
Asclepias: Cherokee; Navajo, Kayenta; Navajo,
　Ramah; Shoshoni
Aster: Okanagan-Colville
Astragalus: Gosiute; Lakota
Atriplex: Navajo; Navajo, Ramah
Bouteloua: Navajo, Ramah
Butomus: Iroquois
Caesalpinia: Zuni
Calochortus: Cheyenne
Carex: Iroquois
Carum: Iroquois
Castanea: Iroquois
Celtis: Meskwaki
Cerastium: Navajo, Ramah
Chamaesyce: Kawaiisu; Navajo, Ramah
Chelidonium: Iroquois
Chimaphila: Cherokee; Rappahannock
Chrysothamnus: Sanpoil
Cicuta: Iroquois; Thompson
Cirsium: Navajo, Ramah
Citrullus: Rappahannock
Clematis: Blackfoot; Dakota; Montana Indian; Nez
　Perce; Sanpoil
Collinsia: Navajo, Kayenta
Collinsonia: Cherokee
Commelina: Navajo, Ramah
Conyza: Potawatomi
Corallorrhiza: Iroquois
Cornus: Iroquois
Corydalis: Navajo, Kayenta
Croton: Diegueño
Cryptantha: Navajo, Kayenta
Cucurbita: Apache, Western; Cahuilla; Coahuilla;
　Shoshoni
Cynodon: Keres, Western
Cyperus: Pima
Dalea: Navajo, Kayenta; Navajo, Ramah
Datura: Cahuilla; Coahuilla; Navajo; Navajo, Ramah
Delphinium: Navajo, Kayenta
Descurainia: Paiute
Dyssodia: Dakota
Echeandia: Navajo, Ramah

Echinacea: Dakota; Omaha; Pawnee; Ponca; Sioux;
　Winnebago
Elymus: Navajo, Ramah
Encelia: Kawaiisu
Equisetum: Blackfoot; Cheyenne; Okanagan-
　Colville
Ericameria: Kawaiisu
Erigeron: Navajo, Ramah
Eriodictyon: Coahuilla
Eriogonum: Navajo, Ramah
Eupatorium: Iroquois
Euphorbia: Navajo, Kayenta
Frasera: Navajo, Kayenta; Navajo, Ramah
Fraxinus: Iroquois
Gaillardia: Blackfoot
Galium: Gosiute
Geum: Blackfoot; Chippewa; Iroquois; Paiute
Glycyrrhiza: Blackfoot; Dakota; Sioux
Grindelia: Flathead; Navajo, Ramah; Pawnee
Gutierrezia: Dakota; Keres, Western; Navajo;
　Navajo, Ramah
Helianthus: Pima
Heuchera: Blackfoot; Shoshoni
Hierochloe: Blackfoot; Karok; Plains Indian
Hybanthus: Iroquois
Hymenopappus: Lakota
Inula: Iroquois; Mohegan
Ipomoea: Keresan; Sia
Ipomopsis: Navajo; Navajo, Ramah; Shoshoni
Iva: Navajo, Kayenta
Juncus: Iroquois
Juniperus: Blackfoot; Dakota; Flathead; Navajo,
　Ramah; Omaha; Paiute; Pawnee; Ponca;
　Thompson
Lachnanthes: Catawba
Lactuca: Cherokee
Larix: Menominee; Potawatomi
Larrea: Coahuilla; Kawaiisu
Lathyrus: Navajo, Ramah; Ojibwa
Lepidium: Cherokee
Leucothoe: Cherokee
Leymus: Thompson
Liatris: Chippewa; Meskwaki; Omaha
Liquidambar: Rappahannock
Lomatium: Blackfoot; Gosiute; Nevada Indian;
　Okanagan-Colville; Oregon Indian; Paiute;
　Shoshoni; Thompson; Ute
Lonicera: Diegueño
Lupinus: Menominee; Thompson
Lycopus: Cherokee
Lygodesmia: Blackfoot; Gosiute
Mahonia: Blackfoot
Maianthemum: Meskwaki
Matricaria: Okanagan-Colville

Witchcraft Medicine

Index of Common Plant Names

Common plant names appearing in the original sources are listed alphabetically and are cross-referenced to the scientific names used in the Catalog of Plants. Plants are identified to the level of species, and a particular common name may apply only to a single subspecies or variety of that species. Word division as used in the original sources has been followed when possible, but indexing often required other word divisions. Some misspellings in the original sources have been corrected, and some editorial conventions have been adopted to facilitate finding names in the index. Unlike scientific names, common plant names do not follow rules of nomenclature. This index is intended as a handy finding tool rather than as a consistently uniform catalog of common names.

Awa: *Piper methysticum*
Awapuhi Kuahiwi: *Zingiber zerumbet*
Aweoweo: *Chenopodium oahuense*
'Awikiwiki: *Canavalia galeata*
Azalea, Cascade: *Rhododendron albiflorum*
Azalea, False: *Menziesia ferruginea*
Azalea, Flame: *Rhododendron calendulaceum*
Azalea, Western: *Rhododendron occidentale*
Bachelor's Button: *Polygala rugelii*
Balloonbush: *Epixiphium wislizeni*
Ball Root: *Orbexilum pedunculatum*
Balm: *Melissa officinalis*
Balm, Western: *Monardella odoratissima*
Balm of Gilead: *Populus balsamifera, P. ×jackii*
Balmony: *Chelone glabra*
Balsam: *Abies balsamea, Balsamorhiza sagittata, Impatiens capensis*
Balsam, Indian: *Lomatium dissectum*
Balsam Apple: *Echinocystis lobata*
Balsam Buds: *Impatiens capensis*
Balsamea, Mexican: *Epilobium canum*
Balsam Herb: *Balsamita major*
Balsam Root: *Balsamorhiza deltoidea, B. hookeri, B. incana, B. sagittata*
Balsam Root, Arrow Leaved: *Balsamorhiza sagittata*
Balsamroot, Deltoid: *Balsamorhiza deltoidea*
Balsamroot, Hairy: *Balsamorhiza hookeri*
Balsamroot, Hoary: *Balsamorhiza incana*
Balsam Root, Hooker's: *Balsamorhiza hookeri*
Bamboo Brier: *Smilax laurifolia*
Bamboovine: *Smilax pseudochina*
Banana, Paradise: *Musa ×paradisiaca*
Baneberry, Red: *Actaea rubra*
Baneberry, Red and White: *Actaea rubra*
Baneberry, White: *Actaea pachypoda*
Bank Flower: *Penstemon ambiguus*
Banner, Golden: *Thermopsis rhombifolia*
Barberry, American: *Berberis canadensis*
Barberry, California: *Mahonia pinnata*
Barberry, Common: *Berberis vulgaris*
Barberry, Desert: *Mahonia fremontii*
Barberry, Dwarf: *Mahonia pumila*
Barberry, Hollyleaved: *Mahonia aquifolium*
Barberry, Red: *Mahonia haematocarpa*
Barberry, Shining Netvein: *Mahonia dictyota*
Barberry, Showy: *Mahonia repens*
Barley, Foxtail: *Hordeum jubatum*
Barley, Wild: *Hordeum jubatum*
Barratt Willow: *Salix scouleriana*
Basketweed: *Rhus trilobata*
Bass-wood: *Tilia americana*
Bay, California Rose: *Rhododendron macrophyllum*
Bay, Red: *Persea borbonia*

Bay, Swamp: *Persea palustris*
Bay, Sweet: *Magnolia virginiana*
Bayberry: *Myrica cerifera*
Bay Flower: *Commelina dianthifolia*
Bayhops: *Ipomoea pes-caprae*
Beach Clover: *Trifolium wormskioldii*
Beachheather: *Hudsonia tomentosa*
Beadruby: *Maianthemum canadense*
Bean, Broad: *Vicia faba*
Bean, Buffalo: *Thermopsis rhombifolia*
Bean, Castor: *Ricinus communis*
Bean, Coral: *Erythrina herbacea*
Bean, Fuzzy: *Strophostyles helvula*
Bean, Ground: *Amphicarpaea bracteata*
Bean, Horse: *Vicia faba*
Bean, Jumping: *Sapium biloculare*
Bean, Mescal: *Sophora secundiflora*
Bean, Mexican Jumping: *Sapium biloculare*
Bean, Screw: *Prosopis glandulosa, P. pubescens*
Bean, Sea: *Mucuna gigantea*
Bean, Slimleaf: *Phaseolus angustissimus*
Bean, Tepary: *Phaseolus acutifolius*
Bean, Wild: *Amphicarpaea bracteata, Phaseolus acutifolius, P. angustissimus, Strophostyles helvula*
Bean Salad: *Streptopus roseus*
Bearberry: *Arctostaphylos alpina, A. nevadensis, A. uva-ursi, Lonicera involucrata*
Beard Tongue: *Penstemon barbatus, P. fendleri, P. fruticosus, P. jamesii, P. linarioides, P. virgatus, Phlox caespitosa*
Beardtongue, Bush: *Keckiella breviflora*
Beardtongue, Cutleaf: *Penstemon richardsonii*
Beardtongue, Eastern Smooth: *Penstemon laevigatus*
Beardtongue, Gilia: *Penstemon ambiguus*
Beard Tongue, Hairy: *Penstemon fruticosus, P. laevigatus*
Beardtongue, James's: *Penstemon jamesii*
Beardtongue, Large: *Penstemon grandiflorus*
Beard Tongue, Sharp Leaved: *Penstemon acuminatus*
Beard Tongue, Small Flowered: *Keckiella breviflora*
Beard Tongue, Torrey: *Penstemon barbatus*
Beardtongue, Upright Blue: *Penstemon virgatus*
Beardtongue, Woodland: *Nothochelone nemorosa*
Bear Root: *Lomatium macrocarpum*
Bear's Food: *Lomatium orientale*
Bear's Foot: *Smallanthus uvedalia*
Beautyberry, American: *Callicarpa americana*
Beaver Tail: *Opuntia basilaris*
Bedstraw, Fendler's: *Galium fendleri*
Bedstraw, Fragrant: *Galium triflorum*
Bedstraw, Licorice: *Galium circaezans*

Bedstraw, Marsh: *Galium tinctorium*

Bedstraw, Northern: *Galium boreale*

Bedstraw, Oneflower: *Galium uniflorum*

Bedstraw, Rough: *Galium asprellum*

Bedstraw, Scented: *Galium triflorum*

Bedstraw, Shining: *Galium concinnum*

Bedstraw, Small: *Galium tinctorium, G. trifidum, G. triflorum*

Bedstraw, Stiff Marsh: *Galium tinctorium*

Bedstraw, Sweet: *Galium triflorum*

Bedstraw, Threepetal: *Galium trifidum*

Beebalm, Mintleaf: *Monarda fistulosa*

Beebalm, Pony: *Monarda pectinata*

Beebalm, Scarlet: *Monarda didyma*

Beebalm, Spotted: *Monarda punctata*

Beebalm, Wildbergamot: *Monarda fistulosa*

Beeblossom, Scarlet: *Gaura coccinea*

Beebrush, Wright's: *Aloysia wrightii*

Beech: *Fagus grandifolia*

Beech Drops: *Epifagus virginiana*

Beefsteakplant: *Perilla frutescens*

Bee Plant: *Cleome serrulata, Scrophularia californica*

Bee Plant, Rocky Mountain: *Cleome serrulata*

Beetleweed: *Galax urceolata*

Bee Weed, Rocky Mountain: *Cleome serrulata*

Beggar Lice: *Hackelia virginiana*

Beggar Louse: *Desmodium paniculatum*

Beggartick, Crowned: *Bidens coronata*

Beggartick, Smooth: *Bidens laevis*

Bellflower: *Campanula parryi, Uvularia sessilifolia*

Bellflower, American: *Campanulastrum americanum*

Bellflower, Bluebell: *Campanula rotundifolia*

Bellflower, Blue Marsh: *Campanula aparinoides*

Bellflower, Parry's: *Campanula parryi*

Bellflower, Small Bonny: *Campanula divaricata*

Bellflower, Tall: *Campanulastrum americanum*

Bellwort: *Disporum smithii, Uvularia grandiflora*

Bellwort, Large Flowered: *Uvularia grandiflora*

Bellwort, Perfoliate: *Uvularia perfoliata*

Bellwort, Sessile Leaved: *Uvularia sessilifolia*

Benne Plant: *Sesamum orientale*

Bergamot, Wild: *Monarda fistulosa*

Betony: *Stachys rothrockii*

Betony, Wood: *Pedicularis bracteosa, P. canadensis, P. racemosa*

Bicknell's Thorn: *Crataegus chrysocarpa*

Big Root: *Balsamorhiza sagittata, Ipomoea leptophylla, Marah oreganus*

Bilberry: *Vaccinium vitis-idaea*

Bilberry, Bog: *Vaccinium uliginosum*

Bilberry, Mountain: *Vaccinium membranaceum*

Bilberry, Red: *Vaccinium parvifolium*

Bilsted: *Liquidambar styraciflua*

Bindweed, Chaparral False: *Calystegia occidentalis*

Bindweed, Field: *Convolvulus arvensis*

Birch, Black: *Betula lenta, B. nigra*

Birch, Bog: *Betula nana*

Birch, Canoe: *Betula papyrifera*

Birch, Cherry: *Betula lenta*

Birch, Downy: *Betula pubescens*

Birch, Glandulose: *Betula pumila*

Birch, Gray: *Betula populifolia*

Birch, Low: *Betula pumila*

Birch, Northern Dwarf: *Betula nana*

Birch, Paper: *Betula papyrifera, B. pubescens*

Birch, Red: *Betula nigra*

Birch, River: *Betula nigra*

Birch, Rocky Mountain: *Betula occidentalis*

Birch, Shrub: *Betula nana*

Birch, Sweet: *Betula lenta*

Birch, Water: *Betula occidentalis*

Birch, Western: *Betula occidentalis*

Birch, Western Paper: *Betula papyrifera*

Birch, White: *Betula papyrifera, B. populifolia*

Birch, Yellow: *Betula alleghaniensis*

Birdrape: *Brassica rapa*

Bird's Beak, Bushy: *Cordylanthus ramosus*

Bird's Beak, Wright's: *Cordylanthus wrightii*

Bird's Foot, Small Leaved: *Amorpha nana*

Biscuitroot, Barestem: *Lomatium nudicaule*

Biscuitroot, Bigseed: *Lomatium macrocarpum*

Biscuitroot, Carrotleaf: *Lomatium dissectum*

Biscuitroot, Desert: *Lomatium foeniculaceum*

Biscuitroot, Fernleaf: *Lomatium dissectum*

Biscuitroot, Nineleaf: *Lomatium triternatum*

Biscuitroot, Northern Idaho: *Lomatium orientale*

Biscuitroot, Nuttall's: *Lomatium nuttallii*

Biscuitroot, Wyeth: *Lomatium ambiguum*

Bishop's Cap: *Mitella diphylla, M. nuda*

Bistort, American: *Polygonum bistortoides*

Bistort, Mountain Meadow: *Polygonum bistorta*

Bitter Ball: *Tagetes micrantha*

Bittercress, Limestone: *Cardamine douglassii*

Bitternut Hickory: *Carya cordiformis*

Bitter Perfume: *Monarda fistulosa*

Bitter Root: *Lewisia spp., Lomatium dissectum*

Bitterroot, Oregon: *Lewisia rediviva*

Bitterroot, Pigmy: *Lewisia pygmaea*

Bittersweet: *Celastrus scandens, Solanum dulcamara*

Bittersweet, Climbing: *Celastrus scandens*

Blackberry: *Empetrum nigrum, Rubus spp.*

Blackberry, Allegheny: *Rubus alleghaniensis*

Blackberry, Arctic: *Rubus arcticus*

Blackberry, California: *Rubus ursinus, R. vitifolius*

Blackberry, Canada: *Rubus canadensis*

Cabbage Palmetto: *Sabal palmetto*

Cactus, Beavertail: *Opuntia basilaris*

Cactus, Brittle Prickly Pear: *Opuntia fragilis*

Cactus, Cane: *Opuntia imbricata, O. whipplei*

Cactus, Chandelier: *Opuntia imbricata*

Cactus, Cholla: *Opuntia whipplei*; see also Cholla

Cactus, Christmas: *Opuntia leptocaulis*

Cactus, Crimson Hedgehog: *Echinocereus coccineus*

Cactus, Cushion: *Escobaria vivipara*

Cactus, Fish Hook: *Mammillaria grahamii*

Cactus, Giant: *Carnegia gigantea*

Cactus, Graham's Nipple: *Mammillaria grahamii*

Cactus, Hedgewood: *Echinocereus coccineus*

Cactus, Many Spined: *Opuntia polyacantha*

Cactus, Nipple: *Mammillaria grahamii*

Cactus, Prickly Pear: *Opuntia engelmannii, O. fragilis, O. phaeacantha, O. polyacantha*; see also Pricklypear

Cactus, Scarlet Hedgehog: *Echinocereus coccineus*

Cactus, Slender: *Opuntia leptocaulis*

Cactus, Sunset: *Mammillaria grahamii*

Cactus, Sweetpotato: *Peniocereus greggii*

Cactus, Turkey: *Opuntia leptocaulis*

Cactus Apple: *Opuntia engelmannii*

Calabash, Long Handled: *Lagenaria siceraria*

Calabazilla: *Cucurbita foetidissima*

Calabrash: *Lagenaria siceraria*

Calamus: *Acorus calamus*

Calla, Wild: *Calla palustris*

Caltrop: *Tribulus terrestris*

Caltrop, California: *Kallstroemia californica*

Camas, Atlantic: *Camassia scilloides*

Camas, Black: *Camassia quamash*

Camas, Blue: *Camassia quamash*

Camas, Common: *Camassia quamash*

Camas, Death: *Zigadenus elegans, Z. venenosus*

Camas, Poison: *Zigadenus venenosus*

Camas, Small: *Camassia quamash*

Camass: see Camas

Camellia, Tea: *Camellia sinensis*

Camomile, Rayless: *Matricaria discoidea*

Camphorweed, Stinking: *Pluchea foetida*

Campion, Bladder: *Silene latifolia*

Campion, Douglas's: *Silene douglasii*

Campion, Drummond's: *Silene drummondii*

Campion, Gregg's: *Silene laciniata*

Campion, Menzies's: *Silene menziesii*

Campion, Mexican: *Silene laciniata*

Campion, Moss: *Silene acaulis*

Campion, Pringle's: *Silene douglasii*

Campion, Scouler's: *Silene scouleri*

Campion, Starry: *Silene stellata*

Campion, White: *Silene latifolia*

Canaigre: *Rumex hymenosepalus*

Cancer Root: *Boschniakia hookeri, Orobanche fasciculata*

Cancer Root, Yellow: *Orobanche fasciculata*

Canchalagua: *Centaurium exaltatum, C. venustum*

Candlewood, American Desert: *Fouquieria splendens*

Candyroot: *Polygala lutea, P. rugelii*

Candytuft, Wild: *Thlaspi montanum*

Cane: *Arundinaria gigantea, Leymus condensatus, Phragmites australis*

Cane, Common: *Phragmites australis*

Cane, Giant: *Arundinaria gigantea*

Cane, Hauve: *Phragmites australis*

Cane, River: *Arundinaria gigantea*

Cane, Switch: *Arundinaria gigantea*

Cane Head: *Sanicula canadensis*

Cane Leaves: *Aletris farinosa*

Cankerweed: *Prenanthes serpentaria*

Caraway: *Carum carvi*

Caraway, Wild: *Perideridia gairdneri*

Cardinal, Red: *Erythrina herbacea*

Cardinal Flower: *Lobelia cardinalis, L. siphilitica*

Carpenter's Square: *Scrophularia marilandica*

Carrion Flower: *Smilax herbacea*

Carrizo: *Phragmites australis*

Carrot: *Lomatium dissectum*

Carrot, Domesticated: *Daucus carota*

Carrot, Wild: *Daucus carota, D. pusillus, Lomatium macrocarpum, Perideridia gairdneri*

Cascara: *Frangula californica, F. purshiana, F. rubra*

Cassena (or Cassine): *Ilex vomitoria*

Cassine, Dahoon: *Ilex cassine, I. vomitoria*

Catberry: *Nemopanthus mucronatus*

Catbriar: *Smilax bona-nox, S. tamnoides*

Cat Brier: *Smilax bona-nox, S. tamnoides*

Catchfly: *Silene acaulis, S. douglasii, S. laciniata, S. menziesii, S. scouleri*

Catchfly, Night Flowering: *Silene noctiflora*

Catchfly, Red Mountain: *Silene campanulata*

Catgut: *Tephrosia virginiana*

Catnip: *Nepeta cataria*

Catnip Noseburn: *Tragia nepetifolia*

Catseye, Brenda's Yellow: *Cryptantha flava*

Catseye, James's: *Cryptantha cinerea*

Catseye, Sanddune: *Cryptantha fendleri*

Catseye, Silky: *Cryptantha sericea*

Catseye, Tawny: *Cryptantha fulvocanescens*

Catseye, Thicksepal: *Cryptantha crassisepala*

Cat's Foot: *Gamochaeta purpurea*

Cat's Foot, Lesser: *Antennaria howellii*

Cat Tail: *Typha angustifolia, T. latifolia*

Cat Tail Flag: *Typha angustifolia, T. latifolia*

Crowfoot, Small Flowered: *Ranunculus abortivus*
Crowfoot, Water Yellow: *Ranunculus flabellaris*
Crownbeard, Golden: *Verbesina encelioides*
Crownbeard, Virginia: *Verbesina virginica*
Crownbeard, White: *Verbesina virginica*
Crownvetch, Purple: *Coronilla varia*
Crow's Foot: *Cardamine diphylla, Ranunculus* spp.; see also Crowfoot
Cucumber, Bur: *Sicyos angulatus*
Cucumber, Guadeloupe: *Melothria pendula*
Cucumber, Indian: *Medeola virginiana*
Cucumber, Oneseed Burr: *Sicyos angulatus*
Cucumber, Wild: *Echinocystis lobata, Marah fabaceus*
Cucumber Tree: *Magnolia acuminata*
Cudweed: *Gnaphalium stramineum*
Cudweed, Glandular: *Corethrogyne filaginifolia*
Cudweed, Lobed: *Artemisia ludoviciana*
Cudweed, Marsh: *Gnaphalium uliginosum*
Cudweed, Smallhead: *Gnaphalium microcephalum*
Cudweed, Winged: *Gnaphalium viscosum*
Cudweed, Wright's: *Gnaphalium canescens*
Culver's Physic: *Veronicastrum virginicum*
Culver's Root: *Veronicastrum virginicum*
Cumin: *Cuminum cyminum*
Cup Plant: *Silphium perfoliatum*
Currant, American Black: *Ribes americanum*
Currant, Black: *Ribes americanum, R. hudsonianum, R. laxiflorum*
Currant, Black Wild: *Ribes americanum*
Currant, Blue: *Ribes bracteosum*
Currant, Buffalo: *Ribes aureum*
Currant, Chaparral: *Ribes malvaceum*
Currant, Cultivated: *Ribes rubrum*
Currant, Golden: *Ribes aureum*
Currant, Hudson Bay: *Ribes hudsonianum*
Currant, Missouri: *Ribes aureum*
Currant, Northern Black: *Ribes hudsonianum*
Currant, Northern Red: *Ribes triste*
Currant, Prickly: *Ribes lacustre*
Currant, Red: *Ribes cereum, R. rubrum, R. triste*
Currant, Rock: *Ribes cereum*
Currant, Skunk: *Ribes bracteosum, R. glandulosum*
Currant, Squaw: *Ribes cereum*
Currant, Sticky: *Ribes viscosissimum*
Currant, Stink: *Ribes bracteosum*
Currant, Swamp: *Ribes lacustre*
Currant, Trailing: *Ribes laxiflorum*
Currant, Wax: *Ribes cereum*
Currant, Western Black: *Ribes hudsonianum*
Currant, Whisky: *Ribes cereum*
Currant, White Flowered: *Ribes laxiflorum*
Currant, Wild: *Ribes aureum, R. cereum, R. glandulosum*

Currant, Wild Black: *Ribes americanum, R. hudsonianum*
Currant, Wild Blue: *Ribes laxiflorum*
Currant, Wild Red: *Ribes rubrum, R. triste*
Currant, Yellow: *Ribes aureum*
Cypress: *Sequoia sempervirens*
Cypress, Heath: *Lycopodium sabinifolium*
Cypress, Piute: *Cupressus nevadensis*
Cypress, Yellow: *Chamaecyparis nootkatensis*
Daggerpod: *Phoenicaulis cheiranthoides*
Dahoon: *Ilex cassine*
Dahoon Cassine: *Ilex cassine, I. vomitoria*
Daisy, Cutleaf: *Erigeron compositus*
Daisy, Easter: *Townsendia strigosa*
Daisy, English (or Lawn): *Bellis perennis*
Daisy, Mesa: *Machaeranthera pinnatifida*
Daisy, Ox Eye: *Leucanthemum vulgare*
Daisy, Paper: *Psilostrophe sparsiflora*
Daisy, White: *Leucanthemum vulgare*
Daisy, Wild: *Erigeron foliosus, Leucanthemum vulgare*
Dandelion: *Malacothrix glabrata, Taraxacum* spp.
Dandelion, Common: *Taraxacum officinale*
Dandelion, Desert: see Desertdandelion
Dandelion, False: *Pyrrhopappus pauciflorus*
Dandelion, Goat: *Pyrrhopappus carolinianus*
Dandelion, Mountain: *Agoseris aurantiaca, A. glauca*
Darning Needles, Devil's: *Clematis virginiana*
Datil: *Yucca baccata*
Day Flower: *Commelina erecta, C. dianthifolia*
Death Camas (or Camass): *Zigadenus elegans*
Death Camas, Foothill: *Zigadenus paniculatus*
Death Camas, Meadow: *Zigadenus venenosus*
Deathcamas, Nuttall's: *Zigadenus nuttallii*
Deer Brush: *Ceanothus integerrimus*
Deer's Ears: *Frasera speciosa*
Deer's Tongue: *Frasera speciosa*
Deer Weed: *Lotus scoparius, Polygonum aviculare*
Deerweed, Common: *Lotus scoparius*
Desert Calico: *Loeseliastrum matthewsii*
Desertchicory: *Pyrrhopappus pauciflorus*
Desertchicory, Carolina: *Pyrrhopappus carolinianus*
Desertdandelion, Fendler's: *Malacothrix fendleri*
Desertdandelion, Smooth: *Malacothrix glabrata*
Desertdandelion, Sowthistle: *Malacothrix sonchoides*
Desert Gourd: *Cucurbita foetidissima*
Desert Parsley, Gray: *Lomatium macrocarpum*
Desertparsley, Great Basin: *Lomatium simplex*
Desertparsley, King: *Lomatium graveolens*
Desert Parsley, Naked: *Lomatium nudicaule*
Desert Plume: *Stanleya pinnata*

Desert Ramona: *Salvia dorrii*
Desert Thorn: *Lycium pallidum, L. torreyi*
Desert Thornapple: *Datura discolor*
Desert Trumpet: *Eriogonum inflatum*
Desert Trumpets: *Linanthus nuttallii*
Devil's Bite: *Liatris scariosa*
Devil's Claw: *Proboscidea althaeifolia, P. parviflora*
Devil's Club: *Oplopanax horridus*
Devil's Darning Needles: *Clematis virginiana*
Devil's Gut: *Cassytha filiformis*
Devilshorn: *Proboscidea althaeifolia*
Devil's Shoestring: *Tephrosia virginiana, Yucca filamentosa*
Devil's Walking Stick: *Aralia spinosa, Oplopanax horridus*
Dewberry: *Rubus canadensis, R. flagellaris, R. hispidus, R. pubescens, R. trivialis, R. ursinus*
Dewberry, Bristly: *Rubus hispidus*
Dewberry, Northern: *Rubus flagellaris*
Dewberry, Pacific: *Rubus vitifolius*
Dewberry, Southern: *Rubus trivialis*
Dewflower, Nakedstem: *Murdannia nudiflora*
Diaper Moss, *Sphagnum* sp.
Dill: *Sanguinaria canadensis*
Dipper Gourd: *Lagenaria siceraria*
Dittany: *Cunila marina*
Dock, Arctic: *Rumex arcticus*
Dock, Bitter: *Rumex obtusifolius*
Dock, Clustered: *Rumex conglomeratus*
Dock, Curly: *Rumex crispus*
Dock, Golden: *Rumex maritimus*
Dock, Great Water: *Rumex orbiculatus*
Dock, Green: *Rumex conglomeratus*
Dock, Mexican: *Rumex salicifolius*
Dock, Narrow Leaved: *Rumex salicifolius*
Dock, Pale: *Rumex altissimus*
Dock, Patience: *Rumex patientia*
Dock, Sand: *Rumex hymenosepalus, R. venosus*
Dock, Sheep Sorrel: *Rumex acetosella*
Dock, Sour: *Rumex acetosa, R. aquaticus, R. arcticus, R. crispus*
Dock, Swamp: *Rumex verticillatus*
Dock, Veiny: *Rumex venosus*
Dock, Water: *Rumex altissimus, R. orbiculatus*
Dock, Western: *Rumex aquaticus*
Dock, Willow: *Rumex salicifolius*
Dock, Winged: *Rumex venosus*
Dock, Yellow: *Rumex crispus*
Dock Root: *Arctium minus*
Dodder, Bigfruit: *Cuscuta megalocarpa*
Dodder, California: *Cuscuta californica*
Dodder, Chaparral: *Cuscuta californica*
Dodder, Common: *Cuscuta gronovii*
Dodder, Compact: *Cuscuta compacta*

Dogbane, Intermediate: *Apocynum ×floribundum*
Dogbane, Spreading: *Apocynum androsaemifolium, A. cannabinum*
Dogbane, Velvet: *Apocynum cannabinum*
Dog Feet: *Disporum trachycarpum*
Dog Fennel: *Anthemis cotula*
Dogfennel, Garden: *Chamaemelum nobile*
Dogfennel, Green: *Matricaria discoidea*
Dog Hobble: *Leucothoe axillaris*
Dogweed: *Thymophylla acerosa*
Dogwood, Alternate Leaved: *Cornus alternifolia*
Dogwood, Bunchberry: *Cornus canadensis*
Dogwood, Creek: *Cornus sericea*
Dogwood, Dwarf: *Cornus canadensis*
Dogwood, Flowering: *Cornus florida, C. nuttallii*
Dogwood, Gray: *Cornus racemosa*
Dogwood, Mountain: *Cornus nuttallii*
Dogwood, Pacific: *Cornus nuttallii*
Dogwood, Panicled: *Cornus racemosa*
Dogwood, Red: *Cornus amomum, C. florida*
Dogwood, Red Osier: *Cornus sericea*
Dogwood, Rough Leaved: *Cornus drummondii*
Dogwood, Round Leaved: *Cornus rugosa*
Dogwood, Silky: *Cornus amomum*
Dogwood, Stiff: *Cornus foemina*
Dogwood, Western: *Cornus sericea*
Doll's Eyes: *Actaea pachypoda*
Doubleclaw: *Proboscidea parviflora*
Dove Weed: *Croton texensis*
Dove Weed, American: *Croton setigerus*
Dragon, Green: *Arisaema dracontium*
Dragon Head: *Dracocephalum parviflorum*
Dragonhead, False: *Physostegia parviflora*
Dragon Root: *Arisaema dracontium*
Dropseed: *Sporobolus cryptandrus*
Dropseed, Prairie: *Sporobolus heterolepis*
Dropseed, Sand: *Sporobolus cryptandrus*
Drops of Gold: *Disporum hookeri*
Drymary, Fendler's: *Drymaria glandulosa*
Duckweed, Star: *Lemna trisulca*
Dudley: *Salix gooddingii*
Dunebroom: *Parryella filifolia*
Durango Root: *Datisca glomerata*
Dustymaiden, Douglas's: *Chaenactis douglasii*
Dustymaiden, Steve's: *Chaenactis stevioides*
Dutchman's Breeches: *Dicentra cucullaria*
Dutchman's Pipe: *Aristolochia californica*
Eardrops, Golden: *Dicentra chrysantha*
Earth Star: *Geastrum* sp.
Eggs, Scrambled: *Corydalis aurea*
Ekaha Kuahiwi: *Asplenium nidus*
Elder, American: *Sambucus canadensis, S. cerulea*
Elder, Blue: *Sambucus cerulea*
Elder, Coastal American Red: *Sambucus racemosa*

Grouseberry: *Vaccinium scoparium*
Guava: *Psidium guajava*
Gum, Black: *Nyssa sylvatica*
Gum, Spruce: *Pinus rigida*
Gum, Sweet: *Liquidambar styraciflua*
Gum Plant: *Grindelia hallii, G. nana, G. robusta, G. squarrosa*
Gum Weed: *Grindelia* spp.
Gumweed, Curlycup: *Grindelia squarrosa*
Gumweed, Curlytop: *Grindelia nuda*
Gumweed, Great Valley: *Grindelia camporum, G. robusta*
Gumweed, Hairy: *Grindelia humilis*
Gumweed, Hall's: *Grindelia hallii*
Gumweed, Idaho: *Grindelia nana*
Gumweed, Pillar False: *Vanclevea stylosa*
Gumweed, Pointed: *Grindelia fastigiata*
Gumweed, Reclined: *Grindelia decumbens*
Gypsyflower: *Cynoglossum officinale*
Gypsyweed: *Veronica officinalis*
Haa: *Antidesma pulvinatum*
Hackberry, Common: *Celtis occidentalis*
Hackberry, Netleaf: *Celtis laevigata*
Hackberry, Rough Leaved: *Celtis occidentalis*
Hackberry, Western: *Celtis laevigata*
Hairybeast Turtleback: *Psathyrotes pilifera*
Hala: *Pandanus tectorius*
Hala-pepe: *Pleomele aurea*
Hame: *Antidesma pulvinatum*
Handsome Harry: *Rhexia virginica*
Hapuu: *Cibotium chamissoi*
Harbinger of Spring: *Erigenia bulbosa*
Hardhack: *Spiraea douglasii, S. tomentosa*
Hard Tack: *Cercocarpus montanus*
Hardweed, Eyelike: *Aster linariifolius*
Harebell: *Campanula rotundifolia*
Harebell, Southern: *Campanula divaricata*
Haresfoot Pointloco: *Oxytropis lagopus*
Hare's Tail: *Eriophorum callitrix*
Harlequinbush: *Gaura hexandra*
Harvestbells: *Gentiana saponaria*
Harvestlice: *Agrimonia parviflora*
Hau-kae-kae: *Hibiscus tiliaceus*
Hauve Cane: *Phragmites australis*
Haw: *Asclepias tuberosa, Crataegus douglasii, C. submollis*
Haw, Black: *Crataegus douglasii, Viburnum lentago, V. prunifolium*
Haw, Dotted: *Crataegus punctata*
Haw, Possum: *Viburnum nudum*
Haw, Red: *Crataegus chrysocarpa*
Hawksbeard, Fiddleleaf: *Crepis runcinata*
Hawksbeard, Longleaf: *Crepis acuminata*
Hawksbeard, Naked Stemmed: *Crepis runcinata*

Hawksbeard, Siskiyou: *Crepis modocensis*
Hawksbeard, Slender: *Crepis atribarba*
Hawkweed: *Hieracium cynoglossoides, H. fendleri, H. pilosella, H. scabrum, H. scouleri, H. venosum*
Hawkweed, Canada: *Hieracium canadense*
Hawkweed, Houndstongue: *Hieracium cynoglossoides*
Hawkweed, Mouseear: *Hieracium pilosella*
Hawkweed, Rough: *Hieracium scabrum*
Hawkweed, Yellow: *Hieracium fendleri*
Hawthorn, Black: *Crataegus douglasii*
Hawthorn, Dotted: *Crataegus punctata*
Hawthorn, Douglas's: *Crataegus douglasii*
Hawthorn, Fireberry: *Crataegus chrysocarpa*
Hawthorn, Hawaii: *Osteomeles anthyllidifolia*
Hawthorn, Littlehip: *Crataegus spathulata*
Hawthorn, Pear: *Crataegus calpodendron*
Hawthorn, Quebec: *Crataegus submollis*
Hawthorn, River: *Crataegus rivularis*
Hay, Red: *Andropogon gerardii*
Hay, Wild: *Bouteloua gracilis*
Hazel: *Corylus americana, C. cornuta*
Headache Weed: *Clematis hirsutissima*
Heal All: *Prunella vulgaris*
Heart Leaf: *Hexastylis arifolia, H. virginica*
Hearts-a-bustin-with-love: *Euonymus americana*
Heart Seed: *Polygonum pensylvanicum*
Heath, Rose: *Chaetopappa ericoides*
Heather, Red Mountain: *Phyllodoce empetriformis*
Heather, Western Moss: *Cassiope mertensiana*
Heather, White Mountain: *Cassiope mertensiana*
Heathgoldenrod, Chaparral: *Ericameria brachylepis*
Heathgoldenrod, Cliff: *Ericameria cuneata*
Heathgoldenrod, Cooper's: *Ericameria cooperi*
Heathgoldenrod, Dwarf: *Ericameria nana*
Heathgoldenrod, Narrowleaf: *Ericameria linearifolia*
Heathgoldenrod, Palmer's: *Ericameria palmeri*
Heathgoldenrod, Parish's: *Ericameria parishii*
Heathgoldenrod, Rabbitbush: *Ericameria bloomeri*
Hedgenettle, California: *Stachys bullata*
Hedgenettle, Great: *Stachys ciliata*
Hedgenettle, Marsh: *Stachys palustris*
Hedgenettle, Rothrock's: *Stachys rothrockii*
Hedgenettle, Smooth: *Stachys tenuifolia*
Hei: *Carica papaya*
Helianthella, Oneflower: *Helianthella uniflora*
Heliotrope, Wild: *Heliotropium curassavicum, Phacelia crenulata*
Hellebore, American False: *Veratrum viride*
Hellebore, American White: *Veratrum californicum*
Hellebore, Indian: *Veratrum viride*

Helleborine, Giant: *Epipactis gigantea*

Hemlock: *Picea glauca, Thuja occidentalis, T. canadensis*

Hemlock, Black: *Tsuga mertensiana*

Hemlock, Canada: *Tsuga canadensis*

Hemlock, Carolina: *Tsuga caroliniana*

Hemlock, Coast: *Tsuga heterophylla*

Hemlock, Crag: *Tsuga caroliniana*

Hemlock, Eastern: *Tsuga canadensis*

Hemlock, Ground: *Lycopodium clavatum, Taxus baccata, T. brevifolia, T. canadensis*

Hemlock, Mountain: *Tsuga mertensiana*

Hemlock, Poison: *Cicuta maculata, Conium maculatum*

Hemlock, Spotted Water: *Cicuta maculata*

Hemlock, Water: see Water Hemlock

Hemlock, Western: *Tsuga heterophylla*

Hemlockparsley, Chinese: *Conioselinum chinense*

Hemlockparsley, Pacific: *Conioselinum gmelinii*

Hemlockparsley, Rocky Mountain: *Conioselinum scopulorum*

Hemp: *Cannabis sativa*

Hemp, Indian: *Apocynum androsaemifolium, A. cannabinum*

Hemp, Mountain: *Apocynum cannabinum*

Hempvine (or Hempweed): *Mikania batatifolia*

Hepatica, Roundlobed: *Hepatica nobilis*

Hepatica, Sharplobe: *Hepatica nobilis*

Herb of the Cross: *Verbena officinalis*

Herb Sophia: *Descurainia sophia*

Hercules's Club: *Aralia spinosa, Zanthoxylum clava-herculis*

Heronbill: *Erodium cicutarium*

Hickory: *Carya alba, C. laciniosa, C. ovata, C. pallida*

Hickory, Bitternut: *Carya cordiformis*

Hickory, Mockernut: *Carya alba*

Hickory, Pignut: *Carya glabra*

Hickory, Sand: *Carya pallida*

Hickory, Shag Bark: *Carya ovata*

Hickory, Shellbark: *Carya ovata*

Hoarhound: *Marrubium vulgare*

Hoarhound, Water: *Lycopus americanus*; see also Water Horehound

Hoarhound, Wild: *Eupatorium pilosum*

Hoary Pea: *Tephrosia purpurea*

Hoarypea, Florida: *Tephrosia florida*

Hoarypea, Sprawling: *Tephrosia hispidula*

Hoary Puccoon: *Lithospermum canescens*

Ho-a-wa: *Pittosporum* sp.

Hobble Bush: *Viburnum lantanoides*

Hognut: *Amphicarpaea bracteata*

Hog Peanut: *Amphicarpaea bracteata*

Hogweed: *Amaranthus retroflexus*

Hogweed, Little: *Portulaca oleracea*

Ho-i-o: *Diplazium meyenianum*

Holdback, James's: *Caesalpinia jamesii*

Ho-le-i: *Ochrosia compta*

Holly, American: *Ilex opaca*

Holly, California: *Heteromeles arbutifolia*

Holly, English: *Ilex aquifolium*

Holly, Mountain: *Ilex aquifolium, Nemopanthus mucronatus*

Holly, Sea: *Eryngium alismifolium*

Holly, Western: *Mahonia aquifolium*

Hollyhock: *Alcea rosea*

Hollyhock, Desert: *Sphaeralcea emoryi*

Honeydew: *Horkelia californica*

Honey Locust: *Gleditsia triacanthos*

Honey Mesquite: *Prosopis glandulosa*

Honeysuckle, American Fly: *Lonicera canadensis*

Honeysuckle, Arizona: *Lonicera arizonica*

Honeysuckle, Bearberry: *Lonicera involucrata*

Honeysuckle, Bush: *Diervilla lonicera*

Honeysuckle, Butters: *Lonicera dioica*

Honeysuckle, Chaparral: *Lonicera interrupta*

Honeysuckle, Coast: *Lonicera involucrata*

Honeysuckle, Dwarf Bush: *Diervilla lonicera*

Honeysuckle, Fly: *Lonicera canadensis, L. oblongifolia*

Honeysuckle, Glaucous: *Lonicera dioica*

Honeysuckle, Johnston's: *Lonicera subspicata*

Honeysuckle, Limber: *Lonicera dioica*

Honeysuckle, Orange: *Lonicera ciliosa*

Honeysuckle, Swamp: *Lonicera involucrata*

Honeysuckle, Swamp Fly: *Lonicera oblongifolia*

Honeysuckle, Twinberry: *Lonicera involucrata*

Honeysuckle, Twining: *Lonicera dioica*

Honeysuckle, Utah: *Lonicera utahensis*

Honohono: *Murdannia nudiflora*

Hop: *Humulus lupulus*

Hopbush: *Dodonaea viscosa*

Hop Hornbeam: *Ostrya virginiana*

Hops: *Humulus lupulus*

Hop Tree: *Ptelea trifoliata*

Hop Vine: *Humulus lupulus*

Horehound, American: *Marrubium vulgare*

Horehound, Water: *Lycopus americanus, L. asper, L. virginicus, Marrubium vulgare*

Horehound, White: *Marrubium vulgare*

Horkelia: *Ivesia gordonii*

Hornbeam: *Carpinus caroliniana*

Hornbean: *Carpinus caroliniana*

Horsebean: *Vicia faba*

Horsebrush: *Tetradymia canescens*

Horsebrush, Hairy: *Tetradymia comosa*

Horsebrush, Mojave: *Tetradymia stenolepis*

Horseflyweed: *Baptisia tinctoria*

Horsehound: *Marrubium vulgare*
Horsemint: *Monarda didyma, M. pectinata, M. punctata, Monardella villosa*
Horsenettle, Carolina: *Solanum carolinense*
Horsenettle, Fendler's: *Solanum fendleri*
Horseradish: *Armoracia rusticana, Rorippa nasturtium-aquaticum*
Horse Tail: *Equisetum arvense, E. byemale, E. laevigatum, E. palustre, E. sylvaticum, E. telmateia*
Horse Tail, Branchless: *Equisetum byemale, E. laevigatum*
Horse Tail, Field: *Equisetum arvense, E. byemale*
Horse Tail, Giant: *Equisetum telmateia*
Horse Tail, Large: *Equisetum byemale*
Horsetail, Marsh: *Equisetum palustre*
Horse Tail, River: *Equisetum laevigatum*
Horse Tail, Small: *Equisetum laevigatum*
Horsetail, Smooth: *Equisetum laevigatum*
Horse Tail, Wood: *Equisetum sylvaticum*
Horse Weed: *Conyza canadensis*
Hound's Tongue: *Cynoglossum grande, C. officinale, C. virginianum*
Huckleberry, Alaska: *Vaccinium ovalifolium*
Huckleberry, Black: *Gaylussacia baccata, Vaccinium ovatum*
Huckleberry, Black Mountain: *Vaccinium membranaceum*
Huckleberry, Blue: *Vaccinium membranaceum, V. ovalifolium*
Huckleberry, California: *Vaccinium ovatum*
Huckleberry, Coast: *Vaccinium ovatum*
Huckleberry, Early: *Gaylussacia baccata*
Huckleberry, Evergreen: *Vaccinium ovatum*
Huckleberry, Fool's: *Menziesia ferruginea*
Huckleberry, Mountain: *Vaccinium membranaceum*
Huckleberry, Oval Leaved: *Vaccinium ovalifolium*
Huckleberry, Red: *Vaccinium ovalifolium, V. parvifolium*
Huckleberry, Thin Leaved: *Vaccinium membranaceum*
Hummingbird: *Castilleja parviflora*
Hummingbird Trumpet: *Epilobium canum*
Hyacinth, Pine: *Clematis baldwinii*
Hyacinth, Wild: *Triteleia grandiflora*
Hydrangea, Ashy: *Hydrangea cinerea*
Hydrangea, Wild: *Hydrangea arborescens*
Hymenopappus, Fineleaf: *Hymenopappus filifolius*
Hymenopappus, Idaho: *Hymenopappus filifolius*
Hymenoxys, Pingue: *Hymenoxys richardsonii*
Hyssop: *Hyssopus officinalis*
Hyssop, Blue Giant: *Agastache foeniculum*
Hyssop, Blue Water: *Bacopa caroliniana*
Hyssop, Bog: *Bacopa caroliniana*

Hyssop, Fragrant Giant: *Agastache foeniculum*
Hyssop, Giant: *Agastache foeniculum, A. nepetoides, A. pallidiflora, A. scrophulariifolia, A. urticifolia*
Hyssop, Lavender: *Agastache foeniculum*
Hyssop, Nettleleaf Giant: *Agastache urticifolia*
Hyssop, New Mexico Giant: *Agastache pallidiflora*
Hyssop, Purple Giant: *Agastache scrophulariifolia*
Hyssop, Water: *Bacopa caroliniana*
Hyssop, Yellow Giant: *Agastache nepetoides*
Icaco Coco Plum: *Chrysobalanus icaco*
Ice Cream, Indian: *Shepherdia canadensis*
'Ie'ie: *Freycinetia arborea*
Ihi-ai: *Portulaca oleracea*
Iliee: *Plumbago zeylanica*
Ilima: *Sida* sp.
Ili-oha Laau: *Conyza canadensis*
Incienso: *Encelia farinosa*
Indian Balsam: *Lomatium dissectum*
Indian Bread Root: *Pediomelum esculentum*
Indian Broom: *Baccharis sarothroides*
Indian Celery: *Lomatium ambiguum, L. nudicaule, L. triternatum*
Indian Cherry: *Prunus ilicifolia*
Indian Coffee: *Senna tora*
Indian Consumption Plant: *Lomatium nudicaule*
Indian Corn: *Zea mays*
Indian Cucumber: *Medeola virginiana*
Indian Cucumberroot: *Medeola virginiana*
Indian Cup: *Sarracenia purpurea*
Indian Cup Plant: *Silphium perfoliatum*
Indian Ginger: *Asarum canadense*
Indian Gum Plant: *Stephanomeria spinosa*
Indian Hellebore: *Veratrum viride*
Indian Hemp: *Apocynum androsaemifolium, A. cannabinum*
Indian Ice Cream: *Shepherdia canadensis*
Indian Lettuce: *Claytonia perfoliata, C. sibirica*
Indian Maize: *Zea mays*
Indian Mulberry: *Morinda citrifolia*
Indian Mustard: *Brassica juncea*
Indian Paint: *Castilleja parviflora, Lithospermum incisum*
Indian Paintbrush: see Paintbrush
Indian Parsley: see Parsley, Indian
Indian Parsnip: *Pteryxia terebinthina*
Indian Pepper: *Saururus cernuus*
Indian Physic: *Porteranthus stipulatus*
Indian Pink: *Spigelia marilandica*
Indian Pipe: *Monotropa uniflora*
Indian Plum: *Oemleria cerasiformis*
Indian Poke: *Veratrum viride*
Indian Posey: *Barbarea vulgaris*
Indian Posy: *Anaphalis margaritacea*

Leek, House: *Sempervivum tectorum*
Leek, Wild: *Allium tricoccum*
Lemita: *Rhus trilobata*
Lenscale: *Atriplex lentiformis*
Leopardbane: *Arnica acaulis*
Lettuce, Bitter: *Lactuca virosa*
Lettuce, Blue: *Lactuca biennis, L. tatarica*
Lettuce, Branch: *Saxifraga pensylvanica*
Lettuce, Canada: *Lactuca canadensis*
Lettuce, Canker: *Pyrola elliptica*
Lettuce, Chalk: *Dudleya pulverulenta*
Lettuce, Garden: *Lactuca sativa*
Lettuce, Indian: *Claytonia perfoliata, C. sibirica*
Lettuce, Miner's: *Claytonia perfoliata, C. sibirica*
Lettuce, Mountain: *Ligusticum canadense*
Lettuce, Prickly: *Lactuca canadensis, L. sativa, L. serriola*
Lettuce, Purple: *Lactuca tatarica*
Lettuce, Rough White: *Prenanthes aspera*
Lettuce, Squaw: *Claytonia perfoliata*
Lettuce, Tall: *Lactuca biennis, Prenanthes altissima*
Lettuce, Tall Blue: *Lactuca biennis*
Lettuce, White: *Prenanthes alba*
Lettuce, Wild: *Claytonia perfoliata, Lactuca canadensis, L. tatarica, L. virosa*
Lettuce, Wire: see Wirelettuce
Lichen, Dogtooth: *Peltigera canina*
Lichen, Flat: *Peltigera aphthosa*
Lichen, Old Man's Beard: *Usnea longissima*
Licorice: *Glycyrrhiza glabra, G. lepidota*; see also Liquorice
Licorice Root: *Glycyrrhiza lepidota*; see also Liquorice Root
Licoriceroot, Canadian: *Ligusticum canadense*
Licoriceroot, Canby's: *Ligusticum canbyi*
Licoriceroot, Celeryleaf: *Ligusticum apiifolium*
Licoriceroot, Fernleaf: *Ligusticum filicinum*
Licoriceroot, Gray's: *Ligusticum grayi*
Licoriceroot, Hultén's: *Ligusticum scothicum*
Licoriceroot, Porter's: *Ligusticum porteri*
Licoriceroot, Scottish: *Ligusticum scothicum*
Life Everlasting, Fragrant: *Gnaphalium obtusifolium*
Lilac: *Syringa vulgaris*
Lilac, Coast: *Ceanothus thyrsiflorus*
Lilac, Wild: *Ceanothus leucodermis*
Lily: *Lilium canadense, Sagittaria latifolia*
Lily, Arrowhead: *Sagittaria latifolia*
Lily, Avalanche: *Erythronium grandiflorum*
Lily, Canada: *Lilium canadense*
Lily, Clinton's: *Clintonia borealis*
Lily, Cluster: see Cluster Lily
Lily, Columbian: *Lilium columbianum*

Lily, Corn: *Clintonia borealis, Veratrum californicum*
Lily, Cow: *Nuphar lutea*
Lily, Crag: *Echeandia flavescens*
Lily, Dogtooth: *Erythronium grandiflorum*
Lily, Easter: *Erythronium oregonum*
Lily, Elk: *Frasera speciosa*
Lily, False: *Maianthemum canadense*
Lily, Fawn: see Fawnlily
Lily, Glacier: *Erythronium grandiflorum*
Lily, Green Banded Mariposa: *Calochortus macrocarpus*
Lily, Leopard: *Fritillaria atropurpurea*
Lily, Lonely: *Eremocrinum albomarginatum*
Lily, Mariposa: see Mariposa; and Mariposa Lily
Lily, Mignonette Scented: *Triteleia grandiflora*
Lily, Orange Red: *Lilium philadelphicum*
Lily, Orangecup: *Lilium philadelphicum*
Lily, Panther: *Lilium columbianum*
Lily, Philadelphia: *Lilium philadelphicum*
Lily, Pine: *Xerophyllum tenax*
Lily, Sage: *Leucocrinum montanum*
Lily, Sand: *Mentzelia albicaulis*
Lily, Sego: *Calochortus gunnisonii, C. macrocarpus*
Lily, Tiger: *Fritillaria atropurpurea, Lilium columbianum*
Lily, Torrey's Crag: *Echeandia flavescens*
Lily, Water: see Water Lily
Lily, Western Wood: *Lilium philadelphicum*
Lily, Wild: *Lilium philadelphicum*
Lily, Wild Yellow: *Lilium canadense*
Lily, Wood: *Lilium columbianum, Lilium philadelphicum*
Lily, Yellow Avalanche: *Erythronium grandiflorum*
Lily, Zephyr: *Zephyranthes sp.*
Lily of the Valley, Wild: *Maianthemum canadense, M. dilatatum*
Linden: *Tilia americana*
Lingon: *Vaccinium vitis-idaea*
Lions Foot: *Prenanthes serpentaria*
Lipfern, Beaded: *Cheilanthes wootonii*
Lipfern, Fendler's: *Cheilanthes fendleri*
Lippa, Wright: *Aloysia wrightii*
Liquoria: *Glycyrrhiza lepidota*
Liquorice: *Glycyrrhiza glabra*; see also Licorice
Liquorice Root: *Hedysarum boreale*; see also Licorice Root
Liquorice Root, Wild: *Glycyrrhiza lepidota*
Littlebrownjug: *Hexastylis arifolia*
Live Forever: *Sedum telephioides, S. telephium*
Liveforever, Chalk: *Dudleya pulverulenta*
Liverleaf: *Hepatica nobilis*
Liverwort, Cone Headed: *Conocephalum conicum*

Lizard's Tail: *Anemopsis californica, Saururus cernuus*
Lobelia, Brook: *Lobelia kalmii*
Lobelia, Great Blue: *Lobelia siphilitica*
Lobelia, Palespike: *Lobelia spicata*
Loco, Haresfoot Point: *Oxytropis lagopus*
Locoweed: *Astragalus allochrous, A. calycosus, A. kentrophyta, A. miser, A. pachypus, A. purshii, Oxytropis campestris, O. lambertii, O. monticola*
Locoweed, American: *Astragalus mollissimus*
Locoweed, Lambert: *Oxytropis lambertii*
Locoweed, Matthew: *Astragalus mollissimus*
Locoweed, Purple: *Oxytropis lagopus, O. lambertii*
Locoweed, Yellowflower: *Oxytropis monticola*
Locust, Black: *Robinia pseudoacacia*
Locust, Bristly: *Robinia hispida*
Locust, Eastern: *Robinia pseudoacacia*
Locust, Honey: *Gleditsia triacanthos*
Locust, New Mexican: *Robinia neomexicana*
London Rocket: *Sisymbrium irio*
Long Trumpet: *Eriogonum nudum*
Loosestrife: *Lysimachia quadrifolia, Lythrum alatum*
Loosestrife, California: *Lythrum californicum*
Loosestrife, Purple: *Lythrum salicaria*
Loosestrife, Spiked: *Lythrum salicaria*
Loosestrife, Tufted: *Lysimachia thyrsiflora*
Loosestrife, Whorled: *Lysimachia quadrifolia*
Lopseed: *Phryma leptostachya*
Lote Bush: *Ziziphus obtusifolia*
Lousewort, Attol: *Pedicularis attollens*
Lousewort, Bracted: *Pedicularis bracteosa*
Lousewort, Canadian: *Pedicularis canadensis*
Lousewort, Dwarf: *Pedicularis centranthera*
Lousewort, Elephanthead: *Pedicularis groen-landica*
Lousewort, Sickletop: *Pedicularis racemosa*
Lovage: *Ligusticum apiifolium, L. canbyi, L. filicinum, L. scothicum*
Love Seed: *Lomatium foeniculaceum*
Lupine, Arctic: *Lupinus arcticus*
Lupine, Beach: *Lupinus albifrons, L. densiflorus, L. polyphyllus, Trifolium wormskioldii*
Lupine, Bigleaf: *Lupinus polyphyllus*
Lupine, Blue: *Lupinus littoralis, L. nootkatensis, L. polyphyllus, L. sericeus*
Lupine, Broad Leaved: *Lupinus polyphyllus*
Lupine, Chinook: *Lupinus littoralis*
Lupine, Dwarf: *Lupinus kingii*
Lupine, False: *Thermopsis macrophylla*
Lupine, Intermountain: *Lupinus pusillus*
Lupine, Kellogg's Spurred: *Lupinus caudatus*
Lupine, King's: *Lupinus kingii*

Lupine, Lyall: *Lupinus lyallii*
Lupine, Mountain: *Lupinus lyallii*
Lupine, Nootka: *Lupinus nootkatensis*
Lupine, Riverbank: *Lupinus rivularis*
Lupine, Rusty: *Lupinus pusillus*
Lupine, Seashore: *Lupinus littoralis*
Lupine, Short Stem: *Lupinus brevicaulis*
Lupine, Silky: *Lupinus sericeus*
Lupine, Silver: *Lupinus albifrons*
Lupine, Silvery: *Lupinus argenteus*
Lupine, Sulphur: *Lupinus sulphureus*
Lupine, Sundial: *Lupinus perennis*
Lupine, Wyeth's: *Lupinus wyethii*
Lyreleaf Greeneyes: *Berlandiera lyrata*
Lythrum, Winged: *Lythrum alatum*
Machaeranthera, Whiteflower: *Machaeranthera canescens*
Madrona (or Madrone, or Madroño): *Arbutus menziesii*
Madwoman's Milk: *Euphorbia helioscopia*
Magnolia, Big-Leaf: *Magnolia macrophylla*
Magnolia, Southern: *Magnolia grandiflora*
Mahogany, American: *Cercocarpus montanus*
Mahogany, Birch Leaf: *Cercocarpus montanus*
Mahogany, Mountain: *Cercocarpus ledifolius, C. montanus*
Mahogany, True Mountain: *Cercocarpus montanus*
Maia: *Musa ×paradisiaca*
Maiden Fern: *Asplenium trichomanes*
Maidenhair, Aleutian: *Adiantum aleuticum*
Maidenhair, California: *Adiantum jordanii*
Maidenhair, Northern: *Adiantum pedatum*
Maidenhair Fern: *Adiantum aleuticum, A. capillus-veneris, A. jordanii, A. pedatum*
Maile: *Alyxia oliviformis*
Maile-kaluhea: *Coprosma* sp.
Maile-kuahiwi: *Alyxia oliviformis*
Maize: *Zea mays*
Ma-ko-u: *Peucedanum sandwicense*
Mallow: *Malva neglecta, M. parviflora, Modiola caroliniana, Sphaeralcea ambigua*
Mallow, Alkali: *Malvella leprosa*
Mallow, American: *Malva neglecta*
Mallow, Bull: *Malva nicaeensis*
Mallow, Cheeses: *Malva neglecta*
Mallow, Common: *Malva neglecta*
Mallow, Copper: *Sphaeralcea angustifolia*
Mallow, Desert: *Sphaeralcea ambigua*
Mallow, False: *Sphaeralcea coccinea*
Mallow, Glade: *Napaea dioica*
Mallow, Globe: see Globemallow
Mallow, Marsh: *Malva moschata*
Mallow, Musk: *Malva moschata*
Mallow, Purple: *Callirhoe involucrata*

Mallow, Purple Poppy: *Callirhoe involucrata*
Mallow, Red Globe: *Sphaeralcea coccinea*
Mallow, Rose: *Hibiscus moscheutos*
Mallow, Scarlet: *Sphaeralcea coccinea*
Mallow Ninebark: *Physocarpus malvaceus*
Mamaki: *Pipturus* sp.
Manawanawa: *Vitex trifolia*
Mandrake: *Podophyllum peltatum*
Manena: *Melicope cinerea*
Manna Grass: *Glyceria obtusa*
Mannagrass, Atlantic: *Glyceria obtusa*
Mannagrass, Water: *Glyceria fluitans*
Man of the Earth: *Ipomoea pandurata*
Man Root: *Ipomoea pandurata, Marah fabaceus*
Manroot, California: *Marah fabaceus*
Manroot, Coastal: *Marah oreganus*
Manroot, Cucamonga: *Marah macrocarpus*
Man Root, Hill: *Marah oreganus*
Man Root, Old: *Marah oreganus*
Manroot, Sierran: *Marah horridus*
Manzanita, Bigberry: *Arctostaphylos glauca*
Manzanita, Blue: *Arctostaphylos viscida*
Manzanita, Eastwood: *Arctostaphylos glandulosa*
Manzanita, Great: *Arctostaphylos glauca*
Manzanita, Green: *Arctostaphylos patula*
Manzanita, Greenleaf: *Arctostaphylos patula*
Manzanita, Hairy: *Arctostaphylos columbiana*
Manzanita, Large: *Arctostaphylos tomentosa*
Manzanita, Mariposa: *Arctostaphylos viscida*
Manzanita, Parry: *Arctostaphylos manzanita*
Manzanita, Pine Mat: *Arctostaphylos nevadensis*
Manzanita, Pointleaf: *Arctostaphylos pungens*
Manzanita, Sticky Whiteleaf: *Arctostaphylos viscida*
Manzanita, Whiteleaf: *Arctostaphylos manzanita*
Manzanita, Woollyleaf: *Arctostaphylos tomentosa*
Ma-o: *Abutilon incanum*
Maple, Big Leaf: *Acer macrophyllum*
Maple, Black Sugar: *Acer nigrum*
Maple, Box Elder: *Acer negundo*
Maple, Broad Leaf: *Acer macrophyllum*
Maple, Douglas: *Acer glabrum*
Maple, Drummond's: *Acer rubrum*
Maple, Dwarf: *Acer glabrum*
Maple, Green: *Acer pensylvanicum*
Maple, Hard: *Acer saccharinum, A. saccharum*
Maple, Manitoba: *Acer negundo*
Maple, Mountain: *Acer spicatum*
Maple, New Mexico: *Acer glabrum*
Maple, Red: *Acer rubrum*
Maple, Rock: *Acer saccharum*
Maple, Rocky Mountain: *Acer glabrum*
Maple, Shrub: *Acer glabrum*
Maple, Silver: *Acer saccharinum*

Maple, Soft: *Acer rubrum, A. saccharinum, A. saccharum*
Maple, Striped: *Acer pensylvanicum*
Maple, Sugar: *Acer saccharinum, A. saccharum*
Maple, Vine: *Acer circinatum*
Maple, White: *Acer alba*
Marbleseed: *Onosmodium molle*
Mariana, Golden: *Chrysopsis mariana*
Marigold, Aztec: *Tagetes erecta*
Marigold, Desert: *Baileya multiradiata*
Marigold, Fetid: *Dyssodia papposa, Pectis angustifolia, P. papposa*
Marigold, Licorice: *Tagetes micrantha*
Marigold, Marsh: *Caltha leptosepala, C. palustris, Ranunculus lapponicus*
Marijuana: *Cannabis sativa*
Mariposa: *Calochortus gunnisonii*
Mariposa, Golden: *Calochortus aureus*
Mariposa, Sagebrush: *Calochortus macrocarpus*
Mariposa, Yellow: *Calochortus aureus*
Mariposa Lily: *Calochortus aureus, C. gunnisonii, C. macrocarpus*
Mariposa Lily, Gunnison's: *Calochortus gunnisonii*
Marshlocks: *Comarum palustre*
Marshmallow, Wild: *Hibiscus moscheutos*
Marshmarigold: see Marigold, Marsh
Marshpennywort: *Hydrocotyle umbellata*
Mastic, False: *Sideroxylon foetidissimum*
Matchbrush: *Gutierrezia sarothrae*
Matchweed: *Gutierrezia microcephala, G. sarothrae*
Matchweed, San Joaquin: *Gutierrezia californica*
Matchwood: *Gutierrezia sarothrae*
Matrimony Vine: *Lycium pallidum*
Matted Crinklemat: *Tiquilia latior*
Mayflower: *Epigaea repens*
Mayflower, Canada: *Maianthemum canadense*
Maypop: *Passiflora incarnata*
Maystar: *Trientalis borealis*
May Weed: *Anthemis cotula*
Mayweed, Disc: *Matricaria discoidea*
Meadow Beauty: *Rhexia virginica*
Meadowparsnip: *Thaspium barbinode*
Meadow Rue, Early: *Thalictrum dioicum, T. thalictroides*
Meadow Rue, Fall: *Thalictrum pubescens*
Meadow Rue, Fendler: *Thalictrum fendleri*
Meadowrue, Fewflower: *Thalictrum sparsiflorum*
Meadow Rue, Flat Fruited: *Thalictrum sparsiflorum*
Meadow Rue, Purple: *Thalictrum dasycarpum*
Meadow Rue, Sierra: *Thalictrum polycarpum*
Meadow Rue, Western: *Thalictrum occidentale*
Meadow Salsify: *Tragopogon pratensis*

Pea, Hoary: *Tephrosia florida, T. hispidula, T. purpurea*

Pea, Partridge: *Chamaecrista fasciculata, C. nictitans, Senna marilandica*

Pea, Scurf: see Scurf Pea

Pea, Wild: *Lathyrus japonicus, L. ochroleucus, L. palustris, L. venosus, L. vestitus, Vicia americana*

Peach, Cultivated: *Prunus persica*

Peach, Desert: *Prunus andersonii*

Peach, Wild: *Prunus andersonii*

Peanut, Hog: *Amphicarpaea bracteata*

Pearl Millet: *Pennisetum glaucum*

Pearly Everlasting: *Anaphalis margaritacea*

Pear, Prickly: see Pricklypear

Pearly Pussytoes: *Antennaria anaphaloides*

Pear Thorn: *Crataegus calpodendron*

Peat Moss: *Sphagnum* sp.

Peavine: *Lathyrus eucosmus*

Peavine, California: *Lathyrus jepsonii*

Peavine, Cream: *Lathyrus ochroleucus*

Peavine, Pacific: *Lathyrus vestitus*

Peavine, Sea: *Lathyrus japonicus*

Peavine, Slenderstem: *Lathyrus palustris*

Peavine, Veiny: *Lathyrus venosus*

Pecan: *Carya illinoinensis*

Pectis, Narrowleaf: *Pectis angustifolia*

Pelotazo: *Abutilon incanum*

Pembina: *Viburnum opulus*

Pencilflower: *Stylosanthes biflora*

Penny Cress: *Thlaspi arvense*

Pennycress, Alpine: *Thlaspi montanum*

Pennyroyal: *Hedeoma nana, H. pulegioides, Mentha arvensis, Piloblephis rigida*

Pennyroyal, American: *Hedeoma pulegioides*

Pennyroyal, Drummond: *Hedeoma drummondii*

Pennyroyal, Mock: *Hedeoma drummondii, H. nana*

Pennyroyal, Mountain: *Monardella odoratissima*

Pennyroyal, Rough: *Hedeoma hispida*

Pennyroyal, Wild: *Piloblephis rigida*

Pennywort: *Obolaria virginica*

Pennywort, Water: *Hydrocotyle umbellata*

Pennyworth: *Obolaria virginica*

Penstemon, Beardlip: *Penstemon barbatus*

Penstemon, Bush: *Penstemon fruticosus*

Penstemon, Colorado: *Penstemon linarioides*

Penstemon, Eaton's: *Penstemon eatonii*

Penstemon, Heartleaf: *Keckiella cordifolia*

Penstemon, Littleleaf Bush: *Penstemon fruticosus*

Penstemon, Mountain Blue: *Penstemon laetus*

Penstemon, Palmer's: *Penstemon palmeri*

Penstemon, Scabland: *Penstemon deustus*

Penstemon, Sharpleaf: *Penstemon acuminatus*

Penstemon, Torrey's: *Penstemon barbatus*

Penstemon, Woodland: *Nothochelone nemorosa*

Peony, American Wild: *Paeonia brownii*

Peony, Western: *Paeonia brownii*

Peony, Wild: *Paeonia brownii, P. californica*

Pepper, Black: *Piper nigrum*

Pepper, Bush: *Berberis canadensis*

Pepper, Cayenne: *Capsicum annuum*

Pepper, Chili: *Capsicum annuum*

Pepper, Indian: *Saururus cernuus*

Pepper, Poor Man's: *Lepidium virginicum*

Pepper, Spur: *Capsicum annuum*

Pepper, Water: *Polygonum hydropiper*

Pepper, Wild: *Capsicum annuum*

Pepper and Salt: *Erigenia bulbosa*

Pepperidge: *Nyssa sylvatica*

Peppermint: *Mentha canadensis, M. ×piperita*

Peppernut: *Umbellularia californica*

Pepper Root: *Cardamine concatenata, C. diphylla*

Peppervine: *Ampelopsis cordata*

Pepperweed, Common: *Lepidium densiflorum*

Pepperweed, Menzies's: *Lepidium virginicum*

Pepperweed, Mountain: *Lepidium montanum*

Pepperweed, Shaggyfruit: *Lepidium lasiocarpum*

Pepperweed, Shining: *Lepidium nitidum*

Pepperwood: *Umbellularia californica*

Periwinkle, Madagascar: *Catharanthus roseus*

Perkysue: *Tetraneuris argentea*

Persicaria, Carey's: *Polygonum careyi*

Persicaria, Dock Leaved: *Polygonum lapathifolium*

Persicaria, Hartwright's: *Polygonum amphibium*

Persicaria, Pennsylvania: *Polygonum pensylvanicum*

Persicaria, Swamp: *Polygonum amphibium*

Persimmon: *Diospyros virginiana*

Peruvian Bark: *Cinchona calisaya*

Peteria, Rush: *Peteria scoparia*

Peyote: *Lophophora williamsii*

Phacelia, Branching: *Phacelia ramosissima*

Phacelia, Silverleaf: *Phacelia hastata*

Phacelia, Varileaf: *Phacelia heterophylla*

Phlox, Clustered: *Phlox caespitosa*

Phlox, Colddesert: *Phlox stansburyi*

Phlox, Desert: *Phlox austromontana*

Phlox, Downy: *Phlox pilosa*

Phlox, Flowery: *Phlox multiflora*

Phlox, Longleaf: *Phlox longifolia*

Phlox, Moss: *Phlox subulata*

Phlox, Slender: *Phlox gracilis*

Phlox, Spiny: *Phlox hoodii*

Pickerel Weed: *Pontederia cordata*

Piedmont Staggerbush: *Lyonia mariana*

Pigeon Berry Poke: *Phytolacca americana*

Pigeonwings: *Clitoria mariana*

Primrose, Hooker's Evening: *Oenothera elata*
Primrose, Pale Evening: *Oenothera pallida*
Primrose, Shortfruit Evening: *Oenothera brachycarpa*
Primrose, Small Evening: *Oenothera perennis*
Primrose, Stemless Evening: *Oenothera triloba*
Primrose, Tansyleaf Evening: *Camissonia tanacetifolia*
Primrose, Tufted Evening: *Oenothera cespitosa*
Primrose, White Evening: *Oenothera albicaulis*
Primrose, Yellow Evening: *Oenothera elata*
Primrosewillow, Carolina: *Ludwigia bonariensis*
Primrosewillow, Savannah: *Ludwigia virgata*
Prince's Pine: *Chimaphila umbellata*
Prince's Pine, Little: *Chimaphila menziesii*
Prince's Pine, Striped: *Chimaphila maculata*
Prince's Plume: *Stanleya pinnata*
Privet, Eastern Swamp: *Forestiera acuminata*
Privet, Wild: *Forestiera pubescens*
Psoralea, Few Flowered: *Psoralidium tenuiflorum*
Psoralea, Silver Leaf: *Pediomelum argophyllum*
Psoralea, Slender Flowered: *Psoralidium tenuiflorum*
Puccoon: *Lithospermum canescens, L. caroliniense, L. incisum, L. ruderale*
Puccoon, Hairy: *Lithospermum caroliniense*
Puccoon, Hoary: *Lithospermum canescens*
Puccoon, Narrow Leaved: *Lithospermum incisum*
Puffball: *Bovista pila, B. plumbea, Bovistella* sp., *Lycoperdon* sp.
Pukiawe: *Styphelia tameiameiae*
Pumpkin: *Cucurbita maxima, C. pepo*
Pumpkin, Field: *Cucurbita pepo*
Pumpkin, Large Pie: *Cucurbita pepo*
Pumpkin, Pumpion: *Cucurbita pepo*
Pumpkin, Wild: *Cucurbita foetidissima*
Puncturevine: *Tribulus terrestris*
Purselane: *Portulaca oleracea*; see also Purslane
Purslane: *Portulaca oleracea*
Purslane, Milk: *Chamaesyce glyptosperma*
Pusley: *Portulaca oleracea*
Pusley, Chinese: *Heliotropium curassavicum*
Pussy Toes: *Antennaria parvifolia, A. rosea, A. rosulata*
Pussytoes, Field (or Howell's): *Antennaria howellii*
Pussytoes, Kaibab: *Antennaria rosulata*
Pussytoes, Pearly: *Antennaria anaphaloides*
Pussy Toes, Pink (or Rosy): *Antennaria rosea*
Pussytoes, Smallleaf: *Antennaria parvifolia*
Pussytoes, Stoloniferous: *Antennaria dioica*
Putty Root: *Aplectrum hyemale*
Pyrola: *Pyrola elliptica*
Pyrola, One Flowered: *Moneses uniflora*
Quack Grass: *Elytrigia repens*

Quail Brush: *Atriplex lentiformis*
Quail Bush: *Atriplex lentiformis*
Quamash: *Camassia scilloides*
Queen Anne's Lace: *Daucus carota, D. pusillus*
Queen of the Meadow: *Eupatorium purpureum*
Queen of the Meadows: *Spiraea salicifolia*
Queen of the Prairie: *Filipendula rubra*
Queen's Cup: *Clintonia uniflora*
Queen's Delight: *Stillingia sylvatica*
Quinine: *Cinchona calisaya*
Quinine, Wild: *Parthenium integrifolium*
Quinine Cherry: *Prunus emarginata*
Rabbitbells: *Crotalaria rotundifolia*
Rabbit Brush: *Chrysothamnus depressus, C. greenei, C. nauseosus, C. parryi, C. viscidiflorus*
Rabbit Brush, Broadscale: *Chrysothamnus nauseosus*
Rabbit Brush, Douglas: *Chrysothamnus viscidiflorus*
Rabbitbrush, Green: *Chrysothamnus viscidiflorus*
Rabbitbrush, Greene's: *Chrysothamnus greenei*
Rabbit Brush, Heavy Scented: *Chrysothamnus nauseosus*
Rabbitbrush, Howard's: *Chrysothamnus parryi*
Rabbit Brush, Little: *Chrysothamnus viscidiflorus*
Rabbitbrush, Parry's: *Chrysothamnus parryi*
Rabbit Brush, Rubber: *Chrysothamnus nauseosus*
Rabbit Brush, Sticky Flowered: *Chrysothamnus viscidiflorus*
Rabbit Bush: *Chrysothamnus nauseosus, C. parryi, C. viscidiflorus*
Rabbitbush Heathgoldenrod: *Ericameria bloomeri*
Rabbit Foot: *Lespedeza capitata*
Rabbit's Foot: *Polypogon monspeliensis*
Rabbit Thorn: *Lycium pallidum*
Raccoon Liver: *Stenandrium dulce*
Ragweed, Ambrosia Leaf Burr: *Ambrosia ambrosioides*
Ragweed, American: *Ambrosia artemisiifolia*
Ragweed, Annual: *Ambrosia artemisiifolia*
Ragweed, Cuman: *Ambrosia psilostachya*
Ragweed, Flatspine Burr: *Ambrosia acanthicarpa*
Ragweed, Giant: *Ambrosia trifida*
Ragweed, Silver Burr: *Ambrosia chamissonis*
Ragweed, Slimleaf Burr: *Ambrosia tenuifolia*
Ragweed, Small: *Ambrosia artemisiifolia*
Ragweed, Western: *Ambrosia psilostachya*
Ragwort, Fendler's: *Senecio fendleri*
Ragwort, Golden: *Senecio aureus*
Ragwort, Seaside: *Senecio pseudoarnica*
Ragwort, Small's: *Senecio anonymus*
Ragwort, Tansy: *Senecio jacobaea*
Ragwort Groundsel: *Senecio multicapitatus*
Ramona: *Salvia dorrii*

Ramp (or Ramps): *Allium tricoccum*
Rape: *Brassica napus*
Rape Mustard: *Brassica rapa*
Raspberry, American Red: *Rubus idaeus*
Raspberry, Arizona Red: *Rubus idaeus*
Raspberry, Black: *Rubus leucodermis, R. occidentalis*
Raspberry, Dwarf: *Rubus arcticus, R. pubescens*
Raspberry, Flowering: *Rubus odoratus*
Raspberry, Grayleaf Red: *Rubus idaeus*
Raspberry, Mountain: *Rubus chamaemorus*
Raspberry, Purple Flowered: *Rubus odoratus*
Raspberry, Red: *Rubus idaeus*
Raspberry, Western: *Rubus leucodermis*
Raspberry, Whitebark: *Rubus leucodermis*
Raspberry, Wild: *Rubus idaeus, R. occidentalis, R. odoratus, R. procumbens*
Raspberry, Wild Black: *Rubus occidentalis*
Raspberry, Wild Red: *Rubus idaeus*
Ratany: *Krameria grayi*
Ratany, Littleleaf: *Krameria erecta*
Ratbane: *Chimaphila umbellata*
Rattan Vine: *Berchemia scandens*
Rattle Box: *Crotalaria rotundifolia, C. sagittalis*
Rattle Pod, American: *Astragalus americanus*
Rattle Pod, Black: *Baptisia bracteata*
Rattle Pod, Little: *Astragalus canadensis*
Rattlesnake Master: *Eryngium aquaticum, E. yuccifolium, Liatris laxa*
Rattlesnake Plantain: *Goodyera oblongifolia, G. pubescens, G. repens*
Rattlesnake Root: *Prenanthes alata, P. alba, P. altissima*
Rattlesnake Weed: *Chamaesyce albomarginata, C. ocellata, Daucus pusillus, Echinacea angustifolia, Hieracium venosum*
Rattle Weed: *Astragalus convallarius, Oxytropis lagopus*
Rattleweed, Many Colored: *Astragalus allochrous*
Redberry: *Rhamnus crocea*
Red Bud: *Cercis canadensis*
Redbug: *Cercis canadensis*
Redcardinal: *Erythrina herbacea*
Red Root: *Ceanothus americanus, Lachnanthes caroliana*
Red Root, Small: *Ceanothus herbaceus*
Redshank: *Adenostoma sparsifolium*
Redwood: *Sequoia sempervirens*
Reed, Bur: *Sparganium eurycarpum*
Reed, Carrizal (or Carrizo): *Phragmites australis*
Reed, Common: *Juncus effusus, Phragmites australis*
Reed, Giant: *Arundo donax*
Reed, Giant Bur: *Sparganium eurycarpum*

Reed, Rood: *Cinna arundinacea*
Reed, Stout Wood: *Cinna arundinacea*
Rein Orchid: see Orchid, Rein
Resurrection Flower: *Lewisia rediviva*
Reverchonia, Sand: *Reverchonia arenaria*
Rhododendron, California: *Rhododendron macrophyllum*
Rhubarb: *Rheum rhaponticum*
Rhubarb, Alaska Wild: *Polygonum alpinum*
Rhubarb, American Wild: *Rumex hymenosepalus*
Rhubarb, Eskimo: *Polygonum alpinum*
Rhubarb, False: *Rheum rhaponticum*
Rhubarb, Indian: *Darmera peltata, Heracleum maximum*
Rhubarb, Wild: *Heracleum maximum, Polygonum alpinum, Rumex crispus, R. hymenosepalus*
Ribbonwood: *Adenostoma sparsifolium*
Ribgrass: *Plantago lanceolata*
Rich Weed: *Collinsonia canadensis, Pilea pumila*
Rockbrake, Sitka: *Cryptogramma sitchensis*
Rock Cress: *Arabis drummondii, A. fendleri, A. puberula*
Rockcress, Drummond's: *Arabis drummondii*
Rock Cress, Early Flowering: *Arabis perennans*
Rockcress, Fendler's: *Arabis fendleri*
Rock Cress, Few Flowered: *Arabis sparsiflora*
Rock Cress, Hoelboell's: *Arabis holboellii*
Rockcress, Perennial: *Arabis perennans*
Rockcress, Sicklepod: *Arabis sparsiflora*
Rockcress, Silver: *Arabis puberula*
Rockcress, Tower: *Arabis glabra*
Rocket, London: *Sisymbrium irio*
Rockgoldenrod, Grassy: *Petradoria pumila*
Rock Harlequin: *Corydalis sempervirens*
Rockjasmine, Pygmyflower: *Androsace septentrionalis*
Rockjasmine, Western: *Androsace occidentalis*
Rockjasmine Buckwheat: *Eriogonum androsaceum*
Rock Spiraea: *Holodiscus discolor, H. dumosus*
Rock Spiraea, Rocky Mountain: *Petrophyton caespitosum*
Rood Reed Grass: *Cinna arundinacea*
Rose, Bald Hip: *Rosa gymnocarpa*
Rose, Bristly Nootka: *Rosa nutkana*
Rose, California Wild: *Rosa californica*
Rose, Carolina: *Rosa carolina*
Rose, Cluster: *Rosa pisocarpa*
Rose, Dwarf: *Rosa gymnocarpa*
Rose, Dwarf Wild: *Rosa virginiana*
Rose, Early Wild: *Rosa blanda*
Rose, French: *Rosa gallica*
Rose, Interior Wild: *Rosa woodsii*
Rose, Nootka: *Rosa nutkana*
Rose, Pasture: *Rosa carolina*

Squirrel Tail Grass: *Hordeum jubatum*
Stag Bush Sloe: *Viburnum prunifolium*
Stagger Bush: *Lyonia mariana*
Stansbury: *Phlox longifolia*
Stansbury Cliffrose: *Purshia stansburiana*
Starflower: *Eriastrum densifolium, Maianthemum stellatum, Trientalis borealis*
Stargrass: *Aletris farinosa*
Stargrass, Yellow: *Hypoxis hirsuta*
Starwort, Tuber: *Pseudostellaria jamesiana*
Steeple Bush: *Spiraea tomentosa*
Stick Leaf: *Mentzelia multiflora, M. pumila, Mentzelia* sp.
Stickseed: *Cryptantha crassisepala, Hackelia floribunda, H. hispida, H. virginiana, Lappula occidentalis, Mentzelia laevicaulis*
Stickseed, Desert: *Lappula occidentalis*
Stickseed, European: *Lappula squarrosa*
Stickseed, Flatspine: *Lappula occidentalis*
Stickseed, Manyflower: *Hackelia floribunda*
Stickseed, Showy: *Hackelia hispida*
Stickseed, Virginia: *Hackelia virginiana*
Stickweed: *Lappula squarrosa*
Stickywilly: *Galium aparine*
Stone Crop: *Sedum divergens, S. lanceolatum, S. rosea, S. spathulifolium, S. stenopetalum*
Stonecrop, Allegheny: *Sedum telephioides*
Stone Crop, Broad Leaved: *Sedum spathulifolium*
Stonecrop, Ditch: *Penthorum sedoides*
Stonecrop, Entireleaf: *Sedum integrifolium*
Stonecrop, Roseroot: *Sedum rosea*
Stonecrop, Spearleaf: *Sedum lanceolatum*
Stonecrop, Wormleaf: *Sedum stenopetalum*
Stoneroot: *Collinsonia canadensis*
Stone Seed: *Lithospermum incisum, L. ruderale*
Straw, Broom: *Andropogon glomeratus*
Strawberry, American: *Fragaria vesca*
Strawberry, Barren: *Waldsteinia fragarioides*
Strawberry, Beach: *Fragaria chiloensis*
Strawberry, Blue Leaved Wild: *Fragaria virginiana*
Strawberry, Broad Petaled Wild: *Fragaria virginiana*
Strawberry, California: *Fragaria vesca*
Strawberry, Coastal: *Fragaria chiloensis*
Strawberry, European Wood: *Fragaria vesca*
Strawberry, Pacific Beach (or Pacific Coast): *Fragaria chiloensis*
Strawberry, Scarlet: *Fragaria virginiana*
Strawberry, Virginia: *Fragaria virginiana*
Strawberry, Wild: *Fragaria chiloensis, F. vesca, F. virginiana*
Strawberry, Wood: *Fragaria vesca*
Stretchberry: *Forestiera pubescens*
String Plant: *Psoralidium lanceolatum*

Sue, Perky: *Tetraneuris argentea*
Sugarberry: *Celtis laevigata*
Sugar Bush: *Rhus ovata*
Sumac, Aromatic: *Rhus aromatica, R. trilobata*
Sumac, Black: *Rhus copallinum*
Sumac, Dwarf: *Rhus copallinum, R. glabra*
Sumac, Flameleaf: *Rhus copallinum*
Sumac, Fragrant: *Rhus aromatica*
Sumac, Ill Scented: *Rhus trilobata*
Sumac, Lemonade: *Rhus trilobata*
Sumac, Poison: *Toxicodendron vernix*
Sumac, Skunkbush: *Rhus trilobata*
Sumac, Smooth: *Rhus glabra*
Sumac, Stag Horn: *Rhus hirta*
Sumac, Sugar: *Rhus ovata*
Sumac, Sweet: *Rhus trilobata*
Sumac, Three Leaved: *Rhus trilobata*
Sumac, Upland: *Rhus glabra*
Sumac, White: *Rhus aromatica, Toxicodendron vernix*
Sumac, Wild: *Rhus trilobata*
Sumac, Winged: *Rhus copallinum*
Sumpweed: *Iva xanthifolia*
Sun Bonnet: *Chaptalia tomentosa*
Sun Brier: *Aralia spinosa*
Sunbright: *Talinum parviflorum*
Suncup, Froststem: *Camissonia multijuga*
Sundew, Pink: *Drosera capillaris*
Sundew, Roundleaf: *Drosera rotundifolia*
Sundrops, Hartweg's: *Calylophus hartwegii*
Sundrops, Smaller: *Oenothera perennis*
Sunflower: *Balsamorhiza* spp., *Helianthus* spp., *Wyethia angustifolia*
Sunflower, Balsam Root: *Balsamorhiza sagittata*
Sunflower, Cusick's: *Helianthus cusickii*
Sunflower, Fewleaf: *Helianthus occidentalis*
Sunflower, Giant: *Helianthus giganteus*
Sunflower, Little: *Helianthella uniflora*
Sunflower, Mountain Bush: *Encelia virginensis*
Sunflower, Nuttall: *Helianthus nuttallii*
Sunflower, Pale Leaved: *Helianthus strumosus*
Sunflower, Parry's Dwarf: *Helianthella parryi*
Sunflower, Prairie: *Helianthus petiolaris*
Sunflower, Saw Tooth: *Helianthus grosseserratus*
Sunflower, Showy: *Helianthus niveus*
Sunflower, Spring: *Balsamorhiza sagittata*
Sunflower, Tall Swamp: *Helianthus giganteus*
Sunflower, Thin Leaved: *Helianthus decapetalus*
Sunflower, Western: *Helianthus anomalus*
Sunflower, Wild: *Helianthus annuus, H. petiolaris, Wyethia angustifolia*
Sunflower, Woolly: *Eriophyllum lanatum*
Supple Jack: *Berchemia scandens*
Surfgrass, Torrey's: *Phyllospadix torreyi*

Swamp Root, American: *Anemopsis californica*
Sweet after Death: *Achlys triphylla*
Sweet Cicely: *Osmorhiza berteroi, O. brachypoda,*
  O. claytonii, O. longistylis, O. purpurea
Sweetcicely, California: *Osmorhiza brachypoda*
Sweet Cicely, Mountain: *Osmorhiza occidentalis*
Sweet Cicely, Smooth: *Osmorhiza longistylis*
Sweet Cicely, Smoother: *Osmorhiza longistylis*
Sweet Cicely, Western: *Osmorhiza berteroi, O. occi-*
  dentalis
Sweet Cicely, Woolly: *Osmorhiza claytonii*
Sweet Clover: *Melilotus indicus, M. officinalis*
Sweet Coltsfoot: *Petasites frigidus*
Sweet Corn: *Zea mays*
Sweet Crabapple: *Malus coronaria*
Sweet Flag: *Acorus calamus*
Sweet Gale: *Myrica gale*
Sweet Grass: *Catabrosa aquatica, Glyceria flui-*
  tans, Hierochloe odorata
Sweet Grass, California: *Hierochloe occidentalis*
Sweet Grass, Common: *Hierochloe odorata*
Sweet Gum: *Liquidambar styraciflua*
Sweetleaf: *Symplocos tinctoria*
Sweetpepperbush: *Clethra acuminata*
Sweet Potato, Wild: *Potentilla nana*
Sweet Shaggytuft: *Stenandrium dulce*
Sweet Shrub: *Calycanthus floridus*
Sweetroot: *Osmorhiza berteroi, Osmorhiza occi-*
  dentalis
Sweetroot, Clayton's: *Osmorhiza claytonii*
Sweetroot, Longstyle: *Osmorhiza longistylis*
Sweetroot, Purple: *Osmorhiza purpurea*
Sweetroot, Western: *Osmorhiza occidentalis*
Sweetroot Springparsley: *Cymopterus newberryi*
Sweetvetch: *Hedysarum boreale*
Sycamore, American: *Platanus occidentalis*
Sycamore, California: *Platanus racemosa*
Sylvan Goat's Beard: *Aruncus dioicus*
Syringa: *Philadelphus lewisii, Syringa* spp.
Tallow Wood: *Ximenia americana*
Tamarack: *Larix laricina*
Tan (or Tan-bark) Oak: *Lithocarpus densiflorus*
Tansy: *Tanacetum vulgare*
Tansyaster, Hoary: *Machaeranthera canescens*
Tansyaster, Lacy: *Machaeranthera pinnatifida*
Tansyaster, Smallflower: *Machaeranthera parvi-*
  flora
Tanseyleaf Aster: *Machaeranthera tanacetifolia*
Tansy Mustard: *Descurainia incana, D. pinnata, D.*
  sophia
Tansy Ragwort: *Senecio jacobaea*
Tararack: *Larix laricina*
Taro: *Colocasia esculenta*
Taro, Giant: *Alocasia macrorrhizos*

Tarragon, Wild: *Artemisia dracunculus*
Tar Weed: *Grindelia squarrosa, Holocarpha*
  virgata, Madia glomerata, Trichostema lanceo-
  latum
Tarweed, Mountain: *Madia glomerata*
Tarweed, Yellowflower: *Holocarpha virgata*
Tassel Flower: *Arnoglossum atriplicifolium*
Tassel Flower, Red: *Dalea purpurea*
Tasselflower Brickellbush: *Brickellia grandiflora*
Tea: *Camellia sinensis*
Tea, Bitter: *Kalmia angustifolia*
Tea, Brigham: *Ephedra fasciculata, E. torreyana*
Tea, Country: *Ledum groenlandicum*
Tea, Desert: *Ephedra californica, E. nevadensis, E.*
  viridis
Tea, Eskimo: *Ledum palustre*
Tea, Hudson Bay: *Ledum palustre*
Tea, Indian: *Aster umbellatus, Ephedra viridis,*
  Ledum groenlandicum
Tea, Jersey: *Ceanothus americanus, C. herbaceus*
Tea, Labrador: see Labrador Tea
Tea, Mexican: *Chenopodium ambrosioides, Ephe-*
  dra viridis
Tea, Mormon: *Ephedra californica, E. fasciculata,*
  E. nevadensis, E. torreyana, E. trifurca, E.
  viridis
Tea, Mountain: *Ephedra viridis*
Tea, Navajo: *Thelesperma megapotamicum*
Tea, New Jersey: *Ceanothus americanus, C.*
  fendleri, C. herbaceus
Tea, Oswego: *Monarda fistulosa*
Tea, Teamster's: *Ephedra antisyphilitica, E.*
  nevadensis
Teaberry: *Gaultheria procumbens*
Teaberry, Eastern: *Gaultheria procumbens*
Tea Plant: *Thelesperma megapotamicum*
Teasel: *Dipsacus fullonum*
Telesonix, James's: *Boykinia jamesii*
Tepary: *Phaseolus acutifolius*
Terrapin Paw: *Prunella vulgaris*
Thelypody, Mountain Mock: *Pennellia micrantha*
Thelypody, Wright's: *Thelypodium wrightii*
Thermopsis, Mountain: *Thermopsis montana*
Thimble: *Rubus odoratus*
Thimbleberry: *Rubus canadensis, R. occidentalis,*
  R. parviflorus
Thimbleweed: *Anemone cylindrica, A. virginiana*
Thistle, American Star: *Centaurea americana, C.*
  melitensis
Thistle, Bull: *Cirsium vulgare*
Thistle, Cainville: *Cirsium calcareum*
Thistle, Canada: *Cirsium arvense*
Thistle, Cotton: *Onopordum acanthium*
Thistle, Eaton's: *Cirsium eatonii*

Thistle, Fewleaf: *Cirsium remotifolium*
Thistle, Field: *Cirsium discolor*
Thistle, Lavender: *Cirsium neomexicanum*
Thistle, Little: *Cirsium altissimum*
Thistle, Maltese Star: *Centaurea melitensis*
Thistle, Mountain: *Cirsium undulatum*
Thistle, New Mexico: *Cirsium neomexicanum*
Thistle, Pale: *Cirsium pallidum*
Thistle, Plumed: *Cirsium undulatum*
Thistle, Rothrock's: *Cirsium rothrockii*
Thistle, Russian: *Salsola australis*
Thistle, Scotch Cotton: *Onopordum acanthium*
Thistle, Scottish: *Cirsium vulgare*
Thistle, Star: *Centaurea americana, C. melitensis*
Thistle, Tall: *Cirsium altissimum*
Thistle, Wavy Leaved: *Cirsium undulatum*
Thistle, Yellow: *Cirsium horridulum*
Thistle, Yellow Spined: *Cirsium ochrocentrum*
Thorn, Bicknell's: *Crataegus chrysocarpa*
Thorn, Pear: *Crataegus calpodendron*
Thorn Apple: *Datura wrightii*
Thornapple, Chinese: *Datura ferox*
Thornapple, Desert: *Datura discolor*
Thornapple, Sacred: *Datura wrightii*
Thorn Bush: *Crataegus rivularis*
Thorn of Christ: *Castela emoryi*
Thorn Skeletonweed: *Stephanomeria spinosa*
Thoroughwort: *Ageratina herbacea*
Thoroughwort, Lateflowering: *Eupatorium serotinum*
Thread Leaf: *Senecio flaccidus*
Threadleaf, Manyflower False: *Schkuhria multiflora*
Threeawn, Poverty: *Aristida divaricata*
Thyme, Wild: *Thymus praecox*
Ti: *Cordyline fruticosa*
Tibinagua: *Eriogonum nudum*
Tickseed, Golden: *Coreopsis tinctoria*
Tickseed, Leavenworth's: *Coreopsis leavenworthii*
Tickseed, Stiff: *Coreopsis palmata*
Tickseed, Tall: *Coreopsis tripteris*
Tickseed, Trefoil: *Desmodium nudiflorum, D. perplexum*
Tick Trefoil, Canada: *Desmodium canadense*
Ticktrefoil, Hawaii: *Desmodium sandwicense*
Tick Trefoil, Illinois: *Desmodium illinoense*
Ticktrefoil, Nakedflower: *Desmodium nudiflorum*
Ticktrefoil, Panicledleaf: *Desmodium paniculatum*
Ticktrefoil, Perplexed: *Desmodium perplexum*
Ticktrefoil, Showy: *Desmodium canadense*
Tickweed: *Coreopsis leavenworthii*
Timbleberry: *Rubus parviflorus*
Tinker's Weed: *Triosteum perfoliatum*
Tiny Mousetail: *Myosurus minimus*

Tiplant: *Cordyline fruticosa*
Toadflax, Bastard: *Comandra umbellata*
Toadflax, False: *Geocaulon lividum*
Toadflax, Yellow: *Linaria vulgaris*
Toadshade: *Trillium sessile*
Tobacco, Aztec: *Nicotiana rustica*
Tobacco, Bigelow's: *Nicotiana quadrivalvis*
Tobacco, Cleveland's: *Nicotiana clevelandii*
Tobacco, Commercial: *Nicotiana tabacum*
Tobacco, Coyote's: *Nicotiana attenuata, N. rustica, N. trigonophylla*
Tobacco, Cultivated: *Nicotiana tabacum*
Tobacco, Desert: *Nicotiana trigonophylla*
Tobacco, Hopi: *Nicotiana attenuata*
Tobacco, Indian: *Lobelia inflata, Nicotiana attenuata, N. quadrivalvis, N. rustica*
Tobacco, Ladies': *Gnaphalium californicum*
Tobacco, Native: *Nicotiana attenuata, N. rustica*
Tobacco, Palmer Wild: *Nicotiana trigonophylla*
Tobacco, Rabbit: *Gnaphalium obtusifolium, Pterocaulon virgatum*
Tobacco, Rabbit's: *Pterocaulon virgatum*
Tobacco, Tree: *Nicotiana glauca*
Tobacco, Wild: *Nicotiana attenuata, N. quadrivalvis, N. rustica, N. trigonophylla*
Tobacco, Woman's: *Antennaria plantaginifolia*
Tobacco, Yaqui: *Nicotiana tabacum*
Tobacco Brush: *Ceanothus velutinus*
Tobacco Root: *Valeriana edulis*
Tolguacha: *Datura wrightii*
Toloache: *Datura wrightii*
Tomatilla: *Lycium pallidum*
Tomatillo: *Lycium pallidum, Physalis philadelphica*
Tomato, Husk: *Physalis pubescens*
Tomato, Wild: *Solanum triflorum*
Tomato Flower: *Rosa acicularis*
Tongue, Beard: *Penstemon barbatus, P. fendleri, P. fruticosus, P. jamesii, P. linarioides, P. virgatus, Phlox caespitosa*
Toothache Tree: *Zanthoxylum americanum*
Tooth Cress, Large: *Cardamine maxima*
Toothwort: *Cardamine diphylla*
Toothwort, Crinkled: *Cardamine diphylla*
Toothwort, Cutleaf: *Cardamine concatenata*
Toothwort, Large: *Cardamine maxima*
Torote Blanco: *Bursera microphylla*
Touch Me Not, Pale: *Impatiens pallida*
Touch Me Not, Spotted: *Impatiens capensis*
Touch Me Not, Wild: *Impatiens capensis, I. pallida*
Touristplant: *Dimorphocarpa wislizeni*
Toyon: *Heteromeles arbutifolia*
Trailplant, American: *Adenocaulon bicolor*
Tree Lichen: *Usnea* sp.
Trefoil, Bird's Foot: *Lotus wrightii*